ZOO & WILD ANIMAL MEDICINE

MURRAY E. FOWLER, D.V.M.

Professor Emeritus, Zoological Medicine
School of Veterinary Medicine
University of California at Davis
Davis, California

R. ERIC MILLER, D.V.M.

Director of Animal Health and Conservation
Saint Louis Zoo, Forest Park
St. Louis, Missouri

ZOO & WILD ANIMAL MEDICINE

Current Therapy 4

W.B. SAUNDERS COMPANY
A Division of Harcourt Brace & Company

Philadelphia   London   Toronto   Montreal   Sydney   Tokyo

W.B. SAUNDERS COMPANY
A Division of Harcourt Brace & Company

The Curtis Center
Independence Square West
Philadelphia, Pennsylvania 19106

Library of Congress Cataloging-in-Publication Data

Zoo and wild animal medicine: current therapy / [edited by] Murray E. Fowler,
R. Eric Miller.—4th ed.
p.   cm.

ISBN 0–7216–8664–8

1. Zoo animals—Diseases.   2. Wildlife diseases.   I. Fowler, Murray E.
   II. Miller, R. Eric.

SF996.Z66   1999   636.089—dc21

DNLM/DLC   97-47281

ZOO AND WILD ANIMAL MEDICINE:
CURRENT THERAPY 4   ISBN 0–7216–8664–8

Printed in the United States of America.

Last digit is the print number: 9   8   7   6   5   4   3   2   1

CONTRIBUTORS

Jack L. Allen, D.V.M.
Senior Veterinarian, San Diego Wild Animal
Park, Escondido, California
*Use of Pulse Oximetry in Monitoring
Anesthesia*

Cheryl S. Asa, Ph.D.
Director of Research, Saint Louis Zoological
Park, St. Louis, Missouri
Contraception

Charlotte Kirk Baer, M.S.
Program Director, Committee on Animal
Nutrition, National Research Council, Board
on Agriculture, Washington, D.C.
*Comparative Nutrition and Feeding
Considerations of Young Columbidae*

Lora Rickard Ballweber, B.S., M.S., D.V.M.
Assistant Professor, Parasitology, College of
Veterinary Medicine, Mississippi State
University, Mississippi State, Mississippi
*Parelaphostrongylus tenuis and
Elaphostrongylus cervi in Free-Ranging
Artiodactylids*

Michael T. Barrie, D.V.M.
Veterinarian, Oklahoma City Zoological Garden,
Oklahoma City, Oklahoma
Chameleon Medicine

John L. Behler, M.Ed.
Curator, Department of Herpetology, Wildlife
Conservation Society, Bronx, New York
*Health Assessment of Chelonians and Release
into the Wild*

Roy G. Bengis, B.V.Sc., M.Sc., Ph.D.
External Examiner—Wildlife Medicine,
University of Pretoria, Faculty of Veterinary
Science, Onderstepoort, South Africa; Africa
Representative, Working Group on Wildlife
Diseases, Office International des Epizooties,
Paris, France
Tuberculosis in Free-Ranging Mammals

Joni B. Bernard, Ph.D.
Adjunct Assistant Professor, Department of
Zoology, Michigan State University, East
Lansing, Michigan
*Vitamin D: Metabolism, Sources, Unique
Problems in Zoo Animals, Meeting Needs*

Joseph T. Bielitzki, M.S., D.V.M.
Chief Veterinary Officer, National Aeronautics
and Space Administration (NASA), Ames
Research Center, Moffett Field, California
*Emerging Viral Diseases of Nonhuman
Primates*

Wendy H. Blanshard, B.V.Sc.
Veterinarian, Sea World Enterprises, Gold Coast,
Queensland, Australia
Diseases of Koalas

Rosemary J. Booth, B.V.Sc.
Senior Veterinarian, Healesville Sanctuary,
Healesville, Victoria, Australia
Diseases of Koalas

Gregory D. Bossart, V.M.D., Ph.D.
Assistant Professor of Pathology, Division of
Comparative Pathology, Department of
Pathology, University of Miami, School of
Medicine, Miami, Florida; Veterinarian,
Miami Seaquarium, Miami, Florida; Medical
Director, Falcon Batchelor Bird of Prey
Center, Miami Museum of Science, Miami,
Florida
Manatee Medicine

Mitchell Bush, D.V.M.
Chief of Veterinary Services, Conservation and
Research Center, National Zoological Park,
Smithsonian Institution, Front Royal, Virginia
*Medical Management of Tree Kangaroos
Diseases of the Callitrichidae*

Paul P. Calle, B.A., V.M.D., Dipl. ACZM
Senior Veterinarian, Wildlife Health Sciences,
Wildlife Conservation Society, Bronx, New
York
*Tuberculin Responses in Orangutans
Anesthesia for Nondomestic Suids*

Richard C. Cambre, D.V.M.
Head, Department of Animal Health, National
Zoological Park, Smithsonian Institution,
Washington, D.C.
Water Quality for a Waterfowl Collection

Terry W. Campbell, B.S., M.S., D.V.M., Ph.D.
Associate Professor of Zoological Medicine, Department of Clinical Sciences, College of Veterinary Medicine and Biomedical Sciences, Colorado State University, Fort Collins, Colorado
Diagnostic Cytology in Marine Mammal Medicine

Scott B. Citino, B.S., D.V.M.
Staff Veterinarian, White Oak Conservation Center, Yulee, Florida
Rotavirus and Coronavirus Infections in Nondomestic Ruminants

Victoria L. Clyde, D.V.M.
Staff Veterinarian, Milwaukee County Zoo, Milwaukee, Wisconsin
Avian Analgesia

Darin Collins, D.V.M.
Associate Veterinarian, Woodland Park Zoological Gardens, Seattle, Washington
Designing an Ideal Animal Shipment

Michael T. Collins, D.V.M., Ph.D.
Professor, Microbiology, School of Veterinary Medicine, University of Wisconsin, Madison, Wisconsin
Paratuberculosis in Zoo Animals

Robert A. Cook, V.M.D.
Chief Veterinarian and Director, Wildlife Health Sciences, Wildlife Conservation Society, Bronx, New York
The Application of Minimally Invasive Surgery for the Diagnosis and Treatment of Captive Wildlife.
Mycobacterium bovis *Infection of Cervids: Diagnosis, Treatment, and Control*

Andrew A. Cunningham, B.V.M.S., MRCVS
Pathologist, London Zoo Regents Park, London, United Kingdom
Scrapie-Like Spongiform Encephalopathies (Prion Diseases) in Nondomesticated Species

William L. Current, B.S., M.S., Ph.D.
Senior Research Scientist, Infectious Diseases Research, Lilly Research Laboratories, Eli Lilly & Co., Indianapolis, Indiana
Cryptosporidium *Species*

Leslie M. Dalton, D.V.M.
Staff Veterinarian, Sea World of Texas, San Antonio, Texas
Diagnosis and Treatment of Fungal Infections in Marine Mammals

Janet L. (Reiter) Dempsey, M.S.
Nutritionist, Saint Louis Zoological Park, St. Louis, Missouri
Advances in Fruit Bat Nutrition

Ellen S. Dierenfeld, B.S., M.S., Ph.D.
Adjunct Associate Professor, Department of Animal Science, Cornell University, Ithaca, New York; Adjunct Research Scientist, Center for Environmental Research and Conservation, Columbia University, New York, New York; Adjunct Associate Professor, Department of Biology, Fordham University, Bronx, New York; Head, Department of Wildlife Nutrition, Wildlife Conservation Society, Bronx, New York
Vitamin E: Metabolism, Sources, Unique Problems in Zoo Animals, and Supplementation
Rhinoceros Feeding and Nutrition

Robert A. Dieterich, D.V.M.
Professor Emeritus, Institute of Arctic Biology, University of Alaska, Fairbanks, Alaska
Brucella suis *Biovar 4 Infection in Free-Ranging Artiodactylids*

Pādraig J. Duignan, B.Sc., M.Sc., M.V.B., Ph.D., MRCVS
Senior Research Fellow in Marine Mammal Pathology, Infectious Diseases and Public Health, Institute of Veterinary, Animal and Biomedical Sciences, Massey University, Palmerston North, New Zealand
Morbillivirus Infections of Marine Mammals

Hym Ebedes, B.V.Sc.
Specialist Scientist, Onderstepoort Veterinary Institute, Onderstepoort, Republic of South Africa
Use of Tranquilizers in Wild Herbivores

Mark S. Edwards, Ph.D.
Nutritionist, Zoological Society of San Diego, San Diego, California
Tapir Medicine

Philip K. Ensley, D.V.M., Dipl. ACZM
Associate Veterinarian, Zoological Society of San Diego, San Diego Wild Animal Park, Escondido, California
Medical Management of the California Condor

Jacques R. B. Flamand, B.A., B.Sc., M.A., V.M.B.
Senior Veterinary Adviser, Wildlife and Domestic Veterinary Programme, Royal Chitwan National Park, Nepal; Researcher, Zoological Society of London, Regent's Park, London, United Kingdom
Medical Aspects of Arabian Oryx Reintroduction

Keven Flammer, D.V.M.
Associate Professor, Companion and Wild Avian Medicine, Department of Companion Animal and Special Species Medicine, College of Veterinary Medicine, North Carolina State University, Raleigh, North Carolina; Associate Professor, Companion and Wild Avian Medicine, Veterinary Teaching Hospital, College of Veterinary Medicine, North Carolina State University, Raleigh, North Carolina
Zoonoses Acquired from Birds

Joseph P. Flanagan, D.V.M.
Senior Veterinarian, Houston Zoological Gardens, Houston, Texas
Snakebite Protocols for Zoos

Joseph J. Foerner, B.S., D.V.M., Dipl. ACVS
Surgeon, Illinois Equine Hospital, Naperville, Illinois
Dystocia in the Elephant

Murray E. Fowler, B.S., D.V.M.
Professor Emeritus, Zoological Medicine, University of California, School of Veterinary Medicine, Davis, California
Plant Poisoning in Zoos in North America

Michelle Willette Frahm, B.S., D.V.M.
Staff Veterinarian, Gladys Porter Zoo, Brownsville, Texas
Medical Management of Duikers

Laurie J. Gage, D.V.M.
Associate Clinical Professor, University of California, Davis, School of Veterinary Medicine (lecturer), Davis, California; Director of Veterinary Services, Marine World Africa USA, Vallejo, California
Radiographic Techniques for the Elephant Foot and Carpus

I. A. Gardner, B.V.Sc., M.P.V.M., Ph.D.
Associate Professor of Epidemiology, School of Veterinary Medicine, University of California, Davis, Davis, California
Validity of Using Diagnostic Tests That Are Approved for Use in Domestic Animals for Nondomestic Species

Della M. Garell, D.V.M.
Staff Veterinarian, Cheyenne Mountain Zoo, Colorado Springs, Colorado
Toxoplasmosis in Zoo Animals

Joseph R. Geraci, B.Sc., V.M.D., Ph.D.
Senior Director, Biological Programs, National Aquarium in Baltimore, Baltimore, Maryland; Research Professor, Comparative Medicine Program, University of Maryland, School of Medicine, Baltimore, Maryland
Toxicology in Marine Mammals

Frank Göritz, D.V.M.
Scientific Co-Worker, Department of Reproduction Management; Senior Veterinarian; and Specialist for Zoo Animals and Wildlife (board certification), Institute for Zoo Biology and Wildlife Research, Berlin, Germany
Use of Ultrasonography in Zoo Animals

Frances M. D. Gulland, V.M.B., M.R.C.V.S., Ph.D.
Director of Veterinary Services, The Marine Mammal Center, Marin Headlands, Sausalito, California
Leptospirosis in Marine Mammals

J. C. Haigh, B.V.M.S., M.Sc., and Dipl. ACZM, FRCVS
Professor, Department of Herd Medicine and Thereogenology, Western College of Veterinary Medicine, Saskatoon, Saskatchewan, Canada
The Use of Chutes for Ungulate Restraint

Craig A. Harms, D.V.M., Dipl ACZM
Graduate Research Fellow, North Carolina State University, College of Veterinary Medicine, Raleigh, North Carolina
Anesthesia in Fish

Darryl J. Heard, B.Sc., B.V.M.S., Ph.D., Dipl. ACZM
Assistant Professor, Department of Small Animal Clinical Science, College of Veterinary Medicine, University of Florida, Gainesville, Florida
Medical Management of Megachiropterans

S. K. Hietala, Ph.D.
Associate Professor of Clinical Immunology,
California Veterinary Diagnostic Laboratory
System, School of Veterinary Medicine,
University of California, Davis, Davis,
California
*Validity of Using Diagnostic Tests That Are
Approved for Use in Domestic Animals for
Nondomestic Species*

Thomas B. Hildebrandt, D.V.M.
Head, Department of Reproduction Management,
and Specialist for Zoo Animals and Wildlife
(board certification), Institute for Zoo Biology
and Wildlife Research, Berlin, Germany
Use of Ultrasonography in Zoo Animals

**Peter H. Holz, B.V.Sc., M.A.C.V.Sc.,
D.V.Sc., Dipl. ACZM**
Associate Veterinarian, Healesville Sanctuary,
Healesville, Victoria, Australia
*The Reptilian Renal-Portal System: Influence
on Therapy*

JoGayle Howard, D.V.M., Ph.D.
Adjunct Professor, Department of Animal and
Avian Science, University of Maryland,
College Park, Maryland; Reproductive
Physiologist, National Zoological Park,
Smithsonian Institution, Washington, D.C.
*Assisted Reproductive Techniques in
Nondomestic Carnivores*

David L. Hunter, B.A., D.V.M.
Adjunct Associate Professor, University of Idaho,
Moscow, Idaho; Wildlife Veterinarian, Idaho
Department of Fish and Game and Idaho
Department of Agriculture, Caldwell, Idaho
Burcellosis Caused by Brucella abortus *in
Free-Ranging North American
Artiodactylids*

Ramiro Isaza, M.S., D.V.M., Dipl. ACZM
Assistant Professor, Department of Clinical
Sciences, College of Veterinary Medicine,
Kansas State University, Manhattan, Kansas
*Designing a Trichostrongyloid Parasite
Control Program for Captive Exotic
Ruminants*

Elliott R. Jacobson, D.V.M., Ph.D.
Professor, Wildlife and Zoological Medicine,
College of Veterinary Medicine, University of
Florida, Gainesville, Florida; Professor and
Service Chief, Wildlife and Zoological
Medicine, Veterinary Medical Teaching
Hospital, University of Florida, Gainesville,
Florida

*Use of Antimicrobial Drugs in Reptiles
Health Assessment of Chelonians and Release
into the Wild*

Donald L. Janssen, D.V.M., Dipl. ACZM
Director, Veterinary Services, San Diego Zoo,
San Diego, California
Tapir Medicine

James L. Jarchow, D.V.M.
Adjunct Associate Professor, Veterinary Science,
University of Arizona, Tucson, Arizona;
Consulting Veterinarian, Arizona-Sonora
Desert Museum, Tucson, Arizona
*Health Assessment of Chelonians and Release
into the Wild*

James M. Jensen, B.S., D.V.M., Dipl. ACZM
Associate Professor, Zoological Medicine,
Veterinary Large Animal Medicine and
Surgery, College of Veterinary Medicine,
Texas A&M University, College Station,
Texas
*Preventive Medicine Programs for Ranched
Hoofstock*

**David A. Jessup, B.S., M.D.V.M., D.V.M.,
Dipl. ACZM**
Associate Researcher, Institute of Marine
Sciences, University of California, Santa Cruz,
Santa Cruz, California; Senior Wildlife
Veterinarian, California Department of Fish
and Game, Marine Wildlife Veterinary Care
and Research Center, Santa Cruz, California
*Paratuberculosis in Free-Ranging Wildlife in
North America
Capture and Handling of Mountain Sheep and
Goats*

Robert L. Johnson, M.D.
Associate Director, Maternal-Fetal Medicine,
Good Samaritan Regional Medical Center,
Phoenix Perinatal Associates, Phoenix,
Arizona
*Fetal Ultrasonography in Dolphins with
Emphasis on Gestational Aging*

Janis Ott Joslin, D.V.M.
Senior Veterinarian, Woodland Park Zoological
Gardens, Seattle, Washington
Designing an Ideal Animal Shipment

Randall E. Junge, M.S., D.V.M., Dipl. ACZM
Adjunct Professor, Department of Medicine and
Surgery, College of Veterinary Medicine,
University of Missouri, Columbia, Missouri;

Staff Veterinarian, St. Louis Zoological Park, Forest Park, St. Louis, Missouri
Diseases of Prosimians

William B. Karesh, D.V.M.
Department Head, Field Veterinary Program, Wildlife Conservation Society, Bronx, New York
Applications of Biotelemetry in Wildlife Medicine

Suzanne Kennedy-Stoskopf, D.V.M., Ph.D., Dipl. ACZM
Visiting Associate Professor, North Carolina State University, College of Veterinary Medicine, Raleigh, North Carolina
Evaluating Immunodeficiency Disorders in Captive Wild Animals
Emerging Viral Infections in Large Cats

Jay F. Kirkpatrick, Ph.D.
Director, Science and Conservation Biology, ZooMontana, Billings, Montana
Contraception in Artiodactylids, Using Porcine Zona Pellucida Vaccination

James K. Kirkwood, B.V.Sc., Ph.D., M.R.C.V.S., C.Biol., Fl.Biol., RCVS Specialist in Zoo and Wildlife Medicine
Visiting Professor, Department of Pathology and Infectious Diseases, Royal Veterinary College, London, United Kingdom; Visiting Research Fellow, Institute of Zoology, Universities Federation for Animal Welfare, South Mimms/Potters Bar, United Kingdom
Scrapie-Like Spongiform Encephalopathies (Prion Diseases) in Nondomesticated Species

Nancy D. Kock, B.S., M.S., D.V.M., Ph.D.
Associate Professor, Department of Veterinary Pathology, University of Zimbabwe, Faculty of Veterinary Science, Mt. Pleasant, Harare, Zimbabwe
Flaccid Trunk Paralysis in Free-Ranging Elephants

George V. Kollias, D.V.M., Ph.D., Dipl. ACZM
Jay Hyman Professor of Wildlife Medicine, Wildlife Health Laboratory, College of Veterinary Medicine, Cornell University, Ithaca, New York; J. Hyman Professor of Wildlife Medicine, Veterinary Medical Teaching Hospital, Cornell University, Ithaca, New York
Health Assessment, Medical Management, and

Prerelease Conditioning of Translocated North American River Otters
Designing a Trichostrongyloid Parasite Control Program for Captive Exotic Ruminants

Terry J. Kreeger, B.S., B.S.V.Sc., M.S., D.V.M., Ph.D.
Adjunct Professor, Department of Veterinary Science, University of Wyoming, Laramie, Wyoming; Adjunct Professor, College of Veterinary Science, University of Minnesota, St. Paul, Minnesota; Supervisor, Veterinary Services, Wyoming Game and Fish Department, Laramie, Wyoming
Chemical Restraint and Immobilization of Wild Canids
Brucellosis Caused by Brucella abortus *in Free-Ranging North American Artiodactylids*

Howard Krum, M.S., V.M.D.
Clinical Associate Professor, Tufts University School of Veterinary Medicine, Grafton, Massachusetts; Department Head, Veterinary Services, New England Aquarium, Central Wharf, Boston, Massachusetts
Medical Management of Sea Turtles in Aquaria

Armin Kuntze, D.M.V., D.Habil.
Private Practice, Ambulance for Wild and Circus Animals, Berlin-Karlshorst, Germany
Oral and Nasal Diseases of Elephants
Poxvirus Infections in Elephants

Nadine Lamberski, D.V.M.
Staff Veterinarian, Riverbanks Zoological Park and Botanical Gardens, Columbia, South Carolina
Nontuberculous Mycobacteria: Potential for Zoonosis

Maria L. Lewis, V.M.D.
Lecturer in Large Animal Ultrasound and Cardiology, University of Pennsylvania, New Bolton Center, Kennett Square, Pennsylvania
Fetal Ultrasonography in Dolphins with Emphasis on Gestational Aging

Irwin K. M. Liu, D.V.M., M.P.V.M., Ph.D.
Professor, University of California, School of Veterinary Medicine, Davis, California; Chief of Service, Veterinary Medical Teaching Hospital, University of California, Davis, Davis, California
Contraception in Artiodactylids, Using Porcine Zona Pellucida Vaccination

Mark Lynn Lloyd, B.S., D.V.M.
Adjunct Assistant Professor of Comparative
Medicine, Tufts University, School of
Veterinary Medicine, Grafton, Massachusetts;
Field Faculty Adviser, Vermont College,
Norwich, Vermont; Adjunct Professor,
Department of Veterinary Technology,
University of Maine, Orono, Maine; Deputy
Director, El Paso Zoo, El Paso, Texas
Crocodilian Anesthesia

Michael R. Loomis, B.S., M.A., D.V.M.
Adjunct Associate Professor in Zoological
Medicine, North Carolina State University
College of Veterinary Medicine, Raleigh,
North Carolina; Chief Veterinarian and
Director, Hanes Veterinary Medical Center,
North Carolina Zoological Park, Asheboro,
North Carolina
*Principles and Applications of Computed
Tomography and Magnetic Resonance
Imaging in Zoo and Wildlife Medicine
Anesthesia for Captive Nile Hippopotamus*

Naida M. Loskutoff, B.S., M.S., Ph.D.
Reproductive Physiologist, Center for
Conservation and Research, Henry Doorly
Zoo, Omaha, Nebraska
*Embryo Transfer and Semen Technology from
Cattle Applied to Nondomestic
Artiodactylids*

**Linda J. Lowenstine, D.V.M., Ph.D., Dipl.
ACVP**
Professor of Veterinary Pathology, Department of
Pathology, Microbiology, and Immunology,
School of Veterinary Medicine, University of
California, Davis, Davis, California; Fellow of
the Zoological Society of San Diego, San
Diego, California
*Health Problems in Mixed-Species Exhibits
Iron Overload in the Animal Kingdom
Intrahepatic Cysts and Hepatic Neoplasms in
Felids, Ursids, and Other Zoo and Wild
Animals*

S. A. Mainka, D.V.M., Dipl. ACZM
Deputy Co-ordinator, International Union for
Conservation of Nature, The World
Conservation Union Species Programme,
Gland, Switzerland
*Giant Panda Management and Medicine in
China*

**Elizabeth J. B. Manning, M.P.H., M.B.A.,
D.V.M.**
Staff, School of Veterinary Medicine, University
of Wisconsin, Madison, Wisconsin
Paratuberculosis in Zoo Animals

James F. McBain, D.V.M.
Corporate Director of Veterinary Medicine, Sea
World of California, San Diego, California
*Diagnosis and Treatment of Fungal Infections
in Marine Mammals*

Helen E. McCracken, B.V.Sc.
Veterinarian, Melbourne Zoo, Parkville, Victoria,
Australia
*Organ Location in Snakes for Diagnostic and
Surgical Evaluation
Periodontal Disease in Lizards*

Rita McManamon, B.A., D.V.M.
Adjunct Associate Professor, Veterinary Teaching
Hospital, Small Animal Medicine and Surgery,
Tuskegee, Alabama; Senior Veterinarian and
Director, Conservation Action Resource
Center, Atlanta-Fulton County Zoo, Inc.,
Atlanta, Georgia
*Veterinarians' Role in Monitoring the
Behavioral Enrichment Standards of the
Animal Welfare Act*

**Tracey McNamara, B.S., D.V.M., Dipl.
ACVP**
Visiting Assistant Professor in Pathology, Albert
Einstein College of Medicine of Yeshiva
University, Bronx, New York; Head,
Department of Pathology, Wildlife
Conservation Society, Bronx, New York
*The Role of Pathology in Zoo Animal
Medicine*

D.G.A. Meltzer, B.V.Sc., M.Sc.
Price Forbes Chair in Wildlife, Faculty of
Veterinary Science, University of Pretoria,
Onderstepoort, Gauteng, Republic of South
Africa
*Medical Management of a Cheetah Breeding
Facility in South Africa*

Dennis A. Meritt, Jr., B.S., M.S., Ph.D.
Associate Adjunct Professor, Department of
Biological Sciences, De Paul University,
Chicago, Illinois
Rodent and Small Lagomorph Reproduction

Erica A. Miller, B.S., D.V.M.
Adjunct Faculty, Department of Clinical
Sciences, University of Pennsylvania School
of Veterinary Medicine, Philadelphia,
Pennsylvania; Veterinarian for Oil Spill
Response and Training, Tri-State Bird
Rescue & Research, Inc., Newark, Delaware
Caring for Oiled Birds

R. Eric Miller, D.V.M., Dipl. ACZM
Adjunct Assistant Professor, Medicine and
Surgery, College of Veterinary Medicine,
University of Missouri, Columbia, Missouri;
Director of Animal Health and Conservation,
Saint Louis Zoo, Forest Park, St. Louis,
Missouri
*Quarantine: A Necessity for Zoo and
Aquarium Animals*
Skin Diseases of Black Rhinoceroses

Richard J. Montali, D.V.M.
Assistant Professor, Division of Comparative
Medicine, Johns Hopkins University School of
Medicine, Baltimore, Maryland; Clinical
Professor of Pathology, George Washington
University School of Medicine, Washington,
D.C.; Associate Adjunct Professor of
Pathology, Uniformed Services University of
the Health Sciences, Bethesda, Maryland;
Head, Department of Pathology, National
Zoological Park, Smithsonian Institution,
Washington, D.C.
Medical Management of Tree Kangaroos
Diseases of the Callitrichidae

Patrick J. Morris, B.S., D.V.M., Dipl. ACZM
Senior Veterinarian, San Diego Zoo, Department
of Veterinarian Services, San Diego,
California
Anesthesia for Nondomestic Suids

Linda Munson, D.V.M., Ph.D., Dipl. ACVP
Associate Professor, Department of Pathology,
Microbiology, and Immunology, School of
Veterinary Medicine, University of California,
Davis, Davis, California
Iron Overload in the Animal Kingdom
Skin Diseases of Black Rhinoceroses

John H. Olsen, B.A., D.V.M.
Director of Veterinary Services, Conservation,
and Science, Busch Gardens Tampa Bay,
Tampa, Florida
Antibiotic Therapy in Elephants

Thomas J. O'Shea, B.S., M.S., Ph.D.
Supervisory Wildlife Research Biologist, U.S.
Geological Survey, Midcontinent Ecological
Science Center, Fort Collins, Colorado
Toxicology in Marine Mammals

Joanne Paul-Murphy, D.V.M., Dipl. ACZM
Assistant Professor, University of Wisconsin,
School of Veterinary Medicine, Madison,
Wisconsin
Avian Analgesia

K. Christina Pettan-Brewer, M.S., D.V.M.
Veterinarian, Independent Consultant, Brazil-
USA Zoo/Wildlife Veterinary Cooperative,
Sparta, New Jersey
*Intrahepatic Cysts and Hepatic Neoplasms in
Felids, Ursids, and Other Zoo and Wild
Animals*

Lyndsey G. Phillips, Jr., D.V.M., Dipl. ACZM
Associate Professor, Department of Medicine and
Epidemiology, University of California, Davis,
School of Veterinary Medicine, Davis,
California
Infectious Diseases of Equids

C. Earle Pope, B.S.A., M.S., Ph.D.
Director of Science, Audubon Center for
Research of Endangered Species, New
Orleans, Louisiana
*Embryo Transfer and Semen Technology from
Cattle Applied to Nondomestic
Artiodactylids*

J. P. Raath, B.V.Sc.
Private Wildlife Consultant Practice, Karino,
Republic of South Africa
Relocation of African Elephants
Anesthesia of White Rhinoceroses
Use of Tranquilizers in Wild Herbivores

Edward C. Ramsay, D.V.M.
Associate Professor, Department of Comparative
Medicine, College of Veterinary Medicine,
University of Tennessee, Knoxville, Tennessee
Anesthesia for Captive Nile Hippopotamus

Bonnie L. Raphael, D.V.M., Dipl. ACZM
Senior Veterinarian, Department of Clinical
Studies, Wildlife Health Sciences, Wildlife
Conservation Society, Bronx, New York
Okapi Medicine and Surgery

Thomas H. Reidarson, D.V.M.
Staff Veterinarian, Sea World of California, San
Diego, California
*Diagnosis and Treatment of Fungal Infections
in Marine Mammals*

**Bruce A. Rideout, D.V.M., Ph.D., Dipl.
ACVP**
Director of Pathology, Zoological Society of San
Diego, San Diego, California
Tapir Medicine

Michael G. Rinaldi, Ph.D.
Professor of Pathology, Medicine, Microbiology,
and Clinical Laboratory Sciences, and

Director, Fungus Testing Laboratory, Department of Pathology, University of Texas Health Science Center at San Antonio, San Antonio, Texas; Chief, Clinical Microbiology Laboratories, and Director, Department of Veterans Affairs Mycology Reference Laboratory, Pathology and Laboratory Medicine Service, Audie L. Murphy Division, South Texas Veterans Health Care System, San Antonio, Texas
Diagnosis and Treatment of Fungal Infections in Marine Mammals

Charles E. Rupprecht, V.M.D., M.S., Ph.D.
Chief, Rabies Section, Viral and Rickettsial Zoonoses Branch, National Center for Infectious Diseases, Centers for Disease Control and Prevention, Atlanta, Georgia
Rabies: Global Problem, Zoonotic Threat, and Preventive Management

Michael J. Schmidt, B.S., D.V.M.
Private Practice, Portland, Oregon
Calving Elephants (Normal)

Amy L. Shima, B.A., B.V.Sc., D.V.M.
Associate Veterinarian, Zoological Society of San Diego, San Diego, California
Sedation and Anesthesia in Marsupials

Kathy Spaulding, D.V.M., Dipl. ACVR
Associate Professor, Radiology, North Carolina State University, Raleigh, North Carolina
Principles and Applications of Computed Tomography and Magnetic Resonance Imaging in Zoo and Wildlife Medicine

Lucy H. Spelman, A.B., D.V.M., Dipl. ACZM
Associate Veterinarian, Department of Animal Health, National Zoological Park, Smithsonian Institution, Washington, D.C.
Vermin Control
Otter Anesthesia

David R. Stoloff, M.S., D.V.M., Dipl. ACVS
Research Fellow, Ethicon, Inc., Somerville, New Jersey
The Application of Minimally Invasive Surgery for the Diagnosis and Treatment of Captive Wildlife

L. Rae Stone, D.V.M.
Veterinarian, Dolphin Quest, Middleburg, Virginia
Fetal Ultrasonography in Dolphins with Emphasis on Gestational Aging

Michael K. Stoskopf, D.V.M., Ph.D., Dipl. ACZM
Professor of Aquatic and Wildlife Medicine and Toxicology, Environmental Medicine Consortium, College of Veterinary Medicine, North Carolina State University, Raleigh, North Carolina
Fish Pharmacotherapeutics

Jay C. Sweeney, V.M.D.
Adjunct Professor, University of Hawaii at Manao, Honolulu, Hawaii
Fetal Ultrasonography in Dolphins with Emphasis on Gestational Aging

Brent Swenson, D.V.M.
Chief Clinical Veterinarian, Yerkes Primate Center, Emory University, Atlanta, Georgia
Great Ape Neonatology

E. Tom Thorne, D.V.M.
Assistant Chief, Services Division, Wyoming Game and Fish Department, Cheyenne, Wyoming
Veterinary Contributions to the Black-Footed Ferret Conservation Program

Forrest I. Townsend, D.V.M.
Veterinarian, Bayside Hospital for Animals, Fort Walton Beach, Florida
Medical Management of Stranded Small Cetaceans
Hand-Rearing Techniques for Neonate Cetaceans

John W. Turner, Ph.D.
Professor, Medical College of Ohio, Department of Physiology and Molecular Medicine, Toledo, Ohio
Contraception in Artiodactylids, Using Porcine Zona Pellucida Vaccination

Duane E. Ullrey, Ph.D.
Professor Emeritus, Department of Animal Science and Department of Fisheries and Wildlife, Michigan State University, East Lansing, Michigan
Vitamin D: Metabolism, Sources, Unique Problems in Zoo Animals, Meeting Needs

Raymund F. Wack, M.S., D.V.M., Dipl. ACZM
Adjunct Associate Professor, Department of Veterinary Clinical Sciences, College of Veterinary Medicine, Ohio State University, Columbus, Ohio; Director of Animal Health, Columbus Zoo, Powell, Ohio
Gastritis in Cheetahs

Michael T. Walsh, B.A., D.V.M.
Adjunct Professor, Department of Small Animal
    Clinical Sciences, College of Veterinary
    Medicine, University of Florida, Gainesville,
    Florida; Staff Veterinarian, Sea World of
    Florida, Orlando, Florida
Manatee Medicine

Christian Walzer, D.M.V.
Zoo Veterinarian, Salzburg Zoo Hellbrunn, Anif,
    Austria
Diabetes in Primates

Sallie C. Welte, B.A., M.A.Ed., V.M.D.
Adjunct Faculty, University of Pennsylvania
    School of Veterinary Medicine, Philadelphia,
    Pennsylvania; Associate Director, Clinic
    Operations, Tri-State Bird Rescue and
    Research, Inc., Newark, Delaware
Caring for Oiled Birds

Brent R. Whitaker, M.S., D.V.M.
Associate Adjunct Faculty, Center of Marine
    Biotechnology, University of Maryland,
    Baltimore, Maryland; Adjunct Professor,
    Virginia/Maryland School of Veterinary
    Medicine, Blacksburg, Virginia; Director of
    Animal Health, National Aquarium in
    Baltimore, Baltimore, Maryland
Preventive Medicine Programs for Fish
Medical Management of Sea Turtles in
    Aquaria

Elizabeth S. Williams, B.S., D.V.M., Ph.D.
Professor, Veterinary Sciences, University of
    Wyoming, Laramie, Wyoming
Veterinary Contributions to the Black-Footed
    Ferret Conservation Program
Paratuberculosis in Free-Ranging Wildlife in
    North America

PREFACE

Medicine and surgery for captive and free-ranging wildlife are becoming more and more sophisticated. The American Association of Zoo Veterinarians and the American Association of Wildlife Veterinarians continue to grow, and presentations at meetings address new areas. The Association of Avian Veterinarians is strong and continues to grow steadily. The literature is expanding almost exponentially. Numerous books are being published on caged bird medicine and surgery, and one book is devoted to ratite medicine and surgery. Veterinarians with interest in herptiles have banded together in the Association of Reptile and Amphibian Veterinarians, and they too have published many fine textbooks to choose from. In the arena of free-ranging wildlife medicine, some of the classic volumes published by Iowa State University Press in the 1970s have been revised, and there is one monograph each on white-tailed deer and Wapiti and red deer.

Zoo & Wild Animal Medicine serves a vital function by bridging the gap between captive and free-ranging wild animal medicine and by fostering a conservation biology ethic. Following the format of the 3rd edition, the 4th edition covers selected topics that have relevance to this period of time. The volume is not all encompassing in terms of the taxa discussed. One hundred ten contributors were selected because of their expertise and interest in a subject. Authorship has not been limited to North American contributors, because it is recognized that many of the animals dealt with are from other countries and because colleagues working in field projects are interrelating with counterparts all over the world. Contributors are from Austria, Australia, Brazil, Canada, Germany, Great Britain, New Zealand, Saudi Arabia, South Africa, the United States, and Zimbabwe. The editors have endeavored to provide contributors with the opportunity to express their individual approach to a topic, within the format and style of the *Current Therapy* concept.

Selected references are associated with each discussion, enabling the reader to delve more deeply into a subject. Most of the material is new to the 4th edition. Where appropriate, citations will direct the reader to a more complete discussion of a taxa in the 2nd edition of *Zoo & Wild Animal Medicine,* which is still in print.

It is the editors' sincere hope that readers will find the text useful as a reference and as a resource for improving the care and understanding of both free-ranging and captive wildlife.

Murray E. Fowler
R. Eric Miller

ACKNOWLEDGMENTS

The editors wish to thank the 110 contributors for their uncompensated contribution to this volume. Thanks are also expressed to the practices and institutions that have supported the contributors and the editors in this effort.

Royalities resulting from the sale of this book are forwarded to the Morris Animal Foundation and are used for research benefiting wild animals.

CONTENTS

◆ **PART I**

GENERAL   2

1   Use of Pulse Oximetry in Monitoring Anesthesia   2
Jack L. Allen

2   The Role of Pathology in Zoo Animal Medicine   3
Tracey McNamara

3   Applications of Biotelemetry in Wildlife Medicine   7
William B. Karesh

4   Quarantine: A Necessity for Zoo and Aquarium Animals   13
R. Eric Miller

5   Designing an Ideal Animal Shipment   17
Janis Ott Joslin
Darin Collins

6   Health Problems in Mixed-Species Exhibits   26
Linda J. Lowenstine

7   The Application of Minimally Invasive Surgery for the Diagnosis and Treatment of Captive Wildlife   30
Robert A. Cook
David R. Stoloff

8   Use of Ultrasonography in Zoo Animals   41
Thomas B. Hildebrandt
Frank Göritz

9   Validity of Using Diagnostic Tests That Are Approved for Use in Domestic Animals for Nondomestic Species   55
S. K. Hietala
I. A. Gardner

10   Evaluating Immunodeficiency Disorders in Captive Wild Animals   58
Suzanne Kennedy-Stoskopf

11   Vitamin D: Metabolism, Sources, Unique Problems in Zoo Animals, Meeting Needs   63
Duane E. Ullrey
Joni B. Bernard

12   Vitamin E: Metabolism, Sources, Unique Problems in Zoo Animals, and Supplementation   79
Ellen S. Dierenfeld

13   Principles and Applications of Computed Tomography and Magnetic Resonance Imaging in Zoo and Wildlife Medicine   83
Kathy Spaulding
Michael R. Loomis

14   Plant Poisoning in Zoos in North America   88
Murray E. Fowler

15   Snakebite Protocols for Zoos   95
Joseph P. Flanagan

16   Tuberculosis in Free-Ranging Mammals   101
Roy G. Bengis

17   Vermin Control   114
Lucy H. Spelman

ZOONOSES   121

18   *Cryptosporidium* Species   121
William L. Current

19   Toxoplasmosis in Zoo Animals   131
Della M. Garell

20   Rabies: Global Problem, Zoonotic Threat, and Preventive Management   136
Charles E. Rupprecht

21   Nontuberculous Mycobacteria: Potential for Zoonosis   146
Nadine Lamberski

22   Zoonoses Acquired from Birds   151
Keven Flammer

◆ PART II

FISH   157

23   Anesthesia in Fish   158
Craig A. Harms

24   Preventive Medicine Programs for Fish   163
Brent R. Whitaker

25   Fish Pharmacotherapeutics   182
Michael K. Stoskopf

REPTILES   190

26   Use of Antimicrobial Drugs in Reptiles   190
Elliott R. Jacobson

27   Chameleon Medicine   200
Michael T. Barrie

28   Crocodilian Anesthesia   205
Mark Lynn Lloyd

29   Medical Management of Sea Turtles in Aquaria   217
Brent R. Whitaker
Howard Krum

30   Health Assessment of Chelonians and Release into the Wild   232
Elliott R. Jacobson
John L. Behler
James L. Jarchow

31   Organ Location in Snakes for Diagnostic and Surgical Evaluation   243
Helen E. McCracken

32   The Reptilian Renal-Portal System: Influence on Therapy   249
Peter H. Holz

33   Periodontal Disease in Lizards   252
Helen E. McCracken

◆ PART III

AVIAN MEDICINE   259

34   Iron Overload in the Animal Kingdom   260
Linda J. Lowenstine
Linda Munson

35   Comparative Nutrition and Feeding Considerations of Young Columbidae   269
Charlotte Kirk Baer

36   Medical Management of the California Condor   277
Philip K. Ensley

37   Water Quality for a Waterfowl Collection   292
Richard C. Cambre

38   Caring for Oiled Birds   300
Erica A. Miller
Sallie C. Welte

39   Avian Analgesia   309
Victoria L. Clyde
Joanne Paul-Murphy

◆ PART IV

MAMMALS   315

40   Contraception   316
Cheryl S. Asa

MONOTREMES AND MARSUPIALS   321

41   Diseases of Koalas   321
Rosemary J. Booth
Wendy H. Blanshard

42   Sedation and Anesthesia in Marsupials   333
Amy L. Shima

43   Medical Management of Tree Kangaroos   337
Mitchell Bush
Richard J. Montali

CHIROPTERA   344

44   Medical Management of Megachiropterans   344
Darryl J. Heard

45   Advances in Fruit Bat Nutrition   354
Janet L. (Reiter) Dempsey

RODENTS AND LAGOMORPHS 361

46 Rodent and Small Lagomorph
Reproduction 361
Dennis A. Meritt, Jr.

PRIMATES 365

47 Diseases of Prosimians 365
Randall E. Junge

48 Diseases of the Callitrichidae 369
Richard J. Montali
Mitchell Bush

49 Emerging Viral Diseases of
Nonhuman Primates 377
Joseph T. Bielitzki

50 Great Ape Neonatology 382
Brent Swenson

51 Veterinarian's Role in Monitoring the
Behavioral Enrichment Standards of
the Animal Welfare Act 387
Rita McManamon

52 Tuberculin Responses in
Orangutans 392
Paul P. Calle

53 Diabetes in Primates 397
Christian Walzer

CARNIVORES 401

54 Emerging Viral Infections in Large
Cats 401
Suzanne Kennedy-Stoskopf

55 Giant Panda Management and
Medicine in China 410
S. A. Mainka

56 Medical Management of a Cheetah
Breeding Facility in South
Africa 415
D. G. A. Meltzer

57 Intrahepatic Cysts and Hepatic
Neoplasms in Felids, Ursids, and
Other Zoo and Wild Animals 423
K. Christina Pettan-Brewer
Linda J. Lowenstine

58 Chemical Restraint and
Immobilization of Wild Canids 429
Terry J. Kreeger

59 Otter Anesthesia 436
Lucy H. Spelman

60 Health Assessment, Medical
Management, and Prerelease
Conditioning of Translocated North
American River Otters 443
George V. Kollias

61 Assisted Reproductive Techniques in
Nondomestic Carnivores 449
JoGayle Howard

62 Gastritis in Cheetahs 458
Raymund F. Wack

63 Veterinary Contributions to the
Black-footed Ferret Conservation
Program 460
Elizabeth S. Williams
E. Tom Thorne

MARINE MAMMALS 464

64 Diagnostic Cytology in Marine
Mammal Medicine 464
Terry W. Campbell

65 Leptospirosis in Marine
Mammals 469
Frances M. D. Gulland

66 Toxicology in Marine Mammals 472
Thomas J. O'Shea
Joseph R. Geraci

67 Diagnosis and Treatment of Fungal
Infections in Marine Mammals 478
Thomas H. Reidarson
James F. McBain
Leslie M. Dalton
Michael G. Rinaldi

68 Medical Management of Stranded
Small Cetaceans 485
Forrest I. Townsend

69 Hand-Rearing Techniques for Neonate
Cetaceans 493
Forrest I. Townsend

70 Morbillivirus Infections of Marine
Mammals 497
Pádraig J. Duignan

71 Fetal Ultrasonography in Dolphins with Emphasis on Gestational Aging 501
L. Rae Stone
Robert L. Johnson
Jay C. Sweeney
Maria L. Lewis

72 Manatee Medicine 507
Michael T. Walsh
Gregory D. Bossart

ELEPHANTS 517

73 Radiographic Techniques for the Elephant Foot and Carpus 517
Laurie J. Gage

74 Calving Elephants (Normal) 521
Michael J. Schmidt

75 Dystocia in the Elephant 522
Joseph J. Foerner

76 Relocation of African Elephants 525
J. P. Raath

77 Antibiotic Therapy in Elephants 533
John H. Olsen

78 Flaccid Trunk Paralysis in Free-Ranging Elephants 541
Nancy D. Kock

79A Oral and Nasal Diseases of Elephants 544
Armin Kuntze

79B Poxvirus Infections in Elephants 547
Armin Kuntze

PERRISODACTYLIDS 551

80 Skin Diseases of Black Rhinoceroses 551
Linda Munson
R. Eric Miller

81 Anesthesia of White Rhinoceroses 556
J. P. Raath

82 Tapir Medicine 562
Donald L. Janssen
Bruce A. Rideout
Mark S. Edwards

83 Rhinoceros Feeding and Nutrition 568
Ellen S. Dierenfeld

84 Infectious Diseases of Equids 572
Lyndsey G. Phillips, Jr.

ARTIODACTYLIDS 575

85 Use of Tranquilizers in Wild Herbivores 575
Hym Ebedes
J. P. Raath

86 Preventive Medicine Programs for Ranched Hoofstock 585
James M. Jensen

87 Designing a Trichostrongyloid Parasite Control Program for Captive Exotic Ruminants 593
Ramiro Isaza
George V. Kollias

88 Embryo Transfer and Semen Technology from Cattle Applied to Nondomestic Artiodactylids 597
C. Earle Pope
Naida M. Loskutoff

89 Rotavirus and Coronavirus Infections in Nondomestic Ruminants 605
Scott B. Citino

90 Paratuberculosis in Zoo Animals 612
Elizabeth J. B. Manning
Michael T. Collins

91 Paratuberculosis in Free-Ranging Wildlife in North America 616
David A. Jessup
Elizabeth S. Williams

92 Brucellosis Caused by *Brucella abortus* in Free-Ranging North American Artiodactylids 621
David L. Hunter
Terry J. Kreeger

93 *Brucella suis* Biovar 4 Infection in Free-Ranging Artiodactylids   626
Robert A. Dieterich

94 Contraception in Artiodactylids, Using Porcine Zona Pellucida Vaccination   628
Irwin K. M. Liu
John W. Turner
Jay F. Kirkpatrick

95 *Parelaphostrongylus tenuis* and *Elaphostrongylus cervi* in Free-Ranging Artiodactylids   631
Lora Rickard Ballweber

96 Anesthesia for Captive Nile Hippopotamus   638
Michael R. Loomis
Edward C. Ramsay

97 Anesthesia for Nondomestic Suids   639
Paul P. Calle
Patrick J. Morris

98 Okapi Medicine and Surgery   646
Bonnie L. Raphael

99 *Mycobacterium bovis* Infection of Cervids: Diagnosis, Treatment, and Control   650
Robert A. Cook

100 The Use of Chutes for Ungulate Restraint   657
J. C. Haigh

101 Scrapie-Like Spongiform Encephalopathies (Prion Diseases) in Nondomesticated Species   662
James K. Kirkwood
Andrew A. Cunningham

102 Medical Management of Duikers   668
Michelle Willette Frahm

103 Capture and Handling of Mountain Sheep and Goats   681
David A. Jessup

104 Medical Aspects of Arabian Oryx Reintroduction   687
Jacques R. B. Flamand

Index   699

PART I

GENERAL

Use of Pulse Oximetry in Monitoring Anesthesia

JACK L. ALLEN

Serial blood gas sampling has been the standard method of monitoring a patient's blood oxygenation. Problems associated with this method include blood vessel trauma from repeated arterial puncture, poor cooperation from the patient, delayed laboratory analysis, and information about the patient only intermittently obtained. In veterinary anesthesia, there is increased acceptance and usage of pulse oximeters as an alternative means of monitoring a patient's blood oxygenation. This is particularly true in the specialty area of zoo and wildlife anesthesia. The pulse oximeter is easy to use, is noninvasive, and provides accurate continuous physiologic information. The wide variety of species and diverse environments in which veterinarians practice make the application of pulse oximetry uniquely suited to zoo and wildlife anesthesia.

PRINCIPLES OF PULSE OXIMETRY

The technology of pulse oximetry is very sophisticated, but the principles of pulse oximetry are simple. Pulse oximeters use two light-emitting diodes (LEDs): red light at approximately 660 nm and infrared light at approximately 920 nm. A photodetector, placed opposite these LEDs across an arterial vascular bed, measures the intensity of transmitted light across the vascular bed.

The differences in the intensity of transmitted light between the two LEDs are caused by the differences in the absorption of light by oxygenated and deoxygenated hemoglobin contained within the vascular bed. The arterial hemoglobin oxygen saturation is computed by the pulse oximeter from the relative amounts of light transmitted to the photodetector. This value is then displayed digitally.[8] In addition, pulse oximeters display the pulse rate.

CLINICAL APPLICATION

Any clinical situation associated with respiratory or circulatory compromise may improve with oxygen saturation monitoring. Pulse oximeters can detect profound arterial desaturation, often without any concurrent abnormalities in heart rate, blood pressure, or respiratory rate.[4] For this reason, they are recommended for monitoring patients during general anesthesia.

Pulse oximetry readings are totally dependent on

the information received from the sensor. Recognized factors that alter sensor readings during zoo and wildlife anesthesia include but are not limited to external light interference, low perfusion, motion artifacts, hypothermia, darkly pigmented skin, thick skin, and excessive hair.[1] Additional although uncommon limitations are electrocautery (which will artifactually decrease the oxygen saturation), intravascular dyes (e.g., methylene blue), and the presence of methemoglobinemia (which leads to overestimation of oxygen saturation).

Transmission oximetry sensors have been used on the tongue, lip, ear, toe, prepuce, and vulva, and reflectance oximetry sensors have been used in the rectum, esophagus, and the oral mucosa.[2, 5–7] Oxygen saturation readings vary with changes in sensor placement.[3] It is important to find a suitable sensor location and leave the sensor in this place throughout the monitoring period. Once the sensor is in place and consistent readings are obtained, accuracy is verified by comparing the displayed oximeter pulse rate with the actual patient's heart rate. These two should be in agreement, and the displayed oxygen saturation reading is true. It is important to monitor oxygen saturation *trends* rather than to focus on any single displayed value. The technology and principles of pulse oximetry are well established. Future contributions will be in the form of creative application of pulse oximetry in zoo and wildlife anesthesia. Contemporary examples include detection of (1) postoperative hypoxemia, (2) pneumothorax, (3) endobronchial intubation, (4) rumen bloating, and (5) monitoring of adequate peripheral perfusion after vascular surgery.

SUMMARY

Pulse oximetry monitoring should be a standard of practice for zoo and wildlife anesthesia. Pulse oximeters are sufficiently accurate and precise that they can be used to monitor oxygen saturation trends in mammals. The application of pulse oximetry in birds, reptiles, and fish is worthy of investigation.

REFERENCES

1. Allen JL: Pulse oximetry: clinical applications in zoological medicine. Proceedings of the Annual Meeting of the American Association of Zoo Veterinarians, South Padre Island, TX, pp 163–164, 1990.
2. Allen JL: Pulse oximetry: everyday uses in a zoological practice. Vet Rec 130:354–355, 1992.
3. Jacobson JD, Miller MW, Mathews NS, et al: Evaluation of accuracy of pulse oximetry in dogs. Am J Vet Res 53(4):537–540, 1992.
4. Kelleher JF: Pulse oximetry. J Clin Monit 5(1):37–62, 1989.
5. Mihm FG, Machado C, Snyder R: Pulse oximetry and end-tidal CO_2 monitoring of an adult elephant. J Zoo Anim Med 19(3):106–109, 1988.
6. Morkel P: Chemical immobilization of the black rhinoceros (*Diceros bicornis*). Proceedings of the Symposium on Rhinos as Game Ranch Animals, Onderstepoort, Pretoria, RSA, pp 128–135, 1994.
7. Raath JP: Anaesthesia of the white rhino. Proceedings of the Symposium on Rhinos as Game Ranch Animals, Onderstepoort, Pretoria, RSA, pp 119–127, 1994.
8. Saint John BE: Pulse oximetry: theory, technology, and clinical considerations. Proceedings of the Annual Meeting of the American Association of Zoo Veterinarians, Oakland, CA, pp 223–229, 1992.

CHAPTER **2**

The Role of Pathology in Zoo Animal Medicine

TRACEY McNAMARA

For many species of animals, zoos serve as their last buffer against extinction. The conservation community intensively manages small populations of animals in zoological institutions through species survival plans (SSPs), taxon advisory groups, and others, in an effort to maximize their reproductive and genetic potential. In view of the limited numbers of animals remaining in certain groups, the critical value of each individual is recognized, and many zoos now employ full-time clinical veterinary staff to provide for the health needs of their collection.

However, of the 172 institutions currently accredited by the American Zoological Association (AZA), only a handful have full-time veterinary pathology support. This is an alarming situation, considering the settings in which zoological animals are found. They are maintained in herds or flocks, in which disease in one individual may spread rapidly to other members of its group. Mixed-species exhibits, although popular with the public, pose the additional threat of interspecies disease transmission. Also, because most zoos are located in large urban parks that contain indigenous fauna, the threat of introduced disease is omnipresent. In many cases, because the practice of zoo medicine is still a relative frontier, the veterinary arsenal of drugs routinely used to prevent disease in domestic animals are simply not available for or are not approved for use in zoo species. In these cases, even when aware of a specific disease threat, veterinarians may have only limited means of preventing the disease, and the best hope of avoiding losses may rest in the rapid detection, through necropsy and histopathology, of the initial or "index" case of what could quickly develop into an epidemic involving many animals. Although diagnosis may not have been established soon enough for the individual undergoing necropsy, the information gained from careful evaluation of that animal may be incorporated into veterinary or curatorial management plans that safeguard the health of the rest of the collection.

For instance, suppose, as is often the case, an animal is simply found dead with no clinical antecedent history. Without the benefit of diagnostic pathology support, the veterinary and curatorial staff are forced to make management decisions in a vacuum on the basis of insufficient information. How is the "exposed" cagemate to be handled? What if it is scheduled to be moved to another part of the zoo? Or, in a more complicated scenario, what if it is supposed to be shipped to another institution? Should the shipment be delayed? Is it necessary to do so? Diagnostic pathology service may provide much-needed answers to the curatorial and veterinary staff and in this way, on a day-to-day basis, play a pivotal role in preventive health programs.

Pathologists may also, through the identification of pathogens and an understanding of their epidemiology, aid curatorial staff in management plans. In many instances, there is no specific treatment or preventive medical measures for the diseases that threaten the health and well-being of zoo animals. In these cases, the best hope of preventing disease lies in decreasing or eliminating exposure of the animals to the organism in question. For example, the identification of an avian tuberculosis problem could translate into a change in exhibit design that would allow for removal and disinfection of soil substrate, thus decreasing exposure to this soilborne pathogen. Another example wherein understanding the transmission cycle of a disease could result in exhibit design changes is that of duck viral enteritis. This virulent herpes infection may cause serious losses in captive waterfowl when they are exposed to migratory waterfowl carrying the virus. In some zoos, this has happened on a seasonal basis because their large ponds and feeding stations prove irresistible to migrating birds, who stop in for a free lunch but, in doing so, introduce this disease with potentially devastating consequences. Armed with a knowledge of the disease and faced with unacceptable losses, some institutions have altered their feeding stations to make them less accessible to wild birds. Some have even gone to the expense of screening off their ponds entirely to prevent further exposure of collection birds to free-ranging waterfowl and have decreased the incidence of this disease problem. Had the disease itself never been identified or understood, these management changes might not have occurred.

Not all of the diseases that threaten zoo animals are of an infectious nature, nor do all of them cause mortality. In some cases, however, if left undiagnosed, they may ultimately have a more serious impact on the collection as a result of their effects on reproductive performance and on viability of young. Nutritional imbalances, genetic disorders, and toxicologic problems may be subtle and difficult to pin down. Identification of such problems requires careful review of all cases, not just sporadically submitted cases, if trends are to be discerned and addressed.

In view of all these concerns, a strong argument can be made for the need for diagnostic pathology service to all zoological collections. As a group, perhaps even more so than their domestic counterparts, zoo animals are in urgent need of accurate and rapid pathology support. Information gained from review and interpretation of surgical biopsy, cytologic, and necropsy material by a pathologist empowers zoo staff to take management steps to halt or prevent disease problems. The zoo community currently expends tremendous effort and resources to ensure the health of the rare and endangered species in their care. Part of that care should include an active pathology program that should be integrated into the multidisciplinary animal care team. Only then will it be possible to ensure that these high-risk animals do not succumb to a preventable disease for simple want of a diagnosis.

On a larger scale, a pathology program will, by necessity, play an increasingly important role in future conservation programs. Professionals in the zoo field know only too well the limitations of current knowledge about the diseases causing problems in zoo animals and their prevalence and potential risks. This lack of information poses a serious problem for conservationists in that reintroduction or translocation programs designed to benefit a species may inadvertently introduce disease to a native population and, in doing so, cause more harm than good. In 1992, concern over the paucity of information was addressed in the International Conference of Implications of Infectious Disease for Captive Propagation and Reintroduction of Threatened Species, which called for "increased monitoring, investigation, and surveillance of disease in captive wildlife in a standardized manner."[3]

Systematic collection of pathology data from as many accredited institutions as possible could well provide answers to the questions that the conservation community hopes to answer. Indeed, the future of health and conservation programs depends on this collection. At present, it is difficult to accomplish this task because there is a shortage of board certified pathologists with an interest in this highly specialized field. In addition, financial constraints faced by most zoological institutions make it impossible for them to pursue pathology programs on a routine basis at this time.

However, the situation is slowly changing. New training programs in the area of zoo and comparative pathology have emerged since 1993, making it possible for more trainees to pursue this career goal. Also, several larger institutions have secured funds to bring on pathology staff. However, even smaller zoological institutions can, and indeed must, have an active pathology component. There are a number of ways in which smaller zoos should enhance their in-house programs and prepare for the future.

THE "NECROPSY"

The 1995 revision of the American Zoological Association (AZA) Accreditation Visiting Committee Handbook[1] specifies only that deceased animals in accredited institutions must be "necropsied whenever possible to determine the cause of death." Evaluation of the definition of "necropsy" is perhaps the best place to launch a uniform pathology program among zoos.

For a Diplomate of the American College of Veterinary Pathology (ACVP), "necropsy" entails a thorough evaluation of all organs, sampling of representative sections of all organs, and fixation in large volumes of properly buffered 10% formalin for histopathologic evaluation, as well as ancillary procedures such as electron microscopy studies, cytologic profiles, bacterial and fungal cultures, and freezing of tissues at $-70°C$ for possible viral isolation or toxicologic or nutritional evaluation. Gross and histologic lesions are documented with photography. Tissues, as well as paraffin blocks and slides, are catalogued and archived for future retrieval. Not only do these procedures increase the likelihood of a successful diagnosis, which is vital to the practice of preventive medicine, but they also establish a reference base that expands knowledge of the disease problems of zoo animals as a whole.

This is the ideal, but the definition of "necropsy" in most zoos is, unfortunately, quite different. Many institutions reserve this intensive a work-up for the few SSP species with specific pathology protocols. Other cases may receive only a "quick peek" at the end of a busy day with limited tissue sampling and even more selective histopathology. Because the majority of zoo necropsies are performed by nonpathologists, it is easy to see how this might happen. Nonetheless, it must be recognized that unless this situation changes, little progress will be made.

The reason why necropsies being performed on some zoo cases are less than optimal is that many clinical veterinarians, on whom the responsibility for necropsy generally falls, have had only limited formal training in necropsy technique and procedures and may feel uncomfortable with this aspect of their jobs. They must, however, become comfortable with it because most institutions will never have a staff pathologist and subsequent histopathologic evaluation of tissues by an outside pathologist will not compensate for an improperly performed postmortem study. Also, because the decision to perform critical ancillary procedures at the time of necropsy is predicated upon correct interpretation of gross observations, clinicians must become well acquainted with gross morbid pathology. Fortunately, a variety of training materials are now available to help reach this goal. All of them are inexpensive and fall within the budgetary means of even small zoological collections.

"ZOO PATHOLOGY" EDUCATIONAL RESOURCES

The University of Georgia produces the International Veterinary Pathology Slide Bank video disc known as "Noah's Arkive." The disc contains more than 30,000 color images of normal and diseased tissues submitted by pathologists and other veterinarians worldwide. It contains a wealth of zoo, exotic, and wildlife cases and is a superb training and reference resource. The accompanying program allows the user to review images on the basis of species, organ system, or specific etiology, either individually or as part of the same search. Plans to make Noah's Arkive available on CD-ROM are under way. For more information or to order the disc, contact Noah's Arkive, The Department of Pathology, College of Veterinary Medicine, The University of Georgia, Athens, GA 30602-7388; phone: 706-542-5837; fax: 706-542-5828; NOAH@CALC.VET.UGA.EDU.

Another resource is available through the Charles Louis Davis, D.V.M., Foundation for the Advancement of Veterinary and Comparative Pathology, which offers videotaped lectures to its members. Many hours of seminars on the pathology of nonhuman primates, reptiles and amphibians, marine mammals, birds, fishes, and free-ranging wildlife are currently available. For further information, contact Dr. Sam Thompson, National Programs Director, Charles Louis Davis, D.V.M., Foundation, 6245 Formoor Lane, Gurnee, IL 60031-4757; phone: 847-367-4359; fax: 847-247-1869; electronic mail: CLDavis@iX.netcom.com.

The Foundation has actively supported the development of the field of zoo and wildlife pathology. In addition to financing symposia, providing scholarships to students with an interest in zoo pathology, and performing fundraising, it has enabled the formation of a consortium of zoo and wildlife pathologists. Their future efforts will be focused on the development of additional educational materials in this field. A collaborative CD-ROM on zoo pathology is planned and will draw on material from zoological institutions with existing pathology programs. Announcements about the availability of this CD-ROM, as well as other training materials, will appear on the following website: http://vetpath1.afip.mil/cldavis/cldavis.html.

Whereas larger institutions may have significant library resources to offer their staff, this may not be true of smaller zoos. Because awareness of a disease problem is the first step to its successful diagnosis, access to pathology literature is a critical component of any health program. Zoos with computers can surf the World Wide Web for references. Even zoos without Internet access can subscribe to commercially available reference databases. One of these, the "Veterinary Librarian," covers not only domestic animal literature but also the zoo literature, including the *Journal of Zoo and Wildlife Medicine* and the *Journal of Wildlife Diseases*. In addition, it includes all the proceedings from the American Association of Zoo Veterinarians (AAZV) annual conferences as well as other meetings. The database is updated biannually and can be used on most computers. It provides an inexpensive and rapid means of scanning the zoo pathology literature and staying current with disease issues. For further information, contact Martin Page, First Move, P.O. Box 215, Littleton, CO 80160; phone: 303-794-3552; fax: 303-795-6276; electronic mail: mpage@unidial.com.

Another source of pathology literature to consider is that available through the University of Utrecht in The Netherlands. European zoo and wildlife pathologists have contributed thousands of citations to the PREX online information service, Department of Laboratory Animal Science database, many of which would not be accessible through routine library searches in the United States. Because so few institutions are actively working on the diseases of zoo animals, it is imperative that what little information is available be accessible and readily shared. A modest subscription fee is required for instant access to a wealth of European zoo pathology literature. To learn more, contact Mr. Theo Bakker, Yalelaan 17, P.O. Box 80166, 3508 TD Utrecht, The Netherlands; phone: 31.30.533158; fax: 31.30.536747; electronic mail: tjg@diva.dgk.ruu.nl.

In addition to access to educational resources, individuals responsible for performing zoo necropsies must be given the opportunity to attend training workshops such as those offered at the AAZV annual meetings.

FUTURE NEEDS

If the conservation community hopes to have meaningful data on which to base future programs, consistency and uniformity of zoo necropsies must be addressed now. In addition, a concerted effort must be made to maximize the amount of information that can be obtained from each necropsy. For many prosectors, this means adopting a more long-term conservation approach to all necropsies.

The death of an animal in a collection is regrettable, but not to learn from it when there are still so many unknowns in the field of comparative medicine is truly wasteful. Questions about comparative anatomy, radiology, endoscopy, and cytology challenge zoo clinicians daily. Pathologists puzzle over comparative gross morbid pathology, comparative histology, and histopathology. In many cases, interpretation of findings in exotic species is hampered by the fact that normal baselines have yet to be established for many of the animals in zoo collections. Many of these problems could be resolved through intensified use of necropsy material.

Each time someone does a perfunctory examination only to verify whether an animal died of head trauma and then simply discards the tissues, many opportunities have been missed. From a practical point of view, unless each organ system is reviewed in a systematic manner, a lesion important to the overall health of the collection, such as a mycobacterial infection, might be missed. If each organ system has not been checked, it is uncertain what may or may not have been present. Haphazard necropsies are dangerous in that they can be misleading and, at worst, lull institutions into a false sense of

security about disease issues. They also contribute little to the overall knowledge about nondomestic species.

Consider all the procedures that could routinely be performed on zoo postmortems. Specimen radiographs could be obtained in each institution in order to create a species-based reference library. This not only would provide valuable information to the individual zoo practitioner but also, if subsequently pooled, could be useful to the entire community. Skeletal preparations could provide insight into surgical procedures or be of use in in-house education programs. In combination with histopathology findings, cytologic studies on both normal and abnormal tissues would make this diagnostic technique a more powerful tool in zoo medicine.

These procedures need not necessarily be performed by already overworked employees and understaffed zoos. To many outside institutions, the necropsy case-load of a local zoo represents a veritable treasure chest of comparative material. Although researchers at nearby medical or veterinary colleges may have limited interest in conservation issues per se, their expertise and access to funds and technology may make it possible to pursue projects that might otherwise be impossible in a zoo setting. More often than not, if a zoo's research interests overlap or complement those of another institution, projects can be conducted at little or no cost and still be of great benefit to zoo animals in general. It is a matter of making the best use of available resources in a pragmatic and yet creative manner.

However, if zoos hope to establish and cultivate these useful collaborations, it is necessary first for them to create banked tissue libraries. This can be accomplished at minimal cost, inasmuch as the purchase of formalin and heat-sealed plastic storage bags does not place an undue burden on even the most meager budget. Failure to bank tissues is shortsighted and self-defeating: On a day-to-day basis, it means that tissues are not available for additional studies that may be recommended by the consulting pathologist. The lack of tissues precludes the ability to take advantage of emerging technologic procedures, such as polymerase chain reaction (PCR), which have greatly increased the diagnostic value of formalinized material. Also, zoos without tissue banks forfeit the possibility of participating in future retrospective studies.

The same argument can be made for frozen tissue banks. Freezers are indeed expensive items, but in view of the number of viral infections that have been described in zoo species since the late 1980s, it must be recognized that the lack of tissues for viral isolation can seriously hamper diagnostic studies.

This is also true of histopathology. Careful gross evaluations are the first and most basic component of any pathology program, but they do have limitations. What is seen at necropsy is only the surface information. Even when seen by an ACVP-certified veterinary pathologist, gross lesions can be difficult to interpret. "White spots" in the liver of a crane as opposed to those in a snake bring to mind entirely different differential diagnoses. In most cases, histopathology *must* be performed for definitive diagnosis.

Unfortunately, the majority of zoos currently find this service beyond their budgetary means. This handicap must be overcome if the conservation community is to get the data that it needs. At present, the majority of information on "zoo pathology" comes from a small number of institutions. There is hope, in the future, of pooling these data and making them available through the pathology module of MedARKS (The Medical Animal Record Keeping System; International Species Information System [ISIS], 12101 Johnny Cake Road, Apple Valley, MN 55124), which is currently being tested in a number of institutions. The power of this database as a clinical and conservation tool will rest in the quality and amount of pathology data ultimately available. When zoos limit themselves to only gross necropsies, they also limit the potential long-term gains of this database.

CONCLUSION

Veterinarians enjoy the reputation of caring for "all creatures great and small" and, in the case of zoo practitioners, this is certainly true. It is also true, however, that in the general veterinary community, zoo species have never received the attention accorded their domestic counterparts because, in the words of George Orwell, "all animals are created equal but some animals are more equal than others."[2] Much of the basic veterinary work on domestic animals done by researchers in the 20th century makes it possible to offer them the highest level of health care. This work, however, still remains to be done on behalf of zoo animals. The impetus for progress will have to come from zoos themselves. Zoo administrators need to acknowledge the integral role that pathology plays in health programs and the necessity of pathology service to their collections, and they need to budget appropriately. Individual zoo clinicians need to make the commitment to do the most complete possible examinations on all necropsies. Until quality diagnostic pathology services are available to all zoos, veterinarians would do well to approach each zoo necropsy as someone would an acre of Brazilian rainforest: something to be treated with a great deal of care, respect and responsibility.

REFERENCES

1. American Zoological Association (AZA): Accreditation Visiting Committee Handbook, rev. ed. Bethesda, MD, AZA Executive Office/Conservation Center, 1995.
2. Orwell G: Animal Farm, Fiftieth Anniversary ed. New York, Harcourt, Brace, Chapter 10, p 149, 1995.
3. Wolff PL, Seal US: Implications of infectious disease for captive propagation and reintroduction of threatened species. J Zoo Wildlife Med 24(3):229–230, 1993.

CHAPTER **3**

Applications of Biotelemetry in Wildlife Medicine

WILLIAM B. KARESH

Remote measurement of biologic data, or biotelemetry, has been widely used since the early 1960s. Applications range from simple automatic counters or weighing devices to complex physiologic monitoring systems for humans and animals in space. Recent technologic advances in electronic miniaturization, programmable microcircuitry, and data transmission methods have improved remote sensing system performance and capabilities. Tens of thousands of radio transmitters have been attached to wild animals since the 1970s and this has led to the refinement of attachment techniques as well as of data collection and storage methods. Table 3–1 lists commonly used approaches for attaching trans-mitters. A number of books and review articles provide good overviews of biotelemetry and include extensive bibliographies.[1, 2, 4, 9] Numerous experienced commercial manufacturers now exist to supply the demand for telemetry equipment (Table 3–2). These companies provide advice on design specifications to meet project needs and on attachment methods used by other researchers for the same or similar species.

The basic telemetry system consists of the transmitter, power supply, antennas, and receiver. Additional components for specific data collection may be added to the transmitter or receiver ends of the system. A wide variety of systems and capabilities are currently

TABLE 3–1. Techniques Used for Attaching Telemetry Equipment to Animals

Fish

Coelomic or intramuscular implants
External tags (fin or body)

Amphibians and Reptiles

Subcutaneous or coelomic implants
Gastric (per os)
Attached with epoxy glue to carapace scutes (chelonians)
Sutured to dorsal scutes (crocodilians)
Backpacks or harnesses

Birds

Coelomic implants with or without external antennas
Leg bands
Backpacks or harnesses
Collars
Petagial tags
Attached with epoxy or other glue to feathers
Sutured to feather shafts
Attached with epoxy glue to maxilla

Mammals

Subcutaneous or abdominal implants
Rumen (per os)
Collars
Ear tags
Bracelet or anklet
Horn implants (rhinoceros)
Attached with glue to pelage (pinnipeds, bats)
Tail peduncle collar with buoy transmitter (manatees)
Nylon bolting to dorsal fin (cetaceans)
Tusk mount (walrus)
Barbed tag (sharks, cetaceans)

---

available, and possible configurations are limited only by basic laws of physics and the financial resources to design and build new systems.

TRANSMITTERS

The transmitter serves as a point source for locating an animal or an object and may also convert collected data to a communication format. Sensors connected to or included in the transmitter package can monitor physiologic data such as temperature, heart rate, blood pressure, body position and movement, or location as determined by geographic positioning system units (GPSs). Remote physiologic monitoring is common in human cardiology, and a wide variety of wildlife applications have been developed for monitoring reproductive physiology, behavioral responses, thermoregulation, and stress.[5, 8, 14, 15] Remote measurement of physiologic data in wildlife allows the acquisition of information while eliminating the effects of human handling or interactions. Transmitted signals may be in any format (AM, FM, VHF, UHF, M-band, etc.). A simple way to indicate a change in sensor information is to vary the pulse rate (beeps per minute). For example, a mercury tilt switch in the collar package senses that the animal lifted its head, and the transmitter then doubles the pulse rate of the signal. Temperature data may be transferred by

use of a continuous scale of temperature versus pulse rates. Another approach is to convert the information to a digital code that is interpreted by software in the receiver unit. This coding of the signal allows for greater variety of information to be transferred and may also allow multiple transmitters to operate on the same frequency.

Circuitry in the transmitter package may be designed to continuously send the collected data or store it for transmission at a later time. Transmitters may be pre-programmed to send data at a set time or day, or they may have a switch that is activated by some external cue. For example, transmitters on marine mammals and turtles frequently have a salt water switch or depth switch that activates the transmitter component when the animal surfaces. Other systems allow for investigators to send a signal to the transmitter package, which instructs it to begin transmitting the stored data. This approach requires that the transmitter package also include a receiver unit that is running at the time of the query. Systems that automatically give a drug injection stored in the collar when signaled by the investigator have been produced but are not commercially available.[10] Relay receiver/transmitters may be used to pick up weak signals and re-send them to more distant locations. This has been useful in work with very small animals or in environments in which signal transmission is poor, such as inside buildings or in mountainous areas.

POWER SOURCES

In most radiotelemetry systems, batteries are used as a power supply. Although battery technology has improved since the 1960s, this component of the system still tends to be the limiting factor in transmitter longevity and package size (weight). Microcircuitry allows the transmitters and sensors to be insignificant in size in comparison to almost any battery. But transmitter design may significantly enhance battery life by reducing power. Several approaches are commonly used: (1) using the minimum signal wattage needed for transmission, (2) reducing the pulse width (length of each pulse) and rate (number of pulses per minute), and (3) programming the transmitter to turn off at regular intervals. These design techniques have led to the availability of 1.5- to 3-g transmitters with a working life of 70 days.

Solar panels attached to the package may be used to recharge batteries during the day. This approach is used to significantly reduce the battery weight in transmitters for some birds. Solar cells may be used without batteries if signal transmission and data collection are needed only during the day. Solar panels are effective only when adequate exposure of the unit to bright sunlight is available and on species in which the panel will stay clean. For this reason, applications of solar panels on diurnal raptors, vultures, and aquatic or semiaquatic birds work well if the units are mounted in a way that they are not covered by feathers.[3] In general, solar systems have limited application for most mammals and reptiles.

TABLE 3–2. Suppliers of Radiotelemetry Equipment

Manufacturer/Supplier	Comments
Advanced Telemetry Systems, Inc. (ATS) 470 1st Avenue North Box 398 Isanti, MN 55040 Phone: 612-444-9267 Electronic mail: 70743.572@compuserve	Wide range of VHF telemetry equipment custom made for all species, including marine applications, physiologic monitoring, and automated data collection
AVM Instrument Co. 2356 Research Drive Livermore, CA 94550 Phone: 510-449-2286	Wide range of VHF equipment for mammals, birds, and fishes, traditionally used by herpetologists
Biotrack, Inc. (United Kingdom) U.S. Representative: Telinject USA 9316 Soledad Canyon Road Saugus, CA 91350 Phone: 805-268-0915 Fax: 805-268-1105	Wide range of VHF equipment, tailpiece transmitter for Telinject darts
Cedar Creek Bioelectronics Lab University of Minnesota Bethel, MN 55005 Phone: 612-434-7361	Specialization in research and development of new technologic methods, automated tracking systems
Custom Electronics 2009 Silver Court West Urbana, IL 61801 Phone/fax: 217-344-3460 Electronic mail: cutomel@aol.com	Custom-made receivers and antennas; various bird transmitters, with a specialty in raptors
Custom Telemetry and Consulting 1050 Industrial Drive Watkinsville, GA 30677 Dan Stonebrenner Phone: 404-769-4067	Specialization in custom-made telemetry packages to meet specific needs of both researcher and animal
F & L Electronics P.O. Box 19 Mahomet, IL 61853 Phone: 217-586-2132 Fax: 217-586-5733	Specialization in small transmitters for birds and fishes, external and implantable, and a range of receivers and antennas
Holohil Systems, Ltd. 112 John Cavanagh Road Carp, Ontario K0A 1L0 Phone: 613-839-0676 Fax: 613-839-0675 Electronic mail: holohil@logisys.com	Wide range of VHF equipment custom made for all species
IMF Technology Gmbh. Grosse Mullroser Strasse 46 15232 Frankfurt, Germany Phone: 49-335-556040 Fax: 49-335-556049	Custom design and manufacture of telemetry systems with a specialty in behavioral and physiologic monitoring; also production of GPS collars and infrared sensing units
Lotek Engineering 115 Pony Drive Newmarket, Ontario L3Y 7B5 Phone: 905-836-6680 Fax: 905-836-6455 Electronic mail: telemetry@lotek.com	Production of GPS telemetry systems with remote downloading capabilities, digital coding for transmitters, and small transmitters for fishes and fisheries management systems

Table continued on following page

TABLE 3–2. Suppliers of Radiotelemetry Equipment *Continued*

Manufacturer/Supplier	Comments
Merlin Systems, Inc. 445 West Ustick Road Meridian, ID 83642 Phone: 208-884-3308 Fax: 208-888-9528 Electronic mail: merlin@cyberhighway.net	Specialize in small VFH transmitters for birds
Microwave Telemetry 10280 Old Columbia Road, Suite 260 Columbia, MD 21046 Phone: 410-290-8672 Fax: 410-290-8847 Electronic mail: microwt@aol.com	Specialization in small satellite transmitter systems for birds, digital coding transmitters, and data collection systems
Minimitter Co., Inc. P.O. Box 3386 Sunriver, OR 97707 Phone: 541-593-8639 Fax: 541-593-5604	Specialization in small telemetry applications and physiologic monitoring systems, automated data collection systems, and software
Service Argos, Inc. 1801 McCormick Drive, Suite 10 Landover, MD 20785 Phone: 301-925-4411 Fax: 301-925-8995 Phone, France: 61-39-4700 Fax, France: 61-75-1014 Phone, Australia: 3-9669-4650 Fax, Australia: 3-9669-4675 Phone, Japan: 3-3779-5506 Fax, Japan: 3-3779-5783	Provision of the required licensing and use privileges; data transfer for Argos satellite system; no provision of any equipment or supplies
Sirtrack, Ltd. Private Bag 1403, Goddards Land Havelock North New Zealand Phone: 64-6-877-7736 Fax: 64-6-877-5422	Specialization in research and development of new telemetry applications, including satellite tracking systems and wide range of VHF transmitters for all species
Smith-Root, Inc. 14014 Northeast Salmon Creek Avenue Vancouver, WA 98665 Phone: 206-573-0202	Specialization in fish transmitters with low frequencies but will custom make transmitters for other applications, fisheries research and management equipment
Starlink, Inc. 6400 Highway 290 East, Suite 202 Austin, TX 78723-1030 Phone: 512-454-5511 Toll-free phone: 800-460-2167 Fax: 512-454-5570 Electronic mail: dfowler@starlingdgps.com	Development and production of satellite, Loran, and automated VHF tracking systems for terrestrial and aquatic environments
Telemetry Systems, Inc. P.O. Box 187 Mequon, WI 53092 Phone: 414-241-8335	Specialization in solar powered transmitters for mammals and birds
Televilt International 711 98 Ramsberg Sweden Phone: 46-581-660-178 Fax: 46-581-660-343	Wide range of VHF equipment; automated tracking and data collection systems and data analysis packages; GPS systems

TABLE 3–2. Suppliers of Radiotelemetry Equipment *Continued*

Manufacturer/Supplier	Comments

Telonics
    932 East Impala Avenue
    Mesa, AZ 85204-6699
    Phone: 602-892-4444
    Fax: 602-892-9139
	Wide range of fixed-design VHF equipment as well as GPS and Argos tracking systems

Titley Electronics, Pty, Ltd.
    P.O. Box 19
    Ballina, New South Wales 2478
    Australia
    Phone/fax: 61-66-866617
    Electronic mail: titley@nor.com.au
	Wide range of VHF equipment; specialized telemetry and ultrasound analysis systems for bats

Wildlife Computers
    16150 Northeast 85th Street, Suite 226
    Redmond, WA 98052
    Phone: 206-881-3048
    Fax: 206-881-3405
	Specialization in dive data recorders and Argos tracking applications for marine vertebrates

Wildlife Materials, Inc.
    R.R. 1
    Giant City Road
    Carbondale, IL 62901
    Phone: 618-549-6330
    Fax: 618-457-3340
	Wide range of VHF equipment and automated data collection; production of a tailpiece transmitter for Cap-Chur darts and collars for psittacines

ANTENNAS AND FREQUENCIES

Both the transmitter and the receiver require antennas. Although this appears to be a simple part of telemetry systems, antenna configurations and radiofrequencies have a tremendous impact on system function. Antenna design (size, configuration, and placement) is based on signal properties, physical limitations for the animals, and the type of information desired. Most transmitters are fitted with omni-directional antennas to maximize signal transmission in all directions. Receivers are equipped with directional antennas either to maximize reception or to determine the location of transmitters; otherwise, omni-directional antennas may be used.

Traditionally, frequencies between 140 and 170 MHz (VHF range) have been used for wildlife applications. This developed as a result of component availability as well as a compromise of signal transmission properties and antenna length. For radio waves, signal transmission is optimized when the length of the antenna is an even multiple of the wave length. Transmitter and receiver antennas are "tuned" by adjusting their length to match the wave length to be used. Because the speed of light (electromagnetic waves) is constant, wave length is inversely proportional to frequency. Higher frequencies have more waves per second and therefore shorter waves. Long waves (low frequencies) travel farther and are attenuated less by physical obstructions; however, they require a long antenna for optimal transmission. Shorter waves (high frequencies) are attenuated easily by objects or moisture, but shorter antennas may be used. Use of low frequencies to max-imize transmission distance is restricted because most animals would not tolerate the length of antenna needed.

Water and even moisture in leaves greatly attenuate high frequencies. For aquatic applications, frequencies in the 40- to 50-MHz range have been used for species such as fishes that can tolerate trailing a long antenna. For animals that never leave the water, ultrasound systems provide a transmission alternative that reduces the length of the antenna needed. For animals that surface or haul out of the water on a regular basis, higher frequencies and shorter antennas may be used to capture airborne signals. Both body fluid and body contact affect transmissions by attenuating signals or acting to de-tune the antenna, much as touching a television or radio antenna does. This effect reduces transmission distance of surgically implanted transmitters and also external transmitters on large mammals. Transmitters that are surgically implanted have one fourth to one third the transmission range that they have before implantation.[7] In theory, coiled antennas commonly used for implantable transmitters have poorer transmission properties than whip antennas, but this has not been documented and possibly the difference is negligible. On the other hand, transmitters with internal coiled antennas are usually easier to surgically implant than are those with whip antennas.

The effect of body mass's attenuating the signal of external or collar transmitters can be simulated by placing the transmitter in contact with a container of water similar in volume to the animal. This provides a more realistic test of transmission distance than does placing the transmitter on a dry, inanimate object. Signals may be improved on externally mounted transmitters by reducing the contact of the distal tip of the antenna with the animal. For example, the tip of the antenna can exit the collar rather than being completely sealed inside if the animal or conspecifics will not damage the antenna. For extremely large-bodied mammals such as elephants, the author uses a counter weight on the collar to prevent the transmitter and antenna from rotating to a position under the animal's head and neck. Transmitter antennas for elephants also have to be enclosed in the collar to protect them, but a spacing material or insulator may be mounted inside the collar to distance the antenna from the animal's body. In the author's experience, transmitters embedded in the horns of rhinoceroses have worked extremely well in comparison with collars used in the same study, and the horn material may provide insulation from the rest of the body.

Newer systems entailing the use of satellite transmissions are also affected by frequency constraints. Satellite systems such as Argos, Inmarsat, and the GPS network operate with frequencies in the 450- to 1600-MHz range. These high frequencies allow for extremely short antennas to be used, but the signals are easily attenuated. Thick forest cover interferes with signal transmission for these systems, despite some of the manufacturers' claims. This fact has limited the application or usefulness in wildlife work to species that are frequently out in the open, but newer GPS components that should improve performance in forest environments are entering the market.

Other factors also affect the transmission distances obtained with radiotelemetry. Vegetation type, soil type, atmospheric and weather conditions, and topography all influence signal transmission. Without prior experience, it is not possible to predict exact performance for a particular site and species. In the 150- to 170-MHz range commonly used in wildlife applications, line-of-sight distance for open environments provides a starting point. The signal may be expected to be detectable if the distances are in a straight line of sight up to 40 km. This would apply to animals in open, dry habitats and when the receiver is in an airplane or at a high point in the terrain. On the other hand, signals from an animal 100 m away and lying down behind a hill may not be detectable. Rocky surfaces or buildings may also reflect radio signals, which results in a false or second-location direction. Distances are typically 300 to 500 m for ground-dwelling animals in thick, wet forest and may be up to 1 km for arboreal species in the same habitat.

RECEIVERS AND DATA COLLECTION

Receivers and data storage units vary with the system or application requirements and may be designed to meet most needs. VHF receivers are commercially available off the shelf and range from simple units that can handle 12 transmitters to more advanced units with programmable scanning, data storage, and computer downloading capabilities. To receive data, only one receiver is necessary. But to determine location of a transmitter, triangulation must be used if a GPS unit is not integrated in the transmitter package. For triangulating a location, a directional bearing must be obtained from two locations separated by a distance that provides an angle (from the animal's point of view) greater than 30 degrees. Custom-designed receiver stations may be used for automated tracking of animals. Other systems provide both receiver and transmitter capabilities that allow for the remote system to be commanded to download information or to change data collection or transmission protocols. Data may also be stored in the collar or unit in the animal and downloaded after the animal is recaptured and the unit is recovered. This may reduce costs and provide excellent data collection in situations in which access to the study animals is reliable.

Satellite receiver systems are available. In the Argos system (Argos, Landover, MD), three circumpolar orbiting satellites can collect data transmitted from land or the ocean surface and can also calculate a location on the basis of the Doppler shift of the signal as the satellite crosses the horizon. In newer systems, GPS units to are used to obtain an accurate location by using geosynchronous orbiting satellites and then transmitting the data via VHF radio communication systems or via the Argos system. Similar data transmission through the use of the Inmarsat system of communications satellites is already widely used for tracking vehicles in commercial fleets, and applications for wildlife tracking are possible. Similar possibilities exist for using cellular phone networks to transfer collected data, but to date, no such systems are on the market.

OTHER CONSIDERATIONS

External transmitter attachments, implantable transmitters, and even recovery from immobilization or surgical procedures affect animals' behavior and physiology. Collars and tags provide a novel stimulus to the animal, to its conspecifics in social interactions, and potentially to predator or prey species.[13] Externally mounted transmitters may interfere with normal mobility and balance, aerodynamics or hydrodynamics, and energy expenditure.[6, 7, 11, 13] All of these effects may not be immediately obvious. For example, a transmitter glued on the feathers of a passerine will have different effects on flight balance, depending on whether it is placed at the base of the tail or on the dorsal thorax. Changes in energy budgets may affect reproductive success.[6] As a general rule, telemetry packages should not exceed 2% of the animal's body weight,[2] and a more conservative approach would use 1% as a maximum.

If possible, transmitter packages should be removed after studies or designed to come off the animal at a future point in time. This is a common practice in avian studies in which transmitters are attached to feathers and for marine mammals in which transmitters are glued to pelage and are lost when the animal molts. Harnesses and backpack mounts may be closed with a biodegradable material such as natural fiber cords or leather to allow the loss of the transmitter package. Collars may also be attached by this method. More typically, they are closed with nuts and bolts that may be made of different metals to facilitate electrolysis and more rapid corrosion. Transmitters that are delivered via a food item or placed directly in the gastrointestinal tract may be made to be passed naturally or removed from the stomach through endoscopy. If surgical implants or internal transmitters are left in the animal, the package design should preclude instrument corrosion or battery leakage.

Effective and safe attachment of transmitters or data storage devices and physiologic monitors is critical for success. Surgical implantation is commonly used in vertebrates. Proper anesthesia and aseptic surgical techniques and principles must be observed in order to maximize the chances of success and to meet the ethical and legal needs of working with animals.[12] For all types of biotelemetry, the impact on the animals to be studied must be considered. There are ethical concerns regarding the short- and long-term impact on the animal, and there are scientific validity issues related to observer or experimental design effects. These concerns must be evaluated and addressed before biotelemetry projects are initiated.

REFERENCES

1. Amlaner CJ (ed): Biotelemetry X. Fayetteville, University of Arkansas Press, 1989.
2. Amlaner CJ Jr, Macdonald DW (eds): A Handbook on Biotelemetry and Radio Tracking. Oxford, UK, Pergamon, 1979.
3. Anderson DE: Longevity of solar-powered radio transmitters on buteonine hawks in eastern Colorado. J Field Ornithol 65:122–132, 1994.
4. Cochran WW: Wildlife telemetry. *In* Schemnitz SD (ed): Wildlife Techniques Management Manual, 4th ed. Washington, DC, Wildlife Society, pp 507–520, 1980.
5. Derrickson KC, Greenberg R, Wolcott T: Heart rate telemetry for small birds. *In* Asa C (ed): Biotelemetry Applications to Captive Animal Care and Research. Bethesda, MD, American Association of Zoological Parks and Aquariums, pp 1–6, 1991.
6. Foster CC, Forsman ED, Meslow EC, et al: Survival and reproduction of radio-marked adult spotted owls. J Wildlife Manage 56:91–95, 1992.
7. Korschgen CE, Maxson SJ, Kuechle VB: Evaluation of implanted radio transmitters in ducks. J Wildlife Manage 48:982–987, 1984.
8. Kreeger TJ, Tester JR, Kuechle VB, Seal US: Measuring heart rate and body temperature via radiotelemetry in wild canids. *In* Asa C (ed): Biotelemetry Applications to Captive Animal Care and Research. Bethesda, MD, American Association of Zoological Parks and Aquariums, pp 37–48, 1991.
9. Mech D: Handbook of Animal Radio-Tracking. Minneapolis, University of Minnesota Press, 1983.
10. Mech D, Gese EM: Field testing the Wildlink capture collar on wolves. Wildlife Soc Bull 20:221–223, 1992.
11. Perry MC: Abnormal behavior of canvasbacks equipped with radio transmitters. J Wildlife Manage 45:786–789, 1981.
12. Reynolds PS: White blood cell profiles as a means of evaluating transmitter-implant surgery in small mammals. J Mamm 73:178–185, 1992.
13. Sorenson MD: Effects of neck collar radio on female redheads. J Field Ornithol 60:523–528, 1989.
14. Thomas PR, Cook RA, Burney DA, et al: Biotelemetric monitoring of physiological function in gaur (*Bos* gaurus). J Zoo Wildlife Med 27:513–521, 1996.
15. Thompson SD: Biotelemetric studies of mammalian thermoregulation. *In* Asa C (ed): Biotelemetry Applications to Captive Animal Care and Research. Bethesda, MD, American Association of Zoological Parks and Aquariums, pp 19–28, 1991.

CHAPTER 4

Quarantine: A Necessity for Zoo and Aquarium Animals

R. ERIC MILLER

Preventive medicine is the most basic aspect of the medical care of captive wildlife.[2] In the zoological park, the adage "An ounce of prevention is worth a pound of cure" is complicated by the difficulty in applying extensive medical treatment to many wild animals and, often, by the animal's innate ability to hide signs until a disease process is well advanced. Quarantine is a basic component of preventive medicine programs in zoos.[4, 5] It is the most fundamental step in the prevention of the spread of disease into an animal collection.

HISTORY

The word *quarantine* is derived from the Latin for "forty," because 40 days was the time period in medieval Venice that human immigrants were kept separated from the general population to limit the spread of bubonic plague. Historically, the quarantine policies of many zoological institutions have been informal and variable. In 1989, however, in recognizing the importance of quarantine, the American Zoo and Aquarium

Association (AZA) requested that its Animal Health Committee draft a written protocol that would be included as part of its requirements for accreditation. The protocol was adopted by the AZA Board of Directors in 1994. Later, in an effort spearheaded by James McBain, DVM, of Sea World, a section was added for marine mammals. Also available from the AZA (AZA Membership Office, Oglebay Park, Wheeling, WV, 26003-1698) is a separate quarantine protocol for fish.

AZA QUARANTINE PROTOCOL

The AZA quarantine protocol recognizes that quarantine cannot be implemented in a preventive medicine vacuum and, to be fully successful, it must be used in conjunction with other preventive medicine programs, including a parasite control program, necropsy program for all deaths, and appropriate vaccination program for each species.[2, 3] Additionally, appropriate quarantine procedures lay a solid foundation for a program that reduces the risk of zoonotic disease spread to personnel in contact with the animals and to the public.[1, 6] Last, although prevention of disease is the primary goal, quarantine also enables zoos and aquariums to establish the baseline health status of new arrivals.

The principles that apply to quarantine for interzoo and wild-to-zoo animal transfers are also crucial for zoo animals moving to the wild in reintroduction projects, and they should be considered in transfers between wildlife areas.

One challenge of the AZA drafting process was to create regulations that were meaningful and detailed, yet allowed institutional veterinarians the flexibility to use their judgment for exceptions. Additionally, the regulations had to reasonably consider the risk of disease versus the risk to the animal (e.g., anesthetizing giraffes for tuberculin testing) and the real capabilities of the institutions (e.g., not all zoos are capable of quarantining an elephant). However, when receiving institutions cannot fully quarantine arriving animals, preshipment testing protocols, such as have been recommended by the Elephant Species Survival Plan, and other procedures may assist in reducing the risk of disease transfer from those animals. Another example is the quarantine of great apes. Although the AZA quarantine protocol requires quarantine for all primates, it also recognizes the limitations of some smaller zoological institutions. The regulations allow isolation of a primate at either the shipping institution (if shipped without contact with other nonhuman primates) or at a primate institution approved by the American Association of Laboratory Animal Science (AALAS).

The regulations were written to be *minimum* standards and they should be adapted to each situation. Those who wish to exceed them are encouraged to do so. The following discussion outlines the specifics of the AZA quarantine protocol for mammals, birds, reptiles, and amphibians.

Facility

Each facility should have a separate quarantine facility that can accommodate mammals, birds, reptiles, am-

phibians, and fish. If there is no such quarantine facility, then newly acquired animals should be isolated from the established collection in such a manner as to prohibit physical contact, prevent fomite transmission, and avoid aerosol and drainage contamination. Such separation should be obligatory for primates, small mammals, birds, and reptiles, and it should be attempted when possible with larger mammals such as large ungulates and carnivores, marine mammals, and cetaceans. If the receiving institution lacks appropriate facilities for isolation of large primates, preshipment quarantine at an AZA- or AALAS-accredited institution may be applied to the protocol of the receiving institution. In such a case, shipment must take place in isolation from other primates. More stringent local, state, or federal regulations take precedence over the recommendations of this report.

Duration

Quarantine for all species should be under the supervision of a veterinarian and should continue for a minimum of 30 days (unless otherwise directed by the staff veterinarian). For mammals, if during the 30-day quarantine period additional mammals of the same *order* are introduced into a designated quarantine area, the 30-day period must begin again. For birds, reptiles, and amphibians, the 30-day quarantine period must be "closed," that is, there can be no introduction of new animals from the same *class*. Therefore, the addition of any new birds into a bird quarantine areas requires that the 30-day quarantine period begin again on the date of the addition of the new birds. The same applies for reptiles and amphibians.

Personnel

A keeper should be designated to care only for quarantined animals, or a keeper should attend quarantined animals only after fulfilling responsibilities for resident species. Equipment used to feed and clean animals in quarantine should be used only with those animals. If this is not possible, then equipment must be cleaned with an appropriate disinfectant (as designated by the veterinarian supervising the quarantine) before use with any other animals.

Institutions must take precautions to minimize the risk of exposure of animal personnel to zoonotic diseases that may be present in newly acquired animals. For example, animal personnel should take disinfectant foot baths, wear appropriate protective clothing and masks, and minimize physical exposure in some species, such as, with primates, by the use of chemical rather than physical restraint. A tuberculin testing and surveillance program must be established for zoo and aquarium employees to ensure the health of both the employees and the animal collection.[1, 6]

Protocol

During the quarantine period, certain prophylactic measures should be instituted. Individual animal fecal samples or representative samples from large numbers of individuals housed in a limited area (e.g., birds of the same species in an aviary or frogs in a terrarium) should be collected at least twice and examined for gastrointestinal parasites. Treatment should be prescribed by the attending veterinarian. Ideally, release from quarantine should depend on obtaining two negative fecal results spaced a minimum of 2 weeks apart, either initially or after parasiticide treatment (although for some parasite infestations, other protocols are necessary). In addition, all animals should be evaluated for ectoparasites and be given appropriate treatment.

Vaccinations should be updated as appropriate for each species.[2, 3] If the animal arrives without a vaccination history, it should be treated as an immunologically naive animal and be given an appropriate series of vaccinations. Whenever possible, blood should be collected and the sera banked. Either a −70°C freezer or a −20°C freezer that is not frost-free should be available to save sera. Such sera could provide an important resource for retrospective disease evaluation.

During the quarantine period, unmarked animals can be permanently identified (e.g., with microchip, tattoo,

ear tag) while they are anesthetized or restrained. Furthermore, whenever animals are restrained or immobilized, a complete physical, including a dental examination, should be performed.

Complete medical records should be kept and available for all animals during the quarantine period. Animals that die during quarantine should have a complete necropsy performed under the supervision of a veterinarian, and representative tissues should be submitted for histopathologic examination.

Procedures

Recommended and required quarantine procedures for each taxonomic group are listed in Table 4–1. These are basic recommendations. If a species is part of a species survival plan (SSP), then the veterinary advisors to that group may also serve as a source of more detailed advice regarding the testing of those species.

Marine mammals may present particular challenges, and this paragraph describes overall recommendations pertaining to their quarantine that do not appear in

TABLE 4–1. Quarantine Testing Requirements and Recommendations by Taxonomic Group

Required	Strongly Recommended
Mammals	
Primates	
Direct and flotation fecal examination	Chest radiographs
A minimun of two negative tuberculin tests using a tuberculin containing at least 1500 units/0.1 ml (e.g., Mammalian Human Isolate, Coopers Animal Health, Kansas City, KS) or other appropriate regimens as necessary for the species in question (e.g., orangutans, New World primates)	Appropriate viral panels (simian immunodeficiency virus, retrovirus type D)
Hemogram/sera chemistry panel	
Culture of feces for salmonella, shigella, *Campylobacter*	
For appropriate species (e.g., Old World monkeys), serology for *Herpesvirus simiae* (Herpes B).	
Hoofstock	
Direct and flotation fecals	Hemogram/sera profile
TB test when possible	Appropriate serology (e.g., leptospirosis, brucellosis, malignant infectious bovine rhinotracheitis (IBR), catarrhal fever, infectious bovine rhinotracheitis, bovine virus diarrhea) and paired titers when possible
	Urinalysis
	Johne's diagnostics if there is history of disease in the herd of origin
	Coggin's test for equids
	Vaccinate as appropriate
Small Mammals/Carnivores	
Direct and flotation fecals	Hemogram/sera profile
Vaccinate as appropriate[2, 3]	Urinalysis
	Appropriate serology tests (e.g., feline infectious peritonitis, feline leukemia virus, feline immunodeficiency virus)
	Heartworm testing in appropriate species
Marine Mammals/Cetaceans	
Hemogram/sera chemistry panel	Direct and flotation fecal examination
Physical examination	Urinalysis
	Blowhole and stool culture and cytology
	Blood zinc levels

Table continued on following page

TABLE 4–1. Quarantine Testing Requirements and Recommendations by Taxonomic Group *Continued*

Required	Strongly Recommended
Pinnipeds	
Hemogram/sera chemistry panel	Direct and flotation fecal examination
Physical examination	Urinalysis
	Morbillivirus titer
	Leptospiral titer
	Heartworm test (if appropriate)
	Stool culture and cytology
	Blood zinc levels
Sirenians	
Hemogram/sera chemistry panel	Direct and flotation fecal examination
Physical examination	Stool culture and cytology
Carnivores (Polar Bear, Sea Otter)	
Direct and flotation fecal examination	Urinalysis
Hemogram/sera chemistry panel	Blood zinc levels
Physical examination	
Vaccination for canine distemper, feline panleucopenia, canine parvovirus, and rabies as deemed necessary by the attending veterinarian	
Birds	
Direct and flotation fecal examinations	Hemogram/sera profile
Evaluate for ectoparasites	Fecal culture for *Salmonella* species
Appropriate serologic tests for psittacosis, and, if positive, confirmation by culture	Fecal Gram's stain
Reptiles/Amphibians	
Direct and flotation fecal examination	Veterinary examination
Evaluate for ectoparasites	Hemogram/sera chemistry panel
	Paramyxoviral titers for viperids, incoming after being quarantined for 30 days
	Full necropsy examination and histopathologic study on all individuals dying while in quarantine

Table 4–1. As discussed for other animals, a facility should be available that can provide for the isolation of newly acquired marine mammals in such a manner as to prohibit cross-contamination including that via untreated water. Ocean pens must be located in a way that prevents the spread of any disease from animal to animal through natural water movement and at a distance from other penned animals deemed adequate by the supervising veterinarian. If a receiving institution does not have appropriate isolation facilities, the staff should arrange for quarantine at an acceptable alternate site or only receive animals that do not require quarantine. Isolation practices should be instituted based on the prior medical history of the newly arrived animals. Isolation is recommended when the animal has one or more of the following characteristics:

1. Recently collected (less than 30 days before arrival).

2. Recently exposed to a new arrival for which an adequate medical history is not available (less than 30 days before arrival).

3. Lack of a documented medical history.

4. Apparent medical problems at the time of arrival.

5. At the direction of the supervising veterinarian.

Otherwise, the general standards for quarantine of marine mammals are similar to those already described in the general section for mammals.

SUMMARY

In addition to disease prevention, the standards described in this chapter have had several related benefits for the zoological community that may not be immediately obvious. Foremost is that they have been instrumental in assisting the AZA in its pursuit of exemptions from disease testing when animals are transferred between AZA-accredited institutions. One example is the exemption from federal requirements for cervid tuberculosis testing because the U.S. Department of Agriculture has accepted that AZA-accredited institutions (1) identify and keep individual records on the animals in their care (critical to tracing them), (2) have animal health programs in place, including the quarantine of new arrivals, and (3) have a veterinarian perform necropsies on all dead animals. These policies are not only advantageous for the animals but they also behoove the zoological community to strictly monitor its own performance in maintaining standards and monitoring disease.

Finally, it is important to re-emphasize that the standards listed above are designed to be minimum standards and those wishing to exceed them are encouraged to do so. It is also anticipated that the protocol will be a changing, "living" document.

REFERENCES

1. Heuschele W, Bredeson-Heuschele C: Zoonotic disease—reducing the risks. 1988 Proceedings of the American Zoo and Aquarium Association, Milwaukee, WI, pp 591–598, 1988.
2. Junge RE: Preventive medicine recommendations. *In* Amand W (ed): Infectious Disease Reviews. Media, PA, American Association of Zoo Veterinarians, 1991, pp 1–15.
3. Miller RE: Immunization of wild animal species against common diseases. *In* Bonagura JD (ed): Current Veterinary Therapy XII. Philadelphia, WB Saunders, 1995, pp 1427–1429.
4. Miller RE: Quarantine procedures for AZA-accredited zoological parks. 1995 Proceedings of the American Association of Zoo Veterinarians, East Lansing, MI, pp 165–172, 1995.
5. Miller RE: Quarantine protocols and preventive medicine procedures for reptiles, birds and mammals in zoos. Rev Sci Off Int Epiz 15:183–189, 1996.
6. Shellbarger WC: Zoo personnel health program recommendations. *In* Amand W (ed): Infectious Disease Reviews. Media, PA, American Association of Zoo Veterinarians, Section 7, 1991.

CHAPTER 5

Designing an Ideal Animal Shipment

JANIS OTT JOSLIN
DARIN COLLINS

Animal shipments are necessary to accomplish some of the basic goals of zoos such as increasing the genetic diversity of the animal collection by bringing in new bloodlines, acquiring new specimens for exhibition, moving surplus animals, and translocating animals between captivity and the wild. Successful shipments result in the transfer of the animals without injury, damage to their health, or inhumane treatment. Successful animal shipments involve effective communication and shared responsibilities among veterinarians, curators, and animal keepers at both the shipping and receiving institutions.

The ideal successful animal shipment is difficult to achieve, but it should be attempted. Transportation is an extremely stressful process, especially on the animal being shipped. The shipment may cause the animal to stop eating, become ill, or even stop its reproductive cycling. Stress is minimized with proper preparation and planning and, sometimes, additional expense. The challenge to everyone involved is to pay attention to details at all levels of this process and to keep the animal's welfare first and foremost. If any time during this process it is determined that it is not in the animal's best interest to continue with the shipment, arrangements should be canceled or rescheduled. The ultimate goal of shipment is to transport the animal humanely so that it arrives at its new institution in the same good condition as it left its previous facility.

To this end, there are many considerations for shipping: the transport container type, size, and design; the physical and psychological needs of the animal; species requirements; regulations; documentation; timing; and coordination and communication. Often, for expedience, regulatory and institutional needs are met but the animal's needs are not given top priority. Zoos are required by the U.S. Department of Agriculture (USDA) Animal Welfare Act (AWA) regulations (7 U.S.C. 2131 et. seq.) to oversee the humane handling, care, treatment and *transportation* of the warm-blooded animals in their care.

PRIMARY TRANSPORT CONTAINERS

Crates

Often, the only preparation that is made for the animal for the shipment is to select the size of the crate to put the animal into for the shipment. The International Air Transport Association (IATA)[5] publishes guidelines that give specific crate design requirements for international shipments. The IATA manual is available through the Publications Assistant, International Air Transport Association, 2000 Peel Street, Montreal, Quebec, Canada H3A 2R4.

Careful thought should be put into choosing the proper crate design. Historically, crates were designed to minimize movement by excitable animals such as hoofstock and large felids during transport, thereby minimizing the risk of injury to the animal. Preventing an animal from turning around may be the best design for these high-strung animals, but this may not be necessary for calmer animals, which may do better in larger containers that allow them to stand, turn around, and lie down in a natural manner. Using the IATA guidelines along with the staff's knowledge of the individual animal's behavior will aid in choosing the best crate.

The crate must be well constructed to withstand damage from other freight, and the joints of wooden crates must withstand damage by the animal from the inside. The doors of the crate must not be able to be accidentally opened from the inside or outside of the crate. According to IATA regulations, heavy crates (i.e., crate plus animal exceed 60 kg) must have forklift spacers that are 5 cm (2 inches) thick and metal bracing must be used to reinforce the crate. There should be handles on the outside of the crate to allow for lifting and spacer bars should extend to 15 cm (6 inches) from the surface of the enclosure to prevent another object from blocking the ventilation ports.

The crate must allow for adequate ventilation. IATA regulations require ventilation ports on three sides of the crate, with most of the ventilation being on the upper part of the container; there are exceptions, depending on the species being shipped. Ventilation apertures should be small enough to prevent the escape of the animal and to prevent the animal from getting any part of its body out of the crate. For smaller species, this may be accomplished by covering and securely attaching a densely woven fabric or mesh over the ventilation ports. Dividers within the container must not preclude adequate ventilation.

Padding may be applied on the inside sides and ceiling of the crate to prevent the animal from injuring itself in shipment. The padding should be tightly attached to the crate to prevent the animal from removing and eating the padding while in transport.

The crate should have a leak-proof bottom with absorbent bedding or a grill with a liquid-proof tray underneath to permit excreta to fall through. The tray must be splash-proof, and the grill space must not be wide enough to trap the limbs of the animal.

The crate must also allow for the feeding and watering of the animal during shipment without the risk of the animal escaping or harming staff. Food and water ports must be clearly marked on the outside of the crate. These containers must be fixed to the inside of the crate, have rounded edges, and be nontoxic. For longer flights, additional food should be sent with the animal for feeding in transit.

Crates must be thoroughly cleaned and disinfected before they are used again. The crate must be examined to ensure that it meets regulatory standards and that it suits the needs of the animal being shipped. It must be checked for structural integrity and to ensure that there are no objects (e.g., wood, nails) projecting into the animal holding area. It must be closely examined to determine that any previous modifications to the crate did not compromise its use (Fig. 5–1). The veterinarian signing the health certificate or the curator should inspect the crate to rule out any problems in advance of shipping so that modifications can be made or another crate is chosen.

Modified plastic pet airline containers can be used for shipping small species of mammals such as lemurs and bush babies. The ventilation areas should be covered by cloth such as burlap to prevent the animals from reaching out of the crates. The doors should be modified so that they cannot be inadvertently opened. This can be done by wiring the door shut or by using a die; threads can be cut onto the top of the metal rods, which act as the closing mechanisms for the crate, so that metal covered nuts can be screwed onto the rods.

Trucks and Trailers

An animal may be shipped loose in the back of a trailer designed for animal transport. Trucks or trailers used for transporting larger species should be clean and well maintained. Trailer tires should be properly inflated and not of excessive wear to maintain proper traction. Wheel bearings and brake linings should be checked before the shipment to be sure they are in good working order. Trailers should have no projections inside the animal area and have enough headroom to allow the animal to stand in a natural position. The flooring must be nonslip and have proper bedding. The inspection doors or windows must allow for the animal to be visually inspected and allow access for feeding and watering during transport without risk of escape or potential injury to the animal or the personnel. There should be a means of illumination of the trailer interior. There should be adequate ventilation in the cargo area and the temperature should be regulated for the comfort of the species being transported. The loading ramp for the trailer should not have gaps where an animal's limb could get caught and it should have solid sides to prevent an animal from falling. The ramp gradient should be such that the animal loads without slipping. The trailer should have a barrier or doors to prevent animals from falling out when the outer door is opened.

The driver should be experienced with hauling animals; the animal's level of comfort depends on the driver's ability to navigate turns and change speed gradually. Adequate rest periods should be scheduled to allow the animal time to eat while the trailer is stopped. Ideally, the trailer should arrive in advance of the departure date. This allows staff time to make any changes that are needed to accommodate loading the animal without difficulty. If the trailer is shipped to the facility well in advance of the shipment, there may be sufficient time for the animal to acclimate to the trailer before the truck arrives to haul the trailer.

THE ANIMAL'S PHYSICAL AND PSYCHOLOGICAL NEEDS

It is important to get the animal acclimated to the shipping container before the shipment. Whenever possible, the animal should be crate trained. This can be accomplished by allowing the animal access to the crate on a daily basis, and, ideally, the animal should be fed solely in the crate. The crate can be bedded with soiled bedding so that the area has a familiar smell to it. Other familiar cage materials (e.g., perching, food bowls) can

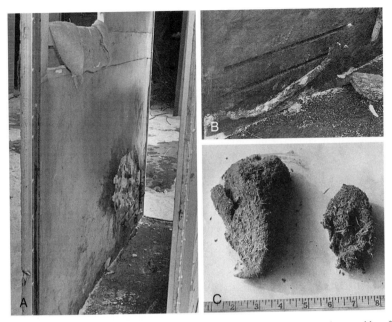

FIGURE 5–1. Crates that are reused must be examined for previous modification, which may be a problem for subsequent shipments. This crate *(A)* was originally built with horizontal vent ports cut in the lower quarter of the back sides of the crate *(B)*. These vent holes were covered with padding inside the crate and with wood on the outside of the crate. An extremely valuable ungulate was put in this crate on the day of shipment without prior crate training; the animal became excited and kicked off the padding with its rear legs, exposing the slots underneath. The animal fractured both rear lateral claws and developed severe capture myopathy. The animal also tore off the padding in the crate and ate several pieces *(C)*, which were found in the rumen of the animal post mortem. The loss of this animal could have been prevented by crate training and replacement of the crate with a suitable container.

be included in the crate to give it a more familiar appeal to the animal. These items must be firmly affixed in the shipping container to prevent them from moving around in the crate and possibly injuring the animal. For smaller animals, the animal's nest box can be placed in the shipping crate to create a familiar environment for the animal.

The crate acclimation process may take up to a month. The decision as to when to ship the animal is best made based on the animal's acclimation to the crate.

All aspects of the shipment must be considered to increase the chance of success. The AWA requires that an experienced employee or attendant of the shipper or receiver accompany shipments of cetaceans, sirenians, pinnipeds, and sea otters. The AWA requires that socially dependent marine mammals must be allowed visual and olfactory contact with one another during transport. This requirement might also be considered for other animals for shipment. Polar bears must have an attendant if the transport period is more than 24 hours. U.S. Fish and Wildlife Service (USF&W) requires a veterinary attendant to accompany a sick or injured animal being transported to the United States only if the primary purpose of the transport is for needed medical attention and the animal can withstand the transportation. The attendant must have access to the animal at all times and have all needed medications readily available. Often, shipments of great apes are accompanied by an attendant, but perhaps other ship-

ments, such as hand-reared hoofstock and other nonhuman primates, would also benefit by the presence of a familiar person. An attendant can only be with the animal in cargo on cargo-only flights or on chartered flights; however, the attendant's presence at loading and unloading and during acclimation to the new facility may be helpful to the animal. One option is to have the recipient zoo send a keeper to the shipping institution to spend a week or more working around the animal to become familiar with the animal's routine and behavior. The recipient zoo keeper could accompany the shipment to the new zoo with or without the animal's regular keeper. Another option is to have the animal be accompanied by its dam or its cagemate, as long as the stress on the companion animal is considered. There are regulations regarding the number of animals and the age and sex of animals that can travel together, but some animals may benefit from visual, auditory, and olfactory contact with a familiar animal in a cage nearby while in transit. This increases the cost of the shipment.

The animal's acclimation period upon its arrival at the new institution should be considered. Often, animals are weaned the day they are shipped, compounding the stress on the animal. If a juvenile animal is to be shipped, then it may be useful to separate it from its dam far in advance of the shipment to prepare it for its eventual isolation during shipment. Such a practice should only be undertaken after taking into account the facilities at the shipping institution for weaning and the personalities of the dam and juvenile animal. If both individuals are likely to pace and vocalize during the separation process, then either the dam or the youngster should be isolated out of visual and hearing range of the other animal.

The specific needs of the individual animal before, during, and after the shipment are best determined by input from the animal keeper caring for the animal being shipped. The quarantine and unit keepers at the receiving institution will want to anticipate the animal's needs before its arrival. The American Association of Zookeepers (AAZK) offers Animal Data Transfer Forms (ADTFs) that allow institutions a format for exchanging information about diet, previous reproductive and medical history, previous enclosure history and design, cleaning and disinfecting procedures, and any personal comments about the animal. The ADTF is available free of charge upon request from AAZK Administrative Offices, 635 SW Gage Boulevard, Topeka, KS 66606. This information should be sent to the receiving institution well in advance of the shipping date.

In most cases, the animal is put on a new or modified diet once it is moved to the new facility. Personnel at both the shipping and the receiving institutions should discuss the issue of diets and determine the best way to make the transition in advance. It is probably best to make the diet transition at the shipping institution so that when the animal arrives at its new zoo, it can be offered a familiar diet. If this cannot be done, then the recipient zoo should be prepared to offer the animal the diet that was offered at the original zoo for several weeks after arrival. Once the animal has acclimated to eating consistently, then a gradual transition from the old diet to the new diet should take place over approximately 1 to 4 weeks. This may mean that the shipping institution needs to supply the animal's current diet along with the shipment to get the animal through the transition period or the diet transition must be coordinated before the animal is shipped.

The use of sedatives and tranquilizers can help minimize the stress of animals during crating and transport. There are several classes of short-acting sedatives that have been used, including diazepinones, alpha$_2$-adrenoceptor agonists, and phenothiazine derivatives. With the advent of long-acting tranquilizers (see Chapter 87), the transport and long-term confinement of exotic animals has greatly decreased mortality rates during shipment.[2, 3] Several of these drugs have antagonist drugs available in case there is an adverse reaction during the sedation. These antagonist drugs should be readily available and the appropriate dosages for these drugs should be indicated in the medical records accompanying the shipment. IATA regulations discourage using tranquilizing drugs for transport because many of the drugs decrease blood pressure, which could be aggravated at high altitudes. In addition, the reaction of various species to drugs cannot always be predicted. The regulations require that, if sedatives are used, the name of the drug and the route and time of administration must be clearly marked on the container and that copies of these documents also be included in the shipping papers. If additional sedatives are given en route, the name of the drug and the route, amount, and time

of administration must be recorded; this information must accompany the shipment. The USF&W has proposed that large crocodilians (more than 180 cm, or 6 feet, in length) that are immobilized for transport to the United States be accompanied by a qualified veterinary technician, trained animal care attendant, or a licensed veterinarian. The name of the drug and the appropriate antidotes should be included in the documents accompanying the shipment.

SPECIES REQUIREMENTS

Each species has specific requirements for shipping containers, feeding, water, nest boxes, and so on. The IATA guidelines address these issues in detail. Certain species require specialized transportation arrangements and preparation.

Reptiles and Amphibians

Snakes and small lizards should be shipped in sealed, long-necked cloth bags made of a sturdy fabric such as cotton or burlap of coarse but sturdy weave that allows ventilation. These bags should be secured in a wooden box lined with Styrofoam. The bags should be secured without the use of nails or staples, which could rip the bags upon removal, or the bags may be placed in individual compartments of the container. Aquatic snakes such as tentacled snakes, elephant trunk snakes, and sea snakes should be transported in damp enclosures as described for amphibians.

Ventilation holes smaller than the snake's head should be made through the Styrofoam and wood. These holes need to be made from the inside out so that there are no splinters protruding into the container, and the holes should be covered with a plastic mesh. If there are several compartments made in the container, then there must be ventilation holes made between the compartments.

There should be metal corners on the outside of the crate to prevent the corners of the crate from being crushed. The top and one or more sides of the crate should say "Live Animal" or "Wild Animal," as appropriate, and the lettering must be at least 1 inch high. It is also advisable to affix labels that state "Avoid Extreme Heat and Cold," "Avoid Direct Sun," "Do Not Tip," and "Only Authorized Personnel May Open This Container."

Poisonous snakes should be double bagged and overhand knotted in the bag. The bag is placed in a Styrofoam enclosure in a wooden box. The top of the bag should be taped down and the tape should be labeled "Venomous" or "Poisonous Snake" with a skull and crossbones appearing in red ink. (Bags containing nonpoisonous snakes should be labeled "Nonpoisonous Snake.") The foam lid should also be labeled with the words "Poisonous Snake" with the accompanying skull and crossbones. Ideally, these are put in a double wooden box clearly labeled "Poisonous Snake" on the outside of each box. The label should include the number of enclosed animals, the common and scientific names, and the antivenom type required to treat bites. The shipper should provide the carrier with the contact information for a snake bite treatment center. Both the shipper and receiver should have antivenom available for the species being transported. The USF&W proposes regulations that venomous reptiles be shipped into the United States in transparent mesh bags with the bag being closed by tying the opening with a knot.

Amphibians may be shipped in tropical fish shipping containers, which have a Styrofoam liner and an outer wooden box. Many species of amphibians may best be shipped in plastic containers placed into the outer wooden box. The plastic container should have air holes punched from the inside of the container outward and the lids should be taped down. The animal may be packed loosely with moist sphagnum moss to prevent the animal from injuring itself and drying out. The moist moss should be rung out so that water does not leak and damage the box but it should be wet enough to maintain humidity for up to 72 hours. Jumping species of amphibians may best be shipped loose in the wooden box with sphagnum moss packed around them. Aquatic amphibians such as *Axolotis*, *Pipa*, and *Xenopus* can be shipped in a primary enclosure of two double-bagged plastic bags filled one third of the way with water and the rest of the way with oxygen.

Reptiles and amphibians are best shipped in warm weather. If they are shipped in cooler weather, then heat packs may be stapled to the lid of the container with newspaper wrapped around the outside of the heat pack to prevent the animal from having direct contact with the heat pack. The wooden box should be closed with screws so that, if the box must be inspected, it can be readily opened and closed.

The proposed USF&W regulations for reptiles going to the United States require the height of this primary enclosure to allow airflow over the animal or its container, with a clearance of 3 cm (1.2 inches) above the highest point of the reptile and 1 cm (0.4 inches) for frogs of 1 cm (0.4 inches) or less in size. More space is needed for larger frogs.

The proposed USF&W regulations would also prohibit the requirement for feeding reptiles and amphibians in transit.

Birds

It is preferable for birds to be sent in individual compartments with adequate food and water. The food and water container must be designed to prevent spillage. A sponge or some other device should be placed in the water container to prevent the bird from drowning. There should be enough height in the crate for the bird to perch with its head upright and its tail clear off the floor. Nonperching birds should be shipped with adequate space so that they can stand. Crates may need additional padding to prevent the birds from injuring themselves. Birds should be shipped only in moderate weather.

According to IATA regulations, during long flights, the cargo compartment lights must be left on to allow birds to feed. Unfledged birds are not permitted to be shipped.

If perching birds are shipped in a group, IATA regulations require that they have wooden perching with sufficient perch space for each bird in the container. The diameter of the perch should allow the bird to have a comfortable, firm grip. The perches should be placed so that droppings do not fall into the food or water containers or onto other birds.

Birds with high metabolism (e.g., hummingbirds) need frequent nectar feedings throughout the shipment. Arrangements should be made ahead of time with zoos en route to provide feedings to accommodate this schedule, or an attendant could accompany the shipment.

IATA regulations recommend that, when shipping flamingos, they may be supported by a body sling to prevent them from falling during flight but which allows them to stand en route. The regulations also allow young ostriches and emus and adult ostriches to be shipped in groups. The IATA regulations require ventilation for ratites to be 20% on all four sides of the crate, which is a variance of the usual regulations.

Mammals

IATA guidelines clearly describe the crate designs for shipment of mammals. In addition, IATA regulations prohibit the shipment of pregnant animals or animals that have given birth within the past 48 hours, unless the animal is accompanied by a written statement by a veterinarian certifying that the animal is fit to travel or that the birth will not occur during the transport. Specifically, the IATA regulation restricts deer from being transported when the horns are in velvet or when they are in heat or in the last 3 months of pregnancy.

USF&W restricts transport to the United States of (1) mammals in the last third of their pregnancy, (2) nursing mammals with young, and (3) unweaned mammals, unless the examining veterinarian certifies in writing that the shipment is for medical treatment and that the animal can tolerate the transport. For nonhuman primates, USF&W allows an established male-female pair, a family group, a pair of immature juvenile animals, or other pairs of animals that have been habitually housed together to be shipped in the same container. A mother and her nursing young can be transported together for medical treatment.

Several articles have been published on transport for marine mammals.[1, 4] The AWA also delineates specific shipping arrangements needed for marine mammals and nonhuman primates. For example, sea otters are temperature sensitive and should be provided with ice for cooling as well as a source of water for drinking. It is best to have a suspended wire floor in the cage to keep their fur as clean as possible during transport.

Small mammals with high metabolic rates should be supplied with adequate amounts of moist fruits and other foods so that they do not become hypoglycemic. These animals should not be shipped in cool weather.

Fishes

Small fishes should be shipped in plastic bags filled with one third water and two thirds oxygen. These bags are placed in a Styrofoam-lined, rigid box, which is leak-proof. Larger fishes, such as sharks, can be shipped in commercial fish boxes in which the water in the container is filtered and bubbled with oxygen during transport. The fishes should be fasted before shipment to decrease nitrogen waste. It is advisable to have an attendant accompany the shipment to monitor the animal and the water quality.[7] These containers must be spill-proof. The containers are placed on plastic sheeting in the cargo hold. It is recommended that fishes be transported under light sedation and that transport fluid be modified to reduce the osmotic gradient between plasma and the transport liquid.[8]

REGULATORY REQUIREMENTS

Shipments must be conducted in accordance with local, state, federal, and international laws governing the movement of animals.[9] Convention on International Trade in Endangered Species (CITES) requirements must be met for shipping endangered species; notification of CITES representatives and wildlife authorities is important for the trade or transport of any animals listed as endangered species.

The USF&W, under the Lacey Act (16 U.S.C. 3371), regulates the humane and healthful transport of wild mammals and birds into the United States. Institutions exporting wild mammals and birds into the United States must have the animals examined and have a health certificate signed by a veterinarian certified as qualified by the national government of the country of export within 10 days before shipment. The health certificate must indicate that the animal has been examined and was found healthy, appears free of any communicable diseases, and is able to be shipped. There are specific regulations pertaining to nonhuman primates, marine mammals, elephants, ungulates, sloths, bats, and flying lemurs, as well as other terrestrial mammals, birds, and insects, and there are proposed regulations for reptiles and amphibians. According to these regulations, if a nursing mother with young, an unweaned mammal unaccompanied by its mother, or an unweaned altricial bird is to be shipped, the shipment must be for medical reasons and it must be accompanied at all times and be accessible to a veterinary attendant during transport. Any sick or injured wild bird or mammal must only be shipped for medical reasons. USF&W restricts any animal with visible external parasites from entering the United States. If two animals are incompatible, they are not to be shipped together or in close proximity. Wild mammals or birds are not accepted for transport to the United States by air carriers more than 6 hours or less than 2 hours before departure. The container design must meet IATA standards, and there must be handholds for lifting and spacer bars on the outside of all walls to ensure that ventilation openings are not blocked by surrounding cargo. The primary enclosure must be thoroughly cleaned and disinfected before each shipment if the crate is reused. The shipping container must have a solid bottom to prevent leakage and there should be fresh absorbent bedding in the crate to absorb and cover excrement, unless the animals are shipped on wire suspended above the solid bottom.

Unless specifically indicated in writing by an examining veterinarian, the USF&W requires that shippers provide information regarding what constituted obvious signs of stress in the species being transported to the United States. It also requires handlers to observe the animals no less than once every 4 hours whenever the cargo hold is accessible and to feed the animals according to the instructions accompanying the animal. The inspection also includes checking that the temperature in the cargo area is within allowable limits, that the crate is not damaged, and that there is adequate ventilation.

Regulations for USF&W for shipments to the United States and IATA indicate that temperatures in the holding area, cargo, or terminal must be a minimum of 12.8°C (55°F) and a maximum of 26.7°C (80°F). When ambient temperature is 23.9°C (75°F) or more, ancillary ventilation must be provided. For penguins and auks, the ambient temperature must be not more than 18.3°C (65°F) and auxiliary ventilation is required when ambient temperature is more than 15.6°C (60°F). For polar bears and sea otters, the ambient temperature cannot exceed 10°C (50°F).

The USF&W proposes that, for reptiles, the ambient temperatures must be a minimum of 21.1°C (70°F) and a maximum of 26.7°C (80°F), and, for amphibians, the temperature cannot be less than 15.6°C (60°F) or more than 21.1°C (70°F).

For shipments within the United States, the AWA requires that ambient temperatures in the holding areas must not be less than 7.2°C (45°F) or more than 29.5°C (85°F) for more than 4 consecutive hours. Animals being transported between holding areas to the aircraft must not be exposed to ambient temperatures of more than 29.5°C (85°F) or less than 7.2°C (45°F) for more than 45 minutes. The veterinarian examining the animal can write a statement that accompanies the animal certifying that the animal is acclimated to temperatures of less than 7.2°C (45°F). The animal cannot be exposed to temperatures lower than those to which the animal is acclimated for more than 45 minutes. This certificate must not be written more than 10 days before shipment.

The crate needs to be marked with the following information:

1. Name, address, and telephone number of a contact person responsible for the shipment
2. Common and scientific name of the animals in the shipment and the number of animals contained therein
3. Appropriate labeling (e.g., "Poisonous" if so indicated)
4. Feeding and watering instructions, including frequency, amount, and type of food and quantity of water required, in writing on the outside of the crate
5. For IATA regulations, at least one "LIVE ANIMAL" label in bright green print on a light background. The label should be 10 × 15 cm (4 × 6 inches) and the lettering should be 2.5 cm (1 inch) high.
6. For IATA regulations, "This Way Up" labels in bright red or black letters on a light background. The labels are to be placed on all four sides if possible. The

label must be 10 × 15 cm (4 × 6 inches); proposed USF&W regulations recommend having labels indicating "Do Not Tip" and "Only Authorized Personnel May Open Container" if appropriate.

The animal cargo area must be maintained to prevent any exhaust fumes and gases from getting to the animal. During any stopovers, the mammal or bird must be observed once every 4 hours. If the cargo space is not accessible during the air transport, then the airline must check the animals at loading and unloading or whenever the cargo space is accessible. The airlines must take adequate precautions to ensure that the animals are not exposed to adverse temperatures. The transport should be done in the most expedient manner with the fewest stopovers possible. The carrier loads the animals last and unloads them first from the airplane. When animals are being transported from animal holding areas to the cargo hold, the carriers must provide adequate shelter from direct sunlight and inclement weather. Animals that are incompatible are not to be shipped together or in close proximity. The shipper needs to verify with the airline if other animals are scheduled on the same flight, to determine whether these animals are compatible from a behavioral or a disease standpoint.

The AWA addresses transport within the United States, and its standards are compatible with the Lacey Act. There are also specifications on shipping delineated in the AWA for nonhuman primates; for example, only one nonhuman primate may be transported in a primary enclosure except for a mother and her nursing infant, an established male-female pair group, or a compatible group of juveniles of the same species that have not reached puberty. The IATA and the AWA regulations specifically delineate the frequency that the animals need to be fed and watered while in transport. Specifically, the AWA stipulates that, for nonhuman primates, the consignor must certify in writing to the carrier that the animal was offered food and water during the 4 hours before shipment and that each nonhuman primate 1 year of age or older must be offered food at least once every 24 hours. Marine mammals shall not be transported for more than 36 hours without being offered food. Special arrangements may need to be made with the air carrier to ensure that these requirements are met.

The Marine Mammal Protection Act (16 U.S.C. 1361 et. seq.) is administered by the USF&W and the National Marine Fisheries Service and delineates the requirements for shipping cetaceans, pinnipeds, polar bears, manatees, and sea otters. The National Marine Fisheries Services must be notified at least 15 days before the transport of the marine mammals.

The Animal Plant and Health Inspection Service (APHIS) division of the USDA also has specific regulations concerning elephants, hippopotamuses, rhinoceroses, and tapirs identified in the regulations in 9 Code of Federal Regulations parts 75, 82, 92, 93, and 94. These animals are required to have a special import permit before entering the United States. There must be a signed health certificate as per the Lacey Act and they must be inspected and treated by a national veterinarian of the exporting country. The animals must be treated for ectoparasites between 3 and 14 days before export and they must remain under the supervision of the veterinarian. There must be no contact with other animals unless they are in the same shipment after treatment. Within 72 hours of loading for transport to the United States, they must be inspected by the veterinarian and found free of any ectoparasites. Upon arrival in the United States, any material from the crate must be removed, sealed in a plastic bag, and incinerated. The shipping crate or the vehicle of transport in the United States must be sealed for transport to the final destination, where, upon unloading, the animal is inspected and treated once if no ectoparasites are found. If there are ectoparasites, then the animal must be treated topically with sprays or dipped until all the ectoparasites are eliminated.

APHIS also regulates the importation and interstate movement of ruminants, swine, birds, and equines as well as animal semen, blood, and serum under USDA/APHIS Authorization Act (21 U.S.C. 101–111 and 134). These regulations designate specific permanent quarantine requirements for ungulates from countries that have rinderpest and foot and mouth disease and swine from African swine fever endemic countries. The shipments must enter the United States through designated ports. The animals must undergo a quarantine overseas in a USDA-approved embarkation quarantine facility before shipment and also must be quarantined in the United States before shipment to a Permanent Post Entry Quarantine (PPEQ) facility. These animals must be shipped in containers that have an official USDA seal applied by a USDA inspector. The pink copy of the ANH Form 17-65C, Permanent Quarantine Record of Zoo Animals, for that animal must accompany the shipment. At the destination, the USDA inspector breaks the seal and supervises the disposition of animal bedding and the cleaning and disinfection of the shipping crate and transport carrier. In transport, there must be provisions made to prevent animal exposure and animal waste dissemination en route. The USDA also regulates the testing of domestic animals for shipment from zoos that maintain ungulates and swine that are being held under PPEQ.

The CITES regulates international trading activities, depending on the level of protection. Both an import permit from the United States and an export permit from the exporting country may be required before the animal can be shipped into the United States. Countries entered and exited while the animal is in transport may require these same permits. The customs veterinarian at the stopover airports in transit can be contacted to verify this requirement. In addition, before exports of CITES Appendix I or II species are allowed, the exporting country must be assured that any living specimen will "be so prepared and shipped as to minimize the risk of injury, damage to health or cruel treatment." CITES has officially supported air transport as the preferred means for the movement of live wild animals and has adopted the IATA animal regulations. The Live Animals Board of IATA meets twice a year and amends its IATA guidelines annually. These guidelines contain specific information for persons handling shipments and for enforcement authorities. For example, the IATA regulations indicate that the animal shipments must be treated as wet cargo and should be placed on plastic sheeting. This prevents spillage from contaminating the cargo hold. It also stops the transfer of cold from the air frame to the crate. The shipment should be located on the plane so that the animal is not affected by outside temperatures when the cargo compartment doors are opened.

Other agencies have regulations for the movement of exotic animals. For example, the National Marine Fisheries Services regulates the transport of marine mammals. In addition, the Centers for Disease Control and Prevention (CDC) registers facilities for importation of nonhuman primates being brought into the United States under the regulations of the U.S. Department of Health, Education and Welfare, Public Health Services (42 U.S.C. part 71). The facility must undergo a lengthy application process including a facility inspection. There are specifications as to how the animal crates are to be transported in the cargo hold. There are specifications on how the crates are to be handled when being unloaded and on the disinfection of the cargo hold after the crate is removed. Any ground transportation of the animal must be in a vehicle that has a separate ventilation system between the animal and the driver. The animal must be quarantined for 31 days after importation, and there are specifications of the testing required and the precautions that staff must take in working around the animals while in quarantine. The registered facility must submit documentation to CDC that all the specifications will be met.

DOCUMENTATION

All the required permits and documentation with the correct number of signed and dated copies must accompany the shipments. The type of documentation required depends on the species being transported and whether the destination is domestic or international. It is helpful to have extra copies of documents available in case the transporter wants additional copies. The drivers of ground transports need to be able to produce the documents required by state and federal inspectors at international or state borders.

For international shipments from the United States, the veterinarian at the shipping institution prepares and signs an international health certificate, and completes a USDA Veterinary Services Form 17-140, which is valid only with the USDA veterinary seal and a signature of the USDA Area Veterinarian in Charge. The health certificate indicates that the animal being shipped is in good health to travel and is free of communicable disease. APHIS Form 7020 (which replaced the VS Form 18-20) should be included for all domestic shipments within the United States, serving as a means to verify that the animal arrived in the condition stated on the health certificate.

The air waybill must be completed before the carrier will accept live animal cargo. Air carriers also require a shipper's certificate that serves as an affidavit that all the information on the air waybill is correct, that the animal is in good health, and that the shipment is not

in violation of international law. It also identifies the species being shipped and indicates that the specific IATA container requirements have been met.

SHIPMENT

The mode of animal transport is typically determined by cost, depending on the species (size and weight) being transported and the distance of the transport. Traditionally, the shipping institution decides on an air carrier or other mode of ground transportation. If possible, transport should be done by air, but only if it is the most expedient means of transport. Shipping by U.S. Postal Service should be avoided. Air shipments require appropriate ground transportation from the zoo to the air carrier by the shipping institution and from the airport to the final destination once the shipment arrives. Crates should be transported in enclosed vehicles to prevent the risk of possible escapes and to avoid temperature fluctuations. Care should be taken to select the route with the fewest number of stops or layovers to minimize any unnecessary handling and possible exposure to climatic changes by the animal. When layovers do occur, there may be commingling of shipments, which increases the risk of disease transfer between highly stressed animals; thus, layovers should be kept to a minimum. The length of time that the animal is kept in the crate must be kept to a minimum.

The animal should be crated just before transport and uncrated immediately upon arrival at the new institution. If the animal is immobilized for crating, it should not leave the zoo grounds until it is standing and determined to be awake and stable enough to transport as determined by the veterinarian certifying the health of the animal. If an animal is transported in a crate while still under the effects of an immobilizing agent, it can easily be jostled around in the crate, attaining a position in which it is unable to breathe adequately, and die. The animal may also become hyperexcited by partial sedation and become hyperthermic. If this is recognized, it is better to wait until the animal appears stable or cancel and reschedule the immediate shipment.

In ground transportation of large animals, it may be necessary to evaluate the route before shipment to be assured that there is enough overhead clearance for electrical transmission lines, tunnels, and overpasses for the vehicle and crate. If there are accompanying vehicles preceding and following the transport vehicle, then all of the drivers should be in contact via radio communication. Depending on local regulations, a special permit may be needed to have an attendant in the back of a van or open truck with the animal. In transporting large animals such as elephants, giraffes, and whales, it may be advisable to notify local police authorities.

A specialized freight forwarder may expeditiously handle all the documentation, supply the shipping container at times, handle and hold an animal during shipment, and make necessary arrangements for transportation between air carriers during layovers. Forwarders should know the best routes and carriers, be aware of governmental regulations, and provide an intimate knowledge of animal shipping, which can prevent problems during the transport. Forwarders may also arrange for insurance coverage, which may be an important consideration for international animal transports because of the extra considerations needed for live animals. Insurance coverage may be extended to include the time periods before and after the actual shipment. Because of their experience, forwarders often have representatives who can meet and coordinate a shipment at the destination of the shipment. This may be an important part of maintaining the welfare of the animal during a transport. Reputable forwarders are registered with the USDA and adhere to the rules and regulations of the AWA and IATA Live Animal Regulations.

Before an international shipment gets underway, scheduling for customs and veterinary clearances must be made with the appropriate individuals. Commercial customs brokers can be helpful in expediting this process and in covering some of the legalities and liabilities at borders. Airlines must be consulted well in advance of the shipment to verify that the dimensions of the container will fit through the cargo door into the cargo hold. Airlines should be contacted 2 to 3 days in advance of the flight to arrange for or confirm that the animal's crate will be the last container put on the plane and the first container removed. Creating good will between the airline personnel and the zoo can greatly enhance the efficiency of the animal shipment. The institutional representatives receiving the animal must be notified in advance and be made aware of the details of the animal's scheduled arrival. They should also be called the day of the shipment to confirm that the animal made the first flight connection. The staff from the shipping institution should not leave the airport until the plane is off the ground. The receiving institution should have someone at the airport before arrival of the shipment to ensure that the animals are off-loaded first and to attend to any immediate or emergency needs of the animal. Veterinarians at institutions en route should be contacted in advance and asked to be on call in case something goes wrong during the shipment.

The shipping institution should monitor weather conditions at the origin, destination, and stops en route. If there is any possibility of significant inclement weather, the shipment should be rescheduled. Shipments of tropical species should not be scheduled during cold winter weather. Shipments should not occur during the Christmas season because animals may be removed at the last minute to handle priority U.S. mail shipments during this time. It is best to avoid shipping on weekends or holidays.

A representative from the receiving institution should notify the shipping institution within 24 hours to report on the animal's shipment. Any unusual findings such as dead or injured animals, damaged crates, or animals that did not arrive as scheduled should be reported to the shipping institution and the carrier. Communication from the receiving veterinarian should be communicated to the shipping veterinarian as it pertains to the animal's condition upon arrival if it is not consistent with information provided in previous communications or as stated on the animal's health certificate. Information about the animal after its quarantine examination should also be communicated to the shipping veterinarian if it is not consistent with the animal's medical history.

PRESHIPMENT TESTING AND MEDICAL HISTORY

It is the responsibility of the shipping institution to determine what tests and permits are needed to ship an animal interstate or internationally. For international shipment, staff at the embassy of the importing country should have the information, or the recipient institution may be able to determine the testing requirements. For interstate shipments, the USDA/APHIS has a regulations retrieval service (RRS) through its National Center for Animal Health Information Systems (NCAHIS) in Fort Collins, CO, with a voice response service (VRS), which contains such information as international regulations and state regulations for the interstate movement of animals, veterinary services, telephone lists for APHIS headquarters, state veterinarian addresses and telephone numbers, certified brucellosis class A– and B–free states, and tuberculosis-free states.

The service is available 24 hours a day at 1-800-545-8732. Once connected to VRS, the caller may choose Emergency Notices, for State Regulations or for Animal Care, for a listing of USDA requirements for the transportation of a list of different species. The state animal health regulations are also available on the World Wide Web at http://www.aphis.usda.gov/vs/sregs. The veterinarian at the receiving institution should also consider the species in question and evaluate the needs for elective preshipment testing in accordance with its own preventive medicine protocols and based on the medical history of the animal to evaluate the suitability of the animal for travel and to consider the possibility of testing to be done at the time of shipment if immobilization is needed for crating.

The animal's full medical history would ideally be forwarded well in advance of the shipment to the receiving institution's veterinarian. Sending the animal's Medical Animal Records (MedARKS) disc may be an efficient means of accomplishing this. Communication between veterinarians to discuss case histories with animals that have chronic illness or ongoing therapies should occur. Copies of pertinent radiographs, video of ultrasound procedures, and other photographic documentation of the animal should be shared well in advance of the animal's shipment. Elective procedures such as permanent identification, application of protective horn guards, sex determination, and photographs should be scheduled accordingly by the shipping institution or performed at the time of crating if sedation is needed for crating. If sedation is not required for shipment, then these procedures should be done well in advance of the shipment.

The veterinarian at the shipping institution must prepare and sign a health certificate. Health certificates for international shipments originating from the United States require the completion of USDA Veterinary Services Form 17-140. The VS Form 17-140 is only valid with the USDA veterinary seal and the signature of the USDA Area Veterinarian in Charge. Proof of required preshipment testing must also accompany the health certificate. The animal being shipped should be in good health, be free of communicable disease, and be in good condition to travel. Animals that are near term pregnant, in estrus, or have antlers in velvet are examples of animals that are not in an ideal condition to be shipped. The health certificate serves as a means to verify that the animal arrived in the condition stated on the health certificate.

QUARANTINE

The quarantine plans should be determined in advance of the arrival of the animal at the zoo.[6] The quarantine keeper should contact the keeper at the shipping zoo to determine whether the quarantine setup, diet, and so forth will meet the individual animal's needs. The quarantine keeper should contact the shipping zoo if there are concerns about how the animal is doing after arrival. The veterinarians at both institutions must communicate if any medical problems arise during or following shipment.

REFERENCES

1. Cornell L: Capture, transportation, restraint, and marking. *In* Fowler ME (ed): Zoo and Wild Animal Medicine, 2nd ed. Philadelphia, WB Saunders, pp 764–770, 1986.
2. Ebedes H: Game ranching in South Africa. *In* Fowler ME (ed): Zoo and Wild Animal Medicine Current Therapy 3. Philadelphia, WB Saunders, pp 112–123, 1993.
3. Ebedes H, Raath JP: The use of long term neuroleptics in the confinement and transport of wild animals. Proceedings of the Joint Conference AAZV/WDA/AAWV, East Lansing, MI, pp 173–176, 1995.
4. Joseph BE, Asper ED, Antrim JE: Marine mammal transport. *In* Dierauf LA (ed): CRC Handbook of Marine Mammal Medicine: Health, Disease and Rehabilitation. Boca Raton, FL, pp 543–551, 1990.
5. Live Animal Regulations, 23rd ed. Montreal, International Air Transport Association, 1996.
6. Miller RE: Quarantine procedures for AZA-accredited zoological parks. Proceedings of the Joint Conference AAZV/WDA/AAWV, East Lansing, MI, pp 165–172, 1995.
7. Stoskopf MK: Environmental requirements and diseases of sharks. *In* Stoskopf MK (ed): Fish Medicine. Philadelphia, WB Saunders, pp 758–763, 1993.
8. Tomasso JR Jr: Environmental requirements and disease of temperate freshwater and estuarine fishes. *In* Stoskopf MK (ed): Fish Medicine. Philadelphia, WB Saunders, pp 240–246, 1993.
9. Vehr KL: Summary of United States wildlife regulations applicable to zoos. *In* Kleiman DG, Allen ME, Thompson KV, et al (eds): Wild Mammals in Captivity: Principles and Techniques. Chicago, The University of Chicago Press, pp 593–599, 1996.

CHAPTER **6**

Health Problems in Mixed-Species Exhibits

LINDA J. LOWENSTINE

The modern zoo focuses on animals as integral parts of their habitats.[10] Mixed-species exhibits educate the public on the complexity of interactions among plants and animals of specific ecosystems. No longer is it acceptable to house animals in sterile, isolated environments. Along with naturalistic exhibits comes a lessened ability to control for variables that influence animal health.

This chapter discusses health problems that may be seen in mixed-species exhibits. Data have been gleaned from necropsies I have performed and through discussions with animal care personnel and clinical veterinarians at several institutions. No systematic survey has been made of institutions with mixed-species exhibits to better document the range and severity of the problems. This sort of survey would be a valuable contribution to captive management and should be undertaken.

TRAUMA

In large mixed-species exhibits of both birds and mammals, trauma is the most frequent and serious health problem. Although trauma may be significant in single-species multiple-animal exhibits, the presence of multiple species compounds the problem. Competition for use of "prime habitat" within an enclosure and establishment of territories surrounding water or food sources can lead to aggressive interactions. Competition for nesting sites or materials as well as for food may result in trauma among avian species. Behavior that signals displeasure in one species may not be appropriately interpreted by another species. Socially inept young animals are particularly at risk. Normal behaviors, such as the rubbing of velvet from antlers or the play of young animals, may be interpreted as challenges by other animals. Although trauma may be the proximate cause of death, a thorough necropsy often reveals underlying disease processes that may have altered the animal's behavior or ability to escape from aggressive exhibit mates, particularly in avian species. Abnormal motion, such as the flopping flight of pinioned or tenectomied birds in field enclosures, may initiate damaging investigative or aggressive behavior from hoofstock. Flight distances may also differ; a spacial arrangement that would be acceptable among individuals within one species may not be acceptable to individuals of another species. Trauma may be self-inflicted when an animal injures itself while fleeing when frightened or when fleeing from an aggressor. Some species that normally live on open plains, such as Saiga antelope (*Saiga tatarica*), do not look for barriers when running and are prone to self-induced injuries. Direct interactions may result in either blunt or sharp trauma from kicking, butting, and use of antlers, horns, or teeth. In addition to suffering fractured limbs and ribs, aspiration pneumonia may result from impact, causing regurgitation and aspiration of ingesta or cud in ruminant animals. Crushing muscle injuries and exertional myopathy may result in myoglobinuria with subsequent lower nephron nephrosis and renal failure.

Traumatic encounters may be minimized by ensuring that the behavioral needs of each species are met, with provision of hiding areas and minimization of obstacles that might cause trauma to running animals. Provision of multiple feeding and watering stations, nesting sites for birds, and "tucking" areas for young of hoofstock prevents congregation of animals. Seasonal variation in aggressive behavior is apparent in deer and some other species. The removal of rutting males or the blunting or capping of horns and antlers may limit the severity of penetrating wounds, but it does not prevent blunt trauma. Similarly, dubbing of canine teeth in primates limits punctures and lacerations, but it does not prevent crushing injuries.

A few species are notorious for being "antisocial." Some individuals of these species may be amiable enough to be housed in mixed-species exhibits, but, for the most part, black rhinoceroses (*Diceros bicornus*), zebras (*Equus grevyi*), and possibly ostriches (*Struthio camelus*) are poorly compatible with other species. Oryx of all species may also be problematic. Even white rhinoceroses (*Ceratotherium simum*), which are more gregarious than their hook-lipped cousins, have a reputation for stepping on newborn animals of other species.

NUTRITIONAL AND DIET-RELATED HEALTH PROBLEMS

Adjusting diets to fit all species and members of large mixed-species exhibits is a true challenge for zoological nutritionists, veterinarians, and curatorial staff. Feeding stations must be of sufficient number and configuration to ensure that some animals are not prevented from eating while others overeat. Deer especially seem prone to obesity, which may lead to a syndrome of fat necrosis. Hard calcified fat pads in the pelvic canal have been associated with fatal dystocias in affected does of species such as Barasingha (*Cervu duvauceli*).

Requirements of trace minerals and other nutrients may differ among species. For example, although picivorous birds such as herons usually need supplementation with vitamin E to prevent nutritional steatosis, vitamin E toxicity has been reported in pink-backed pelicans when fish were supplemented with standard multivitamin tablets.[16] Some species of antelope such as blesbok (*Damaliscus dorcas*) and sable antelope (*Hippotragus niger*) seem prone to development of copper deficiency, especially during pregnancy, even when diets have adequate copper based on data available for other ruminant animals.[5] Competition from other minerals such as molybdenum may play a role. Hypervitaminosis D has been identified in pacas (*Cuniculus paca*) and agoutis (*Dasyprocta aguti*) housed with New World monkeys.[13] It was surmised that the rodents ate New World monkey biscuits, which are high in vitamin D3. In mixed-species aviaries, it is difficult to ensure that low-iron diets are only eaten by birds that need them and iron "intolerant" species, such as toucans and mynahs, may readily consume items not on their menu that are intended for other animals in the exhibit.

INFECTIOUS DISEASES

Infectious diseases are responsible for morbidity and mortality in mixed-species exhibits. Among the most dramatic examples are epizootics caused by viruses, particularly herpesviruses. Outbreaks of malignant catarrhal fever (MCF) have occurred in several facilities.[3] The African form of the disease is caused by acelaphine herpesvirus-1, a gammaherpesvirus, which is carried by wildebeests (*Connochaetes* species). Related viruses are carried by topi (*Damaliscus* species) and hartebeests (*Alcelaphus* species). All these antelope species are of the subfamily Alcelaphinae of the family Bovidae. A North American form of MCF has been associated with sheep and goats (subfamilies Ovinae and Caprinae). Other species of the families Bovidae and Cervidae are highly susceptible to infection. Species involved in outbreaks have included gaur (*Bos gaurus*), Pere David's deer (*Elaphurus davidianus*), muntjac (*Muntiacus* species), and kudu (*Tragelaphus* species), among others. Transmission occurs when virus is shed by carrier species during parturition. Thus, carrier species should not be in breeding situations in direct contact or even close proximity to susceptible species.

Equine herpesvirus-1 is less well appreciated to be a risk to non-equid species, but there have been verified cases in a Bactrian camel (*Camelus bactrianus*), llamas (*Lama glama*), and a Thomson's gazelle (*Gazella thomsoni*).[2, 12] In this most recent report, zebras housed in the same exhibit were thought to have shed the virus. This virus may be shed during the respiratory infection, parturition, or abortion, which occur in infected equids. In addition to infection of domestic horses and zebras, infection of onagers has also been documented. Vaccination of equids does not entirely protect against active infection and it might be advisable to use only seroneg-ative equids in mixed-species exhibits.

Nonhuman primate herpesviruses are well known to cross species lines in mixed-housing situations, even when animals are not in direct contact.[8] *Herpesvirus simiae* (also called B-virus, herpesvirus B, or most recently cercopithecine herpesvirus-1) is carried latently by rhesus and other macaques (*Macaca* species). It is transmitted through biting and scratching, but it can also be aerosolized or carried in dried secretions on surfaces where the virus remains viable for several hours. An outbreak in zoo-housed colobus monkeys has been documented. Macaques housed in mixed-species exhibits should be virus negative by serological testing.

Another group of Old World primate herpesvirus, the simian varicella group (also called Medical Lake macaque virus, deltaherpesvirus, and Liverpool vervet virus), can also cross species.[17] The disease in macaques is often mild and self-limiting, suggesting that ma-caques are the natural hosts. Infection may be fatal in Patas monkeys (*Erythrocebus patas*) and other African cercopithecines. In these animals, disseminated disease includes cutaneous lesions and respiratory disease. To avoid spread of this disease, African and Asian primates should not be mixed.

Squirrel monkeys (*Saimiri sciureus*) are hosts to two herpesviruses capable of infecting other species of New World monkeys, specifically callitrichids and aotids. *Herpesvirus tamarinus* (herpesvirus T, *Herpesvirus platyrrhinae*) causes mild cold sores in squirrel mon-keys but fatal disseminated infection in other species, notably marmosets, tamarins, and owl monkeys (*Aotus* species). *Herpesvirus saimiri* is a gammaherpesvirus that has been shown experimentally to cause lympho-proliferative disease and lymphosarcoma when inocu-lated into marmosets, tamarins, cebus (*Cebus* species), and howler monkeys (*Alouatta* species).[8] Spontaneous infections have occurred in both vivarial and zoological settings. In one outbreak, three black-tailed marmosets (*Callithrix argentata*) housed in an aviary-like exhibit with neotropical birds, brocket deer, and squirrel mon-keys died of lymphoproliferative disease within a year of being placed in the exhibit.[7] *Herpesvirus ateles* is a gammaherpesvirus of spider monkeys (*Ateles* species), which has been shown experimentally to produce dis-ease similar to *H. saimiri* when inoculated into marmo-sets, tamarins, and owl monkeys. Although natural transmission has not been documented for *H. ateles,* spider monkeys as well as squirrel monkeys should not be placed in mixed-species exhibits with other primates.

Avian herpesviruses may also cross species lines. Pacheco's disease virus is thought to be carried by some species of conures, such as patagonian (*Cyanoliseus patagonus*) and nanday conures (*Nandayus nenday*). Devastating outbreaks have occurred in other species of psittacine birds, including New World and Old World species. Infection has also been documented in a toucan that had been housed with macaws.[4] The mode of trans-mission is uncertain, but fecal and respiratory shedding are suspected.

Similarly, some species of tortoises may serve as reservoirs for herpesvirus infections in other species. In one report, South American red-footed tortoises (*Geochelon carbonaria*) remained healthy while co-housed Argentine tortoises (*Geochelon chilensis*) suf-fered a high mortality rate.[11] Other viral diseases that can cross species lines include simian hemorrhagic fe-ver and simian immunodeficiency virus. These primate infections are spread between African and Asian species and emphasize the fact that Asian and African species should not be housed together. Varying susceptibilita to ophidian paramyxovirus infection has been noted among viperids and the infection may be introduced into collections by inapparently infected individuals.[11] Other groups of snakes, such as boids, elaphids, and colubrids, may also become infected.

Sometimes, uninvited species share exhibits with collection specimens. *Mus musculus* is thought to be the vector for "callitrichid hepatitis," which is caused by lymphocytic choriomeningitis virus, an Old World arena virus. Infected rodents, including rats, mice, and squirrels, have been implicated in outbreaks of encepha-lomyocarditis virus infection in zoo animals.

Bacterial diseases are generally less host specific and infections of multiple species in an exhibit usually result from common environmental exposure. However, organisms that may be normal flora for one species may prove hazardous to another. One such example is *Bordetella bronchiseptica,* which may be a normal inhabitant of the rabbit oropharyngeal flora but it is associated with bronchopneumonia in guinea pigs. The status of this agent vis-à-vis other lagomorphs and ro-dents is unknown. Many species of birds such as psitta-cines do not normally carry gram-negative organisms as part of their flora. Colonization by gram-negative bacteria acquired from exhibit mates that carry the or-ganism may result in systemic infection. *Chlamydia psittaci* may be carried chronically by a variety of birds and may cause more significant infection in other avian as well as nonavian species. Fecal contamination of feed and substrates is obviously unavoidable in large exhibits with natural ground cover.

Sometimes, prey or diet items serve as a source of contagion for co-housed species. *Streptococcus zooepi-demicus* septicemia developed in New World monkeys housed in a mixed-species exhibit after ingestion of a horse meat–based diet that was meant for armadillos.[18] Horse meat contamination of diets has also been impli-cated in outbreaks of toxoplasmosis in primates.

Vectors such as feral rodents, English sparrows, and pigeons, which share exhibits with collection animals, may serve as carriers for bacterial pathogens such as *Salmonella typhimurium* and *Salmonella enteritidis, Yersinia pseudotuberculosis,* and *Yersinia enterocolitica.* These infections may subsequently spread among ani-mals on exhibit.

PARASITES

Parasites with direct life cycles and broad host range pose the greatest threat in mixed-species exhibits. Dis-ease potential can vary greatly depending on the host species, intercurrent disease processes, nutritional sta-tus, and stage of host life cycle.

Protozoal parasites with direct life cycles and broad

species tropism include several of the gastrointestinal parasites that can easily contaminate exhibit substrates, water, and foliage. For example, *Balantidium coli* is seldom a pathogen in cercopithecine monkeys unless they are immunosuppressed; however, in great apes, especially gorillas, *Balantidium* is reported to be an important pathogen, causing severe invasive infections. Thus, if monkeys and great apes are housed together, care must be taken not to introduce *Balantidium*. Inapparent amoebiasis is common in both New World and Old World primates, and pathogenicity is usually associated with immune suppression.[1] In colobine monkeys, invasive gastric amoebiasis is a serious problem that may be extremely difficult to eliminate.[14] Giardiasis, hexamitiasis, trichomoniasis, and cryptosporidiosis are all potential infections of mixed exhibits housing primates.

Oroesophageal trichomoniasis may be a problem in mixed aviaries. Infection is relatively common in columbiforms and may spread to passerines or psittacines at feeders and in water sources. Another serious avian protozoanosis is atoxoplasmosis. This apicomplexan protozoan has a complex life cycle that involves gametogony in the intestinal tract followed by infection of monocytes and lymphocytes and subsequent dissemination to lungs, liver, and elsewhere. The species specificity of the organism is in question and some species such as myna seem to be quite susceptible with high losses in nestling and fledgling birds. The life cycle is direct.

Even protozoa with indirect life cycles may be a problem in mixed aviaries. *Plasmodium* species that cause mild infections in North American bird species may pose a serious hazard to other birds, especially penguins, and montane or island passerines, which have no natural resistance. Indoor mixed exhibits may exclude the mosquito vectors, but, in outdoor exhibits, carrier birds must be excluded.

Metazoan parasites of note include those causing disease resulting from aberrant migrations or variation in host response. *Baylisascaris procyonis* and *Baylisascaris columnaris* from raccoons and skunks are well known for their predilection to cause visceral larval migrans in aberrant hosts. Housing New World primates and avian species with shedders can result in losses from cerebral spinal nematodiasis.[9] Similarly the meningeal worm *Parelaphostrongylus tenuis* of white-tailed deer (*Odocoileus virginianus*) can cause fatal neural nematodiasis in other cervids such as moose (*Alces alces*), elk (*Cervus elaphus*), and Pere David's deer.

Heterakis isolonche, a cecal worm of gallinaceous birds, causes much more severe disease in some pheasants such as golden pheasants (*Chrysolophus pictus*) than in other game birds.[7] *Geopetitia aspiculata*, a spirurid nematode, caused devastating widespread infection in multiple species of birds from several different orders at several major zoological collections. Various insects, including those fed as part of the diet, such as crickets, meal worm beetles, and pest species such as cockroaches, apparently acted as intermediate hosts to perpetuate the infection.[6] Cockroaches were also incriminated in the fatal infections of golden lion tamarins (*Leontopithecus rosalia rosalia*) with *Pterygodermatites nycticebi*, a nematode of the slow loris (*Nycticebus*

coucang), when an enclosure vacated by the latter species was used to house the former. These last examples highlight the need for control of insect pests and for thorough periodic cleaning or changing of substrates when possible.

Enteric nematode infestations in hoofstock may affect several different species, and elimination of the infections may be difficult in species that avoid medicated feed or that are more susceptible to infection.[15] Irrigation of pastures to allow grazing may perpetuate the problem by providing a microclimate suitable for parasite development. The desert gazelle species seem to be more susceptible than some of the other antelopes.

Arthropod parasites may also pose a problem in mixed-species housing. In macaques, infestation with the simian lung mite (*Pneumonyssus simicola*) is usually clinically inapparent. In langurs, notably Douc langurs (*Pygathrix nemaeus*), infection can be serious.[7] The mites can be eliminated with the use of ivermectin.

REFERENCES

1. Beaver PC, Blanchard JL, Seibold HR: Invasive amebiasis in naturally infected New World and Old World monkeys with and without clinical disease. Am J Trop Med Hyg 39:343–352, 1988.
2. Bildfell R, Yason C, Haines D, McGowan M: Herpesvirus encephalitis in a camel (*Camelus bactrianus*). J Zoo Wildlife Med 27:409–415, 1996.
3. Castro AE, Heuschele WP: Veterinary Diagnostic Virology. St. Louis, Mosby–Year Book, 1993.
4. Charlton BR, Barr BC, Castro AE, et al: Herpes viral hepatitis in a toucan. Avian Pathology 34(3):787–790, 1990.
5. Dierenfeld ES, Dolensek EP, McNamara TS, Doherty JG: Copper deficiency in captive blesbok antelope (*Damaliscus dorcas phillipsi*). J Zoo Wildlife Med 19:126–131, 1988.
6. French RA, Todd KS, Meehan TP, Zachary JF: Parasitology and pathogenesis of *Geopetitia aspiculata* (Nematoda: spirurida) in zebra finches (*Taeniopygia guttata*): Experimental infection and new host records. J Zoo Wildlife Med 25:403–422, 1994.
7. Griner LA: Pathology of Zoo Animals. San Diego, CA, Zoological Society of San Diego, 1983.
8. Hunt RD: Herpesviruses of primates: An introduction. *In* Jones TC, Mohr U, Hunt RD (eds): Nonhuman Primates I. Berlin, Springer-Verlag, pp 73–93, 1993.
9. Huntress SL, Spraker T: Baylisascaris infection in the marmoset. Proceedings of the Annual Meeting of the American Association of Zoo Veterinarians, Scottsdale, AZ, p 78, 1985.
10. IUDZG—The World Zoo Organization and the Captive Breeding Specialist Group of IUCN/SSC. The World Zoo Conservation Strategy: The Role of Zoos and Aquaria of the World in Global Conservation. Brookfield, IL, Chicago Zoological Society, 1993.
11. Jacobson ER: Viral diseases of reptiles. *In* Fowler ME (ed): Zoo and Wild Animal Medicine. Current Therapy 3. Philadelphia, WB Saunders, pp 153–159, 1993.
12. Kennedy MA, Ramsay E, Diderrich V, et al: Encephalitis associated with a variant of equine herpesvirus 1 in a Thomson's gazelle (*Gazella thomsoni*). J Zoo Wildlife Med 27:533–538, 1997.
13. Kenny D, Cambre RC, Lewandowski A, et al: Suspected vitamin D3 toxicity in pacas (*Cuniculus paca*) and agoutis (*Dasyprocta aguti*). J Zoo Wildlife Med 24:129–139, 1993.
14. Loomis MR, Britt JO, Gendron AP, et al: Hepatic and gastric amebiasis in black and white colobus monkeys. J Am Vet Med Assoc 183:1188–1191, 1983.
15. Mikolon AB, Boyce WM, Allen JL, et al: Epidemiology and control of nematode parasites in a collection of captive exotic ungulates. J Zoo Wildlife Med 25:500–510, 1994.
16. Nichols DK, Wolff MJ, Phillips LG Jr, Montali RJ: Coagulopathy in pink-backed pelicans (*Pelecanus rufescens*) associated with hypervitaminosis E. J Zoo Wildlife Med 20:57–61, 1989.
17. Padovan D, Cantrell CA: Varicella-like herpesvirus infections of nonhuman primates. Lab Anim Sci 36:7–13, 1986.
18. Schiller CA, Wolff MJ, Munson L, Montali RJ: *Streptococcus zooepidemicus* infections of possible horse meat source in red-bellied tamarins and Goeldi's monkeys. J Zoo Wildlife Med 20:322–327, 1989.

CHAPTER 7

The Application of Minimally Invasive Surgery for the Diagnosis and Treatment of Captive Wildlife

ROBERT A. COOK

DAVID R. STOLOFF

The use of rigid endoscopic techniques for minimally invasive surgery (MIS) has gained wide acceptance for selected diagnostic and therapeutic procedures in human[13] and domestic animal medicine.[24] In zoological and wildlife medicine, this technology has had its greatest application in assisted reproduction procedures. It has been underused in many other potential applications.[6, 16] The conditions under which wildlife are maintained in zoological parks require the adaptation of techniques that will reduce postoperative care requirements and shorten recovery period. MIS equipment has been improved dramatically in recent years, allowing broader potential for its use in captive wildlife. In comparison with most traditional open surgical procedures, MIS induces relatively minor tissue trauma, which, in most cases, results in shorter postoperative recovery periods, decreased postoperative care, and fewer postoperative complications. Anesthesia is necessary for conducting most manipulative procedures in wildlife, and, because MIS adds little additional risk, this technique should be considered when diagnostic or therapeutic procedures are indicated.[7]

If the procedure would not be performed using traditional surgical methods, then beginning surgeons probably should not consider using MIS. As the surgeon gains experience, the availability of MIS may prompt earlier intervention, because rapid diagnosis and therapy may lead to an improved prognosis.

HISTORY

The abdominal cavity was first examined endoscopically in the dog in 1901, establishing the use of laparoscopy as a diagnostic tool.[27, 28] This study established the safety of intra-abdominal insufflation pressures of air up to 50 mm Hg and demonstrated the use of insufflation to tamponade abdominal organ bleeding. In 1910, the use of diagnostic laparoscopy was reported in 17 patients with ascites.[21] In 1965, a controlled automatic gas insuf-

flation system, the Wisap CO_2 Pneu-Automatic Insufflator was developed.[32]

In 1918, an insufflation instrument that prevented iatrogenic visceral injury was developed.[14] This device consisted of a short, sharp outer cannula and a longer, round-tipped inner cannula for insufflation, which was spring loaded into the outer cannula. The inner cannula retracted into the outer cannula during tissue penetration and emerged from the cannula after penetration to prevent damage to the viscera. The creation of this device eventually led to the development of the Veress needle.[44]

Most early rigid endoscopies were performed with a cystoscope, which limited the angle of vision to 90 degrees. In 1929, a dual-punch technique was developed with an oblique-viewing lens system that increased the viewing angle to 135 degrees.[26] In 1952, a method of transmitting light from an external source along a quartz rod to the far end of the endoscope was developed.[12] Continued improvements led to the development and manufacture in the 1960s of a modified rod-lens telescope using long quartz rods that were separated by short air spaces. This system doubled the light transmission capacity of the endoscope and resulted in a larger, clearer aperture.[10] Introduction of "cold light" and elimination of incandescent lighting has reduced the risk of iatrogenic injuries.[11] The development of the computer chip television camera, which led to video laparoscopy and the advances in rigid endoscopic instrumentation, has revolutionized the application of MIS procedures.

EQUIPMENT

The basic components of the MIS equipment include a light source, a telescope, a video imaging system, an insufflator, and an irrigation and aspiration instrument (Fig. 7–1). A video recording system, a 35-mm camera with telescope adaptor, and an electrosurgical generator

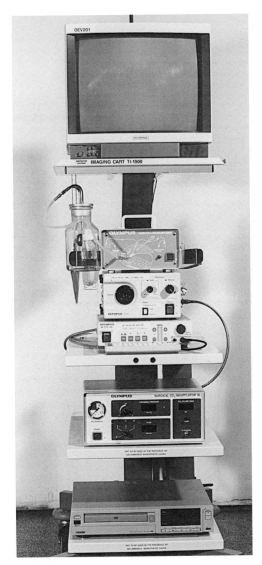

FIGURE 7–1. Minimally invasive surgery equipment kept on a rolling cart for ease of use and storage. (Courtesy of Olympus America, Inc., 2 Corporate Center, Melville, NY 11747-3157.)

are all valuable additions. Selected equipment, instruments, and supply manufacturers are listed in Table 7–1.

Light Source

Having sufficient light to view large, cavernous spaces is essential for the thorough examination of the wildlife patient. A high-intensity xenon light source provides a full spectrum of light, especially for video laparoscopic procedures. The light source should have both manual and automatic intensity control options, enabling the surgeon to operate in a variety of intraoperative lighting conditions. The manual intensity control can be used effectively to visualize less brightly lit areas within a generally bright field.

Telescopes

A wide range of telescopes are being manufactured by a number of companies (Fig. 7–2). For work on the smallest of patients, a human pediatric or fetal laparoscope with a diameter of 1.7 mm may be most appropriate. For slightly larger patients, a 2.7-mm telescope increases light availability as well as field of view. A metal cannula is used with the 1.7-mm telescope. These telescopes are lightweight and provide an excellent field of view. Small laparoscopic trocars or cannulas may be used with these telescopes. Cystoscope sheaths that simultaneously accommodate 1.9-mm or 2.7-mm telescopes and a 3- or 5-French instrument are also available. With these instruments, biopsies can be performed with a single-puncture technique. The 4.0-mm telescopes, often used for arthroscopy, should be considered in small animals that are large enough to accommodate a slightly increased diameter. The length of the telescope should also be considered because working with very small animals can be awkward if the telescope length is excessive.

Larger diameter telescopes are used in large animals. These telescopes increase the field of view and amount of light within the operating field. Telescopes of 5.0 to 10 mm can be used to visualize structures in medium to large and even giant species. With the megavertebrates, it may be preferable to seek out a customized longer-length 10-mm diameter telescope.

Telescopes are available in a variety of viewing angles to accommodate a spectrum of patient sizes and anatomic sites. The 0- and 30-degree-angle telescopes are the most popular in veterinary medicine. Smaller telescopes with a 30-degree angle are used in small cavities. This angle permits the surgeon to rotate the telescope in place while observing a 360-degree panoramic view. In the larger cavities, a large-diameter telescope (i.e., 4 mm or greater) with a 0-degree angle is often used. This telescope allows the operator to view structures without requiring interpretation for the viewing angle. It may be useful to start with a 0-degree telescope if the greatest versatility is needed in a single telescope.

Insufflation

A pneumoperitoneum or insufflation of the coelomic cavity is required to perform the majority of procedures on mammals, amphibians, and reptiles. The chelonia's shell creates a cavity for visualization, but some insufflation may be required. Avian species have a unique air sac system, which precludes the need for insufflation. Distention of the cavity with CO_2 creates a space between the abdominal or coelomic wall and the viscera, permitting visualization and manipulation. A high-flow insufflator that delivers a maximum flow of approximately 9 L/min quickly creates and automatically maintains the intra-abdominal pressure that is preset between 12 and 15 mm Hg. In the megavertebrates, the time required for insufflation can be lengthy because of the excessive free space that must be distended. When multiple ports are used, dramatic reduction in the pneumo-

TABLE 7–1. Selected Product Manufacturers

Circon/ACMI, 300 Stillwater Ave., P.O. Box 1971, Stamford, CT 06904-1971.
Endosurgery telescopes and instruments.

Ethicon, Ethicon Endo-Surgery, Inc., 4545 Creek Road, Cincinnati, OH 45242-2839.
Endosurgery instruments and supplies.

MIST (Minimally Invasive Surgical Technologies), 3310 US 70 West, Smithfield, NC 27577.
Full range of telescopes and endosurgery instruments including 1.7 mm.

Olympus America, Inc., 2 Corporate Center, Melville, NY 11747-3157.
Full range of telescopes, video-imaging system, endosurgery instruments.

Smith and Nephew Endoscopy (Dyonics), 160 Dascomb Road, Andover, MA 01810.
Specializing in arthroscopy telescopes and instruments.

Karl Storz Veterinary Endoscopy-America, Inc., 175 Cremona Drive, Goleta, CA 93117.
Telescopes, endosurgery instruments, and supplies including the 2.7-mm telescope with biopsy port.

United States Surgical Corporation, Norwalk, CT 06856.
Full range of endosurgery instruments and supplies.

Valleylab, Inc., 5920 Longbow Drive, Boulder, CO 80301.
Force 2 electrosurgical generator.

R. Wolf Medical Instruments, 7046 Lyndon Ave., Rosemont, IL 60018.
Telescopes and endosurgery instruments.

peritoneum may result in lengthy delays in the surgical procedure. High-flow insufflators maintain intra-abdominal pressure constantly and provide rapid insufflation when needed during surgery.

Irrigation/Aspiration and Electrosurgical Generator

Depending on the procedure, the availability of both an irrigation/aspiration unit and an electrosurgical generator may prove invaluable. The irrigation/aspiration unit allows for rapid clearing when the surgical field is obstructed by body fluids. The electrosurgical generator is attached to the endoscopic instruments for direct application of cutting or coagulation. Electrosurgery is the primary method used to maintain hemostasis in the endoscopic field. It is also useful to have a multifunctional instrument that has both cautery and aspiration capabilities to reduce the need for instrument exchange and reduce surgical time.

Video Imaging System

When considering multiport, multisurgeon MIS, a video imaging system is essential. A single-chip camera that provides 400 lines of horizontal resolution is attached to a high-resolution rod lens telescope (Fig. 7–3). The video monitor should be large enough to permit all participants to easily view the operative procedure and provide the color, clarity, and degree of resolution captured by the camera (Fig. 7–4). Most commercial monitors provide 350 to 500 lines of horizontal resolution. A video cassette recorder may be used to document the MIS for patient records and teaching purposes.

INSTRUMENTATION AND TECHNIQUE CONSIDERATIONS

The type and quantity of instrumentation used is dictated by the nature of the operative procedure, the size and condition of the patient, and the special anatomic characteristics of the species. The range of telescopes and corresponding instrumentation includes the 1.7-mm pediatric/fetal laparoscopic (14-gauge series, MIST, 3310 US 70 West, Smithfield, NC 27577), the 2.7-, 3.0-, and 4.0-mm arthroscopic, and the 5.0- and 10-mm laparoscopic sizes. In those species in which insufflation

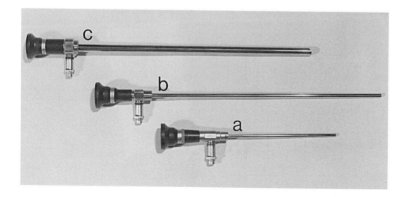

FIGURE 7–2. Rigid fiberoptic telescopes in sizes 2.7 mm *(a)*, 5 mm *(b)*, and 10 mm *(c)*. (Courtesy of Olympus America, Inc., 2 Corporate Center, Melville, NY 11747-3157.)

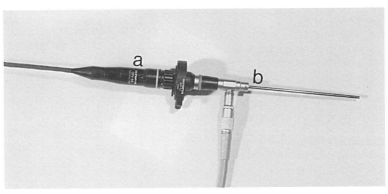

FIGURE 7-3. A digital signal-processing single-chip camera, Olympus OTV-S4. *(a)*, attached to a high-resolution, 0-degreee, 2.7-mm rigid fiberoptic telescope *(b)*. (Courtesy of Olympus America, Inc., 2 Corporate Center, Melville, NY 11747-3157.)

is to be maintained for MIS, the instruments selected must be of appropriate diameter to fill the lumen of the cannula without significant loss of CO_2 and must be of adequate length to afford optimal viewing of the surgical site.

Minimally Invasive Surgery Approach

In wildlife species in which anatomic variations are not well documented, it is advisable to approach the coelomic or abdominal cavities via an open approach or Hasson's technique. In those species in which anatomic landmarks are well understood, a closed approach may be preferred. When there may be multiple adhesions or

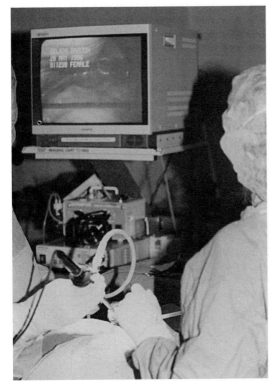

FIGURE 7-4. Surgeons perform MIS while viewing a 20-inch color monitor.

visceral distention, or when the falciform ligament must be excised to facilitate better visibility, an open technique should be used.

Open Technique (Hasson's Technique)

A 1- to 2-cm ventral abdominal incision is made through the skin, subcutaneous tissue, abdominal musculature, and peritoneum. Care is taken to minimize the size of the incision, because an air-tight seal is needed to maintain the pneumoperitoneum. Through the minilaparotomy, the visible portion of the peritoneal or coelomic cavity is inspected. If required to improve visibility, a major portion of the falciform ligament may be excised. One simple interrupted suture is placed through the fascia on either side of the incision. A blunt-tipped trocar is placed into the minilaparotomy and the preplaced sutures on either side of the incision are fixed to the tieposts on the cannula under tension to seal the incision and prevent gas leakage.

Closed Technique

In the closed technique, a Veress needle (Fig. 7–5) is used to puncture and insufflate the abdomen. The Endopath Ultra Veress needle pictured incorporates a spring-loaded blunt stylet, which extends beyond the needle tip (see Fig. 7–5A). An incision approximately 3 mm in length is made through the skin to admit the Veress needle. In preparation for insertion, saline is placed in the drain-down tube (see Fig. 7–5D) of the Veress needle handle and a two-way stopcock valve (see Fig. 7–5E) is closed. The abdominal wall is grasped on either side of the skin incision and lifted to create a space between the viscera and the wall; the Veress needle is inserted through the wall. As the needle begins to penetrate the tissues of the abdominal wall, the safety indicator changes from green to red (see Fig. 7–5 *arrowhead*). After being passed through the peritoneum, the stylet automatically advances forward and the safety indicator returns to green. To check for proper needle placement, the stopcock valve is opened to the atmosphere. If placement is correct, the saline in the drain-down tube flows into the peritoneal cavity causing the ball, which had been floating in the saline, to drop. This procedure is referred to as the *hanging drop test*.

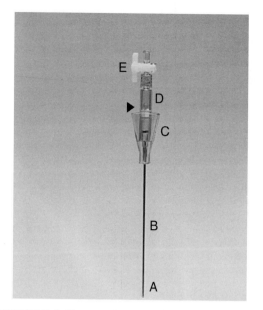

FIGURE 7–5. Veress needle (Endopath Ultra Veress Needle, Ethicon Endo-Surgery, Inc., Cincinnati, OH 45242-2839) with blunt safety stylet (A), needle cannula (B), red/green safety indicator (C), ball float *(arrow)*, down-drain tube (D), and two-way stopcock valve (E).

Additional saline may be placed in the drain-down tube to repeat the hanging drop test.

An aspiration and injection technique can also be used to evaluate the needle placement. A syringe containing 4 to 5 ml of saline is attached to the stopcock. Aspiration is performed and the barrel of the syringe is examined to ensure that no blood, urine, or intestinal contents are present. Approximately 2 ml of saline is then injected into the cavity. The saline should be injected into the abdomen with very little force. Some surgeons prefer to perform the aspiration and injection test before performing the hanging drop test.

The insufflation line is connected to the Veress needle. The insufflator is set at a low-flow rate of 1 to 2 L/min and the insufflation pressure is monitored to ensure that there is no sudden increase in intra-abdominal pressure, which suggests a needle placement problem. Once proper flow is ensured, the flow rate of the insufflator is increased to 9.0 L/min.

Trocars and Cannulas

Surgical trocars with cannulas are used to provide a port for the telescope or other instruments while maintaining the integrity of access into the body cavity (Fig. 7–6). Ranging in size from 1.9 mm outside diameter to 33 mm OD, these devices enable the surgeon to deliver instruments to the surgical site and excise large masses without the need for a laparotomy. Cystoscopes and hysteroscopes are designed to accommodate both a telescope and an operating instrument. With these instruments, biopsies may be performed through a single port. When appropriate, insufflation capabilities of the

cannula can be utilized so as to maintain an expanded cavity of operation. A large trocar and cannula can be placed and then a reducer cap employed so that smaller instruments can be used without loss of insufflation gases.

Disposable guarded trocars are available with safety shields. These trocars require minimal force to penetrate the distended body wall and provide a safety shield to protect the sharp point. The safety shield retracts as it passes through the body wall. After entering the cavity, the safety shield automatically advances and locks, covering the exposed sharp tip. It is advantageous to use a nonconductive cannula to prevent electrical burns if electrosurgical instruments are used. Stability threads secure the position of the cannula and reduce the chance of prematurely dislodging during a surgical procedure (see Fig. 7–5, *arrow*). In very small patients, 1.9-mm or 2.7-mm cystoscopes are used. The metal cystoscope sheath does not have a safety shield for the tip and is not generally used through a trocar. In very small patients, the weight of the telescope alone can present a problem. If the cannula is also used, it too should be very light.

Scissors, Dissectors, and Grasping Forceps

A variety of instruments allow the surgeon to perform a broad range of MIS procedures (Fig. 7–7). The greatest

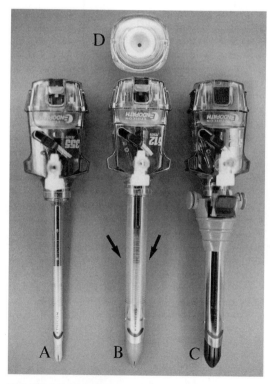

FIGURE 7–6. Five-millimeter (A) and 12-mm (B) Disposable Endopath Dilating Tip Trocar with stability sleeve (Ethicon Endo-Surgery, Inc., 4545 Creek Road, Cincinnati, OH 45242-2839); TriStar blunt-tip trocar (C); and Universal one-seal reducer cap (D).

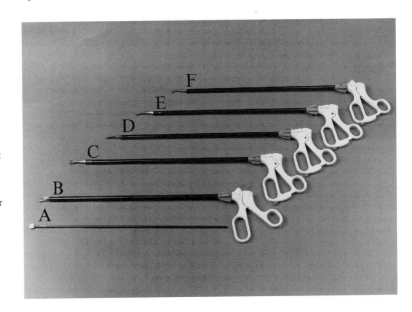

FIGURE 7–7. Ten-millimeter instruments (Endopath, Ethicon Endo-Surgery, Inc., 4545 Creek Road, Cincinnati, OH 45242-2839): Blunt Cherry dissector (A); Metzenbaum scissors (B); Babcock grasper (C); Allis clamp (D); Kelly clamp (E); and right-angle dissector *(F)*.

number of instruments are available for the 5- and 10-mm ports, but as demand increases, the smaller sized products are becoming available. Scissors and dissectors with unipolar cautery allow for tissue dissection while hemorrhage is controlled (Fig. 7–8). Dissectors without unipolar cautery are useful for nontraumatic tissue manipulation. Grasping forceps, such as atraumatic Babcocks, Babcocks, Allis clamps, Kelly clamps, Glassman clamps, lung clamps, and curved Kelly clamps, allow for a variety of tissue handling over an extended surgical field.

Staplers and Electrosurgical Probes

Staplers are combined with linear cutters to facilitate organ biopsy, resection, and mass removal. Multifeed staplers alone are used for the ligation of vessels, and circular staplers along with intraluminal staplers are used for intestinal resection (Fig. 7–9). A variety of monopolar electrosurgical probes (see Fig. 7–9) are available as hooks, spatulas, balls, and bullets and provide the ability to dissect and coagulate tissues where bleeding is most likely to occur.

Suture, Needle Holders, and Retrieval Pouches

Needle holders are designed to work through the operating port and deliver appropriate suture materials with needles into the surgical field for knot placement. Ligatures with pretied extracorporeal knots facilitate ligation of vascular structures and can be used effec-

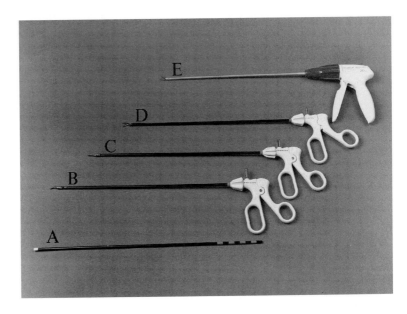

FIGURE 7–8. Five-millimeter instruments (Endopath, Ethicon Endo-Surgery, Inc., 4545 Creek Road, Cincinnati, OH 45242-2839): blunt tip dissector (A); curved dissector with unipolar cautery (B); straight dissector with unipolar cautery (C); curved scissors with unipolar cautery (D); and Ligaclip endoscopic multiple clip applier with rotating shaft (E).

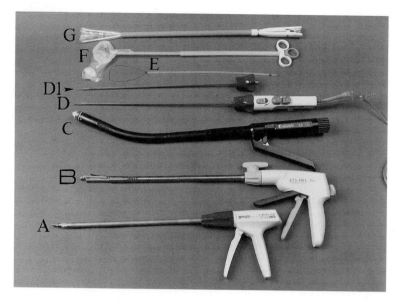

FIGURE 7–9. Ligaclip endoscopic multiple clip applier with rotating shaft (A); Endopath, ETS-Flex articulating endoscopic linear cutter (B); Endopath ILS endoscopic curved intraluminal stapler (C); multipurpose irrigator, aspirator, and electrosurgical instrument (Endopath Probe Plus II) with 5-mm shaft with spatula (D) and hook electrodes (D1); Endoloop Ligature (E); Endopouch specimen retrieval bag (F); and inflatable large organ retractor (G). (Urohealth Systems, Inc, Advanced Surgical, 3050 Redhill Avenue, Costa Mesa, CA 92626).

tively for biopsy procedures (ENDOLOOP ligature, Ethicon Endo-Surgery, Inc., 4545 Creek Road, Cincinnati, Ohio 45242-2839). The ENDOLOOP ligature is placed through one port and a grasper is placed through a second operating port. The grasper is placed through the loop and the tissue to be ligated is grasped. In vascular ligation procedures, the ligature is tightened and the suture is cut adjacent to the knot, leaving approximately a 1-cm tail. In biopsy procedures after tightening the ligature, the tissue is transected and removed through the access port. The suture is then cut. Specimen retrieval pouches facilitate the extraction of dissected tissues through the MIS port site (see Fig. 7–9).

APPROACHES AND ANATOMIC VARIATIONS

The zoo and wildlife veterinarian embarking on surgical intervention is challenged with a broad range of species in four major classes: amphibians, reptiles, birds, and mammals. The anatomic differences between these species requires a unique approach to each and it is recommended that one investigate all possible sources of anatomic information before embarking on an MIS procedure.

Amphibians

Amphibians are best approached in dorsal recumbency. The coelomic cavity is such that a single port can provide visualization of organs including heart, lungs, liver, gall bladder, gastrointestinal tract, urinary bladder, and reproductive organs. A large ventral abdominal vein courses down the ventral midline and should be avoided. Therefore, a para-midline approach is recommended. The thin skin must be carefully incised so as not to create too large an incision.

Transillumination of the body wall reveals vessels

that should be avoided in secondary port placement. Additional ports may add to leakage of insufflation gases and every effort should be made to minimize incision length. The larger amphibians are of great enough size that manipulation and multiport procedures are easily performed. The smaller species limit the instrumentation size and may necessitate single-port procedures.

Most amphibians are egg layers; however, a few species bear live young. In males, the testes lie ventral to the head of the kidneys and the adrenal and distal to the paired fat bodies. The fat bodies are unique in form and are seen as large finger-like projections within the coelomic cavities of frogs and toads. Many amphibians that inhabit terrestrial environments have a large urinary bladder, whereas those that are solely aquatic lack this organ completely. The oviducts of the female lie lateral and distal to the kidneys, with the egg-laden ovaries lying ventral to the oviducts and kidneys. The oviduct is the major reproductive tract organ in the female. Gravid females may have fully half of the coelomic cavity distended with eggs.

Reptiles

The three most commonly encountered groups of reptiles in zoo and wildlife medicine are in the orders testudinata, squamata, and crocodilia. Like the amphibians, a common coelomic cavity houses all of the internal organs with no true diaphragmatic separation. Similar to amphibians and birds, respiratory inspiration does not depend on a negative pressure environment. This is a great advantage during MIS procedures. In general, reptile skin is substantial, with adaptations of bone, scutes, or simply thickened skin present. A large ventral vein courses along the midline of many reptiles; therefore a para-median incision is recommended for port placement in snakes, lizards, and crocodilians.

SNAKES

Because of the unique anatomic adaptations of snakes, laparoscopic visualization of structures is diminished. It is most difficult to perform MIS on snakes. Ribs may extend from the skull to the cloaca, and the rib cage creates a nondistensible cavity. Adaptations to a long, narrow body form limit the free space within the coelom. Because of these restrictions, it is difficult to extend the telescope from the site of entry for any distance. It is better to use alternative imaging modalities, such as radiography or ultrasonography to determine the target organ location for proper port placement. It may be necessary to make multiple entries at different sites simply to view the entire surface of a single organ, such as the liver.

LIZARDS

The lizard species have adapted to a wide range of environments. In some species, the skin may be so thin that it may be traumatized during gentle handling; in other species, it may be so thick that spines can injure the handler.

The lizard is placed in dorsal recumbency and approached dorsally through a ventral para-median incision to avoid the midline abdominal vein. Tenting of the abdominal skin and an open Hasson approach is safer and easier than a blind introduction of a Veress needle (Fig. 7–10). Insufflation is a helpful addition for internal structure visualization; however, in some species, tenting of the overlying skin can provide a similar expansion of the coelomic space without the use of insufflation.

With the telescope directed caudally, a urinary bladder can be visualized in most species. Prominent lobulated fat bodies may impair visibility. Ventral to the bladder sits paired metanephric kidneys deep within the pelvic canal. By manipulating the bladder and intestinal structures, using instruments introduced via a second port, the operator may visualize, proximal to the kidneys, paired gonads and small paired adrenal glands ventral to these structures. Visualization may be assisted

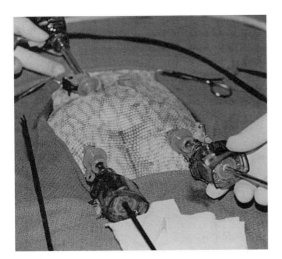

FIGURE 7–10. A Savannah monitor lizard (*Varanus exanthematicus*) in dorsal recumbency with three MIS port placements. The cranial-most cannula *(top)* is the primary telescope site at the initiation of surgery and the port is placed paramedian to avoid the midline vein.

by tilting the animal in a variety of oblique postures. Directing the laparoscope further craniad, the operator may see the liver with the gall bladder on the ventral surface of the right liver lobe when the structure is lifted. Proximal to the liver on the ventral midline sits the heart, and ventral and lateral to the heart are paired lungs.

CHELONIA

The bony carapace and plastron present significant barriers to traditional surgical procedures. In comparison, MIS can be accomplished with relative ease. The most common approach to the coelomic cavity is through the abdominal musculature cranial to the left rear limb with the animal in right lateral recumbency. Using the Hasson technique, incision size must be limited to maintain a seal during insufflation. The urinary bladder may be of significant size and obstruct the field of view. The surgeon may choose to drain the urinary bladder using a laparoscopically guided fine needle suction tip via a second and parallel port. Rotating the animal to dorsal recumbency and moving the urinary bladder to the side, intestinal structures and liver may be visualized. Generally, the right liver lobe is larger than the left. Rotating the animal in a variety of oblique postures facilitates the movement of intestine and liver out of the field. If the liver and intestine are distracted to the down side, lung and heart may be visualized along with the gall bladder on the dorsal side of the liver.

CROCODILIANS

Crocodilians have a body form similar to that of lizards and therefore the approach is much the same, dorsal recumbency with a ventral para-median incision. Incisions should be made between the scales where the skin is more pliable. A Hasson technique followed by insufflation or tenting of the skin is necessary to provide visualization of more distal structures and maneuverability within the coelomic cavity.

Birds

In general, birds are excellent MIS candidates because of their unique respiratory system. The development of air sacs in birds is associated with a complicated subdivision of the body cavity, which appears to promote the efficiency of breathing. Knowledge of the location of the air sacs and their association with the subdivided peritoneal cavities and coelomic viscera are key to successful MIS. Air sac morphology varies among species, but there are great similarities in the more commonly examined members of the Passeriformes, Psittaformes, Columbiformes, Gruiformes, Strigiformes, and Falconformes. There are eight air sacs: one cervical, one clavicular, two cranial thoracic, two caudal thoracic, and two abdominal.[30] In addition, there are five peritoneal cavity partitions: the left and right ventral hepatic peritoneal, the left and right dorsal hepatic peritoneal, and the intestinal peritoneal.[29]

The bird is placed in dorsal left lateral or right lateral recumbency, depending on the organ of interest and its relationship to the adjoining air sacs. With the possible exception of ratites, the avian coelomic cavity does not need to be insufflated to expand the field of view and it is therefore unnecessary to create a tight seal around the laparoscope.

The best approach to the liver of birds is through the ventral midline incision just caudal to the sternum into the paired ventral hepatic peritoneal cavities.[43] A fat pad overlying this ventral hepatic peritoneal cavity may be encountered via this approach. A lateral approach to the liver can be accomplished through the caudal thoracic air sac into the ventral hepatic peritoneal cavity. The incision for the standard lateral approach to the reproductive organs is often extended to examine the liver.

The lung can be approached via the third intercostal space just ventral to the scapula.[43] Intercostal muscles must be bluntly dissected and great care must be taken not to traumatize lung tissues when using this approach. Within the intestinal peritoneal cavity are the proventriculus, intestines, gonads, and supporting structures.

A lateral approach to the caudal thoracic air sac allows visualization of many coelomic cavity structures, including the gonads. With the bird in right lateral recumbency, the wings are extended dorsally and the upper leg is extended and held caudally.[4] The trocar placement is located by palpating the triangle cranial to the musculature of the femur, ventral to the synsacrum, and caudal to the last rib. The site for trocar insertion may also vary depending on species differences. An approach between the seventh and eighth ribs or possibly more cranial is appropriate in some species. From the caudal thoracic air sac viewing craniodorsally, the pericardial sac, heart, lobe of the liver, and caudal lung regions may all be seen. Redirecting the laparoscope to the abdominal air sac and dissecting through it, it may be possible to visualize the proventriculus, edge of the liver, kidney, adrenal gland, spleen, and intestine in addition to the left gonad.[43]

Mammals

Because of the many variations in the 20 orders of mammalia, it is advisable to research anatomic information on the specific nondomestic mammal being considered for MIS before the procedure. In thoracic or abdominal procedures of small to large mammals, excluding many hoofstock and megavertebrates, it is usually advisable to place the animal in dorsal recumbency. If the anatomy is unfamiliar or altered because of body condition or disease, the Hasson technique is preferred to avoid injury to internal organs.

Examination of the otic canals, the oropharyngeal cavity, the larynx, glottis, trachea, and esophagus, and the nasal passages can all be accomplished via MIS depending on the animal's size.

Most nondomestic mammalian MIS procedures closely follow the techniques used in related domestic animals or humans. For example, one would use techniques similar to those used in humans to perform MIS in gorillas or baboons. As well, those techniques used in the domestic dog or cat can be applied when performing an MIS procedure in the tiger.

In general, mammalian species have a complete diaphragm and maintain negative pressure in their pleural space. The exception is in the elephant, in which the lung parenchyma is adhered to the chest wall by fibrous connective tissue and thus there is no negative intrapleural pressure. This adaptation facilitates expansion of the elephant's immense lungs. In all but the elephant, thoracoscopy must follow the same surgical principles applied to surgery of domestic animals. Care must be taken to reestablish negative pressure in the pleural space at the completion of MIS of the thorax.

The megavertebrates in general pose the greatest challenge to the successful performance of MIS. Elephants, rhinoceroses, hippopotamuses, and giraffes are of large enough size as to preclude most MIS procedures. The development of custom made equipment may overcome some of these barriers to success.

PROCEDURES

Many different procedures may be performed using MIS as familiarity with the technique is achieved. The primary port is placed following insufflation via a Veress needle, if appropriate. When distention is not indicated or when anatomic variations necessitate, the Hasson technique is used. In appropriate species, the cavity is then distended. The telescope is inserted and secondary ports are placed in relatively avascular areas of the body wall. When possible, the body wall is transilluminated to reveal vessels traversing the area. To transilluminate the abdominal or coelomic wall, the room lights are dimmed and the lens of the telescope is projected against the body wall. If the wall thickness allows, vessels traversing the abdominal wall are revealed. These vessels are avoided when selecting the site for trocar insertion.

Liver and renal biopsies, as well as biopsies of abdominal or coelomic masses, are performed via an operating port and a second instrument port. A single cannula with an operating port may ease the retrieval of the biopsy specimen in limited spaces. An endoscopic biopsy instrument with unipolar electrocautery is best employed. MIS has been used to perform renal biopsies in tigers (*Panthera* species), cheetahs (*Acinonyx jubatus*),[6] and giant panda (*Ailuropoda melanoleuca*)[5] and liver biopsies in cheetahs.[6]

Extracorporealization has been used extensively, especially in situations in which intracorporeal techniques would significantly increase the length of surgery or in situations that are beyond the expertise of the surgeon. This technique has been used primarily to exteriorize segments of the intestinal tract for visual examination, biopsy, or resection. Exteriorizing segments of the intestinal tract through one small abdominal or coelomic incision site enables the surgeon to rapidly examine the viscera and provide surgical intervention with minimal tissue trauma. To perform this procedure, the diseased segment of bowel is grasped with a pair of atraumatic forceps through a secondary port. The cannula and stability threads (if used) are removed and the intestinal segment is guided through the opening in the abdominal wall. Additional segments of bowel can be withdrawn sequentially through the same incision site. Care is taken to continually return small segments of bowel to the abdominal cavity. If too great an amount of bowel is exteriorized it can be difficult to replace. If intestinal resection and anastomosis are required, intracorporal ligation of the intestinal vasculature is performed before exteriorizing the segment to reduce the need to lengthen the original incision.

MIS can be used to evaluate body orifices such as the buccal and pharyngeal cavities, the trachea (Fig. 7–11), and the auditory canals. The use of laparoscopy has been effective for sex determination of monomorphic birds,[15, 25, 35] including birds of prey.[8] This technique has also been used to examine ovaries of a woodchuck (*Marmota monax*),[47] water buffalo (*Bubalus bubalis*),[22, 23] llamas (*Lama glama*) and alpacas (*Lama pacos*),[41] red deer (*Cervus elaphus*),[1] cheetahs,[6, 46] cyclic jaguar (*Panthera onca*),[6] Bengal tigers (*Panthera tigris*),[6] and fallow deer (*Damma dama*).[46] Oocyte aspiration in the puma (*Felis concolor*)[33] and gorilla (*Gorilla gorilla gorilla*)[31] and embryo collection and transfer in suni (*Neotragus moschatus zuluensis*)[37] have been performed laparoscopically. Intrauterine insemination of Eld's deer (*Cervus eldi thamin*),[34] puma (*Felis concolor coryi*),[2, 17] cheetah,[17, 20] clouded leopard (*Neofelis nebulosa*),[17, 19] ocelot (*Felis pardalis*),[42] and domestic cats[18] has been performed using this technique. Laparoscopy has been used to assist in the diagnosis of endometriosis in rhesus monkeys (*Macaca mulatta*)[38] and in reproductive organ evaluation of gorillas,[45] gelada baboons (*Theropithecus gelada*) (Fig. 7–12), and silvered leaf monkeys (*Presbytis crestatus ultimus*). In addition, it has been used to study spontaneous endometriosis in baboons (*Theropithecus species*).[9]

Intra-abdominal vasectomies in Canada geese (*Branta canadensis*),[36] llamas and alpacas,[3] crab-eating foxes (*Cerdocyon thous*),[6] African lions (*Panthera leo*),[6] Siberian and Bengal tigers,[7] and Rocky Mountain goats (*Oreamno americanus*)[39] have been performed laparo-

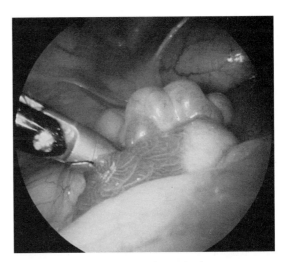

FIGURE 7–12. An MIS assisted reproductive tract evaluation in a gelada baboon (*Theropithecus gelada*). The fimbria in the foreground is gently moved away from the ovaries with a 5-mm closed Kelly clamp to observe dye introduced through a transcervical intrauterine catheter.

scopically. This surgical approach has been used to perform uterine tubal ligations of African lions[40] and Rocky Mountain goats.[5]

Acknowledgment

The authors would like to thank Ms. Diane Gauzman and Dr. Ron Kolata for technical and surgical assistance, Mr. Irwin Baker, Andrew Fleischaker, John Sciabelli, and William Athas for technical support, and Drs. Paul Calle, Bonnie Raphael, and Mark Stetter for their surgical contributions.

REFERENCES

1. Asher GW, Fisher MW, Jabbour HN, et al: Relationship between the onset of oestrus, the preovulatory surge in luteinizing hormone and ovulation following oestrous synchronization of farmed red deer (*Cervus elaphus*). J Reprod Fertil 96:261–273, 1992.
2. Barone MS, Wildt DE, Byers AP, et al: Gonadotrophin dose and timing of anaesthesia for laparoscopic artificial insemination in the puma (*Felis concolor*). J Reprod Fertil 101:103–108, 1994.
3. Bravo PW, Sumar J: Evaluation of intra-abdominal vasectomy in llamas and alpacas. J Am Vet Med Assoc 199(9):1164–1166, 1991.
4. Bush M: Laparoscopy in birds and reptiles. *In* Harrison R, Wildt DE (eds): Animal Laparoscopy. Baltimore, Williams & Wilkins, pp 183–197, 1980.
5. Bush M, Montali RJ, Phillips LG, et al: Anemia and renal failure in a giant panda. J Am Vet Med Assoc 185(11):1435–1437, 1984.
6. Bush M, Seager SWJ, Wildt DE: Laparoscopy in zoo mammals. *In* Harrison R, Wildt DE (eds): Animal Laparoscopy. Baltimore, Williams & Wilkins, pp 169–182, 1990.
7. Bush M, Wildt DE, Kennedy S, et al: Laparoscopy in zoological medicine. J Am Vet Med Assoc 173:1081–1087, 1978.
8. Cooper JE: Metomidate anaesthesia of some birds of prey for laparotomy and sexing. Vet Rec 94:437–440, 1974.
9. Cornillie FJ, D'Hooghe TM, Bambra CS, et al: Morphological characteristics of spontaneous endometriosis in the baboon (*Papio anubis* and *Papio cynocephalus*). Gynecol Obstet Invest 34:225–228, 1992.
10. Cuschieri A, Buess G: Introduction and historical aspects. *In* Cuschieri A, Buess G, Perissat J (eds): Operative Manual of Endoscopic Surgery. New York, Springer-Verlag, pp 1–5, 1992.

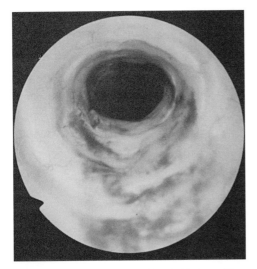

FIGURE 7–11. A view of a fungal tracheitis in a white-winged wood duck (*Carina scutulata*) through a 2.7-mm telescope.

11. Filipi DJ, Fitzgibbons RJ, Salerno GM: Historical review: Diagnostic laparoscopy to laparoscopic cholecystectomy and beyond. *In* Zucker KA (ed): Laparoscopy. St. Louis, Quality Medical Publishing, pp 3–21, 1991.

12. Fourestier M, Gladu A, Vulmiere J: Perfectionnements a l'endoscopie medicale. Realisation bronchoscopique. La Presse Medicale 61:1292–1294, 1952.

13. Gaskin TA, Isobe JH, Mathews JL, et al: Laparoscopy and the general surgeon. Surg Clin North Am 71(5):1085–1097, 1991.

14. Goetze O: Die rontgendiagnostik bei gasgefullter bauchhohle; eine neue methode. Münch Med Wochenschr 65:1275–1280, 1918.

15. Greenwood AG: Avian sex determination by laparoscopy. Vet Rec 112:105, 1973.

16. Harrison RM: Laparoscopy in monkeys and apes. *In* Harrison R, Wildt DE (eds): Animal Laparoscopy. Baltimore, Williams & Wilkins, pp 73–93, 1980.

17. Howard JG, Barone MA, Byers AP, et al: Ovulation induction sensitivity and laparoscopic intrauterine insemination in the cheetah, puma and clouded leopard. Proc Am Soc Androl J Andro 14(Suppl):55(abstract 129), 1993.

18. Howard JG, Barone MA, Donoghue AM, et al: The effect of preovulatory anaesthesia on ovulation in laparoscopically inseminated domestic cats. J Reprod Fertil 96:175–186, 1992.

19. Howard JG, Byers AP, Brown JL, et al: Successful ovulation induction and laparoscopic intrauterine artificial insemination in the clouded leopard (*Neofelis nebulosa*). Zoo Biol 15(1):55–69, 1996.

20. Howard JG, Donoghue AM, Barone MA, et al: Successful induction of ovarian activity and laparoscopic intrauterine artificial insemination in the cheetah (*Acinonyx jubatus*). J Zoo Wildlife Med 23:288–300, 1992.

21. Jacobaeus HC: Uber die moglichkeit die zystoskopie bei untersuchung seroser hohlungen anzuwenden. Münch Med Wochenschr 40:2090–2092, 1910.

22. Jainudeen MR, Bongso TA, Ahmad FB: A laparoscopic technique for in vivo observation of ovaries in the water buffalo (*Bubalus bubalis*). Vet Rec 111:32–35, 1982.

23. Jainudeen MR, Sharifuddin W, Ahmand FB: Relationships of ovarian contents to plasma progesterone concentration in the swamp buffalo (*Bubalus bubalis*). Vet Rec 113:369–372, 1983.

24. Jones BD: Laparoscopy. Vet Clin North Am Small Anim Pract 20(5):1243–1263, 1990.

25. Jones DM, Samour JH, Knight JS: Sex determination of monomorphic birds by fiberoptic endoscopy. Vet Rec 115:596–598, 1984.

26. Kalk H: Erfahrungen mit der laparoskopie (zugleich mit beschreibung eines neuen instrumentes. Zeitschr Klin Med 111:303–348, 1929.

27. Kelling G: Die tamponade der bauchhohle mit luft zur stillung lebensgefahrlicher intestinalblutungen. Münch Med Wochenschr 48:1535–1538, 1901.

28. Kelling G: Uber oesophagoskopie, gastroskopie und kolioskopie. Münch Med Wochenschr 49:21–24, 1902.

29. King AS, McLelland J: Coelomic cavities. *In* King AS, McLelland J (eds): Birds: Their Structure and Function. Philadelphia, Balliére Tindall, pp 79–83, 1984.

30. King AS, McLelland J: Respiratory system. *In* King AS, McLelland J (eds): Birds: Their Structure and Function. Philadelphia, Balliére Tindall, pp 110–144, 1984.

31. Loskutoff NM, Huntress SL, Putman JM, et al: Stimulation of ovarian activity for oocyte recovery in nonreproductive gorillas (*Gorilla*). J Zoo Wildlife Med 22(1):32–41, 1991.

32. Melzer A, Buess G, Cuschieri A: Instruments for endoscopic surgery. *In* Cuschieri A, Buess G, Perissat J (eds): Operative Manual of Endoscopic Surgery. New York, Springer-Verlag, pp 14–36, 1992.

33. Miller AM, Roelke ME, Goodrowe KL, et al: Oocyte recovery, maturation, and fertilization *in vitro* in the puma (*Felis concolor*). J Reprod Fertil 88:249–258, 1990.

34. Monfort SL, Asher GW, Wildt DE, et al: Successful intrauterine insemination of Eld's deer (*Cervus eldi thamin*) with frozen-thawed spermatozoa. J Reprod Fertil 99:459–465, 1993.

35. Prus SE, Schmutz SM: Comparative efficiency and accuracy of surgical and cytogenetic sexing in psittacines. Avian Dis 31(2):421–424, 1987.

36. Raphael BL, Calle PP, Karesh WB, et al: Contraception program at the New York Zoological Society institutions. Proceedings of the Annual Meeting of the American Association of Zoo Veterinarians, Oakland, CA, pp 102–103, 1992.

37. Raphael BL, Loskutoff NM, Howard JG, et al: Embryo transfer and artificial insemination in suni (*Neotragus moschatus zuluensis*). Theriogenology 31(1):244, 1989.

38. Rier SE, Martin RE, Bowman WP, et al: Endometriosis in rhesus monkeys (*Macaca mulatta*) following chronic exposure to 2,3,7,8-tetrachlorodibenzo-p-dioxin. Fundam Appl Toxicol 21:433–441, 1993.

39. Seager SWJ, Foster JW, Marts BS, et al: Semen collection, evaluation, and laparoscopic sterilization of the male and female Rocky Mountain goat (*Oreamnos americanus*). Proceedings of the Annual Meeting of the American Association of Zoo Veterinarians, Louisville, KY, p 183, 1984.

40. Seager SWJ, Foster JW, Marts BS, et al: Laparoscopic sterilization in the female mountain goat. Proceedings of the Annual Meeting of the American Association of Zoo Veterinarians, Louisville, KY, p 184, 1984.

41. Steptoe PC: Laparoscopy in Gynaecology. Edinburgh, Livingstone, p 12, 1967.

42. Swanson WF, Howard JG, Roth TL, et al: Responsiveness of ovaries to exogenous gonadotrophins and laparoscopic artificial insemination with frozen-thawed spermatozoa in ocelots (*Felis pardalis*). J Reprod Fertil 106:87–94, 1996.

43. Taylor M: Endoscopic examination and biopsy techniques. *In* Ritchie BW, Harrison GJ, Harrison LR (eds): Avian Medicine: Principles and Application. Lake Worth, FL, Wingers Publishing, pp 327–354, 1994.

44. Veress J: Neues instrument zur ausfuhrung von brust-oder bauchpunktionen und pneumothoraxbehandlung. Dtsch Med Wochenschr 41:1480–1481, 1938.

45. Wildt DE, Cambre RC, Howard JG, et al: Laparoscopic evaluation of the reproductive organs and abdominal cavity content of the lowland gorilla. Am J Primatol 2:29–42, 1982.

46. Wildt DE, Platz CC, Seager SWG et al: Induction of ovarian activity in the cheetah (*Acinonyx jubatus*). Biol Reprod 24:217–222, 1981.

47. Woolf A, Curl JL: A technique for laparoscopic examination of woodchuck ovaries. J Am Assoc Lab Anim Sci 37(5):664–665, 1987.

CHAPTER 8

Use of Ultrasonography in Zoo Animals

THOMAS B. HILDEBRANDT

FRANK GÖRITZ

The first medical application of ultrasonographic techniques was developed for soft tissue characterization in humans in the 1950s.[4] Subsequently, there has been a dramatic development of ultrasonographic techniques and they have been used in a wide range of applications, including ophthalmology, cardiology, neurology, nephrology, gynecology and andrology, obstetrics, organ transplantation, oncology, orthopedics, and dermatology. The incorporation of sonographic techniques into veterinary medicine began almost 20 years later. "Veterinary ultrasound has grown from an exotic imaging modality in the late 1970s to an essential service at university hospitals and many veterinary practices."[29]

Despite the significant advances made in ultrasonographic applications in human and veterinary medicine, the use of this technology has been limited in zoological and wildlife medicine. O'Grady and colleagues[30] first recommended the use of ultrasonography in zoo animals as a diagnostic tool. Subsequently, several ultrasonographic descriptions of various species were published, but the development of sonographic techniques for use in exotic animals has been sporadic.[1, 5, 27, 37, 39] However, the number of publications involving the use of ultrasonographic techniques in zoo and wild animals has steadily increased since the early 1990s. These studies have focused primarily on mammalian species (69%), secondarily on reptiles (19%), and thirdly on avian species (12%). Fish and amphibian species have been the least represented (<1%) and no publications exist on ultrasonographic imaging in invertebrates.[6]

The advantages of ultrasonography in comparison to other imaging techniques, such as radiography, magnetic resonancy, or endoscopy, are that it

1. Is noninvasive and thereby repeatable
2. Provides real-time visual, reproducible imaging
3. Provides high-resolution characterization of soft tissues
4. Produces sectional images of tissues and organ structures
5. Allows examination of motion and direction (e.g., heartbeat, vascular flow, fetal movement)
6. Allows morphometric measurements of structures in situ (e.g., organs, implants, foreign bodies)
7. Facilitates documentation and preservation of primary data on storable media

8. Is portable and thus compatible with zoo and field studies

However, the application of ultrasonography to zoo and wild animals presents a number of specific difficulties that are not usually problematic in human or classic veterinary medicine.

First, physical or chemical restraint is necessary for performing ultrasonography in most exotic animals. For example, birds of prey must be held by the wings and legs in dorsal recumbency; carnivores must be sedated or anesthetized. However, elephants[13, 30] and rhinoceroses[33] are trainable for transrectal ultrasonography without any pharmacologic or mechanical restraint.

Moreover, certain morphologic features of exotic animals may interfere with ultrasonographic examinations. Acoustic coupling of the ultrasound probe is problematic when the body surface is covered by shells, plates, feathers, or fur. Avian air sacs, thick leathery skin, large subcutaneous fat pads, air-filled intestinal loops, and large body size all decrease the effectiveness of ultrasonographic imaging. In addition, there are relatively few reference data on the sonomorphologic appearance of organs in many taxa, for instance, of kidneys and gonads in fish, amphibians, and birds or of ovaries in elephants. Each investigator may have sonographic experience in only a limited variety of animals. Hence, it is important for the verification of the ultrasound results to perform postmortem ultrasonographic investigations in intact carcasses and isolated organs of interest. Basic information about the internal topography of exotic animals may be available from anatomic descriptions or other high-resolution imaging techniques such as magnetic resonance tomography.[34, 38] Lastly, ultrasound equipment customized for exotic animals requires many additional components in contrast to that used for domestic animals, such as a wide variety of transcutaneous and intraoperative transducers (3.5 to 10.0 MHz), cable extensions for ultrasound probes, animal-specific scan head adapters for transrectal ultrasonography, and battery packs for field investigations. The acquisition of such accessory components needed to establish the capability for ultrasonography in a variety of taxa may cost from $55,000 and more for a zoo veterinarian, a price that may be prohibitive for many zoos. However, with further development of the technology, more affordable units may become available.

Ultrasonography has many important research and diagnostic applications in zoo and wildlife medicine, including in reproduction, oncology, morphology, cardiology, and ophthalmology. In most publications for which this imaging technique has been applied to zoo and wild animals, it has been described in connection with reproduction (Fig. 8–1). This chapter, too, concentrates primarily on applications of noninvasive ultrasonography in reproductive biology.

Reproduction in zoo animals is often less successful than in natural populations, preventing the establishment of self-sustaining captive populations. Infertility caused by reproductive disorders and mismanagement may have a devastating effect on captive breeding programs, especially for endangered species. There is a dearth of knowledge regarding the reproductive anatomy and physiology of many exotic species. The development of techniques for determining sex, defining sexual maturity, evaluating the reproductive tract including gonads, characterizing the reproductive cycle, and monitoring gestation and fetal growth are critical to the success of natural and assisted breeding programs. The recent advancement of endocrinologic assessment techniques has allowed for the generation of basic data regarding reproductive status in many exotic animals. Noninvasive endocrine monitoring, through urine and fecal assays, has gained particular significance in zoo and wild animal management. Gamete collection and analysis has also provided insights into reproductive processes of exotic animals, and has served as the basis for several programs of assisted reproduction.

The potential for the use of ultrasonography as an adjunct approach for noninvasive assessment of zoo and wild animal reproduction has not been fully realized. Ultrasonography is a powerful tool that can reveal detailed information that is not accessible through classical research methods of experimental reproductive biology and endocrinology. It may be used to visualize the structures of the reproductive tract as well as the changes in those structures over time or resulting from pathologic alterations. This chapter discusses ultrasound techniques that have been incorporated into studies of zoo and wild animal reproduction.

SEX DETERMINATION IN MONOMORPHIC SPECIES

Many species show little or no phenotypic or behavioral variation between the sexes, making breeding decisions difficult for animal managers. This problem is especially evident among avian species and has led to the development of several techniques for sex determination in birds. The most common techniques are laparoscopy, which is invasive and requires anesthesia, and genetic evaluation, which requires blood sampling and is species-specific. Ultrasonography, in contrast, provides a noninvasive, accurate technique that can be used to detect gonadal or genital structures in birds.[17] Difficulties encountered during transcutaneous ultrasonography of birds in transmitting through air sacs have been overcome by the development of both transintestinal and transcloacal methods, which use high-resolution, miniaturized probes. The use of either the transintestinal or transcloacal technique depends on the size of the intestine in the species concerned. Transintestinal ultrasonography allows visualization of the gonads and the entire genital tract, whereas the transcloacal technique provides an image of the caudal portions of the genital tract only.[14, 24] The smallest birds that have been examined successfully with a newly developed ultrasound system are common quail (*Coutornix coutornix*). Examples of ultrasonography in various avian species are shown in Fig. 8–2.

Sonographic sex determination is also a valuable tool for several monomorphic fish, amphibian, and reptilian species (Fig. 8–3). Transcutaneous ultrasonography is very effective in most of these species, except for reptiles with very dense scales, such as Komodo dragons. Transintestinal ultrasonography, however, is effective in determining the sex of these animals.[18] Although not as common as in other taxa, variations of monomorphism also occur in some mammals (e.g., beaver, sloths, and spotted hyena).[11, 15] Transrectal ultrasonography has been used successfully to determine sex in some of these species (Fig. 8–4). There have been no published reports on the use of ultrasonography for

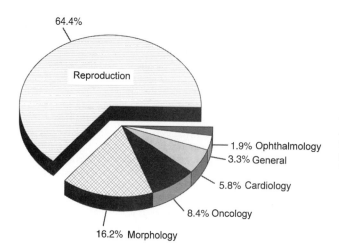

64.4%

Reproduction

1.9% Ophthalmology
3.3% General
5.8% Cardiology
8.4% Oncology
16.2% Morphology

n = 147

FIGURE 8–1. Diagram represents the prevalence of reproduction in applications of imaging ultrasonography in zoo and wild animal medicine, in comparison with all other medical fields.

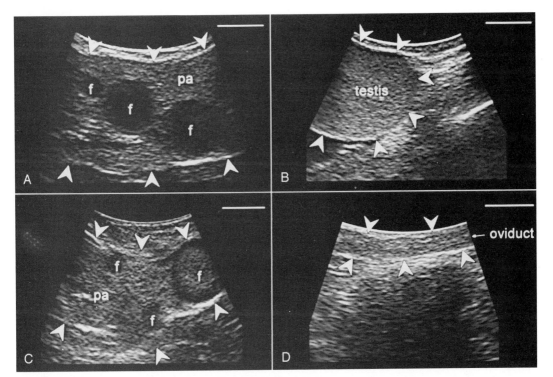

FIGURE 8–2. Sonographic sex determination in birds by imaging the female *(A, C, D)* or male *(B)* internal genital organs with transintestinal *(A–C)* or transcloacal *(D)* sonography. Gonads *(white arrowheads)* of adult female *(A)* and male *(B)* helmet cassowaries *(Casuarius casuarius)*. Also shown are the left ovary *(white arrowheads)* of an adult African marabou *(Leptoptilus crumeniferus) (C)* and the caudal part of the left oviduct *(white arrowheads)* of an adult black-footed penguin *(Spheniscus demersus) (D)*. f, follicle; pa, parenchyma. Scale bar represents 10 mm.

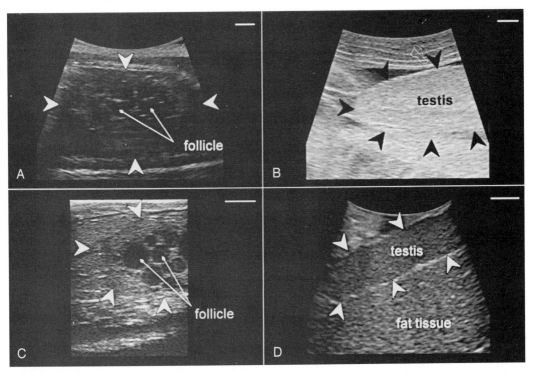

FIGURE 8–3. Sonomorphologic appearance of the gonads in different fish, amphibian, and reptilian species visualized by transcutaneous *(A–C)* or transintestinal *(D)* sonography: active ovary *(A, white arrowheads)* of an adult female arowana *(Osteoglossum bicirrhosum)*; active testis *(B, black arrowheads)* of an adult male Chinese giant salamander *(Andrias davidianus)*; active ovary *(C, white arrowheads)* of an adult female gila monster *(Heloderma suspectum)*; inactive testis *(D, white arrowheads)* of a subadult male Komodo dragon *(Varanus komodoensis)* attached to the corpus adiposum. Scale bar represents 10 mm.

43

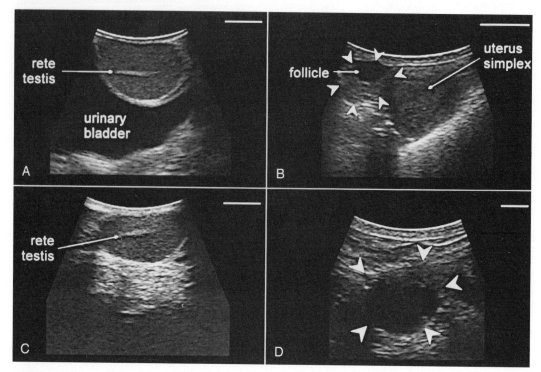

FIGURE 8–4. Sonomorphologic appearance of an intra-abdominal testis *(A)* and female genital tract *(B)* in adult two-toed sloth (*Choloepus didactylus*) visualized by transrectal ultrasonography. The ovary *(white arrowheads)* with a large follicle is located craniolateral to the uterus simplex. In spotted hyena (*Crocuta crocuta*), visualization of the testes *(C)* is possible by transcutaneous ultrasonography in the perineal region. Ovaries can be detected in hyenas by transrectal ultrasonography. The ovary *(D, white arrowheads)* is situated on a large fat pad near the kidney. Scale bar represents 10 mm.

determining the sex of marine invertebrates, but it is possible that this technique will be used in the future.

DETERMINATION OF REPRODUCTIVE STATUS AND CYCLICITY

There are limited data available on sexual maturation and reproductive cyclicity from most species in natural populations. Additionally, zoo animals often show irregular patterns of reproductive activity compared to their wild counterparts. Ultrasonography may be used for distinguishing adult from juvenile animals, both male and female, in species in which sexual maturation is not obvious. For example, the sonographic visualization of the bursa of Fabricius in birds (Fig. 8–5)[14, 17] or the mucus-filled vagina in combination with inactive ovaries in elephants (Fig. 8–6) is indicative of juvenile status. In contrast, ultrasonography may also detect reproductive inactivity in adult and senile animals.[9] The length of the female reproductive cycle can be determined by repeated sonographic examinations over time (Fig. 8–7). Endocrine analyses, particularly noninvasive urine and fecal assays, can provide valuable complementary support for ultrasonographic findings and vice versa.[9] The influence of hormones released during different phases of the cycle on genital tract structure can be examined sonographically to provide insights into proximate mechanisms of reproductive processes. For example, recent findings show that, in the Proboscidea, a nonovulatory peak of luteinizing hormone[26] is correlated with the initiation of follicular growth and a breakdown of the vaginal mucus. Ultrasonography may also detect seasonal changes in size and structure of the testes and accessory glands.

HEALTH ASSESSMENT OF POTENTIAL BREEDERS

Generally, exotic animals show signs of diseases or disorders late in their progression. Sonographic examination of the major thoracic and abdominal organs, such as heart, lung, liver, spleen, kidney, adrenal, and pancreas, may provide useful criteria to appraise the fitness or breeding potential of an animal.[36] Detection of subclinical changes in these organs indicates that a clinically apparent metabolic disorder may occur under the physiologic burden of breeding activity and pregnancy, which could have possible lethal consequences for mother or fetus. Ultrasonography may be used to detect certain pathologic changes in the organs listed in Table 8–1.

Excessive intra-abdominal accumulation of fluid has been detected in a variety of animals by sonographic investigation (Fig. 8–8), which proved to be secondary to subclinical cardiac, hepatic, or renal irregularity as

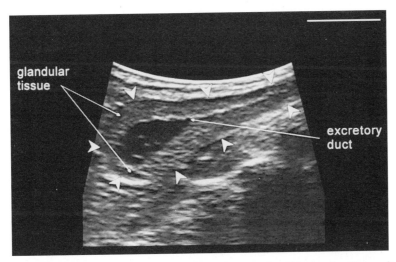

FIGURE 8–5. The well-developed pear-shaped bursa of Fabricius *(white arrowheads)* in a gentoo *(Pygoscelis papua)* is a clear indicator of the juvenile status of this animal. This immunologic organ is situated above the dorsal wall of the cloaca and is detectable by transcloacal sonography. Scale bar represents 10 mm.

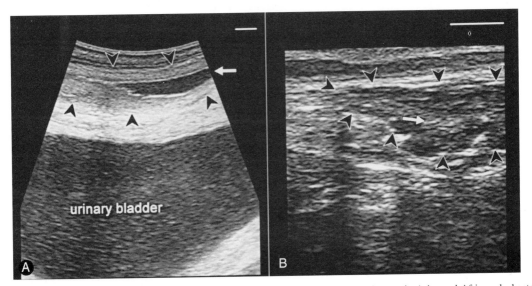

FIGURE 8–6. Transrectal ultrasonography is a practical tool for evaluation of the sexual status in Asian and African elephants *(Elephas maximus, Loxodonta africana)*. The mucus-filled, unfolded vagina *(A, black arrowheads)* associated with inactive ovaries indicates juvenile status in elephants. The prepubertal mucus *(white arrow)* is heavier in comparison to mucus during sexual activity and is characterized by its anechoic appearance. The inactive ovary *(B, white bordered arrowheads)* shows an echoic center (medulla ovarii, *white arrow*) and a hypoechoic periphery (cortex ovarii) with an obvious absence of functional structures (follicles, corpora lutea). Scale bar represents 10 mm.

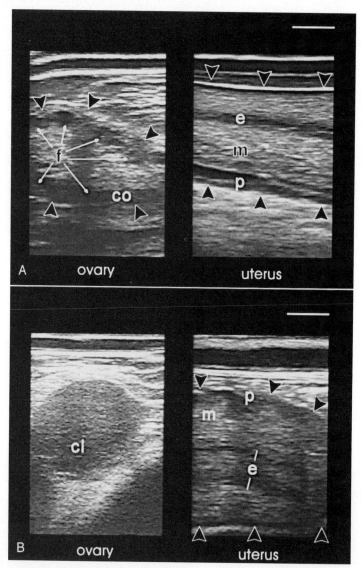

FIGURE 8–7. Sonograms of ovary *(left)* and uterine horn *(right)* of an Asian elephant *(Elephas maximus)* during follicular phase *(A)* and luteal phase *(B)*. The follicular phase is characterized by several growing follicles *(f)* in the cortex ovarii *(co)* and a hypoechoic endometrium *(e)*. During the luteal phase, a large active corpus luteum *(cl)* is obvious on the ovary. The endometrium *(e)* appears enlarged and more echogenic than during the follicular phase. m, myometrium; p, parametrium. *Arrowheads* indicate the organ borders of the ovary or uterus; scale bar represents 10 mm.

TABLE 8–1. Pathologic Changes in the Major Thoracic and Abdominal Organs in Vertebrates

Organ	Pathologic Changes	Ultrasound Application				
		Fish	Amphibians	Reptiles	Birds	Mammals
Heart	Arrhythmia†, enlargement, tumor, pericardial effusion‡, calcified pericardium	tc	tc	tc, te*	tc	tc, te*
Lung	Hydrothorax, fluid lung, superficial abscess or tumor	tc*	tc	tc, te*	tc	tc, te*
Liver	Enlargement, congestion, rupture, cystosis, necrosis, cirrhosis, abscess, calcification, tumor, stasis of the gallbladder and common bile duct, structures in the gallbladder (e.g., parasites, concretion, stones)	tc	tc	tc, ti*	tc, ti*	tc, ti*
Spleen	Enlargement, congestion, rupture, necrosis, calcification, tumor	tc	tc	tc	ti, tc*	tc
Kidney	Congestion, enlargement, atrophy, cystosis, necrosis, gout formation, calcification, rupture, tumor	tc	tc	tc, ti*	ti*	tc, tr*
Adrenal gland	Enlargement, tumor (see Fig. 8–9)	—	tc*	tc*	ti*	tc, ti*
Pancreas	Necrosis, tumor	—	tc*	tc*	ti*	tc, ti*

tc, transcutaneous ultrasonography; te, transesophageal ultrasonography; tr, transrectal ultrasonography; ti, transintestinal ultrasonography.
*Restricted to few species.
†Functional heart diseases are difficult to diagnose in exotic animals because of the lack of reference data.
‡Physiologic appearance in a variety of amphibians and turtles.

well as malignant tumors (Fig. 8–9) in the abdominal cavity. However, in amphibians, turtles, and, interestingly, white rhinoceroses (wild and captive), there is a large amount of physiologic body fluid. Findings regarding the general health of the animal and those specific to the genital tract should be considered when deciding which animals to breed.

PREGNANCY DETECTION AND MONITORING

Pregnancy diagnosis by ultrasonography is described in a large number of wild and zoo animals (viviparous reptiles and mammals, including elephant[10, 20] and rhinoceros[1, 19, 33]) with a single ultrasound examination[5, 7, 16, 30] (Figs. 8–10, 8–11). For a long time, biologists, zoo keepers, and veterinarians have relied on observations of sexual behavior, mating, and birth to determine the average gestation length for different animal species. With these methods, the day of delivery may be estimated. Management and feeding of the gravid animal can be adjusted accordingly. The introduction of imaging ultrasonography to veterinary medicine allows monitoring of the early stages of gestation and fetal development. Measurement of fetal structures and comparison of these findings with reference data[41] allow the stage of gestation to be estimated and the approximate

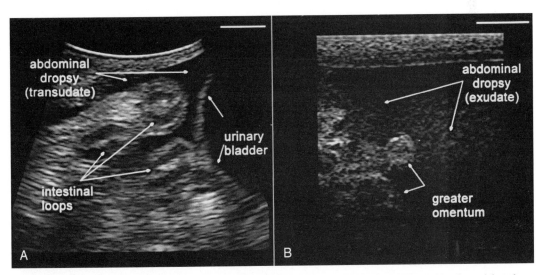

FIGURE 8–8. Abdominal dropsy in an adult female cheetah (*Acinonyx jubatus*) with a renal failure (*A*) and an adult male Asian wild dog (*Cuon alpinus lepturus*) with a hepatoma (*B*). Accumulation of transudate (*a*) caused by passive congestion appears unechoic (*black areas*). Abdominal exudate (*B*) caused by malignant tumors and inflammatory processes appears more cloudy and echoic. The best scan head position for visualizing ascites is near the cranial wall of the urinary bladder. Scale bar represents 10 mm.

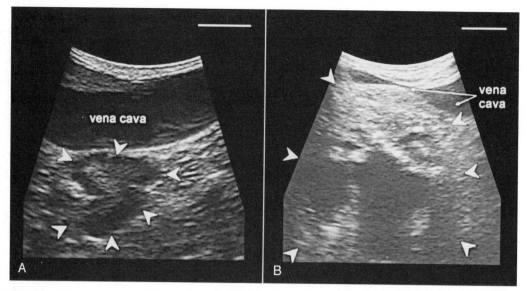

FIGURE 8–9. Normal adrenal gland *(A, white arrowheads)* in a puma *(Puma concolor)* in contrast to an adrenal adenosarcoma *(B, white arrowheads)* in a clouded leopard *(Neofelis nebulosa)* on transrectal ultrasonography. The tumor is characterized by enlargement, irregular surface, and blood-filled cavities *(dark areas)*. The adrenal glands, important endocrinologic organs, are difficult to visualize in most exotic species by transcutaneous ultrasonography. Transintestinal or transrectal ultrasonography (see Table 8–1) improves the detection of these glands cranial to the kidneys near the vena cava caudalis in a large number of species. Scale bar represents 10 mm.

date of delivery to be predicted. Indirect methods of pregnancy determination, such as measurement of progesterone and estrogen metabolites in feces or urine, can be highly informative but are often species-specific because of differences in hormone metabolism and physiology.

Another use for ultrasonography in pregnant animals is fetal sex determination.[3] A definite fetal age, a definite position of fetus, and sufficient amniotic fluid are necessary to determine sex in the fetal animal. Therefore, there are only a few opportunities to perform fetal sex determination successfully (Fig. 8–12). With this method, number, vitality, and developmental stage of the embryo may also be assessed. Transcloacal and transintestinal ultrasonography may be used to image the yolk and ovary in birds or oviparous reptiles. Based on the extent of calcification, a laying term prediction is possible. Because ultrasonography is a noninvasive,

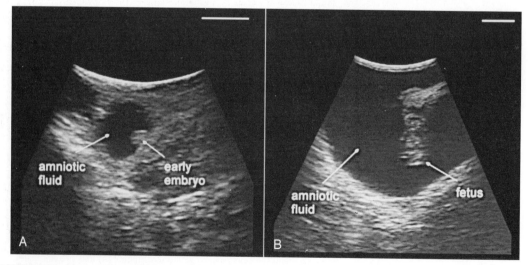

FIGURE 8–10. Sonographic pregnancy detection in European roe deer *(Capreolus capreolus)* by transrectal ultrasonography. Few days after delayed implantation *(A)*, the pregnancy is characterized by rapid accumulation of embryonic fluid and an early embryo. Two weeks later *(B)*, the amount of amniotic fluid is increased and the fetus has a body length of 20 plus or minus 5 mm. Scale bar represents 10 mm.

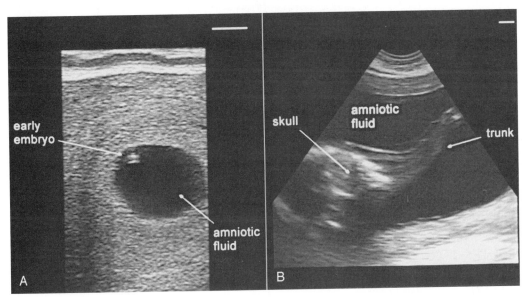

FIGURE 8–11. Imaging of two different stages of pregnancy in an Asian elephant (*Elephas maximus*) with transrectal ultrasonography. *A,* Early pregnancy (3.5 months) is characterized by a round embryonic vesicle containing a small embryo (2 mm). *(B)* In the 28th week of pregnancy, the fetus is well differentiated and has a crown-rump length of 170 plus or minus 10 mm. Scale bar represents 10 mm.

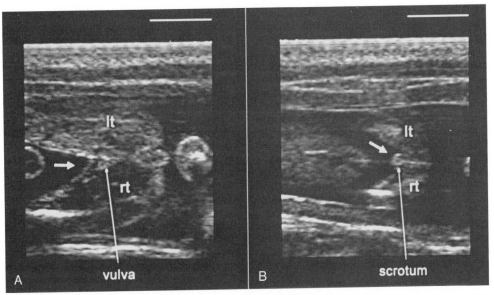

FIGURE 8–12. Prenatal sex determination of approximately 3-month-old female *(A)* and male *(B)* cynomolgus fetus (*Macaca fascicularis*) with transcutaneous ultrasonography. The detection of the vulva *(A)* and scrotum *(B)* in the perineal region *(arrow)* is possible in midterm pregnancy in this small monkey. lt, left thigh; rt, right thigh. Scale bar represents 10 mm.

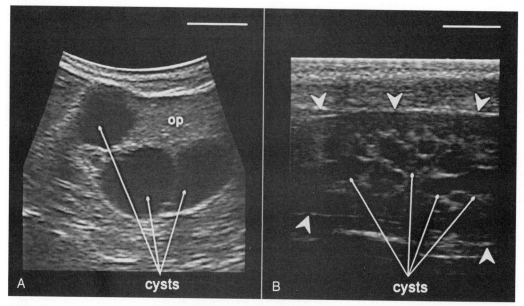

FIGURE 8–13. Cystic ovary *(A)* in a 12-year-old Sumatran tiger *(Panthera tigris sumatrae)* visualized by transrectal ultrasonography. Transcutaneous ultrasound image *(B)* of a uterine horn *(white arrowheads)* in an Asian wild dog *(Cuon alpinus lepturus)* with a cystic endometrium. Cystic degenerations of the female genital tract are frequent in carnivores. op, ovarian parenchyma. Scale bar represents 10 mm.

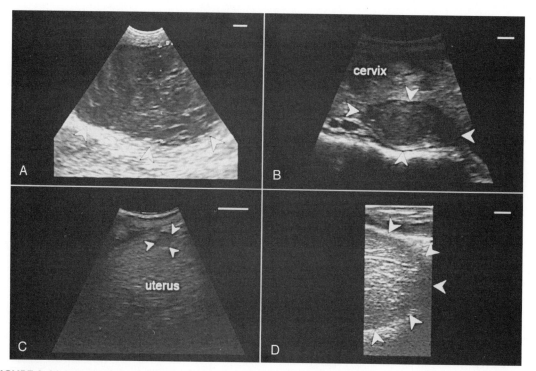

FIGURE 8–14. Leiomyomas *(white arrowheads)* are frequently found in the female genital tract of several mammalian species by transrectal ultrasonography. The influence of these benign smooth muscle tumors for the general health of most individuals is mostly negligible, but they may be an important infertility factor in females. *A,* Vaginal leiomyoma in a Bactrian camel *(Camelus ferus)*; *B,* cervical leiomyoma in an Asian rhinoceros *(Rhinoceros unicornis)*; *C,* uterine leiomyoma in a pygmy hippopotamus *(Choeropsis liberiensis)*; *D,* uterine leiomyoma in an Asian elephant *(Elephas maximus)*. Scale bar represents 10 mm.

direct method that allows imaging of embryonic and fetal morphologic structures, it offers many advantages as a method for pregnancy diagnosis in zoo animals.

DIAGNOSIS OF REPRODUCTIVE DISEASES

Knowledge concerning the appearance of healthy genital structures is necessary for clear recognition of pathologic alterations. Given the wide variability of genital tract structures within vertebrates, this is not always possible. Some pathologic changes, such as ovarian and endometrial cysts (Fig. 8–13) or uterine muscle tumors (Fig. 8–14), are relatively easy to identify. Alterations in the testes, such as calcification, intraparenchymal cysts, or tumors, permits healthy and pathologic structures to be distinguished relatively easily (Fig. 8–15). It is more difficult to distinguish between physiologic uterine fluid and a pathologic condition. For example, purulent endometritis in macaques is not easily distinguished from monthly menstruation fluid.[12]

Based on ultrasound findings in more than 2500 animals from more than 200 species, a remarkable susceptibility to special diseases was found in some species. For instance, there is a high prevalence of leiomyoma in the female genital tract of Asian elephants[13, 22] and in Asian rhinoceros species.[22, 35] In contrast, leiomy-

omas never develop in captive African elephants but they frequently have endometrial cysts. Additional examples are endometriosis[40] in nonhuman primate species and cystic degeneration of ovaries and endometrium in old carnivores,[36] especially in great cats in whom contraception is achieved by progestin implants such as melengestrol acetate.[28]

Assessment of the reproductive capacity of an animal is based on the health of the internal genital tract. It is therefore important to detect pathologic alterations of the inner genital tract and to determine the importance or influence they may have on reproductive performance before forming breeding groups.

IDENTIFICATION OF PRENATAL CONDITIONS

Prenatal conditions include embryonic and fetal death, retardation, and malformation. Generally, lack of fetal heart action and fetal movement, free-floating fetal membranes associated with a loss of fetal integrity, reduction of the volume or increasing echogenicity of fetal fluid, and partial or premature separation of the placenta are clear ultrasonographic signs of a prenatal problems (Fig. 8–16). However, the identification of minor or moderate prenatal conditions is difficult and requires both a high level of experience from the sonog-

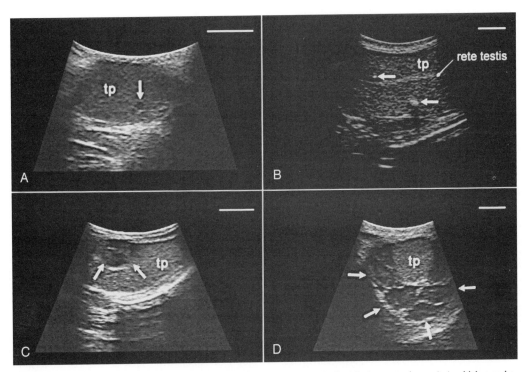

FIGURE 8–15. Ultrasonography reveals pathologic alterations *(white arrows)* of testicular parenchyma *(tp)*, which may be responsible for subfertility in males. Four sonograms demonstrate examples in different species: *A,* single testicular cyst in a gibbon *(Hylobates lar)*; *B,* multiple testicular calcifications in a scimitar oryx antelope *(Oryx gazella dammah)*; *C,* small testicular tumor in an Asian wild dog *(Cuon alpinus lepturus)*; *D,* massive tumor-related destruction of the testis in a Siberian tiger *(Panthera tigris altaica)*. Scale bar represents 10 mm.

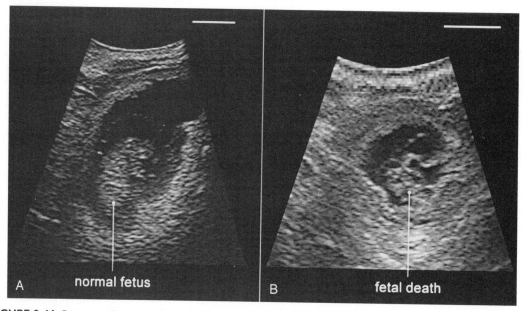

FIGURE 8–16. Sonogram of a normal fetus *(A)* and a fetal death *(B)* in European brown bear (*Ursus arctos*). Fetal death is characterized by cardiac arrest and later by a loss of fetal integrity, floating membranes, and cloudy amniotic fluid. Scale bar represents 10 mm.

rapher and an ultrasound system with high-resolution scan heads. First, an overview of the entire pregnant genital tract (including conceptus/concepti) must be obtained; second, high-frequency ultrasound probes must be used for detailed diagnostic images.

Most pathologic disorders of embryogenesis occur during the time of implantation. Early embryonic death is a frequent event that may be retrospectively detected with ultrasonography and structural changes within the endometrium of the slightly enlarged uterus can be visualized. Changes indicating early embryonic death in placentaria include the detection of an approximately 1 mm large undifferentiated echogenic mark in the uterine lumen (Fig. 8–17) and a corpus luteum on at least one ovary. Embryonic membranes and fluid are frequently still present in the uterus.

In stages of late gestation, fetal growth associated with the formation of scales, thick skin, or fur and increased calcification of the skeleton interferes with good image quality. In megavertebrates, the time frame in which pathologic changes of the fetus are detected is mainly in the first trimester of gestation, although this period may extend until the end of the second trimester. After this period, the fetus sinks to the maternal abdominal wall and is covered by intestinal loops. Changing of the examination position (standing position, lateral recumbency) may be helpful for better visualization of the genital tract. However, the evaluation of the health status of a near-term pregnancy, for instance, in elephants, is sometimes possible without seeing the fetus. The detection of cloudy fluid in the caudal part of the fetus-free uterus in combination with a distinct reduction of the uterine blood vessels indicate a pathologic alteration or death of the fetus.

Growth disorders (e.g., severe retardation) are easily

apparent in multiparous females with healthy and retarded fetuses or by follow-up examinations during gestation. Malformations causing accumulation of fluid such as ascites, cystic kidneys, or hydrocephalus are clearly imaged with ultrasonography. Some abnormalities have been ultrasonographically detected in exotic animals such as twin monster syndrome in Przewalski horse,[21] schistosoma reflexum in red deer, hydrocephalus in marmoset,[5] and anencephaly in bottlenosed dolphin.[2]

The use of ultrasonography in viviparous fish and reptiles or in soft shell eggs is also helpful for assessment of embryonic or fetal health status.

SUPPORT OF ASSISTED REPRODUCTION TECHNIQUES

The portability, relative affordability, and ability to provide high-quality real-time diagnostic information make ultrasonography an ideal supporting tool for assisted reproduction techniques in exotic animals.[25] Ultrasound is a noninvasive imaging technique that can provide imaging guidance for diverse diagnostic procedures (e.g., biopsy, aspiration) and treatments (e.g., laparoscopic ultrasonography-guided cyst puncture, local cancer treatment) in modern veterinary medicine. It can be used to guide the insertion or manipulation of instruments in patients for such procedures as flushing of the uterus or collecting embryos. Ultrasonographically supported embryo collection in the crab-eating macaque (*Macaca fascicularis*) is a nonsurgical way to collect blastocysts from the uterus by transcervical insertion of a two-way catheter (Fig. 8–18).[23]

Artificial insemination in Asian elephants has been

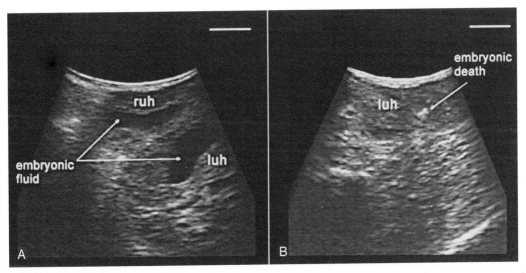

FIGURE 8–17. A normal pregnant uterine horn *(A)* few days after implantation in contrast to an early embryonic death *(B)* in European roe deer *(Capreolous capreolus)*. Typical signs of embryonic loss are a slightly enlarged uterus, absence of embryonic fluid, and a calcification focus at the implantation site *(arrow)*. Early embryonic death is without any clinical symptoms in the mother. This reproductive disorder is detectable by transrectal ultrasonography only by means of a high-frequency transducer. ruh, right uterine horn; luh, left uterine horn. Scale bar represents 10 mm.

performed using ultrasonography to guide a catheter more than 2 m deep into the uterus[31] (see Fig. 8–18). Artificial insemination in roe deer has been performed including the ultrasound monitoring of prostaglandin-induced luteolysis and follicle growth.[8] Similar methods are useful for intrauterine artificial insemination in gorilla and nonhuman primates.

Ultrasonography has also been used to select pregnant and nonpregnant African elephants for performing a contraception project in Kruger National Park, South Africa. Transrectal ultrasonography has been applied in captive European brown bears for monitoring antiprogesterone treatment as a new possibility for contraception in this species.[7]

Transrectal ultrasonographic imaging provides a noninvasive means for locating and measuring male reproductive structures, thus providing a basis for reproductive assessment. For example, the evaluation of the spermatozoa-storing ampullary glands in male elephants has been used for preselection of potential semen

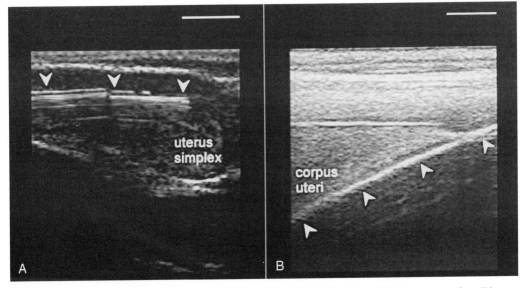

FIGURE 8–18. Intrauterine laying catheters *(white arrowheads)* for nonsurgical embryo collection in cynomolgus *(Macaca fascicularis)* visualized by transcutaneous ultrasonography *(A)* and for artificial insemination in a female Asian elephant *(Elephas maximus)* visualized by transrectal ultrasonography *(B)*. Scale bar represents 10 mm.

donors. The use of transrectal ultrasonography during manually induced ejaculation in elephant bulls[32] was very effective in characterization of the accessory glands and their roles in the ejaculatory process. Ultrasonography may also provide intraoperative orientation for the castration of elephant bulls.

Sonographically assisted follow-up evaluations make it easier to monitor the recovery of animals and to optimize ongoing treatment. Attempts to treat cystic ovaries and uterine myometrial tumors with a gonadotropin-releasing hormone analog have been monitored by transrectal ultrasonography in two female Asian rhinoceroses.

REFERENCES

1. Adams GP, Plottka ED, Asa CS, et al: Feasibility characterizing reproductive events in large nondomestic species by transrectal ultrasonic imaging. J Zoo Biol 10:247–259, 1991.
2. Brook F: Ultrasound diagnosis of anencephaly in the fetus of a bottlenosed dolphin (*Tursiops aduncus*). J Zoo Wildlife Med 25:569–574, 1994.
3. Curran S, Ginther OJ: Ultrasonic diagnosis of equine fetal sex by location of the genital tubercle. J Equine Vet Sci 9:77–83, 1989.
4. Donald I, Macvicar J, Brown TG: Investigation of abdominal masses by pulsed ultrasound. Lancet 1:1189–1191, 1958.
5. Du Boulay GH, Wilson OL: Diagnosis of pregnancy and disease by ultrasound in exotic species. Symp Zool Soc Lond 60:135–150, 1988.
6. Göritz F: Sonographie bei Zoo und Wildtieren. DVM Thesis, Freie University, Berlin, Germany, 1996.
7. Göritz F, Hildebrandt TB, Jewgenow K, et al: Transrectal ultrasonographic examination of the female urogenital tract in nonpregnant and pregnant captive bears (*Ursidae*). J Reprod Fertil Suppl 51:303–312, 1997.
8. Göritz F, Hildebrandt TB, Lengwinat T: Ultrasound guided artificial insemination in roe deer (*Capreolus capreolus*). Reprod Domest Anim 30(6):460, 1996.
9. Göritz F, Hildebrandt TB, Nötzold G, et al: Untersuchungen zum reproduktiven Status und Zyklusgeschehen beim Anoa (*Bubalus depressicornis*) mittels transrektaler Ultrasonographie. Verh ber Erkrg Zootiere 36:107–119, 1994.
10. Göritz F, Hildebrandt TB, Quandt S, et al: Transrectale Ultraschalluntersuchung des Urogenitalsystems beim Afrikanischen Elefanten. Ultraschal Med 16:38, 1995.
11. Göritz F, Hildebrandt TB, Thielebein J: Transrektale Ultraschalluntersuchung beim Faultier. Bildgebung Imaging 61(Suppl 2):98, V1.3, 1994.
12. Hildebrandt TB: Die Ultraschalldiagnostik—ein wichtiges Element bei der Erkennung und Behandlung von Reproduktionsstörungen weiblicher Javamakaken (*Macaca fascicularis*). Z Säugetierkd Suppl 1:29, 1993.
13. Hildebrandt TB, Göritz F: Sonographischer Nachweis von Leiomyomen im Genitaltrakt weiblicher Elefanten. Verh ber Erkrg Zootiere 37:287–294, 1995.
14. Hildebrandt TB, Göritz F, Bosch H, et al: Ultrasonographic sexing and reproductive assessment of penguins. Penguin Conservation 4:6–12, 1996.
15. Hildebrandt TB, Göritz F, Göltenboth R, et al: Sonomorphologische Geschlechtsdiagnose bei der Tüpfelhyäne (*Crocuta crocuta* Erxleben). Fertilität 12:46–50, 1996.
16. Hildebrandt TB, Göritz F, Hermes R, et al: Diagnosis of ovarian activity and pregnancy in roe deer (*Capreolus capreolus*) by transrectal sonography. Reprod Domest Anim 30(6):341, 1996.
17. Hildebrandt TB, Göritz F, Pitra C, et al: Transintestinale Ultraschalluntersuchung bei Wildvögeln. Verh ber Erkrg Zootiere 36:127–139, 1994.
18. Hildebrandt TB, Göritz F, Pitra C, et al: Sonomorphological sex determination in subadult Komodo dragon. Proceedings of the Annual Meeting of the American Association of Zoo Veterinarians, Puerto Vallarto, Mexico, pp 251–254, 1996.
19. Hildebrandt TB, Göritz F, Quandt S, et al: Graviditätsdiagnose beim Breitmaulnashorn mit Hilfe der transrektalen Adaptersonographie. Ultraschall Med 16:68, 1995.
20. Hildebrandt TB, Göritz F, Quandt S, et al: Ultrasonography as a tool to evaluate the reproductive tract in female Asian and African elephants. J Ultrasound Med 15:59, 1996.
21. Hildebrandt TB, Göritz F, Seidel B, et al: Fetale Mißbildung beim Przewalskipferd (*Equus przewalskii*). Verh ber Erkrg Zootiere 35:321–324, 1993.
22. Hildebrandt TB, Ippen R, Kaiser HE, et al: Leiomyomas in the genital tract of captive exotic mammals. Anticancer Res 15:1754, 1995.
23. Hildebrandt TB, Pitra C, Reinsch A: Ultraschallgestützte Embryonengewinnung und Trächtigkeitsuntersuchungen bei *Macaca fascicularis*. Tierärztl Praxis Suppl 1:66–67, 1993.
24. Hildebrandt TB, Pitra C, Sömmer P, et al: Sex identification in birds of prey by ultrasonography. J Zoo Wildlife Med 26:367–376, 1995.
25. Jewgenow K, Blottner S, Göritz, F et al: The application of assisted reproduction in puma (*Felis concolor*). Verh ber Erkrg Zootiere 36:59–67, 1994.
26. Kapustin N, Critser JK, Olson D, et al: Nonluteal estrous cycles of 3-week duration are initiated by anovulatory luteinizing hormone peaks in African elephants. Biol Reprod 55:1147–1154, 1996.
27. Karesh WB: The use of diagnostic ultrasonography in zoo medicine. Proceedings of the Annual Meeting of the American Association of Zoo Veterinarians, Tampa, FL, pp 2–4, 1983.
28. Munson L, Harrenstien L, Haslem CA, et al: Update on diseases associated with contraceptive use in zoo animals. Proceedings of the Annual Meeting of the American Association of Zoo Veterinarians, East Lansing, MI, pp 398–400, 1995.
29. Nyland TG, Mattoon JS: Preface. *In* Nyland TG, Mattoon JS (eds): Veterinary Diagnostic Ultrasound. Philadelphia, WB Saunders, 1995.
30. O'Grady JP, Yeager CH, Thomas W, et al: Practical applications of real time ultrasound scanning to problems of zoo veterinary medicine. J Zoo Anim Med 9:52–56, 1978.
31. Pratt NC, Hildebrandt TB, Göritz F: Non-invasive reproduction assessment and artificial insemination of an Asian elephant. Biol Reprod 89:132, 1996.
32. Price PJ, Bradford J, Schmitt D: Collection and semen analysis in Asian elephants. Proceedings of the American Association of Zoological Parks and Aquariums, Minneapolis, pp 310–313, 1986.
33. Radcliff RW, Osofsky SA: Reproductive applications of transrectal ultrasonography in captive African rhinoceros, and thoughts on in situ use. Proceedings of the Annual Meeting of the American Association of Zoo Veterinarians, Puerto Vallarta, Mexico, pp 42–47, 1996.
34. Rübel A, Kuoni W, Augustiny N: Emerging Techniques: CT scan and MRI in reptile medicine. Semin Avian Exotic Pet Med 3:156–160, 1994.
35. Schaffer NE, Zainal-Zahari Z, Suri MSM, et al: Ultrasonography of the reproductive anatomy in the Sumatran rhinoceros (*Dicerorhinus sumatrensis*). J Zoo Wildlife Med 25:337–348, 1994.
36. Seidel B, Hildebrandt TB, Göritz F: Einsatz bildgebender Verfahren in der Diagnostik von Erkrankungen abdominaler Organe. Verh ber Erkrg Zootiere 36:93–99, 1994.
37. Silverman S: Diagnostic imaging in zoological animals and birds—equipment and techniques. Verh ber Erkrg Zootiere 36:89–92, 1994.
38. Stetter MD, Raphael BL, Cook RA, et al: Comparison of magnetic resonance imaging, computerized axial tomography, ultrasonography, and radiology for reptilian diagnostic imaging. Proceedings of the Annual Meeting of the American Association of Zoo Veterinarians, Puerto Vallarta, Mexico, pp 450–453, 1996.
39. Stoskopf M: Clinical imaging in zoological medicine: A review. J Zoo Wildlife Med 20:396–412, 1989.
40. Swenson RB: Endometriosis in nonhuman primates. *In* Fowler ME (ed): Zoo and Wild Animal Medicine, 3rd ed. Philadelphia, WB Saunders, pp 339–340, 1993.
41. Tarantal AF, Hendrickx AG: Characterization of prenatal growth and development in the crab-eating macaque (*Macaca fascicularis*) by ultrasound. Anat Rec 222:177–184, 1988.

CHAPTER 9

Validity of Using Diagnostic Tests That Are Approved for Use in Domestic Animals for Nondomestic Species

S. K. HIETALA

I. A. GARDNER

Laboratory testing for evidence of exposure to infectious agents is a convenient and efficient means of diagnosis, health monitoring, and surveillance in both nondomestic and domestic species. Although it is a critical and frequently utilized tool in veterinary medicine and animal husbandry, laboratory testing is often performed or results are interpreted without full knowledge of the reliability or the limitations of the specific assays and techniques. To use test results appropriately, it is important to first understand basic principles in performance and evaluation of the specific tests and to recognize the limitations of applying that information across different species. The ability to use diagnostic tests approved for domestic animals in free-ranging and captive wildlife has some critical constraints, including variation in host responses to infectious agents, epidemiology of the disease agent or vectors in different environments, and the intended use of the resulting information. This chapter introduces (1) the principles involved in evaluation and interpretation of tests and (2) the basic constraints and applications of antigen detection and antibody detection tests. Discussion is limited to antigen and antibody detection tests; however, the principles of evaluation and interpretation are similar for clinical chemistry, toxicology, and the other test systems used in veterinary medicine.

EVALUATION AND INTERPRETATION OF LABORATORY TESTS

When laboratory test results are used to assist in management decisions, it is important to determine which tests should be used, the number of different tests to use, and a strategy for interpreting results. To employ laboratory tests effectively, the user must first understand the principles behind performance and interpretation of the assays and must assign some measure of accuracy to the results. Accuracy is characterized by two indices: sensitivity and specificity.

Test sensitivity is the probability that a test correctly identifies as positive the animals that are exposed to the agent in question. Factors that may affect test sensitivity include, but are not limited to, the length of time between exposure and testing, detection limits of the assay used, exogenous or endogenous substances in the sample that may interfere with test performance (e.g., steroids, blocking antibodies, antimicrobials), or biologic variation between field strains and reference strains of viral, bacterial, or parasitic agents.

Test specificity is the probability that a test will identify as negative the animals that are not exposed to the agent in question. Factors affecting specificity include cross-reactions caused by antigenically related or similar agents; the presence of specific or nonspecific antibodies after vaccination; and assay failure resulting from exogenous substances, including bacterial contamination in the sample.

Test results are typically measured on a continuous scale, such as optical densities reported for enzyme-linked immunosorbent assays (ELISAs), or on an ordinal scale, typified by the doubling dilutions reported as serum titers (e.g., 1:4, 1:8, 1:16). The interpretation of any test is based on selection of a cutoff value above which a result is considered positive and below which a result is considered negative. For some tests, a suspicious, intermediate, or uninterpretable range is included to account for overlap of test values among positive and negative populations. Decreasing a test's cutoff value typically increases the sensitivity but decreases the specificity of a test. Increasing the cutoff value of a test has the reverse effect; however, the comparative magnitude of change in sensitivity and specificity will vary, depending on the prevalence of the disease and performance characteristics of the test.[8]

No laboratory test is perfectly sensitive and perfectly specific, and for most assays the true sensitivity and specificity are not known. In theory, the sensitivity and specificity of assays are obtained by testing diverse populations of animals known to include true-positive, false-positive (nonexposed but test results positive), false-negative, and true-negative members (Fig. 9–1). The true exposure status of the animal is determined by means of a gold standard test: generally necropsy results or isolation and identification of the agent in question. All too often, the gold standard used in evaluating a test is not perfectly accurate, and poor sensitivity or specificity can be amplified in defining the accuracy of the test being compared. Because of the technical and logistic difficulties in obtaining appropriate and representative samples from wildlife populations, few tests used in nondomestic species have defined sensitivity and specificity. In many situations, tests approved for use in domestic species have been directly tranferred for use in wildlife, without consideration of potential cross-reacting agents present in the host or environment, differences in immunologic or host susceptibility between species, or potential for assay errors that are based on incompatibility between test components and the species being tested.

In general, the intended use of the test results dictates whether tests are selected on the basis of their sensitivity or specificity. For surveillance or health certification for the purpose of introducing an animal into a disease-free population, tests with high sensitivity are preferred. The risk of introducing an exposed animal with false-negative test results into a naive population usually exceeds the economic benefit or risk of excluding the animal from the population. Tests with high specificity are typically selected for diagnostic purposes or when animals deemed important for maintenance of population genetics would be excluded from reintroduction programs on the basis of false-positive test results. Employing multiple tests or serial testing is an effective means of evaluating a population with low disease prevalence. For serial testing, assays of high sensitivity are selected to screen the population in order to optimize identification of all test-positive members by knowingly including a large proportion of false-positive members, followed by an assay or assays of higher specificity for confirmation of the screening-positive animals. Serial testing is often implemented on the bases of lower cost, of screening assays and of the economic benefits of testing fewer numbers of animals with a more expensive confirmation assay. The blood tuberculosis test (BTB), which is widely used in New Zealand, is an example of multiple assay testing that incorporates three different

assays for evaluation of each animal suspected of having tuberculosis.[4]

The measure of test performance, or the ability of a test result to correctly indicate exposure status in an individual, termed *predictive value,* is determined by test sensitivity, test specificity, and agent prevalence in the population being evaluated. Unlike sensitivity and specificity, which are inherent properties of a test, predictive value varies with changing prevalence in different populations. As prevalence of an agent increases in a population, the predictive value of a positive result increases and the predictive value of a negative result decreases. In the following example, a high prevalence of brucellosis in a population results in a relatively low percentage of false-positive results and a high positive predictive value. The same test applied to a similar population with a low prevalence yields significantly more false-positive results and a low positive predictive value.

Example: *Brucella* screening test, 98% sensitivity and 70% specificity. The prevalences in the two populations are 60% and 1%, respectively. By multiplying true positive and negative animals by the sensitivity and specificity of the test, and using a 2 × 2 table, the difference in predictive value of the same ELISA in the two populations can be seen (Table 9–1).

For wildlife species, there are added difficulties in defining the predictive value of a test on the basis of the epidemiology of diseases in populations under distinctly different management conditions (e.g., free-ranging versus confinement) or in extremely diverse geographic regions. For wildlife, in particular, it is critical to consider that agents not encountered in one environment may occur in another because of altered contact between species or because of management of feed and insect vectors. The prevalence of mycobacterial diseases in confined hoofstock[3] and the occurrence of pseudorabies in captive-fed big cats[2] in comparison with their free-ranging counterparts are examples. Geographic occurrence of specific agents also affects predictive values, as in the serologic cross-reactivity between epizootic hemorrhagic disease and bluetongue virus which causes low predictive values for agar gel diffusion assays in some geographic regions but does not affect the same assay in regions where the insect vector is absent. An understanding of the agent in question, the test, and potential cross-reacting or interfering agents is needed for interpreting any test result. Strategies to improve the positive predictive value of a test used in low-prevalence populations include selective sampling of "high-risk" groups (e.g., those with clinical disease; older animals, if exposure risk is age related), increasing specificity of the test by changing the cutoff for interpretation, using a test with higher specificity, or using appropriate serial testing.[1]

TEST METHODS

Laboratory tests most often used can be classified as antigen detection and antibody detection assays. The antigen detection assays are those that test for the agent directly and include direct examination of tissues or

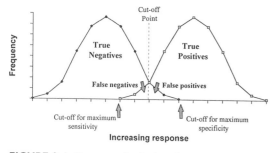

FIGURE 9–1. Frequency distributions for test results in a population that includes exposed (true positive) and unexposed (true negative) animals.

TABLE 9–1. *Brucella* **Screening Test**

Herd	Positive	Negative	Total	Comments
Herd I: size of 100 at 60% prevalence: 60 animals are true positive, 40 are true negative				
Test (+)	59 true positive	12 false positive	71	59 of 71 test-positive animals are correctly classified: positive predictive value = 83%
Test (−)	1 false negative	28 true negative	29	28 of 29 test-negative animals are correctly classified: negative predictive value = 96%
Totals	60	40	100	
Herd 2: size of 100 at 1% prevalence: 1 animal is true positive, 99 are true negative				
Test (+)	1 true positive	30 false negative	31	1 of 31 test-positive animals is correctly classified: positive predictive value = 3%
Test (−)	0 false negative	69 true positive	69	69 of 69 test-negative animals are correctly classified: negative predictive value = 100%
Totals	1	99	100	

fluids for parasites or bacteria, bacterial and virus isolation, and a variety of immunoassays, including ELISA, for detection of the specific agent in host-derived tissues or fluids. Antibody assays rely on detection of serum antibodies as indirect evidence of exposure to a specific agent and are the most widely used of the laboratory tests because of their cost efficiency and relative ease in sample collection and storage.

Antigen Detection Assays

Antigen detection assays tend to be very specific but may lack sensitivity, depending on the stage of disease and tissue distribution of the agent. In general, antigen detection assays are used for confirmation testing. Lack of sensitivity in antigen detection assays can be associated with technical difficulties in propagating an agent in vitro, such as occurs with *Leptospira* species and selected strains of *Mycobacterium paratuberculosis*. In many of these cases, serologic testing becomes the accepted substitute. Sensitivity issues may similarly relate to innate species differences in shedding of an agent: for instance, prolonged and detectable shedding of foot and mouth disease virus in cattle in comparison with llamas, which appear to be resistant to infection and shedding, despite detectable seroconversion.[7] Specificity problems associated with antigen detection assays frequently include laboratory errors in identification of a specific agent. For instance, technical errors in identifying eperythrozoon or anaplasma on improperly prepared blood smears have been implicated as a source of false-positive results. Cross-reactions with related agents, such as gram-negative organisms that cause false-positive reactions with selected *Chlamydia* antigen detection ELISAs,[6] are also concerns for other immunoassay systems. Polymerase chain reaction (PCR) assays which amplify in vitro the genetic material of microbes,

introduce a new concern for test interpretation. PCR amplification increases the sensitivity of antigen detection—in some instances to as little as a single microbe per gram of tissue—but it has not yet been established whether detection at that level correlates to potential for shedding or association with clinical disease for most infectious agents. The ability not only to detect an agent but also to determine the association with disease is critical to wildlife management programs.[5]

Antibody Detection Assays

Depending on the agent and type of assay, serologic assays can be used as screening or confirmatory tests. Because of their relative cost efficiency and comparative ease of sample handling and storage, serologic assays are widely used as the sole test system for surveillance, health certification, and oftentimes diagnostic testing in wildlife. However, assays that depend on detection of antibody tend to be more variable between species than those that detect a microbe directly. It should not be assumed that a serologic test validated for a domestic breed or species will perform equally well in nondomestic animals, because there may be differences in immune responsiveness, potential for exposure to cross-reacting agents, and technical need for species specific reagents in some serologic assays. The use of homologous versus heterologous reagent red blood cells in complement fixation and hemagglutination assays can alter test performance and results, as can the use of antispecies immunoglobulin directed against one species to identify antibody responses of other species, as often occurs when ELISA tests designed and validated for one species are used in another. Although antibovine immunoglobulin will recognize immunoglobulins in the families bovidae, cervidae, and giraffidae, the detection limits and performance characteristics of assays used in breeds or species other than domestic ones has rarely been verified or documented. Competitive ELISAs and ELISAs entailing the use of protein A or protein G are technique modifications that circumvent the need for species-specific anti-immunoglobulin.[9] However, with these as with other tests used in wildlife species, quality assessment and standardization of tests have not been routinely implemented.

For any serologic test, sensitivity is affected by the lag of days to months, depending on the microbe, before detectable levels of antibody are produced after exposure to the agent. Sensitivity is also affected in many serologic assays by antigenic differences between laboratory reference strains and new variants of microbes. Influenza virus variants are a prime example of how quickly an infectious agent can change antigenically, which emphasizes the need for laboratory reference strains to be validated against field isolates. Specificity issues most often associated with antibody detection are related to antigenic cross-reactions and to specific or nonspecific antibodies associated with vaccine or other nonspecific antigenic stimulation as previously noted.

Despite their limitations, laboratory tests continue to be used extensively and effectively in wildlife medicine and management. The key to using the tests and results

most efficiently is an ample understanding of their limitations as well as continued efforts to improve standardization and validation of the tests for the different domestic and nondomestic species.

REFERENCES

1. Gardner IA, Hietala SK, Boyce WM: Validity of using serological tests for diagnosis of diseases in wild animals. Rev Sci Tech Off Int Epiz 15:323–335, 1996.
2. Glass CM, McLean RG, Katz JB, et al: Isolation of pseudorabies virus from a Florida panther. J Wildlife Dis 30:180–184, 1994.
3. Haigh JC: Management practices to minimize infectious and parasitic diseases of farmed and ranched cervids and bison. Rev Sci Tech Off Int Epiz 15:209–226, 1996.
4. Hunter DL: Tuberculosis in free-ranging, semi free-ranging and captive cervids. Rev Sci Tech Off Int Epiz 15:171–181, 1996.
5. Munson L, Cook RA: Monitoring, investigation, and surveillance of diseases in captive wildlife. J Zoo Wildlife Med 24:281–290, 1993.
6. Sanderson TP, Anderson AA: Evaluation of a commercial solid-phase enzyme immunoassay for the detection of ovine *Chlamydia psittaci*. J Vet Diagn Invest 4:192–193, 1992.
7. United States Animal Health Association [USAHA]: Report of the Committee on Infectious Disease of Cattle, Bison, and Llama. Proceedings of the 97th Annual Meeting of the USAHA, Las Vegas, NV, pp 171–185, 1993.
8. Vizard AL, Anderson GA, Gasser RB: Determination of optimum cut-off value of a diagnostic test. Prev Vet Med 10:137–143, 1990.
9. Worley MB: Molecular biology and infectious diseases: present and future trends in diagnosis. J Zoo Wildlife Med 24:336–345, 1993.

CHAPTER 10

Evaluating Immunodeficiency Disorders in Captive Wild Animals

SUZANNE KENNEDY-STOSKOPF

Clinical features associated with immunodeficiency include chronic infection, recurrent infection, unusual infecting agents, incomplete resolution between episodes of infection, or failure to respond to treatment. Anyone ever involved with the medical care of captive wild animals has experienced the frustration of a case that conforms to these criteria. Even more frustrating is the apparent inability to document immunodeficient states in these animals. The zoological medicine literature is full of case reports that conclude that an animal died because it was immunocompromised, with no data to support the assertion.

Immune responses can be divided into two general categories: innate and acquired. Innate or natural immunity provides a rapid response to noxious substances

and includes phagocytosis and complement pathways. Acquired or specific immunity is a slower response mechanism and includes humoral and cell-mediated functions. Although innate and acquired immune responses are intricately interrelated through shared regulatory proteins (cytokines) and cell surface receptor interactions, clues to the defect in immunity are often provided by the type of infection observed. Phagocytic disorders are associated with superficial skin infections or systemic infections with pyogenic organisms. Complement deficiencies are associated with recurrent infections with pyogenic organisms. Humoral immunodeficiency is associated with enhanced susceptibility to gram-negative and pyogenic bacterial infections, whereas cell-mediated immunodeficiency enhances susceptibility to intracellular organisms, which include viruses, protozoa, fungi, and bacteria such as *Mycobacterium, Brucella,* and *Listeria.*

Since the 1980s, significant advances have been made in the development of reagents to characterize the immune systems of domestic animals. In some instances, these advances can benefit nondomestic species, but more often than not, the clinician working with these animals has to rely on tests that are decades old and are not dependent on species-specific reagents. Nonetheless, understanding what tests are available, what their limitations are, and how to evaluate the results is the first step needed if clinical immunology is to become relevant for nondomestic animals.

PRIMARY IMMUNODEFICIENCIES

Primary immunodeficiencies are associated with congenital defects that are frequently inherited. The deficiency may result from an enzymatic defect or a developmental anomaly. The location of the defect determines whether the deficiency will affect phagocytosis, humoral immunity, cell-mediated immunity, or multiple systems. In veterinary medicine, more primary immunodeficiencies are being recognized in economically important species such as horses and in companion species such as dogs. Very few primary immunodeficiencies have been documented in nondomestic species.

Chédiak-Higashi syndrome has been reported in white tigers, killer whales, and Aleutian mink.[7] In people and cattle, the syndrome is inherited as an autosomal recessive condition. Chédiak-Higashi syndrome is associated with a defect in cell structure that results in the production of abnormally large granules in neutrophils, eosinophils, and monocytes and in enlarged melanin granules. Enlarged melanin granules can be observed by examining hair shafts and are responsible for the dilution of hair pigmentation and light-colored irises seen with this syndrome. The abnormally large granules in leukocytes can be readily observed in a stained blood smear. These leukocytes have impaired chemotactic responses and reduced intracellular killing. Natural killer cell function is also abnormal, and as a consequence, affected animals are more susceptible to some viral infections and tumor formation. Platelet function may also be affected and result in bleeding episodes.

The marked deficiency of catalase activity and low erythrocyte adenosine triphosphate (ATP) concentrations in the black rhinoceros are believed responsible for both the mucocutaneous ulcerative disease and acute episodic hemolysis observed in this species.[5] The enzymatic defect, combined with impaired hexose monophosphate shunt metabolism, decreases the ability of black rhinoceros cells to neutralize oxidant stresses. Analogous situations occur in humans and are believed to be adaptive mechanisms for combating malaria.

Juvenile llama immunodeficiency syndrome is a condition affecting llamas less than 3 years of age that is characterized by wasting and low-grade, chronic bacterial infections that fail to respond appropriately to therapy.[2] The exact etiology remains unknown but is probably a primary immunodeficiency. Affected animals have low serum immunoglobulin G (IgG) concentrations, poor vaccination responses to *Clostridium perfringens* C toxoid, and decreased lymphoblastogenesis responses to Protein A, a B cell mitogen, all of which suggest a defect in the humoral immune system, although defects in the innate immune system have yet to be fully explored.

The greatest temptation in zoological medicine is to equate lack of genetic diversity with immunodeficiency. A similar situation is encountered with dog breeds and inbred strains of laboratory mice.[7] Certain breeds of dogs, as well as laboratory mice, exhibit marked differences in susceptibility to certain infectious diseases. The exact genetic defect affecting a specific immune function that results in disease susceptibility is often not known but so far has not been linked conclusively with homozygosity of the major histocompatibility complex (MHC).[8] In mice highly susceptible to intracellular bacteria and parasites, a gene present on chromosome 1 fails to regulate gamma interferon activation of cytotoxic macrophages, thereby allowing the pathogens to replicate efficiently.[8] If the mouse does not encounter any intracellular pathogens during its life span, then phenotypically it appears immunocompetent. Such subtle defects in immune function are associated not only with inbred animals but also with animals within a population, inasmuch as the changes can be caused by pinpoint genetic mutations. This scenario may explain why certain animals within the population at large die quickly during an infectious disease outbreak.

SECONDARY IMMUNODEFICIENCIES

Secondary immunodeficiencies are acquired and are undoubtedly responsible for most suspected instances of immunocompromised conditions in nondomestic species. Common causes of secondary immunodeficiency include infectious agents, environmental contaminants, drugs, neoplasia, advanced age, nutritional status, and failure of colostral transfer.[7] Retroviruses, both the oncoviruses and lentiviruses, are well-recognized etiologies of virus-induced immunosuppression. Malnutrition, in general, is linked to impaired cell-mediated immunity. Vitamin and mineral deficiencies depress specific immune functions. Zinc is especially critical for the proper functioning of the immune system because it affects both cell-mediated and humoral immunity. Failure of passive transfer of maternal antibodies is a well-recognized secondary immunodeficiency of neonatal zoo ungulates and can occur because of inadequate colostrum availability, inadequate intake, or inadequate absorption. Although failure of passive transfer directly affects humoral immunity, the impact of other causes of secondary immunodeficiency may not be so readily apparent. The immune system is, fortunately, quite redundant, and acquired immunodeficiency is seldom an all-or-nothing event. Establishing cause and effect is difficult and frequently perplexing.

EVALUATING IMMUNE FUNCTION

Faced with an animal suffering chronic infections, unresponsive to treatment, or prone to relapses, a veterinarian cannot help but wonder whether the patient is immunocompromised (Table 10–1). Proving it, however, is problematic and quite frustrating. Most commercial laboratories that provide veterinary biomedical services offer very little in the way of immune function assays. Autoimmune panels are available for dogs, cats, and horses, and certain subclasses of immunoglobulins can be measured. Colleges of veterinary medicine are more likely to provide clinical immunology services that can be adapted to nondomestic species, and in some instances, human medical institutions may be of assistance.

The veterinarian should contact the laboratory to determine whether any tests that may be useful are available. Often, certain assays are not performed as a clinical service, but personnel may be able to suggest a research laboratory that may be willing to assist. According to personal experience, research laboratories are more likely to help than are commercial or service laboratories. The veterinarian should be prepared to submit samples from additional unaffected animals of the same species to serve as a basis of comparison. No normal reference values are likely to exist for the species under investigation. Even comparing results from a large felid against domestic cat standards, although admittedly a logical strategy to begin with, can lead to erroneous conclusions. If all members of a species in the collection are affected, then samples from another institution with apparently healthy animals should be solicited. This is usually not a problem if serum samples are required because banked specimens are usually available. However, if fresh peripheral blood leukocytes (PBLs) are required, as in a lymphocyte blastogenesis assay, then multiple immobilizations must be planned so that samples arrive, preferably simultaneously, to eliminate intra-assay variation and at a time when the laboratory can process them, because this assay is labor intensive.

The following tests are offered by the clinical immunology laboratory at North Carolina State University (NCSU) and serve as an example of the kinds of tests that are available for evaluating immunologic parameters that can be adapted to nondomestic species.

Phagocytosis

Phagocytosis can be divided into four stages: chemotaxis, adherence/opsonization, ingestion, and destruction. Defects may occur at any stage. Tests exist to evaluate the various steps of phagocytosis and are not dependent on species-specific reagents as the process of phagocytosis is highly conserved. Oyster heterophils and mammalian neutrophils function similarly in phagocytic assays. However, not all assays for each step of phagocytosis are routinely conducted by veterinary clinical immunology laboratories.

Failure of intracellular killing is the major class of inherited defects in phagocytosis for domestic animals.[7] Intracellular killing occurs through either the respiratory burst pathway or the action of lysosomal enzymes. Nitroblue tetrazolium (NBT) dye reduction test is an assay used to assess intracellular killing. A clear, yellow, water-soluble compound, NBT forms formazan, a deep blue dye, on reduction. Measuring the reduced dye photometrically after extraction from neutrophils correlates with the production of superoxide anion, an early component of the respiratory burst pathway. This assay is no longer offered by the clinical immunology laboratory at NCSU because of poor reproducibility of results and tremendous variation within replicate samples. Other tests available for evaluating intracellular killing include chemiluminescence and measuring such respiratory burst components as hydrogen peroxide and superoxide radical formation. Chemiluminescence is particularly useful for evaluating intracellular killing initially, because all steps in the respiratory burst pathway must be intact before a response can be detected. None of these assays, however, are offered through the clinical immunology laboratory at NCSU partly because the demand for these tests is limited. These assays are available in various research laboratories which illustrates the necessity of seeking the assistance of investigators with specialized interests.

Humoral Immunity

FAILURE OF PASSIVE TRANSFER

The zinc sulfate turbidity test is the fastest and most economic method for diagnosing failure of passive transfer of immunoglobulins in foals.[7] Zinc sulfate, as well as other chemicals such as glutaraldehyde and sodium sulfite, precipitates globulins out of serum. The turbidity of the solution can be read visually or spectro-

TABLE 10–1. Screening for Immunodeficiency Disorders in Captive Wild Animals

Presenting Signs	Suspected Defect	Tests
Recurrent skin infections; systemic infections with pyogenic bacteria	Phagocytosis	Chemiluminescence
Increased susceptibility to gram-negative and pyogenic bacteria	Humoral immunity	Serum electrophoresis immunoglobulin quantitation; B cell quantitation; response to B cell mitogens
Increased susceptibility to intracellular organisms	Cell-mediated immunity	Total lymphocyte count; T cell quantitation (subsets); response to T cell mitogens and specific antigens

photometrically if a standard curve has been previously generated for the species being investigated. In absence of colostral transfer, the solution remains clear. A threshold of 400 mg/dl of IgG must be present before there is a turbid reaction with zinc sulfate. This quantity of IgG is considered protective for foals but may not necessarily be adequate for all exotic ungulates. It has been suggested that a neonate should be considered hypogammaglobulinemic if serum concentrations of gamma globulins are less than 25% of the adult average for that species.[6] Gamma globulins can be measured by serum electrophoresis.

Total protein concentrations are an indirect and quick method of screening for suspected failure of passive transfer of immunoglobulins when other options are not readily available. In calves and lambs, a total protein concentration of less than 4.5 g/dl is suggestive of failure of passive transfer, whereas levels of 4.5 to 5.0 g/dl suggest partial failure of passive colostral transfer.[4]

SERUM ELECTROPHORESIS

Globulin concentrations are determined by subtracting the albumin concentration from the total protein concentration. The globulin fraction includes not only immunoglobulins but various acute-phase proteins, such as haptoglobulin, fibrinogen, C-reactive protein, and ferritin, as well as complement factors, clotting factors, and enzymes. Therefore, an elevated globulin level does not necessarily mean increased immunoglobulin production.

Electrophoretic separation of serum proteins is based on the migration of charged protein particles in an electric field. Globulins move in groups classed as alpha, beta, and gamma globulins. Depending on the species, there may be one or two alpha, one or two beta, and one or two gamma fractions. This variability between species may initially cause some confusion in the attempt to establish normal parameters for nondomestic animals, but at least serum electrophoresis does not require species-specific reagents. In general, acute-phase proteins migrate as alpha and beta globulins, and IgG and other immunoglobulin isotypes migrate as gamma globulins. In some instances, IgM and immunoglobulin A (IgA) extend from the beta$_2$ to the gamma region. Although serum electrophoresis is quantitative for the different globulin fractions, it does not quantify specific immunoglobulins.

QUANTITATION OF IMMUNOGLOBULINS

Radial immunodiffusion is a method frequently used to quantify amounts of specific immunoglobulin isotypes in domestic animals. The assay requires that antiserum to specific immunoglobulin subclasses be available. The antiserum is incorporated into agar. Dilutions of serum are added to wells cut in the agar. A ring of precipitate forms around the test wells, the area of which is proportional to the amount of immunoglobulin present. A standard curve generated by adding known amounts of immunoglobulin to the agar wells enables the calculation of the amount of immunoglobulin in the unknown serum sample. Radial immunodiffusion for quantitation of IgG levels in dogs, cats, horses, cows, and llamas is available. Additional immunoglobulin isotypes can be quantified for some of these species. The ability to apply this technique to nondomestic species depends on whether the antiserum to a particular domestic species IgG cross-reacts with a nondomestic species. For instance, lion IgG can apparently be measured in the same way as domestic cat IgG.

Cell-Mediated Immunity

LYMPHOCYTE BLASTOGENESIS

A number of plant lectins and other substances collectively referred to as mitogens can activate lymphocytes nonspecifically. Among the most frequently used mitogens are concanavalin A (ConA), phytohemagglutinin (PHA), pokeweed mitogen (PWM), and various different bacterial lipopolysaccharides (LPS). According to studies in mice and humans, PHA and ConA activate T lymphocytes, PWM activates primarily B lymphocytes and some T lymphocytes, and LPS activates B lymphocytes, although the efficacy of different sources of LPS varies between species.

The assay requires freshly collected blood in anticoagulant. Lymphocytes are purified by density gradient centrifugation. Cultures are set up in triplicate, usually in microtiter plates, and incubated with various concentrations of mitogens, usually for 72 hours, before the addition of tritiated ^{3}H-thymidine, a nucleoside precursor. Thus the amount of ^{3}H-thymidine incorporation over a period of 18 to 24 hours reflects the rate of DNA synthesis. Tritiated thymidine incorporation is most frequently determined by scintillation counting in a liquid scintillation spectrophotometer. Data is expressed as counts per minute (cpm) or corrected for quenching to disintegrations per minute (dpm). The cpm in control cultures are subtracted from stimulated cpm as a measure of lymphocyte responsiveness. Alternatively, cpm in control cultures are divided into stimulated cpm to yield a ratio commonly referred to as the stimulation index (SI). Ideally, data should be presented and evaluated both ways.

Lymphocyte blastogenesis assays, also referred to as lymphocyte transformation and lymphocyte stimulation, have frequently been performed in nondomestic species to evaluate cell-mediated immune function simply because the test can be conducted. However, a multitude of technical as well as conceptual variables can affect the results of this assay system. These include the concentration of cells, the geometry of the culture vessel, contamination of cultures with nonlymphoid cells or microorganisms, the dose of mitogen, the incubation time of cultures, and the source and amount of serum in the culture medium. Culture time and dose-response kinetics are particularly crucial. In clinical immunology laboratories, these parameters have been established and periodically re-verified for the species that are routinely evaluated. Without such careful controls, it is nearly impossible to observe partial or subtle defects in lymphocyte responsiveness to various disease states. Unfortunately, it is often impossible to collect enough samples from nondomestic species to address all of these concerns. Consequently, results of mitogen stimulation assays in nondomestic animals are frequently ambiguous.

The clinical immunology laboratory at NCSU seldom performs lymphocyte blastogenesis assays even in domestic animals because of the difficulty in interpreting results reliably. In human clinical immunology laboratories, lymphocyte stimulation with mitogens is performed as an initial diagnostic test when primary immune deficiencies are suspected. The lack of responsiveness to a T or B cell mitogen is a quick way to pinpoint a profound defect in either the cellular or humoral immune system.

Lymphoproliferative responses to specific antigens can also be measured to evaluate anamnestic responses. Tetanus toxoid and *C. perfringens* C and D toxoid are examples of antigens used to evaluate lymphocyte responsiveness in animals with known vaccination histories.[1, 2] With certain acquired immunodeficiencies, such as those associated with retroviral infections, lymphoproliferative responses to specific antigens are frequently impaired long before those to mitogens. Differential lymphoproliferative responses to *Mycobacterium bovis* and *Mycobacterium avium* have been used to assess whether an animal has been exposed to a pathogenic or atypical mycobacterium.

FLOW CYTOMETRY

Flow cytometers are instruments capable of analyzing properties of single cells as they pass through an orifice and are illuminated by a laser beam. The interaction between the cells and light can be used to measure physical characteristics, such as size and granularity. Size and granularity can be used to distinguish granulocytic leukocytes, monocytes, and lymphocytes in peripheral circulation. Monoclonal antibodies conjugated to fluorescent dyes that illuminate specific proteins present on cell surfaces can be incubated with cell suspensions that are injected into the flow cytometer in order to recognize and count specific cell subsets. These proteins present on certain populations of cells are referred to as a cluster of differentiation (CD). For instance,

helper T lymphocytes are CD4 positive, and cytotoxic/suppressor T lymphocytes are CD8 positive.

Care must be exercised when evaluating species cross-reactivities of monoclonal antibodies to lymphocyte subsets and extrapolating lymphocyte subset percentages for domestic animals to their nondomestic counterparts. Although the monoclonal antibodies used at NCSU College of Veterinary Medicine to distinguish lymphocyte subsets in the domestic cat are useful for tigers and leopards, additional reagents had to be screened for lions and cheetahs. Although the CD4:CD8 ratio is approximately 1.7 for cats and lions, cats have about twice as many B lymphocytes in circulation as do lions.[3] Flow cytometry data are useful for following trends in cell populations during an infection or during immunosuppressive therapy. A decreased CD4:CD8 ratio as a result of diminished CD4+ cells is suggestive of a compromised immune system but is not a direct measure of immune function.

REFERENCES

1. De Swart RL, Ross PS, Timmerman HH, et al: Impaired cellular immune response in harbour seals (*Phoca vitulina*) fed environmentally contaminated herring. Clin Exp Immunol 101:480–486, 1995.
2. Hutchison JM, Garry FB, Belknap EB, et al: Prospective characterization of the clinicopathologic and immunologic features of an immunodeficiency syndrome affecting juvenile llamas. Vet Immunol Immunopath 49:209–227, 1995.
3. Kennedy-Stoskopf S, Gebhard DH, English RV, et al: Clinical implications of feline immunodeficiency virus infection in African lions (*Panthera leo*): Preliminary findings. Proceedings of the Annual Meeting of the American Association of Zoo Veterinarians, Pittsburgh, pp 345–346, 1994.
4. Mechor GD: Management of neonatal hoofstock. Proceedings of the Annual Meeting of the American Association of Zoo Veterinarians, South Padre Island, TX, pp 221–226, 1990.
5. Paglia DE, Miller RE: Erythrocytic ATP deficiency and acatalasemia in the black rhinoceros (*Diceros bicornis*) and their pathogenic roles in acute episodic hemolysis and mucocutaneous ulcerations. Proceedings of the Joint Conference of the American Association of Zoo Veterinarians and the American Association of Wildlife Veterinarians, Oakland, CA, pp 217–219, 1992.
6. Satterfield WC, O'Rourke KI: Identification and management of hypogammaglobulinemic neonatal nondomestic hoofed stock. Proceedings of the Annual Meeting of the American Association of Zoo Veterinarians, Seattle, pp 112–113, 1981.
7. Tizard IR: Veterinary Immunology, 5th ed. Philadelphia, WB Saunders, 1996.
8. Wiegertjes GF, Stet RJM, Parmentier HK, et al: Immunogenetics of disease resistance in fish: a comparative approach. Dev Comp Immunol 20:365–381, 1996.

CHAPTER 11

Vitamin D: Metabolism, Sources, Unique Problems in Zoo Animals, Meeting Needs

DUANE E. ULLREY

JONI B. BERNARD

METABOLISM

There is evidence that solar irradiation may be responsible for the presence of vitamin D in forms of life from phytoplankton to humans.[43] Nearly all terrestrial vertebrates appear to require a source of vitamin D, whether transferred through the food chain or endogenously synthesized, to support normal calcium and bone metabolism. Why plants and nonvertebrates synthesize vitamin D is less well understood.

The spectrum of irradiance wavelengths that reach the atmosphere of Earth from the sun is from approximately 100 to 3200 nm. Molecules in the atmosphere absorb certain wavelengths, so that the solar spectrum is attenuated when the radiation reaches the surface of Earth. For example, atmospheric ozone and molecular oxygen absorb virtually all ultraviolet (UV) wavelengths shorter than 290 nm, essentially eliminating the UVC range (100 to 280 nm) and 10 nm (280 to 290 nm) of the UVB range (280 to 315 nm). Oxygen, carbon dioxide, and water vapor absorb strongly in the far red and near infrared regions. Thus, the principal solar radiation to which Earth-dwelling creatures are exposed is some UVB (290 to 315 nm), UVA (315 to 400 nm), visible light (400 to 700 nm), and the near infrared (700 to 1000 nm). About 20% of the solar energy reaching the surface of the Earth has wavelengths longer than 1000 nm.[30, 77, 123]

Although exposure to both UVA and UVB produces the erythema characteristic of sunburn and induces the increased melanin pigmentation known as tanning, the UVB range encompasses those wavelengths required for photobiogenesis of vitamin D. This process and subsequent metabolic events have led to classification of vitamin D as a hormone rather than as a nutrient. Provitamin D_3, 7-dehydrocholesterol, in the malpighian layer of the epidermis of human skin, is converted to previtamin D_3 by UV irradiation in the range of 290 to 315 nm, with maximum conversion at 297 $\pm$ 3 nm.[45] Of the wavelengths reaching the surface of Earth that have been studied, 296.7 nm has been reported to be most potent in preventing rickets in rats.[38] Other research has reported peak conversions of 7-dehydrocholesterol to previtamin D_3 at 303 nm in rat skin[111] and at 295 nm in ethanolic solution.[66] Exposure of skin to the sun or to simulated solar irradiance, as opposed to narrow-band irradiation, diminishes the maximum formation of previtamin D_3 to about 15% to 20% of the original amount of 7-dehydrocholesterol, and enhances previtamin D_3 conversion to lumisterol$_3$. A quasiphotostationary state is established between 7-dehydrocholesterol, tachysterol$_3$, lumisterol$_3$, and previtamin D_3 as a result of exposure to longer UV wavelengths.[46, 78, 120] Previtamin D_3, in turn, undergoes thermal isomerization to vitamin D_3 in the skin over a period of hours to days. As previtamin D_3 stores are depleted by thermal isomerization, exposure of cutaneous lumisterol$_3$ and tachysterol$_3$ to solar UV may promote reverse photoisomerization of these compounds to previtamin D_3.[46]

Provitamin D_2, ergosterol, in molds, yeasts, senescent lower leaves of growing plants, and sun-dried cut forage is converted to vitamin D_2 by UVB irradiation. Peak conversion of ergosterol in ethanolic solution was reported at 295 nm.[67] Although ergocalciferol is commonly considered the plant form of vitamin D, some higher plants contain cholecalciferol or cholecalciferol metabolites, as well. For example, both ergocalciferol and cholecalciferol have been isolated from sun-cured, field-grown alfalfa (*Medicago sativa*), although ergocalciferol concentrations were more than 98% of the total.[50] Cholecalciferol was also found in golden oat grass (*Trisetum flavescens*)[103] and orchard grass (*Dactylis glomerata*).[13] Golden oat grass and wild jasmin (*Cestrum diurnam*), *Solanum malacoxylon*, and *Solanum glaucophyllum* are calcinogenic and contain 1,25-dihydroxycholecalciferol in the form of a glycoside.[38, 68, 84, 103, 119, 122] *S. malacoxylon* also contains glycosides of cholecalciferol and 25[OH]D_3.[12]

Although other forms of vitamin D are known, cholecalciferol and ergocalciferol are responsible for most of the vitamin D activity of importance to animals that have been studied. During the 1930s, the structures of ergocalciferol and cholecalciferol were established, and the ability to produce them by UV irradiation of their respective provitamins was demonstrated. They differ in structure only in their side chains as shown in Figure 11–1. Ergocalciferol has a double bond between carbons 22 and 23 and a methyl group on carbon 24, whereas cholecalciferol has neither. Alternative trivial names are calciol for vitamin D_3 and ercalciol for vitamin D_2.

The pure vitamins are white to yellowish powders that are insoluble in water, moderately soluble in fats, oils, or ethanol, and readily soluble in acetone, diethyl ether, or petroleum ether. Crystalline vitamin D_3 is now the international vitamin D standard, with 0.025 μg vitamin D_3 = 1 IU (1 μg vitamin D_3 = 40 IU). The international vitamin D standard originally supplied by the World Health Organization is no longer available. However, 0.025 μg of the USP Cholecalciferol Reference Standard has 1 IU of vitamin D activity.[115]

Vitamin D_3, formed in the skin, is bound to D-binding protein (DBP), enters the circulation, and is transported to the liver where it is converted to 25-hydroxycholecalciferol (25[OH]D_3, or calcidiol). From there, 25[OH]D_3 is transported to the kidney where it is converted to the principal active form, 1α,25-dihydroxycholecalciferol (1,25[OH]$_2D_3$, or calcitriol) or to 24,25-dihydroxycholecalciferol (24,25[OH]$_2D_3$).

The D-binding and D-metabolite–binding transport proteins appear to vary among species.[23, 39–41] Sixty-five mammalian species were found to transport 25[OH]D_3 on an alpha-globulin, whereas seven used albumin.[39] In an earlier study, Edelstein and associates[24] speculated that the apparent dissimilarity between New World and Old World monkeys in the biologic activity of vitamin D_2 and vitamin D_3[56, 71] might be due to a difference in transport proteins. In a New World monkey, the white-fronted capuchin (*Cebus albifrons*) the majority of radioactive cholecalciferol and 25[OH]D_3 was bound to albumin, whereas in an Old World monkey, the red guenon or patas monkey (*Erythrocebus patas*), the majority of 25[OH]D_3 was bound to alpha-globulin. However, Hay and Watson[39] found that among the five New World species they examined, 25[OH]D_3 was transported on alpha-globulin in golden lion tamarins (*Leontodeus rosalia*) and douroucoulis or night monkeys (*Aotus trivirgatus*) and albumin was used in capuchins (*Cebus albifrons*, *Cebus apella*, *Cebus capucinus*). Thus, it was concluded that if there are general differences between New and Old World monkeys in their ability to use vitamin D_2, the explanation does not reside with the difference in electrophoretic mobility of transport proteins. Furthermore, when the affinities of the specific plasma D-binding transport proteins for 25[OH]D_2 and 25[OH]D_3 were studied in 63 vertebrate species, 25[OH]D_2 was bound less efficiently in fish, reptiles, birds, monotremes, and nine mammal species. Binding affinities were equal in 22 mammal species, including the five New World primates (night monkey, three capuchins [*C. capucinus, C. albifrons, C. apella*], common or white ear-tufted marmoset [*Callithrix jaccus*]), and four Old World primates (rhesus macaque [*Macaca mulatta*], olive baboon [*Papio anubis*], red guenon, white-handed gibbon [*Hylobates lar*]) that were studied.[41]

If vitamin D_2 or vitamin D_3 are present in the diet, absorption occurs in the small intestine of rats, chicks, and certain primates, and is stimulated by bile acids and fat. Most of the absorbed vitamin D is associated with chylomicrons in the lymph, is transferred to DBP in the blood, and enters the metabolic pathways as previously described. Absorbed vitamin D_3 is ultimately

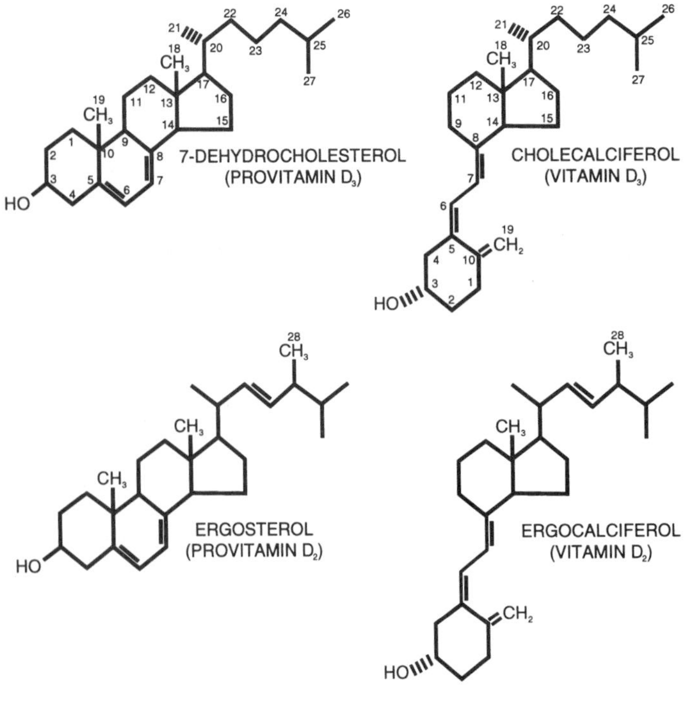

FIGURE 11–1. The structure of 7-dehydrocholesterol, cholecalciferol, ergosterol, and ergocalciferol.

converted to $1,25[OH]_2D_3$, whereas absorbed vitamin D_2 is converted to $1\alpha,25$-dihydroxyergocalciferol ($1,25[OH]_2D_2$; ercalcitriol) or to 24,25-dihydroxyergocalciferol ($24,25[OH]_2D_2$). However, there are species differences in the absorption and metabolism of vitamins D_2 and D_3, and some species may not easily absorb orally presented vitamin D in either form.

Calcitriol has been shown to bind to a specific receptor in the enterocyte nucleus and to induce the formation of Ca^{2+}-binding proteins (CaBP) that promote absorption of Ca^{2+} and phosphate from the intestine. When dietary calcium supplies are insufficient to sustain normal blood Ca^{2+} concentrations, calcitriol in conjunction with parathormone (PTH) induces bone resorption by triggering the differentiation of stem cells to osteoclasts that enhance mobilization of Ca^{2+}. Resorption of Ca^{2+} and phosphate in the distal renal tubule also improves. As blood Ca^{2+} concentrations increase toward normal, PTH secretion wanes and 24,25-dihydroxycalciferol and calcitriol stimulate osteoblasts to make osteocalcin and enhance alkaline phosphatase activity and bone mineralization. In addition to their presence in intestine and bone, nuclear calcitriol receptors have been found in the brain, pituitary, parathyroids, stomach, gonads, dermis, epidermis, monocytes, and activated T and B lymphocytes.[44]

In the case of hypercalcemia, parafollicular C cells in the thyroid or ultimobranchial glands produce calcitonin (CT), which suppresses mobilization of Ca^{2+} and phosphate from bone and may promote excretion of Ca^{2+} and phosphate by the kidneys. During lactation or egg shell production, when Ca^{2+} demand is high, 1α-hydroxylase in the kidneys is stimulated by prolactin, resulting in elevated blood concentrations of calcitriol.

Although these interactions are complex and have been studied in only a few species, the classic functions of vitamin D are to stimulate intestinal uptake of Ca^{2+} and phosphate, and to promote incorporation of these ions into bone. In company with PTH and CT (as well as other hormones), vitamin D maintains plasma Ca^{2+} and phosphate homeostasis and, thus, impacts a variety of soft tissue events such as neuromuscular activity, reproduction, and immune function.[20, 37, 105]

A deficiency of vitamin D may result in hypocalcemia, hypophosphatemia, elevations in plasma alkaline phosphatase activity, declines in plasma osteocalcin concentration,[72] hypotonia, muscle weakness, secondary hyperparathyroidism, defects in bone mineralization (generally characterized as rickets in young and osteomalacia in adults), diminished fertility and neonatal growth, and reduced immune response. A number of human metabolic diseases, such as vitamin D–resistant rickets, hypoparathyroidism, renal osteodystrophy, osteoporosis, and psoriasis have been shown to respond to $1,25[OH]_2D_3$ or its analogs.

Vitamin D in human blood has a half-life of about 24 hours. Thus, serum concentrations tend to reflect the most recent exposure to sunlight or the most recent oral intakes of vitamin D. "Normal" human serum vitamin D values range from 0 to 120 ng/ml (0 to 310 nmol/L).

Circulating 25[OH]D in humans has a half-life of about 3 weeks, and a steady-state value tends to reflect the sum of vitamin D from diet and photobiogenesis over a period of several weeks or months. Concentrations of serum or plasma 25[OH]D are considered particularly useful in assessing the vitamin D status of humans and animals; between 8 and 60 ng/ml (20 to 150 nmol/L) normally circulates in humans, although values after extended exposure to summer sun may be higher.[44] As noted in the following discussion, quite different concentrations may circulate in other species.

The half-life of $1,25[OH]_2D$ in human blood is 4 to 6 hours, with a normal serum range of 16 to 60 pg/ml (38 to 144 pmol/L). Because even very low levels of 25[OH]D are efficiently converted to $1,25[OH]_2D$, a deficient individual who obtains (immediately pretest) a very small amount of vitamin D from food or brief solar exposure can have low, normal, or high serum concentrations of $1,25[OH]_2D$ with low or undetectable concentrations of 25[OH]D. Thus, measures of $1,25[OH]_2D$ are of limited use for identifying vitamin D deficiency, but they can be of considerable value in evaluation of individuals with acquired or inherited disorders of vitamin D metabolism.

SOURCES

Ultraviolet Irradiation (Natural)

Paleontologic evidence indicates that, more than 50,000 years ago, Neanderthal man was afflicted with rickets. The first scientific description of this disease was written in 1645 by Daniel Whistler, but its cause was not clear before the separation and naming of the antirachitic factor (vitamin D) in 1922 by McCollum and colleagues.[79] Earlier suggestions ranged from faulty heredity to syphilis. Ultimately, a study of the worldwide distribution of rickets found a parallel with the lack of sunlight, and Huldschinsky reported in 1919[52] that UV rays were effective in its healing. Air pollution was appreciable during the early industrial revolution, and there were major population shifts to urban settings where sun exposure was limited. These circumstances were exacerbated by the location of many large cities in northern temperate regions where, in winter, indoor living, heavy clothing, short days, and the acute solar zenith angle minimized UV penetration to the skin.

The skin of many mammals is a rich source of the provitamin, 7-dehydrocholesterol (approximately 250 $\mu g/g$ in the rat). The most direct way to ensure that vitamin D needs of most animals is met is to provide regular exposure of the skin to the sun. It has been estimated that exposure of 1 cm^2 of white human skin to direct sunlight for 1 hour results in production of about 10 IU of cholecalciferol. Exposure of the arms and face daily for 10 minutes in optimal light should provide for human needs. However, there are many factors that influence these estimates. For example, thickening and pigmentation of skin reduces penetration of UV into the stratum spinosa and stratum basale of the epidermis, where the highest concentrations of 7-dehydrocholesterol occur, and persons with dark skin may require six times as much UV irradiance as persons with light skin. With aging, human epidermal concentrations of 7-dehydrocholesterol decline and, at age

80 years, concentration is half that of a 20-year-old person.[120]

Although exposure to monochromatic light at 295 nm has been shown to convert 65% to 71% of 7-dehydrocholesterol in skin to previtamin D_3, only about 20% was converted when the same skin was exposed to full-spectrum sunlight.[78] Additional solar irradiation (up to 8 hours) produced no more previtamin D_3, but led to epidermal increases in lumisterol, tachysterol, and 5,6-*trans*-vitamin D_3, biologically inactive forms. This demonstrates that solar wavelengths, other than 295 nm, influence vitamin D biogenesis, and helps explain the absence of D hypervitaminosis even after intensive sunlight exposure.

Animals whose skin is covered by fur, feathers, or scales may experience less UV penetration of the epidermis than animals without these coverings. However, the greatest impediments are artificial barriers between the sky and animals housed in buildings in which walls, roofs, windows, and skylights do not allow penetration of UVB. Direct solar exposure may not be necessary because scattering of solar UVB wavelengths by atmospheric molecules and aerosols has the effect of increasing the diffuse (sky) short-wave component of global (sun plus sky) radiation. Thus, the sky is an important source of natural UVB irradiance, and, although not as energetically intense, sky radiation may have a higher proportion of UVB, compared to visible wavelengths, than direct sunlight.[36] Nevertheless, if UVB wavelengths cannot reach an animal in confinement, if its food does not contain vitamin D, if it does not eat the food, or if it is unable to use dietary vitamin D, rickets or osteomalacia is a likely result.

A number of light-transmitting materials have been examined for their ability to allow penetration of the spectrum from 280 to 600 nm. Window glass was shown not to transmit wavelengths less than 334 nm.[42] Our studies found that polycarbonate and fiberglass did not transmit light of wavelengths less than 370 nm. New vinyl transmitted little light of wavelengths less than 305 nm and, after 3 months of simulated solar exposure, did not transmit light wavelengths less than 360 nm. Milk-white Teflon (E.I. du Pont de Nemours & Co., Wilmington, DE), 5 mils thick, transmitted all wavelengths equally well, but 90-mil Teflon (with sufficient strength for skylight applications) attenuated 295 nm light transmission to less than 1% of transmission through air.

Acrylic polymers differed in their UV transmission, depending on their formulation. New Plexiglas UVT (Rohm and Haas, Philadelphia, PA), 0.25 inches thick, transmitted light at 295 and 300 nm at 57% and 70%, respectively, of light transmitted through air. After 2 years of rooftop solar exposure at the San Diego Zoo (32.5 degrees north latitude), respective light transmissions had declined to 24% and 31%. New Polycast SUVT (Polycast Technology Corp., Stamford, CT), 0.25 inches thick, transmitted light at the above wavelengths at 74% and 81%, respectively. After 2 years of rooftop exposure, light transmission was 52% and 59%.

A reformulated acrylic polymer, Solacryl SUVT, (Polycast Technology Corp., Stamford, CT), 0.25 inches thick, has been found to transmit light at both 295 and 300 nm at 85% of light transmission through air. When incorporated into a double-pane skylight (two 0.25-inch panes separated by 2.5 inches of air), light transmission at 295 and 300 nm was 60% and 64% of light transmitted through air. Independent tests of solarization are not available, but a Solacryl distributor reported that 0.25-inch Solacryl SUVT declined 7 percentage units in light transmission at 295 nm after 1000 hours in a tanning bed application.

Solacryl has been used to advantage in skylights during remodeling of animal housing at several institutions, including the San Diego Zoo and the Toledo Zoo. It is recommended either that there be some outside animal area, allowing unimpeded opportunity for solar exposure, or that this product be considered in new construction or remodeling of buildings designed to house animals inside.

Ultraviolet Irradiation (Artificial)

Commercial lamp manufacturers have attempted to duplicate various aspects of solar irradiance by designing lamps that provide visible light, UVA radiation, UVB radiation, UVC radiation, infrared radiation, or combinations intended to parallel the spectrum of the sun.[61, 77] Lamps emitting UVC radiation are intended for germicidal use and are not considered safe for living organisms. Infrared lamps are used principally for heat. Low-intensity "black lights" emit a high proportion of UVA radiation that induces fluorescence or phosphorescence (creating interesting effects in mineral and marine exhibits). Medical lamps that emit strongly in the shorter visible (blue) wavelengths are sometimes used to irradiate preterm human infants or neonates that are hyperbilirubinemic. Bilirubin is dermally photoisomerized to forms that are more readily excreted. Thus, the likelihood of brain damage from bilirubin deposition in basal ganglia and brain stem nuclei (kernicterus) is reduced. Fluorescent sun lamps that are designed for tanning beds may emit wavelengths in the UVA, UVB, and UVC regions, but are used with plastic shields that absorb most of the UVB and UVC wavelengths. Similar UV-emitting lamps may be used for treatment of psoriasis.

Most lamps are produced for general illumination with visible light. Most incandescent lamps emit mainly long wavelengths and are somewhat deficient in the shorter wavelengths, relative to the spectrum of the sun. The manufacture of fluorescent lamps allows for more flexibility in this regard. The fluorescent lamp is a low-pressure gas discharge source in which light is produced predominantly by fluorescing powders (phosphors). These phosphors are activated by UV energy generated by a mercury arc. The character of emitted light is controlled by the mix of phosphors and the transmitting characteristics of the outer envelope.

Although fluorescent lamps are of several types, only the daylight fluorescent lamp spectrum matches that of sunlight qualitatively. The cool-white and warm-white lamp spectra have higher relative irradiances of blue light than does sunlight, but they have lower relative irradiances of the longer visible wavelengths of sunlight.

Artificial light sources often are chosen for use in indoor animal exhibits with the expectation that they will provide normal-appearing illumination and promote animal health.[75] It is commonly assumed that the wavelength spectra will include some UV light and that the lamps will produce desired photoperiod effects. The cool-white fluorescent lamps that are so frequently used produce photoperiodic effects, but few emit significant radiation at wave lengths less than 400 nm[33] and are thus unsuitable as a source of the UVB wavelengths necessary for vitamin D biogenesis. Although promoted as a full-spectrum lamp, the Vita-Lite (Duro-Test Corporation, North Bergen, NJ) emits negligibly less than 310 nm and does not prevent rickets in growing chickens fed a vitamin D–free diet,[11] nor does it increase plasma 25[OH]D₃ in hospital patients exposed at normal illumination levels for 1 year.[22] However, Neer and associates[98] reported that elderly men with no sunlight exposure or dietary vitamin D had greater calcium absorption when exposed 8 hours per day to 500 footcandles of light from Vita-Lite lamps, as compared to exposure to usual illumination intensities of 10 to 50 footcandles of mixed incandescent and fluorescent lighting. Measures of vitamin D metabolites in the plasma were not made.

We have examined the spectral irradiance, from 250 to 700 nm, of 15 commercial fluorescent lamps and five experimental fluorescent lamps.[9] Included were lamps from Duro-Test Corporation, Energy Savers Unlimited, Inc. (Harbor City, CA), Zoo Med Laboratories, Inc. (San Luis Obispo, CA), General Electric Lighting (Cleveland, OH), Philips Lighting (Somerset, NJ), and Sylvania Lighting (Danvers, MA). None of the lamps emitted significant radiation at wavelengths less than 280 nm, and most emitted no significant radiation less than 320 nm. There is an obvious mercury line in most lamps at 313 nm, but emissions at this wavelength appear to have little antirachitic effect.[65]

The experimental lamps produced by Sylvania Lighting contained a phosphor, identified as 2096, alone or in various proportions with daylight phosphors. Percentages of the irradiance ($\mu W/cm^2$) emitted in UVB, UVA, and visible light regions by lamps containing only phosphor 2096 were 36.3, 59.8, and 3.9, respectively. As a consequence, this lamp was very active in vitamin D biogenesis, but the light emitted was blue and did not provide desirable general illumination. To correct this problem, a reformulated mix of phosphors was used to produce a lamp, designated Sylvania Experimental Reptile lamp, with a correlated color temperature of 5600°K and a color rendering index of 91 (compared to 5600° to 6000°K and 100 for the sun). This lamp produced 78.3 $\mu W/cm^2$ of irradiance at a distance of 61 cm, with a percentage distribution of 9.0, 25.6, and 65.4 in UVB, UVA, and visible regions. Illuminated objects had a normal appearance, biogenesis of vitamin D was supported, and UVB exposure for 8 hours at a distance of 61 cm was within safe limits as established by the National Institute for Occupational Safety and Health.[85] These lamps are not yet commercially available.

None of the other commercially available lamps supplied both significant UVB irradiation and normal illumination. However, by use of two-lamp fixtures containing a Sylvania 350 Blacklight and a daylight lamp, UVB wavelengths required for vitamin D biogenesis can be supplied in reasonable amounts while providing somewhat acceptable general illumination. However, large quantities of UVA also are supplied. Although a weak UVB emitter, the GE Chroma 50 lamp (General Electric Lighting, Cleveland, OH), mounted so that exposure distance was within 30 cm, has been found to offer some protection against rickets in green iguanas (*Iguana iguana*). The Sylvania Design 50 also provides acceptable general illumination, has higher irradiance energy between 290 and 300 nm than the GE Chroma 50, but has not been tested with animals for its antirachitic potential. Illumination for viewing of nocturnal exhibits and modest amounts of UVB might be provided by Sylvania 350 Blacklight lamps, but it is not clear whether nocturnal animals require or can use UVB light, nor has the Sylvania 350 Blacklight been tested in this application.

Vitamin D in Foods

Vitamin D concentrations have been determined in very few foods. A provisional table of values in human foods has been published by the U.S. Department of Agriculture,[53] and some of these values are presented in Table 11–1. However, few samples have been analyzed. Vitamin D activity is influenced by UV exposure, and dietary vitamin D intakes by animals may influence vitamin D concentrations in animal products. Thus, these values should be used with caution. Furthermore, the listed fish liver oils frequently contain concentrations of vitamin A so high that excessive use can lead to vitamin A toxicity.

Studies of the concentrations of vitamin D and vitamin D metabolites in milk are relevant to the needs of nursing mammals. Ergocalciferol, cholecalciferol, 25[OH]D₂, 25[OH]D₃, 24,25[OH]₂D₂, 24,25[OH]₂D₃, 1,25[OH]₂D₂, and 1,25[OH]₂D₃ have all been found in human and cow's milk, but total vitamin D activity is not very responsive to normal solar exposure or to dietary intakes.[48, 69, 112] In fact, it has been found that a 14-fold increase in dietary vitamin D₃ intake caused only a twofold increase in the vitamin D activity in cow's milk.[104] As a consequence, U.S. public health policy requires supplementation with 400 IU vitamin D per quart of fluid cow's milk. If further research reveals that a low concentration of vitamin D is common in the milk of other mammals, it is clear that UVB irradiance is particularly important for nursing infants that do not consume other vitamin D–containing foods.

Herbivores that are confined indoors depend heavily upon sun-cured forages for their vitamin D supply, unless they are otherwise supplemented. The vitamin D concentrations published for alfalfa hay and red clover hay by the National Research Council[91] are 1900 to 2000 IU/kg dry matter, essentially identical to the concentration reported in sun-cured alfalfa by Horst and colleagues.[50] Vitamin D concentrations in mixed legume–grass hays and timothy hays, determined by rat bioassay, ranged from 375 to 3800 IU/kg.[62] When vita-

TABLE 11–1. Vitamin D Concentrations in Human Foods (Wet Basis)

Food	IU/kg Edible Portion
Dairy and Egg Products	
Milk, cow, fluid, fortified*	
Whole, low fat, or skim	400
Milk, cow, whole, fluid, unfortified	
Summer	30
Winter	10
Milk, goat, whole, fluid, unfortified	120
Milk, human, whole, fluid	40
Cheese	
Cheddar	120
Edam	360
Swiss	440
Cream, cow, heavy whipping, fluid	520
Egg, chicken	
Whole, fresh or frozen	520
Whole, dried	1,880
White, fresh	0
Yolk, fresh	1,480
Fats	
Butter	560
Margarine, fortified†	600
Margarine, unfortified	0
Cod liver oil	
Medicinal, regular	167,000
Medicinal, high-potency	400,400
Low-potency	50,000
Commercial, refined	100,000
Dogfish liver oil	24,200
Halibut liver oil	3,680,000
Mackerel oil	1,300,000
Rockfish liver oil	978,000
Sardine oil (Atlantic or Pacific)	3,320
Swordfish liver oil	6,930,000
Tuna liver oil	1,300,000
Fish and Shellfish	
Catfish, channel, fillet, raw	5,000
Cod, fillet, raw	440
Eel, European, fillet, raw	2,000
Flounder, fillet, raw	600
Garfish, fillet, raw	3,400
Halibut, Greenland, fillet, raw	6,000
Herring, Atlantic, fillet, raw	16,280
Mackerel, Atlantic, fillet, raw	3,600
Clams	40
Oysters	3,200
Shrimp	1,520
Meat and Related Products	
Beef	
Kidney	320
Liver	160
Skeletal muscle, lean	120
Vegetables	
Mushrooms	
Chanterelle	840
Morel	1,240
Shitake	1,000
Yellow boletus	1,240

*Fortified so that 1 quart of milk contains 400 IU of vitamin D.
†Values based on label claims.
From Human Nutrition Service: Provisional Table on the Vitamin D Content of Foods. Washington, DC, Nutrient Data Research Branch, Nutrition Monitoring Division, U.S. Department of Agriculture, 1991.

min D assays were conducted on first-cutting alsike clover, ladino clover, red clover, and timothy before sun curing, about 50 IU/kg were found. After sun curing and 6 months of storage, vitamin D concentrations were 180 to 320 IU/kg. The presence of carotenoids in these forages may have suppressed the antirachitic response in the rat bioassay and caused an underestimation of vitamin D activity.[121] Vitamin D_2 concentrations in some animal feeds are shown in Table 11–2.[88]

Oral Vitamin D Supplements

Both vitamin D_2 and vitamin D_3 supplements are sold commercially, but the latter is more generally available as a feed additive because of its widespread use in poultry and livestock feeds. Vitamin D_2 is found in irradiated dried yeast, which may be blended with carriers to produce specified potencies. Some manufacturers produce spray-dried powders containing controlled amounts of vitamin D_3 in a gelatin-dextrin matrix, with ethoxyquin as an antioxidant. Such products have good

stability and are water dispersible. Rovimix D_3 500 and 2000 are spray-dried products of the Roche Chemical Division (Hoffman-La Roche, Inc., Nutley, NJ). They contain minimum potencies of 500 IU and 2000 IU vitamin D_3/kg, respectively. These products are designed for use in drinking water, milk replacers, premixes, base mixes, and complete feeds. This company also produces Rovimix D_3 400, a blend of spray-dried vitamin D_3 in a carrier, with a concentration of 400 IU/kg. It is designed for use in premixes, base mixes, and complete feeds.

25-Hydroxycholecalciferol is available in a free-flowing beadlet through formulation into food-grade, hydrogenated vegetable oil containing butylated hydroxytoluene and citric acid as antioxidants. The formulated beadlet contains 12.5 mg of 25[OH]D_3/g. It is marketed as Hy.D by IsoGen L.L.C. (Naperville, IL). The relative biologic activity of 25[OH]D_3 as compared to that of vitamin D_3 has been estimated for domestic poultry in more than 25 studies. Using criteria such as calcium absorption, plasma calcium, bone ash, bone strength, tibial dyschondroplasia, and egg shell defor-

TABLE 11–2. Vitamin D$_2$ Concentrations in Animal Feeds (Dry Basis)

Feed	IU/kg
Alfalfa	
Fresh	191
Hay, sun-cured, early bloom	1996
Hay, sun-cured, midbloom	1544
Hay, sun-cured, mature	1411
Barley	
Hay, sun-cured	1103
Straw	662
Birdsfoot trefoil	
Hay, sun-cured	1544
Bromegrass	
Hay, sun-cured	1407
Corn	
Distillers grains with solubles, dehydrated	600
Fodder, sun-cured, aerial part with ears	1323
Stover, sun-cured, aerial part without ears	1103
Oats	
Hay, sun-cured	1544
Straw	662
Prairiegrass	
Hay, sun-cured, full bloom	992
Red clover	
Hay, sun-cured, full bloom	1914
Sorghum	
Grain	29
Soybean	
Hay, sun-cured	1059
Sweetclover	
Hay, sun-cured	1874
Timothy	
Hay, sun-cured, midbloom	1985
Wheat	
Hay, sun-cured	1544
Straw	662
Sugarbeet	
Pulp, dehydrated	637

From National Research Council: Nutrient Requirements of Sheep. Washington, DC, National Academy Press, 1985. (IU/mass corrected).

mation, strength, and quality, the relative biologic activity of 25[OH]D$_3$ was one to four times that of vitamin D$_3$.[110] Estimates of the relative toxicity of 25[OH]D$_3$ vary, but the narrowest margin of safety was found when renal tubular calcification was used as an index of toxicity in day-old broiler chicks.[83] Beginning renal tubular calcification was found after 14 days in chicks fed 0.1 mg of 25[OH]$_3$/kg diet (approximately 8000 IU/kg). Other researchers have concluded, based on renal tubular calcification and reduced body weight of broilers, that 25[OH]D$_3$ is five to 10 times more toxic than vitamin D$_3$.[125]

Animals might be individually dosed using tablets or capsules. A tablet containing 200 IU vitamin D$_3$ and 5 mg calcium (from CaCO$_3$) is marketed as Calel-D (Rhone Poulenc Rorer Pharmaceuticals Inc., Collegeville, PA). Capsules containing 0.25 or 0.5 μg 1,25[OH]$_2$D$_3$ for oral administration are marketed as Rocaltrol (Hoffman LaRoche, Inc., Nutley, NJ). Initial dosages used for adult humans are commonly 0.25 μg/day, but optimal dosages should be individually determined.[21]

Vitamin D Injectables

Examination of The Compendium of Veterinary Products,[8] the Physicians GenRx,[21] and the Physician's Desk Reference[99] revealed no commercially available injectables containing only vitamin D$_3$. A number of products are sold that contain both vitamins D and A. The vitamin A concentrations are typically very high and could be counterproductive (and possibly toxic) when administering pharmacologic doses of vitamin D.

An injectable 1,25[OH]$_2$D$_3$ is marketed as Calcijex (Abbott Laboratories, Abbott Park, IL). It contains either 1 μg/ml or 2 μg/ml, and the recommended dosage for humans with renal failure is 0.01 μg/kg body weight, three times per week.

An injectable vitamin D$_2$ preparation is marketed as Calciferol in oil (Schwarz Pharma, Kremers Urban Co., Milwaukee, WI). It contains 500,000 IU/ml.

Crystalline cholecalciferol can be purchased from the Sigma Chemical Company (St. Louis, MO; Catalog No. C-9756) or the U.S. Pharmacopeia (Rockville, MD; USP Cholecalciferol Reference Standard, Catalog No. 13100-9).

UNIQUE PROBLEMS IN ZOO ANIMALS

Vitamin D Deficiency

CARNIVORES

Nutritional and metabolic bone diseases are common problems in many zoo animals,[31] but identification of their cause may be difficult. When carnivores are fed muscle meat without bone, calcium intakes are deficient, calcium-to-phosphorus ratios are markedly inverse (approximately 1:20), and nutritional secondary hyperparathyroidism may result. Excessive vitamin A intakes from the consumption of liver may interfere with vitamin D metabolism, exaggerate bone remodeling, and increase the severity of skeletal changes.

There is developing evidence that some carnivores may have limited ability to use UVB light for cutaneous biogenesis of vitamin D. Skin from domestic dogs and cats had low concentrations of 7-dehydrocholesterol (10% that of rat skin), and UVB irradiation produced no cutaneous increases in vitamin D$_3$ concentration compared to a 40-fold increase in rat skin.[51] This and previous studies with intact dogs indicate that, unlike herbivores and omnivores, dogs and cats are unable to synthesize sufficient vitamin D in the skin and are dependent upon a dietary source. Thus, for these species and perhaps for some related species, vitamin D fulfills the traditional definition of an essential nutrient rather than that of a hormone.

PRIMATES

Primates in captivity have exhibited rickets or osteomalacia on numerous occasions.[5, 18, 27, 31, 80–82, 114, 116] Terms used for the syndrome include *simian bone disease, wooly monkey disease,* and *cage paralysis.* It has been reported more often in young primates than mature ones, and in platyrrhines (New World primates) more often than in catarrhines (Old World primates). Some researchers have proposed that this difference is a consequence of a higher vitamin D requirement in New World primates or of a limited ability to use vitamin D$_2$.[54] However, the suggestion by Freedman and colleagues[31] that it is a failure of conversion of vitamin D$_2$ to vitamin D$_3$ is not consistent with known metabolic pathways.

Relatively few of the extant New World and Old World primate species have been studied. However, evidence that vitamin D$_2$ is less active than vitamin D$_3$ for the studied New World primates is quite convincing. For example, Lehner and associates[71] found that growing squirrel monkeys (*Saimiri sciureus*) fed no vitamin D or vitamin D$_2$ at 1250, 2500, 5000, or 10,000 IU/kg diet grew poorly and showed evidence of rickets. In contrast, squirrel monkeys fed vitamin D$_3$ at 1250, 2500, 5000, or 10,000 IU/kg diet grew equally well and did not show evidence of rickets. Suggestions that New World primates, as a group, have unusually high dietary vitamin D$_3$ requirements are not supported by published research. However, most of that research was not designed to answer the question. Until controlled studies demonstrate elevated requirements in individual primate species or groups of species, the narrow margin of safety of vitamin D in diets for humans[93] and many other species[90] argues against excessive use.

Hunt and coworkers[55] found that fibrous osteodystrophy developed in adult white-fronted capuchins fed purified diets containing 0.8% calcium, 0.46% phosphorus, 12,500 IU vitamin A/kg, and 2000 IU vitamin D$_2$/kg for 2 years. The monkeys were thin, inactive, had distorted limbs, exhibited kyphosis, and had multiple fractures with no evidence of callus formation. Dietary vitamin D$_2$ was replaced with 2000 IU vitamin D$_3$/kg for 5 months. The monkeys improved in appearance and became more active. Previous fractures became resistant to movement, and callus formation was evident radiographically. These workers fed adult cotton-top tamarins (*Saguinus oedipus*), white-lipped tamarins (*Saguinus nigricollis*), and black-chested mustached tamarins (*Saguinus mystax*) a commercial primate diet containing 2200 IU vitamin D_2/kg for 8 to 12 months and observed deficiency signs that were similar but less severe than those exhibited by the capuchins. Healing was initiated by offering 500 IU vitamin D_3 per animal per week. These authors reported anecdotally that they had seen fibrous osteodystrophy in squirrel monkeys fed vitamin D_2, but not in squirrel monkeys or wooly monkeys (*Lagothrix* species) fed vitamin D_3 or exposed to sunlight. They also stated that thousands of rhesus macaques and other *Macaca* species had been fed diets containing only vitamin D_2 without evidence of metabolic bone disease. No information on dietary nutrient concentrations or husbandry was provided.

Vickers[116] described osteomalacia and rickets in capuchins fed a commercial monkey diet containing vitamin D_2 and noted that vitamin D injections (form unspecified) or 2200 IU of vitamin D_3/kg of diet would reverse the disease. Lehner and associates[70, 71] observed bone lesions in squirrel monkeys fed diets containing vitamin D_2 that regressed when vitamin D_3 was substituted for vitamin D_2. These lesions could not be prevented by 10,000 IU of vitamin D_2/kg of diet, whereas as little as 1250 IU (the lowest level tested) of vitamin D_3/kg of diet was effective.

A study was conducted with the objective of studying vitamin E deficiency in juvenile Old World (crab-eating macaque [*Macaca fascicularis*]) and New World (capuchins [*C. albifrons, C. apella*]) monkeys.[7] A purified diet supplying 1000 IU vitamin D_3/kg fed for 2 years resulted in normal growth without evidence of bone lesions in any species.

Rickets has been described in a Bolivian red howler (*Alouatta seniculus*) infant born in an exhibit without sunlight exposure or an artificial UVB light source.[114] The mother was fed a commercial primate diet containing vitamin D_3 plus various fruits and vegetables. The primate diet was not relished, and limited amounts were consumed. The infant nursed exclusively for 5 months, ate little solid food subsequently, and did not choose vitamin D–containing items. The infant howler gradually became less agile, had difficulty grasping its mother, and frequently fell from climbing structures. Radiologic examination revealed deformed and broken bones, as shown in Figure 11–2, and the infant died. Vitamin D_2 concentrations in the plant material consumed by the mother were not available, but even if present, the biologic activity of this form would be limited. Furthermore, if vitamin D_3 intakes were restricted because of poor acceptance of the commercial primate diet, the concentration of this vitamin in the mother's milk may have been low, as it would have been in the milk of humans and cows.

Signs similar to those in the red howler infant also have been seen in juvenile colobus monkeys (*Colobus guereza kikuyuensis*) housed with their mothers in enclosures without UVB exposure.[82] Clinical signs were pronounced in a 10-month-old colobus and included hypocalcemia and hypophosphatemia, reduced activity, and difficulty in climbing, walking, and grasping its

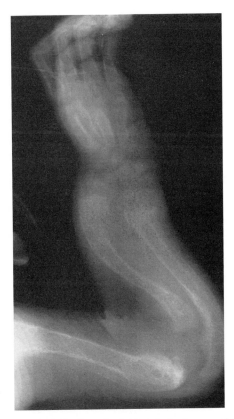

FIGURE 11–2. Radiograph of rickets in the forearm of a nursing Bolivian red howler monkey without solar or artificial ultraviolet light exposure.

mother. Appendicular joints were lax and swollen, and long bones were bowed. Radiographic changes included cupping of the metaphyses, widening of the epiphyseal plates, and thinning of the cortices. Fractures of the distal femoral epiphyses were seen bilaterally. Some bones exhibited fibrous osteodystrophy, and serum alkaline phosphatase activities were elevated. Serum 25[OH]D concentrations were less than the analytical limit of detection (<10 ng/ml). Because of the severity of the lesions, this animal was euthanized. A 6-month-old colobus exhibiting most of the above signs, but of less severity, was injected intramuscularly with 30,000 IU vitamin D_2 in a slow-release suspension, administered weekly for 8 weeks. Improvement in motor skills was noted within 1 week, and increased epiphyseal plate bone density was apparent radiologically at 4 and 8 weeks. One year later, serum 25[OH]D concentration was 13 ng/ml, and radiographs were normal. A 2-month-old colobus exhibiting no obvious clinical signs but having joint laxity and enlargement plus radiographic changes was injected intramuscularly with 15,000 IU vitamin D_2 in a slow-release suspension on two occasions, 1 week apart. It was then moved to an enclosure receiving unfiltered sunlight. At 4 weeks, radiographs were normal, and at 1 year, serum 25[OH]D concentration was 19 ng/ml.

The lactating females, from which these infants were

nursing, received a diet containing about 1500 IU vitamin D_3/kg dry matter and exhibited no signs of vitamin D deficiency. When housed previously in enclosures with direct access to sunlight, no signs of vitamin D deficiency had been seen in adults or in infants. Although colobus milk was not analyzed for vitamin D or its metabolites, it is suspected that it was low in these compounds. Thus, infant colobus that nurse exclusively for many months or eat little vitamin D–containing solid food would be at particular risk of deficiency in the absence of sunlight or artificial UVB irradiation.

Subsequent to the described cases of rickets in colobus, UVB-transmitting skylights (Solacryl SUVT, Polycast Corp.) were installed in the exhibit. Since that installation, an infant colobus has been raised to 2 years of age with no clinical signs of rickets.

An attempt has been made to establish serum norms for 25[OH]D in cotton-top tamarins so that incipient vitamin D deficiency might be detected before the appearance of clinical disease.[102] Blood was collected from 18 wild cotton-top tamarins in Colombia, South America. The mean serum concentration of 25[OH]D was 76 ng/ml with a range of 25 to 120 ng/ml. Juveniles had a higher mean value (95 ng/ml) than adults (69 ng/ml), and the mean value in nonpregnant females was higher (88 ng/ml) than in pregnant females (53 ng/ml). Power and colleagues[102] suggested that their unpublished data and those of Shinki and associates[108] and Yamaguchi and coworkers[124] infer a high probability of acute bone problems in captive common marmosets when serum 25[OH]D concentrations are less than 20 ng/ml.

The range of serum 25[OH]D values reported by other researchers in captive callitrichids is wide, with a concentration as high as 600 ng/ml in a common marmoset.[124] Five-fold higher plasma $1,25[OH]_2D_3$ concentrations have been reported in a New World species than in an Old World species, and an end-organ resistance to this hormone has been inferred.[1, 108] Gacad and Adams[32] used a B-lymphoblastoid cell line from the common marmoset in an in vitro study and found that the rank order of steroid binding was as follows: $25[OH]D_3 > 1,25[OH]_2D_3 \geq$ estradiol = progesterone = testosterone. However, the binding factor was a 58-kD protein, distinct from the nuclear $1,25[OH]_2D_3$ receptor, and had two to three orders of magnitude less affinity for $1,25[OH]_2D_3$. The functions of this binding protein are unknown, but the authors speculated that it would be useful in intercepting high levels of vitamin D metabolites, such as $1,25[OH]_2D_3$ glycosides from plants that coevolved in the same geographic region (e.g., as in *S. glaucophyllum*), or nonvitamin D steroids that might otherwise be harmful. Considering what is known of the dietary habits of the common marmoset, consumption of *S. glaucophyllum* by this primate seems unlikely. A nocturnal New World primate, the night monkey also exhibits this binding protein, but at a much lower level.

It is common for captive New World primates to be fed much higher dietary vitamin D_3 levels than Old World primates. Marmosets and tamarins are often fed commercial diets containing 7000 to 22,000 IU vitamin D_3/kg dry matter. Whether such high values are necessary needs to be established. Such high vitamin D levels may produce signs of hypervitaminosis D in Old World primates[64] and frank toxicity in pacas (*Cuniculus paca*) and agoutis (*Dasyprocta aguti*) that consume primate diets dropped on the floor of multispecies exhibits containing New World primates.[63]

REPTILES

Metabolic bone disease is one of the most common disorders seen in green iguanas (*Iguana iguana*).[5, 29] Anorexia, paraplegia, apparent thickening of the limbs, and softening and increased flexibility of long bones may be evident. Radiographic evidence of fractures, fibrous osteodystrophy, thin bone cortices, wide osteoid seams, poorly mineralized trabeculae, and hypocalcemic tetany may be seen in advanced cases or at necropsy.

Studies with green iguanas at the National Zoological Park, Washington, D.C.,[10] revealed that diets formulated to contain 1.4% calcium, 0.7% phosphorus, and 2000 IU vitamin D_3/kg did not support normal calcium metabolism. Some animals died and were found at necropsy to have soft tissue calcification, signs that have been seen in vitamin D toxicity in mammals and birds. Similar signs have been reported by Wallach[118] and a diagnosis of hypervitaminosis D made in green iguanas fed fresh vegetables and greens with a vitamin and mineral supplement. However, the dietary, medical, and pathologic records were not sufficiently quantitative to justify the diagnosis. The vitamin D concentration of the diet used at the National Zoological Park was confirmed both by chemical analysis and rat bioassay, and although levels of vitamin D were higher than in the usual diets formulated for domestic livestock and poultry, it seemed unlikely that vitamin D toxicity should result. Further examination revealed that plasma $25[OH]D_3$ concentrations were less than 5 ng/ml, compared to a mean of 150 ng/ml (highest > 400 ng/ml) in the plasma of captive iguanas kept outdoors in Costa Rica. Radiographs revealed a high incidence of long bone fractures, and these bones were reduced in ash and calcium. Retrospective examination of plasma calcium levels revealed that they were highly variable compared to the narrow range seen in male iguanas in Costa Rica. Thus, it appeared that these iguanas had limited ability to use dietary vitamin D_3. Subsequent exposure of some of these iguanas to a Sylvania fluorescent lamp containing 35% 2096 phosphor and 65% daylight phosphor for 12 hr/day resulted in plasma $25[OH]D_3$ concentrations of 300 to 500 ng/ml. These iguanas were able to regulate their distance from the lamp from 5 to 70 cm, but they were provided no shaded area.

An additional study was conducted with hatchling green iguanas that had been fed a diet containing 1.5% calcium, 0.7% phosphorus, and 2000 IU vitamin D_3/kg dry matter but without exposure to UVB light for 6 months.[9] At the end of that period, there was clinical and radiologic evidence of rickets in all the iguanas, and they were assigned to either a single oral dose of vitamin D_3 suspended in corn oil (8.5 IU/g body weight) plus 12 hr/day of exposure to GE Cool White fluorescent lamps or to 12 hr/day of exposure to a fluorescent Sylvania Experimental Reptile lamp. All lamps were mounted 61 cm above the floor of the reptile enclosures, allowing the iguanas to regulate their distance between 30 and 61 cm, but there was no completely shaded area. Mean daily dietary dry matter intake was 0.7% of body weight. Thus, the single oral dose provided the equivalent of more than 1,200,000 IU of vitamin D_3/kg of dietary dry matter or the amount of vitamin D_3 that would have been consumed in 600 days by the iguanas exposed to the UVB-emitting Sylvania Experimental Reptile lamp (assuming no change in absolute daily intake). Mean serum 25[OH]D concentrations on day 0 were 18 and 15 ng/ml for the oral dose and UVB lamp treatments, respectively, and were not different. On day 7, the respective values had increased to 184 and 136 ng/ml but were still not different. On day 21, serum 25[OH]D concentrations had declined to 141 ng/ml for the oral dose treatment and had continued to increase to 412 ng/ml for the UVB lamp treatment. This difference was statistically significant ($p<0.005$) and remained so at day 35, when respective serum 25[OH]D concentrations were 68 and 424 ng/ml. Bone mineral content increased in both groups as estimated by radiographic bone densitometry, and callus formation was seen in the region of radiologically defined fractures and in other bone regions where there may have been microfractures that could not be visualized by radiography. However, there was no evidence of soft tissue mineralization, nor was there any evidence of ocular or cutaneous pathology, as determined by ophthalmologic and histologic examination. Whereas a single massive oral dose of vitamin D_3 resulted in some absorption, the amount retained was not sufficient to sustain "normal" serum 25[OH]D concentrations to 5 weeks. It seems unlikely that dietary concentrations of vitamin D_3 considered safe for animals with known dietary requirements would be sufficient to meet the vitamin D needs of green iguanas. If, in fact, those needs can be met by diet, definition of the dietary requirement awaits further research.

When green iguanas were housed in indoor multispecies exhibits (18-foot ceilings with tropical plantings) at the National Zoological Park, which included 12 hours of illumination per day from weak UVB-emitting lamps (GE Chroma 50) mounted on the ceiling, some of the iguanas exhibited lethargy, anorexia, and loss of ability to cling to perches.[106] At necropsy, widespread soft tissue mineralization was observed, suggestive of vitamin D toxicity in mammals. The presence of broken bones was initially attributed to the trauma of falling. However, serum levels of 25[OH]D_3 in the surviving iguanas ranged from 7 to 36 ng/ml, very low compared to the greater than 400 ng/ml level found in healthy iguanas housed outdoors at the Honolulu Zoo, Honolulu, Hawaii. It appeared that affected iguanas may have chosen to live in territories remote from or not illuminated by the lamps. As a consequence, even though the iguana diet contained about 3000 IU vitamin D_3/kg, neither the diet nor UVB exposure was sufficient to meet vitamin D needs.[5] It was concluded that it is not appropriate to assume that soft tissue calcification, without other evidence, is pathognomonic of vitamin D toxicity (see discussion by Feldman[26] and Kenny et al.[63]).

The distance between the iguanas and the lamps may have been critical. The amount of radiant energy reaching a subject is inversely related to the square of the distance from the source. When weak UVB emitters (GE Chroma 50 or GE Chroma 50 plus GE BL 40 black lights) on a 12-hours light, 12-hours dark schedule were mounted no more than 46 cm from the bottom of cages containing green iguanas, the animals were healthy and had serum 25[OH]D_3 levels of more than 225 ng/ml.[3]

The conversion of previtamin D_3 to vitamin D_3 in the skin of reptiles is temperature dependent, as demonstrated in the savanna monitor lizard (*Varanus exanthomaticus*)[113] and the green iguana.[47] When green iguana skin was incubated in vitro at temperatures of 5°C and 25°C, the time required for a 50% conversion of previtamin D_3 to vitamin D_3 was 72 hours and 8 hours, respectively. Thus, the location and use of basking sites may influence this process. It has been suggested that the panther chameleon (*Chamaeleo pardalis*) may select basking sites on the basis of need for UVB.[59, 60] A natural solar basking site would provide both UVB and warmth. In an artificial environment using fluorescent lamps that are both cool and weak UVB emitters, it may be helpful to encourage basking in proximity to the lamps by locating a heat source in the immediate vicinity. Cutaneous conversion of 7-dehydrocholesterol to previtamin D_3 would be promoted by the UVB, and thermal isomerization of previtamin D_3 to vitamin D_3 would be promoted by the heat source.

Leopard geckos (*Eublepharus macularius*) developed normally even when the diet was the only source of vitamin D_3, but day geckos (*Phelsuma madagascariensis*) and Komodo dragons (*Varanus komodoensis*) required UV light for normal bone structure and calcium metabolism.[3] In a second study of 255 days,[5] leopard geckos fed crickets containing about 0.85% calcium and 720 IU vitamin D_3/kg (dry basis) had well-developed, well-mineralized bones, in the absence of UVB exposure. These nutrient concentrations are not typical for crickets but were achieved by maintaining them on diets containing about 8% calcium and 70,000 IU vitamin D_3/kg for 48 to 72 hours before they were fed to the geckos.[2, 4] The day geckos fed these fortified crickets, without UVB exposure, grew poorly, did not survive beyond 110 days, and had soft pliable bones at necropsy. Thus, there seems to be a fundamental difference in vitamin D metabolism between this basking species and the nocturnal leopard gecko.

The insectivorous, heliophilic lizard *Sceloporus occidentalis* appeared not to require UVB irradiation in a 10-week study, but the data were equivocal.[34]

Vitamin D metabolism in chelonians is poorly understood. It has been found that the thyroxin-binding protein in plasma of the turtle *Trachemys scripta* also is the DBP.[73, 74]

Adult desert tortoises (*Gopherus agassizii*) housed in outdoor pens in the Mojave desert at the Desert Tortoise Conservation Center, Las Vegas, NV, had a mean serum 25[OH]D concentration of 8.2 ng/ml ($n=14$), with a range of less than 5 ng/ml ($n=3$) to 16.5 ng/ml ($n=1$) (Bernard and Oftedal, unpublished). Juvenile desert tortoises and African spurred tortoises (*Geochelone sulcata*) housed indoors and fed diets containing about 2000 IU vitamin D_3/kg had serum concentrations of 25[OH]D that were less than 5 ng/ml without evidence of pathology.[9] When the juvenile desert tortoises were orally dosed with 20,000 IU each of vitamin D_2 and vitamin D_3, or when the juvenile African spurred tortoises were orally dosed with 8.5 IU of vitamin D_3/g body weight, there were no measurable responses in serum concentrations of 25[OH]D.

OTHER SPECIES

Early studies suggested that domestic chickens discriminate against vitamin D_2 (10% the activity of vitamin D_3),[95] whereas other farm animals do not. Studies have established that the domestic pig, cow, and horse also discriminate against vitamin D_2, but not to the same extent as the chicken. The mechanism of discrimination is still a subject of debate. However, Horst and colleagues[49] developed data suggesting that discrimination may be a consequence of enhanced clearance of 25[OH]D_2 and 1,25[OH]$_2D_2$ as well as lower absorption of vitamin D_2 from the intestine.

Differences in plasma concentrations of vitamin D metabolites have been found among a variety of species.[49] The low concentrations of 25[OH]D found in the horse and rabbit appear related to the unique manner in which these species regulate calcium metabolism. Unlike other species that modulate calcium absorption in the intestine, horses and rabbits appear to modulate calcium excretion by the kidney. Calcium excretion in urine is positively correlated with dietary calcium consumption, and horses and rabbits appear to have a very low requirement for vitamin D, although El Shorafa and associates[25] described rickets in juvenile ponies that were deprived of sunlight and dietary vitamin D for 5 months.

Mole rats (*Heterocephalus glaber* and *Cryptomys damarensis*) also have very low or undetectable serum concentrations of 25[OH]D (<5 ng/ml),[15, 16] and sunlight exposure of the damara mole rat (*C. damarensis*) or oral dosing of either mole rat species with vitamin D_3 had no effect on calcium and inorganic phosphorus balance,[17, 101] although serum 25[OH]D_3 and 1,25[OH]$_2D_3$ concentrations did increase. Mole rats appear to have no vitamin D receptors in the skin, but 1,25[OH]$_2D_3$ receptors are present in the intestine and kidneys.[107] No source of vitamin D has been found in the wild for the damara mole rat.[109] Nevertheless, dietary calcium absorption may range from 86% to 97%, with the excess excreted in the urine.[100] However, the naked mole rat (*H. glaber*) had lower fecundity when fed a vitamin D–deficient diet in captivity.[14]

Amphibians that have been studied appear to require vitamin D,[19] and the toad *Xenopus laevis* transports cholecalciferol and 25[OH]D_3 attached to alpha-lipoproteins.[24] Skin of the frog *Rana temporaria* at 25°C in vitro, converted previtamin D_3 to vitamin D_3 as efficiently as green iguana skin or human skin.[47]

Vitamin D Toxicity

Although several farm animal species have been shown to tolerate high short-term dietary intakes of vitamin D_3, the safe upper levels for periods of exposure greater than 60 days may, in many instances, be only 4 to 10 times the minimal dietary requirement.[90] Toxicity has been demonstrated in children consuming 45 μg (1800 IU) vitamin D_3/day and who have a recommended dietary allowance of 10 μg (400 IU) vitamin D_3/day.[93] Because 10 μg (400 IU) of vitamin D_3 would be supplied by 1 quart of milk, fortified at current levels, it is clear that inappropriate use of supplements can lead to toxicity. The issue is greatly complicated by current limited knowledge of the needs of most species found in the zoo.

Excess dietary or parenteral vitamin D tends to increase serum 25[OH]D and promotes increased calcium and phosphorus absorption, increased bone resorption, systemic alkalosis, elevated serum phosphorus, hypercalcemia, soft tissue calcification, hypercalciuria, and nephrolithiasis. The signs and their severity vary with species and circumstances, such as the type of vitamin D (D_2 or D_3), size of the dose, route and period of administration, and other components of the diet (e.g., high vitamin A reduces toxicity). Treatment should include immediate withdrawal of vitamin D, but the extended half-life of plasma 25[OH]D_3 may delay a response. A prompt reduction in dietary calcium helps relieve the hypercalcemia. Other medical measures also have been used.[63, 90]

Daily oral doses of 50,000 to 100,000 IU of vitamin D_3 produced hypervitaminosis D in squirrel monkeys and white-fronted capuchins, whereas similar amounts of vitamin D_2 did not.[57] The syndrome in squirrel monkeys included hypercalcemia, hyperphosphatemia, uremia, and death within 20 to 55 days, with no significant metastatic calcification and minimal nephrocalcinosis. The capuchins died within 52 to 89 days and exhibited widespread metastatic calcification, including mineralization in the kidneys, aorta, lung, myocardium, stomach, and various tissue arteries and arterioles. Bone lesions were not seen in either species.

When daily oral doses of 50,000 to 200,000 IU of vitamin D_3 were given to rhesus monkeys, hypercalcemia developed and the monkeys died within 16 to 160 days; nephrocalcinosis was apparent at necropsy.[58] The same dosages of vitamin D_2 to rhesus monkeys produced no deaths, although hypercalcemia was seen without soft tissue calcification.

Rhesus monkeys fed a commercial primate diet containing 6600 IU vitamin D_3/kg (furnishing 1000 to 1200 IU/day) had normal serum concentrations of calcium, inorganic phosphorus, and PTH, but serum 25[OH]D concentrations were considered high (mean ± SD, 188 ± 94 ng/ml).[6]

Free-ranging rhesus monkeys, maintained on Cayo Santiago by the Caribbean Primate Research Center in Puerto Rico, were fed a commercial high-protein monkey diet containing 8200 IU vitamin D_3/kg to complement wild foods.[117] However, the monkey density was so high that this commercial diet comprised most of their food. Sera from 48 monkeys (six from each sex in each of four age classes) were analyzed for 25[OH]D. Group means ranged from 143 to 230 ng/ml and were considered high. Serum concentrations of 1,25[OH]$_2$D were variable but also very high, and the authors suggested that, if the higher concentrations of this metabolite were sustained in individual monkeys, changes could occur in calcium and phosphorus metabolism that might partially explain the incidence of calcium pyrophosphate dihydrate crystal deposition arthropathy in this colony.

A study of the differences between four species of nonhuman primates in their response to vitamin D_2 and vitamin D_3 included a comparison of serum 25[OH]D concentrations.[76] Consumption of a commercial diet containing 6000 to 6600 IU vitamin D_3/kg resulted in mean 25[OH]D values of 96, 144, 88, and 148 ng/ml in the serum of crab-eating macaques, rhesus macaques, night monkeys, and squirrel monkeys, respectively. After transfer to a diet containing 1500 IU vitamin D_3/kg for 5 months, respective serum 25[OH]D concentrations were 44, 68, 56, and 60 ng/ml. There was no hypercalcemia, parathormone suppression, or azotemia, which would be suggestive of hypervitaminosis D, on the commercial diet, but, based on the lack of biochemical and histologic evidence of vitamin D deficiency in rhesus macaques fed diets containing 1500 IU of vitamin D_2 or vitamin D_3/kg, the researchers suggested that the commercial diet providing 6000 to 6600 IU vitamin D_3/kg was providing excessive amounts of this nutrient for this species.

Gray and coworkers[35] offered brown lemurs (*Lemur fulvus*) a commercial diet containing 6600 IU vitamin D_3/kg plus fresh fruit, and a "supplement" containing oats, soy flour, eggs, wheat germ, evaporated milk, sugar, and bananas. Mean serum calcium concentrations were 10.6 mg/dl, and mean serum 25[OH]D concentrations were about 29 ng/ml. Because of the opportunity to make variable food choices, it was not possible to directly relate diet composition to biochemical measures in individuals that appeared to be outside a normal range. Nevertheless, the researchers suggested that some lemurs were hypercalcemic and had elevated levels of 25[OH]D and 1,25[OH]$_2$D, possibly because of episodic intoxication with vitamin D from the commercial diet.

Pacas (*C. paca*) and agoutis (*D. aguti*), housed in mixed-species exhibits at three zoos, died with extensive soft tissue mineralization, including mineralization in the kidneys, which led to renal failure.[63] New World primates shared the exhibits, and zoo personnel reported that dropped primate diets had been consumed by the affected animals. Data supplied by the manufacturers of these diets indicated that they contained from 7000 to 22,000 IU vitamin D_3/kg dry matter. Analyses of blood from four moribund pacas revealed reduced packed red cell volume and elevations in serum calcium, inorganic phosphorus, urea nitrogen, and creatinine. Histologic examination of affected paca tissues confirmed extensive mineralization of the kidneys, heart, major blood vessels, stomach, intestinal tract, liver, spleen, and skeletal muscle. Serum vitamin D metabolites were not analyzed, but a provisional diagnosis of vitamin D toxicity was made.

MEETING NEEDS

In nature, animals appear to have evolved different strategies for meeting their vitamin D needs, dependent upon the environment in which they live, their food selections, and other aspects of their behavior. Those with regular exposure to the sun have the potential options of getting vitamin D from cutaneous photobiogenesis or from their food. Some species, such as most farm animals, appear able to do both. Animals that sunbask, such as green iguanas, day geckos, and Komodo dragons seem very dependent upon UVB irradiation, even when fed dietary vitamin D concentrations that are adequate for other species. Carnivores, such as the domestic dog and cat, whose natural diet would include animal tissues high in vitamin D, have largely lost the ability to produce vitamin D by cutaneous photobiogenesis. Nocturnal animals and animals living underground must derive vitamin D needs from their diets or may have no vitamin D requirement at all.

When animals are confined in zoos and aquariums, consideration must be given to the special needs that are a result of their evolutionary history. Modern exhibits include design features that make them appear natural to the general public, and a visit to a zoo or aquarium is a much more esthetically pleasing experience than in the days of barred cages and bare aquarium tanks. Nevertheless, the restrictions of space and funding make it virtually impossible to simulate an ecosystem exactly. The issue is complicated further by exhibiting animals at latitudes far removed from their natural habitat. Tropical animals that are exhibited in temperate regions may require inside housing much of the year because of low tolerance to cold and the dangers of ice underfoot. Arctic animals exhibited in tropical and subtropical regions may require inside housing because of low tolerance to heat. For those animals that use dietary vitamin D sources, such confinement poses little problem. However, for those that depend on solar irradiance, including UVB, special accommodations must be made.

The most certain means of providing the UVB wavelengths required for cutaneous biogenesis of vitamin D is to provide solar exposure in an exhibit that includes an outdoor area or that incorporates UVB-transmitting plastic (such as Solacryl SUVT) into walls or roofs of the exhibit building. An alternative would be use of UVB-emitting lamps in the exhibit. However, most commercially available fluorescent lamps emit no or very little UVB. Although not likely to be entirely satisfactory, because of unnatural color rendition, a two-lamp fixture equipped with a Sylvania Design 50 and a Sylvania 350 Blacklight offers some theoretic advantage for use in a basking area to which animals are attracted by heat or other exhibit design features.

Although some zoo and aquarium animals are known to use dietary vitamin D, quantitative requirements have been estimated only for a few primates. Extrapolation of requirements for other nutrients from data on related species has previously proven useful, and authors of the National Research Council Nutrient Requirement series[87–89, 91, 92, 95–97] concluded that domesticated farm animals, dogs, cats, and laboratory animals (total of 18 species of mammals and birds) have a dietary vitamin D requirement in the range of 200 to 1200 IU/kg dry matter. Some of the values are estimates, based upon evidence that they are sufficient but without evidence that they represent minimal need. Proposed vitamin D requirements for rainbow trout range from 1600 to 2400 but are 250 to 1000 IU/kg dietary dry matter for channel catfish.[94] Most of the above requirement estimates were based on use of vitamin D[3], although in some cases, the form of vitamin D was not identified.

The work of Lehner and associates[71] made it clear that the form of vitamin D used in setting the requirement is important when they found that 1250 IU of vitamin D[3]/kg diet was adequate for growing squirrel monkeys, whereas 10,000 IU of vitamin D[2]/kg of diet was not. The National Research Council[86] recommended 2000 IU vitamin D[3]/kg diet (presumably 90% dry matter) for nonhuman primates, and the research of Flurer and Zucker[28] indicated that this was optimal for Callitricidae. However, unpublished observations that 3000 IU vitamin D[3]/kg dietary dry matter may not maintain bone mineralization in multiparous female common marmosets have been reported.[5] Much more research is needed to set vitamin D requirements for primates with certainty, and interrelationships between vitamin D and the supply and bioavailability of dietary calcium and phosphorus also must be considered.

Commercial primate diets vary widely in their specified vitamin D concentrations, with stated values for "complete" diets ranging from 1200 to 22,000 IU/kg dry matter. Products marketed for New World primates are generally higher than those for Old World primates, with the former commonly containing 7000 to 22,000 IU vitamin D[3]/kg dry matter whereas the latter contains commonly 7000 IU vitamin D[3]/kg dry matter or less. A dry flavored powder containing gelatin, to be mixed with water, cooled, and allowed to gel, is marketed for marmosets. Product specifications state that it contains 30,000 IU vitamin D[3]/kg dry product. Inappropriate use of some of these products could lead to toxicity both in primates and in other animals sharing a multispecies exhibit.

For the species for which there is no information, vitamin D needs can only be speculated upon. Large numbers of psittacines and passerines have been raised in confinement on diets providing 2000 IU vitamin D[3]/kg or less. Ruminant animals and terrestrial hindgut fermenting animals typically consume sun-cured hays and vitamin D–fortified pellets, but frequently have some access to the sun. Carnivores are fed diets containing animal tissues that supply vitamin D, and these diets often are fortified further. Some insectivorous animals (tarsiers [*Tarsius* species] and certain reptiles) benefit when food insects, such as crickets, are allowed access to high calcium, high vitamin D insect diets before they are consumed as food. Reptiles and amphibians exhibit some unique features of calcium regulation,[19] and, for some, solar irradiance is vital and dietary vitamin D is unimportant.

Based on the research to date and extrapolation from known values in domestic species, it seems likely that the vitamin D needs of most zoo and aquarium animals (that can use a dietary source) can be met by 2200 IU or less vitamin D[3]/kg dietary dry matter. Whether Callitrichids are an exception awaits further reports.

Routine additions of vitamin D supplements to diets

that are formulated to be nutritionally complete are not recommended because of the danger of toxicity. The incorporation of vitamin D supplements into mixtures of vitamin D–deficient foods that can be differentially selected may result in a range of problems from inadequate to excessive intakes of vitamin D. Prevention of vitamin D deficiency and intoxication, through thoughtful exhibit design, attention to nutrient requirements, and appropriate dietary husbandry, is likely to be significantly more successful than attempts at treatment.

REFERENCES

1. Adams JS, Gacad MA, Baker AJ, et al: Diminished internalization and action of 1,25-dihydroxyvitamin D[3] in dermal fibroblasts cultured from New World primates. Endocrinol 116:2523–2527, 1985.
2. Allen ME: Nutritional aspects of insectivory. Ph.D. dissertation, Michigan State University, 1989.
3. Allen ME, Bush M, Oftedal OT, et al: Update on vitamin D and ultraviolet light in basking lizards. Proceedings of the American Association of Zoo Veterinarians, Pittsburgh, pp 314–316, 1994.
4. Allen ME, Oftedal OT: Dietary manipulation of the calcium content of feed crickets. J Zoo Wildl Med 20:26–33, 1989.
5. Allen ME, Oftedal OT, Horst RL: Remarkable differences in the response to dietary vitamin D among species of reptiles and primates: is ultraviolet B light essential? *In* Holick MF, Jung EG (eds): Biologic Effects of Light 1995. Berlin, Walter de Gruyter, pp 13–30, 1995.
6. Arnaud SB, Young DR, Cann C, et al: Is hypervitaminosis D normal in the rhesus monkey? *In* Norman AW, Schaefer K, Grigoleit HG, et al (eds): Vitamin D: A Chemical, Biochemical and Clinical Update. Berlin, Walter de Gruyter, 1985, pp 585–586.
7. Ausman LM, Hayes KC: Vitamin E deficiency anemia in Old and New World monkeys. Am J Clin Nutr 27:1141–1151, 1974.
8. Bennett K (ed): The Compendium of Veterinary Products, 2nd Ed. Port Huron, MI, North American Compendium Inc., 1993.
9. Bernard JB: Spectral irradiance of fluorescent lamps and their efficacy for promoting vitamin D synthesis in herbivorous reptiles. Ph.D. dissertation, Michigan State University, 1995.
10. Bernard JB, Oftedal OT, Barboza PS, et al: The response of vitamin D-deficient green iguanas (*Iguana iguana*) to artificial ultraviolet light. Proceedings of the American Association of Zoo Veterinarians, Calgary, Alberta, pp 147–150, 1991.
11. Bernard JB, Watkins BE, Ullrey DE: Manifestations of vitamin D deficiency in chicks reared under different artificial lighting regimes. Zoo Biol 8:349–355, 1989.
12. Bills CE: Vitamin D. II. Chemistry. *In* Sebrell WH, Harris RS (eds): The Vitamins, vol 2. New York, Academic Press, pp 149–173, 1967.
13. Boland RL: Plants as a source of vitamin D[3] metabolites. Nutr Rev 44:1–8, 1986.
14. Buffenstein R, Jarvis JVM, Opperman LA: Vitamin D metabolism and expression in chthonic naked mole rats [Abstract]. J Bone Min Res 3:S119, 1988.
15. Buffenstein R, Sergeev IN, Pettifor JM: Vitamin D hydroxylases and their regulation in a naturally vitamin D-deficient subterranean mammal, the naked mole rat (*Heterocephalus glaber*). J Endocrinol 138:59–64, 1993.
16. Buffenstein R, Skinner DC, Yahav S, et al: Effect of oral cholecalciferol supplementation at physiological and supraphysiological doses in naturally vitamin-D deficient subterranean damara mole rats (*Cryptomys damarensis*). J Endocrinol 131:197–202, 1991.
17. Buffenstein R, Yahav S: Cholecalciferol has no effect on calcium and inorganic phosphorus balance in a naturally cholecalciferol-deplete subterranean mammal (the naked mole rat (*Heterocephalus glaber*). J Endocrinol 129:21–26, 1991.
18. Bullock BC, Bowen JA: Rickets and osteomalacia in squirrel monkeys [Abstract]. Fed Proc 25:533, 1966.
19. Dacke CG: Calcium Regulation in Sub-Mammalian Vertebrates. London, Academic Press, 1979.
20. DeLuca HF: The vitamin D story: a collaborative effort of basic science and clinical medicine. FASEB J 2:224–236, 1988.
21. Denniston PL Jr (ed): Physicians GenRx. Riverside, CT, Denniston Publishing, 1995.

22. Devgun MS, Patterson CR, Cohen C, et al: Possible value of fluorescent lighting in the prevention of vitamin D deficiency in the elderly. Age Aging 9:117–120, 1980.
23. Edelstein S: Vitamin D binding proteins. *In* Harris RS, Diczfalusy E, Munson PL, et al (eds): Vitamins and Hormones, vol 32. New York, Academic Press, pp 407–428, 1974.
24. Edelstein S, Lawson DEM, Kodicek E: The transporting proteins of cholecalciferol and 25-hydroxycholecalciferol in serum of chicks and other species. Biochem J 135:417–426, 1973.
25. El Shorafa WM, Feaster JP, Ott EA, et al: Effect of vitamin D and sunlight on growth and bone development of young ponies. J Anim Sci 48:882–886, 1979.
26. Feldman F: Soft tissue mineralization: roentgen analysis. Curr Probl Diagnostic Radiol 15:161–240, 1986.
27. Fiennes RN: Problems of rickets in monkeys and apes. Proc R Soc Med 67:309–314, 1974.
28. Flurer CI, Zucker H: Evaluation of serum parameters relevant to vitamin D status in tamarins. J Med Primatol 16:175–184, 1987.
29. Fowler ME: Metabolic bone disease. *In* Fowler ME (ed): Philadelphia, WB Saunders, pp 69–90, 1986.
30. Frederick JE, Snell HE, Haywood EK: Solar ultraviolet radiation at the earth's surface. Photochem Photobiol 50:443–450, 1989.
31. Freedman MT, Bush M, Novak GR, et al: Nutritional and metabolic bone disease in a zoological population: a review of radiologic findings. Skeletal Radiol 1:87–96, 1976.
32. Gacad MA, Adams JS: Specificity of steroid binding in New World primate B95-8 cells with a vitamin D-resistant phenotype. Endocrinol 131:2581–2587, 1992.
33. Gehrmann WH: Ultraviolet irradiances of various lamps used in animal husbandry. Zoo Biol 6:117–127, 1987.
34. Gehrmann WH, Ferguson GW, Odom TW, et al: Early growth and bone mineralization of the iguanid lizard, *Sceloporus occidentalis* in captivity: is vitamin D_3 supplementation or ultraviolet B irradiation necessary? Zoo Biol 10:409–416, 1991.
35. Gray TK, Lester GE, Moore G, et al: Serum concentrations of calcium and vitamin D metabolites in prosimians. J Med Primatol 11:85–90, 1982.
36. Green AES, Cross KR, Smith LA: Improved analytical characterization of ultraviolet skylight. Photochem Photobiol 31:59–65, 1980.
37. Halloran BP, DeLuca HF: Effect of vitamin D deficiency on fertility and reproductive capacity in the female rat. J Nutr 110:1573–1580, 1980.
38. Haussler MR, Wasserman RH, McCain TA, et al: 1,25-Dihydroxyvitamin D_3-glycoside: identification of a calcinogenic principle of *Solanum malacoxylon.* Life Sci 18:1049–1056, 1976.
39. Hay AWM, Watson G: The plasma transport proteins of 25-hydroxycholecalciferol in mammals. Comp Biochem Physiol 53B:163–166, 1976.
40. Hay AWM, Watson G: The plasma transport proteins of 25-hydroxycholecalciferol in fish, amphibians, reptiles and birds. Comp Biochem Physiol 53B:167–172, 1976.
41. Hay AWM, Watson G: Vitamin D_2 in vertebrate evolution. Comp Biochem Physiol 56B:375–380, 1977.
42. Hess A, Pappenheimer AM, Weinstock M: A study of light waves in relation to their protective action in rickets. Proc Soc Exp Biol Med 20:14–16, 1922.
43. Holick MF: Phylogenetic and evolutionary aspects of vitamin D from phytoplankton to humans. *In* Pang PKT, Schreibman MP (eds): Vertebrate Endocrinology. Fundamentals and Biomedical Implications. Orlando, FL, Academic Press, pp 7–43, 1989.
44. Holick M: The use and interpretation of assays for vitamin D and its metabolites. J Nutr 120:1464–1469, 1990.
45. Holick MF, Adams JS, Clemens TL: Photoendocrinology of vitamin D: the past, present and future. *In* Norman AW, Schaefer K, Herrath Dv, et al (eds): Vitamin D, Chemical, Biochemical and Clinical Endocrinology of Calcium Metabolism. Berlin, Walter de Gruyter, pp 1151–1156, 1982.
46. Holick MF, MacLaughlin JA, Doppelt SH: Regulation of cutaneous previtamin D_3 photosynthesis in man: skin pigment is not an essential regulator. Science 211:590–592, 1981.
47. Holick MF, Tian XQ, Allen M: Evolutionary importance for the membrane enhancement of the production of vitamin D_3 in the skin of poikilothermic animals. Proc Natl Acad Sci USA 92:3124–3126, 1995.
48. Hollis BW, Greer FR, Tsang RC: The effects of oral vitamin D supplementation and ultraviolet phototherapy on the antirachitic sterol content of human milk. Calcif Tissue Int 34(suppl):S52, 1982.
49. Horst RL, Koszewski NJ, Reinhardt TA: Species variation of vitamin D metabolism and action: lessons to be learned from animals. *In* Norman AW, Shaefer K, Grigoleit H-G, et al (eds): Vitamin D. Molecular, Cellular and Clinical Endocrinology. Berlin, Walter de Gruyter, pp 93–101, 1988.
50. Horst RL, Reinhardt TA, Russell JR, et al: The isolation and identification of vitamin D_2 and vitamin D_3 from *Medicago sativa* (alfalfa plant). Arch Biochem Biophys 231:67–71, 1984.
51. How KL, Hazewinkel HAW, Mol JA: Dietary vitamin D dependence of cat and dog due to inadequate cutaneous synthesis of vitamin D. General Comp Endocrinol 96:12–18, 1994.
52. Huldschinsky K: Heilung von Rachitis durch kuntsliche Hohensonne. Dtsch Med Wochenschr 14:712–713, 1919.
53. Human Nutrition Information Service: Provisional Table on the Vitamin D Content of Foods. Washington, DC, Nutrient Data Research Branch, Nutrition Monitoring Division, U.S. Department of Agriculture, 1991.
54. Hunt RD, Garcia FG, Hegsted DM: Vitamin D requirement of New World primates (abstr). Fed Proc 25:545, 1966.
55. Hunt RD, Garcia FG, Hegsted DM: A comparison of vitamin D_2 and D_3 in New World primates. I. Production and regression of osteodystrophia fibrosa. Lab Anim Care 17:222–234, 1967.
56. Hunt RD, Garcia FG, Hegsted DM, et al: Vitamin D_2 and D_3 in New World primates: influence on calcium absorption. Science 157:943–945, 1967.
57. Hunt RD, Garcia FG, Hegsted DM: Hypervitaminosis D in New World monkeys. Am J Clin Nutr 22:358–366, 1969.
58. Hunt RD, Garcia FG, Walsh RJ: A comparison of the toxicity of ergocalciferol and cholecalciferol in rhesus monkeys (*Macaca mulatta*). J Nutr 102:975–986, 1972.
59. Jones JR: Ultraviolet-B radiation and vitamin D in chameleon husbandry: an experimental study. Proceedings of the 19th Annual International Herpetological Symposium, Denver, 1995.
60. Jones JR, Ferguson GW, Gehrmann WH: Differential behavioral responses to ultraviolet light based on nutritional state regarding vitamin D. Proceedings of the 98th Annual Meeting of the Texas Academy of Sciences, Baylor University, 1995.
61. Kaufman JE, Christensen JF (eds): Light sources. *In* IES Lighting Handbook (Reference Volume). New York, Illuminating Engineering Society of North America, pp 8–1 to 8–68, 1984.
62. Keener HA: The effect of various factors on the vitamin D content of several common forages. J Dairy Sci 37:1337–1345, 1954.
63. Kenny D, Cambre RC, Lewandowski A, et al: Suspected vitamin D_3 toxicity in pacas (*Cuniculus paca*) and agoutis (*Dasyprocta aguti*). J Zoo Wildl Med 24:129–139, 1993.
64. Knapka JJ, Barnard DE, Bayne KAL, et al: Nutrition. *In* Bennett BT, Abee CR, Henrickson R (eds): Nonhuman Primates in Biomedical Research: Biology and Management. San Diego, Academic Press, pp 211–248, 1995.
65. Knudson A, Benford F: Quantitative studies of the effectiveness of ultraviolet radiation of various wavelengths in rickets. J Biol Chem 124:287–299, 1938.
66. Kobayashi T, Hirooka M, Yasumura M: Effect of wavelength on the ultraviolet irradiation of 7-dehydrocholesterol. Vitamins (Japan) 50:185–189, 1976.
67. Kobayashi T, Yasumura M: Studies on the ultraviolet irradiation of provitamin D and its related compounds: III. Effect of wavelength on the formation of potential vitamin D_2 in the irradiation of ergosterol by monochromatic ultraviolet rays. J Nutr Sci Vitaminol 19:123–128, 1973.
68. Krook L, Wasserman RH, McEntee K, et al: *Cestrum diurnum* poisoning in Florida cattle. Cornell Vet 65:557–575, 1975.
69. Kunz C, Niesen M, Lilienfeld-Toal HV, et al: Vitamin D, 25-hydroxy-vitamin D and 1,25-dihydroxy-vitamin D in cow's milk, infants formulas and breast milk during different stages of lactation. Int J Vit Nutr Res 54:141–148, 1984.
70. Lehner NDM, Bullock BC, Clarkson TB, et al: Biological activity of vitamins D_2 and D_3 fed to squirrel monkeys [Abstract]. Fed Proc 25:533, 1966.
71. Lehner DEM, Bullock BC, Clarkson TB, et al: Biological activity of vitamins D_2 and D_3 for growing squirrel monkeys. Lab Anim Care 17:483–493, 1967.
72. Lian JB, Carnes DL, Glimcher MJ: Bone and serum concentrations of osteocalcin as a function of 1,25-dihydroxyvitamin D_3 circulating levels in bone disorders in rats. Endocrinol 120:2123–2130, 1987.
73. Licht P: Thyroxine-binding protein represents the major vitamin D-binding protein in the plasma of the turtle, *Trachemys scripta.* Gen Comp Endocrinol 93:82–92, 1994.

74. Licht P, Moore MF: Structure of a reptilian plasma thyroxine-binding protein indicates homology to vitamin D-binding protein. Arch Biochem Biophys 309:47–51, 1994.

75. Logan T: Experiments with Gro-lux light and its effects on reptiles. Int Zoo Yrbk 9:9–11, 1969.

76. Marx SJ, Jones G, Weinstein RS, et al: Differences in mineral metabolism among nonhuman primates receiving diets with only vitamin D₃ or only vitamin D₂. J Clin Endocrinol Metab 69:1282–1290, 1989.

77. McKinlay AF: Artificial sources of UVA radiation: uses and emission characteristics. *In* Urbach F (ed): Biological Responses to Ultraviolet Radiation: A Symposium. Kansas City, Vandermor Publications, pp 19–38, 1992.

78. MacLaughlin JA, Anderson RR, Holick MF: Spectral character of sunlight modulates photosynthesis of previtamin D₃ and its photoisomers in human skin. Science 216:1001–1003, 1982.

79. McCollum EV, Simmonds N, Becker JE, et al: Studies on experimental rickets: XXI. An experimental demonstration of the existence of a vitamin which promotes calcium deposition. J Biol Chem 53:293–312, 1922.

80. Meehan TP, Crissey SD, Langman CB, et al: Vitamin D related disease in infant primates. Proceedings of the American Association of Zoo Veterinarians, Puerto Vallarta, Mexico, pp 91–93, 1996.

81. Miller RM: Nutritional secondary hyperparathyroidism in monkeys. *In* Kirk RW (ed): Current Veterinary Therapy IV. Philadelphia, WB Saunders, pp 407–408, 1971.

82. Morrisey JK, Reichard T, Lloyd M, et al: Vitamin D-deficiency rickets in three colobus monkeys (*Colobus guereza kikuyuensis*) at the Toledo Zoo. J Zoo Wildl Med 26:564–568, 1995.

83. Morrissey RL, Cohn RM, Empson RN Jr, et al: Relative toxicity and metabolic effects of cholecalciferol and 25-hydroxycholecalciferol. J Nutr 107:1027–1034, 1977.

84. Napoli JL, Reeve LE, Eisman JA, et al: *Solanum glaucophyllum* as a source of 1,25-dihydroxy vitamin D₃. J Biol Chem 252:2580–2583, 1977.

85. National Institute for Occupational Safety and Health: Criteria for a Recommended Standard.... Occupational Exposure to Ultraviolet Radiation. Washington, DC, US Department of Health, Education, and Welfare, 1972.

86. National Research Council: Nutrient Requirements of Nonhuman Primates. Washington, DC, National Academy Press, 1978.

87. National Research Council: Nutrient Requirements of Dogs. Washington, DC, National Academy Press, 1985.

88. National Research Council: Nutrient Requirements of Sheep. Washington, DC, National Academy Press, 1985.

89. National Research Council: Nutrient Requirements of Cats. Washington, DC, National Academy Press, 1986.

90. National Research Council: Vitamin Tolerance of Animals. Washington, DC, National Academy Press, 1987.

91. National Research Council: Nutrient Requirements of Dairy Cattle. Washington, DC, National Academy Press, 1989.

92. National Research Council: Nutrient Requirements of Horses. Washington, DC, National Academy Press, 1989.

93. National Research Council: Recommended Dietary Allowances. Washington, DC, National Academy Press, 1989.

94. National Research Council: Nutrient Requirements of Fish. Washington, DC, National Academy Press, 1993.

95. National Research Council: Nutrient Requirements of Poultry. Washington, DC, National Academy Press, 1994.

96. National Research Council: Nutrient Requirements of Laboratory Animals. Washington, DC, National Academy Press, 1995.

97. National Research Council: Nutrient Requirements of Beef Cattle. Washington, DC, National Academy Press, 1996.

98. Neer RM, Davis TRA, Walcott A, et al: Stimulation by artificial lighting of calcium absorption in elderly human subjects. Nature 229:255–257, 1971.

99. PDR: Physician's Desk Reference. Montvale, NJ, Medical Economics, 1996.

100. Pitcher T, Buffenstein R, Keegan JD, et al: Dietary calcium content, calcium balance and mode of uptake in a subterranean mammal, the damara mole-rat. J Nutr 122:108–114, 1991.

101. Pitcher T, Sergeev IN, Buffenstein R: Vitamin D metabolism in the damara mole rat is altered by exposure to sunlight yet mineral metabolism is unaffected. J Endocrinol 143:367–374, 1994.

102. Power ML, Oftedal OT, Savage A, et al: Assessing vitamin D status of callitrichids: baseline data from wild cotton-top tamarins (*Saguinus oedipus*) in Colombia. Zoo Biol 16:39–46, 1997.

103. Rambeck WA, Weiser H, Zucker H: A vitamin D₃ steroid hormone in the calcinogenic grass *Trisetum flavescens*. Z Naturforsch 42c:430–434, 1986.

104. Reeve LE, Jorgensen NA, DeLuca HF: Vitamin D compounds in cow's milk. J Nutr 112:667–672, 1982.

105. Reinhardt TA, Hustmyer FG: Role of vitamin D in the immune system. J Dairy Sci 70:952–962, 1987.

106. Richman LK, Montali RJ, Allen ME, et al: Paradoxical pathologic changes in vitamin D deficient green iguanas (*Iguana iguana*). Proceedings of the Joint Conference of the American Association of Zoo Veterinarians, Wildlife Disease Association, and American Association of Wildlife Veterinarians, East Lansing, MI, pp 231–232, 1995.

107. Sergeev IN, Buffenstein R, Pettifor JM: Vitamin D receptors in a naturally vitamin D-deficient subterranean mammal, the naked mole rat (*Heterocephalus glaber*): biochemical characterization. Gen Comp Endocrinol 90:338–345, 1993.

108. Shinki T, Shiina Y, Takahashi N, et al: Extremely high circulating levels of 1α,25-dihydroxyvitamin D₃ in the marmoset, a New World monkey. Biochem Biophys Res Commun 114:452–457, 1983.

109. Skinner DC, Moodly G, Buffenstein R: Is vitamin D₃ essential for mineral metabolism in the damara mole rat (*Cryptomys damarensis*)? Gen Comp Endocrinol 81:500–505, 1991.

110. Soares JH Jr, Kerr JM, Gray RW. 25-Hydroxycholecalciferol in poultry nutrition. Poultry Sci 74:1919–1934, 1995.

111. Takada K, Okano T, Tamura Y, et al: A rapid and precise method for the determination of vitamin D₃ in rat skin by high-performance liquid chromatography. J Nutr Sci Vitaminol 25:385–398, 1979.

112. Takeuchi A, Okano T, Tsugawa N, et al: Effects of ergocalciferol supplementation on the concentration of vitamin D and its metabolites in human milk. J Nutr 119:1639–1646, 1989.

113. Tian XQ, Chen TC, Allen M, et al: Photosynthesis of previtamin D₃ and its isomerization to vitamin D₃ in the *Savanna monitor* lizard. *In* Norman AW, Bouillon R, Thomasset M (eds): Vitamin D, a Pluripotent Steroid Hormone: Structural Studies, Molecular Endocrinology and Clinical Applications. Berlin, Walter de Gruyter, pp 893–894, 1994.

114. Ullrey DE: Nutrition of primates in captivity. *In* Benirschke K (ed): Primates: The Road to Self-Sustaining Populations. New York, Springer-Verlag, pp 823–835, 1986.

115. USP/NF: The United States Pharmacopeia, 23rd ed (The National Formulary, 18th ed). Rockville, MD, United States Pharmacopeial Convention, Inc., 1995.

116. Vickers JH: Osteomalacia and rickets in monkeys. *In* Kirk RW (ed): Current Veterinary Therapy III. Philadelphia, WB Saunders, pp 392–393, 1968.

117. Vieth R, Kessler MJ, Pritzker KPH: Serum concentrations of vitamin D metabolites in Cayo Santiago rhesus macaques. J Med Primatol 16:349–357, 1987.

118. Wallach JD: Hypervitaminosis D in green iguanas. J Am Vet Med Assoc 149:912–914, 1966.

119. Wasserman RH, Corradino RA, Krook LP, et al: Evidence for 1,25-dihydroxycholecalciferol [1,25-(OH)₂D₃]-like substances in the domestic plant *Cestrum diurnum* (abstr). Fed Proc 34:893, 1975.

120. Webb AR, Holick MF: The role of sunlight in the cutaneous production of vitamin D₃. Annu Rev Nutr 8:375–399, 1988.

121. Weits J: The antivitamin D factor in roughages. Netherlands J Agr Sci 2:32–36, 1954.

122. Worker NA, Carillo BJ: "Enteque seco," calcification and wasting in grazing animals in the Argentine. Nature 215:72–74, 1967.

123. Wurtman RJ: The effects of light on man and other mammals. Annu Rev Physiol 37:467–483, 1975.

124. Yamaguchi A, Kohno Y, Yamazaki T, et al: Bone in the marmoset: a resemblance to vitamin D-dependent rickets, type II. Calcif Tissue Int 39:22–27, 1986.

125. Yarger JG, Quarles CL, Hollis BW, et al: Safety of 25-hydroxy-cholecalciferol as a source of cholecalciferol in poultry rations. Poultry Sci 74:1437–1446, 1995.

Vitamin E: Metabolism, Sources, Unique Problems in Zoo Animals, and Supplementation

ELLEN S. DIERENFELD

The pathophysiology and lesions associated with vitamin E deficiency are similar between domestic and exotic species, as detailed in recent reviews.[4, 6] However, a number of variables contribute to relevant interpretation and assessment of vitamin E nutrition in zoo animals. Even though biochemical mechanisms have not been experimentally determined for most zoo species, rapid advances in knowledge of the transport mechanisms for vitamin E in laboratory models provide speculative evidence. Hepatic discrimination in distribution of stereoisomers of vitamin E as well as differences in lipoprotein fractions of the blood may underlie comparative differences in animal response to vitamin E supplementation. Furthermore, applied feeding management suggests that dietary concentrations required to mitigate clinical signs of deficiency appear to differ between zoo animals and domestic counterparts. These implied requirement data are supported by limited information on the levels of vitamin E quantified in diet ingredients. Feed concentration of vitamin E appears to be the single most important variable affecting vitamin E status, although other nutrient interactions including level and type of dietary fat, antagonisms with other fat-soluble compounds, and oxidant stressors must also be considered. Thus, the assessment of vitamin E status (i.e., circulating levels of vitamin E), although relatively easy to obtain, is subject to variability from differences in diet, unknown animal physiology, and sample handling, storage, and analytical procedures. Nor do circulating levels of vitamin E reflect overall vitamin E status; storage tissue concentrations would provide a more useful measure of adequacy, but are unknown for most exotic species.

ABSORPTION AND TRANSPORT

Traber and coworkers[20] provide an excellent and comprehensive overview of mechanisms of tocopherol absorption, transport, and delivery. Dietary vitamin E is absorbed in association with fat, and it is transported via chylomicrons to the liver and other tissues. Thus, low levels of dietary lipid may inhibit availability simply because there is a lack of suitable uptake. In addition, diseases or metabolic states that limit fat digestive processes (including any of the stages of emulsification, solubilization within bile salt micelles, uptake by the enterocyte, encasement within chylomicrons, and secretion into circulation) may also affect the absorption of vitamin E.

Efficiency of absorption of tocopherol can be influenced by numerous factors in the diet as well as the physiologic state of the animal, depending on the amount and form given, vitamin E status of the individual, whether the dosage is offered as a bolus or gradually, and dietary lipid complement. Monoglycerides and triglycerides appear to stimulate the absorption of tocopherol to a greater degree than unsaturated fatty acids. Medium-chain triglycerides enhance absorption more so than long-chain triglycerides, and retinoic acid and long-chain polyunsaturated fatty acids (PUFAs) reduce absorption (the latter at least in part because of oxidation in vivo).[20] Impaired pancreatic function as well as liver disease or biliary obstruction, which results in lowered intestinal bile salt concentration, also impact efficiency of absorption.

Once absorbed by passive diffusion into the small intestinal enterocyte, the micellized tocopherol is incorporated into chylomicrons and secreted via the lymphatics into the bloodstream. Vitamin E is transported in the blood plasma lipoproteins and erythrocytes, with no evidence of a carrier protein, and is delivered to the tissues by any of at least three pathways:

1. Chylomicrons are catabolized by lipoprotein lipases into remnants, which are taken up by the liver and secreted discriminantly back into the bloodstream within very low density lipoproteins (VLDLs). This hepatic discrimination mechanism appears responsible for differences in incorporation of various tocopherol stereoisomers (alpha tocopherols ≥ gamma tocopherols) into VLDL, mediated by a hepatic tocopherol-binding protein (TBP). Genetic disorders that affect TBP (either lack of a gene or defective gene) may

underlie familial predisposition to vitamin E deficiency symptoms observed in humans and livestock,[6] but these have not been evaluated in adequate detail. Preliminary data to determine the presence of TBPs in zoo rhinoceros livers suggest species differences (Walker et al., unpublished), which may influence metabolism of this nutrient.

2. Adipose and muscle, or other tissues with lipoprotein lipase activity (regulated by energy requirements), may obtain tocopherol from circulation directly.

3. Tissues with LDL receptors (regulated by cholesterol requirements) may receive tocopherol via membrane transfer from high-density lipoprotein (HDL) and low-density lipoprotein (LDL) carriers.[16, 20] In tissues lacking both lipoprotein receptors and lipoprotein lipase activity (e.g., erythrocytes), spontaneous transfer and exchange may occur. HDLs may also have a role in delivery of tocopherol to the nervous system. Known differences in plasma lipoprotein distribution among species[2, 14] may govern the predominant pathway in different species, but further investigation is needed.

SOURCES OF VITAMIN E

Biologic activity of vitamin E is found naturally in two groups of compounds found in plant materials, the tocopherols and tocotrienols,[18] constituting a chromanol head group with a phytyl side chain. These active compounds differ in the number and positions of methyl groups in the aromatic ring and in the structure of the side chain. The most biologically active form of vitamin E is alpha tocopherol; the natural alpha tocopherol is designated RRR-alpha tocopherol, and the synthetic compound (a mixture of up to eight stereoisomers each with its own activity) is designated all-rac-alpha tocopherol. The National Research Council has stipulated, for dietary purposes, that vitamin E activity be expressed as RRR-alpha tocopherol equivalents (alpha-TE). One alpha-TE is defined as the activity of 1 mg of RRR-alpha tocopherol; total alpha-TE of mixed forms are estimated with conversion factors.[18] If synthetic all-rac-alpha tocopherol is present, the milligrams of the compound present should be multiplied by 0.74; natural-source alpha tocopherol has more relative biologic value than the synthetic mixture in all species examined to date.

Dietary Supplements

A number of pharmaceutical products for use as dietary additives are available commercially. Combination vitamin E and selenium preparations should not be used as a primary vitamin E supplement; they should be given only if selenium status is tenuous or clearly deficient. Acetate and succinate esters of vitamin E are often used as vitamin E sources in commercial supplements because they are more stable to oxygen than the free tocopherols. Bioavailability data comparing esterified tocopherols (both natural and synthetic) with free or micellized alcohols fed to ruminant animals have led to somewhat conflicting reports. Plasma (but not other tissue) concentrations increased more rapidly following administration of the alcohol in both cattle and sheep, but overall treatments were not significantly different.[13, 15]

A water-soluble vitamin E preparation (d-alpha tocopheryl polyethylene glycol 1000 succinate, or TPGS), which was developed as a therapeutic treatment for children with cholestatic liver disease who do not absorb oral vitamin E,[19] has been promoted as a supplement for zoo elephants and rhinoceroses.[17] Although the product has been shown to be effective for elevating tissue tocopherol concentrations in human and tissue culture studies, the rationale for its use in exotic species is unclear. Although plasma levels of vitamin E are low in elephants and rhinoceroses compared with other hoofstock,[4, 6] inhibited absorption of vitamin E has not been clearly documented. Because absorption of vitamin E is commensurate with lipid uptake, ensuring functional fat digestion may be a prudent initial step in understanding metabolism in these species. Furthermore, bioavailability of TPGS was shown to be lower than orally administered all-rac tocopherol acetate fed to sheep in controlled studies.[12] Intracellular hydrolysis of the TPGS is required to release free tocopherol to tissues, and it is a slow process in vitro. Evaluating the efficacy of hydrolysis of this compound and its incorporation into tissues (apart from blood) of endangered species should be undertaken. Horses fed TPGS demonstrated significantly higher circulating tocopherol concentrations in plasma samples that had been saponified compared with unsaponified matched samples, suggesting that TPGS had not been cleaved to release free tocopherol.[10] A similar plasma profile is seen in matched blood samples (n = 5) collected from zoo elephants and rhinoceroses fed this product, with saponified samples averaging twofold to threefold higher than unsaponified samples (Dierenfeld, unpublished observations). Presumably, the TPGS reaches target tissues, but labeled treatment studies would clarify this issue. Finally, regardless of whether this is the most effective method of administering vitamin E, long-term toxicity of chronic absorption of the carrier molecule—PEG 1000—should be monitored; excretion is known to be quite low (1.7% of the oral dose).[19]

Food Sources and Zoo Diets

The vitamin E concentration in animal fats is generally less than that of plant oils, but the lower PUFA content of most carnivore diets in comparison with that of herbivores contributes to a lower requirement for supplemental dietary vitamin E. In addition, the vitamin E in animal fats is almost exclusively alpha tocopherol, as opposed to a significant amount of gamma tocopherol in some edible oils, the latter of which has only 10% the biologic activity.[18] Vitamin E activity in produce items, seeds, nuts, and oils consumed can readily be found in human and livestock food composition tables, but whole prey represents an entire category of foodstuffs for which compositional data are not widely available.

Vitamin E deficiency is not widespread among mammalian carnivores in general; however, muscular degeneration and fat necrosis have been reported in seals and sea lions fed fish-based diets not supplemented with vitamin E.[6] In addition, cases of vitamin E deficiency in carnivorous reptiles and birds fed unsupplemented diets containing high levels of PUFAs are numerous.[4, 6] Levels of 100 IU vitamin E/kg fish (up to 400 IU/kg dry matter [DM]) have been suggested as necessary to prevent deficiencies in piscivorous species. The vitamin E content of several whole fish species commonly used in zoo and aquarium diets is found in Table 12–1. Although quite variable, concentrations of vitamin E measured in these prey are often less than dietary recommendations, indicating a need for external supplementation, particularly if fish are stored for any length of time such that lipid oxidation occurs.

Although specific requirements for vitamin E have not been established for exotic carnivores, National Research Council (NRC) recommendations of 20 to 80 mg/kg DM appear adequate for zoo canids and felids. Most whole vertebrates listed in Table 12–1 contain vitamin E concentrations within that range and thus would appear to supply adequate levels of this nutrient. Free-ranging prairie dogs, included for comparison, supply the staple food of the black-footed ferret and provide the only existing data on naturally occurring levels of this nutrient in whole rodents. Species and

diet effects on ultimate vitamin concentration of whole vertebrate prey appear more significant than sex or age,[3] except in pinkie (neonatal) rats, which seem to accumulate vitamin E.[8] Specific effects of differences in vitamin concentration of prey species on health and reproduction of consumers remain to be investigated.

Vitamin E concentrations in invertebrate prey have been examined in even less detail than vertebrate prey; however, vitamin E deficiency in strictly insectivorous species has not been reported. Perhaps concentrations quantified in prey are adequate or perhaps other diet ingredients supply this nutrient, because very few species are fed solely insects. Dietary manipulations have a significant effect on subsequent vitamin E content of prey insects. Comparison with free-living prey species may provide useful guidelines for evaluating nutritional adequacy of diets.

Vitamin E concentrations in green plants used in zoo feeding programs have also been summarized.[5] In general, levels of this nutrient measured in fresh forages (approximately 50 to 200 mg/kg DM) are considerably higher than in dried forages (<35 mg/kg DM) used in most zoos, and they are higher than NRC recommendations (15 to 80 mg/kg) for livestock species used as models for exotic species. Low dietary levels almost certainly contribute to the high incidence of vitamin E deficiency documented among zoo herbivores,[4, 6] but a number of interactions must also be considered.

TABLE 12–1. Vitamin E Concentrations (Average Plus Ranges) Measured in Whole Prey Items Used in Zoos and Aquariums

Species	n	Vitamin E Activity (IU/kg DM)	Range
Fish			
Herring	29	74.4	18–222
Mackerel	10	141.3	126–209
Capelin	29	116.3	41–414
Smelt (6 species)	14	164.1	87–332
Spearing	7	166.7	67–570
Trout, rainbow	15	236.1	159–462
Other vertebrates			
Mice	57	46.2	40–69
Rats	41	190.0	119–470
Guinea pigs	6	24.2	15–30
Prairie dogs	100	53.8	48–67
Rabbits	8	18.1	10–66
Chicks	10	258.7	83–434
Chickens	8	30.4	51–67
Quail	18	44.7	26–115
Toad	5	341.5	232–622
Frog	7	82.2	51–96
Invertebrates			
Mealworms	18	25.7	12–38
Crickets	14	75.3	29–122
Waxworms	5	509	277–741
Aquatic invertebrates			
Krill	5	51.7	26–120
Clams	5	49.1	27–55
Squid	16	57.2	27–376

From Refs. 3, 5, 8 and Wildlife Conservation Society, unpublished data.

NUTRIENT INTERACTIONS

A main determinant of the requirement for vitamin E is intake of PUFAs, which, over time, is reflected in tissue PUFA concentrations of nonruminant animals. PUFAs are concentrated in the cell membrane and sequester vitamin E in amounts commensurate with their own concentration and degree of unsaturation.[9] Seasonal variation in circulating vitamin E concentrations of hoofstock (both free-ranging and zoo species) has been attributed to possible differences in PUFA content of forages consumed,[4, 6] with freshly emerging plants containing much higher levels of PUFAs and, consequently, depleting body stores of this nutrient. Although this hypothesis has been inferred from studies with livestock, there are no published data combining both dietary composition and herbivore vitamin E status that substantiate this hypothesis in exotic species.

Other fat-soluble nutrients, including vitamins A, D, and K as well as carotenoids, have been shown to interact with vitamin E.[9] Excess vitamin A decreases the uptake and deposition of vitamin E and carotenoids,[1, 11] and beta carotene may have an indirect effect through its capacity to increase vitamin A in the serum and liver, thereby promoting the antagonism of vitamin A toward vitamin E. Specific vitamin E toxicity has not been documented, but excessive dietary levels of vitamin E have been associated with abnormal bone mineralization, clotting abnormalities, and poor reproduction in avian species,[6] suggesting that antagonisms with other fat-soluble vitamins may be reciprocal. Simultaneous assessment of both dietary and physiologic concentrations of the fat-soluble nutrients in relation to each other would increase current understanding of these interactions.

Iron and other transition metals can cause membrane damage by catalyzing the decomposition of lipid hydroperoxides to yield free radicals, which can lead to further tissue peroxidation.[9] This peroxidation caused by iron-catalyzed formation of free radicals consumes vitamin E as an antioxidant in vivo; other minerals used as cofactors in antioxidant enzyme systems can also be integrally related to vitamin E status. The role of selenium as a component of the antioxidant glutathione peroxidase describes a specific enzyme system rather than the more general antioxidant function of vitamin E. In most field cases of selenium-responsive diseases in animals, a response is also seen to the administration of (much less potentially toxic) vitamin E or a biologically active synthetic antioxidant. Selenium deficiency in domestic animals appears to result primarily from an increased vitamin E requirement in the presence of low selenium status, often aggravated by deterioration of vitamin E during feed storage.[9] Thus selenium status must be assessed before the use of selenium (in combination or singly) in response to potential antioxidant imbalance disease syndromes. In at least one documented case with exotic birds,[7] increased feed selenium led to decreased vitamin E status, with possible lowered reproductive output. Anecdotal data in elephants also suggest that elevated dietary selenium has led to lower vitamin E status (Wildlife Conservation Society, unpublished).

ASSESSMENT OF STATUS

Dietary requirements for vitamin E have not been established for most zoo species, and measurements of tissue concentrations of this nutrient are rare. Consequently, clinical symptoms and pathologic lesions provide diagnostic tools, and blood samples provide the primary basis for quantitative evaluation of vitamin E status. Circulating plasma concentrations of vitamin E are similar between comparable groups of animals,[4, 6] but wide variability exists both within and among animal species, and limitations of the use of serum samples as a diagnostic tool are recognized.[21] Future emphasis must be placed on understanding physiologic differences in fat metabolism or distribution among species and on more comprehensive quantification of fat-soluble vitamin and overall antioxidant status.

REFERENCES

1. Blakeley SR, Mitchell GV, Young ML, et al: Effects of β-carotene and related carotenoids on vitamin E. *In* Packer L, Fuchs J (eds): Vitamin E in Health and Disease. New York, Marcel Dekker, pp 63–68, 1992.
2. Chapman M: Comparative analysis of mammalian plasma lipoproteins. *In* Segrest J, Albers J (eds): Plasma Lipoproteins. Part A. Preparation, Structure and Molecular Biology. Orlando, Academic Press, pp 70–143, 1986.
3. Clum NJ, Fitzpatrick MP, Dierenfeld ES: Effects of diet on nutritional content of whole vertebrate prey. Zoo Biol 15:525–537, 1996.
4. Dierenfeld ES: Vitamin E deficiency in zoo reptiles, birds, and ungulates. J Zoo Wildl Med 20:3–11, 1989.
5. Dierenfeld, ES: Enhancing zoo diets through native foods analysis. Proceedings of the Cornell Nutrition Conference for Feed Manufacturers, Rochester, NY, pp 63–69, 1994.
6. Dierenfeld ES, Traber MG: Vitamin E status of exotic animals compared with livestock and domestics. *In* Packer L, Fuchs J (eds): Vitamin E in Health and Disease. New York, Marcel Dekker, pp 345–370, 1992.
7. Dierenfeld ES, Sheppard CD, Langenberg J, et al: Vitamin E in cranes: Reference ranges and nutrient interactions. J Wildl Dis 29:98–102, 1993.
8. Douglas TC, Pennino M, Dierenfeld ES: Vitamins E and A, and proximate composition of whole mice and rats used as feed. Comp Biochem Physiol 107A:419–424, 1994.
9. Draper HH: Interrelationships of vitamin E with other nutrients. *In* Packer L, Fuchs J (eds): Vitamin E in Health and Disease. New York, Marcel Dekker, pp 53–62, 1992.
10. Filizola do Nascimento M: The influence of vitamin E supplementation on blood alpha-tocopherol concentration of horses. M.S. thesis, Cornell University, 1994.
11. Frigg M, Broz J: Relationships between vitamin A and E in the chick. Int J Vit Nutr Res 54:125–134, 1984.
12. Hidiroglou M, Ivan M: Plasma α-tocopherol profiles in sheep after oral administration of d-l_z-α-tocopherol acetate and D-α-tocopheryl polyethylene glycol-1000 succinate. Res Vet Sci 51:177–179, 1991.
13. Hidiroglou N, Laflamme LF, McDowell LR: Blood plasma and tissue concentrations of vitamin E in beef cattle as influenced by supplementation of various tocopherol compounds. J Anim Sci 66:3227–3234, 1988.
14. Leat WMF, Northrop CA, Buttress N, et al: Plasma lipids and lipoproteins of some members of the order Perissodactyla. Comp Biochem Physiol 63B:275–281, 1979.
15. Ochoa L, McDowell LR, Williams SN, et al: α-Tocopherol concentrations in sheep and tissues of sheep fed different sources of vitamin E. J Anim Sci 70:2568–2673, 1992.
16. Packer L: Vitamin E is nature's master antioxidant. Sci Am Sci Med 1:54–63, 1994.
17. Papas AM, Cambre RC, Citino SB, et al: Efficacy of absorption of various vitamin E forms by captive elephants and black rhinoceroses. J Zoo Wildl Med 22:309–317, 1991.
18. Sheppard AJ, Pennington JAT, Weihrauch JL: Analysis and distribution of vitamin E in vegetable oils and foods. *In* Packer L, Fuchs

J (eds): Vitamin E in Health and Disease. New York, Marcel Dekker, pp 9–31, 1992.
19. Traber MG, Thellman CA, Rindler MJ, et al: Uptake of intact TPGS (*D*-α-tocopheryl polyethylene glycol 1000 succinate) a water-miscible form of vitamin E by human cells in vitro. Am J Clin Nutr 48:605–611, 1988.
20. Traber MG, Cohn W, Muller DPR: Absorption, transport, and delivery to tissues. *In* Packer L, Fuchs J (eds): Vitamin E in Health and Disease. New York, Marcel Dekker, pp 35–51, 1992.
21. Ullrey DE, Allen ME: Identification of nutritional problems in captive wild animals. *In* Fowler ME (ed): Zoo and Wild Animal Medicine, 3rd ed. Philadelphia, WB Saunders, pp 38–41, 1993.

CHAPTER **13**

Principles and Applications of Computed Tomography and Magnetic Resonance Imaging in Zoo and Wildlife Medicine

KATHY SPAULDING

MICHAEL R. LOOMIS

Obtaining complete histories, performing physical examinations, diagnosing disease, and treating zoo animals and wildlife present unique challenges to the attending clinician. These challenges are coupled with a vast diversity of species, each with its own distinctive characteristics and diseases, the often limited availability of normal comparative animals, the need to handle and chemically sedate fractious or frightened and fragile animals, and the value of endangered species. The selection of the most informative, noninvasive diagnostic modality to image these animals is important. The utility of frequently available diagnostic modalities such as radiography is often compromised by overlying skeleton, air sacs, or epidermal scales characteristic of various animals. Computed tomography (CT) and magnetic resonance imaging (MRI) are modalities that offer tomographic imaging, providing excellent structural and physiologic information not available by other means.[4, 13] These modalities are rapidly becoming part of the information gathering methods used to diagnose disease and further study these unique animals. The availability, capabilities, and use of these modalities are rapidly changing and will become more of a standard in the diagnostic arsenal.

COMPUTED TOMOGRAPHY

CT imaging was introduced in 1972. Tremendous changes and strides have since occurred and are contin-uing to take place for this rapidly developing diagnostic modality. Increased speed in the acquisition of images allows for a moving organ such as the heart to be imaged beat by beat. Image resolution has been improved, and contrast enhancement and three-dimensional reconstruction of the image have been introduced. Many veterinary colleges and referral specialty practices routinely offer CT scanning as part of their diagnostic portfolio. Many local community hospitals avail their equipment and expertise for imaging animals. This modality is complementary to and augments diagnostic radiology, MRI, ultrasonography, and nuclear medicine. It has become a useful ancillary aid as a noninvasive method of imaging and of providing important information for the diagnosis and treatment of zoo animals or wildlife and for investigating anatomy, physiology, and pathophysiology of unfamiliar, unusual, or endangered species.

CT combines x-rays and computers in the production of cross-sectional anatomic images. The CT scanning depends on detection of the x-ray attenuation properties of the tissues, which are dependent on atomic number and physical density of the tissue. The basic concept is that a thin cross-sectional slice of the body (like a thin piece of bread out of the entire loaf) is imaged from multiple angles by a very small x-ray beam. The x-ray tube is on one side of the body and the x-ray detectors are on the opposite side. Multiple emissions by the x-ray tube and subsequent detections by the x-ray detectors are made. The different tissues of the body attenuate the x-ray beam to varying degrees. The remaining energy of the transmitted photons through the body obtained by the detector is measured for each slice. The detectors convert this information into digital electronic signals, which are analyzed by a computer and given a numerical assignment. The CT image is composed of small squares (pixels), each having its own numerical assignment. Each pixel is then assigned a shade of gray based on the amount of attenuation of the x-rays by the tissues in the slice imaged (its number). This gray shade can be manually manipulated to enhance or optimize specific tissues. These numbers are often used to identify a specific tissue type, or a specific organ or structure. The type of tissue can be identified by its unit number. For example, a mass containing fluid or fat may be identified by its number. Through computer manipulation, reconstruction of the combined multiple images can be performed in planes other than that of the original image. A compilation of the signals by computers is used to reconstruct the thin section of the body part imaged into a recognizable cross-sectional tomographic anatomic image. Each slice is not influenced by body parts outside the selected slice thickness. Multiple, sequential images allow sectioning through an entire organ or body.

Contrast agents are often used in combination with the CT study to further evaluate the vascular characteristics of a lesion or an organ. Three-dimensional reconstruction of the two-dimensional information is becoming available for surface remodeling and rotation in space and is especially useful in evaluating complicated bony regions such as the head, spine, and pelvis.

Reports of uses of CT in zoo and wildlife species are rapidly expanding. The most common reported uses involve imaging soft tissue protected by bone such as neural tissue. Frequent areas of imaging include nasal passages, brain, spinal cord, both axial and appendicular skeleton, visceral organs including the kidneys, liver, gastrointestinal tract, pancreas, retroperitoneum, lungs, air sacs, mediastinum, and heart. CT imaging is often used for tumor staging and as a follow-up for evaluation of therapy.

Whereas there are many advantages to CT imaging, disadvantages also exist. There is relatively low differentiation of specific soft tissues when compared to MRI and ultrasound imaging. The imaged body is exposed to ionizing radiation. There are interfering artifacts produced, especially when there are metallic objects present or when imaging soft tissue adjacent to bone. The equipment is not universally accessible and available for use in exotic and wildlife species. The cost of acquisition, access, or maintenance of the equipment is high. Technical assistance to use unfamiliar equipment is needed. The animals must be still throughout the procedure, which often necessitates the use of anesthesia or an appropriate fixation device. The animals usually must be transported out of a familiar, secured, and protected environment to the place where the equipment is located. The table supporting the animal as it is transported through the gantry has a weight limit of about 350 pounds. The table must be adapted for heavier animals. The gantry size also limits the size of the

animal imaged. For example, the head and part of the cranial cervical spine on an adult male gorilla could be imaged, but the larger size of the remainder of the body preclude it from fitting through the gantry. Incomplete data are acquired if the slices chosen are too far apart or too thick, or if an improper window setting is chosen. When tissues of marked opacity disparity are adjacent to each other, volume averaging occurs and erroneous numbers and thus inappropriate gray shades may be assigned. Other artifacts may make bone appear thicker or may disallow imaging in specific areas because of surrounding bone (e.g., caudal skull). Infrequently, animals have an adverse reaction to the iodine-based contrast agents. There is an increased risk of morbidity and mortality when anesthetizing animals that are excited or sick.

MAGNETIC RESONANCE IMAGING

MRI and CT are similar in that images produced are in a cross-sectional format. However, the information gained, method of acquisition, and principle of production are completely different. MRI is accomplished through the response of nuclei with odd protons or neutrons in the nucleus (especially hydrogen) and a specific magnetic spin resulting from excitation from radio frequency electromagnetic waves. When exposed to an external magnetic field, protons collectively behave like small magnets. As they are exposed to radio waves, they develop spinning patterns, like a child's toy top. The hydrogen nucleus is excited by the radio frequency waves, followed by recovery of the nucleus to its original state. The analysis of how they recover and return to their natural state forms the basis for MRI.[8, 9, 15]

MRI has greater sensitivity in subtle soft tissue types than radiographs, ultrasound, or CT. MRI can be used to identify small alterations in tissue types, resulting in exquisite images of soft tissue. Some tissue characterization and actual element identification may be made. Motion blurring may be avoided by triggering the image with an electrocardiogram. Ionizing radiation is not involved.

However, MRI is not suitable for bone imaging because regions of bone appear dark where no signal is generated. MRI is not universally available, and there is a high cost for acquiring and maintaining the equipment and work area. Technical assistance is necessary to maintain the equipment. Animals must be immobile for the study, so most animals must be anesthetized. Anesthesia must be done without the use of any metal near the magnet in the machine. When the animal is within the coil of the magnet, there is limited access to the animal for monitoring.

MRI can be used to image any soft tissue within the body. It has applications both in diagnosis and in research. Common applications of MRI in zoo and wildlife animals include evaluating soft tissue changes within the central nervous system, examining the soft tissues of various joints, and studying blood flow with and without contrast agents. It has been used in the diagnosis of cerebral infarction in aged rhesus monkeys and of bacterial sinusitis in the Mongolian gerbil. It has been used in the study of the normal eye of the owl and of the developing yolk of an avian egg.[1, 3, 7, 10, 14]

Both CT and MRI are valuable forms of imaging. Each has its own unique uses and features. Each can add greatly to the diagnosis and prognosis of individual case management as pet owners elect to provide more extensive diagnostic and therapeutic care to their pets and valuable endangered species are given more access to these diagnostic modalities. Both modalities offer valuable opportunities to study endangered species, assist in diagnosis of disease, and obtain valuable scientific information.[2, 6, 11, 12]

◆ CASE STUDIES

Case 1: Lowland Gorilla

An 18-year-old male gorilla had drainage of purulent material from the left ear canal and a draining fistula caudal and ventral to the left ear. On the basis of these findings, a preliminary diagnosis of mastoiditis was made.[5] A CT scan was performed to confirm the diagnosis and determine the extent of involvement. Expansive bony proliferation nearly completely obliterating the left mastoid air space was identified on the CT study. This was consistent with chronic mastoiditis with osteomyelitis extending from the mastoid air space to the sagittal crest and involving the zygomatic arch (Fig. 13–1).

The gorilla weighed 450 pounds. Because the gantry table for the CT machine is rated for 350 pounds, modifications to the table were made by the manufacturer in order for the gantry to operate properly.

The infection progressed and did not respond to antibiotic therapy. The gorilla died from meningoencephalitis.

Case 2: San Esteban Island Chuckwalla

Severe posterior paresis acutely developed in an adult male San Esteban Island chuckwalla. Although

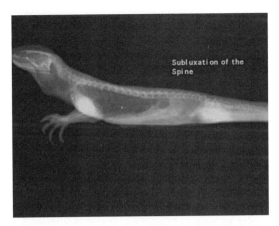

FIGURE 13–2. Lateral horizontal beam radiograph of a San Esteban Island chuckwalla showing a suspicious step deformity.

the rear legs and tail were flaccid, he could move them in response to painful stimuli. His cloacal sphincter tone was normal. A preliminary diagnosis of transverse myelopathy was made. Spinal radiographs were made. A step deformity of the spine was identified. A CT scan was performed to further examine this area. Three-dimensional reconstruction of the CT image was performed to further show the lesion. A vertebral subluxation was confirmed (Figs. 13–2, 13–3).

Case 3: Blue and Gold Macaw

A 12-year-old female blue and gold macaw had abdominal enlargement of 1 month's duration. Radiographs of the abdomen were made. Distention of the coelomic cavity was present. There were caudal displacement of the intestinal tract and marked loss of serosal detail. A mass was suspected (Fig. 13–4). A multilobulated mass was identified on the ultrasound examination (Fig. 13–5). A soft tissue round mass extended into the fluid compartment. The mass occupied the majority of the caudal coelomic cavity. The origin of the cystic mass was not determined. Fluid accumulation was suspected. The coelomic fluid was aspirated and a dark brown serous modified transudate was removed. CT was performed to ascertain the origin and extent of the mass. The soft tissue mass seen on the ultrasound extended into a large coelomic cystic structure. The mass protruded from the liver. A celiotomy and liver biopsy were performed. The bird went into cardiac arrest during recovery from the liver biopsy. Cystic biliary adenocarcinoma was confirmed by histopathologic study (Fig. 13–6).

Case 4: Hyacinth Macaw

An adult, female hyacinth macaw had an enlarging mass on the skull. Activity of the bird had been decreasing for 2 weeks. The bird's mate had been feeding her. Survey radiographs and a CT examina-

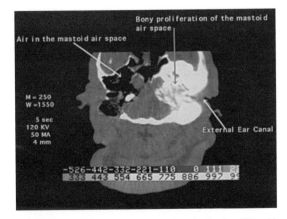

FIGURE 13–1. Chronic mastoiditis in a lowland gorilla with extensive bony proliferation and obliteration of the mastoid air space.

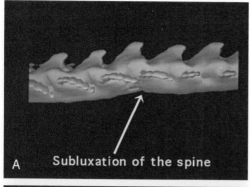

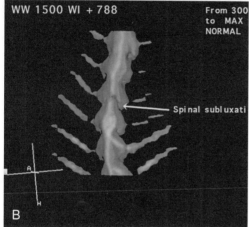

FIGURE 13–3. Three-dimensional reconstruction of a computed tomography image of the chuckwalla in Figure 13–2 showing vertebral subluxation.

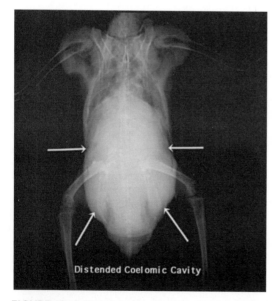

FIGURE 13–4. Ventral-dorsal radiograph of a blue and gold macaw showing distention of the coelomic cavity, loss of serosal detail, and caudal displacement of the intestinal tract.

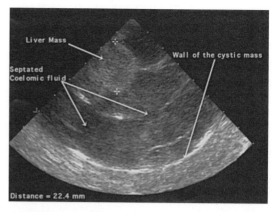

FIGURE 13–5. Ultrasonogram of macaw in Figure 13–4 showing a multilobulated mass.

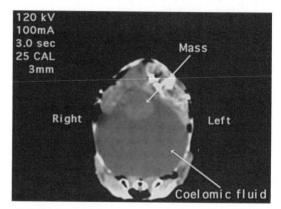

FIGURE 13–6. Computed tomography image of macaw in Figure 13–4 showing a mass protruding from the liver.

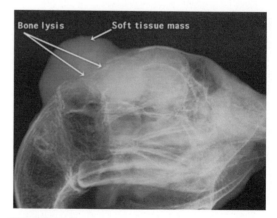

FIGURE 13–7. Lateral radiograph of a hyacinth macaw with an enlarging mass on the skull showing lysis of underlying calvaria.

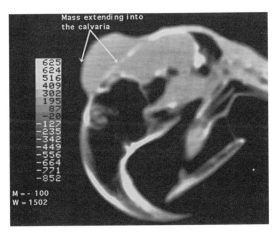

FIGURE 13–8. Computed tomography image of macaw in Figure 13–7 showing extension of the mass into the calvaria.

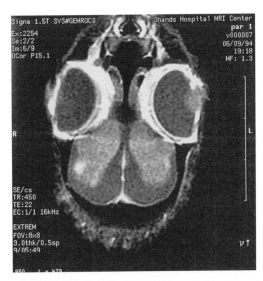

FIGURE 13–11. Magnetic resonance image of the brain of an Amazon parrot showing focal lesions in the brain. (Courtesy of Dr. Juergen Schumacher.)

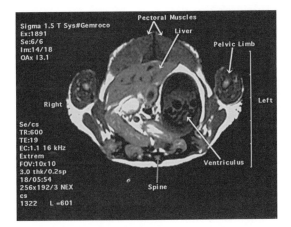

FIGURE 13–9. Magnetic resonance image of the coelomic cavity of a normal pigeon. (Courtesy of Dr. April Romangnano.)

tion were done to ascertain the extent of the disease. A soft tissue mass with underlying lysis of the calvaria were seen. The mass extended through the right periorbital sinus. An aggressive, infiltrating tumor was found. Histopathologic study confirmed a fibrosarcoma. The bird was euthanized (Figs. 13–7, 13–8).

Case 5: Pigeon

The anatomy of the coelomic cavity of a normal pigeon is evident on the MRI study (Fig. 13–9).

Case 6: Pigeon

Normal anatomy of the brain of a pigeon is delineated by the MRI study of the skull (Fig. 13–10).

Case 7: Amazon Parrot

MRI of the brain of an Amazon parrot *(Amazona farinosa farinosa)*. The adult mealy Amazon had a history of repetitive seizures of unknown origin. A radiographic survey of the bird was normal. Focal lesions in the brain were seen on the MRI study. At necropsy, a nonsuppurative meningoencephalitis was diagnosed. The vacuolated neuropil and mononuclear perivascular cuffs accounted for the MRI findings. A viral cause was suspected (Fig. 13–11).

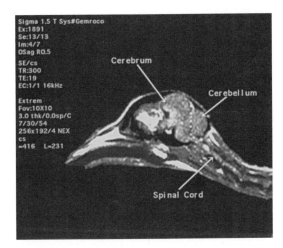

FIGURE 13–10. Magnetic resonance image of the brain of a normal pigeon. (Courtesy of Dr. April Romangnano.)

REFERENCES

1. Allen KL, van Bruggen N, Cooper JE: Detection of bacterial sinusitis in the Mongolian gerbil *(Meriones unguiculatus)* using magnetic resonance imaging. Vet Rec 132:633–635, 1993.
2. Brouwers MEL, Kamminga C, Klooswijk AIJ, et al: The use of computed tomography in cetacean research. Airsac determination of *Lagenorhynchus albirostris*, Part 1. Aquatic Mammals 16.3:145–155, 1990.

3. Falen SW, Szeverenyi NM, Packard DS, et al: Magnetic resonance imaging study of the structure of the yolk in the developing avian egg. J Morphol 209:331–342, 1991.
4. Hudson LC, Cauzinille L, Kornegay JN, Tompkins MB: Magnetic resonance imaging of the normal feline brain. Vet Radiol Ultrasound 36(4):267–275, 1995.
5. Iverson WO, Popp JA: Meningoencephalitis secondary to otitis in a gorilla. JAVMA 173(9):1134–1136, 1978.
6. Jenkins JR: Use of computed tomography (CT) in pet bird practice. Proceedings of the Association of Avian Veterinarians, Chicago, pp 276–279, 1991.
7. Morgan RV, Donnell RL, Daniel GB: Magnetic resonance imaging of the normal eye and orbit of a screech owl (Otus asio). Vet Radiol Ultrasound 35(5):362–367, 1994.
8. Patton JA, Kulkarni MV, Craig JK, et al: Techniques, pitfalls and artifacts in magnetic resonance imaging. Radiographics 7(3):505–519, 1987.
9. Pusey E, Lufkin RB, Brown RKJ, et al: Magnetic resonance imaging artifacts: Mechanism and clinical significance. Radiol Clin North Am 6(5):891–911, 1986.
10. Raiti P, Haramati N: MR of bowel using mineral oil as a contrast agent: A viable option in reptiles with long transit times. Proceedings of the Association of Reptilian and Amphibian Veterinarians, Pittsburgh, p 59, 1994.
11. Rübel A, Kuoni W, Augustiny N: Emerging techniques: CT scan and MRI in reptile medicine. Semin Avian Exotic Pet Med 3(3):156–160, 1994.
12. Stoskopf M: Clinical imaging in zoological medicine: A review. J Zoo Wildl Med 20(4):394–412, 1989.
13. Thomson CE, Kornegay JN, Burn RA, et al: Magnetic resonance imaging—A general overview of principles and examples in veterinary neurodiagnosis. Vet Radiol Ultrasound 20(4):396–412, 1989.
14. Uno H, Richardson R, Houser WD: Cerebral infarction in aged rhesus monkeys and magnetic resonance imaging. Am J Primatol 20(3):239–240, 1990.
15. Villafana T: Fundamental physics of magnetic resonance imaging. Radiol Clin North Am 26(4):701–715, 1988.

CHAPTER 14

Plant Poisoning in Zoos in North America

MURRAY E. FOWLER

Although plant poisoning is not a common problem in zoos, it is readily preventable with planning and attention to landscaping. Many ornamental and landscape plants contain chemicals that may be harmful to one or more species of animals. Some larger zoos employ a horticultural staff with professional expertise in maintaining the flora of the zoo. However, not all horticulturalists or landscape architects are knowledgeable about the myriad species of plants that may pose a potential threat to herbivorous animals. Zoo veterinarians should review plans for new landscape plantings and periodically inspect plantings in or around herbivore enclosures. Zoo veterinarians may likewise not have sufficient background to identify dangerous plantings. This chapter provides the zoo veterinarian with concepts, principles, and resources for dealing with potential plant poisoning in a collection of captive wild animals.

Why are poisonous plants found in zoos? Many plants that contain poisons are beautiful or fulfill the purpose of the landscaper. Additionally, to enhance a geographic feeling, foreign plants are used, and little may be known about them in North America. Poisoning caused by plants usually requires a unique combination of circumstances that are rarely met. A given plant may be considered safe because there is a history of no cases of poisoning, but circumstances may occur that

precipitate a poisoning. Examples of such changes include the following:

- An animal escapes and begins to forage on its own.
- A storm fells trees into, or leaves or branches are blown into an enclosure.
- A patron feeds nearby plant material to an animal.
- A new animal is introduced into an enclosure.

Problems may arise under the following circumstances:

1. Inappropriate plantings are made in newly constructed facilities or fill dirt contains weed seeds. For example, a small zoo completed a lovely lemur island. Within 10 days, two lemurs died and another became seriously ill from eating the leaves and fruits of hairy nightshade Solanum sarrachoides, an endemic weed. It is desirable that when landscaping is finished in a new or refurbished enclosure that watering or irrigation is used to germinate any seeds present in the soil so plants may be identified before animals are introduced.

2. Personnel may fail to heed warnings about known poisonous plants. For example, patches of tree tobacco Nicotiana glauca were identified in a hoofstock enclosure in a safari park. Even though the recommendation

was made to remove the plants immediately, a month later it was reported that three giraffes had died of tree tobacco poisoning at that park.

3. Untrained personnel may be assigned to collect browse for feeding. For example, I have seen a zoo employee collect prunings of yellow oleander *Thevetia peruviana*, thinking it was acacia.

4. Animals that are natural browsers are at special risk in open facilities such as safari parks, game farms, animal reserves, breeding farms, or holding areas. A thorough botanical survey should be conducted before freeing animals into large areas containing native vegetation. Such surveys should be conducted seasonally to aid in the recognition of shrubs and herbaceous plants. Species such as wild or choke cherry (*Prunus* species), mountain laurel (*Leucothoe davisiae*), azaleas and rhododendrons (*Rhododendron* species), scrub oaks (*Quercus* species), lantana (*Lantana camara*), and rattlebox (*Crotalaria* species) should be eliminated. Browser animals such as aoudads (*Ammotragus lervia*) may denude a shrubby enclosure in a short time even though they are provided with adequate hay. Other browsers include some marsupials, some primates, elephants, black rhinoceroses, deer, camelids, giraffe, sheep and goats, and many other artiodactylids.

5. Special attention should be given to forages obtained from commercial suppliers. Baled, cubed, or pelleted hay may be processed from hay containing poisonous plants. Keepers may be able to identify some poisonous plants in baled hay, but any incorporated into cubes or pellets cannot be identified. Thus, the integrity of the supplier must be relied upon to deliver quality feeds. Plants of concern include fiddleneck (*Amsinckia intermedia*), tansy ragwort (*Senecio jacobaea*), and groundsel (*Senecio vulgaris*). Concentrates and supplement feeds should also be checked for quality because fungal contaminated seeds may contain mycotoxins. The species of poisonous weeds in hays may be a regional matter, but plants containing pyrrolizidine alkaloids are particularly hazardous because the delayed hepatotoxic effects may occur 6 to 12 months later and the connection to a forage ingestion may not be easy.

6. Planters inside the public area for winter viewers may include ornamental plants that may be picked by zoo patrons and offered to animals. Potted plants to be avoided include oleander (*Nerium oleander*), yew (*Taxus* species), philodendrons (*Philodendron* species), and dumbcane (*Dieffenbachia* species).

AVOIDING PLANT POISONING

1. Know what plants are in the zoo.
   a. Take inventory of the following:
      (1) Trees and shrubs
      (2) Perennial plants
      (3) Weeds growing in or around enclosures
      (4) Planted beds
      (5) House plants in offices and buildings
   b. Take periodic (particularly seasonal) walks through the zoo to check for unsuitable plant growth.

2. Be particularly watchful when garden clubs volunteer to do plantings or donate plants to the zoo.
3. Establish a policy that only one person approves all plants that come into the zoo.
4. Develop a plan for replacement of known poisonous plants, trees, or shrubs with more suitable plants. This must be done judiciously and with the degree of risk taken into consideration. Regionally popular trees may contain poisonous substances, but the poisoning risk may be slight. For instance, it would not be appropriate to cut down 100-year-old oak trees because there is a slight risk of tannin poisoning.

POTENTIALLY DANGEROUS PLANTS

Tables 14–1 to 14–4 list plants that should not be planted in a zoo, those that may be planted with caution, and those that may be planted freely. The tables are intended as a guide and do not include all poisonous species.

SOURCES OF INFORMATION ABOUT POISONOUS PLANTS

The bibliography at the end of this chapter is a resource for additional information on plants and plant poisoning. Even though a large number of plants appear on lists of dangerous plants, particularly in literature for humans, there is little concern for plants that cause allergic dermatitis in humans. Many plants are so listed because they are perpetuated on lists compiled more than 100 years ago from circumstantial evidence. A recent toxic plant survey has been published by the Association of Zoological Horticulture and the American Association of Zoo Veterinarians; however, it also lists many plants that contain no known toxic substances and have never been involved in livestock or companion animal poisoning. The compiler of the survey reported information submitted by respondents and did not editorialize. It is evident that there is a vital need for education of zoo personnel on matters of plant poisoning. Of particular concern is that no distinction is made between plants containing a poisonous substance and plants that may produce mechanical injury. It should also be understood that the ingestion of quantities of any plant material that has not been a part of the regular diet of an animal may cause a transient digestive upset, including mild gastroenteritis or even a severe impaction. This does not mean that the plant is poisonous.

COPING WITH POISONOUS PLANTS

All animals, wild or domestic, cope with chemical substances (secondary plant compounds [SPC]) in plants by using one or more of the following strategies: avoidance, dilution, degradation, or detoxification.

TABLE 14-1. Suitability of Plants for Landscaping Zoos

Category	Common Name	Scientific Name	Toxin	Toxic Part of the Plant
Deciduous trees and shrubs that should not be planted	Kentucky coffee tree	*Gymnocladus doica*	Alkaloid, cystisine	All parts
	Chinaberry, pride of India, bead tree, umbrella tree	*Melia azedarach*	Unknown	Fruits
	Chinese tallow tree	*Sapium sebiferum*	Saponin	Seeds
	Castorbean, palma christi	*Ricinus communis*	Albumitoxin, ricin	Seeds primarily
	Horse chestnut, buckeye	*Aesculus* species	Coumarin glycoside	Leaves, seeds, twigs, bark
Deciduous trees that should be planted with caution*	Golden shower, senna	*Cassia fistula*	Cathartic	Foliage
	Black walnut	*Juglans nigra*	Glycoside	Foliage and husk of fruit
	English walnut	*Juglans regia*		
	Golden-chain tree	*Laburnum* species	Alkaloid, cystisine	Seeds and pod pulp
	Cherry, plum, peach	*Prunus* species	HCN	Foliage, pits
	Wild black cherry	*Prunus serotina*	HCN	Foliage, especially if wilted or frosted
	Japanese pagoda tree, Chinese scholar tree	*Sophora japonica* and other species	Alkaloid	Seeds
	Black locust, false acacia	*Robinia pseudoacacia*	Phytotoxin	Foliage and bark
	Red maple	*Acer rubrum*, possibly other species	Unknown	Leaves
	Oak, deciduous	*Quercus* species	Tannins	Frosted foliage and acorns
Narrow-leafed evergreen trees or shrubs that should not be planted	Yew, Japanese yew, English yew	*Taxus* species	Taxine, an alkaloid	Foliage, seeds
	Oleander	*Nerium oleander*	Oleandrin, a steroidal glycoside	All parts of the shrub
	Yellow oleander, Yellow-be-still tree	*Thevetia peruviana*	Digitalis-like glycoside	All parts of the shrub
Broad-leafed evergreen trees or shrubs that should not be planted	Mountain laurel	*Kalmia latifolia*	Andromedotoxin, glycoside	Foliage
	Black laurel, leucothoe	*Leucothoe* species	Same	Same
	Rhododendron	*Rhododendron* species	Same	Same
	Andromeda, floribunda	*Pieris* species	Same	Same
	Catalina cherry	*Prunus lyonii*	Cyanide	Foliage, pits
	Holly-leaf cherry	*Prunus ilicifolia*		
	Acacia, golden wattle	*Acacia* species	Most of the acacias are nontoxic, but one must know the species	Foliage

Category	Common name	Scientific name	Toxic principle	Toxic part
Broad-leafed evergreen trees and shrubs that should be planted with caution*	Box, boxwood	*Buxus* species	Alkaloids	Foliage
	Croton	*Croton* species	Irritant oil	Foliage
	Daphne, spurge laurel	*Daphne* species	Glycoside	Foliage
	Euphorbias, spurges	*Euphorbia* species	Irritant oil	Foliage
	St. John's wort, gold flower, aaronsbeard	*Hypericum* species	Glycoside, hypericin	Foliage
	Privet	*Ligustrum* species	Glycoside	Berries, leaves
	Oaks, nondeciduous	*Quercus* species		Leaves, stems
	Dumbcane, dieffenbachia	*Dieffenbachia sequine*	Protein-like substance	Foliage
Vines and ground cover that should not be planted	Clematis, travelers's joy, Virgin's bower	*Clematis* species	Alkaloidal glycoside	Foliage
	Ivy, English ivy	*Hedra helix*	Saponin glycoside	Foliage, fruits
	Morning glory	*Ipomea* species	Unknown	Foliage
	Lantana	*Lantana* species	Hepatotoxin	Foliage, fruits
	Matrimony vine	*Lycium halimifolium*	Unknown	Foliage
	Moonseed	*Menispermum canadense*	Unknown	Foliage
	Monostera, Swiss cheese plant, ceriman, Mexican breadfruit	*Monostera* species	Protein-like toxin	Foliage
	Creeper, Virginia creeper, Boston ivy	*Parthenocissus* species	Unknown	Foliage, fruits
	Philodendron	*Philodendron* species	Protein-like toxin	Foliage
	Mexican flame vine	*Senecio* species	Pyrrolizidine alkaloids	Foliage, seed
	Goldcup chalice vine, cup of gold, trumpet plant	*Solanum* species	Steroidal glycosides	Foliage, seed
		Solandra species		
	European bittersweet	*Solanum dulcamara*	Steroidal glycoside	Foliage, fruits
	Carolina jessamine, yellow jessamine	*Gelsemium sempervirens*	Alkaloids	Foliage, roots
	Sweet pea, rough pea	*Lathyrus odoratus* and others species	Neurolathrogen	Primarily seeds, but also foliage
	Wisteria	*Wisteria* species	Glycoside	Primarily seeds
	Lily of the valley	*Convallaria majalis*	Cardioglycoside	Foliage
	Autumn crocus	*Colchicum autumnale*	Alkaloid, colchicine	Leaves

*Trees and shrubs in this group have been reported as poisonous to one or more species of animal. Perhaps one growth stage (foliage, fruits, seeds) of the plant is poisonous. Animal access must be guarded against.

91

TABLE 14–2. Poisonous Species of the Heather (Ericaceae) Family*

Common Name	Scientific Name
Mountain laurel, ivy-bush, bank laurel	*Kalmia latifolia*
Sheep laurel, wicky, lambskill	*Kalmia angustifolia*
Mountain fetter-bush, staggerbush, Mountain pieres, flame of the forest, andromeda	*Pieres floribunda*
Dog laurel, fetter-bush	*Leucothoe racemosa*
Black laurel	*Leucothoe davisiae*
Labrador tea	*Ledum granulosum*
Evergreen rhododendron, great laurel	*Rhododendron maximum* or *Rhododendron catawbiense*
Azalea	*Rhododendron* species
California rosebay	*Rhododendron occidentale*
Western azalea	*Rhododendron californicum*

*All these shrubs contain the same poisonous substance (andromedotoxin), which causes the same general syndrome in all species of animals (i.e., coughing, choking, retching, vomiting, grinding the teeth, colic, rolling, groaning, recumbency, depression, refusal to eat, stumbling and prostration).

Avoidance

Zoo animals may use avoidance if fed adequately and allowed to adjust to plants slowly; however, it is a misconception that poisonous plants are always bitter or unpalatable and that they will be avoided. It is not uncommon to walk through a herbivorous animal enclosure and observe plants that are known to be poisonous to one or more species of livestock. There are many situations that break down the inhibitions to eat harmful plants, including introducing animals into an enclosure that has been vacant for some time, allowing growth of undesirable plants, changing the species of animal in an enclosure, feeding insufficient amounts of palatable forage, or releasing new animals into an enclosure when they are hungry.

Some wild animals develop avoidance behavior by learning from parents or siblings. These may be crucial skills that captive wild animals reintroduced into the wild may not have been able to acquire.

Dilution

Free-ranging herbivores usually eat a large variety of plants. Such a diet tends to dilute the toxic agent from any one plant. Because as many as 40% of the species of plants in the habitat of a herbivore may contain one or more SPCs, dilution is an important means of coping with poisonous plants. Zoo herbivores may not have to deal with dilution because they are often fed a single type of hay as a standard diet.

Degradation

The third strategy for coping is degradation of SPCs in the digestive tract. Degradation may be a chemical reaction or involve the action of gastrointestinal microorganisms. The complex microflora and fauna in the rumen of ruminant herbivores not only assist in the digestive process but also assist in degradation of SPCs. Specific microorganisms may be required to degrade such substances as oxalates. If a zoo animal has never ingested small amounts of oxalates, oxalate degrading microflora may not be present, or they may occur in such small numbers that an otherwise nontoxic dose may be dangerous.

Detoxification

Once a toxic agent is absorbed from the gastrointestinal tract, the body must either excrete the substance unchanged, sequester it into a nonactive storage site, detoxify it by molecular rearrangement, or suffer the ill

TABLE 14–3. Herbaceous Weeds and Shrubs that Should Be Eliminated from Enclosures and Planted Areas

Common Name	Scientific Name
Tree tobacco, any of the wild tobaccos	*Nicotiana glauca* and other species
Foxglove, purple foxglove	*Digitalis purpurea*
Nightshades	*Solanum* species
Jimson weed, Jamestown weed	*Datura stramonium*, other daturas
Poison hemlock	*Conium maculatum*
Koa haola, lead tree	*Leucaena leucocephala*
Poke weed, Poke	*Phytolacca americana*

TABLE 14–4. Trees and Shrubs that May Be Planted Freely Within a Zoo

Common Name	Scientific Name
Deciduous Broad-Leafed Trees and Shrubs*	
Maples (except red maple), box elder	*Acer* species
Tree of heaven, ailanthus	*Ailanthus altissima*
Silk tree, mimosa	*Albizia* species
Alder	*Alnus* species
Orchid tree, bouhinia, Mt. ebony	*Bauhinia varigata*
Birches	*Betula* species
Hornbeams	*Carpinus* species
Pecan, hickory	*Carya illinoensis*
Catalpa, Indian bean	*Catalpa* species
Hackberry	*Celtis* species
Redbud, judastree	*Cercis* species
Dogwood	*Cornus* species
Hawthorn	*Crataegus* species
Persimmon	*Diospyros* species
Russian olive	*Elaeagnus augustifolia*
Beeches	*Fagus* species
Fig trees	*Ficus* species
Ashes	*Fraxinus* species
Honey locust	*Gleditsia* species
Jacaranda, green ebony	*Jacaranda* species
Crape myrtle	*Lagerstroemia indica*
Larch	*Larix decidua*
Sweet gum, liquidambar	*Liquidambar styraciflua*
Tulip tree, yellow poplar	*Liriodendron tulipifera*
Magnolia, cucumber tree	*Magnolia* species
Apple, crabapple	*Malus* species
Mulberry	*Morus* species
Pepperidge, black tupelo, sour gum	*Nyssa sylvatica*
Paulownia, empress tree	*Paulownia tomentosa*
Pistache, Chinese pistache	*Pistachio chinensis*
Plane tree, sycamore, buttonball, buttonwood	*Plantanus* species
Poplars, cottonwoods, aspen	*Populus* species
Mesquite, honey mesquite	*Prosopis* species
Pear, flowering pear, gallery pear	*Pyrus callerynana* and *Pyrus* species
Willows	*Salix* species
Sassafras	*Sassafras albidum*
Mountain ash	*Sorbus* species
Tree lilac	*Syringa amurensis*
Linden, basswood	*Tilia* species
Elms	*Ulmus* species
Narrow-Leafed Evergreen Trees and Shrubs†	
Firs	*Abies* species
Norfolk pine	*Arauicaria heterophyla*
Cedars, deodar and others	*Cedurs* species
Cypress	*Chamaecyparis* species
Cypress	*Cypressus* species
Junipers, pfitszers	*Juniperus* species
Incense cedar	*Libocedrus decurrens*
Dawn redwood	*Metasequoia glyptostrodoides*
Coastal redwood	*Sequoia sempervirens*
Giant sequoia	*Sequoia giganteum*
Spruces	*Picea* species
Pines	*Pinus* species. There is some concern about *Pinus ponderosa* causing abortion in parkland habitat.
Podocarpus, fern podocarpus	*Podocarpus* species
Douglas fir	*Pseudotsuga menziesii*
Bald cypress	*Taxodium distichum*
Arbor vitae	*Thuja* species
Hemlock	*Tsuga* species

Table continued on following page

TABLE 14–4. Trees and Shrubs that May Be Planted Freely Within a Zoo *(Continued)*

Common Name	Scientific Name
Broad-Leafed Evergreen Trees or Shrubs	
Abelia	*Abelia* species
Strawberry tree	*Arbutus unedo*
Manzanita, bearberry	*Arctostaphylos* species
Barberry	*Berberis* species
Bottlebrush	*Collistemon* species
Camellia	*Camellia* species
Beefwood, she oak, Australian pine	*Casuarina equisetifolia*
California lilac, mountain lilac	*Ceanothus* species
Camphor tree	*Cinnamomum caphora*
Orange, lemon, lime, grapefruit	*Citrus* species
Cotoneaster	*Cotoneaster* species
Loquat	*Eriobotrya japonica*
Eucalyptus, gum trees	*Eucalyptus* species
Eugenia	*Eugenia* species
Euonymus	*Euonymus* species
Aralia	*Fatsia japonica*
Pineapple guava	*Feijoa sellowiana*
Gardenia	*Gardenia jasminoides*
Laurel, sweet bay	*Laurus nobilis*
Oregon grape, holly	*Mahonia repens*
Heavenly bamboo, sacred bamboo	*Nandia domestica*
Olive	*Olea european*

This is not an exhaustive list of trees or shrubs that may be used freely in zoo landscaping, but provides a foundation upon which to build. Additional information may be obtained from the bibliography.

*Many of the trees and shrubs in this group may be used for browse; however not all are equally palatable.

†Trees and shrubs in this group are not usually used for browse.

effects caused by the toxicant. All vertebrates have general detoxification pathways that deal with many different toxicants, such as alkaloids, glycosides, saponins, or tannins. Detoxification is accomplished by oxidation, reduction hydrolysis, esterification, N-dealkylation, and conjugation. Besides the general mechanism, species may develop a specific detoxification system to deal with unique toxins.

Much detoxification is carried out by hepatic microsomal enzyme activity. More limited microsomal activity takes place in the kidney, intestinal mucosa, lungs, and skin. Some detoxification mechanisms are inherent, but others depend on prior exposure to a toxicant. Only minimal quantities of a particular enzyme are present unless the enzyme system has been stimulated by prior exposure. This is called the "pump priming effect." Zoo animals may not have had an opportunity to "prime the pump," and they may be vulnerable to accidental exposure to a toxicant.

The efficiency of microsomal enzyme systems may also depend on age, size, sex, and reproductive status of an animal. Young animals have less fully developed microsomal enzyme systems than older animals. Older animals may also have more materials to draw from for conjugation. Sex hormones may either enhance or diminish the effects of various toxins. Cortisol increases the capacity for detoxification by microsomal enzymes.

BIBLIOGRAPHY

Sources for Identification

The USDA Cooperative Extension Service in each state or the botany department at state universities frequently publishes a booklet on poisonous plants. Curators at botanical gardens are also knowledgeable about local plants.

Regional Books

Blohm HL: Poisonous Plants of Venezuela. Cambridge, MA, Harvard University Press, 1962.

Everist SL: Poisonous Plants of Australia. Sydney, Australia, Angus and Robertson, 1981, revised edition.

Forsyth AA: British poisonous plants [Bulletin 161]. London, England, Her Majesty's Stationery Office, Ministry of Agriculture, Fisheries and Food, 1968.

Fuller TC, McClintock E: Poisonous Plants of California. Berkeley, CA, University of California Press, 1986.

Gessner O, Orzechowski G: Gift-und Arzneiflanzen von Mitteleuropa (Medical Botany, Pharmacology and Poisonous Plants of Central Europe). Heidelberg, 1974.

Hogan EL (ed): Sunset Western Garden Book, 5th ed. Menlo Park, CA, Sunset Publishing Company, 1990.

Hulbert LC, Oehme FW: Plants Poisonous to Livestock, 3rd ed. Manhattan, Kansas State University Printing Service, 1968.

Kellerman TS, Coetzer JAW, Naude TU: Plant Poisoning and Mycotoxicosis of Livestock in Southern Africa. Cape Town, South Africa, Oxford University Press, 1982.

Kingsbury JM: Poisonous Plants of the United States and Canada. Englewood Cliffs, NJ, Prentice-Hall, 1964.

Schmutz EM, Freeman BN, Reed RE: Livestock-Poisoning Plants of Arizona. Tucson, AZ, University of Arizona Press, 1968.

Tokarnia CH, Doebereiner J, da Silva MF: Plantas Toxicas da Amazonia (Poisonous plants of the Amazon). Manaus, Amazonas (Brazil), INPA, 1979.

Verdcourt B, Trump EC: Common Poisonous Plants of East Africa. London, Collins, 1969.

Watt JM, Breyer-Brankwijk MG: The Medicinal and Poisonous Plants of Southern and Eastern Africa. Edinburgh, Scotland, E & S Livingstone, 1962.

General Information on Poisoning

Anonymous: Toxic Plant Hotline. Animal Poison Control Center. Toxicology Hotline, University of Illinois, College of Veterinary Medicine, Urbana, IL. Telephones: 1-800-672-1697 or 217-333-3611.

Cheeke PR (ed): Toxicants of Plant Origin, Vol I. Alkaloids. Boca Raton, FL, CRC Press, 1989.

Cheeke PR (ed): Toxicants of Plant Origin, Vol II. Glycosides. Boca Raton, FL, CRC Press, 1989.

Cheeke PR (ed): Toxicants of Plant Origin, Vol III. Proteins and Amino Acids. Boca Raton, FL, CRC Press, 1989.

Cheeke PR (ed): Toxicants of Plant Origin, Vol IV. Phenolics. Boca Raton, FL, CRC Press, 1989.

Cheeke P, Shull LR: Natural Toxicants in Feeds and Poisonous Plants. Westport, CT, AVI Publishing, 1985.

Fowler ME: Toxicities in exotic and zoo animals. Vet Clin North Am Small Anim 5:685, 1975.

Fowler ME: Plant Poisoning in Small Companion Animals. St. Louis, Ralston Purina, 1981.

Fowler ME: Plant poisoning in free-living wild animals—a review. J Wildl Dis 19:34, 1983.

Fowler ME: Plant poisoning in pet birds and reptiles. *In* Kirk RW (ed): Current Veterinary Therapy IX (Small Animal Practice). Philadelphia, WB Saunders, pp 737–743, 1986.

Graf AB: Exotica, Series 3, 10th ed. (Pictorial Cyclopedia of Exotic Plants from Tropical and Near-Tropic Regions). East Rutherford, NJ, Roehrs Company, 1980.

James LF, Keeler RF, Bailey EM Jr, et al (eds): Poisonous Plants. Proceedings of the Third International Symposium. Ames, Iowa State University Press, 1992.

Wall V (compiler): 1992 Toxic Plant Survey. Media, PA, Association of Zoological Horticulture and American Association of Zoo Veterinarians, 1992.

CHAPTER 15

Snakebite Protocols for Zoos

JOSEPH P. FLANAGAN

Accidental human exposure to venoms from captive venomous reptiles is a risk in any zoological facility maintaining these specimens in its display, research, or breeding collections. Veterinarians are likely to be the only staff in zoological institutions with any medical training other than basic first aid or cardiopulmonary resuscitation (CPR). It is therefore important for veterinarians treating venomous species to educate themselves in the prevention and first aid treatment of envenomation.

Many zoological facilities routinely maintain species not native to the local area. It is therefore important to work with local hospital emergency room personnel to educate them concerning the presence of exotic venomous species at the zoological facility. Zoo staff should advise emergency room personnel of the zoo's emergency snakebite procedures and where a supply of antivenom for the species of snakes is kept in the facility. The hospital may look upon the zoo as a resource should there be a bite from an exotic venomous snake in the local community for which they need treatment materials (antivenom) not normally stocked in the hospital pharmacy. The hospital may also call upon zoo staff to assist in the identification of local and exotic snakes involved in bite cases from the community.

Successful response to bites by venomous species depends on knowledge and preparation. Safe handling techniques, proper equipment, well-trained staff, and good planning are critical to the prevention of such incidents. These same elements are essential in response if and when an accidental bite does occur. Staff should be trained in procedures to use in the event of a bite from a venomous snake, and practice drills should be conducted regularly. Routine practice helps staff members familiarize themselves with emergency procedures and allows for regular review and updating of protocols as treatment regimens are revised.

PREVENTION

Institutions maintaining venomous reptiles have an obligation to their staff, visitors, and animals to operate in a safe manner and to be prepared in the event of any emergency. Venomous species of animals should not be maintained unless the institution is prepared to meet the financial commitments involved with adequate staffing, maintenance of cages, restraint, and treatment equipment, and with maintenance of a current antivenom inventory. In addition, protocols for staff training in routine handling measures and response to envenoma-

TABLE 15–1. Before a Bite

Practice safe animal handling and husbandry techniques
Write an emergency snakebite procedure
Establish alarm or warning system
Teach procedures to staff potentially involved in bites or emergency response
Consult with hospital emergency personnel concerning presence of exotic species at zoo
Procure AZA Antivenom Index
Maintain antivenom inventory
Maintain emergency equipment
Practice emergency response procedures
Review procedures regularly

tion should be in effect before staff members work with venomous species (Table 15–1).

All cages should be labeled with cage cards identifying the species of snake, number of specimens in the enclosure, whether the species is venomous or not, and which antivenom is appropriate in the event of envenomation (Fig. 15–1). Caging facilities should allow for visibility of all animals enclosed. Keepers servicing display or holding cages should be able to identify the location and posture of each animal without entering the enclosure. Housing areas should allow adequate space for staff to remove animals from their enclosures and handle them from a safe distance. Some species of snakes can strike out to approximately half their body length. A "safe" working distance is generally considered to be one body length of the animal being handled.[7]

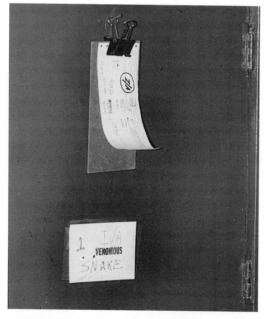

FIGURE 15–1. The cage card should identify the species of snake, number of specimens in the enclosure, whether the species is venomous or not, and which antivenom is appropriate.

If an animal requires physical handling, proper restraint procedures should be used at all times. Staff should be trained in restraint procedures with nonvenomous species before working with venomous specimens. Staff working with venomous species maintained in zoo quarantine or hospital facilities separate from the main collection should have similar training and be well trained in response to emergency scenarios.

Without exception, a minimum of two persons trained in the emergency treatment of envenomation should be present during the handling of any venomous animal. A number of restraint devices are available and are identified in their use elsewhere.[4] Physical restraint for veterinary examination or treatment often requires access to the oral cavity. This is safely carried out with snake hooks and Pilston tongs. These can be used to guide the animal into a clear plastic tube or squeeze box for restraint. If an animal is removed from an enclosure, the immediate area in which animals are restrained should be free of obstacles and hiding places in order to prevent the animal from escaping the handler's control. Handlers should identify escape routes for themselves and not become trapped. Specific circumstances may determine the specific method of restraint used. A snake hook or shift box may be all that is needed to transfer an animal into a new enclosure. A shield or squeeze box may be used if an animal needs an injection, or a clear plastic tube may be utilized for injections as well as for access to the oral cavity for examination, oral medication, or tube feeding. Physically "pinning" down the snake with a hook or sponge and transferring to manual restraint increases the risk to both handler and animal.

ANTIVENOM

No venomous snake should be maintained by an institution without prior acquisition of a suitable antivenom for use in the event of a bite from that specimen. Antivenoms are manufactured against the venoms of most venomous snakes throughout the world. In case an antivenom is not manufactured for a particular species, institutions must weigh the relative value of education or conservation purposes against the relative danger of a bite from that species. The two types of antivenom manufactured in the United States can be used against bites from all native venomous snakes (Wyeth Laboratories Inc., Marietta, PA). No antivenom is available for the venomous lizards in the genus *Heloderma*.

An Antivenom Index[1] is published by the American Zoo and Aquarium Association (AZA). This index is a useful guide to the types of antivenom recommended for use in treatment of bites by most species kept by zoological facilities. It also lists sources of antivenom and current phone numbers of persons who could act as consultants in the event of envenomation from exotic species of snakes. A current copy of the index should be kept by all facilities maintaining venomous reptiles. As new venomous snakes are acquired, reference should be made to the index in order to stock the most appropriate antivenoms.

Many antivenoms are manufactured in foreign countries for use against bites from snakes in their region. Acquisition of antivenom from such sources can be difficult because of export or importation restrictions of the countries involved. Procedures for importation of antivenoms to the United States are found in the Antivenom Index. Once antivenom is acquired, the instructions for its use are usually written in the language of the country of origin. Physicians require translation of the instructions before administering antivenom to a patient. If antivenom instructions are available only in a foreign language, translation should occur immediately upon receipt at the facility, not after a bite has occurred.

Antivenom should be stored in a controlled environment at approximately 4°C. It should not be exposed to temperature fluctuations and should never be frozen. A simple method of storage is to use clear plastic boxes with a code letter or number clearly visible when the refrigerated storage area is opened (Fig. 15–2). The code is used to match the antivenom with the species of animal for which it is suited. The expiration date of each antivenom should be clearly marked on the storage box, and inventory should be checked and renewed on a regular basis. Each snake in the collection should have an individual identification card (cage card). On the card of venomous species should be a clear notation of the type of antivenom recommended for use in the event of a bite from that specimen. The use of a code letter or number on the cage card to match against the antivenom in the storage area makes retrieval of the proper antivenom more efficient in the event of an emergency (Fig. 15–3).

EFFECTS OF VENOM

Venom is the secretion of modified salivary glands. It is used in the capture and digestion of prey. Venom is composed of a variety of proteins and enzymes that vary from species to species and may even vary within a species across a geographic range.[3] Venoms of different species of snakes have varying types of activity based largely on the species' usual prey. The venoms of vipers, pit vipers, and some elapids generally have the localized effect of tissue necrosis. The systemic effects include hypotension, hemorrhagic diathesis, hypersensitivity, and generalized myonecrosis. The venom of elapid snakes such as coral snakes, cobras, and sea snakes has more neurotoxic activity. Most venoms have a mixture of elements with varying neurotoxic, hemorrhagic, and necrotizing effects. Toxic effect depends on the species of snake, strength of the venom, the quantity and location of venom injection, and the size and health of the victim. Death is not a common sequela of bites from most venomous species and in the United States occurs in fewer than 1% of cases when medical care is started within 1 to 2 hours. World wide, approximately 10% of bites from venomous snakes result in death.[3, 6] However, permanent injury or death may occur in untreated or inappropriately treated cases. Rapid and appropriate treatment may lead to full recovery, but in some cases, death or permanent damage such as scarring, impaired function, or abnormal sensation may result in spite of excellent care.[6] Consequently, first aid efforts vary on the basis of the specifics of each case. The most important feature of any first aid effort is immediate transport to a medical facility where definitive care can be given.

COMMUNICATION

As previously mentioned, staff should work with venomous reptiles only when at least two fully trained persons are present. In the event of a bite, the second person will be available to take emergency actions. Upon being bitten, the victim should immediately advise his or her coworker (assistant) of the occurrence of a bite, the species of snake involved, and the area of the body bitten. The snake should be secured, and the victim should remove the animal's cage card from the

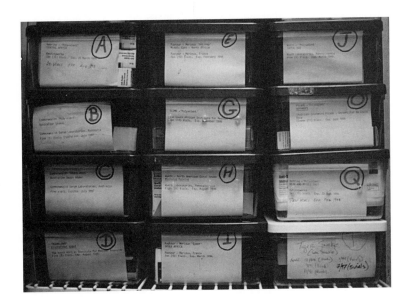

FIGURE 15–2. Antivenom should be stored at a controlled temperature near 4°C. Each type should be clearly marked with a code letter that matches it to the species of snakes for which it is used. Inventory should be "in date" and in adequate supply to treat a bite if needed.

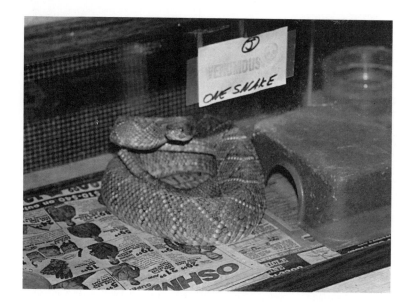

FIGURE 15–3. Letter codes on the cage card clearly identify the type of antivenom to use from the storage area.

enclosure and keep it during transport to the hospital. This can be used should the victim become unconscious, and it will act as a cross reference to the type of antivenom to be removed from the storage area for use in the hospital emergency room if required.

The assistant must then immediately contact an additional person ("contact") who must act as an information hub. The contact may be another keeper in the animal area, a person who normally acts as a switchboard operator, other office personnel, or an administrator. This contact should be given all available information, including who was bitten, by what species of animal, the location of the bite on the individual, and the individual's condition. The assistant is then freed to provide first aid efforts to the victim. Upon notification, the contact will call for emergency assistance to summon an ambulance or similar emergency transportation. The contact will also need to notify the designated hospital emergency room that a snakebite has occurred, what species was involved, and that the victim will be arriving soon. If an ambulance is called, an escort should be available to lead the vehicle from the entrance of the facility directly to the site where the envenomation occurred. Others to be notified should include the zoo director, appropriate curatorial or supervisory staff, and possibly public relations personnel.

Notification of coworkers and administrative personnel can be made through the use of an alarm system. Hard-wired systems have been developed to indicate the location where the alarm was sounded (Fig. 15–4). Depending on the location of venomous reptiles within the zoological facility and their relative distance to other buildings and/or personnel, other more inexpensive or available notification methods could be used to indicate that a bite has occurred and the location of the incident. These methods could entail the use of whistles, two-way radios, telephone lines, or other available means.

EMERGENCY FIRST AID

The exact treatment and handling of an envenomation varies with the species of animal involved and the

distance to the hospital (Table 15–2). No variation should be allowed on the basis of a subjective assessment of the "severity" of the bite. The victim should not wait to see whether the bite was a "dry bite" or only a small amount of venom was injected. The most important action in the event of a bite from a venomous

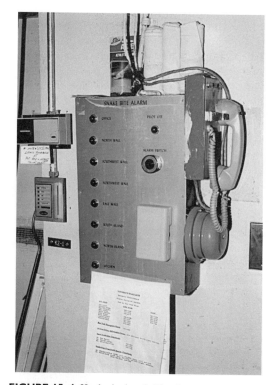

FIGURE 15–4. Hard-wired snakebite alarms can show the location where the bite occurred and have an audible signal that can be heard at a great distance. Emergency first aid equipment can be stored in the area of the alarm for convenience.

TABLE 15–2. Venomous Snakebite First Aid Equipment

Stretcher
Self-adherent elastic wrap (minimum 4 rolls)
Splints (various sizes for arm or leg use)
A copy of institutional snakebite procedures
Eyewash stations
Insect sting kit
Venom suction device ("The Extractor")

TABLE 15–4. Assistant Response

Stay calm
Notify contact for emergency transportation
Get antivenom from storage
Assist victim with immobilization of bitten limb
Stay with victim until assistance arrives

snake is that everyone involved should stay calm. The second most important action is to move the victim immediately to medical care. The risk of immediate death from the bite of a venomous snake is extremely small and would result from the intravenous injection of venom by a highly toxic species or an allergic reaction on the part of the victim. In most cases, there is plenty of time to get the victim to medical assistance with little risk to life or limb, but there should be no delay in transport to hospital care.

After notifying the assistant, the victim should immediately grab the cage card, attempt to secure the snake, and then remove jewelry and potentially restrictive clothing. Swelling of the bitten limb occurs through the local effects of many types of venom. Rings, bracelets, watches, and other restrictive materials could cut off circulation as the appendage swells (Table 15–3).

The spread of venom can be slowed through the use of passive immobilization (Table 15–4). In the case of bites from non-elapid snakes, the bitten extremity should be splinted to reduce activity, thus reducing the rate of lymphatic transport of the venom. The splint should not constrict the limb but rather immobilize it while the victim is transported. The limb should be kept at or below the level of the heart. Physical activity of the victim should be restricted as much as possible. A stretcher should be used if possible to carry the victim from the site of the bite to the ambulance or emergency vehicle. A tourniquet or ice could cause further damage from ischemia or by compounding the local necrotizing effects of the venom and should not be used.[5]

In the case of bites from certain species of elapid snakes, in which swelling of the limb and local tissue necrosis is limited or not expected, an improved method of slowing the distribution of venom involves Sutherland's pressure/immobilization technique. The method consists of firmly wrapping the entire extremity with an elastic bandage and then splinting (Fig. 15–5). The rationale is to confine the venom to the area of the bite until the victim arrives at a medical facility. The extremity is unwrapped only after an intravenous line is established and antivenom is available. This method should not be used for species whose venom causes significant local necrosis, such as vipers, pit vipers, and some elapids.[5] The wrap should be placed on the affected limb in a distal to a proximal manner, approximately as tight as if being applied to a sprain.

The victim should then be transported on a stretcher to a hospital emergency room for treatment. The appropriate antivenom should accompany the victim to the emergency room along with a copy of the AZA Antivenom Index.[4]

Medical opinion varies on the use of direct suction at the site of envenomation. In a study of the efficacy of "The Extractor" (Sawyer Products, P.O. 7036, Long Beach, CA 90807), it was shown to remove up to 34% of the venom after 30 minutes of application if applied immediately after the bite was inflicted (Fig. 15–6).[5] A delay in the use of suction of even a few minutes can significantly reduce the quantity of venom removed. If performed, suction should be applied over the site of the bite immediately, but only if medical care is at least 30 minutes away. Under no circumstances should incisions be made at the site of the bite wound.

TABLE 15–3. Bite Victim Response

Stay calm
Secure or kill snake
Grab "cage card"
Notify assistant
Remove jewelry and restrictive clothing
Immobilize affected limb and keep lower than heart
Wait quietly for assistance
Get transported on stretcher to nearest hospital emergency room

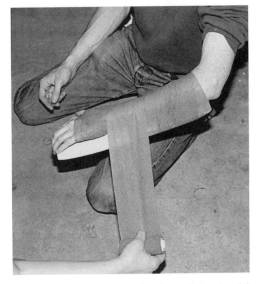

FIGURE 15–5. Pressure immobilization technique involving self-adhering elastic wrap and splinting to immobilize the bitten limb and inhibit the spread of venom.

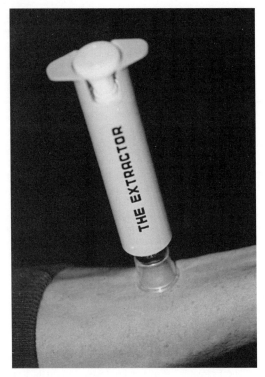

FIGURE 15–6. The extractor can be used if hospital treatment is more than 30 minutes away. It exerts approximately one atmosphere of negative pressure and can remove a quantity of venom if applied within minutes of a bite from a venomous snake.

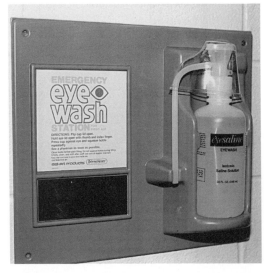

FIGURE 15–7. Eyewash stations should be used whenever venom contaminates the eye or conjunctival membranes.

If signs of anaphylactic shock (such as difficult breathing, laryngeal swelling, or low blood pressure) are present before the arrival of emergency medical aid, treatment may be necessary. Premeasured amounts of epinephrine found in insect sting kits (Anakit Hollister-Stier, Miles Inc., Pharmaceutical Division, Spokane, WA 99207) can be used and should be located in snakebite emergency first aid kits.

Under certain circumstances, venom may contaminate the eye and conjunctival membranes. Some pit vipers may strike and release venom before contact with a solid object, flinging venom into the air at the handler. In other cases, such as with spitting cobras, venom may be deliberately directed at the face and eyes of the handler. Venom should be immediately wiped from the face and away from the eyes. The eyes should be copiously irrigated with sterile saline solution, available at conveniently located eyewash stations wherever venomous snakes are maintained (Fig. 15–7). The victim should then go for treatment at a hospital emergency room.

BITES FROM VENOMOUS LIZARDS

Lizards in the genus *Heloderma* are the only types of lizard that are venomous. The genus has two species, both of which are popular zoo exhibit animals. There is no antivenom available for the bites from these lizards. Emergency first aid should consist of removal of jewelry and restrictive clothing and performing immediate suction, if possible, over the fang puncture sites, using the Sawyer venom extractor. The affected limb should be immobilized to reduce the rate of systemic spread of the venom.[1] The victim should be transported immediately to a hospital emergency room for treatment and monitoring.

REFERENCES

1. Boyer DM: The Antivenom Index. Bethesda, MD, American Zoo and Aquarium Association and the American Association of Poison Control Centers, 1994.
2. Dart RC, McNally JT, Spaite DW, Gustafson R: The sequelae of pitviper poisoning in the United States. *In* Campbell J, Brodie E (eds): Biology of the Pitvipers. Tyler, TX, Selva, pp 395–404, 1992.
3. Fowler ME: Veterinary Zootoxicology. Boca Raton, FL, CRC Press, 1994.
4. Fowler ME: Restraint and Handling of Wild and Domestic Animals, 2nd ed. Ames, IA, Iowa State University Press, 1995.
5. Hardy DL: A review of first aid measures for pitviper bite in North America with an appraisal of Extractor™ Suction and stun gun electroshock. *In* Campbell J, Brodie E (eds): Biology of the Pitvipers. Tyler, TX, Selva, pp 405–414, 1992.
6. Keyler DE: Venomous snake bite. *In* Tenth Annual Proceedings of the Association of Zoo Veterinary Technicians, pp 61–63, 1990.
7. Peterson KH: Personal communication. Houston, TX, Houston Zoo.

CHAPTER 16

Tuberculosis in Free-Ranging Mammals

ROY G. BENGIS

Pathogenic mycobacteriosis has been recorded as a cause of significant morbidity and mortality in *captive* mammals, birds, reptiles, amphibians, and fish, with some reports dating back to the latter decades of the 19th century. Wildlife collections in zoological gardens and primate colonies worldwide have been plagued by this chronic infectious disease, which has been well documented and has been the subject of many publications. This chapter, however, will deal with mycobacteriosis and, more specifically, bovine tuberculosis (BTB) in *free-ranging mammals*, which themselves may be indigenous, feral, or exotic in a particular ecosystem.

BTB is a chronic progressive bacterial disease, generally characterized by the development of pyogranulomatous lesions in the lungs and lymph nodes of the victim but with the potential to spread to almost any organ. This disease is rapidly emerging as one of the most significant infectious diseases of free-living mammals in many parts of the world today and is of grave concern to conservationists, wildlife veterinarians, wildlife managers, and regulatory bodies.

ETIOLOGY

Although sporadic cases of mycobacteriosis caused by *Mycobacterium avium* and some of the environmental saprophytic (atypical) mycobacteria have been reported, these opportunistic infections appear to be incidental and, in general, noncontagious in free-ranging mammalian populations. Virtually all cases of progressive, contagious tuberculosis reported in wild or feral populations have been due to infection with *Mycobacterium bovis*, the etiologic agent of BTB. *M. bovis* is one of the three closely related species of *Mycobacterium tuberculosis* complex, which can also cause tuberculosis in humans.

M. bovis isolates may be differentiated into numerous strains by means of a variety of sophisticated molecular biologic techniques, including polymerase chain reaction (PCR), restriction endonuclease analysis (REA), and restriction fragment length polymorphism (RFLP, which is DNA fingerprinting). This strain differentiation relies mainly on DNA polymorphism driven by mobile DNA (insertion sequences) and short repetitive DNA elements that are abundantly present in *M. tuberculosis*–complex bacteria.[58–60] The importance of strain differentiation lies in the field of molecular epidemiology for determining the sources or relationships of outbreaks, as well as their spatial and temporal spread.

RECORDED FREE-RANGING WILDLIFE HOST RANGE OF BOVINE TUBERCULOSIS

Tuberculosis caused by *M. bovis* has been reported in many free-ranging wildlife populations in geographically and climatologically diverse parts of the world (Table 16–1).

EPIZOOTIOLOGY AND TRANSMISSION

Source of Infection

Historically, BTB appears to have been a European disease of cattle that was disseminated to many countries on other continents during the colonial era, with the shipping of European breeds of cattle to these colonies for agricultural purposes, or to "upgrade" the native cattle breeds. These infected cattle then became an important source of infection for native livestock and, in turn, for free-ranging wildlife sharing pasture and habitat in those countries. Thus contact with infected domestic cattle or people was essential initially for the disease to establish itself in wildlife.[55] Three different scenarios have been identified once a wildlife population becomes infected.

Outbreaks of tuberculosis in free-ranging kudu,[1a, 30a, 38, 45, 48, 61] buffalo,[30a] lechwe antelope,[20, 21] water buffalo,[28] and bison,[22, 52a, 53] which all belong to the family Bovidae and have gregarious habits, become endemic. The infection persistently cycles in these populations, and these species appear to have the ability to become true maintenance hosts for *M. bovis*. The same pattern may apply in certain infected cervid populations.[1, 5, 41]

In contrast, lions, cheetahs,[31] wart hogs,[67] duiker,[38] feral pigs,[8, 15, 16, 43] hedgehogs,[35] and feral cats[14] appear to be "spill-over" hosts that have become incidentally infected, and there is limited possibility for the disease to persist in the population without an external source of reinfection. In support of this statement, McInerney and colleagues[39] reported that the prevalence of BTB in

TABLE 16–1. Free-Ranging Wildlife Species in Which Tuberculosis Has Been Recorded

Common Name	Genus and Species	Country	Reference
Greater kudu	*Tragelaphus strepsiceros*	South Arica	Paine et al, 1928[45]
		South Africa	Thornburn and Thomas, 1940[56]
		South Africa	Weber and van Hoven, 1992[61]
		South Africa	Bengis et al, in press[2]
Common duiker	*Sylvicapra grimmia*	South Africa	Paine et al, 1928[45]
American buffalo	*Syncerus caffer*	Uganda	Giulbride et al, 1963[23]
			Thurlbeck et al, 1965[57]
			Woodford, 1982[66]
		South Africa	Bengis et al, 1996[2]
Kafue lechwe	*Kobus leche bafuensis*	Zambia	Gallagher et al, 1972
Eland	*Taurotragus oryx*	Zambia	Kraus et al, 1990[32]
Warthog	*Phacochoerus aethiopicus*	Uganda	Woodford, 1982[67]
Lion	*Panthera leo*	South Africa	Keet et al, 1996[31]
Cheetah	*Acinonyx jubatus*	South Africa	Keet et al, 1996[31]
Chacma baboon	*Papio hamadryas*	South Africa	Keet et al, 1996[31]
Olive baboon	*Papio cynocephalus anubis*	Kenya	Tarara et al, 1985[52]
Black rhinoceros	*Diceros bicornis*	South Africa	Keep and Basson, 1973[30]
Impala	*Aepyceros melampus*	South Africa	De Vos et al, 1977[11]
White-tailed deer	*Odocoileus virginianus*	U.S.A.	Belli, 1962[1]
		U.S.A.	O.I.E. Report, 1996[43]
American Bison	*Bison bison*	Canada	Tessaro et al, 1990[53]
Elk	*Cervus canadensis*	U.S.A.	O.I.E. Report, 1995[42]
Feral swine	*Sus scrofa*	Hawaii	Essey et al, 1981[16]
		Australia	Corner et al, 1981[8]
		Italy	O.I.E. Report, 1996[43]
Axis deer	*Cervus axis axis*	Hawaii	Sawa et al, 1974[50]
Possum	*Trichosurus vulpecula*	New Zealand	Ekdahl et al, 1970[14]
Red deer	*Cervus elaphus*	New Zealand	Nugent and Lugton, 1995[41]
Ferrets	*Mustelo putorius furo*	New Zealand	Lugton et al, 1995[35]
Hedgehogs	*Erinaceus europaeus*	New Zealand	Lugton et al, 1995[35]
Water buffalo	*Bubalus bubalus*	Australia	Letts, 1964[34]
Wild boar			
Badger	*Meles meles*	England	Unknown, 1975
		Ireland	Unknown
Roe Deer	*Capreolus capreolus*	United Kingdon	O.I.E. Report, 1996[43]

feral pigs in the northern territories of Australia decreased from 47.7% to 6.2% after a dramatic depopulation of *M. bovis*–infected cattle and buffalo in the area.

The third scenario is one that has been described extensively in several medium- to high-density but less gregarious small nonungulate mammals and marsupials, such as badgers[6, 6a, 40a] in England and Ireland and possums[14, 29, 46, 47, 63] in New Zealand. These species also appear to be able to persistently maintain infection in their populations and become true reservoir hosts. This maintenance potential appears to be related to close and frequent intraspecific contact and to effective excretion routes of the organism.[63]

The situation with regard to BTB in baboons is controversial. Sapolsky and Else[49] and Tarara and associates[52] reported that horizontal transmission of disease between baboons appears to be minimal. This is in contrast to both the situation reported in captive primates and the preliminary data available from an outbreak of BTB in a troop of baboons in the Kruger National Park, South Africa, where disease appeared to be rapidly progressive in the individual as well as in the troop (Keet and Bengis, 1996, unpublished observations).

Thus in several regions of the world, infected wildlife maintenance hosts have now become endemically infected and represent important sources of infection for both domestic livestock and other wildlife species.

Transmission

In the original classical BTB situation in cattle, transmission was generally by aerosol (droplet) infection between individuals in close proximity; that is, BTB was a "nose-to-nose," density-dependent disease. The need in Europe to house livestock in barns during the inclement winter months and changes in farming practices (intensive dairy systems and feedlots) in the developing and developed world all facilitated transmission of this disease. In the less developed world, where it is necessary to kraal the cattle at night in enclosures to protect them from predators or discourage theft, aerosol transmission of infection would also be facilitated. Vertical (in utero) and pseudovertical (via nursing or grooming) transmission also occur but are less usual transmission modes.

In African buffalo, water buffalo, bison, and lechwe, most tuberculous lesions are found in the head nodes and thoracic organs, which indicates classical aerosol transmission between herd members, as is seen with cattle.

In predators that feed on infected carcasses, infection would be expected to take place via the digestive tract, as has been reported in zoo lions,[18] ferrets,[7] and domestic cats[10] and where gastrointestinal and hepatic lesions were most commonly encountered.

Contrary to expectations, in the three lions and two cheetah diagnosed with BTB in the Kruger National Park, the lesions were limited to lungs.[31] There are two possible explanations for this anomaly:

1. Direct intraspecific horizontal aerosol transmission from other pride members would occur during activities such as panting, grooming, or feeding (competitive growling and fighting over food).

2. Large predators frequently suffocate their prey by biting through and occluding the larynx/trachea or by biting over the muzzle to occlude the mouth and nostrils. In both situations, a prey animal with open pulmonary lesions could conceivably infect the predator during its agonal gasping struggles.

In baboons it is difficult to determine the site of the primary complex, as lesions compatible with both alimentary and respiratory infection routes are frequently encountered, and both or either may be involved. Thereafter, in this species, rapid hematogenous spread then occurs with miliary dissemination to many organs and sites. The presence of both mesenteric and renal lesions in these generalized cases makes fecal and urinary transmission feasible.

In cervids, the respiratory route appears to be the most important, inasmuch as lesions of the head nodes, tonsils, and thoracic organs are most frequently encountered.[5] Experimentation by Mackintosh and Griffin,[37] however, demonstrated that in farmed deer, primary infection of the tonsils appears to be the primary route, after which infection spreads to the medial retropharyngeal lymph node.

In possums and badgers, frequent intraspecific contact related to medium- to high-density populations and sequential den sharing and communal sett use, respectively, pulmonary infection is common, and aerosol spread is a major route of intraspecific transmission in both species.[63] In addition, in possums, tuberculous lymph node abscessation with fistulous tract formation results in external contamination with an infectious mucopurulent discharge. This may result in infection being passed on horizontally (during fighting or mating) to other possums or pseudovertical transmission (during nursing or grooming) to offspring. This infected discharge may also infect cattle through environmental contamination of food or water or through close contact (direct sniffing or mouthing) by curious cattle.

In badgers, superficial tuberculous skin lesions (abscesses, bite wounds), renal and mesenteric lesions may result in horizontal intraspecific spread through direct contact or indirect interspecific spread by environmental contamination with infectious exudate, feces, and urine. Badgers are implicated in 90% of new cattle cases of tuberculosis in southwest England.[6]

In kudu, *M. bovis* infection occurs via the oral, nasal, or cutaneous routes. The lymph nodes of the head appear to become infected first, and Thorburn and Thomas[56] theorized that because the parotid lymph nodes (which are assumed to drain the aural and upper head structures) are frequently affected and clinically enlarged and visible, these kudu, which shared range with infected cattle, scarified the skin around their ears by scratching at ticks and irritating horn flies, with their contaminated hind hooves. The shared range was very dense, and cattle and kudu were forced to use the same narrow footpaths, which were possibly contaminated by infected coughing cattle with open tuberculous lesions. Another possibility is that the very large ears of the kudu, which are relatively smooth and hairless on the inside of the pinna, frequently become scratched as they browse on thorn trees. These breaks in the epidermis then become contaminated by exudate from fistulating abscessed parotid lymph nodes of infected kudu browsing at the same level. Similarly, leaves contaminated by this exudate may be eaten by other kudu. This second transmission mode appears more likely, because identical lesions have been seen in five kudu in the greater Kruger National Park complex (Bengis and Keet, 1996, unpublished findings), which is a more open woodland/savannah in which confinement to narrow footpaths is not a feature, and buffalo, at much lower stocking rates, are the original source of infection (proved by molecular typing of the strain). In kudu, the infection then usually spreads to the thoracic organs, and extensive lesions involving lungs, lymph nodes, and pleura are common.

Thus, in summary, *M. bovis* infection may be transmitted by respiratory droplet infection or acquired from eating contaminated vegetation, material, or carcasses; drinking contaminated water; or contact with infectious exudates. Differences in route of transmission may be very significant, because fewer organisms are required for transmission by the respiratory than by the oral route in many species. Vertical (intrauterine) and pseudovertical transmission (through infected milk) may also occur but appear to be rare events.

Population at Risk

From the literature, it is apparent that *M. bovis* has an extremely wide potential host range. In captive wildlife, *M. bovis* infection has been reported in a wide variety of species from many taxa. All free-ranging mammals are potentially at risk if they come into contact with any infected host or its infective excretions, secretions, or exudates. A newly infected species then has the potential itself to become a reservoir host or a "dead-end" spill-over host, depending on its population density; social structure; feeding, mating, and territorial behavior; and habits.

SEXUAL PREDILECTION

No sexual predilection for *M. bovis* infection was recorded from more than 400 African buffalo randomly sampled during tuberculosis sampling in the Kruger National Park from 1992 to 1996. Hein and Tomasovic[28] similarly recorded no statistically significant sexual difference in tuberculosis prevalence among 11,322 water buffalo randomly slaughtered in the Northern territories of Australia. Gallagher,[20] however, reported an overall tuberculosis infection rate of 27% in males, in contrast to 41% in females, among randomly sampled Kafue lechwe in Zambia. He ascribed this to the added stresses of pregnancy and lactation in females and to the fact that the herds of females generally prefer the moister marsh edges for grazing, where mycobacterial survival in the environment may be enhanced. Lugton and associates,[35] in their study of wild ferrets in New Zealand, state that "there was a trend for more males than females to be infected" in a random sample of this species. This was ascribed to horizontal transmission through bite wounds during fighting among males. Similarly, Jackson and colleagues[29] reported that male possums (at two different sampling sites in New Zealand) were more frequently infected than were females (relative risk, 1.78), which differed from a finding in a previous longitudinal study population.

AGE PREDILECTION

As would be expected in a chronic progressive disease, a definite correlation exists between the age and infection rate in an infected population because the older the animal, the longer the exposure to infection. This has been demonstrated in African buffalo in South Africa[12] and Kafue lechwe in Zambia.[20] In New Zealand, Lugton and associates, in a study involving wild ferrets, noted that the relative risk of mature vs immature infection was 4.3 thus confirming this almost universal observation.[36] Also in New Zealand, Nugent and Lugton[41] reported that in a random sample of 65 deer, tuberculosis was present in 50% of the adults but not in any of the 10 fawns examined. In Australia, the selective harvesting of mature animals reduced the BTB prevalence in feral water buffalo from 16.4% to 1.7% over a period of 19 years.[28]

There are, however, certain exceptions, and these are usually related to the following scenarios:

1. Rapid progression of the disease in a particular species, with early development of "open" infectious lesions. This appears to be important in possums and baboons, in which the other important behavioral prerequisite, frequent intraspecific contact, is present.

2. Pseudovertical transmission from dam to infant during contact, grooming, and nursing. Once again, this is illustrated most dramatically in possums, in which draining fistulous tracts contaminate the fur of the dam and also in which up to 12% of tuberculous females have been recorded to have lesions in the mammary glands.[29]

3. A situation in which extremely high tuberculosis prevalence rates are present in a gregarious species. This has been documented in South Africa (Raath and Bengis, unpublished results), where, in an African buffalo herd with a random sample prevalence rate of 92%, all of the four calves sampled were found to be infected.

Prevalence and Mortality Rates

Prevalence rates of BTB in free-ranging wildlife vary greatly and depend on transmission rate, which in turn is a function of immunologic susceptibility, pathogen excretion and secretion rates, social structure in the target species, and behavioral vulnerability to infection. Prevalence rate estimates are usually based on the presence of macropathologic lesions, but true prevalence rates can be determined only after histopathologic studies and culture have also been completed. Another problem with interpretation of prevalence rate estimates is that in wildlife they are frequently based on a "once off" ad hoc sample of a population that may or may not have been randomly collected and represent just a window in the time course of the epidemic curve of the disease. In view of these limitations, BTB prevalence estimates were reported for certain populations of free-ranging wildlife (Table 16–2).

Mycobacterium bovis is generally an alien pathogen in these ecosystems, and some of the hosts listed appear to be immunologically naive and to have no innate resistance to infection; hence prevalence rates climb to more than 90% in possums and African buffalo, with reported progressive pathology and eventual death.

Mortality rates are difficult to assess in free-ranging wildlife, because so few carcasses become available for necropsy, particularly in uninhabited and extensive ecosystems in which coverage is difficult and predators and scavengers are common. This, coupled with the fact that BTB is usually a slow, insidious disease in most species and may take months or even years to progress from primary infection to generalized disease and death, make estimations of mortality rate difficult. The best estimates may be obtained from random samples of an infected population, in which it is assumed that all individuals with generalized disease or extensive caseating tuberculous pneumonia will die in the short term, and this is expressed as a percentage of the total sample. Using this assumption, Gallagher and colleagues determined that the tuberculosis related mortality rate among Kafue lechwe in the Lochinvar National Park would be in the region of 20% at the then current prevalence rate of 36%.[21] Similarly, De Vos and associates[12] reasoned that a 10% mortality rate could be expected in buffalo herds in the Kruger National Park, which had a disease prevalence of 65%, and Tessaro and colleagues suggested a tuberculosis-related mortality rate of 4% to 6% in bison in Wood Buffalo National Park, in which the prevalence of infection was found to be between 12% and 32%.[53]

To fine-tune these assumptions, it would be necessary to determine the time course from primary infection to death, after experimental infection of the species concerned by a natural route.

Survival of the Organism

Wilesmith (1991)[62a] reported survival of *M. bovis* in badger excreta from 3 to 14 days in summer and 28 to 70 days in winter in Great Britain. Duffield and Young[13] reported survival for 4 weeks in artificial conditions,

TABLE 16–2. Prevalence of Bovine Tuberculosis in Certain Free-Ranging Populations

Common Name	Country	Prevalence Rate	Remarks
Lechwe antelope	Zambia	36%	Random sampling
African buffalo	Uganda	10%	Random sampling
African buffalo	South Africa	3%–92%	Different herds, random sampling
Chacma baboons	South Africa	48%	Random sampling
Anubis baboon	Kenya	40%	Random sampling
Bison	Canada	33.4%	Random cull
Water buffalo	Australia	1.7%–16.4%	1964–1978; prevalence decreased as result of selective harvesting
Feral pigs	Australia	0.25%–19%	1976–1992; prevalence decreased as result of destocking of definitive hosts
Feral pigs	Italy	14%	Hunter kills
Ferrets	New Zealand	27%–88%	Random samples from different regions
Badgers	United Kingdom	6.5%	Random sampling
Possums	New Zealand	2.1%–93%	Random sampling, different sites
Wild deer	New Zealand	37%	Random sampling

kept in the shade or darkness at typical north Queensland, Australia, temperatures, but not exposed to direct sunlight. They[13] also reported that under field conditions in north Queensland, *M. bovis* survived in feces and soil in the shade for at least 1 week, but no longer than 2 weeks.

CLINICAL SIGNS

In general, and with few exceptions, clinical signs of infection with *M. bovis* become manifested only once the disease has progressed to an advanced stage. The insidious, slowly progressive nature of this disease and the lack of accompanying clinical signs in early and moderate cases are the frustrating hallmarks of a disease whose presence is usually not even suspected until the first positive necropsy is performed.

Clinical signs in advanced cases have been described in many species and include anorexia with resultant listlessness, weakness, depression, progressive emacia-

tion, and staring hair coat. In species with long hair, it may be difficult to appreciate the degree of emaciation from a distance. When advanced pulmonary disease is present coughing, reduced exercise tolerance and progressive dyspnea may be seen.

The few species in which animals may show certain definite clinical signs while apparently in generally good health are as follows:

1. Free-ranging kudu: BTB-infected animals frequently show mumps-like swellings below the ear and sometimes extending ventrally behind the ramus of the mandible (Fig. 16–1).[1a, 30a, 56] These swellings are a result of tuberculous abscessation of the parotid lymph nodes and may also frequently involve the retropharyngeal and cervical nodes. The swellings may be unilateral or bilateral and may form fistulating tracts draining to the exterior.

2. Possums: BTB-infected animals frequently develop draining fistulous tracts from infected superficial lymph nodes in the intermediate stages of disease. The

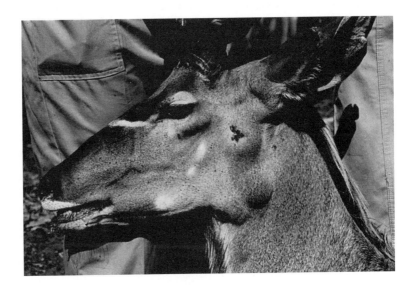

Figure 16–1. Tuberculous lymphadenitis in a greater kudu.

deep axillary and inguinal nodes are most commonly involved, and 31% of tuberculous possums were reported by Jackson and colleagues[29] to have open sinuses.

3. Occasionally, external swellings caused by enlarged lymph nodes, sometimes with draining abscesses, have been reported in wild axis deer[50] and in bison.[52a] Visible subcutaneous swellings or fistulas that result from pleural abscesses that penetrate the thoracic or abdominal wall have been reported in elk.[51a]

Other nonspecific clinical signs that have been recorded are poorly healing skin wounds in lions and badgers, areas of alopecia in lions and cheetah, and corneal opacities in lions and kudu.[31] Posterior paresis as a result of tuberculous spondylitis have been seen in a young baboon and an adult buffalo bull (Keet and Bengis, unpublished observations).

PATHOGENESIS

It is beyond the scope of this chapter to include an indepth treatise on the pathogenesis of *M. bovis*. However, to summarize,[54] tubercle bacilli enter the host via the respiratory, digestive, or percutaneous route. After exposure, *M. bovis* is ingested by phagocytes in the terminal bronchioles, lamina propria of the gastrointestinal tract, or dermis and subcutis. These phagocytes are then carried by lymphatic circulation to the regional lymph nodes or by general circulation to other sites and organs. After ingestion of the bacillus, the mononuclear macrophages attempt to kill the organism; however, virulent tubercle bacilli possess the ability to resist or escape killing. Also, their intracellular location protects the bacilli from bactericidal components in serum. The bacilli then multiply and destroy the phagocytes, and other phagocytes are recruited into the area to ingest the increasing number of tubercle bacilli. A small cluster of cells referred to as a *granuloma* develops. Cellular responses attempting to control the disease result in the accumulation of large numbers of phagocytes and finally the formation of a macroscopic lesion referred to as a *tubercle*. Ten to fourteen days later, cell-mediated immune (CMI) responses develop, increasing the capacity of macrophages to kill the intracellular bacilli. The CMI responses are mediated by T lymphocytes, which release lymphokines that attract, immobilize, and activate additional blood-borne mononuclear cells at the sites where virulent mycobacteria or their products are present. The cellular hypersensitivity that develops contributes to cell death and tissue destruction (caseous necrosis).

Thereafter, in some instances, liquefaction and cavity formation result from enzymatic action, and rupture of these cavities (which may contain many bacilli) allows the organism access to the airways, lymphatic vessels, or blood stream, facilitating aerosol transmission bacterial metastasis to lymph nodes or other distant sites. Only by lysing macrophages whose infection has gotten out of control and creating an inflammatory response is it possible for the tissues to dilute out the invading organisms to a level that can be resisted by new infiltrating, activated mononuclear phagocytes. In many cases, however, fibrous tissue development in the dynamics of granuloma formation probably contribute to the localization of lesions. Thus granuloma formation is an attempt by the host to localize the disease process and to allow inflammatory and immune mechanisms to destroy the bacilli. It must be remembered that no matter how effective this encapsulation appears to be, and even if the lesion appears to be regressing and is surrounded by well-organized connective tissue, such lesions may contain viable bacilli in a dormant focus.

Depending on the success of this immune response, which appears to vary from species to species, the infection may become localized to the primary complex, may have limited spread with secondary localization, or may become progressive and, at worst, develop into overwhelming generalized or miliary disease.

Unfortunately, in most documented studies of BTB in wildlife, *progressive* disease appears to be the rule and not the exception.

PATHOLOGY

Gross Pathology

The major differences in gross pathology among different wildlife species suffering from BTB are related to the distribution of lesion sites and the degree of encapsulation, caseation, liquefaction, and mineralization (nature of the exudate) of the lesions (Table 16–3).

The classical well-known macropathologic picture (distribution of lesions and nature of exudate), as is seen in tuberculous cattle, has been described in some wild bovids such as bison, African buffalo, and water buffalo, and occasionally in cervids.

The macroscopic lesions in general consist of focal to multifocal pyogranulomata in the affected organ. In the lungs, multifocal lesions may become confluent, resulting in large areas of consolidation. The pyogranulomata usually contain a caseous necrotic exudate, which may become liquefied or inspissated. Encapsulation and calcification of the lesions is a regular feature. In more generalized cases in cattle, wild bovids, and cervids, granulomata are numerous on the serosa of the pleura (Fig. 16–2) and peritoneum, forming typical smooth, encapsulated, pearl-like nodules.

There are, however, some definite differences with regard to the gross appearance of tuberculous lesions. The pulmonary lesions in lions appear as ill-defined, firm, rubbery areas of consolidation. No caseation is present, but the cavities present in the lesions contain an opaque, mucoid exudate.[31] Similarly, in ferrets, caseation is rarely seen and the necrotic foci present in these lesions are generally coagulative or liquefactive. Subpleural pale, discoid-shaped plaques are also frequently found in this species.[7, 35] In kudu[2a, 30a] and cervids, affected lymph nodes are markedly enlarged, thin-walled, and turgid, containing creamy, liquid exudate. In the lungs of African buffalo and Kafue lechwe, focal to multifocal caseous granulomata that frequently form confluent areas of consolidation are most commonly found in the bases of the diaphragmatic lobes (Fig. 16–3).

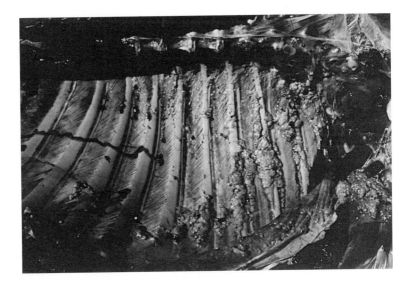

Figure 16–2. Tuberculous pleuritis in a greater kudu.

TABLE 16–3. Frequency Distribution of Tuberculous Lesion Sites in Different Species

Species	Head Nodes	Thoracic Organs	Gastrointestinal Tract	Peripheral Nodes	Other Sites
African Buffalo	+ +	+ + +	+	+	
			—	—	—
Water Buffalo	+ +	+ + +	+ +	+	+ +
Bison	+ + +	+ +	+	+	+ +
Cervids	+ + +	+ + +	+ +	+	
					—
Baboons	+	+ + +	+ +	+	+ + +
Lions	—	+ + +	(+ +)	—	—
Cheetahs	—	+ + +	—	—	—
Possums	+	+ + +	+ +	+ + +	+ +
Badgers	+ + +	+ + +	+ +	+ +	+ +
Ferrets	+ +	+ +	+ + +	+ +	+ + +
Feral Pigs	+ + +	—	—	—	—
Lechwe	+	+ + +	+ +	+ +	—

Symbols: − = unreported; + = rare; + + = common; + + + = frequent; ( ) = reported in captive animals.

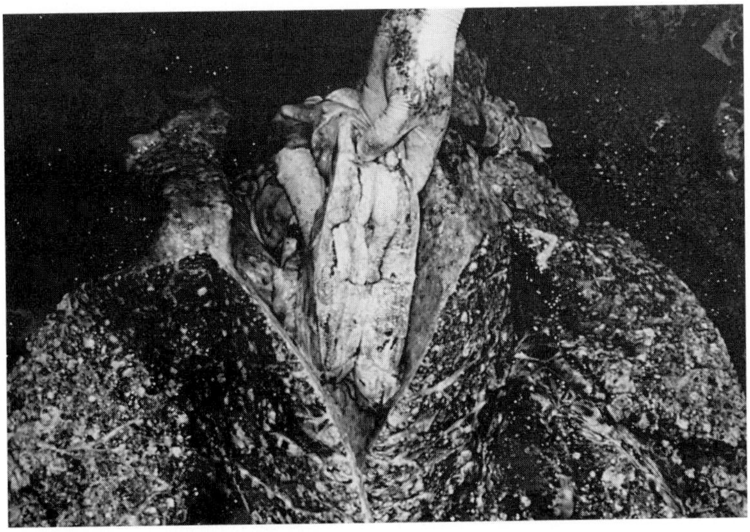

Figure 16–3. Advanced pulmonary tuberculosis in a Cape buffalo: lungs and bronchial lymph nodes.

In baboons, pulmonary lesions normally consist of multifocal to confluent granulomatous pneumonia, with caseation and cavitation (Fig. 16–4). In this species, there appears to be an accelerated progression of the disease, with miliary hematogenous spread to many organs and focal to multifocal granulomata frequently in the spleen, kidneys, and liver. Splenic lesions in this species were a consistent finding in all 19 positive cases in which necropsies were performed in the Kruger National Park (Keet and Bengis, unpublished observations). In possums, the peripheral lymph nodes have the highest prevalence of tubercular lesions, and the respiratory tract is the second most frequent site of tubercular pathology. In this species, the exudate is of a more fluid, mucoid consistency.

Histopathology

Microscopically, in most species, the lesions have the appearance of typical pyogranulomata, consisting of a connective tissue capsule, a peripheral mantle of lymphocytes mixed with epithelioid macrophages, and modest numbers of Langhans'-type giant cells.[17] Central zones are characterized by large areas of caseous or liquefactive necrosis, containing substantial populations of neutrophils and widely scattered foci of mineralized debris. The degree of encapsulation and mineralization appears to be related to the age of the lesion and indirectly to the host's resistance and immune competence. With Ziehl-Neelsen staining, acid-fast organisms are usually scanty and located in the necrotic centers and within the layer of macrophages. In contrast, numerous acid-fast bacilli are usually present in and around the necrotic tissue in baboons and possums.[7, 31]

In ferrets, microscopic granulomatous foci were present in the livers of 94% of infected animals, although gross hepatic lesions had not been observed in any of them. Histologic lesions were also present in the gastrointestinal tract of 76% of ferrets, but multinucleate giant cells were not observed in this species.

DIAGNOSIS

Postmortem Diagnosis

A presumptive postmortem diagnosis depends on the presence of characteristic macroscopic lesions, which may be substantiated and confirmed by

1. Demonstration of acid-fast bacilli in impression smears or exudates.
2. Typical histopathologic picture.
3. Culture, isolation, and identification of the pathogen.
4. PCR techniques.

All necropsy cases in which suspect granulomatous inflammatory lesions are present should be investigated for tuberculosis. Confirmational isolation and identification of the organism are mandatory for a diagnosis, and when possible, typing of the pathogen is useful for follow-up epidemiologic studies.

Antemortem Diagnosis

Although the antemortem diagnosis of BTB in wild mammals has been most widely used in captive wildlife, there is definite application for these diagnostic tests in free-ranging wildlife for nonlethal surveys and also for screening herds from which individuals or groups are to be obtained for translocation or genetic enrichment programs. Unfortunately, the current antemortem diagnostic tests lack the specificity and sensitivity for screening individuals in a population. The results of these tests can, at best, be interpreted only on a herd basis if certification for zoo–sanitary regulatory requirements is the objective.

Tuberculin skin testing, which relies on a delayed tissue hypersensitivity reaction, has been used extensively and refined for domestic cattle. This test in free-ranging wild mammals is difficult to execute, frequently inaccurate, and notoriously difficult to interpret, for the following reasons.

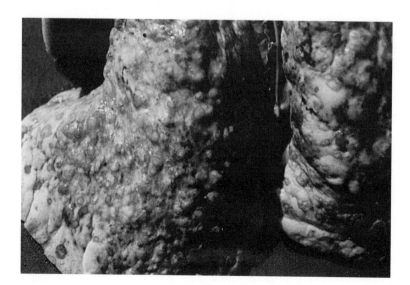

Figure 16–4. Advanced tuberculosis of a baboon lung.

The Animal Factor

1. A double immobilization, with its attendant risks, is usually required for satisfactory restraint, execution, and reading of the test.

2. Newly captured animals out of free-ranging populations are often highly stressed during their adaptation periods in captivity. Such stress and the initial catabolic state in these animals during adaptation to new surroundings and strange diets additively raise endogenous cortisol levels, which may attenuate the local delayed hypersensitivity reaction on which this antemortem test is based.[62]

3. Baseline data, to assist in interpretation of the results and to decide on cutoff points for each species, are often unavailable.

The Antigen Factor

Various antigens ranging from rough "old" tuberculins to highly purified protein derivatives (PPDs) have been used with varying results. This results in problems with interpretation caused by lack of standardization. The ensured long-term availability of any one of these antigens, as well as their potency standardization are empirical.

Skin Site

The site for effective intradermal injection and the feasibility of accurate skinfold measurements also vary from one species to the next. Pachyderms such as elephant, rhinoceros, hippopotamus, buffalo, and giraffes are particularly difficult subjects. In the more hairless species, in which there is no shave area to identify the injection sites, it is important to mark these sites with a long-lasting indelible ink circle.

Sensitivity of the Test

In wildlife, as in cattle, problems are also encountered in early infections as well as in so-called "anergic" cases with advanced disease in which test results are negative. These false-negative results are the most serious obstacle to tuberculosis-free certification.

Specificity of the Test

Frequently, wild animals with certain habitat or environmental preferences are exposed to large numbers of atypical mycobacteria, resulting in cross-sensitization to standard tuberculin antigens. This is particularly true in aquatic and mud-wallowing species, such as the African and Asian pachyderms, and may result in frequent false-positive reactions. A simultaneous, balanced, comparative avian tuberculin skin test may assist in the interpretation of this type of reaction.

In spite of all of these potential pitfalls, successful tuberculin skin testing has been reported in deer with a sensitivity of 70% and specificity of 99% with the comparative cervical test[10a]) and in free-ranging African buffalo with a sensitivity of 77.5% and a specificity of 92.5%.[46a]) It remains essential that an interpretation key be developed to address the inverse relationship of sensitivity and specificity. This test remains the mainstay of most tuberculosis testing in captive and farmed wildlife of many species, and intradermal sites commonly used are eyelid or abdominal skin (primates) and cervical or tailfold skin in ungulates.

Another drawback of the skin test is that with the exception of a 10-day post-testing window period, retesting of suspicious or inconclusive animals should be delayed for 60 to 90 days because of post-test suppression of skin reactivity.

In Vitro Cellular Immunodiagnostic Assays

The first of these tests, the lymphocyte transformation assay, was developed as an alternative to skin testing.[44] Although it was useful in research and diagnosis,[26] practical limitations in handling and performance speed generally precluded its widespread use.

Subsequent recognition of the cytokines and their role in tuberculosis immunology has led to the development of an in vitro assay for gamma interferon as an indicator of tuberculosis.[64] This assay was demonstrated by Wood and associates[65] to have superior sensitivity and specificity in comparison with the single intradermal tuberculin test in cattle, and similar results were reported by Griffin and Cross[26] in farmed deer. Unfortunately, this test makes use of specific monoclonal antibodies that detect only bovine (including buffalo), caprine, and ovine gamma interferon. Evaluation of this test in free-ranging African buffalo[46a]) has yielded encouraging results.

It is hoped that diagnostic kits based on this principal will be developed to address the problem of tuberculosis diagnosis and screening in wild pachyderms, felids, suids, and many other species. The beauty of this test is that only a single heparinized blood sample is needed, and no antigens are injected into the animal, so that a retest can be performed at any time. One drawback is that the blood sample must be processed within 8 hours of sampling. This processing involves the 16- to 24-hour incubation (at 37°C) of three aliquots of the blood sample in the presence of bovine PPD, avian PPD, and phosphate buffered saline, respectively. Thereafter, the plasma supernatant is drawn off and can be frozen away for later analysis.

Serodiagnostic Tests

A variety of serodiagnostic assays have been developed for tuberculosis, but results showed considerable variation in sensitivity and specificity.[25] These assays appear to be of limited value because of the dominance of cell-mediated rather than humoral responses to this disease. Humoral responses are generally weak and slow to develop, frequently reaching significant levels only in advanced cases of disease, especially when cell-mediated immunity has broken down and anergy develops. Mycobacterial organisms contain antigens that are widely shared among species, and animals that have recurrent contact with environmental mycobacteria may develop low levels of immune sensitization, which might explain the lack of specificity found with serodiagnostic testing.

Thus the use of tests that measure humoral antibody levels (e.g., the various enzyme-linked immunosorbent assay [ELISA] systems) are not used for routine tuberculosis testing or screening. They may, however, have application in identifying anergic animals and may be useful in a post–skin test antibody response test, because it has been shown that exposure to tubercular antigens during tuberculin testing increases humoral antibody levels in tuberculous animals.[27, 33]

Differential Diagnosis

The presence of any chronic granulomatous or pyogranulomatous lesion at necropsy should alert the clinician to the possibility of mycobacteriosis. Numerous other infectious agents, particularly the higher bacteria and systemic fungi, can cause lesions that are macroscopically difficult to distinguish from tuberculous lesions. These differential diagnoses include actinomycosis, actinobacillosis, nocardiosis, pseudotuberculosis, epizootic lymphangitis, blastomycosis, cryptococcosis, histoplasmosis, coccidioidomycosis, fusiformis nodosus and sporotrichosis, to name a few. Certain neoplasms involving the lungs, lymph nodes, and serous membranes may also be confused with tuberculous lesions. In general, etiologic differentiation is possible only by histopathology with special staining techniques or by culture and isolation when appropriate.

Veterinary Public Health Concerns

Of all the bacterial diseases, tuberculosis is still the leading cause of human morbidity and mortality in many developing countries.[40] It is the leading infectious killer of adults in the world, accounting for more than 3 million deaths annually. The contribution of *M. bovis* to the number of clinical cases in developing countries is unknown, because most diagnoses are made on radiographic or acid-fast positive sputum samples, and treatment is instituted without culture and identification of the causative organism. *M. bovis*, as the cause of human tuberculosis, is therefore probably grossly underreported, inasmuch as mycobacteriologic examinations employed in many laboratories fail to differentiate between *M. bovis* and *M. tuberculosis*. At the beginning of the 20th century, in the pre-pasteurization era, it was estimated that 40% of all human tuberculosis cases were caused by *M. bovis* with a predilection for extra pulmonary sites. For example, in Great Britain in 1937, *M. bovis* was responsible for 85% of primary abdominal tuberculosis, 50% of cervical lymphadenitis, 49% of tuberculous lupus, 25% of tuberculous meningitis, and 20% of bone and joint tuberculosis. However, occupational or sociologic exposure to aerosols containing infectious material can result in pulmonary infectious disease in humans. The advent of the human immunodeficiency virus (HIV) panzootic is a strong predisposing factor to the development of postprimary tuberculosis in dually infected persons.[24] It is therefore probable that HIV infection will also predispose to the reactivation of disease caused by *M. bovis*.

In the changing nature of human tuberculosis caused by *M. bovis*, there are indications that a cattle-to-human link may now be epidemiologically augmented by human-to-cattle and human-to-human transmission. In several developing countries in Africa where *M. bovis* infection is present in domestic livestock, local customs—such as the drinking of raw or soured unpasteurized milk, as well as close physical association with infected animals in which livestock share shelter with people, as is practiced by certain pastoral ethnic groups—may play a key role in the transmission of this disease. With regard to wildlife, numerous populations of indigenous, exotic, and feral wildlife are known to be infected with BTB; wherever these animals or their carcasses are handled, a finite risk of zoonotic transmission exists. Thus with game capture exercises, culling operations, clinical treatment of wild animals, or abattoir processing operations, suitable sanitary precautions should be observed if tuberculosis is known or suspected to be present in that wildlife population. There are several instances in which tuberculous animals among captive wildlife have infected their keepers. In a report from the Audubon Park Zoo in New Orleans,[9] 7 of 24 zookeepers exposed to a Southern white rhinoceros (*Ceratotherium simum*) that died of severe *M. bovis* pneumonia became infected.

Control and Treatment

The control of BTB in *free-ranging* wildlife is an extremely difficult, almost impossible task unless drastic measures are instituted. Wildlife managers should strive at all costs to prevent introduction of the disease by preventing contact with domestic livestock or translocation of infected wildlife into a tuberculosis-free conservation area.

Once introduced, and if a sylvatic maintenance host is present in that ecosystem, the disease will be almost impossible to eradicate without extreme measures.

The decision about which option to implement for the control or attempted eradication of this disease will depend on the status of the free-living maintenance host concerned: that is, is it an indigenous species, is it a free-ranging exotic species, or is it a free-ranging feral species? The ecologic considerations and public opinion become much more relevant in dealings with an infected indigenous population. Some case histories illustrate this point:

In Australia, where *feral* water buffalo became a free-ranging tuberculosis maintenance host in the Northern Territories, the decision was made to attempt to depopulate this area, and subsequently hundreds of thousands of these buffalo were killed and processed. Feral cattle in the same area were also depopulated. This program appears to have come a long way to reaching its goal in that the monitoring of an associated (nonmaintenance host) indicator species, the feral pig, has shown a dramatic decrease in tuberculosis prevalence from 19% in 1976 to 0.25% in 1992[39] since the numbers of infected bovids have been reduced.

In New Zealand, population control of the possum and possibly the ferret has been an accepted practice to protect the national cattle herd from these free-ranging *exotics* and to support the national BTB eradication scheme.[44, 46]

On Molokai, Hawaii, *M. bovis* disappeared from

both wild deer and feral swine following "focal depopulation" of these species and depopulation of infected cattle. Focal depopulation is the depletion of affected animal species in selected areas by sustained hunting and trapping until evidence of disease is no longer present.

As animals are removed from an affected area, individuals from outside migrate into the area, attracted by the improved food supply. Consequently, animal populations remain fairly constant throughout the process.[15, 16] This type of success relies, of course, on accurate identification of infected foci.

In these situations, depopulation, be it by hunting, shooting, trapping, or poisoning, appears to have been acceptable to conservationists and most members of the public, because exotic species are being controlled, which generally is to the benefit of the habitat and indigenous wildlife. Additional population control techniques, such as chemical or immunosterilization and contraception, are currently being investigated in the problem areas. With tuberculosis in an indigenous species that has become a maintenance host to this alien organism, such as African buffalo and antelopes in Africa, bison in Canada, and badgers in England and Ireland, control of the disease becomes a lot more complex and emotional. The presence of this disease in an indigenous wildlife population carries certain inherent implications:

1. It may reach prevalence and subsequently mortality rates that may negatively affect the population dynamics of the host species. In the Kafue lechwe, which is an endemic species in Zambia, mortality rates of 20% from BTB infection were estimated by Gallagher and colleagues.[20, 21] In the Kruger National Park, the prevalence of BTB in several buffalo herds now exceeds 60%, and a random sample from one herd had a prevalence rate of 92%.

2. It may "spill over" into other species and may even pose a threat to rare and endangered species. In the Kruger National Park, BTB has now spilled over into lions, cheetah, baboons, and kudu.

3. It is a potential new source of infection for neighboring domestic livestock.

4. It has zoonotic implications, particularly in conservation areas or where wild animals are harvested for human consumption.

5. It may result in regulatory constraints being placed on translocation of other sympatric species in the conservation area, resulting in that area's becoming a "conservation island." This is particularly disturbing when a moratorium may be placed on the translocation of rare and endangered species, because of the presence of tuberculosis and the absence of reliable antemortem screening tests for the disease. A case in point is that of free-ranging black and white rhinoceros in Africa, where 90% of the remaining natural populations reside in two conservation areas that currently have a high prevalence of BTB in their buffalo herds.

The options available for addressing this disease problem are as follows:

Option 1. Laissez faire—do nothing. In the light of the implications mentioned, this may be irresponsible or shortsighted.

Option 2. Minimal interference—in which no control efforts are initiated but active intensive monitoring and epidemiologic research are undertaken. This option allows researchers to study the disease dynamics and monitor the potential impact on the population as well as spillover into other species. This is a very important aspect that has frequently been neglected in the past. Many of the outbreaks reported in the 1960s to 1980s were "once off" surveys, which are indicative of the status of the disease during a particular time. A better understanding of tuberculosis disease dynamics with attendant predictive value would have been available for several free-ranging species had regular monitoring been implemented. This option is the minimum that should be done.

Option 3. Limited intervention—to buy time. This is appropriate for preventing spread to known disease-free herds of the same species. In the African buffalo tuberculosis outbreaks in Queen Elizabeth National Park[66] and Kruger National Park,[2, 12] there existed definite areas where the buffalo herds were tuberculosis free. In order to prevent spread of infection to these herds, depopulation of buffalo at the interface between the diseased and disease-free herds to effectively create a buffalo-free zone may achieve this goal. In Uganda, a natural barrier in the form of a dense forest appears to have assisted in this separation. Similarly, in Canada, where tuberculosis-infected wood/plains buffalo hybrid herds in Wood Buffalo National Park could encroach on disease-free, genetically pure wood buffalo herds, the creation of a buffalo-free corridor between the two may be a viable option.

A second indication for this limited intervention would be if a few infected foci were identified in a generally tuberculosis-free area. This would be a strong motivation to extirpate infected herds by means of focal depopulation.[2]

Another indication for limited intervention would be to reduce spill over of infection into other species. Here the focal depopulation of all known high-prevalence herds could feasibly reduce the amount of gross environmental contamination and chance of spread to satellite species. All these scenarios would, however, entail the destruction of significant numbers of animals, which, even if justifiable, would not be very popular among some environmentalists and members of the public. The advantage of these methods would be to contain the infection and retain the disease-free status of segments of the population. This would be a valuable tool to use until an effective vaccine or better option becomes available.

Option 4. This option is the most drastic and involves the total depopulation of infected herds in a conservation area, with the idea of repopulating the area with disease-free animals after a suitable time period. This option would probably receive little support from conservationists and the public.

Option 5. This option involves test and slaughter and obviously is applicable only to small, finite populations of rare or endangered species for which a sensitive and specific antemortem test is available.

Vaccination and Treatment

In the long term, the most appealing and popular control measure would be vaccination with progressive reduction in the susceptibility to infection of the target species. The bacille Calmette-Guérin (BCG) is the basis of a tuberculosis vaccine that has been most widely used in humans and domestic livestock throughout many countries of the world, but its use is illegal in the United States. It is originally an *M. bovis* isolate with low pathogenicity. The use of BCG in tuberculosis control programs in cattle and humans in many parts of the world have met with varying success. Much of this variability has been ascribed to the dose and route of administration. Immunologic advances have indicated that low-dose administration appears to result in better "immune locking," resulting in improved responses in the appropriate T lymphocyte population and, in turn, in better protection in cattle and deer. It also appears that oral, intratracheal, and intranasal administration of BCG in cattle, and in some cases in possums, gave equal or superior protection in comparison with the subcutaneous route.[3]

Another vaccine candidate, *Mycobacterium vaccae,* has yielded promising results when given orally to badgers in a trial in Ireland.[51] This same organism has shown promise as an immunostimulant in humans. In other species, however, vaccines produced with this organism have so far proved disappointing in their ability to protect against challenge.[43] The only other attractive candidate vaccine is one that has been developed from the vole bacillus, *Mycobacterium microti.* Results from a British Medical Research Council trial yielded results comparable with those of BCG.

The global epidemic of tuberculosis in humans compounded by the current HIV pandemic have focused the attention of researchers in many countries on the development of alternative new generation vaccines. New approaches include the development of a BCG recombinant, rationally attenuated *M. bovis* vaccine, subunit vaccines, DNA vaccines, and heterologous host vectors for protective mycobacterial antigens.

Vaccine application to free-ranging wildlife depends on the recommended route of administration. Although various projectile systems such as drop-out darts and biobullets are available for long-range remote injection of large mammals, these would be an expensive and time-consuming option. It would be more practical to administer the vaccine by means of baits, drinking water, or aerosol sprays from helicopters, or to have it spread by or as a self-replicating agent throughout a target herd. These last alternatives could be contemplated only if the environmental safety of the vaccine in target and nontarget species has been thoroughly investigated.

In the final analysis, the development and practical administration of a safe and effective vaccine for BTB remains a long-term solution for controlling this disease in a free-ranging population.

Treatment of free-ranging mammals with antituberculous drugs is not practical because of the long treatment period required for using multiple drug therapy. It has been successfully used only in small groups of animals from endangered species that have been captured and confined for the treatment period.[19]

Domestic Animal Health Concerns

In many countries in the world, active BTB eradication schemes in domestic cattle have been successfully implemented and executed at great cost over a number of years. This has resulted in eradication of the disease in some countries or has brought the prevalence rate down to fractional levels, so that eradication appears attainable in the near future. The specter of new sylvatic maintenance hosts for BTB in such countries is a nightmare for the veterinary regulatory and public health authorities. This bleak situation already exists in the United States, Canada, New Zealand, Australia, Western Europe, and South Africa. The control of BTB in free-ranging wildlife will remain a challenge for many years to come and necessitates focused research funding and effort.

REFERENCES

1. Belli LB: Bovine tuberculosis in white tailed deer. Can Vet J 3:356–358, 1962.
1a. Bengis RG, Keet DR, Michel AL, Kriek NPJ: Tuberculosis, caused by *Mycobacterium bovis,* in a kudu (*Tragelaphus strepsiceros*) from a commercial game farm in the Malelane area of the Mpumalanga Province, South Africa. Onderstepoort J Vet Res, in press.
2. Bengis RG, Kriek NPJ, Keet DF, et al: An outbreak of bovine tuberculosis in a free-living African buffalo (*Syncerus caffer–Sparrman*) population in the Kruger National Park: a preliminary report. Onderstepoort J Vet Res 63:15–18, 1996.
3. Buddle B, Aldwell F, Wedlock N: Vaccination of cattle and possums against bovine tuberculosis. Proceedings of the Otago Conference on Tuberculosis in Wildlife and Domestic Animals, University of Otago, Otago, Dunedin, New Zealand, pp 111–115, 1995.
4. Buddle B, Monaghan M, Hewinson G, et al: Report of the meeting of an OIE ad hoc Group on Bovine Tuberculosis Control in Developing Countries, Paris, 10–21 February 1996. Paris, Office International des Epizooties, 1996.
5. Carter CE: Tuberculosis control in the New Zealand deer industry. Proceedings of a Symposium on Bovine Tuberculosis in Cervidae, Denver, pp 61–65, 1991.
6. Clifton-Hadley R, Cheeseman CL: *Mycobacterium bovis* infection in a wild badger (*Meles meles*) population. Proceedings of the Otago Symposium on Tuberculosis in Wildlife and Domestic Animals, University of Otago, Otago, Dunedin, New Zealand, pp 260–263, 1995.
6a. Clifton-Hadley RS, Wilesmith JW, Stuart FA: *Mycobacterium bovis* in the European badger (*Meles meles*): epidemiological findings in tuberculous badgers from a naturally infected population. Epidemiol Infect 111:9–19, 1993.
7. Cook M, Wobeser G, Luton I: Comparative pathology of *Mycobacterium bovis* infection in possums and ferrets. Proceedings of the Otago Conference on Tuberculosis in Wildlife and Domestic Animals, University of Otago, Otago, Dunedin, New Zealand, pp 232–235, 1995.
8. Corner LA, Barret RH, Lepper WD, et al: A survey of mycobacteriosis of feral pigs in the Northern Territory. Australian Veterinary Journal, 57:537, 1981.
9. Dalovisio JR, Stetter M, Mikota-Wells S: Rhinoceros' rhinorrhea: cause of an outbreak of infection due to airborne *Mycobacterium bovis* in zookeepers. Clin Infect Dis 15:598–600, 1992.
10. Dannenberg AMJ: Pathogenesis of pulmonary tuberculosis in man and animals. *In* Montali RJ (ed): Proceedings of the Symposium on Mycobacterial Infections in Zoo Animals. Washington, DC: Smithsonian Institution Press, pp 165–175, 1978.
10a. de Lisle GW, Corrin KC, Carter CE: Ancillary tests for detecting

tuberculosis in farmed deer. Proceedings of the Deer Branch of the New Zealand Veterinary Association, Course No. 1, pp 9–12, 1984.

11. De Vos V, McCully RM, Van Niekerk CAW: Mycobacteriosis in the Kruger National Park. Koedoe 20:1–9, 1977.

12. De Vos V, Raath JP, Bengis RG, et al: The epidemiology of bovine tuberculosis in the Kruger National Park, South Africa. Proceedings of the Otago Conference on Tuberculosis in Wildlife and Domestic Animals, University of Otago, Otago, Dunedin, New Zealand, pp 255–259, 1995.

13. Duffield BJ, Young DA: Survival of *Mycobacterium bovis* in defined environmental conditions. Vet Microbiol 10:193–197, 1985.

14. Ekdahl MO, Smith BO, Money BL: Tuberculosis in some wild and feral animals in New Zealand. New Zealand Veterinary Journal 18:44–45, 1970.

15. Essey MA: Follow up survey of feral swine for *Mycobacterium bovis* infection on the Hawaiian island of Molokai. Proceedings of the Annual Meeting of the United States Animal Health Association, vol 87, pp 589–595, 1983.

16. Essey MA, Payne RL, Himes EM, Luchsinger D: Bovine tuberculosis surveys in axis deer and feral swine on the Hawaiian island of Molokai. Proceedings of the Annual Meeting of the United States Animal Health Association , vol 85, pp 538–549, 1981.

17. Essey MA, Vantium JS: *Mycobacterium bovis* infection in captive Cervidae: an eradication program. *In* Thoen CO, Steele JH (eds): *Mycobacterium bovis* Infection in Animals and Humans. Ames, Iowa State University Press, pp 145–157, 1995.

18. Eulenberger K, Elze K, Schuppel KF, et al: Tuberkulose und ihre bekampfung bei primaten und feliden im Leipziger Zoologischen Garten von 1951–1990. Erkrankungen der Zootier, Verhandelungsbericht des 34 Internasionale Symposium uber die Erkrankungen der Zoo- und Wildtiere, Santander, Spain, pp 7–15, 1992.

19. Flamand JRB, Greth A, Haagsma J, Griffin F: An outbreak of tuberculosis in a captive herd of Arabian oryx (*Oryx leucoryx*): diagnosis and monitoring. Vet Record 134:115–118, 1994.

20. Gallagher J: Handling lechwe antelope for vaccination and tuberculin testing. Vet Record 90:367, 1972.

21. Gallagher J, Macadam I, Sayer J, Van Lavieren JP: Pulmonary tuberculosis in free-living lechwe antelope in Zambia. Trop Animal Health Prod 4:204–213, 1972.

22. Gates CC, Melton DA, McLeod R: Cattle diseases in Northern Canadian bison: a complex management issue. Poster presentation at Ungulés/Ungulates 91 Conference, Section: Population: Pathology and Mortality Factors. pp 547–550, 1991.

23. Giulbride PDL, Rollison DHL, McAnulty EG, et al: Tuberculosis in the free living African (Cape) buffalo (*Syncerus caffer*, Sparrman). J Comp Pathol Theriol 73:337–348, 1963.

24. Grange JM: Human aspects of *Mycobacterium bovis* infection. *In* Thoen CO, Steele JH (eds): *Mycobacterium bovis* Infection in Animals and Humans. Ames, Iowa State University Press, pp 29–46, 1995.

25. Grange JM, Laszlo A: Serodiagnostic tests for tuberculosis: a need for assessment of their operational predictive accuracy and acceptability. Bull WHO 68(5):571–576, 1990.

26. Griffin JFT, Cross JP: Diagnosis of tuberculosis in New Zealand farmed deer: an evaluation of intradermal skin testing and laboratory techniques. Irish Vet J 42:101–107, 1986.

27. Hanna J, Neill SD, O'Brien JJ: Vet Microbiol 13:243–249, 1992.

28. Hein WR, Tomasovic AA: An abbatoir survey of tuberculosis in feral buffaloes. Aust Vet J 57:543–547, 1981.

29. Jackson R, Cooke M, Coleman J, et al: Transmission and pathogenesis of tuberculosis in possums. Proceedings of the Otago Conference on Tuberculosis in Wildlife and Domestic Animals, University of Otago, Otago, Dunedin, New Zealand, pp 228–231, 1995.

30. Keep ME, Basson PA: Mycobacteriosis in a black rhinoceros (*Diceros bicornis* Linnaeus 1758). J South Afr Vet Assoc 3:285–288, 1973.

30a. Keet DF, Kriek NPJ, Bengis RG, Michel AL: Tuberculosis in buffaloes (*Syncerus caffer*) in the Kruger National Park. Spread of the disease to kudu (*Tragelaphus strepsiceros*). Onderstepoort J Vet Res, in press.

31. Keet DF, Kriek NPJ, Penrith M-L, et al: Tuberculosis in buffaloes (*Syncerus caffer*) in the Kruger National Park: spread of the disease to other species. Onderstepoort J Vet Res 63:239–244, 1996.

32. Krauss H, Roettcher D, Weiss R, et al: Wildlife as a potential source of infection in domestic animals—studies on game in Zambia. Unknown source, pp 42–57, 1990.

33. Lepper AWD, Pearson CW, Outteridge PM: Assessment of the bentonite flocculation test for detecting tuberculosis in cattle. Aust Vet J 49:445–450, 1973.

34. Letts GA: Feral animals in the Northern Territory. Aust Vet J 40:84, 1964.

35. Lugton I, Johnstone A, Wobeser G, et al: *Mycobacterium bovis* infection in New Zealand hedgehogs (*Erinaceus europaeus*). Proceedings of the Otago Conference on Tuberculosis in Wildlife and Domestic Animals, University of Otago, Otago, Dunedin, New Zealand, pp 287–289, 1995.

36. Lugton I, Wobeser G, Morris R, Caley P: A study on *Mycobacterium bovis* infection in wild ferrets. Proceedings of the Otago Conference on Tuberculosis in Wildlife and Domestic Animals, University of Otago, Otago, Dunedin, New Zealand, pp 239–242, 1995.

37. Mackintosh CG, Griffin JFT: *In* Proceedings of the New Zealand Veterinary Association Deer Group, vol 10, pp 297–304, 1993.

38. Martinaglia G: A strain of *Mycobacterium tuberculosis* from giraffe and further observations of *M. tuberculosis* from the koodoo and the duiker. 16th Report of the Director of Veterinary Services and Animal Industry, Union of South Africa, p 143, 1930.

39. McInerney J, Small K, Caley P: Prevalence of *Mycobacterium bovis* in feral pigs in the northern territory. Proceedings of the Otago Conference on Tuberculosis in Wildlife and Domestic Animals, University of Otago, Otago, Dunedin, New Zealand, pp 252–254, 1995.

40. Meslin FX, Cosivi O: World Health Organization. *In* Thoen CO, Steele JH (eds): *Mycobacterium bovis* Infection in Animals and Humans. Ames, Iowa State University Press, pp 22–25, 1995.

40a. Nolan A, Wilesmith JW: Tuberculosis in badgers (*Meles meles*). Vet Microbiol 40:179–191, 1994.

41. Nugent G, Lugton I: Prevalence of bovine tuberculosis in wild deer in the Hauhungaroa range, North Island, New Zealand. Proceedings of the Otago Conference on Tuberculosis in Wildlife and Domestic Animals, University of Otago, Otago, Dunedin, New Zealand, pp 273–275, 1995.

42. Office Internationale d'Epizooties: O.I.E. Report of the Working Group on Wildlife Diseases, Paris, June 13–15, 1995.

43. Office Internationale d'Epizooties: O.I.E. Report of the Working Group on Wildlife Diseases, 1996.

44. Outteridge PM, Lepper AWD: The detection of tuberculin-sensitive lymphocytes from bovine blood by uptake of radio-labelled nucleosides. Res Vet Sci 14:296–305, 1973.

45. Paine R, Martinaglia G: Tuberculosis in wild buck living under natural conditions. J South Afr Med Assoc 1:87, 1928.

46. Pannet G: Possum control in the Wellington region: how successful has it been? Proceedings of the Otago Conference on Tuberculosis in Wildlife and Domestic Animals, University of Otago, Otago, Dunedin, New Zealand, pp 294–296, 1995.

46a. Raath JP, et al: Evaluation of the comparative intradermal skin test and the in vitro gamma interferon assay for the ante mortem diagnosis of bovine tuberculosis in free ranging African buffalo (*Syncerus caffer*) in the Kruger National Park. In preparation.

47. Roberts M: Tuberculosis control in possums: culling or vaccination? Proceedings of the Otago Conference on Tuberculosis in Wildlife and Domestic Animals, University of Otago, Otago, Dunedin, New Zealand, pp, 222–224, 1995.

48. Robinson EM: A note on strains of tuberculosis from the Cape kudu. Onderstepoort J Vet Res Animal Industry 19:23, 1944.

49. Sapolsky RM, Else JG: Bovine tuberculosis in a wild baboon population: epidemiological aspects. J Med Primatol 16:229–235, 1987.

50. Sawa TR, Thoen CO, Nagoa WT: *Mycobacterium bovis* infec-tion in wild axis deer in Hawaii. J Am Vet Assoc 1965:998–999, 1974.

51. Stanford JL: Should it be cows that we are vaccinating? Proceedings of the Annual Conference on the National Federation of Badger Groups, pp 59–63, September 11–13, 1992.

51a. Stumpff CD: Epidemiological study of an outbreak of bovine tuberculosis in confined elk herds. Proc US Anim Health Assoc 86:528–537, 1982.

52. Tarara R, Suleman MA, Sapolsky R, et al: Tuberculosis in wild olive baboons, *Papio cynocephalus anubis* (Lesson) in Kenya. J Wildlife Dis 21(2):137–140, 1985.

52a. Tessaro SV: A descriptive and epizootiologic study of brucellosis and tuberculosis in bison in northern Canada. PhD thesis, University of Saskatchewan, 1988.

53. Tessaro SV, Forbes LB, Turcotte C: A survey of brucellosis and tuberculosis in bison in and around Wood Buffalo National Park, Canada. Can Vet J 31:174–180, 1990.

54. Thoen CO, Bloom BR: Pathogenesis of *Mycobacterium bovis*. *In*

Thoen CO, Steele JH (eds): *Mycobacterium bovis* Infection in Animals and Humans. Ames, Iowa State University Press, pp 3–14, 1995.

55. Thoen CO, Himes EM: Tuberculosis. *In* Davis JW, Karsted LH, Trainer DP (eds): Infectious Diseases of Wild Animals. Ames, Iowa State University Press, pp 263–274, 1981.

56. Thorburn JA, Thomas AD: Tuberculosis in the Cape kudu. J South Afr Vet Med Assoc 11(1):3–10, 1940.

57. Thurlbeck WM, Butas CA, Mankiewicz EM, Laws RM: Chronic pulmonary disease in the wild buffalo (*Syncerus caffer*) in Uganda. Am Rev Respir Dis 92:801–805, 1965.

58. Van Sooligen D, De Haas PEW, Hermans PWM, Groenen PMA: Comparison of various repetitive DNA elements as genetic markers for strain differentiation and epidemiology of *Mycobacterium tuberculosis*. J Clin Microbiol 31:1987–1995, 1993.

59. Van Sooligen D, Hermans PWM, De Haas PEW, et al: The occurrence and stability of insertion sequences in *Mycobacterium tuberculosis* strains: evaluation of IS-dependent DNA polymorphism as a tool in the epidemiology of tuberculosis. J Clin Microbiol 29:2578–2586, 1991.

60. Van Sooligen D, Hermans PWM, De Haas W, Van Embden JDA: Insertion element IS1081 associated restriction fragment length polymorphism in *Mycobacterium tuberculosis* complex species: a reliable tool for recognizing *Mycobacterium bovis* BCB. J Clin Microbiol 30:1772–1777, 1992.

61. Weber A, Van Hoven W: Tuberculosis of the parotid salivary gland in a kudu. *Tragelaphus strepsiceros.* Koedoe 35(1):119–122, 1992.

62. Whipple D, Bolin C: Effect of stress on comparative cervical skin test reponses in cattle. Proceedings of the Otago Conference on Tuberculosis in Wildlife and Domestic Animals, University of Otago, Otago, Dunedin, New Zealand, pp 310–312, 1995.

62a. Wilesmith JW: Ecological and epidemiological findings from a prospective study of a naturally infected badger population. Symposium on Tuberculosis (publication No. 132), Palmerston North, New Zealand, Massey University, Veterinary Continuing Education, pp 89–111, 1991.

63. Wobeser G: Involvement of small wild animals in bovine tuberculosis. Proceedings of the Otago Conference on Tuberculosis in Wildlife and Domestic Animals, University of Otago, Otago, Dunedin, New Zealand, pp 267–269, 1995.

64. Wood PR, Corner LA, Plackett P: Development of a simple, rapid in vitro cellular asssay for bovine tuberculosis based on the production of gamma interferon. Res Vet Sci 49:46–49, 1990.

65. Wood PR, Corner LA, Rothel JS, et al: Field comparison of the interferon-gamma assay and the intradermal tuberculin test for the diagnosis of bovine tuberculosis. Aust Vet J 68(9):286–290, 1991.

66. Woodford MH: Tuberculosis in wildlife in the Ruwenzori National Park, Uganda (Part I). Trop Animal Health Prod 14:81–88, 1982.

67. Woodford MH: Tuberculosis in wildlife in the Ruwenzori National Park, Uganda (Part II). Trop Animal Health Prod 14:155–160, 1982.

CHAPTER 17

Vermin Control

LUCY H. SPELMAN

In this discussion, *vermin* refers to vertebrate pests, or unwanted birds and mammals, found in zoos or wildlife parks. Vermin contribute to economic losses. They consume and contaminate foods, prey on collection animals, and detract from the visitor experience by damaging plants and buildings. Vermin can also transmit infectious diseases to collection animals. The resulting morbidity and mortality increase the caseload for the veterinary staff and carry zoonotic risk. For many of these diseases, treatment is unrewarding, and control depends on prevention (Table 17–1). Despite the fact that licensed animal facilities are required to maintain a pest control program (Animal Welfare Act, Part 3, Section 3), relatively little has been published on vermin control in zoo or wildlife parks.[3, 4, 9]

INTEGRATED PEST MANAGEMENT

General

The most successful pest control programs employ the general strategy of integrated pest management (IPM).[3,

[8, 9] The goal of IPM is to reduce pest numbers to a tolerable level through methods that are least disruptive to the environment. The pest is first identified and its natural history is reviewed (i.e., feeding patterns, reproductive cycles). Control measures are then selected from the following categories: exclusion, habitat management, sanitation, removal (trapping, baiting, relocation, or euthanasia), and repellents. In a zoo or wildlife park, the veterinary staff should oversee any method involving chemical agents or animal handling. Whenever possible, nontoxic and nonlethal solutions should be sought for vertebrate pest control. Consultation with commercial pest control companies that emphasize "least toxic" methods may be extremely helpful (e.g., Bio-Integral Resource Center (BIRC), Berkeley, CA 94707; phone: 510-524-2567).

Communication among keepers, pest control staff (if present), and veterinary staff is essential to the success of IPM.[3] Keepers are the first line of defense, and they should be trained to monitor pest numbers. This includes daily patrol of fence lines for tracks, droppings, signs of burrowing, digging, and so forth. The program is coordinated by a pest control officer (the veterinarian

TABLE 17–1. Examples of Infectious Diseases Potentially Transmitted by Vermin

Disease	Pest Species	Zoo Species
*Balisascaris procyonis**	Raccoons	Primates Ratites Turkeys
Canine distemper virus	Raccoons, feral dogs	Red panda, black-footed ferret Canids Large felids (lions, tigers, jaguar, puma)
*Chlamydia psittaci**	Columbiforms	Psittacine birds
Lymphocytic choriomeningitis virus	Rodents (mice)	Callitrichids
Mycobacterium species *avium** *bovis*	Birds (especially waterfowl) Deer	Marsupials, primates Artiodactylids (e.g., camel) Perissodactylids (e.g., rhino)
Paraelaphostrongylus tenuis	White-tailed deer (Intermediate host: snail)	Artiodactylids (oryx, reindeer, sable)
Sarcocystis species	Feral mammals (Intermediate host: cockroach)	Psittacine birds
Rabies virus*	Raccoons, skunks, bats, feral dogs or cats	All
*Toxoplasma gondii**	Feral cats	Marsupials Psittacine birds

*Zoonotic.

in some cases) who receives input from the keepers and devises a control plan. The pest control officer updates the area supervisors and veterinary staff with regard to problem areas and scheduled measures (e.g., trapping, baiting). Both the pest control officer and the keepers may be licensed to apply pesticides. Most states offer certifying examinations for pesticide application in accordance with U.S. Environmental Protection Agency (EPA) guidelines and with state and local regulations.

Exclusion and Habitat Management

Physical barriers are the first step in vermin control. General examples include perimeter fencing, roofing, netting, below-ground fencing, and properly sealed doors and windows. The next step is to eliminate harborages by blocking or removing burrows, pruning foliage (e.g., fruit trees that attract birds or rodents), preventing access to false ceilings or cement block, and sealing gaps around pipes and electrical wires (especially important in dealing with rodents). For exclusion and habitat management measures to succeed, the identity and the biology of the pest must be known. Most small mammals and birds may be identified through visual or physical evidence (droppings, nests, tracks, trails, burrows, damaged structures, gnaw marks). Additional useful information includes habitat and food preferences (feeding frequency and pattern), water requirements, reproductive cycle (seasonality, fecundity), social habits, home range, and physical abilities. Although structural modifications may be the most expensive aspect of vertebrate pest control, they are long lasting (and ideally are built into the design of new exhibits).

Sanitation

Food storage bins should be well sealed and elevated above ground. Stored feed bags or hay should be arranged in rows with adequate space between them to facilitate detection of a pest problem and placement of baits or traps when necessary. In addition to vigilant cleaning of animal areas, uneaten food should be recovered as frequently as possible. Ideally, foodstuffs are not offered until midmorning and uneaten portions are removed before dark. Food for human consumption should not be kept in animal areas. Common areas (e.g., picnic tables, concession stands) should be regularly cleaned, and public feeding of waterfowl, squirrels, and other pest species should be discouraged.

Trapping

The risk of secondary toxicity and nontarget toxicity from baiting is especially high in zoo and wildlife parks. Therefore, trapping is preferred over baiting for removal of vertebrate pests, with the exception of severe rodent overpopulation. One advantage of trapping is that pests are clearly identified. However, proper trap placement and surveillance are labor intensive, and trapping limits pest numbers only when combined with appropriate exclusion measures. Dead-fall or snap traps are commonly used for rodents, but most other species are live-trapped. Several companies provide a wide selection of trap types (e.g., Tomahawk Live Trap Company, P.O. Box 323, East Mohawk Drive, Tomahawk, WI 54487; phone: 800-272-8727; their catalog includes a list of recommended baits for common species).

Live-trapped animals must be relocated or humanely euthanized. It is essential that each institution develop a policy for removal of vertebrate pests that incorporates the concerns of managers, veterinarians, keeper staff, and local wildlife officials. In general, state wildlife agencies regulate trapping and translocation of all species other than feral dogs, cats, and squirrels. In many cases, euthanasia of wild animals is permitted only through special exceptions granted by federal, local, and state wildlife agencies. In the development of this policy, several questions should be considered. For example, what are the risks of disease transmission to species in the relocation site? The recent spread of rabies along the eastern United States has been attributed to translocation of raccoons from Florida. After relocation, will the animal attempt to return (and be killed during attempts to cross the highway)? Will it be able to adapt to its new surroundings, or will it die of starvation? Will it disrupt the ecosystem at the translocation site? Some institutions relocate all live-trapped animals; others screen some for infectious diseases before relocation; and others euthanize all trapped vertebrates.

Baiting

Baiting should be undertaken as the last resort if exclusion, sanitation, and trapping fail to control the problem or if pest numbers are high and infectious disease threatens the collection. Various sedative and deterrent baits have been designed for birds, but most baits for mammals are designed to be lethal. Baiting has serious disadvantages, which include toxin resistance (e.g., to warfarin), untargeted toxicity (small mammals, birds), and secondary toxicity (e.g., brodifacoum), which may even occur through invertebrate intermediate hosts (e.g., cockroaches).[7] In addition, carcasses can be difficult to recover from burrows or building spaces and can attract more pests as they decay.

A few general statements can be made regarding toxic baits. Only clearly labeled "bait stations" should be used, and each should be designed to allow access only to the target species. For example, bait stations for rodents should have two openings, located on opposite sides of the box, that allow animals to see an escape route as they enter. All stations should be clearly labeled and secure. Ideally, bait maps are constructed for each area of the zoo or park. All stations should be regularly monitored by keepers and pest control staff to determine the species of pest visiting and the efficacy of the selected agent. If necessary, nontarget species can be baited away from the area.

Repellents

Alternatives to toxic baits include taste, sound, and visual repellents. Various chemical taste preparations that may discourage browsing by rabbits or deer or pilfering by birds are available, but most are unsuccessful over the long term because they require regular and repeated application. Sound or visual repellents are also regarded as generally ineffective and may disturb collection animals. Commercial pest control companies continue the search for nontoxic methods of pest control, and several new strategies (e.g., pheromones) appear promising. In fact, many of these companies advertise extensively on the World Wide Web, which can serve as an alternative source of ideas.

Other Methods

Biologic control may work in specific situations with careful monitoring. For example, the American roadrunner (*Geococcyx californiana*) may be used to control house sparrows (*Passer domesticus*) in an aviary exhibit, but this predator may also eat other small birds. Contraception is the best means of vertebrate pest control, but practical methods have yet to be developed. Hormonal implants (levonegesterol in skunks)[1] and contraceptive vaccines (porcine zona pellucida [PZP] vaccine in wild ungulates)[6, 11] have proved effective, but these techniques are expensive and labor intensive. Several oral contraceptive agents (boric acid, immunocontraception) have great potential for feral rodent and rabbit control.[5, 10]

RODENTS

Mice and Rats

Common rat species include the larger Norway rat (also known as the sewer or white rat, *Rattus norvegicus*), and the roof rat (also known as the ship or black rat, *Rattus rattus*). As a rule, for every rat seen at night, there are at least five or more in the vicinity. Because rats prey on mice, controlling a rat problem may reveal a mouse problem. It is also useful to remember that rats, unlike mice, require water and prefer to nest near a water source.

The house mouse (*Mus musculus*) can be found living indoors regardless of season. In comparison, the "wild" mice species (e.g., deer mouse, *Peromyscus* species; meadow mouse or vole, *Microtus* species; and harvest mouse, *Reithrodontomys* species) inhabit buildings primarily during the winter. Mice are extremely prolific; females produce, on average, a litter of 6.7 young every 20 days (87 per year).

In general, rodents have poor vision but exceptional senses of smell and touch.[2, 8] They are skillful climbers, jumpers, and swimmers and can fit through any opening the size of their heads or larger (>0.5 cm for mice, >1.3 cm for rats). Rodents are habitual, following the same pathways between food source and nesting site. Therefore, they are extremely wary of new objects such as traps and baits. Rats may train their young to avoid bait stations, or they may eventually use them as nest boxes. Although detection of a rodent problem is usually not difficult, species identification is essential for successful control. For example, traps should be placed high on rafters for roof rats but along baseboards for Norway rats. Successful control of wild mice requires blocking entry sites and removing sources of shelter, in addition to trapping, whereas removing food sources and nesting material are more important for control of house mice.

Rodent control depends on exclusion, removal of food sources, and an efficient trapping program. Entry sites may be identified by sprinkling a patch of nontoxic powder (flour, chalk, talcum) around suspect holes and examining the area for tracks. Physical modifications should include plugging all active exit and entry sites, installing metal kickplates on doors, screening drains, and placing guards to prevent movement along pipes and wires. In addition, trees and shrubs should be pruned to maintain a gap of at least 1 m between the foliage and ledges or roof tops. Ground cover and shrubs along buildings should also be pruned to expose the lower 45 cm of trunk to facilitate inspection and discourage burrowing and hiding. As always, garbage and uneaten food should be regularly removed from exhibit areas.

Because mice and rats habitually travel along edges, trapping is highly successful with proper trap placement. Snap traps are used most often, although live traps and glue boards may also be used. A common error in setting snap traps is to set too few: in an active area, a sufficient number of traps is 5 to 10. Traps should be set in groups of three, with the triggers against the walls to discourage jumping. If food is readily available, traps are more effective without bait. When bait is used, prebaiting the traps for several days before setting them allows the opportunity to switch baits if necessary (e.g., rolled oats and peanut butter, or a nonfood item such as cotton for nesting material.) If the remaining population appears to become trap shy, the traps should be removed for 1 week and then tried again. Gloves should be worn when the traps are handled, to avoid human smells. For field mice, the traps should first be buried in the soil and grass to remove odors and then placed similarly outside along runways. Glue boards are not as effective as snap traps and are considered inhumane by many people (mice often struggle and die of dehydration), but they may be useful in areas where placement of snap traps is difficult.

Baiting should be used only if trapping and rodent-proofing measures are unsuccessful. Baiting should be restricted to indoor areas, away from exhibits containing rodents or rodent-eating birds, mammals, and reptiles. Outdoor baiting should be used only when pest numbers are very high, because rodents may cache food and increase the risk of secondary toxicity. Commonly available baits and their general features are presented in Table 17–2. Whenever possible, first-generation anti-coagulants (D-Con, Final) should be used. Among the chemicals responsible for secondary toxicity, bradicoum (D-Con II, Talon) has been a significant problem for wild and captive raptors. If the risk of secondary toxicity is high, zoo or park personnel should consider vitamin D_3 (Quintox), zinc phosphide (Ridall), or brometha-lin (Assault, Vengeance) over the second-generation anticoagulants (D-Con II, Talon, Contrac).

Ground Squirrels, Moles, and Gophers

Ground squirrels, moles, gophers, and other burrowing rodents are readily captured by means of special underground traps. These species should not be baited, because the risk of secondary toxicity is high. Fumigation is another alternative and can also be used for mice and rats. Only underground burrow networks outside of animal exhibit areas should be treated. A variety of toxic and nontoxic commercial products are available, and fumigation is most effective when the soil is moist (see Table 17–2). Burrows should first be checked for commensal animals such as snakes and burrowing owls.

Tree Squirrels

Tree squirrels (*Sciurus* species) are capable of consuming large amounts of bird food (up to 3 kg per week) and may chew through aviary netting to access food sources. They also debark trees and consume fruits and flowers. Tree squirrels can be identified by their chewing pattern (several small holes) and droppings, which are larger and more cone-like in shape than those of rats. Live-trapping with peanut butter or fruit as bait is effective. Double-ended traps should be used although some squirrels are fast enough to escape before the second door closes. As with control measures for mice and rats, trees and shrubs should be pruned. Collars or steel spikes can be placed around trees or ledges to prevent access. A single strand of electric wire along the top fence line also discourages climbing.

SMALL MAMMALS (OMNIVORES)

Most small mammal pests are nocturnal omnivores (raccoons, opossums, skunks), and most are females looking for a den or food for their young. These pests may be identified by direct observation or by their behavior (e.g., structural damage, predation). For example, in the case of egg or bird predation, raccoons typically pull off the head of small birds and may eat the entrails; skunks crush one end of an egg (and may leave their odor behind) or eat only small portions of an adult bird; and opossums steal the whole egg (as do snakes) but rarely eat a whole bird.

General control measures for these species are similar: preventing access to food (by tightening garbage can lids), discouraging digging (by using a buried wire mesh fence), blocking areas under stairways or porches, pruning trees, using sheet metal barriers to prevent climbing, and trapping nuisance animals. Both raccoons (*Procyon lotor*) and opossums (*Didelphis virginiana*) can be trapped easily. Skunks are best controlled by exclusion, and there are important behavioral differences among species (e.g., the striped skunk, *Mephitus mephitus*, digs, whereas the spotted skunk, *Spilogale putorius*, climbs). Once a skunk den is identified, the animals should be observed at night until they leave the burrow, and then the entry/exit sites should be sealed.

TABLE 17–2. Commonly Available Rodenticides

Rodenticide	Features	Risk of Secondary Toxicity
First-Generation Anticoagulants		
Warfarin (D-Con, others) Diphacinone (Ditrac) Chlorphacinone (Rozol)	Widely used, low toxicity; no bait shyness so no prebaiting needed; death within 4–9 days, resistance increasing	Possible
Second-Generation Anticoagulants		
Broadifacoum (D-ConII, Talon) Bromadiolone (Contrac, Maki)	One dose may be lethal; resistance has not been documented; long biologic half-life	Moderate
Single-Dose Toxins		
Zinc phosphide (Ridall, ZP Rodent Bait) Vitamin D_3 (Quintox)	Rodents tend to be bait shy; high toxicity	Moderate
Fumigants		
Carbon dioxide Cyanide Magnesium or aluminum phosphide Other (least toxic): sulfur, sawdust	Useful in small spaces, especially with moist soil	Safest of all

If skunks are to be live-trapped, the trap should be covered because the skunks are less likely to spray if they cannot see a target.

The relatively high incidence of rabies in small mammals, especially in raccoons and skunks, is a critical factor in the decision of whether to relocate or euthanize these animals. For example, at the National Zoological Park (Washington, D.C.), rabies testing is performed on all dead raccoons recovered on the zoo grounds. Live-trapped raccoons exhibiting signs of illness are euthanized for rabies testing. Healthy raccoons are immobilized, tagged, fitted with a transponder, and relocated to a wooded area several miles away. Raccoons that return to zoo grounds are designated nuisance animals and are euthanized.

BATS

Among the more common pest species of bat are the little brown bat (*Myotis lucifugus*) and the big brown bat (*Eptesicus fuscus*). Urine and fecal debris are the usual reasons for eliminating a bat roost. However, it may be wise to remember the beneficial traits of bats, which include preying on several species of pest insects (wasps, mosquitos, and moths). Bats may be observed at dawn and dusk or can be detected by the presence of their feces, which readily disintegrate into tiny, shiny fragments of insect pieces (in contrast to mouse droppings, which remain formed). The only means of controlling bats is exclusion. Effective bat proofing requires placement of a fine mesh (1.25 cm or less) over entry and exit sites, so that the netting serves as a one-way exit, or by caulking. Despite heavy marketing, ultrasonic devices are ineffective. Open spaces can be filled with fiberglass insulation, which apparently discourages

bats from roosting. Sticky repellents placed around the entry or exit site may also work. Moth flakes (naphthalene) in sufficient amounts have been used successfully to deter bats, but they must be reapplied frequently, and their toxic fumes are potentially carcinogenic.

LARGE MAMMALS (CARNIVORES)

Common pest species include feral or domestic dogs and cats, coyotes, and foxes; less common are bobcats and mountain lions. Successful control of these species depends on a cooperative effort among zoo staff, local animal control officers, and wildlife officials. Options include trapping (for small cats, dogs, and foxes) and immobilization through remote injection (for coyotes, dogs, and large cats). A protocol that clearly states who is responsible for each control measure should be in place. For example, the designated role of the zoo veterinarian may be to respond to nuisance animals within immediate animal areas or to any animal that is potentially dangerous, diseased, or injured. For animals found in parking lots or service areas, local officials may be contacted directly.

DEER

Deer are perceived by some people as pests, by others as pets, and by still others as potential sport. The main species are the white-tailed deer (30 *Odocoileus virginianus* subspecies) and the western mule deer (11 *O. hemionus* subspecies). Deer typically forage in the early morning and late afternoon and can have a home range of up to 40 hectares. Although generally obvious when in high numbers, deer can be detected by their gnaw marks on trees (rough cuts, in contrast to the sharp cuts made by rabbits), rub marks, and browse selection (they prefer smaller twigs but if hungry will stand on their hind limbs to eat larger twigs).

Several habitat management measures can be attempted to control nuisance deer. Cultivated buffer zones that extend 365 m or longer from cover or woodlands can be established. Diversionary plots of alfalfa or clover can be planted, or the deer can be encouraged to eat unpalatable brush by spraying it with molasses (which also helps remove unwanted vegetation). Resistant ornamental foliage, such as American holly, lilac, black locust, onions, garlic, and dill can be planted (but if deer are starving, they will eat anything). Repellents have limited usefulness on ornamentals (e.g., a hanging bar of soap, such as Hinder) and are also overridden if the animals are starving. Other chemical repellents reported to be successful in some cases are human hair, hot sauce, predator scents, blood meal, and egg solids (Deer Away).

Fencing can exclude deer but is not always affordable or esthetically acceptable. The most effective fence is a complete perimeter fence taller than 2.4 m and built tight to the ground. Other options include a five-strand, 1.5-m wire fence with the top strand electrified, or a 1.5-m fence angled at 45 degrees to the ground. Single-strand electrical wire or electrical tape can also be used but requires regular maintenance and is not weather resistant. Wire cylinders can also be used for tree guards. Reproductive control with the PZP vaccine has been shown to be highly effective in deer, as well as in other wild ungulates, but the technique is expensive and labor intensive.[6, 11] Hunting remains the most direct solution for deer overpopulation.

PIGEONS, SPARROWS, AND STARLINGS

Pigeons (*Columba livia*), English (house) sparrows (*Passer domesticus*), and common (European) starlings (*Sturnus vulgaris*) are probably the most obvious and common bird problem in zoos, especially in urban areas. These birds are especially numerous during the cooler months. Habitat modification is extremely helpful in controlling bird numbers and should include pruning trees, netting off roosting sites or netting over exhibit bird pens, and eliminating overhangs and ledges from buildings. Screening material must be less than 2 cm to keep out sparrows. Mechanical repellents can also be used to prevent roosting: wire prongs or sheet metal spikes can be placed along ledges or under eaves. Sticky repellents are less effective and harden with age. Fishing line, piano wire, or grounded electrical wire can be tightly stretched at appropriate intervals (4 to 6 m) to discourage either roosting or feeding. Feeders can be redesigned to discourage pilfering by birds.

A continuous trapping program with rotation of trap sites placed in nonpublic areas can be very effective. Large traps with a narrowing funnel entry site work well for pigeons; top-opening traps, for crows, blackbirds, and starlings; and funnel or elevator-type traps, for sparrows. A decoy bird with food and water left in the trap increases trap efficiency. It may be helpful to prebait the traps for 1 week and to bait surrounding areas. Traps can be moved to other prebaited areas to avoid trap shyness. Zoo or park personnel should always check for legally banded pigeons. No federal permits are required for trapping or scaring these bird species, but local laws may apply. Nest destruction (with the use of long poles) is also effective but must be repeated every 10 to 14 days.

Auditory exclusion devices (shell crackers, propane exploders) are effective only if directed at the birds as they roost for the night and only if used within 7 days of the birds' arrival. Scare eye-spot balloons may ward off starlings (as well as jays and crows), but pigeons and sparrows readily become accustomed to both visual and auditory devices.

Numerous bird baits are available. It is important to warn zoo and park personnel to look for dead birds when using lethal baits. Soporifics (grains soaked in alcohol) were the original bird bait, allowing the drunken birds to be collected for consumption. Starlicide (3-chloro-4-methylbenzenamine) bait has been used successfully for starlings and has a low risk of secondary toxicity, but this toxin may affect nontarget species. The chemical Avitrol (4-aminopyridine) apparently induces fright and has been used most successfully for gulls and pigeons. A number of other chemical repellents, such as insecticides, are commonly used to protect food crops but carry a much higher risk of affecting nontarget species and can be safely used only for large roosts of birds.

WATERFOWL

Despite their widespread recognition as urban pests, Canada geese (*Branta canadensis*) and nondomestic ducks remain highly valued during the hunting season. These species are protected in North America under the Migratory Bird Treaty Act of 1918, and a permit is required to trap, hunt, kill, or sell them. Control of nuisance waterfowl, especially geese, depends on discouraging public feeding, preventing nesting, and preventing molting flocks from forming. Geese return to nest at the site where they first learned to fly and continue to return to that location year after year (for up to 30 years). Just before molting, geese tend to flock together. The result is a large group of flightless birds that spend the next 4 to 6 wks congregated in one location and produce large amounts of residue (feathers, feces) and noise.

Nesting can be prevented by planting dense ground cover around water and in grassy areas to break up congregations of birds. If new zoo exhibits are designed, islands surrounded by water should be avoided whenever possible. Nests can be destroyed and eggs addled, but to be effective, these measures must be done repeatedly. Turf repellents such as methylanthranilate (ReJexit) are variably effective. Harassment techniques can be used to break up flocks before the molt. Options include streamers, strobe lights, "eye" balloons or kites, and fake swan or eagle scarecrows. Cannons and pyrotechnics (two-shot shotgun shells) are more likely to be irritating to all than to be successful and must be fired repeatedly.

Removal methods for waterfowl, arranged in association with local wildlife officials, include capture and relocation or increased hunting. Cannon net trapping has been used successfully. Alphachloralose (a sedative) has been registered for use with the U.S. Department of Agriculture (USDA) as a waterfowl capture drug for urban environments.[11-13] However, questions again arise with regard to the effectiveness of this approach, in view of the tendency for waterfowl, especially geese, to repeatedly return to the same nesting site. Many experts recommend euthanasia rather than relocation. Special hunting seasons are another alternative but require public acceptance and coordination with local, state, and federal wildlife officials.

RAPTORS, HERONS, AND EGRETS

Carnivorous birds may be responsible for significant losses of chicks or small birds, rodents, reptiles, and fishes. The species involved is often identified by its pattern of predation. For example, owls preying on birds typically take only the head, whereas other raptors leave plucked feathers and talon marks. Like waterfowl, these species are protected, and permits are required for trapping, hunting, or removal. Therefore, control measures are limited to netting over bird enclosures or wire stands stretched over fish ponds.

REFERENCES

1. Bickle CA, Kirkpatrick JF, Turner JW: Contraception in striped skunks with Norplant implants. Wildl Soc Bull 19(3):334–338, 1991.
2. Buckle AP, Smith RH (eds): Rodent Pests and Their Control. Wallingford, UK, CAB International, 1994.
3. Collins D, Powell D: Applied pest control at Woodland Park Zoological Gardens. Proceedings of the Annual Meeting of the American Association of Zoo Veterinarians, Puerto Vallarta, Mexico, pp 290–295, 1996.
4. Fitzwater W: Chasing the snake out of Eden. Pest Control, 60–72, 1991.
5. Holland MK: The use of viral vectored immunocontraception for feral pest control in Australia. Proceedings of the Joint Conference of the American Association of Zoo Veterinarians/Wildlife Disease Association/American Association of Wildlife Veterinarians, East Lansing, MI, pp 43–54, 1995.
6. Kirkpatrick JF, Lin IK, Turner JW, Bickle CA: Chemical and immunological fertility control in wildlife. Proceedings of the American Association of Zoo Veterinarians, Oakland, CA, p 32, 1992.
7. Littrell EE: Effects of field vertebrate pest control on nontarget wildlife. Proceedings of the Vertebrate Pest Conference, University of California, Davis, vol 14, pp 59–61, 1990.
8. Olkowski W, Daar S, Olkowski H: Common-Sense Pest Control (BIRC). Newtown, CT, Taunton Press, 1991.
9. Pursley WE: Methods of pest control and how they can be applied in zoological or aquarium settings. American Association of Zoological Parks and Aquariums Regional Proceedings, Omaha, NE, pp 427–429, 1993.
10. Trienan KA, Chapin RE: Development of testicular lesions in F344 rats after treatment with boric acid. Toxicol Appl Pharm 107:325–335, 1991.
11. Turner JW, Kirkpatrick JF, Irwin KM: Effectiveness, reversibility, and serum antibody titers associated with immunocontraception in captive white-tailed deer. J Wildl Manage 60(1):45–51, 1996.
12. Woronecki PP: Philosophies and methods for controlling nuisance waterfowl populations in urban environments. Proceedings of the American Association of Zoo Veterinarians/American Association of Wildlife Veterinarians, Oakland, CA, p 51, 1992.
13. Woronecki PP, Dolbeer RA, Seamans TW: Use of alpha-chloralose to remove waterfowl from nuisance and damage situations. Proceedings of the Vertebrate Pest Conference, University of California, Davis, vol 14, pp 343–349, 1990.

Magazines/Publications

Common Sense Pest Control Quarterly. Bio-Integral Resource Center (BIRC), P.O. Box 7414, Berkeley, CA 94707 (phone: 510-524-2567). Back issues available, e.g., "Managing Pest Birds"; "Opossums as Pests"; "Managing Canada Geese."

The IPM Practitioner. 10 issues. Bio-Integral Resource Center (BIRC), P.O. Box 7414, Berkeley, CA 94707 (phone: 510-524-2567). (Back issues are available; e.g., "1997 Directory of Least-Toxic Pest Control Products.")

Pest Control Magazine. 12 issues. Advanstar Communications, 7500 Old Oak Blvd., Cleveland, OH 44130.

Pest Management. National Pest Control Association, 8100 Oak Street, Dunn Loring, VA 22027.

ZOONOSES

CHAPTER 18

Cryptosporidium Species

WILLIAM L. CURRENT

Organisms of the genus *Cryptosporidium* are small coccidian parasites that infect the microvillous region of epithelial cells lining the digestive and respiratory organs of vertebrates. Recognized and named in 1910 by the American parasitologist E. E. Tyzzer,[38, 39] these small (2- to 6-μm, depending on stage of life cycle), obligate intracellular protozoans remained for 70 years little more than a biomedical curiosity. Before 1980, infections with species of *Cryptosporidium* were considered rare in animals, and in humans they were believed to be the result of a little-known opportunistic pathogen of immunodeficient individuals outside its normal host range. Beginning in 1982, the concept of these protozoan parasites changed; they are now considered to be important, widespread causes of diarrheal illness in humans and in some domesticated and wild animals.

The role of *Cryptosporidium parvum* as an enteropathogen of humans is now well established. In immunocompetent persons, *C. parvum* may cause a short-term (3- to 20-day) diarrheal illness that resolves spontaneously. However, in the immunocompromised patient, cryptosporidiosis often causes a life-threatening, prolonged, cholera-like illness. There is currently no proven effective therapy for cryptosporidiosis; thus the finding of this parasite in the immunocompromised host, especially patients with the acquired immunodeficiency syndrome (AIDS), usually carries a poor prognosis.

Cryptosporidium species are also important pathogens of many wild and domesticated vertebrates, including captive and free-ranging wildlife. After brief discussion of the taxonomy and life history of *Cryptosporidium* species, the pathogenesis, management, and diagnosis of cryptosporidiosis in animals are addressed. A more thorough understanding of *Cryptosporidium* species and cryptosporidiosis can be obtained from several papers and reviews[3, 7, 9, 10, 17, 34] and from two books.[15, 18]

THE ETIOLOGIC AGENTS OF CRYPTOSPORIDIOSIS

Small protozoans assigned to the genus *Cryptosporidium* have a close taxonomic relationship with the other true coccidia—*Isospora belli, Sarcocystis* species, and *Toxoplasma gondii*—that infect human beings and to *Eimeria* species and *Isospora* species that infect other mammals and birds. All of these organisms are obligate intracellular protozoans assigned to the phylum Apicomplexa (unicellular organisms that possess an apical complex typically composed of one or more polar rings, rhoptries, micronemes, and usually a conoid), class Conoidasia (presence of a complete conoid composed of a hollow, truncated cone), subclass Coccidiasina (gamonts

121

usually develop intracellularly), order Eucoccidiorida (which possess merogony, gamogony, and sporogony), and suborder Eimeriorina (the true coccidia that lack syzygy, produce microgametocytes with many gametocytes, and have stationary zygotes). There are two families of true coccidia, the Eimeriidae and the Cryptosporidiidae, that contain members that often parasitize enteric sites in vertebrates. The family Cryptosporidiidae contains a single genus: *Cryptosporidium*. All known species are homoxenous (have only one host in the life cycle) and have endogenous stages with a unique "feeder organelle" that develop just beneath the host cell membrane rather than deep within the cell. Microgametes of *Cryptosporidium* are unusual among the coccidia in that they lack flagella. Oocysts contain four naked sporozoites not surrounded by a sporocysts wall; hence the genus name is derived from *crypto* (hidden) and *sporidium* (sporocyst).

Most species of *Cryptosporidium* named in the biomedical literature after Tyzzer's[38] description of the genus were done so with the assumption that these coccidia were as host specific as the (taxonomically) closely related species of *Eimeria* infecting mammals and birds. However, cross-transmission studies conducted in the early 1980s demonstrated little or no host specificity for "species" of *Cryptosporidium* isolated from mammals. The lack of host specificity exhibited by mammalian isolates prompted some researchers to consider *Cryptosporidium* as a single species genus. A more realistic approach was presented by Levine,[31] who consolidated the 21 parasites named at that time into four species: one each for those infecting fishes (*C. nasorum*), reptiles (*C. crotali*), birds (*C. meleagridis*), and mammals (*C. muris*). Current information indicates that this consolidation is not entirely correct. *Cryptosporidium crotali* is now considered to be a species of *Sarcocystis*, a genus of coccidian parasites found

commonly in snakes. Eight species of *Cryptosporidium* are currently considered valid, four of which occur in mammals, and several additional isolates will probably be assigned names in the future (Table 18–1). On the basis of oocyst morphology, *C. parvum*, not *C. muris*, is associated with almost all well-documented cases of cryptosporidiosis in mammals.[41] Thus the species with oocysts measuring 4 to 5 μm that produces clinical illness in humans and other mammals should be referred to as *C. parvum* or as *Cryptosporidium* species if there is not enough morphologic, life-cycle, and/or host specificity data to relate it to Tyzzer's original description.[39]

LIFE HISTORY

Currently, more is known about the life history and structure of developmental stages of *C. parvum* than about those of any other member of the genus. Studies[11] of different isolates (calf and human) of *C. parvum* in suckling mice revealed that the life cycle of this parasite (Fig. 18–1) is similar to that of other true coccidia (e.g., *Eimeria* and *Isospora* species) infecting mammals in that it can be divided into six major developmental events: excystation, the release of infective sporozoites; merogony, the asexual multiplication within host cells; gametogony, the formation of microgametes and macrogametes; fertilization, the union of microgametes and macrogametes; oocyst wall formation, to produce an environmentally resistant stage that transmits infection from one host to another; and sporogony, the formation of infective sporozoites within the oocyst wall.

The life cycle of human and calf isolates of *C. parvum* differs somewhat from that of other monoxenous coccidia such as *Eimeria* and *Isospora* species, the parasites usually referred to as the "typical coccidia." Each intracellular stage of *C. parvum* resides

TABLE 18–1. Recognized Species of *Cryptosporidium* that Infect Vertebrates*

| Species | Host(s) | Oocyst Size (μm) | | Site of Infection and Clinical Signs |
		Range	Mean	
C. parvum	Mammals (>80 species)	4.5–5.4 × 4.2–5.0	5.0 × 4.5	Small and large intestine: diarrhea; biliary tree
C. muris	Mice, rats	7.5–9.8 × 5.5–7.0	8.4 × 6.3	Cholecystitis; upper respiratory tract: bronchitis
C. species (muris?)	Cattle	6.6–7.9 × 5.3–6.5	7.4 × 5.6	Digestive glands of stomach
C. wrari	Guinea pigs		5.4 × 4.6	Small and large intestines: diarrhea
C. felis	Cats		5.0 × 4.5	Small and large intestines: diarrhea
C. baileyi	Chickens	6.0–7.5 × 4.8–5.7	6.2 × 4.6	Respiratory epithelium: pneumonia and airsacculitis; cloaca and bursal epithelium: poor weight gain?
C. meleagridis	Turkeys	4.5–6.0 × 4.2–5.3	5.2 × 4.6	Small intestine: diarrhea
C. species	Quails	4.5–6.0 × 3.6–5.6	5.2 × 4.6	Small intestine and cloaca: diarrhea
C. species	Ostriches	3.0–6.1 × 3.3–5.0	4.6 × 4.0	Site of infection unknown; may cause diarrhea in young birds
C. serpentis	Reptiles		6.0 × 5.4	Gastric mucosa: gastric hyperplasia and anorexia
C. nasorum	Fishes	Not available		Intestine: anorexia and emaciation?

*These are species that the author believes to be valid, on the basis of published studies.

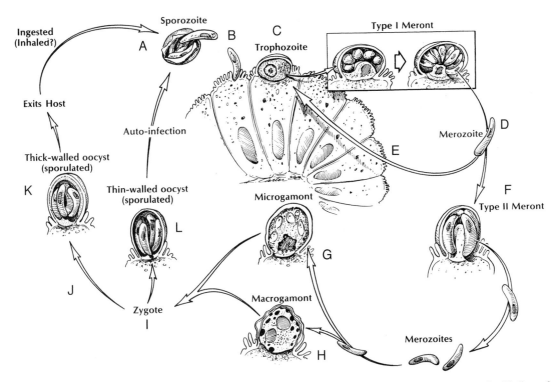

FIGURE 18–1. Diagrammatic representation of the proposed life cycle of *C. parvum* as it occurs in the mucosal epithelium of an infected mammalian host. After excysting from oocysts in the lumen of the intestine *(A)*, sporozoites *(B)* penetrate into host cells, and develop into trophozoites (which are uninucleate meronts) *(C)* within parasitophorous vacuoles confined to the microvillous region of the mucosal epithelium. Uninucleate meronts *(C)* undergo asexual divisions (merogony) to form merozoites. After being released from type I meronts, invasive merozoites *(D)* enter adjacent host cells *(E)* and form additional type I meronts (recycling of type I meronts) or form type II meronts *(F)*. Type II meronts do not recycle but enter host cells to form the sexual stages: microgamonts *(G)* and macrogamonts *(H)*. Most (approximately 80%) of the zygotes *(I)* formed after fertilization of the microgamont by the microgametes (released from microgamont) develop into environmentally resistant, thick-walled oocysts *(J)* that undergo sporogony to form sporulated oocysts *(K)* containing four sporozoites. Sporulated oocysts released in feces are the environmentally resistant life cycle forms that transmit the infection from one host to another. A smaller percentage of zygotes (approximately 20%) do not form a thick, two-layered oocyst wall; they have only a unit membrane surrounding the four sporozoites. These thin-walled oocysts *(L)* represent autoinfective life cycle forms that can maintain the parasite in the host without repeated oral exposure to the thick-walled oocysts present in the environment. The life cycle of *Cryptosporidium baileyi*, infecting chickens, differs from the one shown in that this parasite has an additional (type III) meront that is derived from type II merozoites.

within a parasitophorous vacuole confined to the microvillous region of the host cell, whereas comparable stages of *Eimeria* or *Isospora* species occupy parasitophorous vacuoles deep (perinuclear) within the host cells. Oocysts of *C. parvum* undergo sporogony while they are within the host cells and are infective when released in the feces, whereas oocysts of *Eimeria* or *Isospora* species do not sporulate until they are passed from the host and exposed to oxygen and temperatures below 37°C. Studies with experimentally infected mice have also shown that approximately 20% of the oocysts of *C. parvum* within host enterocytes do not form a thick, two-layered, environmentally resistant oocyst wall. The four sporozoites of this autoinfective stage are surrounded only by a single-unit membrane. Soon after being released from a host cell, the membrane surrounding the four sporozoites ruptures and these invasive forms penetrate into the microvillous region of other enterocytes and reinitiate the life cycle. Approxi-

mately 80% of the oocysts of *C. parvum* found in enterocytes of suckling mice were similar to those of *Eimeria* and *Isospora* species in that they developed thick, environmentally resistant oocyst walls and were passed in the feces. Thick-walled oocysts are the life cycle forms that transmit the infection from one host to another.

The presence of autoinfective, thin-walled oocysts and type I meronts that can recycle are believed to be the life cycle features of *C. parvum* that are responsible for the development of severe infections in hosts exposed to only a small number of thick-walled oocysts and for persistent, life-threatening disease in immunodeficient persons who are not exposed repeatedly to these environmentally resistant forms. Light microscopic and ultrastructural features of some of the developmental stages of *Cryptosporidium* in enterocytes of the experimentally infected host are shown in Figures 18–2 to 18–4. Additional details of the life history and ultra-

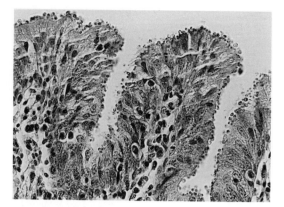

FIGURE 18–2. Light photomicrograph of a histologic section (stained with hematoxylin and eosin) of the cloaca of a chicken heavily infected with *Cryptosporidium baileyi*. Numerous developmental stages of *C. baileyi* can be seen within the brush border of the enterocytes.

structure of *Cryptosporidium* species have been published.[9–13, 15, 18]

CLINICAL FEATURES AND PATHOGENESIS

Mammals Infected with *Cryptosporidium parvum*

CLINICAL FEATURES

At least 79 species of mammals belonging to nine orders have been reported as suitable hosts for *C. parvum*.[34] *Cryptosporidium parvum* is a parasite primarily of the lower small intestine of humans and neonate mammals and is responsible for almost all (>99%) well documented cases of diarrheal illness caused by cryptosporidiosis.[41]

The most common clinical feature of cryptosporidiosis in immunocompetent and immunocompromised humans is diarrhea, the symptom that most often leads to diagnosis. Characteristically, the diarrhea is profuse and watery; it may contain mucus, but rarely blood and leukocytes. Both the duration of symptoms and the outcome typically vary according to immune status of the patient. In severely immunocompromised persons such as patients with AIDS, the illness is usually prolonged and life-threatening, whereas in most immunocompetent persons the illness is short term with complete, spontaneous recovery. In AIDS patients, *C. parvum* also infects the gallbladder and biliary tree epithelium and can cause acalculous cholecystitis. There have been several reports of tracheal and bronchial infections that resulted in bronchitis.[7, 10, 13]

Severe, profuse diarrhea is also the most common clinical feature of cryptosporidiosis in many domesticated and wild mammals, especially animals less than 4 weeks of age. Calves, sheep, goats, deer, horses, and a number of exotic ruminants have been reported to have severe cryptosporidial diarrhea; a list of host species can be found in the review paper of O'Donoghue.[34] The main presenting sign of cryptosporidiosis in the young of these animals is profuse diarrhea with shedding of infective oocysts (up to 10^7/g of feces). Varying degrees of dullness, anorexia, fever, and wasting can occur. Similar clinical features have been reported in some nonhuman primates infected with *C. parvum*. In most of these animals, cryptosporidiosis is characterized by high morbidity but low mortality. In cases of high mortality, confounding factors such as environmental stress (e.g., cold), inadequate nutrition, or co-infection with other enteropathogens (e.g., rotavirus or enterotoxigenic *Escherichia coli*) are usually identified.

Diarrheal illness caused by cryptosporidiosis has been reported but is less common in dogs, cats, raccoons, rabbits, pigs, and rodents. It appears that these mammalian hosts may often have asymptomatic infections of *C. parvum* and that they may serve as potential reservoir hosts.[15, 18]

PATHOGENESIS

Intestinal infections of *C. parvum* are relatively unremarkable histopathologically. Microscopically, the endogenous life cycle forms are observed in the epithelium, usually without obvious damage to host cells except that cells may be low columnar or cuboidal and microvilli may be absent at the site of parasite attachment (see Figs. 18–3, 18–4). Intestinal lesions include mild to severe villus atrophy, blunting and fusion of villi, and inflammatory changes marked by mild to moderate infiltration of plasma cells, neutrophils, mac-

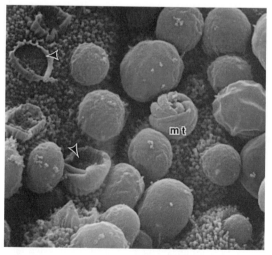

FIGURE 18–3. Scanning electron micrograph showing numerous developmental stages of *Cryptosporidium* in the microvillous region of the intestinal mucosa. Each parasite is contained within a parasitophorous vacuole that bulges out from the microvillous region of the enterocyte. Some merozoites of a mature type I meront (mt) are exposed as a result of a portion of the parasitophorous vacuole membrane's being removed during processing. *Arrowheads* point to craters in the mucosal surface formed by empty vacuoles that remain after the parasites are released.

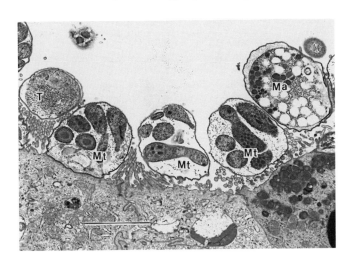

FIGURE 18–4. Transmission electron micrograph of developmental stages of *Cryptosporidium parvum* within parasitophorous vacuoles bulging from the microvillous region of ileal enterocytes of an experimentally infected mouse. Macrogametes (one labeled Ma) contain the characteristic amylopectin granules near the center and wall-forming bodies near the periphery. One trophozoite (T) (uninucleate meront) and three meronts (Mt) with merozoites can be seen. Line represents 5 μm.

rophages, and lymphocytes into the subepithelial lamina propria.[10, 15, 27]

At present, the pathophysiologic mechanisms of *Cryptosporidium*-induced diarrhea are poorly defined. Studies in germ-free calves monoinfected with *C. parvum* suggest that malabsorption and impaired digestion in the small bowel coupled with malabsorption in the large intestine are major factors responsible for diarrhea in calves with cryptosporidiosis.[27] Similar malabsorption, attributed to parasite-induced villus damage, has also been reported in a neonatal pig model.[5] This malabsorption and impaired digestion may result in an overgrowth of intestinal microflora, a change in osmotic pressure across the gut wall, and an influx of fluid into the lumen of the intestine. Malabsorption and impaired digestion have also been reported in humans infected with *C. parvum*.

The secretory (often described as cholera-like) diarrhea common to most immunodeficient humans with cryptosporidiosis is suggestive of a toxin-mediated hypersecretion into the gut; however, the author is not aware of reports establishing that *C. parvum* possesses enterotoxin. Studies reporting changes in electrical potential of rabbit and human ileum after exposure to *C. parvum* extracts suggest, but do not establish, the presence of enterotoxins.[25]

Cattle Infected with *Cryptosporidium* Species (*C. muris*–Like)

CLINICAL FEATURES AND PATHOGENESIS

A species of *Cryptosporidium* whose oocysts are slightly smaller than those of *C. muris*, described by Tyzzer in 1912,[39] is the agent of a disease known as abomasal (gastric, peptic gland) cryptosporidiosis (see Table 18–1). This organism produces lesions of dilation of peptic glands in the abomasum of calves and adult cattle. Infected cattle may shed oocysts in their feces for 4 to 6 months or more. A severely affected abomasum may weigh 2 to 3 times more than an abomasum

from a noninfected bovine of the same age and size. Histologic examination of such heavy infections often reveals that most peptic glands contain numerous developmental stages of the parasite; one report[2] described all glands as being full of developing parasites. In such severely parasitized cattle, lower weight gains (a decrease of up to 33%) have been noted in comparison with noninfected penmates.[2]

The prevalence and distribution of the *C. muris*–like species in cattle and its overall role as an agent causing economic loss to the bovine industry remain undefined. The parasite has been reported from calves and/or adult cattle in Washington state, Idaho, Nevada, California, and Alabama. Using an acid-fast staining technique with a sensitivity of approximately 86% of that provided by Sheather's sugar flotation, Anderson reported that 54 of 1216 (4.4%) feeder cattle in eight lots in Idaho had *C. muris*–like oocysts in their feces. The same diagnostic procedure revealed that approximately 1.6% of the 12,069 samples obtained from calves and cows in 21 dairy herds in Idaho, Nevada, and California contained *C. muris*–like oocysts. Additional studies are needed to more clearly define the impact of this parasite on beef and dairy production. Additional features of *Cryptosporidium* infections in cattle can be found in the published work of Anderson.[1, 2]

BIRDS INFECTED WITH *CRYPTOSPORIDIUM* SPECIES

Species of *Cryptosporidium* have been observed in the enteric, respiratory, and renal epithelium of numerous species of birds.[34] Within the enteric tract, endogenous stages of the parasites have been reported in the salivary glands, proventriculus, small intestine, cecum, colon, cloaca, and bursa of Fabricius. In the respiratory tract and oculonasal tissues, parasites have been observed in the nasal chamber, palatine cleft, turbinates, infraorbital sinuses, conjunctiva, larynx, trachea, all levels of the bronchi, and the air sacs. Within the excretory tract, developmental stages of *Cryptosporidium* species have been found in the ureters, collecting ducts, collecting tubules, and distal convoluted tubules. At the time of this writing, there are at least two valid species of *Cryptosporidium* infecting birds (see Table 18–1), and there are undoubtedly other species that have not been described. What little is known about the clinical features and pathogenesis of *Cryptosporidium* species infecting chickens, turkeys, quails, and ostriches is outlined as follows.

Cryptosporidium baileyi Infecting Chickens

Cryptosporidium baileyi is apparently restricted to the respiratory tract and distal gastrointestinal tract (cecum, distal colon, cloaca, and bursa of Fabricius). Respiratory disease is observed most commonly and is more severe than the intestinal disease. Clinical signs consist of respiratory distress characterized by lethargy, rales, coughing, sneezing, and/or dyspnea. The lumens of organs of the respiratory tract contain a mucocellular exudate consisting of exfoliated epithelial cells, macrophages, heterophils, lymphocytes, plasma cells, and developing parasites. Accumulation of this exudate results in both pneumonia and airsacculitis. Additional details of the clinical features and pathogenesis of *C. baileyi* infections have been published.[12, 30, 32]

Cryptosporidium meleagridis Infecting Turkeys

Intestinal cryptosporidiosis may result in moderate to severe diarrhea and, in some cases, mortality. Postmortem examination of *Cryptosporidium*-infected turkeys with diarrhea revealed a small intestine that was pale and contained cloudy, mucoid exudate. Villi were moderately atrophic, crypts were hyperplastic, and infected segments of the small intestine contained a mixed mucosal inflammatory infiltrate. Additional details of the clinical features and pathogenesis of *C. meleagridis* infections in turkeys have been published.[24, 36]

Cryptosporidium Species Infecting Quails

Natural or experimental cryptosporidiosis (intestinal and respiratory) has been reported from the bobwhite and the common quail. Clinical signs and pathogenesis are similar to those reported earlier for *C. baileyi* infections in chickens; however, infection in quails is not with *C. baileyi*. Intestinal disease usually results in high mortality among birds from hatch to 12 days of age. Diarrhea may appear as a clear to brown fluid, or it may be white and watery. Villus atrophy, sloughed villi, and detached enterocytes are prominent histopathologic features. Additional details of the clinical features and pathogenesis of *Cryptosporidium* species infecting quails have been published.[15, 29]

Cryptosporidium Species Infecting Ostriches

A species of *Cryptosporidium* whose oocysts are structurally distinct (see Table 18–1) from those of *C. baileyi*, *C. meleagridis*, and *Cryptosporidium* species infecting quail has been reported[19, 20] in ostriches imported to Canada from Africa. At the time of this writing, it was not clear whether this parasite causes morbidity or mortality in ostriches. In adult birds, no clinical signs have been associated with the presence of oocysts in feces.[19, 20] However, the author has had personal communication from veterinarians in Texas and Arizona who claimed that diarrhea and death was associated with *Cryptosporidium* infection in young (2- to 4-week-old) ostriches. On the basis of these anecdotal reports, cryptosporidiosis should be considered in the differential diagnosis of diarrheal illness in young ostriches.

Reptilian Cryptosporidiosis

Cryptosporidium species infections have been reported in more than 57 reptilian species, including 40 species of snakes (boids, colubrids, elapids, and viperids), 15 species of lizards (agamids, gekkonids, chamaeleonids, helodermatids, lacertids, teiids, and varanids), and two species of tortoises (both testudinids).[34] Morphometric analysis[40, 42] of oocysts from snakes and lizards revealed at least five morphologic types of oocysts, one of which conforms to previous descriptions of *C. serpentis* (see Table 18–1).

The clinical course of cryptosporidiosis in snakes is markedly different from that in mammals and birds. In snakes, *Cryptosporidium* species localize in the gastric mucosa. Although oocysts may be passed in the feces for many months or even years, cryptosporidiosis is most often diagnosed because of clinical signs that may include anorexia, persistent or intermittent postprandial regurgitation, lethargy, firm midbody swelling, and progressive weight loss. Microscopic lesions consist of hyperplasia and hypertrophy of gastric glands, concomitant atrophy of the glandular cells, edema of the submucosa and lamina propria, reduction in luminal diameter, and inflammation of the gastric mucosa. Most reported cases in lizards involved subclinical gastric infections, and both reports of tortoises describe clinical signs of gastritis and regurgitation.[34, 40, 42]

EPIZOOTIOLOGY

Studies of experimental infections in laboratory and farm animals clearly demonstrate that *Cryptosporidium* species are transmitted by environmentally resistant oocysts that are fully sporulated and infective at the time they are passed in feces.[10] As long as the thick, two-layered wall remains intact, *Cryptosporidium* species oocysts are very resistant to common disinfectants and can survive for months if kept cold and moist. Exposure of oocysts to high concentrations of disinfectants such as ammonia, hydrogen peroxide, and chlorine may reduce the number of viable oocysts but rarely result in elimination of the source of infection. The most effective ways of reducing the number of oocysts in the environment is by heat ($>60°C$) or desiccation.

Infections with *Cryptosporidium* have been recorded in more than 170 different host species, approximately half of which are mammals, originating from more than 50 countries ranging in location from tropical to temperate zones throughout the world.[34] Human-to-human transmission is common, and transmission from farm and companion animals to humans is also well documented. Contaminated water and food are known sources of infections for susceptible mammalian hosts; large waterborne outbreaks of human cryptosporidiosis have been reported in North America and Europe.[10, 26, 33] Because numerous mammalian species can be infected with *C. parvum*, there is a large potential zoonotic reservoir. One such potential reservoir is infected calves, which release large amounts of watery feces containing numerous oocysts (up to 10[7]/mL of watery feces) into the environment. Runoff land contaminated by infected calves may introduce large numbers of oocysts into watersheds.[35] Such a scenario, coupled with failure of a water treatment plant, was postulated by some authors to be responsible for a waterborne outbreak in which more than 400,000 persons in Milwaukee had water diarrhea caused by cryptosporidiosis.[33]

The highly transmissible nature of *C. parvum* was demonstrated in studies of healthy volunteers who developed cryptosporidial diarrhea after ingestion of 30 to 1000 oocysts; the median infective dose calculated by linear regression was 132 oocysts.[16] It appears that the risk of acquiring cryptosporidiosis can be high when there is exposure to fecal contamination from infected mammals. However, there is no evidence that species of *Cryptosporidium* other than *C. parvum* can infect humans.

TREATMENT AND MANAGEMENT OF CRYPTOSPORIDIOSIS

Chemotherapy

Despite numerous years of investigations using animal and in vitro models to evaluate agents[6] and the administration of a vast array of chemotherapeutic, immunomodulary, and palliative agents to AIDS patients,[37] a consistently effective, approved therapy for human cryptosporidiosis is still lacking. A formidable list of approximately 100 ineffective compounds has been generated as a result of largely anecdotal attempts to control this life-threatening disease in immunocompromised patients.[37] Since the 1980s, controlled treatment trials have been conducted but have not succeeded in identifying agents efficacious against this infection. A compilation of the agents evaluated for anticryptosporidial activity in animal models and humans has been published.[6, 37] Virtually all traditional anticoccidial compounds failed to eliminate infections when administered at nontoxic levels. The most active compounds appear to be the ionophores (alborixin, halofuginone, lasalocid, and maduramicin), the aminoglycoside paromomycin, the nucleoside analog arprinocid, and the macrolide azithromycin. However, none of these compounds have proved to be effective agents for the treatment of cryptosporidiosis in animals.

Management

In the absence of an effective treatment, management to prevent outbreaks and supportive measures for infected animals appear to be the only logical ways to intervene.

Measures for controlling outbreaks of calf cryptosporidiosis on the farm, as outlined by Angus,[4] may also be applicable to some captive animals. These measures, listed as follows, are equally applicable to other enteric infections, which is important because multiple-agent outbreaks that include *Cryptosporidium* are usually more common than monoinfections with this parasite. In addition to the knowledge that oocysts are environmentally resistant and refractive to commercial disinfectants (which is not true for bacterial and viral enteropathogens) and that clinical disease can be deferred by individual penning from birth in sterilized pens or hutches, the following principles based on the experiences of veterinary scientists should be adopted:

1. Calf rearing should be on an "all-in, all-out" basis.
2. Individual pens should be stringently cleaned and disinfected between batches of calves.
3. Calves should be born and raised in a clean, dry environment.
4. Ideally, newborn calves should be penned individually for 2 to 3 weeks.
5. Sick calves should be removed immediately from the company of healthy calves.
6. Attendants of healthy calves should be different from those of sick calves.
7. Attendants should keep boots, protective clothing, and so forth, as free from feces as possible.
8. Utensils should be heat sterilized—if possible, daily.
9. Vermin, farm dogs, and cats should be controlled.
10. Colostrum management and nutrition should be satisfactory.
11. Appropriate prophylactic measures against other agents, such as rotavirus or enterotoxogenic *E. coli* K99+ vaccines, should be employed.

Even on the best managed farms, not all of these control measures may be possible. Adopting these measures to the management of wild captive animals may be even more difficult. In general, any procedure that reduces fecal-oral contamination should be adopted. Maintaining animals, especially the young, in warm, dry, clean environments is important. Also, if an animal becomes infected, it is important to isolate it from noninfected animals and to make sure that it receives adequate fluids and nutrients. Adequate fluids in the form of milk or milk replacers is usually sufficient; however, electrolyte rehydration solutions may be of value.

DIAGNOSIS OF *CRYPTOSPORIDIUM* INFECTIONS

Before 1980, human cryptosporidiosis was diagnosed by histologic examination of biopsy specimens from the intestinal mucosa. Routine hematoxylin and eosin staining can be used to visualize the developmental stages of the parasite as dark, basophilic, spherical bodies 2 to 5 μm in diameter (depending on stage in life cycle) in the brush border of mucosal epithelium. Transmission electron microscopy can be used to confirm the diagnosis. Such invasive, expensive, and time-consuming procedures are no longer required for the diagnosis of cryptosporidiosis, because a variety of techniques have been developed to identify *Cryptosporidium* species oocysts in feces and other body fluid specimens.[8, 21, 22] Oocysts, usually released in large numbers from the infected epithelium, can be identified in stool specimens that represent a sampling of the entire intestinal tract or in sputum or respiratory aspirates that represent a sampling of the entire respiratory tract. Biopsy specimens may be of some value in determining the site of infection and defining lesions associated with the parasite.

PRESERVATION AND STORAGE OF SPECIMENS CONTAINING OOCYSTS

Most diagnostic specimens examined for oocysts are stool samples; however, other fluids such as sputum should be handled the same way. For the diagnosis of cryptosporidiosis, stool specimens should be submitted as fresh material or in 10% formalin or sodium acetate–acetic acid–formalin (SAF) preservatives. If parasites are not going to be used for subsequent experimental purposes, fixed specimens are recommended because of biohazard considerations. Fresh or preserved stool specimens can be examined as wet mounts, or they can be concentrated or stained, as outlined later, to aid in the visualization of *Cryptosporidium* species oocysts.

Potassium dichromate solution ($K_2Cr_2O_7$, 2% to 2.5% w/v in water) is used routinely as a storage medium to preserve oocyst viability; it is not a fixative. When stored at 4°C in $K_2Cr_2O_7$, *Cryptosporidium* species oocysts remain viable for at least 3 months, and some may retain infectivity for up to 12 months.[10] Because the percentage of viable oocysts begins to decrease after 3 months of cold storage, it is advisable to generate fresh oocysts every 3 to 4 months. Some researchers prefer to store oocysts of *Cryptosporidium* species in balanced salt solutions supplemented with antibiotics because chromium is an environmental contaminant requiring special disposal and handling procedures. Hank's balanced salt solution (HBSS), containing penicillin (10,000 U), streptomycin (10 mg), amphotericin B (0.05 mg), and nystatin (500 U/ml), is recommended for the storage of *Cryptosporidium* species oocysts and also for the storage of sporocysts of *Sarcocystis* species.[8]

IDENTIFICATION OF OOCYSTS

Two general approaches have been used widely to identify *Cryptosporidium* species oocysts in stools or body fluid specimens. Concentration techniques are used routinely in the research laboratory, whereas staining techniques, before or after concentration of oocysts, are used more often in the clinical microbiology labora-

tory.[8, 10, 21] Because *Cryptosporidium* species oocysts are similar in size and shape to some yeast cells, considerable experience is required in order to obtain accurate results with concentration and/or staining techniques. Useful stool concentration techniques include sedimentation of oocysts with the use of formalin-ether and formalin-ethyl acetate and flotation of oocysts in Sheather's sugar solution, in zinc sulfate solution (1.18 or 1.2 specific gravity), or in saturated sodium chloride solution (1.27 specific gravity).

Sheather's Sugar Flotation

Sheather's sugar flotation, perhaps the most useful concentration procedure in the research and veterinary diagnostic laboratory, is outlined as follows.[8]

1. If the stool specimen is not fluid, it may be necessary to dilute it with water before it is strained through cheesecloth to remove large particulate material. Mix thoroughly approximately 1 ml of fecal or sputum suspension with 10 ml of Sheather's sugar solution (sugar, 500 g; water, 320 ml; phenol, 6.5 g) in a 15-ml centrifuge tube. A cap should be placed on the tube to prevent aerosol formation.

2. Centrifuge at 500 × gravity for 10 minutes, obtain a sample from the surface of the flotation medium (this can be done easily by using a wire loop or Pasteur pipette), place it on a microscope slide, add a coverslip, and examine microscopically.

3. Sheather's sugar flotation combined with phase-contrast microscopy is an excellent procedure for identifying oocysts and for distinguishing oocysts from contaminating yeast cells.[10, 21] *C. parvum* oocysts appear as bright, birefringent, 4.5- to 5.5-μm spherical bodies containing one to four dark granules (Fig. 18–5b). With good-quality, phase-contrast, oil immersion objectives, the four sporozoites surrounding the centrally located oocyst residuum are often seen. Oocysts of other species of *Cryptosporidium,* such as *C. muris* or *C. baileyi,* are of a different size and shape but otherwise appear similar to those of *C. parvum* (see Table 18–1). Contaminating yeast cells do not appear as bright, birefringent bodies, do not contain dark granules or sporozoites, and sometimes have small budding cells on their margin. When viewed with brightfield microscopy, oocysts are often difficult to distinguish from yeast cells. When viewed with brightfield microscopy, *C. parvum* oocysts appear as 4.5- to 5.5-μm translucent, spherical bodies containing one to four dark granules. With some microscopes, these oocysts often appear light pink. Yeast cells do not have the characteristic granules and are not pink. After approximately 15 minutes in the hyperosmotic Sheather's solution, some oocysts begin to collapse, and the percentage of collapsed oocysts increases with time. Collapse of the oocysts usually involves a folding in of the oocyst wall along the oocyst wall suture.

Acid-Fast Staining

Most recommended stains for *Cryptosporidium* species oocysts cannot be performed on stools preserved in

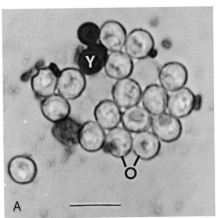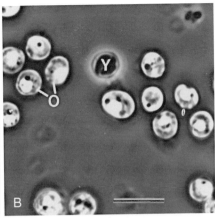

FIGURE 18–5. Light micrographs of oocysts of *Cryptosporidium parvum*. *A*, Brightfield micrograph of negative-stained oocysts appear bright and birefringent against a dark staining background. Fecal debris, yeast (Y), and bacteria all stain darkly. *B*, Phase-contrast micrograph demonstrating bright, birefringent appearance of oocysts, which contain one to four dark granules, and four sporozoites surrounding the centrally located oocyst residuum. Contaminating yeast cells (Y) do not appear as bright, birefringent bodies, do not contain dark granules or sporozoites, and sometimes have small budding cells on their margin. Line represents 10 μm.

polyvinyl alcohol (PVA) fixative. The routine stains (trichrome, iron hematoxylin) used for stool diagnosis of other parasites are not helpful for the identification of *Cryptosporidium* species oocysts. The most widely used staining techniques for demonstrating *Cryptosporidium* species oocysts in fecal specimens are based on the acid-fast staining properties of the oocyst wall. Several acid-fast stains have been used in hot or cold procedures and modified by incorporation of dimethyl sulfoxide. It appears that reported differences in acid-fast stains and methods represent personal preference rather than marked differences in sensitivity and specificity.[21, 22] The most commonly used acid-fast procedure is the modified Kinyoun cold technique, described as follows.[8]

1. With a wooden applicator stick or a disposable culture loop, spread the specimen on a microscope slide and allow to air dry.
2. Fix in absolute methanol for 5 to 10 minutes, and air dry.
3. Cover the smear with modified Kinyoun acid-fast stain (fuchsin-carbol, Harleco, Gibbstown, NJ) for approximately 2 minutes.
4. Rinse briefly in tap water (some authors prefer 50% ethanol), cover the smear with decolorizing solution (10% H_2SO_4), incubate for approximately 1 minute, and then rinse briefly in tap water.
5. Cover the smear with counterstain (light green SF yellowish stain, Harleco; or methylene blue, 0.3 g/100 mL deionized water), incubate for approximately 1 minute, rinse in tap water, air dry, and observe microscopically.
6. For optimal staining with this procedure, staining, decolorizing, and counterstaining times are determined empirically. Also, it is important that fecal smears are not too thick, so as to ensure adequate penetration of the reagents.
7. When stained properly, oocysts are 4.5 to 5.5

μm, red, spherical bodies against a green or blue (depending on counterstain) background. Oocysts stain red with varying degrees of intensity, whereas most fecal debris and yeast cells take up the color of the background stain.

Negative Staining

The negative staining procedure originally described by Heine[28] is also useful for detecting oocysts in fecal specimens. This procedure has the advantage of requiring less preparation time and fewer steps than the Kinyoun technique but does not result in the production of a permanent slide. The procedure works best on fresh fecal specimens, but it will give satisfactory results with specimens fixed in 10% formalin. The author does not know whether specimens preserved in other fixatives lend themselves to negative staining. A modification of the original negative-staining procedure has been published[14] and is described as follows.

1. With a wooden applicator stick, mix thoroughly on a microscope slide equal volumes (5 to 10 μl) of feces and modified Kinyoun's carbol fuchsin stain. (The stain is prepared by dissolving 4.0 g of basic fuchsin in 100 mL deionized water plus 20 ml of 95% ethanol. After the stain is dissolved, add slowly 8 ml of liquefied phenol.)
2. As soon as the smear has air dried, add a drop of immersion oil directly to the smear. Place a coverslip on top of the immersion oil, and observe with a brightfield microscope.
3. The characteristic bright, birefringent appearance of *Cryptosporidium* species oocysts against a dark staining background occurs because the oocyst wall is not stained during this procedure and is impervious, preventing entry of the stain and loss of water from the interior of the oocyst (Fig. 18–5*a*). Fecal debris, yeast, and bacteria all stain darkly. Often the stain collects

around the outside of the oocyst as the smear dries, resulting in dark rings around bright oocysts. After approximately 15 minutes in immersion oil, the oocysts begin to collapse.

Immunofluorescent Antibody Stains

Most humans and animals with cryptosporidiosis pass enough oocysts in their stools so that most of the concentration and/or staining techniques described in the literature (several are outlined earlier) are adequate for detection and diagnosis. However, more sensitive techniques are sometimes needed to detect oocysts in specimens that contain few parasites and large amounts of debris. These specimens include fecal samples from asymptomatic carriers and filtrates from surface or drinking water samples. Both polyclonal and monoclonal antibodies specific to *C. parvum* can be used in direct or indirect immunofluorescent assays to detect oocysts in these specimens. A commercially available immunofluorescent diagnostic kit (Merridian Laboratories, Cincinnati, OH) entails use of a monoclonal antibody specific to the oocyst wall of *C. parvum*. The utility of immunofluorescent assays has been addressed by Garcia and colleagues.[23]

IDENTIFICATION OF ENDOGENOUS STAGES

Routine histologic methods can be used to detect endogenous stages of *Cryptosporidium* species in specimens of mucosal epithelium, but identification of different life cycle stages can be difficult.[10] Transmission electron microscopy facilitates identification of developmental stages of *Cryptosporidium* species that reside within parasitophorous vacuoles confined to the microvillous region of epithelial cells.[11] To identify stages of *Cryptosporidium* species in fresh mucosal scrapings, in cultured cells, or in the chorioallantoic membrane of chicken embryos, a light microscope equipped with high-quality phase-contrast or Nomarski interference contrast (NIC) optics is best. The author prefers NIC optics for this purpose. If NIC or phase-contrast optics are not available, brightfield microscopy can be used to identify some of the developmental stages of *Cryptosporidium* species in stained mucosal smears.[30]

REFERENCES

1. Anderson BC: Patterns of shedding of cryptosporidial oocysts in Idaho calves. J Am Vet Med Assoc 178:982–984, 1981.
2. Anderson, BC: Abomasal cryptosporidiosis in cattle. Vet Pathol 24:235–238, 1987.
3. Angus KW: Cryptosporidiosis in man, domestic animals and birds: a review. J R Soc Med 76:62–70, 1983.
4. Angus KW: Cryptosporidiosis in ruminants. *In* Dubey JP, Speer CA, Fayer R (eds): Cryptosporidiosis of Man and Animals. Boca Raton, FL, CRC Press, pp 83–104, 1990.
5. Argenzio RA, Liacos JA, Levy ML, et al: Villous atrophy, crypt hyperplasia, cellular infiltration and impaired glucose-Na absorption in enteric cryptosporidiosis of pigs. Gastroenterology 98:1129–1140, 1990.
6. Blagburn BL, Soave R: Prophylaxis and chemotherapy: human and animal. *In* Fayer R (ed): *Cryptosporidium* and Cryptosporidiosis. Boca Raton, FL, CRC Press, pp 113–130, 1997.
7. Crawford, FG, Vermund SH: Human cryptosporidiosis. CRC Crit Rev Microbiol 16:113–159, 1988.
8. Current WL: Techniques and laboratory maintenance of *Cryptosporidium*. *In* Dubey JP, Speer CA, Fayer R (eds): Cryptosporidiosis of Man and Animals. Boca Raton, FL, CRC Press, pp 31–50, 1990.
9. Current WL, Blagburn BL: *Cryptosporidium*: Infections in man and domesticated animals. *In* Long PL (ed): Coccidiosis of Man and Domesticated Animals. Boca Raton, FL, CRC Press, pp 155–185, 1990.
10. Current WL, Garcia LS: Cryptosporidiosis. Clin Microbiol Rev 4:325–358, 1991.
11. Current WL, Reese NC: A comparison of endogenous development of three isolates of *Cryptosporidium* in suckling mice. J Protozool 33:98–108, 1986.
12. Current WL, Upton SJ, Haynes TB: The life cycle of *Cryptosporidium baileyi* n. sp. (Apicomplexa, Cryptosporidiidae) infecting chickens. J Protozool 33:289–296, 1986.
13. Current WL, Reese NC, Ernst JV, et al: Human cryptosporidiosis in immunocompetent and immunodeficient persons: studies of an outbreak and experimental transmission. New Engl J Med 308:1252–1257, 1983.
14. Current WL: Human cryptosporidiosis. N Engl J Med 309:1326–1327, 1983.
15. Dubey JP, Speer CA, Fayer R (eds): Cryptosporidiosis of Man and Animals. Boca Raton, FL, CRC Press, 1990.
16. Dupont HL, Chappell C, Sterling C, et al: The infectivity of *Cryptosporidium parvum* in healthy volunteers. N Engl J Med 332:855–859, 1995.
17. Fayer R, Ungar BLP: *Cryptosporidium* spp. and cryptosporidiosis. Microbiol Rev 50:458–483, 1986.
18. Fayer R (ed): *Cryptosporidium* and Cryptosporidiosis. CRC Press, Boca Raton, 1997.
19. Gajadhar AA: *Cryptosporidium* species in imported ostriches and consideration of possible implications for birds in Canada. Can J Vet 34:115–116, 1993.
20. Gajadhar AA: Host specificity studies and oocyst description of a *Cryptosporidium* sp. isolated from ostriches. Parasitol Res 80:316–319, 1994.
21. Garcia LS, Current WL: Cryptosporidiosis: clinical features and diagnosis. CRC Clin Rev Clin Lab Sci 27:439–460, 1989.
22. Garcia LS, Bruckner DA, Brewer TC, Shimizu RY: Techniques for the recovery and identification of *Cryptosporidium* oocysts from stool specimens. J Clin Microbiol 18:185–190, 1983.
23. Garcia LS, Brewer TC, Bruckner DA: Fluorescent detection of *Cryptosporidium* oocysts in human fecal specimens by using monoclonal antibodies. J Clin Microbiol 25:119–121, 1987.
24. Goodwin MA, Steffens WL, Russell ID, Brown J: Diarrhea associated with intestinal cryptosporidiosis in turkeys. Avian Dis 32:63–67, 1988.
25. Guarino A, Canani RB, Pozio E, et al: Enterotoxic effect of stool supernatant of *Cryptosporidium*-infected calves on human jejunum. Gasteroenterol 106:28–32, 1994.
26. Hayes EB, Matte TD, O'Brien TR, et al: Large community outbreak of cryptosporidiosis due to contamination of a filtered public water supply. N Engl J Med 320:1372–1376, 1989.
27. Heine J, Pohlenz JFL, Moon HW, Wood GN: Enteric lesions and diarrhea in gnotobiotic calves monoinfected with *Cryptosporidium* species. J Infect Dis 150:768–775, 1984.
28. Heine J: Ein einfadche Nachweismethode Fur Kryptosporidien im Kot. Zentralbl Veterinaermed Reihe B 29:324–327, 1982.
29. Hoerr FJ, Current WL, Haynes TB: Fatal cryptosporidiosis in quail. Avian Dis 30:421–425, 1986.
30. Latimer KS, Goodwin MA, Davis MK: Rapid cytologic diagnosis of respiratory cryptosporidiosis in chickens. Avian Dis 32: 826–830, 1988.
31. Levine ND: Taxonomy and review of the coccidian genus *Cryptosporidium* (Protozoa, Apicomplexa). J Protozool 31:94–98, 1984.
32. Lindsay DS, Balgburn BL, Sundermann CA, Giambrone JJ: Effect of broiler chicken age on susceptibility to experimentally induced *Cryptosporidium baileyi* infection. Am J Vet Res 49:1412–1414, 1987.
33. MacKinzie WR, Hoxie NJ, Proctor ME, et al: A massive outbreak in Milwaukee of *Cryptosporidium* infection transmitted through the public water supply. N Engl J Med 331:161–167, 1994.

34. O'Donoghue PJ: *Cryptosporidium* and cryptosporidiosis in man and animals. Int J Parasitol 25:139–195, 1995.

35. Ongerth JE, Stibbs HH: Identification of *Cryptosporidium* oocysts in river water. Appl Environ Microbiol 53:672–676, 1987.

36. Slavin D: *Cryptosporidium meleagridis* (sp nov). J Comp Pathol 65:262–266, 1955.

37. Soave R: Treatment strategies for cryptosporidiosis. Ann N Y Acad Sci 616:442–451, 1990.

38. Tyzzer EE: An extracellular coccidium, *Cryptosporidium muris* (gen et sp nov) of the gastric glands of the common mouse. J Med Res 23:487–516, 1910.

39. Tyzzer EE: *Cryptosporidium parvum* (sp nov) a coccidium found in the small intestine of the common mouse. Arch Protistenkd 26:394–412, 1912.

40. Upton SJ: *Cryptosporidium* spp. in lower vertebrates. *In* Dubey JP, Speer CA, Fayer R (eds): Cryptosporidiosis of Man and Animals. Boca Raton, FL, CRC Press, pp 149–156, 1990.

41. Upton SJ, Current WL: The species of *Cryptosporidium* (Apicomplexa, Cryptosporidiidae) infecting mammals. J Parasitol 71:625–629, 1985.

42. Upton SJ, McAllister CT, Freed PS, Barnard SB: *Cryptosporidium* spp. in wild and captive reptiles. J Wildl Dis 25:20–30, 1989.

CHAPTER 19

Toxoplasmosis in Zoo Animals

DELLA M. GARELL

INCIDENCE

Toxoplasmosis gondii has a worldwide distribution. Virtually all vertebrate species are susceptible to infection.[2, 17, 30, 35, 37] In many species, infection may be common, but clinical disease is rare. However, there does appear to be a unique susceptibility to clinical and even fatal toxoplasmosis in certain taxonomic groups such as Australian marsupials[4, 13, 20, 26, 29, 31, 32, 34] (especially macropods) and New World primates (especially squirrel monkeys).[1, 7, 28] Prosimians, particularly ring-tailed lemurs (*Lemur catta*) also appear to be extremely sensitive.[1, 5, 14] It may be that marsupials and prosimians are more susceptible to severe toxoplasmosis because of their reduced evolutionary exposure to felids, the family of animals that are capable of transmitting the parasite.[9]

Domestic and exotic felids are the only known definitive hosts of this parasite and as such are the only animals capable of completing the parasite's enteroepithelial life cycle and shedding the oocysts in their feces.[11, 18, 22, 30, 31] Approximately 30% of domestic cats in the United States are seropositive for *T. gondii*. Felid hosts commonly acquire the parasite from ingesting wild rodents or birds that contain the tissue cysts of *T. gondii*.[18]

ETIOLOGIC AGENT AND TRANSMISSION

The etiologic agent, *T. gondii*, is an obligate intracellular coccidian parasite. There are three infectious stages: (1) sporozoites in fecal oocysts; (2) invasive tachyzoites from ingested sporozoites; and (3) tissue-encysted bradyzoites.[9]

Transmission is via three possible routes: (1) ingestion of feline fecal matter contaminated with sporulated oocysts (sporogeny occurs in deposited feces after 24 to 96 hours); (2) congenital (transplacental) infection; and (3) ingestion of tissue cysts in uncooked muscle, liver, or other tissues.[12] Carnivores, especially if housed outside, may be exposed through ingestion of infected rodents and birds. A common means of exposure for noncarnivores is through ingestion of hay or grain contaminated with infective oocysts from feline feces[17] (Fig. 19–1).

In Felidae the prepatent period is 3 to 10 days after ingestion of tissue cysts and 20 to 34 days after ingestion of sporulated oocysts in fecal matter.[18] Millions of oocysts may be shed by felines for 1 to 2 weeks during primary infection. This initial infection is commonly associated with diarrhea and usually occurs in kittens soon after weaning. During subsequent reinfection, cats shed oocysts in lower numbers briefly or do not shed at all. Reinfections are usually subclinical and lead to the carrier state.[18]

At least 24 hours must pass before fecal oocysts sporulate and become infective. They may remain infective under favorable conditions (moist soil) for 18 months or more.[18] Freezing may reduce oocyst viability somewhat.[8]

PATHOGENESIS

After a susceptible host ingests tissue cysts or fecal oocysts, the acute clinical signs are caused by intestinal

POSTULATED TRANSMISSION OF TOXOPLASMA GONDII IN ZOOS

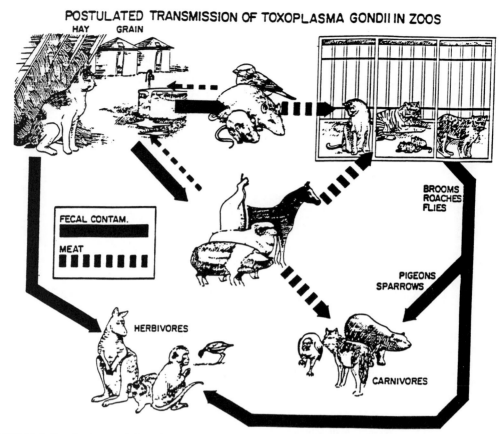

FIGURE 19–1. Postulated transmission of toxoplasmosis in zoos. Infective oocysts are spread by feline fecal contamination and via fomites. Tissue cysts contained in meat or prey are an additional source of infection for carnivores. (From Frenkel JK: Protozoan diseases of zoo and captive mammals and birds. *In* Montali RJ, Migaki G (eds): Comparative Pathology of Zoo Animals. Washington, DC, Smithsonian Institution Press, pp 329–342, 1980.)

necrosis caused by tachyzoites. The organism spreads via blood or lymph to many organs. *T. gondii* has affinity for the central nervous system (CNS), lung, pancreas, lymphoid system, liver, heart, adrenal, and ocular tissue.[9]

Acute disseminated infections may be fatal, particularly in highly susceptible species. However, in mature cats and most other species, including humans, the disease is usually mild.[9] The immune system gradually slows tachyzoite replication, and by the third week, cyst formation occurs in tissues.[12] If the host is subsequently immunosuppressed, the released bradyzoites may initiate a reactivation and clinical relapse.[19]

CLINICAL FINDINGS

Clinical manifestation is variable in different species and may include sudden death. Signs may be localized as in ocular involvement (retinitis, uveitis), CNS involvement, or pneumonia, or they may be generalized. Depression, anorexia, fever, dyspnea, diarrhea, emesis, icterus, and ataxia are all possible signs.[12] Clinical signs and laboratory abnormalities depend on the organ system or systems affected. Hepatitis, pneumonia, myocar-

ditis, myositis, encephalitis, pancreatitis, and lymphadenitis are commonly noted. Alanine aminotransferase (ALT), aspartate aminotransferase (AST), and creatine phosphokinase (CPK) levels may be elevated, depending on organ involvement.[12] Australian marsupials and certain primate species often acquire overwhelming infection with *T. gondii* and may die peracutely.[4, 26, 32]

DIAGNOSTIC PROCEDURES

Serology

The detection of antibodies in serum suggests previous or current infection by *T. gondii*. Serologic tests available include the following: (1) methylene blue dye binding (MBD); (2) indirect immunofluorescent antibody (IFA); (3) indirect hemagglutination; (4) enzyme-linked immunosorbent assay (ELISA); (5) direct and modified agglutination tests (DAT, MAT); and (6) latex agglutination (LA).[23, 38]

The MBD test is considered the gold standard in humans, but it is not validated as such in other species. It also requires the use of live *T. gondii* organisms and is therefore rarely used diagnostically today.[33] IFA is accurate and may be adapted to detect immunoglobulin M or G (IgM, IgG) separately or in combination, but only for a limited number of domestic species in which the species-specific conjugate has been developed. The ELISA is more sensitive than the commercially available kits for LA or indirect hemagglutination assays, but at this time it has been validated only with domestic cat and dog serum.[25] However, the ELISA appears to accurately detect antibody in nondomestic cat serum as well.[21] The presence of IgM in serum is most consistent with recent infection, but testing for specific anti-*Toxoplasma* IgM is available only for feline species (domestic and nondomestic). The ELISA for detection of IgM and IgG in feline serum has been validated by Western blot immunoassay and can also be used to detect antibodies in aqueous humor or cerebrospinal fluid from cats and dogs with suspected ocular or CNS involvement. ELISA testing may be performed by Dr. Michael R. Lappin, Diagnostic Laboratory, Colorado State University, Fort Collins, CO 80523 (phone: 303-221-4535).

The DAT as first developed lacked sensitivity and specificity. The modified DAT (MAT) results correlate well with those of the MBD and IFA tests.[33] The conventional MAT detects only IgG, but it is a very specific and sensitive test for *T. gondii* in any species.[15] It can also be modified to detect IgG antibodies specific to acute infection.[10] Dubey and Thulliez[15] found that the MAT was more sensitive than the MBD, IHA, or LA tests in detecting *T. gondii* antibodies. The MAT is not commercially available in the United States; however, Dr. J. P. Dubey is interested in zoological serum samples for MAT analysis and he will perform this test. He should be contacted, before samples are sent, at the Parasite Biology and Epidemiology Laboratory, Livestock and Poultry Sciences Institute, Agricultural Research Service, U. S. Department of Agriculture, Beltsville, MD 20705 (phone: 301-504-8128).

A commercially available LA test (Toxotest-MT, Tanabe USA, Inc., 7930 Convoy Ct., San Diego, CA 92111; phone: 619-571-8410) has been used with serum from multiple nondomestic species. Results from domestic cats, nondomestic cats, and domestic dogs suggest that this assay may be more sensitive than the IHA kit in detecting anti-*Toxoplasma* IgG in serum.[25, 33] Until a more sensitive serological test for toxoplasmosis in nondomestic species is readily available, the ease of performance, ease of interpretation, and availability of the LA test make it a good non–species-specific assay.

Titer magnitude and significance varies with the species tested and the assay used. Serology laboratories provide positive cut-off values (usually >1:1024). A single high IgG titer documents exposure to *T. gondii* but does not confirm active infection, inasmuch as some domestic cats have IgG titers higher than 1:1000 for up to 29 months after infection.[15] Paired IgG titers measured 2 to 3 weeks apart with the same test (and, preferably, run at the same time) that show at least a serial fourfold rise in IgG are indicative of active infection.[12]

Necropsy

There may be no abnormal findings at gross necropsy. If lesions are present, there are usually visible necrotic foci in the liver, spleen, or kidneys or small, white, nodular foci in the lungs.[4] Histopathologically, cellular necrosis is the predominant lesion, especially in the liver, lymph nodes, lungs, CNS, and muscle.[12]

Toxoplasma gondii may be demonstrated in tissue by light and electron microscopy, immunohistochemical staining, bioassay, tissue antigen ELISA, or polymerase chain reaction (PCR) analysis. These tests are *T. gondii*–specific and most are available in these laboratories: (1) Dr. Michael R. Lappin, Diagnostic Laboratory, Colorado State University, Fort Collins, CO 80523 (phone: 303-221-4535); (2) Dr. J. P. Dubey, Parasite Biology and Epidemiology Laboratory, Livestock and Poultry Sciences Institute, Agricultural Research Service, U.S. Department of Agriculture, Beltsville, MD 20705 (phone: 301-504-8128); and (3) Dr. Sharon Patton, Clinical Parasitology Laboratory, University of Tennessee, Knoxville, TN 37901 (phone: 615-974-5645). The laboratories may be contacted directly regarding tissue preparation for specific testing procedures. The PCR method of detection of *T. gondii* is a more recent development. It is very specific and sensitive but also expensive, prone to contamination, and not widely available at this time.[21, 27]

CLINICAL MANAGEMENT

No treatment is effective in eliminating infection with *T. gondii*. However, most protocols do arrest the multiplication of the organism. Clindamycin hydrochloride is considered to be the drug of choice for the treatment of clinical toxoplasmosis in dogs and cats.[9, 12] It may be administered orally or parenterally at 10 to 15 mg/kg every 8 or 12 hours for 4 weeks.[9, 15, 23] The reported *Clostridium difficile* enteric overgrowth that may cause severe ulcerative colitis in humans has not been reported in dogs, cats, or other species.[12] Clindamycin has good tissue distribution. It crosses the blood-brain barrier in animals infected with toxoplasmosis. Clindamycin has been used successfully for the treatment of CNS toxoplasmosis in people, mice, and domestic cats.[9, 16, 23]

Clinical signs should start to improve within the first week of treatment, although some permanent damage may have occurred, especially to the CNS. Personal clinical experience with glaucoma and exposure keratitis secondary to anterior uveitis in two Bennett wallabies may indicate that response to standard glaucoma therapy and parenteral clindamycin is good, if the infection is localized to the ocular tissues.

Another chemotherapeutic that has been used successfully is the synergistic combination of sulfonamides (sulfadiazine or triple-sulfas) at 30 to 60 mg/kg PO every 12 hours with pyrimethamine at 0.25 to 0.5 mg/kg PO every 12 hours.[9, 12] Megaloblastic anemia may develop during pyrimethamine use. Because these drugs are antifolates, the patient should receive folinic acid supplementation (5.0 mg/day) or brewer's yeast (100 mg/kg/day) to counteract any bone marrow suppression.[9, 12] Hemograms should be monitored for anemia, leukopenia, and thrombocytopenia. Pyrimethamine is also unpalatable and teratogenic. Trimethoprim sulfdiazine alone may be effective in cats at 15 mg/kg PO every 12 hours,[23] but it reportedly is ineffective therapeutically for severe ocular toxoplasmosis in dogs.[3] Drugs with fewer side effects that may be less effective but are relatively safe for long-term therapy are chloramphenicol and tetracycline or doxycycline.[12]

Because toxoplasmic encephalitis is a common complication of human immunodeficiency virus (HIV) infection in people,[24] newer drugs and combinations are being developed and tested (e.g., clarithromycin-pyrimethamine, roxithromycin, spiromycin, azithromycin, and A-56268).[6, 16] No therapeutic agents eliminate *T. gondii,* and so disease may recur at times of stress or immunosuppression.

PREVENTION

A common source of *T. gondii* exposure in herbivores may be contaminated hay, straw, or grain.[17] Cats and kittens are commonly found in barns where hay is stored. Kittens shed extremely high numbers of oocysts after their first exposure to infected prey, and weanling kittens may therefore be the predominant source of forage contamination. Efforts should be made to rid hay barns of cats and/or to have catproof hay storage areas. If this is difficult on a large scale, at least the portion of hay or straw provided to the species most susceptible to severe forms of toxoplasmosis should be kept away from cats.

The only effective prevention at this time is to reduce or eliminate exposure to feline feces and uncooked meat. For carnivores, this means excluding access for the consumption of wild mammals and birds. Examples of some strategies are eliminating stray cats or preventing feral cats from entering exhibits and hay storage areas; pest control; and routine examination of exotic cat fecal samples. The processed raw horse meat diet commonly fed as feline and canine diets in zoos is usually stored frozen, which significantly reduces the viability of any *T. gondii* cysts present, although it still may present a small risk.[8]

In outbreak situations, it may be advisable to place individual animals at risk on a prophylactic protocol of therapeutic levels of trimethoprim-sulfadiazine or clindamycin.

ZOONOTIC POTENTIAL

Toxoplasmosis is a zoonotic disease. In various geographic regions of the United States, 20% to 70% of the human population have antibodies to *T. gondii* (i.e., are latently infected).[9, 18] Usual sources of infection are feline fecal matter (commonly found in garden soil, sand boxes, or litter boxes) and uncooked meat. Postnatal infections in immunocompetent people are usually asymptomatic or produce mild flu-like signs (myalgia, sore throat, fever, lymphadenopathy) that are self-limiting.[9]

Prenatal infection is serious; abortion, encephalitis, blindness, or mental retardation of the fetus may result. In women latently infected with *T. gondii* before con-

ception, fetuses are not usually at risk for disease.[9] In immunocompromised people, especially those with acquired immunodeficiency syndrome (AIDS), a fatal reactivation of a latent *T. gondii* infection can develop.[24] Toxoplasmic encephalitis is one of the most common causes of encephalitis in the United States, primarily in patients with AIDS.[24]

It may be prudent for any zoo employee who is immunocompromised or of childbearing age and who will be exposed to uncooked meat or feline fecal matter to have a toxoplasmosis antibody titer determined at the pre-employment examination and when ill or before becoming pregnant. Disposal of all feline fecal matter and thorough cleaning of contaminated tools before oocyst sporulation (i.e., every 24 hours) help to reduce exposure.[18] Employees who are immunocompromised or pregnant and at risk of infection should take special protective measures (e.g., frequent hand washing; wearing disposable gloves and footwear; or, ideally, arranging a temporary job reassignment).

FUTURE DIRECTIONS

A vaccine for cats that prevents oocyst shedding upon repeat exposure to *T. gondii* has been developed. The vaccine is currently undergoing further testing for potential marketing.

A lemur-specific *T. gondii* antibody assay is being developed. Also, a tissue antigen ELISA is being studied in multiple species at Colorado State University. (Contact Dr. Michael R. Lappin, 303-221-4535, for availability of testing).

Several types of vaccines have been formulated and trialed in various species. A *Hammondia hammondi* based vaccine appears to protect Tammar wallabies from clinical disease upon initial infection with *T. gondii*; however, tissue cysts are still formed.[36] The tissue cysts may pose a significant risk of disease from reactivation of the latent infection. A commercially available attenuated *T. gondii* (S48) vaccine marketed for sheep and goats (Toxovax; AgResearch, Wallaceville, New Zealand) underwent trials in Tammar wallabies and appears to induce fatal toxoplasmosis in naive animals.[26] A temperature sensitive strain (ts-4) of *T. gondii* used to vaccinate opossums induced a serologic response; however, protection against infection was not determined.[33] Preliminary trials with the ts-4 vaccine in naive wallabies suggest that it may be safe in this species (personal communication, Patrick Morris, DVM, San Diego Zoo, San Diego, CA). Further trials and challenges are indicated for the ts-4 strain vaccine.

REFERENCES

1. Borst GHA, van Knapen F: Acute acquired toxoplasmosis in primates in a zoo. J Zoo Animal Med 15:60–62, 1984.
2. Burns R, Williams ES, O'Toole D, et al: Toxoplasmosis in black-footed ferrets (*Mustela nigripes*) at the Louisville Zoo. Proceedings of the American Association of Zoo Veterinarians, St. Louis, MO, p 48, 1993.
3. Bussanich MN, Rootman J: Implicating toxoplasmosis as the cause of ocular lesions. Vet Med 80:43–51, 1985.
4. Canfield PJ, Hartley WJ, Dubey JP: Lesions of toxoplasmosis in Australian marsupials. J Comp Pathol 103:159–167, 1990.

5. Chang J, Kornegay RW, Wagner JL, et al: Toxoplasmosis in a sifaka. *In* Montali RJ, Migaki G (eds): The Comparative Pathology of Zoo Animals. Washington, DC, Smithsonian Institution Press, pp 347–352, 1980.

6. Chang HR, Pechere JF: In vitro effects of four macrolides (roxithromycin, spiramycin, azithromycin [CP-62,993], and A-56268) on *Toxoplasma gondii*. Antimicrob Agents Chemother 32(4):524–529, 1988.

7. Cunningham AA, Buxton D, Thomson KM: An epidemic of toxoplasmosis in a captive colony of squirrel monkeys (*Saimiri sciureus*). J Comp Pathol 107:207–219, 1992.

8. Dubey JP: Effect of freezing on the infectivity of *Toxoplasma* cysts to cats. J Am Vet Med Assoc 165:534–536, 1974.

9. Dubey JP, Beattie CP: Toxoplasmosis of Animals and Man. Boca Raton, FL, CRC Press, 1988.

10. Dubey JP, Carpenter JL: Histologically confirmed clinical toxoplasmosis in cats: 100 cases (1952–1990). J Am Vet Med Assoc 203(11):1556–1566, 1993.

11. Dubey JP, Gendron-Fitzpatrick AP, Lenhard AL: Fatal toxoplasmosis and enteroepithelial stages of *Toxoplasma gondii* in a pallas cat (*Felis manul*). J Protozool 35:528–530, 1988.

12. Dubey JP, Greene CE, Lappin MR: Toxoplasmosis and neosporosis. *In* Greene C (ed): Infectious Diseases of the Dog and Cat. Philadelphia, WB Saunders, pp 818–834, 1990.

13. Dubey JP, Hedstrom O, Machado CR, et al: Disseminated toxoplasmosis in a captive koala (*Phascolarctos cinereus*). J Zoo Wildl Med 22(3):348–350, 1991.

14. Dubey JP, Kramer LW, Weisbrode SE: Acute death associated with *Toxoplasma gondii* in ring-tailed lemurs. J Am Vet Med Assoc 187:1272–1273, 1985.

15. Dubey JP, Thulliez P: Serologic diagnosis of toxoplasmosis in cats fed *Toxoplasma gondii* tissue cysts. J Am Vet Med Assoc 194:1297–1299, 1989.

16. Fernandez-Martin J, Leport C, Morlat P, et al: Pyrimethamine-clarithromycin combination for therapy of acute *Toxoplasma* encephalitis in patients with AIDS. Antimicrob Agents Chemother 35(10):2049–2052, 1991.

17. Frenkel JK: Protozoan diseases of zoo and captive mammals and birds. *In* Montali RJ, Migaki G (eds): Comparative Pathology of Zoo Animals. Washington, DC, Smithsonian Institution Press, pp 329–342, 1980.

18. Frenkel JK, Dubey JP: Toxoplasmosis and its prevention in cats and man. J Infect Dis 126(6):664–673, 1972.

19. Frenkel JK, Nelson BM, Arias-Stella J: Immuno-suppression and toxoplasmic encephalitis. Human Pathol 6:97–111, 1975.

20. Hartley WJ, Dubey JP, Spielman DS: Fatal toxoplasmosis in koalas (*Phascolarctos cinereus*). J Parisitol 76(2):271–272, 1990.

21. Hyman JA, Johnson LK, Kirk CL, et al: Polymerase chain reaction, histological, and ultrastructural diagnosis of disseminated toxoplasmosis in a squirrel (*Sciurus carolinensis*). Proceedings of the American Association of Zoo Veterinarians, St. Louis, MO, p 407, 1993.

22. Jewel ML, Frenkel JK, Johnson KM, et al: Development of *Toxoplasma* oocysts in neotropical Felidae. Am J Trop Med Hyg 21:512–517, 1972.

23. Lappin MR: Feline toxoplasmosis: interpretation of diagnostic test results. Semin Vet Med Surg (Small Animals) 11(3):154–160, 1996.

24. Lappin MR, Jacobson ER, Kollias GV, et al: Comparison of serologic assays for the diagnosis of toxoplasmosis in nondomestic felids. J Zoo Wildl Med 22(2):169–174, 1991.

25. Lappin MR, Powell CC: Comparison of latex agglutination, indirect hemagglutination, and ELISA techniques for the detection of *Toxoplasma gondii*–specific antibodies in the serum of cats. J Vet Intern Med 5:299–301, 1991.

26. Luft BJ, Remington JS: AIDS commentary: toxoplasmic encephalitis. J Infect Dis 157(1):1–6, 1988.

27. Lynch MJ, Obendorf DL, Statham P, et al: Serological responses of tammar wallabies (*Macropus eugenii*) to inoculation with an attenuated strain of *Toxoplasma gondii*. Proceedings of the American Association of Zoo Veterinarians, St. Louis, MO, pp 185–187, 1993.

28. MacPherson JM, Gajadhar AA: Sensitive and specific polymerase chain reaction detection of *Toxoplasma gondii* for veterinary and medical diagnosis. Can J Vet Res 57:45–48, 1993.

29. McKissick GE, Ratcliffe HL, Koestner A: Enzootic toxoplasmosis in caged squirrel monkeys (*Saimiri sciureus*). Pathol Vet 5:538–560, 1968.

30. Miller DS, Mitchell GF, Biggs B, et al: Disease and small populations: Toxoplasmosis and ocular pathology in the eastern barred bandicoot (*Perameles gunni*). Proceedings of the American Association of Zoo Veterinarians, St. Louis, MO, pp 183–184, 1993.

31. Miller NL, Frenkel JK, Dubey JP: Oral infections with *Toxoplasma* cysts and oocysts in felines, other mammals, and birds. J Parasitol 58(5):928–937, 1972.

32. Obendorf DL, Munday BL: Toxoplasmosis in wild Tasmanian wallabies. Aust Vet J 60:62, 1963.

33. Patton S, Funk RS: Serological response of the opossum (*Didelphis virginiana*) to a temperature-sensitive mutant (ts-4) of *Toxoplasma gondii*. J Parasitol 78(4):741–743, 1992.

34. Patton S, Johnson SL, Loeffler DG, et al: Epizootic of toxoplasmosis in kangaroos, wallabies, and potaroos: possible transmission via domestic cats. J Am Vet Med Assoc 189:1166–1169, 1986.

35. Patton S, Rabinowitz A, Randolph S, et al: A coprological survey of parasites of wild neotropical Felidae. J Parasitol 72:517–520, 1986.

36. Reddacliff GL, Parker SJ, Dubey JP: An attempt to prevent acute toxoplasmosis in macropods by vaccination with *Hammondia hammondi*. Aust Vet J 70:33–35, 1993.

37. Stover J, Jacobson ER, Lukas J, et al: *Toxoplasma gondii* in a collection of nondomestic ruminants. J Zoo Wildl Med 21:295–301, 1990.

38. Wilson M, Ware DA, Juranek DD: Serologic aspects of toxoplasmosis. J Am Vet Med Assoc 196(2):277–281, 1990.

Rabies: Global Problem, Zoonotic Threat, and Preventive Management

CHARLES E. RUPPRECHT

Zoo professionals should be concerned about rabies because it is an acute, fatal encephalomyelitis, a reportable disease, and an obvious occupational hazard. In addition, it persists as one of the oldest recognized zoonoses that still results in tens of thousands of human deaths[32] and is geographically widespread. This entity, caused by rabies virus and a number of related *Lyssaviruses,* abounds on all inhabited continents (Table 20–1). Although no warm-blooded vertebrates are known to be resistant to experimental infection, mammals are the only principal hosts. Natural infections have spanned the taxonomic gamut from armadillos[31] to zebras,[53] but distinctive reservoirs are limited to specific representation among the Carnivora and Chiroptera. Partly because of the global distribution and horrific reputation of this re-emerging malady, multiple attributes of *Lyssaviruses* are receiving increasing attention, more than a century after Pasteur.

APPLIED TAXONOMY AND MICROBIOLOGY

Taxonomically, the viruses that cause rabies belong to the family Rhabdoviridae. The genus *Lyssavirus* includes rabies virus and a group of antigenically and genetically related viruses that represent the penultimate neurotropic agents. Rabies viruses and these so-called rabies-related viruses were previously defined on the bases of morphology, serology, and the ability to cause encephalitis in laboratory animals. Currently, monoclonal antibodies (Mabs) and genetic sequencing[50] can differentiate rabies viruses from others in the genus. Such basic laboratory techniques have been essential to studies in viral taxonomy and phylogeny and have provided useful insights into the distribution and perpetuation of different viral variants. At least six other

TABLE 20–1. Global Disease Surveillance: Examples of Countries and Political Units Reporting No Recent Cases of Rabies*

Region	Countries
Africa	Cape Verde; Congo; Libya; Mauritius; Reunion; Seychelles
Americas	
North	Bermuda; St. Pierre and Miquelon
Caribbean	Anguilla; Antigua and Barbuda; Bahamas; Barbados; Cayman Islands; Dominica; Guadeloupe; Jamaica; Martinique; Montserrat; Netherlands Antilles (Aruba, Bonaire, Curacao, Saba, St. Maarten, and St. Eustatius); St. Christopher (St. Kitts) and Nevis; St. Lucia; St. Martin; St. Vincent and Grenadines; Tobago; Turks and Caicos Islands; Virgin Islands
South	Uruguay
Asia	Bahrain; Hong Kong; Japan; Malaysia (Malaysia-Sabah); Maldives; Qatar; Singapore; Taiwan
Europe	Cyprus; Denmark; Faroe Islands; Finland; Gibraltar; Greece; Iceland; Ireland; Malta; Netherlands; Norway (mainland); Portugal; Spain (except Ceuta/Melilla); Sweden; United Kingdom (Britain and Northern Ireland)
Oceania	American Samoa; Australia; Cook Islands; Fiji; French Polynesia; Guam; Hawaii; Indonesia (with exception of Java, Kalimantan, Sumatra, and Sulawesi); Kiribati; New Caledonia; New Zealand; Niue; Papua New Guinea; Solomon Islands; Tonga; Vanuatu

*Bat rabies may exist in some areas that are reportedly free of terrestrial rabies, and some classifications may be considered provisional. This list is based on data from the following publications and other information provided to the Centers for Disease Control and Prevention:

(1) World Health Organization: World Survey of Rabies 30 (for 1994); Division of Emerging and Other Communicable Diseases Surveillance and Control, Geneva, 1996.

(2) WHO Collaborating Centre for Rabies Surveillance and Research: Rabies Bulletin Europe, vols. 1 and 2, 1996.

(3) Pan American Health Organization: Epidemiological surveillance of rabies in the Americas, 1994, vol 25 (Nos. 1–12), 1995.

distinct lyssaviruses related to rabies are tentatively recognized (Table 20–2).

Being enveloped, lyssaviruses do not persist well outside the mammalian host. Survival time depends partly on the nature and amount of infectious material, such as dense brain tissue or a thin film of saliva. Viral isolation from infected tissue is readily performed by the intracerebral inoculation of laboratory rodents or by cell culture propagation. Lyssaviruses are rapidly inactivated by many lipid solvents, by exposure to fixatives such as formalin, by strong acids and bases, by most detergents, by heat, and by ultraviolet radiation, including that in sunlight. Repeated freezing and thawing typically leads to a loss of infectivity. Viruses may remain infective for years under special laboratory conditions (e.g., sterile support media at $-70°C$).

Rabies virus is the only lyssavirus with nearly cosmopolitan distribution and the only one found to date in the New World. Nonrabies lyssaviruses are often considered microbiologic curiosities, typically restricted to the Old World. Aside from occasional isolations, their epizootiology is poorly understood. Although traditional rabies vaccines provide broad cross-reactivity against all known field isolates of rabies virus, this action does not necessarily extend to the nonrabies lyssaviruses, such as Mokola virus or Lagos Bat virus. The ease of modern transportation of wildlife from tropical locations may enable these agents to spread in

TABLE 20–2. Currently Recognized Members of the *Lyssavirus* Genus, Family Rhabdoviridae

Lyssavirus	Reservoirs	History
Rabies virus	Found on all continents, except Australia and Antarctica. Enzootic and sometimes epizootic in a variety of mammalian species, including canids, mustelids, viverrids, and New World insectivorous and hematophagus bats; >50,000 human cases/year, primarily in areas of uncontrolled domestic dog rabies.	Clinical disease described in ancient documents. During the late 19th century, Pasteur attenuated virus through serial passage and desiccation, to vaccinate humans and domestic animals. Inclusions in nerve cells described by Negri in 1903. Immunofluorescent test for diagnosis developed in the 1950s. Monoclonal antibodies (Mabs) for variant characterization produced in the late 1970s and genetic sequencing in the 1980s.
Lagos bat virus	Unknown but probably fruit bats, with spillover infection to domestic animals. Virus isolated in Nigeria, South Africa, Zimbabwe, Central African Republic, Senegal, and Ethiopia. No known human deaths.	Isolated in 1956 from Nigerian fruit bats (*Eidolon helvum*) on Lagos Island, but not characterized until 1970; initially diagnosed as rabies, but weak immunofluorescence led to suspicion of "rabies-related" viruses, later confirmed with Mabs. Marginal cross-protection with rabies vaccines.
Mokola virus	Unknown but probably an insectivore or a rodent. Cases identified in Nigeria, South Africa, Cameroon, Zimbabwe, Central African Republic, and Ethiopia. Spillover infection to domestic animals and at least 2 humans.	First isolated from *Crocidura* shrews trapped near Ibadan, Nigeria, in 1968. Like Lagos bat virus, not characterized until 1970, when evidence of infection was appreciated only by poor reaction with antirabies diagnostic reagents. No known cross-protection with currently licensed rabies vaccines.
Duvenhage virus	Unknown but probably insectivorous bats. Cases identified in South Africa, Zimbabwe, and Senegal. No cases in domestic animals, but 1 human fatality.	First identified in 1970 in a man bitten by a bat in South Africa. Negri bodies detected, but immunofluorescence tests led to suspicion of "rabies-related" virus, confirmed by antigenic typing. Marginal vaccine cross-protection.
European bat virus 1 (EBVI)	European insectivorous bats (probably *Eptesicus serotinus*). One confirmed human case in 1985. No known domestic animal cases.	Although suggested as early as 1954, firm identification not attempted until 1985, with >400 bat cases identified to date. Marginal cross-protection with rabies vaccines.
European bat virus 2 (EBV2)	European insectivorous bats (probably *Myotis dasycneme*). At least 1 human death, but no known domestic animal cases.	Isolated from a Swiss bat biologist who died in Finland in 1985. Limited surveillance suggests that it is less common than EBV1. Marginal cross-protection with rabies vaccines.
Australian bat virus	Probably Australian fruit and insectivorous bats. At least 1 human death, but no known domestic animal cases documented to date.	Identified from a black flying fox (*Pteropus alecto*) in 1996 from New South Wales. Limited surveillance suggests that the virus is more widespread. Cross-protection with rabies vaccines.

unexpected manners. Moreover, the discovery of an apparently new lyssavirus in Australia,[23] a continent previously believed to be free of these agents, has increased concern over the true significance of nonrabies lyssaviruses.

Australian investigations of an unrelated zoonotic agent, equine morbillivirus (EMV),[35] implicated native pteropid bats as a potential reservoir of EMV and stimulated further studies to delineate the role of Megachiroptera in this emerging infectious disease. Surveillance for EMV unexpectedly uncovered an ill bat suffering from a nonsuppurative encephalitis, with rabies virus–like inclusions in the central nervous system (CNS). The index case was a flying fox obtained in May 1996 in New South Wales, although earlier cases dated back to at least 1995, according to retrospective inquiries. At least 40 isolates have already been obtained among fruit and insectivorous bat species, from Darwin to Melbourne. One human case has also been reported.[1] A 39-year-old woman from Rockhampton became ill in October 1996, was hospitalized, required ventilatory support, became comatose, and died several days later. The patient was a wildlife caretaker who had been exposed to a number of bats and terrestrial mammals, but no definitive source could be confirmed. The broad distribution and species involvement suggest that this virus is established as an indigenous agent, rather than reflective of a recent outbreak.

Initial reports of this rabies-like illness associated with Australian Megachiroptera in the spring of 1996 prompted a collaborative investigation[47] with the Australian Animal Health Laboratory. Mouse brain passaged material originating from an infected black flying fox (*Pteropus alecto*) was obtained for a number of virologic comparisons. The tentatively entitled pteropid bat virus (PBV) isolate produced typical signs of acute encephalitis within 2 to 3 weeks of inoculation of laboratory rodents. The PBV antigens in cell culture and rodent brain tissues cross-reacted with commercial reagents commonly used for routine rabies virus diagnosis. Both immunofluorescent and immunohistochemical assays detected typical inclusions in fixed animal brain tissue. Sequence and Mab analysis indicated that the PBV had taxonomic affinities to the genus *Lyssavirus*. Although this PBV appeared unique in comparison with all other lyssaviruses examined, it more closely resembled the type species of the genus, rabies virus, than all previously characterized agents. Human rabies immunoglobulin neutralized the PBV at levels comparable with that observed for rabies virus, and human sera from individuals immunized with licensed human rabies vaccines neutralized the PBV to a similar extent as rabies virus; it did not have the same effect on a distantly related lyssavirus, Mokola. Similarly, laboratory rodents immunized with rabies vaccines were completely protected against challenge with the PBV, but not with Mokola virus. These preliminary data suggest that current diagnostic reagents will detect infection and that rabies vaccines may offer protection against this new lyssavirus, whose larger public health role, veterinary significance, and geographic distribution remain to be determined. This discovery adds yet another pressure on bat populations already in global decline and region-ally part of the diets of many indigenous Pacific human populations.

A PRIMER OF BASIC PATHOGENESIS

No major changes have occurred in the basic understanding of the classical schema of rabies virus pathogenesis[14] since the 1970s. The disease is caused by entry of virus into a wound, usually inflicted by the bite of a rabid animal and only infrequently by a scratch or through mucosal exposure (e.g., licking, ingestion). Aerosolization has resulted in infection only under unique environmental circumstances. Viremia is unimportant, as is any consideration of invertebrate vectors. Viral reproduction is believed similar to that of other negative-stranded RNA viruses. Attachment to cell membranes is thought to occur through a conformational change in the G protein and receptor-mediated fusion (putatively thought to be related to acetylcholine[3] or other protein-based receptors).

After adsorption, virions penetrate the cell cytoplasm within vesicles, fuse with lysosomes, uncoat, and initiate primary transcription, protein synthesis, and replication of genomic RNA. Viral assembly of individual components, and virion budding from the infected cell surface, may occur by an inverse process of initial attachment. Virus may replicate locally in muscle tissue, but such activity is not an absolute pathogenetic requirement before direct nervous system infection.[48] Centripetal spread of virus occurs within the axoplasm of motor and sensory nerves. Incubation periods can vary from days to years[51] but are usually less than 3 months. Despite intense study, the precise location, capacity, and mechanism by which lyssaviruses can exist during prolonged incubation periods are unresolved. No reliable antemortem method is available to diagnose rabies during the incubation period, before clinical signs. Once the CNS is infected, rapid centrifugal viral dissemination occurs along neuronal pathways to a variety of organs, but urine, feces, most glandular secretions, and reproductive fluids are not generally regarded as infectious. Transplacental transmission has been documented on only very rare occasions. Salivary glands are primary exit portals of infectious virus for transmission.

Host response to infection may include both nonspecific inflammatory and specific immune mechanisms. However, much of what is suspected to occur in vivo is a broad extrapolation from experimental rodent models and fixed rabies viruses or human rabies cases. Exposure may or may not lead to infection, production of viral progeny, and detectable immune responses. Rabies virus neutralizing antibodies (VNA) may be detected at illness onset, but usually do not occur until late in the disease. Rabies VNA in the cerebrospinal fluid (CSF) are usually a reliable indication of infection but also may not be detectable. The nature of immune responses to infection may be unpredictable: either detrimental or protective.[14] For example, administration of rabies immunoglobulin alone immediately after rabies exposure may actually prolong the incubation period, as may immunosuppression. In contrast, vaccination alone during the incubation period may produce an "early death" phenomenon, in which vaccinated animals die earlier than nonvaccinated animals. Postexposure administration of both immunoglobulin and vaccine[9] is usually completely protective. Nevertheless, no administration of any biologic agents is therapeutic when administered after onset.

Diagnosis is a conundrum for the practitioner because the initial clinical signs of rabies, such as fever, malaise, and inappetence, are subtle and nonspecific. No unique syndromes have been documented for zoo mammals in comparison with domestic counterparts. Paresthesia may occur at the presumed entry of virus. During the acute neurologic phase in humans, hydrophobia (contractions of throat muscles after attempts to swallow water) may occur but has not been described in other animals. Paresis may begin in the bitten limb and progresses to complete flaccid paralysis. Either "furious" or "dumb" rabies may occur. Death usually results from cardiac or respiratory failure. Although rabies is considered invariably fatal, recovery, usually with severe neurologic sequelae, has been documented, albeit infrequently.

Despite hyperacute onset, dramatic behavioral alterations, and an extremely high rate of fatality, pathologic alterations are relatively mild.[14] Typically, gross lesions are lacking, other than minor cerebral edema and meningeal congestion. Microscopically, inflammatory CNS infiltration, consisting mostly of mononuclear cells, may be present. Perivascular cuffing, neuronophagia, and neuronal necrosis are modest in comparison to extensive viral antigen distribution. Likewise, microscopic identification of the eosinophilic intracytoplasmic pathognomic viral inclusions (Negri bodies) in Purkinje and pyramidal cells (less often in basal and peripheral ganglia), typically detected in only 50% to 75% of specimens, do not reflect pathogen dissemination. Spongiform change, selectively affecting the neurophil and neuronal cell bodies of the thalamus and cerebral cortex, has also been documented but is generally inadequate as a primary explanation of mortality. Pathophysiologic dysfunction of critical neurologic activities, rather than conventional structural disruption, may be the ultimate explanation to apparent viral virulence.

THE EPIDEMIOLOGIC TRIAD REVISITED

Familiarity with the natural history of rabies in the United States[30] by region may allow zoo professionals the opportunity to make better management decisions concerning the prevention of this disease, which has not remained static because of changes in the agents, hosts, and their environmental interactions. Since the 19th century, the epizootiology of rabies in the United States has changed significantly. Currently, more than 90% of all reported animal rabies cases occur in wildlife. As an example of a recent peak, the 9495 animal rabies cases reported during 1993 were previously exceeded only in 1946, when the domestic dog was the major host.

The increase in wildlife rabies since 1950 is partially related to changes in human demographics, animal translocations, ecologic alterations, and viral adaptations.[45] Rabies epizootics tend to be characterized by compartmentalization of virus in a single major host.[52] Although other mammals may be infected through contact with these primary reservoirs, such cases are usually sporadic. Once viruses become established within a particular mammalian population, transmission events can perpetuate for centuries. For example, in the North American prairie region, skunks have long persisted as an important reservoir; rabies was so common in the late 19th century that canvas sheets were marketed with tents as protection for campers from nocturnal attacks by these "phobey cats." Historically, rabies has also been enzootic for decades in Arctic (*Alopex lagopus*) and red fox (*Vulpes vulpes*) populations of Alaska and New England, respectively, and in raccoon (*Procyon lotor*) populations of the southeastern states. The translocation of infected raccoons from the southeast to the mid-Atlantic region during the late 1970s led to an intensive rabies outbreak[44] that continues to the present but now stretches from Maine to Florida. Similar concerns attend the potential spread of a newly recognized outbreak among coyotes in south Texas,[18] where the virus was previously enzootic among unvaccinated free-ranging dogs. Translocation[11, 20, 37] of infected coyotes from this Texas nidus might have devastating consequences, akin to that observed in the raccoon rabies epizootic.

From these few examples emerges a basic understanding that rabies is a disease composite among certain hosts with enhanced vagility and that viral spillover to the other mammalian species that they encounter (including domestic animals and humans) is only incidental. Mammals may serve as both reservoirs and vectors that perpetuate the disease, such as bats, dogs, foxes, raccoons, skunks and other mustelids, mongooses and other viverrids, and so forth, or as significant vectors but nonreservoirs. Some carnivores[15, 29, 30, 38, 49, 54, 56] such as wolves, wild dogs, jackals, bears, and pinnipeds fit this latter category, wherein rabies originates from vulpine or domestic canine sources, rather than from unique variants. Similarly, although cases of rabies have been reported among a variety of felids[5, 7, 24, 30, 53]—including lions, tigers, leopards, cheetahs, pumas, bobcats, ocelots, and domestic cats—and although these animals are very effective disease vectors, they are not regarded as reservoirs per se; rather, the disease originates as spillover cases. Last, there is a rabies category of mammalian "victim," in which animals die of overt trauma without the usual opportunity for secondary case development. Notable examples[16, 25, 30, 33, 36, 39, 53] are marsupials, primates, insectivores, rodents, lagomorphs, and ungulates. However, even presumed "victim" species may be substantially involved on occasion, as documented by the thousands of rabies deaths witnessed among kudu, presumably from peculiar animal-to-animal transmission in South Africa.[27, 53]

The epizootiology of rabies is complex in part because of the preservation of mammalian biodiversity.[55] When viral populations are sequestered in such hosts, accumulated mutations create distinctive variants that can be identified by molecular techniques. Antigenic and genetic analysis has identified a great biodiversity of rabies viral variants, each associated with a particular host; in mammalian carnivores, these have relatively discrete geographic boundaries that can be displayed on surveillance maps.[30]

Although the relative risk of rabies acquisition is substantially lower for zoos located outside of major raccoon, skunk, fox, dog, and coyote epizootic areas, the probability is not zero (except in rabies-free areas). Overlaying the disease in terrestrial mammals are multiple, independent cycles among insectivorous bats, also with distinct viral variants; however, specific geographic boundaries cannot be easily defined for bat rabies.[30, 50, 52] Variants associated with particular bat species can be found throughout a migratory range, which may extend over large areas. For example, rabies virus of freetail bats (*Tadarida brasiliensis*) shows minimal sequence variation in samples collected in Florida, Alabama, Texas, New Mexico, Nevada, Colorado, and California. Similarly, samples from the silver-haired bat (*Lasionycteris noctivagans*) in New York, Wisconsin, Washington, Colorado, and California are all nearly identical. Except for Hawaii, all areas of the United States represent a mosaic of different bat species affected by rabies, each transmitting distinct variants. In comparison with that of terrestrial carnivores, the epizootiology of bat rabies is poorly understood. Since the index bat rabies report in 1953, 600 to 1000 cases have been reported annually in the United States. Of bats submitted to diagnostic laboratories, typically only 5% to 15% are rabid. In addition, the occurrence of bat rabies appears largely independent of rabies in terrestrial carnivores, although viral spillover to animals besides bats does occur occasionally. Several features of bat rabies are unique, and the disease accounts for an increasing proportion of rabies virus transmitted to people.

Information gathered from rabies deaths in humans[46] may have some relevance to the zoo environment. Although rabies in humans is rare in the United States, it is also underdiagnosed. Annual human fatalities decreased from more than 100 cases at the end of the 19th century to only 1 to 2 in the 1970s. In the 1940s to 1950s, most cases in humans resulted from the bite of a rabid dog, whereas from 1980 to 1996, 17 of the 32 cases of rabies diagnosed in humans in the United States resulted from infection with rabies virus variants associated with bats. Only 1 of these 17 human rabies cases had a clear history of exposure from bat bite, although many patients had presumed bat contact. Moreover, in 12 of the 17 bat-associated human cases, the variant identified was associated with the silver-haired bat (*L. noctivagans*), a solitary, migratory species, uncommonly submitted for rabies diagnosis, having a preferred habitat of old-growth forest. These human patients may not have been aware of the risk associated with bat bite or may not have realized they had been bitten by bats, in which even apparently limited contact may result in transmission.

For example, in 1995, a bat killed in a child's room was later retrieved and was found to have been rabid, but only after the patient had become moribund. The child was asleep when the bat was found, but no bite was evident. Some bat rabies virus variants may possess

biologic characteristics[34] that support infectious transmission, even with minimal bites. Documentation of conventional bite exposures leading to bat-transmitted rabies may be hampered by the limited injury inflicted by a bat bite, in comparison with lesions inflicted by carnivores, or by circumstances that hinder accurate recall. Therefore, human rabies postexposure prophylaxis may be appropriate in situations in which there is reasonable probability that a bite or scratch occurred, such as when a sleeping individual awakes to find a bat in the room, or if an adult witnesses a bat with a previously unattended child, even in the absence of demonstrable contact.

The information from such "cryptic" human rabies deaths may have application in the rare instances of rabid zoo animals in non-enzootic rabies areas, in which bat contact would be difficult to rule out. Such unexpected rabies cases should be submitted for typing of the isolate in question for potential association as to suspected viral origin.

TO VACCINATE, OR NOT?

The issue of rabies vaccination of exotic captive mammals is somewhat controversial. Although rabies vaccines are not specifically approved for use in any wild or exotic animals,[12] and although there have been no definitive studies to demonstrate efficacy in these animals in the prescribed manner for which rabies vaccines are licensed for domestic animals in the United States, decisions based on reasonable expectations may be warranted. Within the context of doing no harm, vaccination of zoo mammals may thereby be considered the discretionary use of a biologic agent by a veterinarian. Zoos or research institutions may wish to establish vaccination programs in an attempt to protect various stock. However, such activities do not always augment the practice of public health.[9]

Several fundamental developments have occurred since Pasteur's epic vaccination of Joseph Meister. During the 20th century, the overall quality of veterinary vaccines changed considerably, and since the early 1980s, technical improvements in vaccine production have resulted in highly potent, economic, adjuvanted cell culture rabies vaccines for domestic animals; these vaccines have gradually dominated the market because of their safety and efficacy.[6, 40] More recent focus has been on the production of vaccines varying by substrate, virus strain, concentration process, inactivation method, adjuvant type, and storage phase. Currently, these vaccines encompass more than 28 different products in the United States alone.[12] In addition, rabies viral genes have been experimentally expressed in a number of prokaryotic and eukaryotic systems for vaccination of many species.[26, 42, 43]

Nevertheless, will current biologic agents be used to successfully vaccinate typical zoo species? Much has to be extrapolated from domestic animals. In regard to vaccine efficacy, to achieve licensure for use in small carnivores, such as dogs or cats, a rabies vaccine must protect 85% or more of test animals against severe laboratory rabies challenge in which at least 80% of unvaccinated controls die. For many licensed rabies vaccines, the minimum duration of immunity has been extended from 1 to at least 3 years[12]; data indicate that animals younger than 3 months of age may be protected, even in the presence of apparent interference from maternal immunity.[13] Of course, rabies vaccination by itself is not 100% effective. Between 9% and 14% of rabid dogs diagnosed in the United States during 1971–1973, 1980–1983, and 1988 were reportedly previously vaccinated.[19, 22] Closer examination of the 1988 rabies surveillance data revealed that of the rabid dogs with any history of vaccination during their lifetime, all but one had an expired vaccination. The sole dog with a current vaccination had received only a single dose of vaccine, between 3 and 6 months of age. Thus, no dogs had a current vaccination and a history of more than a single vaccination in their lifetime, which should be remembered in the coherent design of zoo rabies vaccination programs.

Failure rates of rabies vaccination in the United States, even under field conditions, are demonstrably low, substantiating the importance of subsequent vaccinations. Besides noncompliance with revaccination, rabies vaccines may be rendered impotent if they are stored inappropriately, administered improperly, or if the recipient responds in a rare, unpredictable manner (e.g., as a result of underlying immunosuppression).[26] These scenarios are not expected with healthy, well-supervised, vaccinated zoo stock. In practice, documented rabies vaccine failures are uncommon, usually occurring in a young animal with only a single immunization, often with no follow-up of a recommended booster after known exposure. A rabid young wolf hybrid,[28] likely infected by a skunk approximately 6 months after primary rabies vaccination, does not necessarily signify the failure of rabies immunization in an exotic animal; rather, this scenario underscores the recommendation for an immediate vaccine booster administration after any suspected rabies exposure in a currently vaccinated animal and does not extend to animals exposed before vaccination under viral incubation. An animal that has received a minimum of two prior vaccinations and a booster after any known viral exposure is presumably very well protected. It is unlikely for a vaccinated animal to die of anything but an extreme challenge under field conditions, such as multiple, severe bites to the head. This scenario is unlikely in most zoos, but not impossible, especially in some safari-parks, where lesions of unknown origin, if noticed, could result from animal bites.

By removal of strays and application of herd immunity through mass vaccination, dog rabies has been nearly eliminated in the United States, from the more than 9000 cases at the beginning of the 20th century, when the majority of rabid dogs in the United States were not vaccinated and were poorly supervised, to only 146 by 1995. Not only is canine rabies in the United States relatively rare and sporadic among an estimated population of more than 50 million domestic dogs, but it is also geographically restricted, in that the majority of cases originate from a rather small area at the Texas-Mexico border.[30] At least 25 states and the District of Columbia did not report any rabid dogs during 1995. Thus vaccination is effective not only in the individual but in the population.

The specific nature of the disease is also an issue for the consideration of relative risk in zoo mammals. Because rabies viruses appear compartmentalized to various mammalian reservoirs in different geographic areas,[30] the epidemiologic risks are not equal. Although in theory all mammals may be basically susceptible to different rabies viruses, in practice it is quite unusual to find viruses freely circulating in a host to which they are not well adapted. For example, it is unusual to detect bat rabies virus in a skunk or fox rabies virus in a raccoon, because the opportunity for viral shedding in the saliva of an infected animal and serial transmission to another are usually reduced for variants not adapted to that primary host.[14, 55] Ultimate explanations may rest at the level of specific cell receptors, required biochemical milieu to support viral replication, or other factors that differ between mammalian species and the peculiar requirements needed for optimal viral variant propagation.[3] Inequities in relative susceptibility of different hosts to diverse variants may exist.

These facets appear to present a particularly poor opportunity for primary infection of a vaccinated zoo mammal with a nonadapted rabies variant that would subsequently result in the transmission and perpetuation of a rabies outbreak. Although wildlife rabies may be relatively common in regard to its distribution and abundance in the United States, the comparative risk for its establishment through transmission among exotic animals is not expected to be epidemiologically equivalent, for example, to that in areas where dog rabies is endemic and control programs for dogs are poorly maintained.

Features related to animal husbandry and veterinary care also alter exposure and relative susceptibility to rabies. In most cases, rabies occurs in unvaccinated, free-ranging animals that are usually exposed to a conspecific. Zoo mammals are in several ways different from the general wildlife population at large. The number of such animals is far lower than those of indigenous wildlife and domestic species. Routine care, conditioning, and handling ensure that the animal is healthier and more tractable than the average wild or feral counterpart. Supervised veterinary care assists in the promotion and selection of extremely healthy animals before release from quarantine. Because immune responsiveness to rabies vaccines appears to have an underlying genetic component, the likelihood of a "nonresponder" species or individual should be greatly reduced, inasmuch as the animal otherwise would have been likely to acquire a number of chronic or debilitating illnesses that would limit its success as a profitable zoo candidate for exhibition, research, or propagation.

Behavior of infected animals should be such that acute personality changes or paralysis from rabies would likely be detected, in view of the extent of husbandry and observation. Rabies in a properly vaccinated zoo mammal would be an extremely unlikely event (as indicated by current rabies surveillance) because zoo mammals are strong candidates for responding to immunization with a potent rabies vaccine and, if infected with rabies, should be discovered readily under daily scrutiny. In general, because rabies is rare in well-supervised vaccinated animals, such zoo mammals by definition would be at a much smaller risk of infection than would the population of that species at large.

Use of a rabies vaccine with a 3-year duration of immunity should probably be encouraged because of its potency. The probability of an ideal immune response should increase with subsequent vaccinations, as should comparative protection against rabies. For example, in a review of approximately 200 reports of rabid dogs in Texas[19] (an area of historical risk because of foci of freely circulating canid-adapted viruses) during 1991–1994, five cases of vaccination failures were discovered, of which only a single dog had received at least two vaccinations with a product having a recommended booster interval of 3 years.

Antibody responses after rabies vaccination usually peak within 4 to 6 weeks. In the remote instance that a zoo mammal was incubating rabies, vaccination may increase the likelihood for a shorter, more acute "early death" period. Conversely, in a naive unvaccinated animal, incubation periods may extend 6 months or more. For example, of five dogs in Texas vaccinated during incubation, all died of rabies within 23 days.[19]

Should VNA titers be determined in zoo species? "Protective titers" cannot be defined and a diagnostic function cannot be attributed to rabies serologic activity in vaccinated animals. Serologic study may be useful in antemortem diagnosis, but only in nonvaccinated animals. In a nonvaccinated animal, a rise in antibody titer in serial serum samples is indicative of infection. Most vaccinated zoo mammals would have pre-existing antibody and should respond to booster vaccination with a rise in titer. Serologic tests cannot easily differentiate between anamnestic responses of a vaccinated animal and primary responses of an infected animal, and antibody titers alone do not indicate protection against rabies. The presence of VNA is only one aspect of the immune response in a vaccinated animal. Despite strong evidence that VNA after vaccination indicates an effective immunization and a lessened chance of infection, antibody alone is not solely protective; otherwise post-exposure management of previously vaccinated animals would depend only on their absolute titer. In many vaccine trials, antibody-negative animals also withstand challenge, and some antibody-positive animals die.[41, 43] Licensed rabies biologic agents will probably elicit antibody responses in properly vaccinated, immunocompetent zoo animals and should at a minimum protect a majority of animals against a severe challenge with rabies virus.

Routine serologic testing for rabies antibody does not appear necessary for properly vaccinated zoo mammals. There is no compelling reason for it for clinical management, beyond academic interest. Serologic testing is a method of demonstrating that an animal is responding immunologically to a foreign substance, such as the complex proteins in a rabies vaccine. Detection of antibody responses after potent rabies vaccination is highly predictable. For example, examination of sera from 1265 domestic animals vaccinated under laboratory conditions with rabies vaccines intended for

licensure demonstrated that in approximately 96% of animals, a titer developed.[6] These laboratory data are supported by observations from the field. In the Philippines,[8] after four different types of commercial inactivated rabies vaccine were used, more than 80% of dogs examined 6 months after vaccination had VNA (ranging as high as 93% for one product); in Peru,[17] approximately 97% of randomly selected dogs, vaccinated with a single, commercial adjuvanted inactivated product, maintained VNA 12 months after vaccination. In view of the rigors necessary for exhibition or research, it would be unusual for a zoo mammal to not respond with VNA to multiple vaccinations with current rabies vaccines, especially in comparison with domestic animals in developing countries that received only a single vaccination under less than ideal circumstances (e.g., questionable nutritional status, veterinary care).

Once a decision has been made to vaccinate, it is probably neither economically practical nor justified on public health grounds to vaccinate all zoo mammals; some, such as insectivores, bats, and rodents, may be maintained in indoor enclosures with little to no opportunity for exposure. However, vaccination may be considered for animals that are particularly rare, are valuable, or may have frequent potential contact with free-ranging reservoirs, especially in epizootic areas. If born at the zoo, all candidate mammals could be vaccinated against rabies at 3 months of age and revaccinated annually. Regardless of the age at initial vaccination and the use of either an annual or a triennial product, a second vaccination should be given at least 1 year later. If a previously vaccinated animal is overdue for a booster, it should be revaccinated with a single dose of vaccine and placed on an annual schedule, regardless of the type of vaccine originally used.

To ensure proper use of the biologic agents in exotic species, use of rabies vaccines should be restricted to a licensed veterinarian. In theory, vaccines with a 3-year duration of immunity could be applied annually. Regardless of product, all vaccines should be otherwise administered in accordance with the specifications of the product label or package insert (with recognition that the majority of zoo mammals will not be listed). If administered intramuscularly, the vaccine should be given in an area of muscle mass suitable to accommodate the volume and to avoid adipose tissue deposition, such as at a single site in the thigh. Accidental inoculation of personnel during administration of animal rabies vaccines constitutes no rabies hazard because all recommended biologic agents are inactivated.[12]

Clearly, modern cell culture vaccines are extremely potent. Results of comparative vaccination trials with a wide variety of taxonomically disparate species support the view that mammalian response to rabies vaccine is a conserved immunologic attribute. For example, current rabies products provide demonstrable efficacy for species in at least six mammalian families.[12] Use of such products already intended for domestic carnivores or hoofstock would follow by extrapolation. In addition, preliminary review of the serologic responses of a number of exotic species to rabies vaccination[42] does not reveal clear significant overall differences in comparison with domestic animals. These combined inferences suggest that zoo mammals should respond in an appropriate manner, as do their domestic relatives.

PUBLIC HEALTH CONCERNS AND MANAGEMENT

Rabies vaccination is not the sole issue related to the public health significance of zoo animals. At present, federal and state animal import regulations are generally considered insufficient to prevent the introduction of rabid animals.[39] Besides federal concerns, the conditional admission of any exotic animals may also be subject to state and local laws. At a minimum, all mammals imported from countries (see Table 20–1) with endemic rabies should be quarantined. Wildlife may be incubating rabies when initially captured; therefore, wild-caught mammals should be quarantined for a minimum of 180 days before exhibition.

Rabies in humans may be completely prevented either by eliminating all exposure to rabid animals or by providing exposed persons with local treatment of wounds, combined with appropriate passive and active immunization.[9] Employees who work directly with zoo mammals should consider pre-exposure rabies immunization. Pre-exposure immunization (Tables 20–3, 20–4) of employees may reduce the need for euthanasia of captive animals and greatly simplifies postexposure management of humans (Table 20–5). The rationale for recommending pre-exposure and postexposure rabies prophylaxis can be found in the recommendations of the Immunization Practices Advisory Committee.[9]

Obviously, zoo animals should be excluded from direct human contact, and the public should be warned not to handle zoo animals. Medicolegal consequences of a bite may be severe. "Do not touch/feed the animals" signs may be highlighted effectively if they also include a short, imaginative notice of the likelihood that zoo mammals that bite or otherwise expose people may be considered for euthanasia and rabies diagnosis. The educational value of any "hands on" experiences should be balanced with the need for personal protection (such as hand washing).

There are a variety of related issues when people are potentially exposed to rabies from nondomestic species. Bites of certain exotic carnivores, especially canids, often tend to be deep and multiple and frequently involve severe wounds to the head, lessening the chances for successful prophylaxis. Currently, a domestic dog, cat, or ferret involved in human exposure can be quarantined and observed over a 10-day period; if the animal remains healthy, rabies postexposure prophylaxis in humans may be avoided. However, in contrast to the experience with canine rabies, the subtle behavioral alterations and associated clinical manifestations indicative of viral encephalitis may not be as readily apparent in rabid exotic animals. Finally, there are no laboratory-based studies of the comparative pathogenesis and viral shedding periods in most zoo animals. Rabies pathogenesis, including viral excretion, may depend on the dose, the route and strain of virus, and the species of biting animal. Thus, because of the insubstantial epizootiologic, clinical, and pathogenetic information associated with rabies in exotic animals, public health officials have oftentimes maintained recommendations for euthanasia of such animals involved in human exposure, regardless of vaccination status.

A person bitten by any wild or exotic mammal should immediately report the incident to a physician, who can evaluate the need for prophylaxis, in consultation with local or state health authorities. Management depends partially on the animal species, the circumstances of the bite, the epidemiology of rabies in the area, the biting animal's history and current health status, and the potential for exposure to rabies. For particularly rare, endangered, or threatened species, euthanasia may not be mandatory, if the animal is completely healthy and the bite was provoked, such as may occur with zoo staff or with a public that continually finds novel ways to breach seemingly impenetrable barriers; if the animal has not been knowingly exposed to a potential rabies reservoir during the past 6 months; if local surveillance does not support a high potential for rabies occurrence; if the animal is currently vaccinated against rabies; or if the exposed person voluntarily elects rabies postexposure prophylaxis.

Captive zoo mammals not completely excluded from all contact with rabies vectors can become infected either by the bite or (rarely) the nonbite routes. From surveillance and experimental data, all species of mammal are believed to be susceptible; hence, any zoo mammal bitten or scratched by an animal known to be rabid or by a wild carnivore or a bat that is not available for testing should be regarded as having been exposed to rabies. Any unvaccinated zoo mammals exposed to rabies could be either euthanized immediately or provided any necessary wound care and placed in strict isolation for at least 6 months. This exposed individual may be vaccinated 1 month before being released from isolation. This is intended to produce a vaccinated animal at the end of the quarantine period and is not performed as a rationale for postexposure prophylaxis,

---

TABLE 20–3. Human Rabies Pre-Exposure Immunization

Pre-exposure immunization consists of three doses of human diploid cell vaccine (HDCV), purified chick embryo cell (PCEC) vaccine, or rabies vaccine adsorbed (RVA), 1.0 ml, IM (i.e., deltoid area), one each on days 0, 7, and 21 or 28.

ONLY HDCV may be administered by the intradermal (ID) route (0.1 ml ID on days 0, 7, and 21 or 28).

If an individual will be taking chloroquine or mefloquine for malaria chemoprophylaxis, a three-dose rabies vaccination series should be completed before initiation of antimalarials. If this is not possible, the IM dose/route should be used. Administration of routine booster doses of vaccine depends on relative exposure risk category.

IM, intramuscular.

Adapted from ACIP: Rabies prevention—United States, 1991. Recommendations of the Immunization Practices Advisory Committee (ACIP). MMWR 40 (RR-3):1–19, 1991.

TABLE 20–4. Human Rabies Risk Categories: Criteria for Pre-Exposure Immunization

Exposure Category	Nature of Risk	Typical Populations	Pre-Exposure Regimen
Continuous	Virus present continuously, often in high concentrations. Aerosol, mucous membrane, bite, or nonbite exposure possible. Specific exposures may go unrecognized.	Rabies research laboratory workers.* Rabies biologics production workers.	Primary pre-exposure immunization course. Serology every 6 months. Booster immunization when antibody titer falls below acceptable level.*
Frequent	Exposure usually episodic with source recognized, but exposure may also be unrecognized. Aerosol, mucous membrane, bite, or nonbite exposure.	Rabies diagnostic laboratory workers,* spelunkers, veterinarians, and animal control and wildlife workers in rabies-epizootic areas. Certain travelers to foreign rabies-epizootic areas.	Primary pre-exposure immunization course. Serologic study or booster immunization every 2 years.
Infrequent (greater than population at large)	Exposure nearly always episodic with source recognized. Mucous membrane, bite, or nonbite exposure.	Veterinarians and animal control and wildlife workers in areas of low rabies endemicity. Veterinary students.	Primary pre-exposure immunization course. No routine booster immunization or serologic study.
Rare (population at large)	Exposure always episodic. Mucous membrane or bite exposure with source recognized.	U.S. population at large, including individuals in rabies-epizootic areas.	No pre-exposure immunization.

*Judgment of relative risk and extra monitoring of immunization status of workers is the responsibility of the supervisor (see U.S. Department of Health and Human Service's Biosafety in Microbiological and Biomedical Laboratories, 1993). Acceptable antibody level is a 1:5 titer (complete inhibition in RFFIT at 1:5 dilution). Boost if titer falls below 1:5.

Adapted from ACIP: Rabies prevention—United States, 1991. Recommendations of the Immunization Practices Advisory Committee (ACIP). MMWR 40 (RR-3):1–19, 1991.

which, except for humans, is not routinely practiced in naive, exposed animals. Individually vaccinated zoo mammals with expired vaccinations need to be evaluated on a case-by-case basis with regard to postexposure management. It seems prudent that animals with current vaccinations be revaccinated immediately and observed for at least 90 days for any signs of associated illness.

During isolation, zoo animals should be observed closely and be evaluated by a veterinarian at the first sign of illness. Any rabies-like illness in the animal should be reported immediately to the local or state health department. If signs suggestive of rabies develop, the animal should be promptly euthanized and its head safely removed and shipped under refrigeration (not fixed or frozen) for examination by a qualified laboratory designated by the local or state health department. Depending on local diagnostic policies and the size of the species in question, officials should modify the precise necropsy and shipping plan accordingly. Neither tissues nor milk from a rabid or suspect rabid animal should be used for local zoo animal consumption. There should be few scenarios in which this would even be a consideration. However, because pasteurization and cooking temperatures normally inactivate rabies virus, the accidental consumption of pasteurized milk or properly cooked tissue by other animals does not usually constitute a rabies exposure.

Ideally, animals found in contact with a rabid or suspect rabid animal should also be regarded as having

been potentially exposed to rabies. However, this may be problematic, especially for multispecies or group housing enclosures. In practice, it is somewhat rare to have more than one rabid animal affected at a time from a point source or to likely observe herbivore-to-herbivore transmission; therefore, it may not be necessary to quarantine the rest of a collection in contact with a suspected carrier, unless they have evidence of concurrent exposure, such as lesions. Nevertheless, diligent observations for signs of rabies should be practiced over the next 6 months.

Can population management of noncaptive mammals be successfully utilized to further lessen the threat of rabies to a zoo? Control of rabies among wildlife and feral animals is difficult. Vaccination of free-ranging wildlife or selective population reduction may be useful in some situations, but success depends on local circumstances. Large-scale, persistent programs for trapping or poisoning wildlife alone are not economically justified in reducing wildlife rabies reservoirs.[21] However, limited short-term humane control, including the elimination of food and shelter resources, in well-defined high-contact areas (zoo picnic grounds, adjoining woodlots) may be indicated for the reduction in density of selected high-risk wildlife or stray domestic species, especially with an impending rabies outbreak. Any stray domestic animals that are trapped may be held for several days, to allow owners time to reclaim lost pets. Besides the removal of strays, oral vaccination

TABLE 20–5. Human Rabies Postexposure Immunization

First Aid
All postexposure prophylaxis should begin with immediate thorough cleansing of all wounds with soap and water.

Persons Not Previously Immunized
Human rabies immune globulin (HRIG), 20 IU/kg body weight, one half infiltrated at bite site (if possible), remainder IM; five doses of HDCV, PCEC, or RVA, 1.0 ml IM (i.e., deltoid area), one each on days 0, 3, 7, 14, and 28.

Persons previously immunized:*
Two doses of HDCV, PCEC, or RVA, 1.0 ml, IM (i.e., deltoid area), one each on days 0 and 3, HRIG should not be administered.

---

*Criteria include pre-exposure immunization with HDCV, PCEC, or RVA; prior postexposure prophylaxis with HDCV or RVA; previous immunization with any other type of rabies vaccine (either pre- or postexposure) and a documented history of a positive antibody response to the prior vaccination.

Adapted from ACIP: Rabies prevention—United States, 1991. Recommendations of the Immunization Practices Advisory Committee (ACIP). MMWR 40 (RR-3):1–19, 1991.

of free-ranging wild carnivores[2, 4, 45] is another strategy that may be considered in a balanced rabies prevention plan. Knowledgeable federal, state, and local wildlife, agricultural, and health agencies should be consulted for coordination of any proposed vaccination or population reduction programs.

It is not feasible or desirable to control bat rabies by reduction of local bat populations. Often this leads to a greater public health problem by the presence of dead and dying bats, which may increase the potential for human and animal exposures. Alternatively, bats may be excluded from animal enclosures and surrounding structures to prevent direct association. Such structures could then be made bat-proof by sealing entrances used by bats, at a time when bats and their offspring may be absent.

Issues related to most zoonoses, such as rabies, are contentious and emotionally charged. Officials must deliberate the consequences of euthanizing valuable animals against the risks inherent with an invariably fatal illness. Advanced comprehensive development of objective disease prevention and management plans, reflective of public health priorities and conservation needs, may minimize reactive policies and forestall a public relations nightmare[10] in the zoo environment.

REFERENCES

1. Allworth A, Murray K, Morgan J: A human case of encephalitis due to a lyssavirus recently identified in fruit bats. Comm Dis Intell 20:504, 1996.
2. Aubert MF, Masson E, Artois M, et al: Oral wildlife rabies vaccination field trials in Europe, with recent emphasis on France. *In* Rupprecht CE, Dietzschold B, Koprowski H (eds): Lyssaviruses. New York, Springer-Verlag, pp 219–243, 1994.
3. Baer G, Shaddock J, Quirion R, et al: Rabies susceptibility and acetylcholine receptor. Lancet 335:664–665, 1990.
4. Baer GM: Oral rabies vaccination: an overview. Rev Infect Dis 10(Suppl 4):S644–S648, 1988.
5. Berry H: Surveillance and control of anthrax and rabies in wild herbivores and carnivores in Namibia. Rev Sci Tech 12:137–146, 1993.
6. Bunn T: Canine and feline vaccines, past and present. *In* Baer GM (ed): The Natural History of Rabies. Boca Raton, FL, CRC Press, pp 415–425, 1991.
7. Bwangamoi O, Rottcher D, Wekesa C: Rabies, microbesnoitiosis and sarcocystosis in a lion. Vet Rec 127:411, 1990.
8. Carlos ET: Control of rabies in the Philippines by canine vaccination. Proceedings: Symposium on Rabies Control in Asia, Jakarta, Indonesia, Fondation Marcel Merieux, pp 139–156, 1993.
9. Centers for Disease Control and Prevention: Rabies Prevention—United States, 1991. Recommendations of the Immunization Practices Advisory Committee (ACIP). MMWR 40(RR–3):1–19, 1991.
10. Centers for Disease Control and Prevention: Mass treatment of humans exposed to rabies—New Hampshire, 1994. MMWR 44:484–486, 1995.
11. Centers for Disease Control and Prevention: Translocation of coyote rabies—Florida, 1994. MMWR 44:580–581, 587, 1995.
12. Centers for Disease Control and Prevention: Compendium of animal rabies control, 1997. MMWR 46(RR–4):1–9, 1997.
13. Chappuis G: Development of rabies vaccines. *In* Beyon PH, Edney ATB (eds): Rabies in a changing world. London, British Small Animal Veterinary Association, pp 49–59, 1995.
14. Charlton KM: The pathogenesis of rabies and other lyssaviral infections: recent studies. *In* Rupprecht CE, Dietzschold B, Koprowski H (eds): Current Topics in Microbiology and Immunology, vol 187. New York, Springer-Verlag, pp 95–120, 1994.
15. Cherkasskiy B: Roles of the wolf and the raccoon dog in the ecology and epidemiology of rabies in the USSR. Rev Infect Dis 10(Suppl 4):S634–S636, 1988.
16. Childs JE, Colby L, Krebs JW, et al: Surveillance and spatiotemporal associations of rabies in rodents and lagomorphs in the United States, 1990–1994. J Wildl Dis 33:20–27, 1997.
17. Chomel B, Chappuis G, Bullon F, et al: Mass vaccination campaign against rabies: are dogs correctly protected? the Peruvian experience. Rev Infect Dis 10(Suppl 4):S697–S702, 1988.
18. Clark KA, Neill SU, Smith JS, et al: Epizootic canine rabies transmitted by coyotes in south Texas. J Am Vet Med Assoc 204:536–540, 1994.
19. Clark KA, Wilson PJ: Postexposure rabies prophylaxis and preexposure rabies vaccination failure in domestic animals. J Am Vet Med Assoc 208:1827–1830, 1996.
20. Davidson WR, Appel MJ, Doster GL, et al: Diseases and parasites of red foxes, gray foxes, and coyotes from commercial sources selling to fox-chasing enclosures. J Wildl Dis 28:581–589, 1992.
21. Debbie JG: Rabies control of terrestrial wildlife by population reduction. *In* Baer GM (ed): The Natural History of Rabies, 2nd ed. Boca Raton, FL, CRC Press, pp 477–484, 1991.
22. Eng TR, Fishbein DB: Epidemiologic factors, clinical findings, and vaccination status of rabies in cats and dogs in the United States in 1988. J Am Vet Med Assoc 197:201–209, 1990.
23. Fraser GC, Hooper PT, Lunt RA, et al: Encephalitis caused by a lyssavirus in fruit bats in Australia. Emerg Infect Dis 2:327–331, 1996.
24. Frye FL, Cucuel JP: Rabies in an ocelot. J Am Vet Med Assoc 153:789–790, 1968.
25. Gopal T, Rao BU: Rabies in an Indian wild elephant calf. Indian Vet J 61:82–83, 1984.
26. Hanlon CA, Niezgoda M, Shankar V, et al: A recombinant vaccinia-rabies virus in the immunocompromised host: oral innocuity, progressive parenteral infection, and therapeutics. Vaccine 15:140–148, 1997.
27. Hubschle O: Rabies in the kudu antelope (*Tragelaphus strepsiceros*). Rev Infect Dis 10(Suppl 4):S629–S633, 1988.
28. Jay MT, Reilly KF, Debess EE, et al: Rabies in a vaccinated wolf-dog hybrid. J Am Vet Med Assoc 205:1729–1732, 1719, 1994.
29. Kat PW, Alexander KA, Smith JS, et al: Rabies and African wild dogs in Kenya. Proc R Soc Lond B Biol Sci 262:229–233, 1995.
30. Krebs JW, Strine TW, Smith JS, et al: Rabies surveillance in the United States during 1995. J Am Vet Med Assoc 209:2031–2044, 1996.
31. Leffingwell LM, Neill S: Naturally acquired rabies in an armadillo (*Dasypus novemcinctus*) in Texas. J Clin Microbiol 27:174–175, 1989.
32. Meslin F-X, Fishbein DB, Matter HC: Rationale and prospects for rabies elimination in developing countries. *In* Rupprecht CE, Dietzschold B, Koprowski H (eds): Current Topics in Microbiology

and Immunology, vol 187. New York, Springer-Verlag, pp 1–26, 1994.

33. Miot MR, Sikes RK, Silberman MS: Rabies in a chimpanzee. J Am Vet Med Assoc 162:54, 1973.

34. Morimoto K, Patel M, Corisdeo S, et al: Characterization of a unique variant of bat rabies responsible for newly emerging human cases in North America. Proc Natl Acad Sci USA 93:5653–5658, 1996.

35. Murray K, Rogers R, Selvay L, et al: A novel morbillivirus pneumonia of horses and its transmission to humans. Emerg Infect Dis 1:31–33, 1995.

36. Nair S, Dighe P, Nanavati A: Role of bandicoots in rabies transmission. Indian J Med Res 67:347–353, 1978.

37. Nettles VF, Shaddock JH, Sikes RK, et al: Rabies in translocated raccoons. Am J Publ Health 69:170–179, 1979.

38. Odegaard O, Krogsrud J: Rabies in Svalbard: infection diagnosed in arctic fox, reindeer and seal. Vet Rec 109:141–142, 1981.

39. Richardson J, Humphrey G: Rabies in imported nonhuman primates. Lab Animal Sci 21:1083, 1971.

40. Rupprecht CE, Charlton KM, Artois M, et al: Ineffectiveness and comparative pathogenicity of attenuated rabies virus vaccine for the striped skunk (*Mephitis mephitis*). J Wildl Dis 26:99–102, 1990.

41. Rupprecht CE, Dietzschold B: Perspectives on rabies virus pathogenesis. Lab Invest 57:603–606, 1987.

42. Rupprecht CE, Hanlon CA, Hamir A, et al: Oral wildlife rabies vaccination: development of a recombinant virus vaccine. Transactions of the 57th North American Wildlife and Natural Resources Conference, Washington, DC, Wildlife Management Institute, pp 439–452, 1992.

43. Rupprecht CE, Hanlon CA, Niezgoda M, et al: Recombinant rabies vaccines: efficacy assessment in free-ranging animals. Ondersterpoort J Vet Res 60:463–468, 1993.

44. Rupprecht CE, Smith JS: Raccoon rabies: the re-emergence of an epizootic in a densely populated area. Semin Virol 5:155–164, 1994.

45. Rupprecht CE, Smith JS, Fekadu M, et al: The ascension of wildlife rabies: a cause for public health concern or intervention? Emerg Infect Dis 1:107–114, 1995.

46. Rupprecht CE, Smith JS, Krebs J, et al: Current issues in rabies prevention in the United States: health dilemmas, public coffers, private interests. Publ Health Rep 111:400–407, 1996.

47. Rupprecht CE, Smith JS, Yager PA, et al: Preliminary analysis of a new lyssavirus isolated from an Australian fruit bat [Abstract]. 7th Annual International Meeting on Advances Towards Rabies Control in the Americas, Atlanta, GA, p 19, 1996.

48. Shankar V, Dietzschold B, Koprowski H: Direct entry of rabies virus into the central nervous system without prior local replication. J Virol 65:2736–2738, 1991.

49. Sillero-Zubiri C, King A, MacDonald D: Rabies and mortality in Ethiopian wolves (*Canis simensis*). J Wildl Dis 32:80–86, 1996.

50. Smith JS: New aspects of rabies with emphasis on epidemiology, diagnosis, and prevention of the disease in the United States. Clin Microbiol Rev 9:166–176, 1996.

51. Smith JS, Fishbein DB, Rupprecht CE, et al: Unexplained rabies in three immigrants in the United States. N Engl J Med 324:205–211, 1991.

52. Smith JS, Orciari LA, Yager PA: Molecular epidemiology of rabies in the United States. Semin Virol 6:387–400, 1995.

53. Swanepoel R, Barnard BJ, Meredith CD, et al: Rabies in southern Africa. Ondersterpoort J Vet Med 60:325–346, 1993.

54. Taylor M, Elkin B, Maier N, et al: Observation of a polar bear with rabies. J Wildl Dis 27:337–339, 1991.

55. Wandeler AI, Nadin-Davis SA, Tinline RR, et al: Rabies epidemiology: some ecological and evolutionary perspectives. *In* Rupprecht CE, Dietzschold B, Koprowski H (eds): Current Topics in Microbiology and Immunology, vol 187. New York, Springer-Verlag, pp 1–26, 1994.

56. Weiler G, Garner G, Ritter D: Occurrence of rabies in a wolf population in northeastern Alaska. J Wildl Dis 31:78–82, 1995.

CHAPTER **21**

Nontuberculous Mycobacteria: Potential for Zoonosis

NADINE LAMBERSKI

The prevalence of tuberculous and nontuberculous disease in the human population has been rising since 1985. This increase has been in association with the increase in human immunodeficiency virus (HIV) infections.[4] Of the 50 species of mycobacteria that have been identified, more than half of these species have caused disease in patients with acquired immunodeficiency syndrome (AIDS); however, many also have caused disease in immunocompetent persons.[4, 28]

Tuberculosis has long been recognized as a pathogen of both humans and animals. The disease is caused by infection with one of two mammalian tubercle bacilli: *Mycobacterium tuberculosis* or *Mycobacterium bovis*.

Tuberculosis is transmitted directly from host to host and is a zoonotic disease.[5, 14, 28, 29]

Although nontuberculous mycobacteria were first recognized in the late 1800s, these organisms were not reported as a cause of human disease until the mid-1950s.[34] Before 1980, infections from nontuberculous mycobacteria were infrequent and usually affected immunocompetent children in the form of chronic cervical lymphadenitis. Since then, nontuberculous mycobacteria have become a common cause of opportunistic infections in people with AIDS.[4] In fact, 45% of patients with advanced AIDS have concomitant systemic nontuberculous mycobacterial infections.[7] The number of nontuberculous mycobacteria isolates has been increasing, possibly as a result of heightened tuberculosis surveillance, increased numbers and survival time of immunocompromised patients, and improved microbiologic and molecular diagnostic methods.[30]

Mycobacterial disease caused by nontuberculous mycobacteria has been reported in mammals, birds, reptiles, amphibians, and fishes. Many of these infections have been reported in captive as well as free-ranging animals. Nontuberculous mycobacteria have also been isolated from animals without evidence of disease and are thought to colonize the respiratory tract and the gastrointestinal tract in various species.[28]

Nontuberculous mycobacteria are ubiquitous in the environment. Although many species could be considered potential pathogens, their presence in clinical samples does not always indicate disease. Disease development is related to species susceptibility, the immune status of the host, the numbers and virulence of the organism, and the route of exposure.[27]

MYCOBACTERIUM AVIUM COMPLEX (MAC)

The *Mycobacterium avium* complex (MAC) consists of slow-growing acid-fast bacilli composed of two major species: *Mycobacterium avium* and *Mycobacterium intracellulare*. MAC also is referred to as MAI (*Mycobacterium avium–intracellulare*), which emphasizes the difficulty in distinguishing between the two species.[9, 34] *Mycobacterium scrofulaceum* is similar to *M. avium* and *M. intracellalare*, and these three organisms in combination may be referred to as the MAIS complex.[34]

This group of nontuberculous mycobacteria has been further classified by seroagglutination, and many have been confirmed through the use of DNA probes. Serotypes 1 to 6, 8 to 11, and 21 represent *M. avium* strains; serotypes 7, 12 to 20, 23, and 25 are *M. intracellulare* strains; and serotypes 41 to 43 are *M. scrofulaceum*. Serotypes 24 and 26–28 are unresolved.[8, 31, 34] Serotypes 1, 4, and 8 are most frequently isolated from AIDS patients in the United States.[34] Serotypes 1, 2, 3, and 8 have been frequently isolated from birds, and serotypes 1, 2, 4, 8, and 23 have been isolated from mammals.[8, 13, 28, 31] MAC is an important pathogen in animals as well as in humans. Water has been identified as the source of human infection; however, the genetic diversity of *M. avium* strains recovered from AIDS patients and the presence of *M. avium* in animals and various environmental samples are suggestive of additional reservoirs.[1]

Strains of MAC have been associated with a variety of mycobacterial diseases in humans, including pulmonary disease, childhood lymphadenitis, and disseminated infection in patients who have AIDS. MAC is the most common disseminated bacterial infection in patients with AIDS in the United States, resulting in significant morbidity and mortality.[34] Patients with pulmonary disease from MAC usually have underlying chronic pulmonary disease such as chronic obstructive pulmonary disease, inactive or active tuberculosis, bronchiectasis, pneumoconiosis, chronic aspiration pneumonia, or bronchogenic carcinoma. However, in one report, pulmonary disease caused by MAC was documented in 21 patients with normal immune function in the absence of underlying disease. In this report, the majority of patients affected were elderly white women in good health whose illnesses were dominated by a productive cough with gradual radiographic progression of multiple small nodules. In seven patients, the pathogens were identified on the basis of recurrent positive acid-fast stains and cultures of sputum. Early specimens were thought to represent clinically unimportant colonization by nonpathogenic organisms. Four of the 21 patients died as a result of the disease.[24] MAC infections are difficult to treat, because strains of MAC tend to be resistant to most antituberculosis drugs.[34]

As for other species of nontuberculous mycobacteria, colonization of the respiratory tract by MAC can occur without causing invasive disease. These organisms may be found in patients with normal-appearing lungs, as well as in patients with pulmonary disease. Disease development is usually related to underlying lung abnormality.[28] Infection is distinguished from colonization on the basis of the persistence of symptoms and the repetitive isolation of the organism.

M. avium, first described in 1890 as a pathogen in chickens, has been reported as a naturally acquired infection in a variety of avian and mammalian species, including anseriforms, columbiforms, gallinaceous birds, gruiforms, passerines, psittacines, raptors, carnivores, marsupials, nonhuman primates, and ungulates.[8, 17, 31] Clinical signs usually include chronic wasting but vary in accordance with the species affected and the organ system involved, as well as with the extent and duration of infection.[31] Transmission occurs primarily through ingestion of contaminated feces or soil, but inhalation of the organism can also occur. In addition, cutaneous infections have been reported.[8, 31] In birds, the main portal of entry is the intestinal tract with colonization of the intestinal mucosa. Bacteremia can occur, and the lack of lymph nodes in birds facilitates the hematogenous spread within the host. In some avian species, lesions develop only in the lungs.[8] MAC is a major cause of death in captive marsupials, but this organism also has been isolated from individuals without evidence of infection. Clinical signs include weight loss, pneumonia, osteomyelitis, abscesses, and neurologic abnormalities.[3] The disease in nonhuman primates tends to cause chronic diarrhea and weight loss; however, the organism has also been isolated from clinically normal primates.[11, 17, 28]

MYCOBACTERIUM KANSASII

Other species of nontuberculous mycobacteria, such as *Mycobacterium kansasii*, can be pathogens under certain conditions. Disseminated *M. kansasii* infections usually occur in patients with advanced HIV infections.[21, 34] The high frequency of pulmonary symptoms in these cases suggest that the lung is the portal of entry for *M. kansasii*. This is in contrast to MAC, in which the gastrointestinal tract is the major site for dissemination. *M. kansasii* is not found in soil but is occasionally found in water samples.[34] A fatal *M. kansasii* infection involving the lymph nodes, liver, and lungs has been reported in a llama. Sporadic reports of infection of other ungulates exist in the literature.[15]

RAPIDLY GROWING MYCOBACTERIA

Rapidly growing mycobacteria (RGM) are often considered to be nonpathogenic commensal species. The first known case of lung disease caused by RGM was reported in 1933, and a small number of additional cases have been documented since then. According to a 1993 review of 154 cases of pulmonary disease caused by RGM, 21 of the patients died from progressive lung disease. Patients were predominantly nonsmoking, white females usually residing at some time in their life along the gulf or southern Atlantic coasts. Cough was the most common presenting sign, and the illness was slowly progressive. The most frequent underlying diseases include previous mycobacterial disease, cystic fibrosis, and gastroesophageal disorders with chronic vomiting. However, nearly one third of the patients had no underlying disorder. The majority of isolates were *Mycobacterium abscessus* (formerly called *M. chelonae* subspecies *abscessus*) and *Mycobacterium fortuitum*. The similarity of the clinical syndromes produced by MAC and RGM suggest a common pathogenicity or host susceptibility.[10]

M. chelonae, another species of rapidly growing mycobacteria that was originally isolated from a turtle, tends to be more drug resistant than *M. fortuitum*, although both organisms are resistant to many standard antituberculosis drugs. *M. fortuitum* is often isolated as a contaminant. Both organisms have produced injection site abscesses, infections of traumatic wounds, keratitis, sternal osteomyelitis after cardiac surgery, wound infection after silicone breast prostheses, catheter-related infections, disseminated and localized infections in dialysis patients, prosthetic valve endocarditis, and disseminated infections with skin lesions in immunocompromised hosts.[32, 34] Pyoderma caused by *M. chelonae* has been reported in a manatee, and pulmonary disease from *M. fortuitum* and *M. chelonae* has been reported in a grey seal.[33]

M. chelonae infection of soft tissue has been acquired from contact with a pet dog. It was not determined whether the haircoat was colonized with the mycobacteria or whether it served as a fomite for the transmission of the organism. *M. chelonae* is thought to be widely distributed in the environment, although no specific environmental reservoirs have been identified.[20]

FASTIDIOUS MYCOBACTERIA

The fastidious mycobacteria are slow-growing species of nontuberculous mycobacteria. Among these, *Mycobacterium genavense*, *Mycobacterium haemophilum*, and *Mycobacterium malmoense* have been described as clinically significant mycobacteria. The isolation of these organisms has been delayed because of their par-

ticular metabolic requirements. These mycobacteria are probably ubiquitous environmental organisms that infect a small proportion of exposed humans or animals.[23]

M. genavense has been found in patients with advanced HIV infections. Chronic illness is characterized by fever, diarrhea, and marked weight loss. The gastrointestinal tract is the primary site of infection and reservoir from which this organism invades other tissues.[23] A similar organism has been isolated from an immunocompetent woman with lymphadenitis. As for other species of nontuberculous mycobacteria, *M. genavense* can colonize the intestinal tract of persons not infected with HIV.[2, 7, 23]

M. genavense has been a reported cause of mycobacteriosis in 27 birds from one zoo and in several privately owned birds. Although large numbers of organisms were found in the intestines, the lungs, liver, and spleen also were involved. The source of infection has not been determined, but contaminated water is suspected.[13, 23, 25]

M. haemophilum can cause generalized infections as well as severe infections of skin, respiratory tract, and bone. Infections are usually in immunocompromised patients; however, *M. haemophilum* has been reported as a cause of perihilar or cervical lymphadenitis in immunologically competent children.[32]

M. malmoense is a respiratory pathogen in patients with or without pre-existing lung disease. Disseminated disease has been seen in patients with other underlying diseases. The source of infection is presumed to be the environment.[32]

Mycobacterium simiae was first isolated from a rhesus macaque in 1965 and rarely has been associated with human disease. The organism has a unique geographic distribution, including Israel, Cuba, and the southern United States, mostly Texas.[32] It has also been isolated from sphagnum vegetation of the coastal southern region of Madagascar.[30] *M. simiae* has been associated with chronic lung infections in patients with previous tuberculosis or malignancy. Bone, bone marrow, kidney, and peritoneal infections have been reported. The organism has been cultured from other sites, including skin, urine, lymph node, and brain. The majority of these isolates are a result of colonization and not infection.[30, 32]

MISCELLANEOUS NONTUBERCULOUS MYCOBACTERIA

Mycobacterium marinum, a nontuberculous mycobacterium that lives in an aquatic environment (fresh and salt water), commonly causes granulomas in fishes.[9] *M. marinum* grows at a lower temperature (30° to 33°C) than do many other species of mycobacteria.[34] This organism can cause granulomatous skin infections in people who handle fishes or come in contact with aquaria. Lymphatic or local spread is possible, and the disease has progressed to the joints in a few reported cases.[26, 32] Humans become infected if mildly traumatized areas of skin are exposed to contaminated water. Only a few cases have been reported among HIV-infected patients. All reported cases involved aquaria as the source of infection. Several of these were disseminated infections, and some were unresponsive to antituberculous therapy.[9] *M. marinum* infection also has been reported in a manatee.[29, 33]

Mycobacterium xenopi was first isolated from a South American toad and has been found as a contaminant in hot-water generators and storage tanks, resulting in respiratory tract colonization in the hospital environment. The pathogenicity of this organism is difficult to assess.[32, 34]

An organism similar to *Mycobacterium paratuberculosis* has been isolated from a few human patients with Crohn's disease; however, the significance of these findings and the possible pathogenic role of this organism in inflammatory bowel disease has not been determined.[28]

SAPROPHYTES WITH LOW PATHOGENIC POTENTIAL

Mycobacterium terrae has caused pulmonary disease, arthritis, and tenosynovitis in humans.[34] *Mycobacterium gordonae* contaminates piped water supplies and can also contaminate bronchoscopes in a hospital setting. It can colonize the respiratory tract without causing disease; however, it has been a reported cause of localized and disseminated infections.[32, 34] *Mycobacterium flavescens* (previously considered to be nonpathogenic) has caused pulmonary disease and synovitis in humans.[34] *Mycobacterium smegmatis* is rarely associated with human disease but can cause skin and soft tissue infections.[32] *M. smegmatis* also has caused a disseminated infection in a sea lion.[33] Other species reported to cause disease in humans are *Mycobacterium szulgai*, *Mycobacterium ulcerans*, and *Mycobacterium asiaticum*.[6, 34]

DIAGNOSIS

The diagnosis of a mycobacterial infection is based on clinical signs, demonstration of acid-fast rods in tissues or in cytologic preparations by direct microscopy, and identification of cultured mycobacteria by biochemical tests. High-performance liquid chromatography (HPLC), however, is an integral component of mycobacteria speciation in many laboratories and may replace biochemical testing. Radiometric culturing techniques also can be used, such as the BACTEC 460 radiometric system (Becton Dickinson Instrument Systems, Sparks, MD), followed by DNA probe analysis or probe analysis of specimens applied to mycobacterial growth from solid cultures. Probes sensitive for MAC, *M. avium*, *M. intracellulare*, *M. kansasii*, *M. gordonae*, and *M. tuberculosis* complex, which includes *M. bovis*, have been developed (AccuProbe; Gen-Probe, San Diego, CA). In addition, polymerase chain reaction (PCR) tests are being developed to identify organisms in biopsy, necropsy, fecal, and other clinical specimens.[12, 19] Finally, serologic diagnosis of mycobacterial infections in birds is being investigated.[22]

ZOONOTIC CONCERNS

Close contact between employees, particularly keepers, and animals in zoos and animal parks is thought to promote zoonotic disease transmission via aerosols, fomites, and infected food and water.[29] Animals are the reservoirs of zoonotic agents. However, many microorganisms, including nontuberculous mycobacteria, are shared by animals and humans, the reservoir being the environment.[14] Although geographic variability exists, nontuberculous mycobacteria are present in animals, plants, soil, dust, foodstuffs, and water.[9, 17, 34]

In contrast to tuberculosis, the nontuberculous mycobacterioses are not transmitted host to host but are usually acquired from the environment by mechanisms not well understood.[34] The interaction of the agent (numbers, virulence, route of exposure) with the host (degree of susceptibility) and the environment they share determines whether transmission of an agent and subsequent infection will occur. This classic interaction is particularly important in the pathogenesis of nontuberculous mycobacteria, inasmuch as these organisms are potential pathogens under certain conditions.[14] The risk of transmission of nontuberculous mycobacteria between animals and humans appears to be low, since most infections are reported in immunocompromised hosts. In addition, immunosuppressive therapy, defects in cellular immunity (other than AIDS), and/or concurrent disease can be predisposing factors.[16, 24]

Mycobacteria are difficult to eliminate because of the organism's ability to survive in the soil.[28] Mycobacteria have been found to remain infectious in soil for up to 7 years.[8, 9] MAC organisms are recovered more frequently and in higher numbers from acidic soils (pH, 5.0 to 5.5) that have high levels of organic matter and grow best at warm temperatures (43°C).[18] This type of environment is very similar to many naturalistic exhibits in zoos. Shedding of nontuberculous mycobacteria from an infected or colonized animal host occurs primarily in feces and can cause contamination of the soil or water. Large numbers of organisms can build up in the exhibit over time, especially if more than one individual are shedding organisms and if the soil is not routinely removed from the exhibit. In addition, relocation of animals from one institution to another and the concomitant transfer of the animals' endogenous microflora could introduce novel mycobacteria into the new environment.

For these reasons, an understanding of how nontuberculous mycobacteria are transmitted is necessary in order to prevent exposure of these potential pathogens to a susceptible host. In addition, the education of animal care, horticulture, and other zoo staff members may be necessary to prevent overreaction to or complacency in the presence of an opportunistic pathogen. Inhalation of infectious aerosols, ingestion of contaminated material, inoculation of organisms through puncture wounds, and contamination of breaks in the skin may result in transmission of the organism and may lead to disease development.[34] Animal keepers in zoos or wildlife parks may come in contact with these organisms during the routine servicing of exhibits, particularly when hosing enclosures. Preventive measures include (1) opportunistic screening of animals for the presence of nontuberculous mycobacteria; (2) wearing face masks or face shields to guard against ingestion and/or inhalation of aerosolized organisms during hosing; (3) wearing gloves to prevent the introduction of organisms through breaks in the skin; (4) practicing good personal hygiene, including frequent hand washing; (5) using foot baths or dedicating shoes for use in zoo exhibits; and (6) using tuberculocidal disinfectants.

REFERENCES

1. Bono M, Jemmi T, Bernasconi C, et al: Genotypic characterization of *Mycobacterium avium* strains recovered from animals and their comparison to human strains. Appl Environ Microbiol 61:371–373, 1995.
2. Bosquee L, Bottger EC, De Beenhouwer H, et al: Cervical lymphadenitis caused by a fastidious mycobacterium closely related to *Mycobacterium genavense* in an apparently immunocompetent woman: diagnosis by culture-free microbiological methods. J Clin Microbiol 33:2670–2674, 1995.
3. Bush M, Montali RJ, Murray S, et al: The diagnosis, treatment and prevention of tuberculosis in captive Matschie's tree kangaroos (*Dendrolagus matschiei*). Proceedings of the Annual Meeting of the Joint Conference of the American Association of Zoo Veterinarians/Wildlife Disease Association/American Association of Wildlife Veterinarians, East Lansing, MI, pp 312–314, 1995.
4. Cleary KR, Batsakis JG: Mycobacterial disease of the head and neck: current perspective. Ann Otol Rhinol Laryngol 104:830–833, 1995.
5. Dalovisio JR, Stetter M, Mikota-Wells S: Rhinoceros' rhinorrhea: cause of an outbreak of infection due to airborne *Mycobacterium bovis* in zookeepers. Clin Inf Dis 15:598–600, 1992.
6. Dawson DJ, Blacklock ZM, Ashdown LR, et al: *Mycobacterium asiaticum* as the probable causative agent in a case of olecranon bursitis. J Clin Microbiol 33:1042–1043, 1995.
7. Dumonceau JM, Fonteyne PA, Realini L, et al: Species-specific *Mycobacterium genavense* DNA in intestinal tissues of individuals not infected with human immunodeficiency virus. J Clin Microbiol 33:2514–2515, 1995.
8. Gerlach H: Bacteria. *In* Ritchie BW, Harrison GJ, Harrison LR (eds): Avian Medicine: Principles and Application. Lake Worth, Wingers Publishing, pp 971–975, 1994.
9. Glaser CA, Angulo FJ, Rooney JA: Animal-associated opportunistic infections among persons infected with the human immunodeficiency virus. Clin Infect Dis 18:14–24, 1994.
10. Griffith DE, Girard WM, Wallace RJ Jr: Clinical features of pulmonary disease caused by rapidly growing mycobacteria. Am Rev Respir Dis 147:1271–1278, 1993.
11. Hatt JM, Guscetti F: A case of mycobacteriosis in a common marmoset (*Callithrix jacchus*). Proceedings of the Annual Meeting American Association of Zoo Veterinarians, pp 241–243, 1994.
12. Herold CD, Fitzgerald RL, Herold DA: Current techniques in mycobacterial detection and speciation. Crit Rev Clin Lab Sci 33:83–138, 1996.
13. Hoop RK, Bottger EC, Ossent P, et al: Mycobacteriosis due to *Mycobacterium genavense* in six pet birds. J Clin Microbiol 31:990–993, 1993.
14. Hugh-Jones ME, Hubbert WT, Hagstad: Zoonoses: Recognition, Control, and Prevention. Ames, Iowa State University Press, 1995.
15. Johnson CT, Winkler CE, Boughton E: *Mycobacterium kansasii* infection in a llama. Vet Rec 133:243–244, 1993.
16. Kiehn TE, Edwards FF, Brannon P, et al: Infections caused by *Mycobacterium avium* complex in immunocompromised patients: diagnosis by blood culture and fecal examination, antimicrobial susceptibility tests, and morphological and seroagglutination characteristics. J Clin Microbiol 21:68–173, 1985.
17. King NW Jr: *Mycobacterium avium–intracellalare* infection. *In* Jones TC, Mohr U, Hunt RD (eds): Nonhuman Primates. New York, Springer-Verlag, pp 57–63, 1993.
18. Kirschner RA, Parker BC, Falkinham JO III: Epidemiology of infection by nontuberculous mycobacteria. Am Rev Respir Dis 145:271–275, 1992.
19. Kox LFF: Tests for detection and identification of mycobacteria. How should they be used? Respir Med 89:399–408, 1995.
20. McKinsey DS, Dykstra M, Smith DL: The terrrier and the tendinitis [Letter]. New Engl J Med 332:338, 1995.
21. Parenti DM, Symington JS, Keiser J, et al: *Mycobacterium kansasii* bacteremia in patients infected with human immunodeficiency virus. Clin Inf Dis 21:1001–1003, 1995.
22. Phalen DN, Grimes JE, Phalen SW, et al: Serologic diagnosis of mycobacterial infections in birds (a preliminary report). Proceedings of the Annual Meeting of the Association Avian Veterinarians, pp 67–73, 1995.
23. Portaels F, Realini L, Bauwens L, et al: Mycobacteriosis caused by *Mycobacterium genavense* in birds kept in a zoo: 11-year survey. J Clin Microbiol 34:319–323, 1996.
24. Prince DS, Peterson DD, Steiner RM, et al: Infection with *Mycobacterium avium* complex in patients without predisposing conditions. New Engl J Med 321:863–868, 1989.
25. Ramis A, Ferrer L, Aranaz A, et al: *Mycobacterium genavense* infections in canaries. Avian Dis 40:246–251, 1996.
26. Ries KM, White GL: Atypical mycobacterial infection caused by *Mycobacterium marinum* [Letter]. New Engl J Med 322:633, 1990.
27. Thoen CO: Tuberculosis and other mycobacterial diseases in captive wild animals. *In* Fowler ME (ed): Zoo and Wild Animal Medicine, 3rd ed. Philadelphia, WB Saunders, pp 45–49, 1993.
28. Thoen CO, Williams DE: Tuberculosis, tuberculoidoses, and other mycobacterial infections. *In* Beran GW (ed-in-chief): Handbook of Zoonoses, Section A: Bacterial, Rickettsial, Chlamydial, and Mycotic, 2nd ed. Boca Raton, FL, CRC Press, pp 41–59, 1994.
29. Thompson PJ, Cousins DV, Gow BL, et al: Seals, seal trainers, and mycobacterial infection. Am Rev Respir Dis 147:164–167, 1993.
30. Valero G, Peters J, Jorgensen JH, et al: Clinical isolates of *Mycobacterium simiae* in San Antonio, Texas. Am J Respir Crit Care Med 152:1555–1557, 1995.
31. VanDerHeyden N: Update on avian mycobacteriosis. Proceedings of the Annual Meeting of the Association Avian Veterinarians, pp 53–59, 1994.
32. Watt B: Lesser known mycobacteria. J Clin Pathol 48:701–705, 1995.
33. Wells SK, Gutter A, Van Meter K: Cutaneous mycobacteriosis in a harbor seal: attempted treatment with hyperbaric oxygen. J Zoo Wildl Med 21:73–80, 1990.
34. Wolinsky E: Other mycobacterioses. *In* Wyngaarden JB, Smith LH Jr, Bennett JC (eds): Cecil Textbook of Medicine, 19th ed. Philadelphia, WB Saunders, pp 1742–1745, 1992.

CHAPTER 22

Zoonoses Acquired from Birds

KEVEN FLAMMER

A number of diseases can be acquired from birds. The more common ones are bacterial, but the list includes those with viral, fungal, and parasitic causes.[6, 11, 15, 20, 21] Despite the potential risk, the incidence of human illness acquired from birds is low. Only chlamydiosis and salmonellosis are reported with any frequency. Awareness of avian zoonoses is important, however, because veterinarians are often the first health workers to identify zoonotic diseases. In addition, contact between birds and susceptible people has increased. Birds are popular pets, and the increased incidence of human acquired immunodeficiency syndrome (AIDS) and use of birds for pet-facilitated therapy for the elderly has brought birds in close contact with a human population that is more susceptible to opportunistic infection.

Most avian zoonoses are transmitted via the fecal-oral or respiratory route, and transmission to people can be reduced by simply practicing good hygiene. Avian owners and caretakers should wear separate clothing in the aviary and wash their hands after cleaning cages or handling birds. Aerosol production should be reduced by avoiding use of high-pressure hoses, vigorous sweeping, and unfiltered vacuum cleaners for primary cleaning. Avian caretakers should wear a dust mask in areas where there is high aerosol production and hearing protection if birds are noisy. If a zoonosis is suspected, a respirator and eye goggles can be worn for additional protection. Protective gear should also be worn during necropsies, or the bird should be examined under a hood. In view of the low incidence, it is probably not necessary to serologically screen personnel for avian zoonoses, unless a specific problem is encountered.

Reducing avian disease in the aviary also decreases human risk and can be accomplished by practicing good husbandry. Newly acquired birds should be quarantined for a minimum of 30 days and tested for the diseases common to the particular species. Cloacal swabs may be cultured for pathogenic bacteria and specific cultures performed for salmonella. Although tests are not 100% accurate, psittaciforms and columbiforms should be screened for chlamydiosis by antigen and/or antibody tests. Fecal parasite examinations can help identify birds with giardia, cryptosporidia, and other parasites. Birds in the resident collection should be fed fresh food, and special care should be extended when animal products are fed. Spilled food should be collected before it spoils, or the birds should be housed in wire bottom cages that allow spilled food to exit the cage. Water and food bowls should be located in areas that discourage the birds from defecating in them. Rodents and aviary vermin can be controlled by implementing an effective pest control program. Finally, all dead birds should undergo necropsy to determine the cause of death. Good record keeping aids in identifying problems as they occur so that appropriate control steps can be implemented.

DISEASE DESCRIPTIONS

Brief summaries of most reported and potential avian zoonoses are provided in Tables 22–1 to 22–3. Additional information is provided below for the diseases of greatest significance. Several reviews provide more complete descriptions of avian zoonoses.[6, 11, 15, 20, 21]

Bacterial Diseases

Chlamydiosis, salmonellosis, campylobacteriosis, and pseudotuberculosis are the most frequently reported avian bacterial zoonosis. Yersiniosis and erysipelas occur in people, but mammals are more likely to be the source of infection. *Mycobacterium avium* of avian origin, *Escherichia coli*, and *Listeria* species can potentially cause human infection but have rarely been reported. Pathogenic strains of *Pasturella* species, *E. coli*, *Pseudomonas* species, and *Vibrio* species could be passed between birds and people, but the risk is low if good hygiene is practiced.

CHLAMYDIOSIS (PSITTACOSIS)

Chlamydia psittaci is an obligate intracellular pathogen that can potentially infect all birds and is particularly common in psittacines (parrots), pigeons, and doves.[18] Clinical signs in birds are nonspecific and include diarrhea, respiratory signs, and generalized illness. Many infected birds are subclinical carriers and show no signs. Infectious particles are shed in the feces and in ocular and oral secretions. People acquire the disease by inhalation of aerosolized fecal debris; person-to-person transmission is extremely rare. The incubation period is approximately 1 to 2 weeks. In people, psittacosis causes a flu-like syndrome and an atypical pneumonia, with occasional cardiac and neurologic effects. Symp-

TABLE 22-1. Diseases Transmitted from Birds to Humans

Disease	Etiology	Bird Reservoirs	Major Signs in Birds	Transmission	Major Signs in Humans	Occurrence
Psittacosis	*Chlamydia psittaci*	All birds, especially psittacines and columbiforms	Generalized illness	Respiratory, fecal-oral	Flu-like syndrome, pneumonia	Occasional
Salmonellosis	*Salmonella typhimurium*	All birds; most common in waterfowl and galliforms	Gastroenteritis, septicemia	Fecal-oral	Fever, diarrhea	Occasional
Campylobacteriosis	*Campylobacter jejuni*	Many species: poultry, scavengers (gulls, crows), wild birds; rare in psittacines	Enteritis, hepatitis	Fecal-oral	Gastroenteritis	Occasional
Pseudotuberculosis	*Yersinia pseudotuberculosis*	Many orders; columbiforms are common hosts	Gastroenteritis, hepatitis	Fecal-oral, transplacental	Acute mesenteric lymphadenitis, fever, gastroenteritis, erythema nodosum	Sporadic
Erysipelas	*Erysipelothrix rhusiopathiae*	Most common in turkeys and waterfowl; occurs in psittacines	Peracute death; some show lethargy, weakness	Direct contact or fomite transmission	Cutaneous nodule	Rare; seen in poultry food/carcass handlers
Miscellaneous bacteria	*Escherichia coli, Vibrio* species, *Pseudomonas* species, *Pasturella* species	All birds	Depend on bacteria and site of infection	Direct, fomite, inhalation, fecal-oral, wound infection	Depend on bacteria and site of infection	Rare
Dermatophytosis	*Trichophyton gallinae, Microsporum gypseum,* others?	Many species	Usually subclinical; may cause skin lesions	Direct contact with infected feathers, skin, or nest	Swollen, erythematous round plaques	Rare
Newcastle's disease	*Paramyxovirus* species	Aerosolized vaccine; poultry; other birds if involved in large outbreaks	Gastrointestinal and neurologic signs; high mortality rate	Aerosol	Sinusitis and conjunctivitis; occasional flu-like syndrome	Rare
Influenza	*Orthomyxovirus* species, Influenza type A	Poultry, waterfowl, many wild bird species, psittacines	Usually asymptomatic	Aerosol	Respiratory	Rare; birds serve as reservoirs.

152

TABLE 22–2. Diseases with Potential but Undocumented Transmission from Birds to People

Disease	Etiology	Bird Reservoirs	Signs in Birds	Transmission	Major Signs in Humans	Occurrence
Mycobacteriosis	*Mycobacteria avium* *M. genavense*	All birds, especially waterfowl and gallinaceous birds	Wasting disease	Respiratory, fecal-oral	Respiratory, wasting disease	Unknown; avian strains rarely infect people
Rabies	*Lyssavirus* species	Birds are rarely infected	Not reported	Contaminated wound	Neurologic	Not reported; transmission by contaminated raptor possible
Giardiasis	*Giardia lamblia*	Many, including domestic, wild, and pet birds	Diarrhea, malabsorption; in many birds, are subclinical	Fecal-oral	Diarrhea, malabsorption	Transmission from avian source not reported
Cryptosporidiosis	*Cryptosporidium* species	Many, including gallinaceous birds, waterfowl, passerines, and psittacines	Enteritis or respiratory signs	Fecal-oral	Diarrhea, vomiting, abdominal pain	Transmission from avian source not reported; birds shed low numbers of parasites

toms can be quite severe if treatment (usually with tetracycline, doxycycline, or erythromycin) is delayed. Clinical signs of *C. psittaci* infection and results of some serologic tests are easily confused with a nonzoonotic form of human chlamydiosis caused by *Chlamydia pneumoniae*.[5] Recovery after treatment is usually rapid and complete, but immunity is of short duration, and reinfection is possible.

SALMONELLOSIS

Salmonella organisms are commonly carried by domestic, pet, and wild birds and may be infectious in people.

Salmonella typhimurium is the most common species.[16] Salmonellosis occurs in all birds but is particularly common in gallinaceous birds, waterfowl, and sea gulls. Infected birds may show clinical signs of generalized illness, lameness and gastroenteritis, and sudden death, or they may show no signs at all. Salmonella is transmitted to people through fecal contamination of fomites, food, or water. Gastroenteritis usually occurs in 6 to 72 hours after exposure, and adults usually recover in less than 1 week. Antibiotics are usually not prescribed because it is believed that they may prolong the carrier state and encourage microbial resistance.[24] Salmonellosis is diagnosed by fecal culture.

TABLE 22–3. Environmentally Transmitted Diseases Associated with Bird Contact

Disease	Etiology	Bird Reservoirs	Signs in Birds	Transmission	Major Signs in Humans	Occurrence
Aspergillosis	*Aspergillus fumigatus*	Many species, especially gallinaceous birds, waterfowl, and raptors	Respiratory disease, wasting	Infected birds are not contagious; source is environmental; inhalation at necropsy is a potential route	Pulmonary granulomatous disease	Not reported
Histoplasmosis	*Histoplasma capsulatum*	Blackbirds, starlings, pigeons, poultry	None	Inhalation of fungal spores; fungus is shed in droppings and proliferates in feces-enriched soil	Three syndromes: pulmonary, chronic cavitary, and disseminated	Occasional
Cryptococcosis	*Cryptococcus neoformans*	Pigeons	None	Inhalation of fungal spores from feces contaminated environment	Respiratory infection, meningitis	Occasional
Allergic alveolitis	Inhaled feather dander and/or bird feces	All birds; most cases associated with pigeons and pet birds	None	Inhalation of feather dander and/or bird feces	Acute, subacute, and chronic forms; dry cough, dyspnea, reduced pulmonary function, weight loss	Occasional
Hearing loss	Loud vocalizations	Loud birds, especially the larger psittacines	None	Noise	Hearing loss	Occasional
Pulmonary cancer	Mechanism unknown	Cohabitation with pet birds	None	Unknown	Primary pulmonary carcinoma	Occurrence questionable

CAMPYLOBACTERIOSIS

Campylobacter jejuni is a gram-negative, non–spore-forming, motile rod. It is commonly carried by many birds, including galliforms, columbiforms, waterfowl, scavenging birds (e.g., crows and gulls), wild birds, petrels, and flamingos.[6] It is rare in psittacines and other pet birds. Infected birds may show signs of hepatitis and enteritis, but infection is usually subclinical. People are usually infected through ingestion of contaminated food, and campylobacteriosis causes abdominal pain, followed by diarrhea, vomiting, and fever.[22] It is diagnosed by paired serum titers or by demonstrating the organism on fecal culture or dark field microscopy. Recovery in adults is usually spontaneous in 7 to 10 days; infection in infants and compromised adults may be fatal.

PSEUDOTUBERCULOSIS

Yersinia pseudotuberculosis is the cause of pseudotuberculosis and is a common cause of mortality in both pet and zoological birds in Europe.[4, 14] The incidence in other regions of the world is sporadic. Toucans and canaries are particularly susceptible to infection. Avian clinical signs include peracute hemorrhagic pneumonia in toucans and enteritis, splenomegaly, and wasting disease in other species.[6] Transmission is via the fecal-oral route, and the incubation period in humans is 1 to 3 weeks. Clinical signs in humans include mesenteric lymphadenitis and hepatic enlargement.[23]

Yersinia enterocolitica organisms, the cause of yersiniosis, are found in birds that inhabit areas contaminated by human sewage. The risk that infected birds pose for people is unknown but is presumably low.

MYCOBACTERIUM

Studies with genetic probes have shown that avian strains of *M. avium* rarely infect people.[2] Although the incidence of *M. avium* infection in patients with AIDS has increased since the 1980s, the strains causing infection are thought to be of environmental, not avian, origin. More precise speciation of mycobacteria has also revealed that *M. genavense* is a common cause of avian mycobacterial infections. *M. genavense* causes infection in people, but the significance of *M. genavense* as a zoonotic agent is currently unknown.[12a] Because the zoonotic risk of avian mycobacterial infections is unknown, care should be taken to prevent human exposure. Avian mycobacteriosis is more completely described in Chapter 21.

Fungal Diseases

Fungal diseases are rarely transmitted from bird to human. Dermatophytes can be found on bird feathers and nesting material and occasionally cause localized skin infections in people. Aspergillosis is a common cause of mortality in raptors, waterfowl, and arctic and antarctic birds. It is possible for a person to inhale aspergillus spores during a necropsy, but environmental sources of infection are more likely. Although not zoonoses in the classical sense, histoplasmosis and cryptococcosis are environmentally transmitted fungal diseases that proliferate in soil contaminated by bird droppings and are therefore acquired through human contact where birds live.

HISTOPLASMOSIS

Histoplasma capsulatum organisms grow in soil enriched by bird droppings and are most commonly found in the lowlands of the Ohio, Missouri, and Mississippi river valleys.[1] Birds are protected from infection by their higher body temperature but shed fungal spores in their feces. Roost sites of blackbirds, starlings, pigeons, and poultry have been linked to human outbreaks. People are infected when spores are aerosolized and inhaled. Most human infections are asymptomatic, but approximately 10% of infected people develop influenza-like symptoms and pulmonary disease. Infection can be prevented by wearing respirators when avian fecal debris is cleaned from contaminated areas.

CRYPTOCOCCOSIS

Cryptococcus neoformans is a yeast-like organism that is commonly found in soil contaminated by pigeon droppings.[1] Like *Histoplasma*, *Cryptococcus* organisms rarely cause avian disease but accumulate in soil at pigeon roost sites and infect people when spores in the environment are aerosolized and inhaled. Pulmonary disease, or a disseminated form that may include meningitis, can develop in infected people.

Viral Diseases

Avian viral diseases are rarely directly transmitted from birds to humans. Newcastle's disease has been transmitted this way, and there is potential for transmission of rabies and influenza. Birds serve as reservoirs for the viral encephalitides caused by Eastern and Western equine encephalitis virus, but these diseases are transmitted by mosquitoes and are not zoonoses in the true sense.[21]

NEWCASTLE'S DISEASE

This illness is caused by a paramyxovirus infection that occurs most frequently in poultry. Viscerotrophic velogenic strains cause disease in many avian species, including psittacines.[10] Signs in birds are strain dependent and highly variable. Infection in people is rare and occurs most frequently in poultry workers and in persons exposed to aerosolized live vaccine. Clinical signs in people include sinusitis and conjunctivitis.[7]

RABIES

Birds are generally resistant to rabies infection, and transmission of rabies from bird to humans has not been documented, but the potential for transmission exists. Rabies has been experimentally transmitted to a number of avian species.[10] Raptors recently exposed to rabies-infected prey could potentially transmit the virus by mechanical means.

INFLUENZA A

Influenza viruses are carried by many wild birds, particularly waterfowl, but bird-to-person transmission is not well documented. Influenza strains from birds may recombine with human strains and produce new virulent strains for people.[21]

Parasitic Diseases

Most avian parasites are not transmissible to mammals. Toxoplasmosis is common in poultry and pigeons and could potentially infect people if infected flesh were eaten, but freezing and cooking kill the toxoplasma oocyst, and birds are therefore not considered an important source of human infection. Cryptosporidiosis and giardiasis commonly infect both birds and people, but it is currently unclear whether parasite strains of avian origin are infectious in people.

CRYPTOSPORIDIOSIS

Cryptosporidium organisms are coccidian parasites that infect many animal species.[19] Avian infection has been documented in galliforms, waterfowl, psittacines, and passerine birds. Clinical signs of infection include enteritis, respiratory problems, and stunted growth of juvenile birds.[8] Adult birds may be subclinical carriers. Transmission occurs when infectious oocysts in bird feces are ingested by a susceptible host. In people, cryptosporidiosis causes severe gastroenteritis with fever, vomiting, diarrhea, and abdominal pain. The zoonotic potential of avian strains of this parasite is unknown. No bird-to-human transmission has been documented, and strains from quail and pheasant were not transmissible to mammalian hosts.[19] Birds shed low numbers of oocyst; therefore, even if avian strains are zoonotic, it is unlikely that they are an important source of human infection.[6]

GIARDIASIS

Giardia lamblia organisms infect many mammalian and avian species. Clinical signs in birds include diarrhea and feather and skin abnormalities; some infected birds show no clinical signs. Transmission is via the fecal-oral route. Infection in people causes diarrhea and malabsorption.[17] There are no documented reports of transmission from avian sources, so the zoonotic potential of avian giardiasis is unknown.

Problems Associated with Bird Contact

ALLERGIES

Human allergies to contact with feather dander and avian fecal material are relatively common. Symptoms include runny eyes, clear nasal discharge, and sneezing.

Sensitivity to feather dander can be diagnosed by skin testing, and hypersensitivity can be treated by allergen injection, or symptoms can be controlled with antihistamine drugs. More severe signs are seen with allergic alveolitis (also called pigeon lung disease, bronchiolitis, and allergic interstitial pneumonitis).[9, 12] Acute disease occurs after exposure to a large amount of avian antigen, and symptoms include coughing, dyspnea, and fever. Subacute disease occurs with long-term exposure to antigen, and a dry cough and progressive dyspnea are the major clinical signs. Prognosis for recovery from the acute and subacute forms is good if sources of the allergen are removed. The chronic form results from prolonged exposure to antigen, which may cause irreversible lung disease. Signs include progressive dyspnea, dry cough, and weight loss. Pulmonary function is decreased as a result of a reduction of vital lung capacity and impairment of oxygen diffusion across the alveolar-capillary junction. Pulmonary changes include interstitial granulomas and fibrosis. Symptoms can be reduced by avoiding further contact with the antigen, but the fibrosis may be irreversible. Avian caretakers can reduce exposure to antigen by wearing dust-filtering masks when cleaning cages. Electrostatic filters and negative ion generators may also reduce the amount of aerosolized antigen.

HEARING LOSS

Many birds, particularly the large psittacines, are capable of producing loud sounds. Avian caretakers should wear hearing protection when working in noisy areas.

LUNG CANCER

A single epidemiologic report, published in 1992, linked pet bird ownership with an increased incidence of primary lung cancer in people.[13] The validity of this study was questioned,[3] and no further reports have collaborated the results. However, the question has been raised and warrants further study.

REFERENCES

1. Ajello L, Kaplan W, Padhye A: Mycotic and actinomycotic zoonoses. *In* Steele JH (ed): CRC Handbook Series in Zoonoses, vol II (Section A). Boca Raton, FL, CRC Press, pp 469–489, 1980.
2. Angulo FJ, Glaser CA, Juranek DD, et al: Caring for pets of immunocompromised persons. J Am Vet Med Assoc 205:1711–1718, 1994.
3. Angulo FJ, Millikan RC, Malmgren R: Question link between human lung cancer and pet bird exposure [Letter]. J Am Vet Med Assoc 202(9):1345, 1993.
4. Borst GHA, Buitelaar M, Poelma FG, et al: Yersinia pseudotuberculosis in birds. Vet Bull 47:507–509, 1977.
5. Bourke SJ, Carrington D, Frew CE, et al: A comparison of the seroepidemiology of chlamydial infection in pigeon fanciers and farmers in the UK. J Infection 25(suppl. 1):91–98, 1992.
6. Carpenter JW, Gentz EJ: Zoonotic diseases of avian origin. *In* Altman RB, Clubb SL, Dorrestein GM, Quesenberry K (eds): Avian Medicine and Surgery. Philadelphia, WB Saunders, pp 350–363, 1997.
7. Chang PW: Newcastle disease. *In* Steele JH (ed): CRC Handbook Series in Zoonoses, vol II (Section B). Boca Raton, FL, CRC Press, pp 261–274, 1981.
8. Clubb SL, Cray C, Greiner E, et al: Cryptosporidiosis in a psittacine nursery. Proceedings of the Association of Avian Veterinarians, Tampa, FL, pp 177–186, 1996.

9. Davies D: Bird fanciers disease. BMJ (Clin Res) 287:1239–1240, 1983.

10. Gerlach H: Viruses. *In* Ritchie BW, Harrison GJ, Harrison, LR (eds): Avian Medicine, Principles and Application. Lake Worth, FL, Wingers Publishing, pp. 862–948, 1994.

11. Harris JM: Zoonotic diseases of birds. Vet Clin North Am (Sm Animal Pract) 21:1289–1298, 1991.

12. Johnson-Delaney CA: Alveolitis (pigeon breeder's lung) in pet bird owners. Proceedings of the Association of Avian Veterinarians, Seattle, pp. 213–215, 1989.

12a. Hoop RK, Bottger EC, Pfyffer GE: Etiological agents of mycobacteriosis in pet birds between 1986 and 1995. J Clin Microbiol 34:991–992, 1996.

13. Kohlmeier L, Arminger G, Bartolomycik S, et al: Pet birds as an independent risk factor for lung cancer. Case-control study. BMJ 305:986–989, 1992.

14. Mair NS: Yersiniosis in wildlife and its public health implications. J Wildl Dis 9:65–71, 1973.

15. McCluggage DM: Zoonotic disorders. *In* Rosskopf WJ, Woerpel RW (eds): Diseases of Cage and Aviary Birds. Baltimore, Williams & Wilkins, pp 535–547, 1996.

16. Meier JE: Salmonellosis and other bacterial enteritides in birds. *In* Kirk RW (ed): Current Veterinary Therapy VIII. Philadelphia, WB Saunders, pp 637–640, 1983.

17. Meyer EA, Jarroll EL: Giardiasis. *In* Steele JH (ed): CRC Handbook Series in Zoonoses, vol II (Section C). Boca Raton, FL, CRC Press, pp 25–40, 1982.

18. National Association of State Public Health Veterinarians: Compendium of chlamydiosis (psittacosis). J Am Vet Med Assoc 206:1874–1879, 1995.

19. O'Donoghue PJ: *Cryptosporidium* infections in man, animals, birds, and fish. Aust Vet J 62:253–258, 1985.

20. Ritchie BW, Dreesen DW: Avian zoonoses: proven and potential diseases. Part I. Bacterial and parasitic diseases. Compend Collect 10(6):26–31, 1988.

21. Ritchie BW, Dreesen DW: Avian zoonoses: proven and potential diseases. Part II. Viral, fungal, and miscellaneous diseases. Compend Collect 10(6):26–31, 1988.

22. Shane SM, Montrose MS: The occurrence and significance of *Campylobacter jejuni* in man and animal. Vet Res Comm 9:167–198, 1985.

23. Stovell PL: Pseudotubercular yersiniosis. *In* Steele JH (ed): CRC Handbook Series in Zoonoses, vol II (Section A). Boca Raton, FL, CRC Press, pp 209–256, 1980.

24. Williams LP Jr: Salmonellosis. *In* Steele JH (ed): CRC Handbook Series in Zoonoses, vol II (Section A). Boca Raton, FL. CRC Press, pp 11–34, 1980.

PART II

FISH

CHAPTER 23

Anesthesia in Fish

CRAIG A. HARMS

Anesthesia facilitates procedures such as restraint for examination, transportation, diagnostic sampling, and surgery on fish. Because many of these procedures are more easily performed out of the water, a condition objectionable to most fish, effective restraint is essential. Chemical immobilization is usually less stressful and traumatic than physical restraint for many minor procedures; for major procedures, the use of an anesthetic agent is required. When necessary, overdose of anesthetic agents is an acceptable means of euthanasia.

GENERAL CONSIDERATIONS

Water quality is an important consideration in all aspects of fish medicine, including anesthesia.[3, 9] Physical and chemical parameters of the anesthesia water should closely match those of the aquarium or pond water. Because anesthetic agents tend to cause respiratory depression, adequate aeration or oxygenation is necessary, particularly when multiple fish are to be anesthetized in the same water. Dissolved oxygen concentrations should be maintained between 6 and 10 ppm. Prolonged exposure to excessively high dissolved oxygen concentrations achievable by administering pure oxygen can lead to gill damage. Because some waterborne anesthetic agents markedly reduce pH, addition of buffers may be

required to avoid inducing acidosis. Water temperature has a direct effect on metabolic rate, and therefore affects the rates of induction and recovery, with higher temperatures speeding both.

In preparation for anesthetizing fish, stressors on the fish should be minimized.[3] Relaxed fish experience a smoother induction than aroused fish. Food should be withheld for at least one feeding cycle before anesthesia. Although aspiration pneumonia is not a hazard for fish, regurgitation can clog gill rakers (sestonosis) and foul the water. Withholding food also reduces production of nitrogenous wastes, an important consideration when sedating fish for transport. For waterborne anesthesia, water and containers for induction, maintenance, and recovery should all be prepared ahead of time. This involves selecting containers of adequate volume and with no toxic chemical residue, adjusting water quality parameters to approximate optimal conditions for the fish (e.g., adding cold packs to reduce temperature for cold-water fishes), and premixing the desired concentrations of anesthetic. When dealing with multiple individuals of an unfamiliar species, the entire anesthetic procedure should be carried through to recovery on one fish before proceeding to the rest, because species variability in susceptibility to anesthetics, as well as varying water conditions, may necessitate adjustment of induction or maintenance doses. Fish should be handled carefully to avoid abrasions or loss of protective mucus. During prolonged out-of-water procedures, The fish's skin should be kept moist and its eyes protected. Soft open-cell foam, saturated with water and with a V-slot cut to accommodate the fish, helps with positioning, maintains moisture where in contact with the fish, and allows water to flow through for collection. Covering the eyes or darkening the room can help calm a fish that is incompletely immobilized.

Anesthetic effects in fish have been staged in varying schemes by different authors.[9] All schemes are gauged by activity, reactivity to stimuli, equilibrium, muscle tone, respiratory rate, and heart rate. Broad stages include sedation, narcosis or loss of equilibrium, and anesthesia, and each stage may be further subdivided into light and deep planes. Not all stages are observed with every anesthetic agent or route of delivery in all fish. An excitement phase may be observed and may necessitate covering the tank to prevent leaping fish from escaping the water and injuring themselves in a fall. Starting at the low end of the recommended dose range and working up to the desired effect is advisable when anesthetizing an unfamiliar species of fish; however, when working with a species whose tolerance for an anesthetic is known, then using a higher dose for induction and switching to a lower maintenance dose results in a much smoother and more rapid induction.

DELIVERY METHODS

Anesthetics may be delivered by any of the usual routes of administration: orally (PO), parenterally (intravenously [IV], intramuscularly [IM], or intraperitoneally [IP]), or by inhalation (topical to gills, absorption, bath, waterborne). Oral administration of anesthetic agents, however, is rarely used in fish medicine, because precise dosing is difficult and there is uncertainty regarding rate and degree of absorption.

IV administration of anesthetics to fish has been studied in research settings; however, for practical reasons, parenteral administration is usually IM or IP in clinical settings. The parenteral mode is best suited for larger fish, for which injection site trauma is less of a hazard. Parenteral administration is also well suited for larger volume aquariums, where adding waterborne anesthetics to the entire tank is impractical, and confinement and capture of the fish in a smaller volume of water is problematic. Injections may be made by hand syringe, pole syringe, or dart. A Hawaiian sling may be modified to serve as a dart delivery system for large fish, although injection site trauma and scale loss are hazards.[9] IM administration of anesthetics is the most practical route for large fish in large aquariums; however, the effects of most IM agents examined to date in teleosts are generally restricted to immobilization suitable for minor procedures only. IM anesthetic administration has been more satisfactory in elasmobranchs. Major procedures in both groups may require subsequent inhalation anesthesia. Respiratory support (directing a stream of well-aerated water over the gills) may

be necessary during immobilization with injectable anesthetics.

Waterborne anesthesia is the most widely used route of anesthetic administration for fish. For bath treatment, the drug can be brought to the desired concentration in water containing the fish, or the fish can be placed in an induction tank containing anesthetic. For short procedures lasting less than 5 minutes, this may be all that is necessary. The fish may be removed from the water for the necessary manipulations and either be returned to the anesthesia tank to extend the procedure or be moved to recovery water when the task is completed.

For longer out-of-water procedures, following removal from the induction tank, water must be delivered in continuous flow to the gills. This can be achieved by a non-recirculating or recirculating system. In a non-recirculating system (the equivalent of a non-rebreathing or Bain system) the anesthetic–water mix is held in a reservoir bag or tank and is conveyed through appropriately sized tubing into the fish's mouth and over the gills. Used water is collected to keep the work area from flooding, but it is not recycled to the fish. This system works well for small fish. A simple design uses empty IV fluid bags as reservoirs and a drip set for delivery, with flow rate being regulated by the drip set clamp.[5]

A recirculating system is well suited to large fish, where economics make conservation of anesthetic and water (e.g., inland salt water) a concern. Numerous recirculating systems have been described,[2, 7] but the basic idea is that anesthesia water from a reservoir is delivered to the gills and is collected and returned repeatedly to the fish. The simplest recirculating system has the operator returning collected water by hand directly to the fish (a turkey baster works well) or to an elevated reservoir for siphoning to the fish. When a power supply is available, less labor intensive designs use pumps to return water to the fish (Fig. 23–1). More complex designs can incorporate a flow meter and valves to control flow. Minimum effective flow rate during fish anesthesia has not been specifically determined, although flow rates from 1 to 3 L min^{-1} kg^{-1} have been used successfully. Monitoring the fish's anesthetic depth is the best guide for determining adequate flow. Excessive flow rates can result in alimentary anesthetic delivery and gastric dilatation.

A common difficulty of waterborne anesthesia systems is adjusting anesthetic concentrations as the depth of anesthesia varies. One simple method for coping with this design deficiency is to prepare appropriate volumes of anesthetic-free water and more concentrated anesthetic solution. These solutions can be delivered to the gills directly using a suitably sized syringe, based on the condition of the fish. Similarly, in Figure 23–1, the submersible pump can be transferred between tanks with and without anesthetic. It is also possible to design a low-volume recirculating system that allows the infusion of water or concentrated anesthetic solution to regulate the anesthetic concentration in a more rapid and controlled manner.

In continuous flow systems, the flow should be normograde (in the oral cavity and out the opercular open-

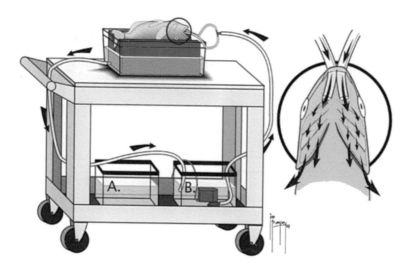

FIGURE 23–1. Recirculating system for delivery of waterborne anesthetic to fish. Submersible pump located in anesthesia water *(B)* can be moved to anesthetic-free water *(A)* if necessary. *Arrows* indicate direction of water flow. *Inset:* Proper direction of water flow into mouth, across gills, and out opercular slits. (From Lewbart GA, Stone EA, Love NE: Pneumocystectomy in a Midas cichlid. J Am Vet Med Assoc 207:320, 1995.)

ing) to achieve optimal gas and anesthetic exchange (see Fig. 23–1). During oral surgery, flow can be reversed if necessary to allow surgical access, but retrograde flow nullifies the normal countercurrent exchange mechanism and may damage the gills.[8]

Bath treatments and recirculating systems used for multiple sequential fish anesthesia procedures eventually become depleted of anesthetic as anesthetic-laden fish are taken out of the bath or off the system. Ammonia concentrations increase as more fish-hours are logged. Both factors eventually necessitate a change of water and anesthetic. Time for change can be assessed by monitoring induction time and anesthetic depth or by direct measurement of water quality. Increasing protein concentration from fish slime causes foaming in aerated water, providing a visual indication of deteriorating water quality.

ANESTHETIC AGENTS

Many compounds have been used as fish anesthetics. Some of the more commonly used or readily available are listed in Table 23–1.

Waterborne Anesthetics

TRICAINE METHANESULFONATE

Tricaine methanesulfonate (MS-222, Finquel) is the most widely used fish anesthetic and is the only one currently approved for use in food fish in the United States. It is a benzocaine derivative with a sulfonate radical, which accounts for its water solubility and increased acidity over the parent compound.[3] Administered as a waterborne solution, tricaine is absorbed across the gill epithelium and is biotransformed in the liver and probably kidney.[1] It is cleared primarily through the gills as the free and acetylated form, with additional metabolites being eliminated in the urine and bile. Tricaine is conveniently administered as a premixed stock solution of 10 g/L (10,000 ppm).[9] The stock solution is unstable in light and should be kept in a dark container. Shelf life may be extended by refrigeration or freezing. Because tricaine solutions are acidic (stock solutions can be as low as pH 3), they should be buffered before administration to fish. Saturation with sodium bicarbonate buffers the stock solution to between pH 7.0 and 7.5.[9] Other buffers (imidazole, sodium hydrogen phosphate, sodium hydroxide) may also be used.[2, 3] Oily residues in buffered stock solutions indicate the presence of a desulfonation product and decreased potency.[9] Although generally considered a safe anesthetic, margins of safety for tricaine are narrower for young fish in warm, soft water, and there is variation across species.[9] Recovery from short procedures is rapid (less than 10 minutes if properly dosed), with prolonged recoveries (up to 6 hours) from longer procedures.

QUINALDINE SULFATE

Quinaldine sulfate is an alternative to tricaine, popular because of the perception of a wider margin of safety with imprecise dosing (i.e., the sprinkle-to-effect method) in some species. It is not approved for use in food fish. Quinaldine sulfate is a highly water-soluble powder. Like tricaine, quinaldine sulfate in solution is strongly acidic and should be buffered. It may also be conveniently administered as a 10 g/L stock solution.[9] Unlike tricaine, it is not metabolized by fish and is excreted entirely unchanged. Because it does not eliminate all reflex responses, quinaldine sulfate may not be suitable for major or delicate surgery.[3]

METOMIDATE

Metomidate is a nonbarbiturate imidazole hypnotic[3, 9] (not to be confused with another imidazole, medetomidine, an alpha₂-adrenergic receptor agonist that can be used with ketamine as an injectable anesthetic). Metomidate is available under the trade name Marinil in Canada, but it is not yet licensed in the United States, although it is available for investigational use. It is readily water soluble and should be stored in tight light-protected containers. Metomidate does not result in increased cortisol typically observed with other anesthetics, most likely because of a metabolic blockade of cortisol synthesis.[9] Some fish anesthetized with metomidate turn very dark transiently. Muscle fasciculations occur at low doses. Metomidate is poorly analgesic in mammals, so by itself it may not be suitable for major surgery, although it is useful for sedation and for minor procedures. Gouramis are believed to be very sensitive to metomidate,[2] and use in cichlids in water of pH less than 5 is contraindicated.

Injectable Anesthetics

KETAMINE AND COMBINATIONS

Ketamine is an injectable short-acting dissociative anesthetic. It can be used alone or in combination with *medetomidine*, which has the advantage of reversibility with *atipamezole*.[12] When administered IM, high doses are required in many teleost species, with incomplete anesthesia resulting, making it more appropriate as an aid to restraint rather than as a substitute for waterborne anesthesia during major procedures. Elasmobranchs are more susceptible than teleosts to the effects of ketamine. *Xylazine* administered concurrently with ketamine reduces muscle spasms that can occur in sharks.[11] Respiratory support may be required with ketamine use.

LIDOCAINE

Lidocaine as an immersion anesthetic yields variable results,[3] but has application as an injectable local anesthetic in fish, alone or in combination with other agents administered at sedative or immobilizing doses. Care must be taken not to overdose small fish with local injections.

Miscellaneous Agents

CARBON DIOXIDE

Carbon dioxide has been used from various sources (Alka-Seltzer, sodium bicarbonate, CO_2 gas) for fish

TABLE 23–1. Fish Anesthetic Dosages*

Agent	Dose
Waterborne Anesthetics	
Tricaine methanesulfonate (MS-222)	
Anesthesia induction	100–200 mg/L
Anesthesia maintenance	50–100 mg/L
Sedation	15–50 mg/L
Quinaldine sulfate	
Anesthesia induction	50–100 mg/L
Anesthesia maintenance	15–60 mg/L
Metomidate (Marinil)	
Transport tranquilization	0.06–0.20 mg/L
Light sedation	0.5–1 mg/L
Heavy sedation	2.5–5 mg/L
Anesthesia	5–10 mg/L (10–30 mg/L for some species)
Injectable Anesthetics	
Lidocaine	
Local anesthesia	$\leq$1–2 mg/kg total dose
Ketamine	
Immobilization	66–68 mg/kg intramuscularly (IM) (teleosts)/12–20 mg/kg IM (sharks)
Ketamine/medetomidine	
Immobilization	1–2 mg/kg ketamine/50–100 μg/kg medetomidine IM
Reversal	Atipamezole 200 μg/kg IM
Ketamine/xylazine	12–20 mg/kg ketamine/6 mg/kg xylazine IM (sharks)
Miscellaneous Anesthetics (for use only if preferred agents not available)	
CO_2 (Alka-Seltzer, sodium bicarbonate, CO_2 gas)	
Anesthesia	
CO_2 gas	120–150 mg/L
$NaHCO_3$	500 mg/L
Alka-Seltzer	1 tablet/L
Isoflurane, Halothane	
Anesthesia	0.5–2 ml/L added directly to water or vaporize and dissolve to effect
Ethanol	
Anesthesia	1%–1.5% in water
Euthanasia	>3% in water

*See text for important notes on dosing. These doses should not be considered suitable for all species, nor for all conditions. When working with unfamiliar anesthetic agents or fish species, start with low doses and low numbers of fish. (Adapted from Harms CA, Bakal RS: Techniques in fish anesthesia. J Small Exotic Anim Med 3:21, 1995.)

anesthesia, apparently with some success.[4] The use of CO_2 has many disadvantages, however. Concentrations in water are difficult to control, oxygen must be maintained at high levels,[3] and blood gases and acid–base balance are markedly altered compared to when other anesthetics are used.[6] The primary advantage of using carbon dioxide, in food animal situations, is the lack of tissue residues of regulatory concern. In clinical situations, however, it should be considered an anesthetic or euthanasia agent of last resort.

ISOFLURANE AND HALOTHANE

Isoflurane and halothane are readily available in veterinary clinics and may be used for fish anesthesia, either by direct addition to water or by vaporizing and bubbling through the water.[3, 4] However, anesthetic levels are difficult to control, localized areas of higher concentrations may occur and result in overdose, and volatilization constitutes a hazard to personnel. Volatile anesthetics are not recommended for use in fish.

ETHANOL

Ethanol is another anesthetic or euthanasia agent of last resort. Anesthetic depth is variable and difficult to control.[3] In nonclinical situations, however, it is sometimes available when other agents are not.

MONITORING TECHNIQUES

A variety of parameters may be monitored visually or palpably during anesthesia induction and maintenance.[3, 9] Respiration (opercular movement) is probably the most important reference of anesthetic depth. Others include loss of equilibrium, jaw tone (which may be present in the absence of opercular movement), color of fin margins (broad pale fin margins, possibly caused by hypoxia or hypotension, indicate excessive depth), response to touch or surgical stimuli, and gill color (primarily as an indication of blood loss). Dead fish can retain good gill color.

Although pulse is not readily palpable in fish, under favorable conditions (thin pliable body wall, comparatively large heart), heart beats can be observed directly. Heart rate can also be monitored by Doppler flow probes placed over the heart, cardiac ultrasonography, or electrocardiogram (ECG). Use of subcutaneous needle electrodes for the ECG minimizes trauma, reduces the chance of grounding out the ECG signal by contact with a wet external surface, and improves the signal quality. Smaller fish may have an ECG undetectable by ordinary ECG equipment. If standard lead placement fails to elicit a detectable signal, a base-apex (dorsoventral) orientation may work.

Attempts to use pulse oximetry in fish have not been encouraging. Blood gases can be measured directly in sufficiently large fish. The dorsal aorta at the roof of the mouth is the only readily accessible sampling site where oxygenated arterial blood can be obtained with certainty, but this may be detrimental in some fish with relatively small vessels (laceration or thrombosis of the

dorsal aorta can be fatal). In some species with unusual oropharyngeal anatomy, even this site is not accessible.

Even though fish are sometimes difficult to monitor directly, especially small fish, the anesthesia water is easily accessible. Little effort is required to ensure that temperature (thermometer) and dissolved oxygen (DO meter) are maintained in appropriate ranges.

RECOVERY AND RESUSCITATION

Recovery and resuscitation are occasionally indistinct. If opercular motions cease or if other signs indicate that depth of anesthesia is too great, anesthetic-free water should be directed across the gills. This can also be done toward the end of a long surgery to hasten recovery. The recovery tank should be well aerated and free of anesthetic agents. When returning a fish to the recovery tank, the fish may be faced into gentle water flow from the filter/aerator. Larger fish can be held with the mouth open and pulled forward, directing water across the gills. A syringe may be used to push water across the gills of smaller fish. Pulling the fish backward should be avoided; it results in greatly reduced efficiency of gas and anesthetic exchange, and may damage the gill filaments.[2] Jaw tone and opercular movement should be monitored. Jaw tone and even biting can precede return of opercular movement. Once the fish begins breathing on its own, it is best left alone, even if it is unable to maintain a normal position, because the recovery can then proceed with less stress. Until the fish is fully recovered (and periodically thereafter), the light level should be reduced and respiration, motion, and equilibrium should be monitored. During recovery, some fish go through an erratic porpoising phase and should be prevented from escaping the tank.

It is sometimes difficult to determine immediately whether a fish has died. Resuscitation attempts should not be abandoned prematurely, because respiratory arrest (lack of opercular motion) can precede cardiac arrest by an extended period of time. Doppler flow probes or cardiac ultrasonography can be useful in detecting heart beats in very bradycardic patients.

Postoperative pain management is underinvestigated in fish. Indeed, the analgesic efficacy even of commonly used fish anesthetics remains somewhat conjectural.[10] Teleost nervous systems do produce opiate-like compounds, however, suggesting that opioids could induce some degree of analgesia. Butorphanol administered at 0.1 mg/kg IM as a single dose immediately following surgery in a limited range of teleosts has produced no evident adverse effects, although beneficial effects are undetermined.

EUTHANASIA

Euthanasia may be accomplished by an overdose of any of the anesthetic agents discussed. Larger fish that cannot easily be transferred to a bath treatment may have the anesthesia solution poured directly over the gills.[2] To be certain the euthanasia is complete, once the fish is deeply anesthetized, cranial concussion, spinal transection, or exsanguination should be performed.

Acknowledgments

I thank Dr. Robert S. Bakal for his input on system design and monitoring, and Dr. M. Andrew Stamper for manuscript review.

REFERENCES

1. Allen JL, Hunn JB: Fate and distribution studies of some drugs used in aquaculture. Vet Hum Toxicol 28(suppl 1):21–24, 1986.
2. Brown LA: Anesthesia in fish. Tropical Fish Medicine: Vet Clin North Am Small Anim Pract 18:317–330, 1988.
3. Brown LA: Anesthesia and restraint. *In* Stoskopf MK: Fish Medicine. Philadelphia, WB Saunders, pp 79–90, 1993.
4. Gratzek JB: Aquariology: The Science of Fish Health Management. Morris Plains, NJ, Tetra Press, p 232, 1992.
5. Harms CA, Bakal RS, Khoo LH, et al: Microsurgical excision of an abdominal mass in a gourami (*Colisa labiosa*). J Am Vet Med Assoc 207:1215–1217, 1995.
6. Iwama GK, McGeer JC, Pawluk MP: The effects of five fish anaesthetics on acid-base balance, hematocrit, blood gases, cortisol, and adrenaline in rainbow trout. Can J Zool 67:2065–2073, 1988.
7. Lewbart GA, Stone EA, Love NE: Pneumocystectomy in a Midas cichlid. J Am Vet Med Assoc 207:319–321, 1995.
8. Moyle PB, Cech JJ Jr: Fishes: An Introduction to Ichthyology. Englewood Cliffs, NJ, Prentice-Hall, pp 43–44, 1982.
9. Stoskopf MK: Anesthesia of pet fishes. *In* Bonagura JD (ed): Kirk's Current Veterinary Therapy XII. Philadelphia, WB Saunders, pp 1365–1369, 1995.
10. Stoskopf MK: Pain and analgesia in birds, reptiles, amphibians, and fish. Invest Ophth Vis Sci 35:775–780, 1994.
11. Stoskopf MK: Shark diagnostics and therapeutics: a short review. J Aquaricult Aquat Sci 5:33–43, 1990.
12. Williams TD, Christiansen J, Nygren S: A comparison of intramuscular anesthetics in teleosts and elasmobranchs. Proc Int Assoc Aquat Anim Med 24:6, 1993.

CHAPTER 24

Preventive Medicine Programs for Fish

BRENT R. WHITAKER

Many of the diseases and deaths commonly seen in captive fish are avoidable. The development of a comprehensive preventive medicine program, fine tuned to meet the needs of both the facility and the fishes kept, is a worthwhile investment of time, energy, and finances. Whether the fish are exotic species destined for display or food animals eventually to be harvested, the basic principles of disease avoidance, control, and monitoring remain the same.

When creating a preventive medicine program, it is most important to develop *reasonable* goals after considering the facilities, equipment, and personnel available. Every program should address the establishment and maintenance of animal records, quarantine procedures, environmental concerns, nutritional concerns, vaccination protocols, sanitation practices, and methods of disease surveillance. The veterinarian should involve individuals in the development of the preventive medicine program who will eventually be responsible for its implementation and execution. Doing so adds significantly to the quality of the program and is likely to lead to a greater level of compliance.

ANIMAL RECORDS

Well-organized, informative records provide an archive of useful information. Records formats range from handwritten files to computer files. Word processing programs require little expertise and time to develop a system for keeping animal records. The creation of a database program, however, requires greater forethought, time, and an understanding of computer programming, but it has the potential to provide more powerful searches and detailed reports. Both methods allow the input of both written text, as well as photographs, video, and audio, which can be useful in identifying individual fishes and in following the progression of a clinical case.

A variety of record topics such as food, mortality, water quality, medical, quarantine, and general husbandry should be applied to each group of fish and, where practical, to individual animals. Methods of individual identification among fish include unique markings, implantation of pit tags, freeze branding (elasmobranchs), and the less desirable spaghetti tag. Food records document the type, frequency, and amount of nutrients consumed. Fish typically eat 1% to 3% of their body weight daily, although this amount varies greatly among species, with some animals requiring much greater amounts of food to sustain their metabolic needs. It is common practice for aquaculture facilities to periodically weigh groups of fish to determine weight gain for food fed, enabling them to readjust diets to achieve maximum production economically. A sudden decrease in food consumption often precedes an obvious outbreak of disease and is sufficient cause to carry out a full examination of three to 10 fish from the group. Infestation of marine fish with the external protozoan *Cryptocaryon irritans*, for example, frequently causes a decline in nutritional intake 3 to 5 days before observation of the classic "white spot" lesions. Progressive anorexia, if noted early, allows the practitioner time to make the diagnosis through a skin scrape and gill biopsy, as well as to instigate an appropriate therapy that minimizes the loss of animals or decrease in production.

Water quality records should include an assessment of water temperature, pH, salinity, dissolved oxygen, alkalinity, ammonia, nitrite, and nitrate. Other additives, such as copper sulfate, should be tested for and all water changes documented. If ozone is used as a disinfectant (see Sanitation, Disinfection, and Sterilization), the oxidation reduction potential (ORP) should be monitored continuously by a controller capable of reducing delivery of the oxidant as levels exceed 400 mv. Hospital, quarantine, and newly set-up tanks should be tested daily until it is evident that the biologic filter is active and the system is stable. At that time, it is possible to reduce sampling to a weekly or biweekly schedule.

Deaths documented and graphed over time enable the identification of tanks experiencing animal loss greater than that which would be expected from attrition. Important data such as tank identification, date of mortality, species, and suspected cause of mortality are typically included. If a diagnosis of disease is made at a later date, mortality records are updated.

Medical records are essential, especially when a diagnosis is made and subsequent treatment prescribed. With growing concern by the Food and Drug Administration (FDA) on the use of chemotherapeutics in fish, it makes good sense to keep detailed and accurate records. Whether they represent an individual or group of fish, these records should reflect the practitioner's interpretation of history, examination, findings, assessment, and clinical plan. Details of medication use, including identification of the fish, the name of the drug and amount to be given, route of application, and duration of treatment, must be recorded. Each entry should be initialed by the attending veterinarian. When trained husbandry staff are to provide treatment, an appropriate form including the written prescription and daily instructions should be provided and kept on or near the tank. Those responsible for the treatment must then confirm successful completion of the task; report whether or not the animals are eating; increase surveillance of water quality, noting any abnormal water quality parameters; and provide any other relevant comments.

General husbandry records should be kept by persons caring for the fish on a daily basis. These should include comments on the behavior and apparent health of the animals, the addition or removal of animals from a tank, the biomass present within a given tank, as well as the amount and frequency of water changes. Other pertinent information should also be recorded including any previous disease diagnoses, the addition of new animals within the last 60 days, significant changes in environmental parameters, observations of social interaction, and the use of medications or other supplements. In many cases, these records also contain food and mortality information.

Quarantine records should include information such as the species and number of animals obtained, source of animals, date of arrival, tank identification, medications administered, food intake, water changes made, deaths, diagnosis of disease, and any other important observations. Monthly reports generated from all quarantine records not only allow an identification of trends but also allow the modification of quarantine protocols as needed.

QUARANTINE

The establishment of a quarantine program for newly acquired fish and invertebrates is an essential component of the preventive medicine program. The goal is to ensure that only healthy, well-adapted animals are placed into established populations. Standards for the quarantine of fish have been recommended by the American Zoo and Aquarium Association and provide an excellent foundation upon which to build a program tailored to the specific needs of a facility. Other references that are useful when developing a quarantine program include Herwig,[14] Blasiola,[3] Whitaker,[32, 34] Stoskopf,[29] and Whitaker et al.[35]

To be successful, a quarantine program requires teamwork between medical and husbandry staff. Tanks used for quarantine fish should be well removed from those housing established animals. Adequate space for each species must be provided to maintain excellent water quality and reduce aggression among tank mates. Removable decor provides ample hiding places, but can be readily moved to allow cleaning or the rapid capture of specimens. Strict hygiene practices minimize the risk that disease will be spread to other tanks or workers. Individual filtration should be provided for each quarantine unit, which may constitute one or more tanks. All animals sharing filtration, however, must be considered to be part of the same quarantine group because of the potential of passing waterborne pathogens. Separate equipment such as nets, filters, and siphons should be used for each system. When equipment must be shared, proper disinfection is essential (see Sanitation, Disinfection, and Sterilization). Workers should thoroughly wash hands and arms with a disinfectant soap before and after working in a quarantine tank.

Most fish entering quarantine are highly stressed. This is especially true for wild-caught fish, which must acclimate to the captive environment and diet. It is helpful to offer newly captured fish foods native to their natural environment while slowly introducing them to a more practical captive diet. Stress in fish produces a hormonal cascade, resulting in adaptive physiologic changes. Under natural conditions, the stressor and subsequent changes are usually brief, such as that experienced by the flounder evading a hungry predator. Prolonged stress such as that experienced by new arrivals, however, typically leads to a depletion of energy stores, loss of osmoregulatory function, and a decreased ability to fight opportunistic pathogens that are ubiquitous in their environment.[31] Bacterial, fungal, viral, and parasitic infections are therefore frequently seen in quarantine fish (Fig. 24–1). Because osmoregulatory function is impaired by stress, newly acquired marine fish are often placed in water of reduced salinity (16 to 25 ppt), whereas salt is often added to tanks holding freshwater species (2 to 10 ppt). The speed and extent to which salinity is altered depend on the values that are tolerated by the species. In comparison to wild-caught animals, captive-born fish experiencing the same stress response readily recover, reducing the likelihood that the physiologic changes will persist long enough to become maladaptive.

The quarantine period should last a minimum of 30 days, although this is often extended to 40 days or more because of the outbreak of disease or failure of the fish to feed well within the first week after arrival. Figure 24–2 shows computer-generated forms that can be modified for each group of fish entering quarantine. Through the use of these forms, general health of the group and response to therapeutics are easily followed. New arrivals are closely examined for evidence of disease. In cases of sensitive or small fish, this examination may consist only of a visual assessment to note the condition of the fins, respiratory rate, coloration, clarity of the eyes, and general behavior. The examination of larger fish and aquaculture species should also include a skin scrape, fin clip, and gill biopsy (Fig. 24–3) of three or more fish. This is especially important if fish are "flashing" (rubbing their body on the substrate or decor), have an elevated respiratory rate, are producing excessive amounts of mucus, or are showing other signs of disease. If bacterial septicemia is suspected, a blood sample should be collected for culture in tryptic soy broth. Specific treatments may be eliminated, added, or realigned, depending on findings of the clinical examination and previous experience.

As soon as possible, most species of fish are encouraged to eat a gelatin food. Once accepted, this provides an excellent route to provide medications without compromising the nitrifying bacteria responsible for biologic filtration. The decision to use chemotherapeutics

prophylactically is based on the likelihood that the fish are harboring potential pathogens such as ciliated and flagellated protozoans, monogenetic trematodes, cestodes, nematodes, and crustaceans. Recently caught fish may benefit by the addition of a broad-spectrum antibiotic, such as furazone-green, thus providing protection against stress-related bacterial illness that may be seen within approximately 14 days of arrival. Captive-born species or specimens purchased from a local pet shop that have already acclimated are less likely to require administration of an antibiotic. Unfortunately, the indiscriminate and improper use of chemicals, including antibiotics, in fish is widespread in the aquatic animal industry. Therefore, a full treatment history should be collected when purchasing fish from a collector or pet shop so that the quarantine program can be modified accordingly.

When selecting chemotherapeutics, their effects on the fish as well as their potential to harm life support performance, resulting in poor water quality, should be considered. Furthermore, there have been few scientific studies to guide the clinician in use of these drugs with fish. Dose, route, frequency, and duration are therefore empirically derived. Medications and dosages used successfully in quarantine for nonfood fishes at the National Aquarium in Baltimore are listed in Table 24–1.

Invertebrates and plants should also be quarantined a minimum of 30 days separate from any fish. Plants can transfer infective protozoal cysts or snails, which serve as intermediate hosts to numerous parasites of fishes. Countless outbreaks of parasitic disease have been attributed to the recent addition of invertebrates such as anemones, live rock, and corals. These animals serve as excellent vectors for parasitic cysts, which hatch and infect any fishes present. Eliminating the vertebrate host for a period of 30 days usually prevents the completion of parasitic life cycles, thus protecting the collection.

ENVIRONMENTAL CONSIDERATIONS

Fish have evolved specific physiologic mechanisms that enable them to survive in a great variety of environments. When fish are brought into captivity, it is crucial that the environmental requirements of individual species be considered. Improper environmental conditions are often the cause of death, either directly as the result of accumulated toxins such as ammonia, or indirectly through a stress-mediated reduction in immunologic function that culminates in disease. Suboptimal conditions may also lead to diminished growth rate and decreased levels of reproduction.[33] Environmental parameters to be considered include water quality, lighting, social structure, and the presence of excess noise.

Water Quality

Water quality parameters that should be monitored routinely include temperature, pH, dissolved oxygen, total and un-ionized ammonia, nitrite, nitrate, and any other

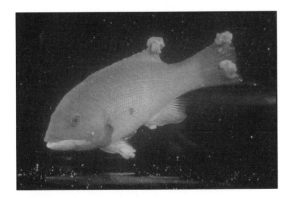

FIGURE 24–1. Lymphocystis, an iridovirus infection, is one of the commonly seen diseases in stressed fishes, especially new arrivals. (Photographed by George Grall, National Aquarium in Baltimore.)

FISH QUARANTINE

ARRIVAL DATE:	SOURCE:	QF
NO. OF FISH / SPECIES:		TANK NO.:
		VOL. (GAL.):

COMMENTS:

Date:

Treatment Day	1	2	3	4	5	6	7	8	9	10	11	12	13	14	15	16	17	18	19	20	21	22	23	24	25	26	27	28	29	30	31	32	33	34	35	36	37	38	39	40
Furazone Green	FG	FG	FG	FG	FG	FG	FG	FG	FG	FG																														
Copper-begin													CU	CU	CU	CU																								
Copper-therapy																	CU	CU	CU	CU	CU	CU	CU	CU	CU	CU	CU	CU	CU	CU	CU	CU	CU	CU	CU	CU				
Panacur								P	P															P	P															
Metronidazole																												MZ	MZ	MZ	MZ	MZ								
Praziquantal																																			PZ	PZ	PZ			
Carbon-ON											CB																											CB		
Carbon-OFF												CB																												CB
Water Change (%)																																								
Salinity (changes)																																								
Mortalities (no.)																																								
Food Intake (G,M,P)																																								

COMMENTS:

RELEASE DATE: BY:

DESTINATION:

A

QUARANTINE NOTES

MORTALITIES:

DATE	NO.	FISH	DATE	NO.	FISH	DATE	NO.	FISH	DATE	NO.	FISH

TREATMENTS / OBSERVATIONS / ROUNDS NOTES:

DATE	COMMENTS

B

FIGURE 24-2. Quarantine forms should be simple in design, easy to use, and able to archive large amounts of data in a small space. *A*, This form, used by the National Aquarium in Baltimore for the quarantine of marine fish, is a computer spread sheet that can be customized for each new group of fishes upon their arrival. Treatments are marked-out with an "X" as they are completed. *B*, Mortalities, as well as important observations and treatment changes are documented using this form. (From the National Aquarium in Baltimore.)

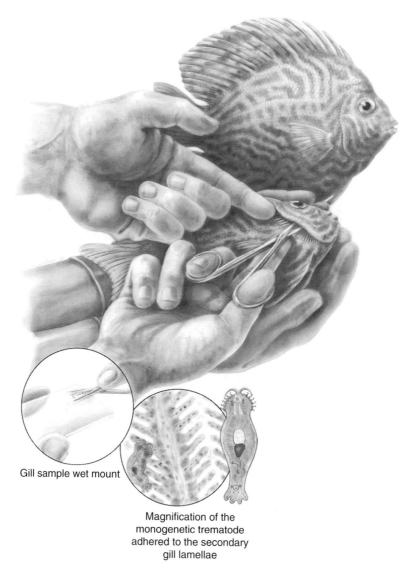

Gill sample wet mount

Magnification of the
monogenetic trematode
adhered to the secondary
gill lamellae

FIGURE 24–3. A gill biopsy requires only a small amount of tissue to survey for ectoparasites and damage to the lamellae. Excessive bleeding is rare, but can be stopped by using hemostats to quickly crush the tissue at the site of hemorrhage. (Drawn by Mark Wieber, Johns Hopkins University.)

chemicals, such as copper, that may be added to the water. If ozone, a powerful oxidant capable of reducing nitrogenous waste and destroying potentially pathogenic organisms, is used, then the oxidation-reduction potential (ORP) must also be measured.

As poikilothermous animals, fish depend on water temperature to maintain metabolic function. Some are able to tolerate a wide range of temperatures, whereas others have more specific requirements. Sudden changes or inappropriate temperatures can be detrimental for many species, causing decreased immune function, reduced digestion, and the inability to metabolize and utilize medications. Proper salinity, the measure of ionic concentration, is also important because fish have developed osmoregulatory mechanisms required to survive in their preferred environment.

Oxygen is needed by fish, nitrifying bacteria, and heterotrophic organisms responsible for the degradation of organic material. Increased temperature, increased salinity, or decreased atmospheric pressure reduces the ability to maintain dissolved oxygen in water. Increased opercular movement is indicative of respiratory distress resulting from hypoxia, septicemia, or damage to the gills. Gas bubble disease (Fig. 24–4) is recognized by the presence of air emboli within the tissues of the fish. It is most often caused by supersaturation of the water with air that has been forced into solution by cavitating pumps. Leaks within pipework or a low water level within the sump often provide a route for the addition of large amounts of air that are subsequently pressurized and forced into solution. Supersaturation can be avoided by designing the filtration system so that degassing automatically occurs. This can be accomplished by pumping water up to a biofilter located above the tank and allowing it to cascade down over media before returning to the tank. Additionally, returning water above the surface as a spray encourages the release of any excess gas, including carbon dioxide (which can cause a reduction in pH).

Ammonia, nitrite, chlorine, chloramines, ozone, and heavy metals such as copper and lead are all potential toxins. Ammonia is excreted by fish and produced by the breakdown of organic matter. It is typically measured as total ammonia nitrogen (TAN); however, it is the un-ionized form (NH_3) that is most toxic. Maintaining a lower pH and temperature favor the less toxic form of ammonia (NH_4^+) (Table 24–2). Excess nitrite, capable of causing methemoglobinemia, may be prevented in freshwater fish by adding salt to the system (6 parts chloride to 1 part nitrite) because chloride competes for the same binding site as nitrite. Maintaining an active nitrogen cycle through efficient biologic filtration is the best way to ensure that ammonia is rapidly converted to nitrite, and subsequently to relatively harmless nitrate.[33, 34] Care must be taken when antibiotics, dyes, and other chemicals are used because

TABLE 24–1. Medications to Consider for Use During Quarantine

Medication	Primary Indication	Route	Dose	Comments
Furazone Green (Dyna-Pet, Campbell, CA)	Broad-spectrum antibiotic used to prevent or treat bacterial disease in highly stressed fishes	Added to the water	Dose according to manufacturer's instructions	Activated carbon removes drug.
Oxytetracycline	Broad-spectrum antibiotic used to prevent or treat bacterial disease	Gel food PO	7 mg/g food SID 10 days 70 mg/kg SID 10–14 days	There is a detrimental effect on biofilter if used as a bath; there is growing resistance to this drug.
Metronidazole (Flagyl, Martec Pharmaceutical Inc., Kansas City, MO)	Flagellate protozoans such as *Hexamita*	Gel food Live brine shrimp	6.25–18 mg/g food 5 days Bathe live brine in 625 mg/100 ml of water for 15–20 minutes immediately before feeding for 5 days	Drug also acts as antibacterial; perform large water change following treatment.
		Bath	250 mg/10 gal water for 8 hours	
Fenbendazole*	Nematodes	Gel food	2.5 mg/g food for 2 days; repeat in 14 days	Drug is safe and effective anthelmintic with wide range of safety; it may be given for 3 consecutive days without adverse affects, although the sudden death of a large burden of nematodes can cause tissue damage or intestinal blockage.
		PO	50 mg/kg for 2 consecutive days; repeat in 14 days	
		Live brine shrimp	Bathe live brine shrimp in 400 mg/100 ml water for 15–20 minutes immediately before feeding; feed 2 consecutive days; repeat in 14 days	
Praziquantel (Droncit, Bayer†)	Trematodes, cestodes, and some acanthocephalans	Gel food	5–12 mg/g food fed for 3 consecutive days	Wide range of dosages have been reported to be safe and effective in fishes; while in bath, fishes should be monitored closely for signs of toxicity including lethargy, incoordination, and equilibrium loss.
		Live brine shrimp	Bathe live brine shrimp in 400 mg/100 ml water for 15–20 minutes immediately before feeding; feed 3 consecutive days	
		Bath	2–10 mg/L for up to 4 hours	
Malachite green	Protozoans, fungi	Bath	0.15–0.20 ppm every 3 days for 3 treatments	A 20%–50% water change is performed before each treatment; fine-scaled fishes such as tetras do not tolerate drug well and require use at half strength. Handle drug with care because it is mutagenic and teratogenic to humans.
Malachite green/ formalin	Protozoans, fungi	Bath	0.15 ppm malachite green plus 25 ppm formalin every 3 days for 3 treatments	As for malachite green; formalin is a potential carcinogen as well to humans.
Citrated copper sulfate	External protozoans, some monogeneans	Continuous bath	0.2 ppm for 14–21 days	Drug is safest used in marine systems. Use copper test kit daily; invertebrates, elasmobranches, and some teleosts are very sensitive to copper. Remove copper with activated carbon.

PO, per os.
*Panacur, Hoechst-Roussel Pharmaceutical, Somerville, NJ.
†Bayer Corporation, Shawnee Mission, KS.

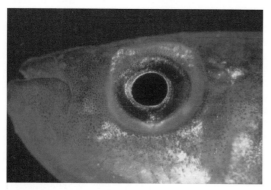

FIGURE 24–4. Air emboli in the conjunctiva of a killifish may be the result of supersaturation of the water with air. (Photographed by George Grall, National Aquarium in Baltimore.)

highly dependent upon pH and salinity and may therefore shift rapidly. For further information about the use of copper, refer to Cardeilhac and Whitaker[5] and Noga.[25] In older homes and buildings, copper and lead may leach from pipes, causing toxicity. This can be avoided by running the water for an extended period of time before its use in the aquarium system.

Periodic water changes, approximately 20% every 2 weeks, are used to remove nitrogenous waste, replenish buffers, and supply the macroelements and microelements required by fish. Goiter, for example, has been observed in fish that lack sufficient iodine in the water (Fig. 24–5). The inability to maintain the pH of the water without the extensive addition of buffers may also be indicative of depleted macroelements including calcium and magnesium. I have seen decreased immunologic ability, hypertrophy of "gill lamellae," and death of salt water teleosts and elasmobranchs exposed to chronic imbalances of calcium, magnesium, nickel, potassium, and sodium. Chlorine and chloramines are added to municipal water supplies for disinfection and must be removed before use in aquaria. These oxidizers are detrimental to fish because they cause damage to the gill lamellae and, at higher levels, they destroy blood cells and disrupt oxygen transfer by oxidizing hemoglobin to a steady state.[28] Dechlorination is achieved by passing water through activated carbon, aerating it overnight in a barrel, or using commercially available dechlorinators containing sodium thiosulfate. Chloramines, a combination of chlorine and ammonia, are dangerous to aquatic animals and more difficult to eliminate.[3] In addition to the chlorine component, ammonia must also be removed. This can readily be accomplished by circulating all new water through a

they may cause sudden death of the microbes responsible for biofiltration. For this reason, water in tanks receiving chemical treatment should be tested daily.

Heavy metals, such as citrated copper sulfate, may be deliberately added to tank water to control external parasites or algae growth. Therapeutic levels of copper (0.18 to 0.20 ppm) may cause anorexia or decreased immune function, and they are toxic to some species of fish and many invertebrates. The likelihood of toxicity can be minimized by adding doses of copper slowly over a period of several hours with a goal of reaching therapeutic levels in 3 days. A reliable copper test kit is essential and is best used at least twice daily because the equilibrium between free and bound copper is

TABLE 24–2. Percent of Total Ammonia in Un-Ionized Form for 10° to 30 C° and pH 6 to 8.5

Temperature °C	pH					
	6.0	6.5	7.0	7.5	8.0	8.5
10	.0186	.0589	.186	.586	1.83	5.56
11	.0201	.0637	.201	.633	1.97	5.99
12	.0218	.0688	.217	.684	2.13	6.44
13	.0235	.0743	.235	.738	2.30	6.92
14	.0254	.0802	.253	.796	2.48	7.43
15	.0274	.0865	.273	.859	2.67	7.97
16	.0295	.0933	.294	.925	2.87	8.54
17	.0318	.101	.317	.996	3.08	9.14
18	.0343	.108	.342	1.07	3.31	9.78
19	.0369	.117	.368	1.15	3.56	10.5
20	.0397	.125	.369	1.24	3.82	11.2
21	.0427	.135	.425	1.33	4.10	11.9
22	.0459	.145	.457	1.43	4.39	12.7
23	.0493	.156	.491	1.54	4.70	13.5
24	.0530	.167	.527	1.65	5.03	14.4
25	.0569	.180	.566	1.77	5.38	15.3
26	.0610	.193	.607	1.89	5.75	16.2
27	.0654	.207	.651	2.03	6.15	17.2
28	.0701	.221	.697	2.17	6.56	18.2
29	.0752	.237	.747	2.32	7.00	19.2
30	.0805	.254	.799	2.48	7.46	20.3

Adapted from Emerson K, Russo RC, Lund RE, Thurston RV: Aqueous ammonia equilibrium calculations: effect of pH and temperature. J Fish Res Board Can 32(12):2379–2383, 1975.

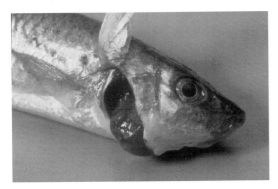

FIGURE 24–5. The operculum of this fish has been retracted, revealing an enlarged thyroid gland. Dietary and environmental deficiencies, or the presence of goitrogenic substances, may result in thyroid hyperplasia. (Photographed by George Grall, National Aquarium in Baltimore.)

canister filter charged with an ammonia-absorbing substrate, such as clinoptilolite, and activated carbon at least 24 hours before use.

Light

Proper photoperiod, spectrum, and intensity of light play an important role in maintaining the health of fish. The failure of timers regulating photoperiod has been associated with anorexia and the onset of parasitism in goldfish at the National Aquarium in Baltimore. Reproductive cycles of many fish are also known to be closely related to photoperiod.[18] Determining photoperiod may be particularly challenging for fish on display or kept in work areas where operating hours are in conflict with their natural daily cycle. Every effort should be made to provide fish with a consistent photoperiod wherein changes are implemented slowly over time.

Metal halide lights provide a spectrum of light required for the growth of many corals. To be effective, these lights need to be placed relatively close to the surface of the water, thus requiring fans and proper ventilation of the area to prevent unwanted warming of the water. Because the quality of light diminishes with age, these bulbs should be replaced every 6 months. Anecdotal reports suggest that natural sunlight may also help prevent and heal head and lateral line disease seen commonly in tangs and other marine teleosts (Fig. 24–6). It is unclear whether this is a direct effect of the sunlight or the consumption of algae that grows as a result of the natural light.

Social Structure

Interspecies and intraspecies aggression can lead to the onset of disease or to death. This is best avoided by understanding the behavioral demeanor of a species and its social structure. For example, wrasses tend to live alone or in pairs and can be aggressive toward other wrasses[21] as well as toward other fishes. Wrasses can change their sex from female to male, showing a great diversity of associated color patterns,[23] which may tempt hobbyists to keep more than is desirable in the space available. To avoid trauma or the onset of stress-related disease, only one sexually mature male, referred to as an alpha, terminal, or supermale, should be housed with a small number of females. As seen with wrasses, the social structure of a group of fish may change as animals mature. It is therefore important to plan for the future and dedicate space from the beginning that is adequate to meet the needs of the fish as it grows.

Adding new fish to an existing population may also disrupt established territories, resulting in elevated levels of stress and fighting. In some cases, it may be advantageous to add new fish at night or rearrange the decor just before an introduction. If an established and dominant fish is seen traumatizing newly added fishes, it sometimes helps to remove the aggressor just before the introduction of new animals. Once the new additions have settled in, the dominant fish can be reintroduced.[13]

Noise Pollution

Noise from pumps, filters, chillers, and other machinery may also provide stress for some fishes. Many fish are known to have auditory capabilities. The impact of noise on aquaculture species is suspected to be significant and is currently under investigation. It therefore makes good sense to isolate noise-producing equipment as far as possible from environments housing fishes.

Environmental Enrichment

Environmental enrichment is very important for many species of fish. Every attempt should be made to re-create a natural environment for the species kept. The challenge becomes even greater when mixing multiple species together. A survey of the literature and correspondence with knowledgeable individuals is strongly suggested before a person acquires a species for the first time. Clown fish, for example, do best when kept with anemones, with which they form a symbiotic rela-

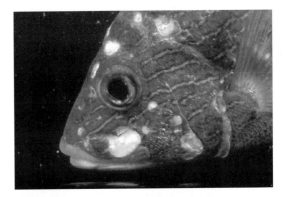

FIGURE 24–6. Natural sunlight and proper diet may play an important role in the prevention of ulcerated epidermal lesions associated with head and lateral line disease. (Photograph by George Grall, National Aquarium in Baltimore.)

tionship. Providing coral, rock, and other decor is not only pleasing to the aquarist but allows fish to find hiding places. In addition, live rock also provides many fish with a tasty variety of algae and invertebrates. Environmental enrichment contributes greatly to the reduction of stress and therefore disease.

NUTRITIONAL CONSIDERATIONS

Fish may be herbivorous, omnivorous, or carnivorous. Anatomically, each has a digestive tract modified to maximize both digestion and assimilation of a particular diet, thus providing the metabolic energy and nutrients required. For this reason, in many mixed species exhibits, the fish must be fed a variety of foods. Commercial pellets or flake food, gelatin diets, fish, grass shrimp, brine shrimp, clams, squid, algae, blackworms, and vegetables are commonly fed to captive fish.

Keeping fish healthy and robust requires an understanding of their basic nutritional requirements. Rock beauties (*Holacanthus tricolor*) for example, are sold commercially, but rarely do well in captivity because of their preferred diet of sponges. These animals are often thought to be grazing over the rocks and decor when they are actually starving to death. Other fish such as salmonids, which are fed high-fat diets, may become obese, resulting in an unhealthy fatty infiltration of the liver.[26] Appetite is an excellent indicator of fish health. A decline of intake over 2 to 5 days is significant and must not be ignored. When this occurs, several animals should be thoroughly examined and water quality parameters evaluated in an effort to determine the cause.

Food fed to fish must be of excellent quality, showing no signs of rancidity or other contamination. Many foods are frozen, extending shelf life and disrupting parasitic life cycles. The thawing of frozen products should occur in a refrigerator, with food being kept chilled until shortly before feeding. Allowing foods to thaw in water encourages the loss of water-soluble nutrients and should be discouraged. For this same reason, many fish benefit by small amounts of food fed frequently so that the food does not sit in the tank longer than 15 minutes before being consumed. Vitamin-enhanced gelatin foods are excellent because they can be quickly thawed, grated into any size needed, with minimal leaching of nutrients or incorporated medications. Flake and pelleted foods are often processed at high temperatures that may destroy vitamins and other nutrients. These products are frequently enhanced with vitamins and therefore the date of processing should be noted to ensure the feed is fresh when used. Both shelf life and storage conditions affect vitamin content of these foods.

When feeding fish, there are several important considerations to ensure good health. Fish are often fed 1% to 3% of their body weight, although individual animals occasionally require greater amounts of food than would be expected for the species. Those animals with extraordinary metabolic needs typically have chronic weight loss despite separation from the group and a hardy appetite. In such cases, increasing the amount of diet

offered by 5% to 10% every other day and monitoring body weight weekly are often rewarding. As poikilothermous animals, fish decrease their need for caloric intake as declining water temperatures slow metabolic pathways. Species of fish that experience a seasonal change in water temperature should therefore be fed accordingly. When feeding fish, the nutrient contributions of organisms present in their environment should be considered, minimizing the amount of food that must be offered as excess nutrients must be broken down and undergo nitrification. In recirculatory systems with a large number of fish or a compromised biofilter, a carefully controlled reduction in feeding for a short period of time may be necessary to correct poor water quality. This course of action must not be used on a continuous basis as a substitute for inadequate filtration because starvation or the outbreak of disease is likely to occur.

Marine fish acquire much of their fresh water from the foods that they eat. Prolonged periods of anorexia may therefore contribute to their dehydration. Many marine fish, especially elasmobranchs, can be encouraged to eat by providing fresh water via stomach tube every two to three days. After two to three administrations, several small fish or shrimp are blended with the water to produce a watery gruel.

The energy requirement for fish is less than that of warm-blooded animals because they do not generate their own internal body temperature, they exert little energy to maintain position and move, and they lose less energy in protein catabolism and excretion of nitrogenous wastes.[20] Caloric needs increase with growth, reproduction, physical exertion, and other conditions that influence metabolic demands.

Numerous vitamin and mineral deficiencies are documented in captive fish (Tables 24–3 and 24–4). Clinical signs associated with nutritional deficiencies are often nonspecific and include poor growth, loss of color, exophthalmos, anorexia, anemia, and ascites. Many fish require omega-3 fatty acids found in the oils of fish that consume marine and freshwater algae. Nonspecific signs of deficiency include reduced growth rate, tissue edema, fatty degeneration of the liver, decreased hemoglobin in red blood cells, fin erosions, and increased susceptibility to disease. Loss of consciousness or shock syndrome seen in excited rainbow trout is avoided by providing omega-3 fatty acids in their diet.[26, 27]

Improper or extended storage of foods can lead to the oxidation of lipids, reducing its nutritive value and causing the formation of pro-oxidative compounds that are toxic to fish.[20] Frozen fish, used to feed marine teleosts and elasmobranchs, typically contain 20% to 25% polyunsaturated fatty acids, which readily become rancid over time or when handled improperly.[11, 20] Vitamin E, an antioxidant that is important to cell membrane stability and function as well as immune function,[2] should therefore be supplemented to diets containing frozen fish. Similarly, thiaminase found in the tissues of most fish used for food destroys thiamine, increasing the likelihood of central nervous system disorders in animals consuming them. The routine addition of thiamine (25 to 35 mg/kg fish feed) and vitamin E (100 IU/kg fish feed) to diets containing frozen fish has been recommended for marine mammals[11] and makes good

TABLE 24–3. Clinical Findings Associated with Vitamin Deficiency in Fish

Vitamin	Symptoms
Fat Soluble	
Vitamin A	Ascites, edema, exophthalmia, hemorrhagic kidneys, poor growth, depigmentation, corneal thinning, retinal degeneration
Vitamin D	Poor growth, tetany of white skeletal muscle, impaired calcium homeostasis
Vitamin E	Reduced survival; poor growth; ascites; ceroid in liver, spleen, and kidney; exophthalmia; pericardial edema, poor growth, red blood cell fragility, variable-sized erythrocytes, anemia, nutritional muscular dystrophy
Vitamin K	Anemia, coagulation time prolonged, lipid peroxidation
Water Soluble	
Vitamin B	
Pantothenic acid	Clubbed gills, prostration, loss of appetite, necrosis of jaw, barbels, and fins, flared opercula, gill exudate, lethargy, poor growth
Riboflavin	Poor appetite, anemia, poor growth, corneal vascularization, cloudy lens, photophobia, darkened coloration, hemorrhage in eyes, striated constrictions of abdominal wall, abdominal pigmentation of the iris
Thiamine	Poor appetite, muscle atrophy, convulsions, instability and loss of equilibrium, edema, poor growth
Biotin	Loss of appetite, lesions on colon and skin, muscle atrophy, dark coloration, death, poor growth, spastic convulsions, erythrocytic fragmentation, ascites
Pyridoxine	Loss of appetite, ascites, ataxia, convulsions, rapid and gasping breathing, flexing of opercles, rapid onset of rigor mortis, weight loss, nervous disorders, anemia
Folic Acid	Anemia, anorexia, ascites, dark coloration, exophthalmia, fragility of caudal fin, lethargy, pale gills, poor growth
Cyanocobalamin	Anorexia, low hemoglobin, fragmentation of erythrocytes, macrocytic anemia
Choline	Poor growth, poor food conversion, hemorrhagic kidney and intestine
Inositol	Poor growth, distended stomach, increased gastric emptying time, skin lesions, anorexia
Niacin	Loss of appetite, lesions on colon, jerky motion, edema of stomach and colon, muscle spasms while resting, poor growth, lethargy, photophobia, swollen gills, high mortality rate
Vitamin C (ascorbic acid)	Anorexia, impaired collagen production, impaired wound healing, scoliosis, lordosis with dislocated vertebrate and focal hemorrhage, poor growth, ocular lesions, hemorrhagic skin, liver, kidney, intestine, and muscle

(Data from references 12 and 20.)

sense for fish as well. Supplementation with ascorbic acid is also important because many fish cannot synthesize this vitamin that aids in wound repair, bone formation, and resistance to disease. Channel catfish, for example, have been shown to be more susceptible to the bacterium *Edwardsiella ictaluri* when fed diets deficient in vitamin C,[20] whereas rainbow trout fed 5 to 10 times the growth requirement showed improved humoral antibody production when challenged with *Vibrio anguillarum*.[22] To be safe, the addition of a multivitamin is also prudent when preparing diets for teleosts, elasmobranchs, and invertebrates.

Many ions including calcium, zinc, iodine, selenium, sodium, chloride, and potassium are obtained by fish from their diet or the water in which they live. Serious imbalances or deficiencies of macroelements within the water can lead to increased disease and mortality rates. Samples from large aquariums, where infrequent water changes are performed, should be analyzed monthly with an atomic spectrophotometer to determine the presence of macroelements. In some cases, corrections can be made by directly adding the appropriate amount of minerals to the water.

Thyroid hyperplasia or goiter is a common disorder observed in captive sharks. A pathognomonic swelling of the thyroid gland and the lack of dietary supplementation with calcium iodate or potassium iodide is sufficient to make a presumable diagnosis. This condition is readily treated and subsequently prevented by providing sharks with 10 mg/kg body weight potassium iodine once weekly[30] or calcium iodate in their food. Mazurri (PMI Feeds, St. Louis, MO) has developed a multivitamin for elasmobranchs that provides 250 mg calcium iodate for each half pound of food fed.

VACCINATIONS

In recent years, there have been efforts to develop vaccinations for many of the viral, bacterial, and parasitic diseases that commonly affect aquaculture and aquarium fish. Research efforts have resulted in vaccines that provide better protection, longer periods of immunity, and improved methods of administration.[24] In the past, for example, the vaccination of fish for vibriosis led to apparent immunosuppression, allowing the onset of bacterial infection before protective immunity could be established. Recent findings, however, show that the concurrent administration of a long-lasting amoxicillin at the time of vaccination appears to be protective.[15] Currently, very few vaccines are commercially available for fish. Of these, enteric red-mouth (*Yersinia ruckeri*) and vibriosis (*Vibrio anguillarum*, *Vibrio ordalii*, and *Vibrio salmonicida*) are highly efficacious, whereas that for furunculosis (*Aeromonas salmonicida*) offers limited protection.[7, 8] Newman[24]

TABLE 24–4. Summary of Mineral Activities and Symptoms of Deficiency in Fish

Mineral Element	Principal Metabolic Activities	Associated Deficiency Symptoms
Calcium	Bone and cartilage formation; blood clotting; muscle contraction; cell membrane permeability; calcium and phosphorus metabolic activities closely related	Anorexia; poor mineralization of bone; skeletal deformities (lordosis); reduced growth and feed conversion
Phosphorus	Bone formation; important constituent of cell membranes; necessary for energy-producing reactions in cell; essential to muscle and nervous tissue metabolism	Those listed for calcium; decreased hematocrit in catfish
Magnesium	Enzyme cofactor extensively involved in the metabolism of fats, carbohydrates, and proteins; essential to skeletal tissue metabolism and neuromuscular transmission	Loss of appetite; poor growth and skeletal deformities; tetany; cataracts; increased mortality rate
Sodium	Primary monovalent cation of intercellular fluids; involved in acid-base balance and osmoregulation	Not defined in fish because of abundance in environment and foods in water; inability to osmoregulate at very low concentrations for most saltwater teleosts and elasmobranchs, resulting in death
Potassium	Primary monovalent cation of intracellular fluid; involved in nerve action and osmoregulation	Not defined in fish because of abundance in environment and foods
Chloride	Primary monovalent anion in cellular fluids; component of digestive juice (HCl); acid-base balance	Not well defined in fish because of abundance in environment and foods
Sulfur	Integral part of sulfur amino acids and collagen; involved in detoxification of aromatic compounds	Not well defined in fish
Iron	Essential constituent of heme compounds such as hemoglobin and myoglobin; constituent of heme enzymes including cytochromes, peroxidases, catalases; essential to other compounds such as transferrin, ferritin, and flavin	Microcytic hypochromic anemia; poor growth; diarrhea
Copper	Component of heme in hemocyanin found in mollusks and crustaceans; associated with cytochrome oxidase, involved in electron transport chain and ceroloplasmin; component of lysyl oxidase, which promotes cross-linking of elastin and oxidase, and dopamine beta-hydroxylase needed for catecholamine production; cofactor in tyrosinase needed for melanin production and ascorbic acid oxidase	Not well defined for fish; poor growth; cataract formation
Manganese	Cofactor for arginase and certain other metabolic enzymes; involved in bone formation and erythrocyte regeneration	Poor growth; skeletal abnormalities; poor hatchability of eggs
Cobalt	Metal component of cyanocobalamin (B_{12}). Prevents anemia; involved in C_1 and C_3 metabolism	Not well defined in fish; possible anemia
Zinc	Component of many metalloenzymes regulating metabolic processes involving protein, carbohydrate, and lipid metabolism; essential for insulin structure and function; cofactor of carbonic anhydrase	Not well defined in fish; cataracts; decreased growth; fin and skin erosions; reduced hatchability of eggs
Selenium	Component of glutathione peroxidase, which protects membranes from oxidative damage by destroying hydrogen peroxide and hydroperoxides; protects against heavy metal toxicity	Poor growth; together with vitamin E deficiency can result in muscular dystrophy in fish
Iodine	Constituent of thyroxine; regulates oxygenases and reductases	Thyroid hyperplasia
Molybdenum	Cofactor of xanthine, oxidase hydrogenases and reductases	Not well defined in fish
Chromium	Involved in collagen formation and regulation of the rate of glucose metabolism	Not well defined in fish
Fluorine	Component of bone apatite	Not well defined in fish

(Data from references 17 and 20.)

provides an excellent review of bacterial vaccines. Efforts to develop a vaccine for cryptocaryon have met with limited success. There are several companies that will attempt to produce custom autogenous vaccines from an infectious agent provided by the client.

The following factors must be considered before determining to use a vaccine: the magnitude of animal loss if the vaccine is not used, the ease of obtaining the fish for inoculation and potential loss of animals resulting from the procedure, the most efficacious route of vaccine administration, and the overall cost in manpower and supplies. Environmental conditions and the general health of the fish also have a significant impact on the successful establishment and duration of protective immunity. Unlike mammals, fish are more dependent upon on nonspecific defense mechanisms than on specific immune responses to combat disease. Even though fish injected with a bacterin may maintain specific antibody titers beyond a year, their nonspecific defense mechanisms may be shortlived.[2]

Vaccines are commonly administered via immersion, injection, or feed. Oral administration has not been as successful for some vaccines as other routes. Injection offers the highest level of protection when used concurrently with adjuvants, but it can be labor intensive as well as stressful to the fish. Immersion of fish in a vaccine bath reduces the level of stress on the animals yet still produces high levels of protection. Because the fish must be caught and placed in a bath, dip, or shower, this commonly used aquaculture technique is not feasible for most aquarium fish. Exposure of fish by adding the vaccine directly to the tank or raceway can be done with some vaccines, although the level and duration of immunization may be less than that obtained by other methods.[24] The protection afforded by oral inoculation, which would work well with aquarium fish, has been disappointing.[16]

The use of immunostimulants, adjuvants, and vaccine carriers to protect fish against disease is under investigation. Immunostimulants increase the uptake of vaccines and singularly may enhance nonspecific defense mechanisms, preventing high mortality rates if applied just before disease outbreaks. This is most effective in diseases that are cyclical and therefore predictable. When mixed with a vaccine, adjuvants induce a greater level of specific immune responses as well as stimulate nonspecific defenses. Their use may reduce the dose of vaccine needed, increase absorption efficiency, cause sustained release and life of antigen, and allow the use of vaccines in colder temperatures. Vaccine carriers may aid the uptake and efficacy of bacterins.[2]

The use of vaccines in aquaculture to protect against disease makes good sense, although further research is needed to provide a greater number of safe, efficacious, and economically sound products. In large aquaria, however, the routine administration of a vaccine currently provides questionable benefit. Improving the protective immunity provided by oral vaccines against bacteria such as *Aeromonas hydrophila* and *Vibrio* species, as well as developing methods to protect animals against commonly observed protozoal infections, would be especially beneficial to many aquarium fish.

SANITATION, DISINFECTION, AND STERILIZATION

Sanitation refers to those measures taken to promote health, whereas disinfection implies a destruction of pathogenic microorganisms and their toxins or vectors. Sterilization refers to the destruction of all microorganisms in or about an object.[19] Developing a program that ensures proper attention is given to sanitation, disinfection, and sterilization protects not only fish but also human workers. Practices commonly used to reduce the risk of infection to fish and humans include adequate water treatment and proper hygiene when handling animals or working in their tanks.

Several methods are currently used to remove potential pathogens and toxins from water to reduce the likelihood of illness. These include ozone, ultraviolet light, and activated carbon. Ozone is a powerful oxidant capable of reducing nitrogenous waste, destroying potentially pathogenic organisms, and removing suspended organic materials that can cause turbidity. It is one of the best options available to improve water quality and prevent the outbreak of disease. Improper use of this gas, however, can lead to oxidation of tissues and death in the fish. Every precaution must be taken to ensure that no residual ozone be allowed to contact the fish. Excessive ozonization of water is suspected when ORP levels approach 500 mv, the water is crystal clear, and the characteristic smell of ozone, reminiscent of a heavily used photocopy machine, is present. Clinical signs of intoxication may include the sudden death of apparently healthy fish, respiratory distress, lethargy, incoordination, or a change in coloration indicative of severe stress. Ozone should not be applied directly to the main tank, but is better used injected into a contact chamber such as a protein skimmer or baffle board contacter, where dose, contact time, and flow rate of the water can be varied.[1] Proper degassing before the return of water to the main system is essential to ensure the safety of the animals.

Ultraviolet light has long been used and can be very effective at reducing bacterial populations within water that is free of suspended solids. Strict attention must be paid to match the appropriate ultraviolet light system to the amount of water that must be treated. The rate of water flow and distance of the pathogen from the bulb are critical factors. Bulbs should be changed every 6 months because their effectiveness rapidly declines with use despite the fact that they continue to produce light. Routine cleaning of the bulb is also necessary to maximize irradiation of pathogens. In effect, the name "ultraviolet light sterilizer" is a misnomer because it implies that all microorganisms are killed. This is highly unlikely under most applications and tends to invoke a false sense of security in persons purchasing these expensive systems. Constant attention and a program of preventive maintenance for the ultraviolet light sterilizer is necessary to achieve the desired results. When combined with ozonization, ultraviolet sterilization is most effective. In addition, the combination of both systems results in some level of protection being provided if either system fails.

Activated carbon has long been used in conjunction with other methods of chemical filtration to remove potential toxins and pathogens from water. It is relatively cheap and is easily placed into canister, bucket, or rapid sand filters. When adding medications to water, the use of activated carbon must be discontinued because it readily removes most chemicals.

Where possible, tanks should be designated as quarantine, hospital, or general holding. Separate equipment

TABLE 24–5. Commonly Used Disinfectants

Disinfectant	Use	Dose	Advantages	Disadvantages
Sodium hypochlorite—chlorine	Net dips; general disinfection of tanks and equipment	1%–2% Solution for 15–20 minutes; prepare daily for maximum effect	Inexpensive and readily available; kills most bacteria, viruses, and fungi	Very toxic to fish Inactivated by organic debris Inactivated by heat Readily destroys nets in a short period of time Less effective in hard water
Sodium hydroxide and teepol	Powerful disinfectant used in earthen, concrete, and butyl-lined ponds; fiberglass tanks and equipment; footbaths	1% Sodium hydroxide mixed with 1% teepol; apply 1 gallon/ 2 m^2 to dried earthen ponds and allow to stand several days, then fill and flush with fresh water for several days. Dips—renew when pH goes below 11	Kills bacteria, viruses, protozoa; organics do not inactivate; detergent teepol enhances penetration into soil and concrete	Extremely caustic—wear protective clothing, including self-contained breathing apparatus Corrosive to metals
Iodophores	General disinfection of nets and other equipment Footbaths Disinfection of eggs	General disinfection: 250 ppm available iodine Net dip and equipment—soak for 15–20 minutes Treatment of salmonid eggs—100 ppm of iodophor compound buffered to a pH of 6–7.5	Less destructive to nets Effective against bacteria, fungi, and viruses, including infectious pancreatic necrosis, viral hemorrhagic septicemia, and infectious hematopoietic necrosis Not affected by hard water	Rapidly inactivated by organic debris Stains surfaces, clothing, and equipment Extremely toxic to fish Some strains of *Pseudomonas* are resistant Inactivated by sunlight and heat
Quaternary ammonium compounds (Roccal-D)	Disinfection of equipment and tanks Net dips Foot baths	Use according to manufacturer's recommendation; prepare daily	Effective against bacteria and many viruses Cost effective	Not effective against fungi, bacterial spores, or mycobacteria Inactivated by high levels of organic debris *Pseudomonas* tends to be resistant
Chlorhexidine gluconates	Disinfection of equipment Foot baths	Use according to manufacturer's recommendation; prepare daily	Effective against many bacteria, fungi, and viruses Causes little corrosion of materials	Not effective against many gram-negative bacteria including *Pseudomonas* Not effective against bacterial spores or mycobacteria Does not kill hydrophilic viruses Organic debris reduces effectiveness Expensive
Alcohols	Disinfection of equipment and tanks	70% Ethyl alcohol sprayed onto cleaned surfaces and allowed to stand a minimum of 20 minutes	Broad-spectrum disinfectant effective against lipophilic and hydrophilic viruses Currently the disinfectant of choice against atypical mycobacteria Inexpensive and readily available	Fumes may be irritating and are flammable

(Data from references 6 and 10.)

such as nets, filters, airstones, heaters, and siphons should be available for each system. When equipment must be shared, disinfectant baths made daily are effective in preventing the spread of potential contagion (Table 24–5). To achieve disinfection, most disinfectants require that equipment be left to soak in an active solution for a minimum of 15 to 20 minutes. For this reason, more than one set of tools should always be available. Following the disinfectant bath, equipment is rinsed with fresh water and allowed to dry, providing

further insurance that potential pathogens are eliminated. Formalin should not be used for net disinfection because of its potential toxic and carcinogenic effects to workers.

Aquatic environments should also be kept clean of organic debris. Organic matter such as decaying plant material and uneaten food should be removed daily. Most importantly, ill or dead fish must be removed immediately before they are consumed by tank mates.

Foot baths placed at the entrance to the animal

facility as well as hospital, quarantine, general holding, and food preparation areas are recommended to prevent the potential spread of infective agents via footware. These baths should contain a disinfectant, such as sodium hydroxide, that is not readily inactivated by organic debris.[10] Foot baths should be changed daily or more frequently if needed.

Typically, the transmission of disease between animals and humans is referred to as zoonosis. Many bacteria with zoonotic potential have been isolated from fish. Those most commonly found are listed in Table 24–6. A veterinary medical surveillance program including the identification of potentially zoonotic pathogens as well as the development of health and safety protocols minimize the risk of human infection. Proper hygienic practices are essential in maintaining good human health. Table 24–7 lists precautions that can be taken to reduce the likelihood of zoonotic infection.

DISEASE SURVEILLANCE

Disease surveillance is an important component of every preventive medicine program. Fish should be assessed on a daily basis for changes in behavior and condition. Close scrutiny of records and communication with persons providing daily care for the fish is essential to success. If recognized early, warning signs such as a reduction in food intake, abnormal behavior (e.g., failing to remain with the group), increased respiratory effort, increased mucus production, and rubbing on the substrate and decor can be immediately investigated. An easily performed skin scrape and gill clip (see Fig. 24–3) allows the rapid identification of external parasites, as well as some bacterial, fungal, and viral infections. When bacterial septicemia is suspected, blood should be collected aseptically for culture and a complete blood count. Although fish pathogens typically take 2 to 5 days to grow at an optimal temperature of 25°C, examination of blood smears may readily show the presence of bacteria or blood parasites. If the patho-

TABLE 24–6. Bacterial Pathogens of Fish with Zoonotic Potential

Aeromonas hydrophila
Atypical mycobacteria
   Mycobacterium fortuitum
   Mycobacterium marinum
   Mycobacterium chelonae
Campylobacter species
Edwardsiella tarda
Enterotoxic *Escherichia coli*
Erysipelothrix species
Legionella pneumophila
Pseudomonas species
Salmonella species
Vibrio parahemolyticus
Vibrio vulnificus
Vibrio fluvialis
Yersinia enterocolitica

TABLE 24—7. Suggested Practices to Reduce the Risk of Zoonotic Infection

Animal Care Staff

Any open wounds are covered preferably using a bandage or water-tight gloves.
Proper hygiene—personnel wash well after handling animals or working in their environment; when handling fish, powder-free latex gloves should be worn.
Immunosuppressed individuals should minimize exposure to fish and tank water.
Ill employees should not come in contact with animals or animal environments.
Proper first aid is administered immediately if injury occurs.

Laboratory Staff

Protective clothing such as laboratory coats are worn while working in the laboratory.
All open wounds are covered.
Proper hygiene—personnel wash well after handling samples; powder-free latex gloves are recommended and essential during necropsy.
Biologic hoods are used when working with microbes.
Immunosuppressed individuals should avoid exposure to potential pathogens.
Ill employees should not work with potentially pathogenic samples.
There should be no eating or drinking in the laboratory.
Food is not stored in the same refrigerator as biologic samples.
Proper first aid is administered immediately if injury occurs.

Divers in Large Aquaria

All divers should receive an annual physical examination.
Proper first aid is administered immediately if injury occurs.
Divers must be informed of possible zoonotic diseases as they are identified.
Immunosuppressed or ill individuals should avoid exposure to potential pathogens.

gen is identified early, a well-planned and proper therapeutic regimen can be developed that minimizes the loss of fish.

A complete and timely necropsy of fish that die or appear moribund is an essential component of disease surveillance. Specimens should be submitted in a small amount of tank water and examined as quickly as possible because populations of parasites and bacteria may change after death of the fish. A skin scrape and gill clip should be collected and viewed immediately because many external parasites are short-lived or abandon the host once death has occurred. A thorough gross examination, including the assessment of squash preparations from each organ, often provides the investigator with valuable information. These are prepared by collecting a small portion of tissue on a glass slide and then squashing it gently with a cover slip. When appropriate, cultures should be taken from the liver, kidney, spleen, and brain. Tissues including gill, skin, skeletal muscle, brain, heart, swim bladder, liver, gall bladder, spleen, stomach, intestine, head and posterior kidney, and gonad are collected for histopathologic study. Specimens are best preserved by placing them in 10% buffered formalin. Alternatively, some laboratories prefer the use of Bouin's solution for 24 hours followed by 70%

TABLE 24–8. General Anatomy of the Fish and Commonly Associated Diseases

Tissue	Location	Function	Disease
Gills	Bilaterally located beneath the operculum, just caudal to the mouth	Respiration, osmoregulation, and excretion. Oxygen is absorbed and CO_2 excreted. Ammonia is excreted via the gills. Chloride cells are present and assist in osmoregulation and mineral balance	Protozoa (*Costia, Oodinium, Ichthyophthirius,* trichodinids, *Scyphidia, Trichophrya, Cryptocaryon, Chilodonella),* monogenea, crustacia, bacteria (*Flexibacter,* BKD), fungal (branchiomycosis), epitheliocystis
Skin	External covering including scales, epidermis, dermis, and hypodermis	Osmotic, immunologic, and physical barrier	Protozoa (*Costia, Oodinium, Tetrahymena, Epistylus, Uronema, Ichthyophthirius, Cryptocaryon,* trichondinids, *Scyphidia, Trichophrya, Chilodonella,* myxospora, microsporidea), monogenea, digenetic metacercaria, leeches, crustacea (*Argulus, Lernea),* bacteria (*Aeromonas, Vibrio),* viral (*Lymphocystis),* fungal (*Saprolegnia)*
Brain	Bony skeleton of head	Controls voluntary and involuntary functions	Bacterial abscesses (*Edwardsiella tarda),* viral (herpes virus of channel catfish), myxosporeans such as *Myxobolus cerebralis* in salmonids
Heart	Cranial coelom adjacent to gills and anterior to liver	Two-chambered organ that circulates blood	Larval tapeworms, granulomas, bacterial infection
Liver	Brownish-red organ in the anterior coelom	Metabolic functions—assists digestion, filtration, and storage	Myxospora, metacercaria of digenetic trematodes, encysted nematodes, cestodes, bacteria (BKD, PKD, mycobacterial granulomas), viral (IHN, CCVD)
Gall bladder	Associated with the liver	Holds bile and enzymes for the digestion of food; larger in anorexic fish	Hexamita and spironucleus, sporozoans (marine fish)
Spleen	Found caudal to the liver in the region of the stomach	Site of red blood cell production and storage. Filtration of blood. Melanomacrophage centers increase in number under conditions of chronic stress or disease	Bacterial (mycobacterial granulomas, BKD), viral (IHN)
Swim bladder	Glistening white sac in dorsal coelom	Buoyancy and balance	Nematodiasis, bacterial infection, myxosporidia
Gastrointestinal	Coelomic cavity	Digestion and absorption of nutrients. Length and structure varies with diet	Protozoa (*Hexamita, Cryptobia, Oodinium, Opalina,* coccidia), monogenea, digenea, cestodes, nematodes, thornyheaded worms, bacterial granulomas (*Mycobacteria, Nocardia),* fungal (*Saprolegnia, Candida),* viral (IPN, IHN, CCVD)
Kidney			
Head kidney	Anterior to air sac and dorsal to heart just caudal to head	Blood cell production	
Posterior kidney	Posterior dorsal aspect of coelom adjacent to vertebral column	Excretory function	Protozoa, myxosporidia (*Mitrospora, Sphaerospora),* bacterial (granulomas—*Mycobacterium, Nocardia;* acute septicemia—*Aeromonas, Vibrio, Pseudomonas;* BKD), fungal (*Ichthyophonus)*
Gonads	Organs not readily identified in immature fish. Testes associated with distal large intestine. Eggs may fill a good portion of the coelomic cavity.	Reproduction	Microsporidea (*Plistophora ovariae),* coccidia, bacteria (*Mycobacterium, Nocardia),* systemic fungal infections (*Ichthyophonus)*
Skeletal muscle	Substantial muscle mass along backbone and caudal to coelom	Movement of fish	Protozoa (microsporidia—*Plistophora hyphessobryconis* of neon tetras and angelfish, myxospora), digenetic metacercaria, nematode larvae

BKD, bacterial kidney disease; CCVD, channel catfish virus disease; IHN, infectious hepatic necrosis; PKD, proliferative kidney disease.
Adapted from Whitaker BR: Quarantine and post mortem examination. Proceedings of the North American Veterinary Conference, Orlando, FL, pp 635–637, 1992.

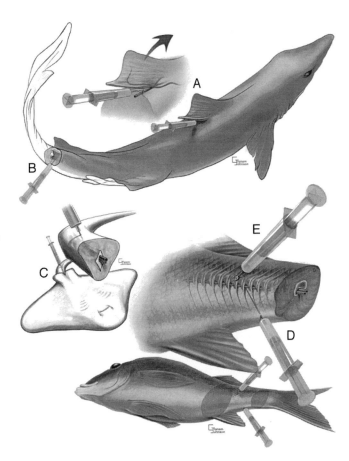

FIGURE 24–7. Phlebotomy sites: Minimal restraint is needed to obtain a slow but steady blood draw from vessels at the base of the dorsal fin *(A)*. Blood may also be obtained from sharks, rays, and fish using a ventral approach to the caudal tail vein *(B,C,D)*. On larger fish, the lateral approach to the caudal vein may simplify the procedure and minimize tissue trauma *(E)*. (Drawn by Graham Johnson, Johns Hopkins University, 1996.)

isopropyl alcohol because it provides decalcification, especially important when small whole fish are submitted, in addition to excellent fixation. Table 24–8 provides a list of commonly found pathogens.

Upon entering and before exiting quarantine, several fish from each group should be thoroughly examined for signs of disease. At a minimum, a skin scrape and gill clip should be performed on a reasonable percentage of the population. If large numbers of commercial or schooling fishes are concerned, it makes good sense to carry out a full necropsy on 3 to 5 randomly selected fish. When purchasing aquaculture species, health certification by a reputable laboratory may reduce the risk of importing disease.

The performance of routine physical examinations of select fish should also be considered. The potential benefit of information gained must be weighed against any potential danger to the fish or personnel. The examination should begin with observation of the fish through the tank glass to gain an appreciation of the animals' behavior and ability to maintain equilibrium. With proper facility design, available equipment, and knowledgeable staff, some fish, including many sharks, can safely be collected for examination. Once the fish are restrained in a well-oxygenated holding container, a complete physical examination can be carried out, which should include a thorough assessment of the skin

and scales, the eyes, the gills, the oral cavity, the teeth, the coelom, and genitourinary apparatus. Blood is collected for a complete blood count and serum chemistries from the caudal coccygeal vessel in teleosts and elasmobranchs. This can be approached either ventrally or, in larger fishes, laterally. Blood may also be collected from the base of the dorsal fin in elasmobranchs (Fig. 24–7). Alcohol should *not* be used to clean the site because it can be very caustic to their tissues. Fish cells are fragile and rupture easily, producing "smudge cells," which make interpretation of the sample difficult. Steps that help reduce the number of smudge cells include using ethylenediaminetetraacetic acid (EDTA) as an anticoagulant, avoiding the discharge of blood through the needle into a vacuum tube, and preparing blood smears immediately after collection by using clean glass slides. Adding 10 to 20 μl of bovine albumin to a separate EDTA Microtainer (microliter brand tube, Becton Dickinson) before the addition of 200 to 300 μl of blood may be helpful if the aforementioned methods do not yield acceptable results. This tube is used for the preparation of blood smears only; all other complete blood count parameters are performed on the tube containing EDTA without albumin. A May-Grunwald/Wright-Giemsa stain (Table 24–9) produces excellent cellular definition, easing interpretation. A summary of fish blood cell morphology and function is presented in

TABLE 24–9. May-Grunwald/Wright-Giemsa Stain

Preparation of Stains

May-Grunwald stock solution—Dissolve 0.25 g May-Grunwald stain in 100 ml methanol and allow to stand for 1 week. Filter prior to use.

Wright-Giemsa working solution—Mix Wright-Giemsa stain with distilled water at a ratio of 1 part Wright-Giemsa stain to 5 parts water.

Carry Out on a Slide Rack

Step 1: Flood slide with May-Grunwald stock solution for 3 minutes.

Step 2: Without rinsing, add equal volumes May-Grunwald stock solution and distilled water for 10 minutes.

Step 3: Without rinsing, flood slide with Wright-Giemsa working solution for 15 minutes.

Carry Out in Coplin Jars

Step 4: Distilled water for 3 dips
Step 5: Acetone for 3 dips
Step 6: Xylene or other clearing agent for 3 dips
Step 7: Xylene or other clearing agent for 3 dips

Adapted from National Aquarium in Baltimore: Protocol for May-Grunwald/Wright Giemsa Stain for Blood Smears.

TABLE 24–10. The Morphology of Fish Blood Cells Prepared with Wright's Stain and Their Associated Functions

Cell Type	Morphologic Characteristics	Function	Comments
Erythrocyte	*Mature cells:* oval to ellipsoid in shape; central oval to round nucleus with dark purple, densely clumped chromatin; nonhomogeneous pale eosinophilic cytoplasm *Immature cells:* rounded; central nucleus with smooth to reticulated chromatin; small amount of basophilic cytoplasm	Transport oxygen and carbon dioxide	Size and number vary among species. There is slight to moderate polychromasia and anisocytosis is normal.
Lymphocyte	Small with round or irregular shape; great nuclear-to-cytoplasmic ratio; dark purple nucleus with coarse chromatin clumping; homogeneous thin blue cytoplasm	Cellular and humoral immunity, antigenic stimulation leads to immunoglobulin production and T-lymphocyte activation	Most lymphocytes found are small and mature although immature cells and plasma cells may also be present; stress may cause lymphopenia.
Granulocytes	Dogfish *(Scyliorhinus canicula)* G1—Eccentric, irregular, nonlobed nucleus; round to oval eosinophilic granules G2—Indented to lobed nucleus; small heterogeneous cytoplasmic granules G3—Lobed nucleus; eosinophilic rod-shaped cytoplasmic granules G4—Elongated cell; moderately eosinophilic cytoplasmic granules Goldfish Neutrophil (heterophil)—eccentric lobed nucleus; pale gray cytoplasm with small gray to pale pink granules Eosinophil—smaller and rounder than neutrophil; eccentric round to bilobed nucleus; pale blue cytoplasm with pale spherical or rod-shaped granules	Migrate to sites of inflammation; phagocytic; exhibit chemokinetic responses; eosinophic staining of fish granulocytes does not imply function and morphology similar to that of mammalian eosinophils	Granulocytes of teleosts and elasmobranchs should be considered as separate types of cells. In dogfish, G1 is most common followed by G4; the G4 cell may be a reactive thrombocyte; there is great species variation among elasmobranchs with some granulocyte types not present; the existence of basophils in fish is controversial.
Monocytes	Large cell lacking distinct cellular margins because of pseudopodia; eccentric round to lobed nucleus fills less than 50% of cell volume; chromatin coarsely granular to reticulated and lacking thick clumping; abundant blue-gray cytoplasm; no granules; occasionally vacuolated	Phagocytic; migrate to areas of inflammation where they develop into macrophages; macrophages are phagocytic and secrete interleukin, interferon, prostaglandin, and leukotriene; actively trap antigen	There is a low number in peripheral blood.
Thrombocytes	Round, fusiform, or elongated in shape; nucleus stains dark purple with dense chromatin	Coagulation of blood	Clumping is commonly seen on smears.

(Data from reference 4.)

Table 24–10. Because normal values are lacking for most fish, routine sampling of healthy animals allows a compilation of values that can be used for comparison.

The use of sentinel fish provides advanced warning of disease onset that may affect the entire collection. Criteria for the selection of these animals are that they are susceptible to the diseases of concern and are easily captured for assessment. Finely scaled, slow-moving fish such as the porcupinefishes, puffers, burrfish and boxfishes are great additions to an aquarium because they are often the first to become affected by external parasites. Evidence of infection includes decreased appetite and the appearance of cloudy eyes as copious amounts of mucus are produced.

Acknowledgments

The author gratefully acknowledges the support of the National Aquarium in Baltimore and all of the aquarists who have provided the opportunity to gain valuable insight not readily available in published texts. Together he and they have learned, and continue to learn, how to provide quality health care for the fishes in their charge. Also, the author wishes to extend his deepest gratitude to librarian Susie Ridenour, who performed the literature searches and collected relevant references. Her enthusiasm, dedication, and excellence are an inspiration to all who worked on this chapter. All photographs were taken by National Aquarium photographer George Grall. Medical illustrations were contributed by Erica Denison and Michael Wieber, students of the Johns Hopkins Art as Applied to Medicine. Their diligence and attention to detail are second to none. Jill Arnold, Roger Williams, Chris Andrews, Bruce Hecker, and Perry Hampton provided critical review of the manuscript and many helpful suggestions. Finally, sincere thanks to Cara Magistrelli, who kept the medical department on track while preparing several of the tables for this chapter.

REFERENCES

1. Aiken A: Use of ozone to improve water quality in aquatic exhibits. Int Zoo Year Book 34:106–114, 1995.
2. Anderson DP: Immunostimulants, adjuvants, and vaccine carriers in fish: applications to aquaculture. Annu Rev Fish Dis 2:281–307, 1992.
3. Blasiola GC: Diseases of ornamental marine fishes. *In* Gratzek JB, Matthews JR (eds): Aquariology: The Science of Fish Health Management—Master Volume. Morris Plains, NJ, Tetra Press, pp 275–300, 1992.
4. Campbell TW, Murru F: An introduction to fish hematology. *In* Practical Exotic Animal Medicine, The Compendium Collection. Trenton, Veterinary Learning Systems, pp 223–229, 1996.
5. Cardeilhac PT, Whitaker BR: Copper treatments: uses and precautions. Vet Clin North Am Small Anim Pract 18:435–448, 1988.
6. Clipsham R: Environmental preventive medicine; food and water management for reinfection control. Proceedings of the Annual Conference Association of Avian Veterinarians, Phoenix, AZ, pp 87–105, 1990.
7. Ellis AE: Current aspects of fish vaccination. Dis Aquat Org 4:159–164, 1988.
8. Ellis AE: Fish Vaccination. New York, Academic Press, 1988.
9. Emerson K, Russo RC, Lund RE, Thurston RV: Aqueous ammonia equilibrium calculations: effect of pH and temperature. J Fish Res Board Can 32(12):2379–2383, 1975.
10. Finlay J: Disinfectants in fish farming. Fish Mgmt 9(1):18–21, 1978.
11. Geraci JR: Nutrition and nutritional disorders. *In* Fowler ME (ed): Zoo and Wild Animal Medicine, 2nd ed. Philadelphia, WB Saunders, pp 760–764, 1986.
12. Halver JE: The vitamins. *In* Halver JE (ed): Fish Nutrition. New York, Academic Press, pp 32–109, 1989.
13. Hecker B: Personal communication, 1996.
14. Herwig N: Handbook of Drugs and Chemicals Used in the Treatment of Fish Diseases. Springfield, IL, Charles C Thomas, 1979.
15. Inglis V, Robertson D, Miller K, Thompson KD, Richards RH: Antibiotic protection against recrudescence of latent *Aeromonas salmonicida* during furunculosis vaccination. J Fish Dis 19:341–348, 1996.
16. Kennedy-Stoskopf S: Immunology. *In* Stoskopf MK (ed): Fish Medicine. Philadelphia, WB Saunders, pp 149–159, 1993.
17. Lall SP: The minerals. *In* Halver JE (ed): Fish Nutrition. New York, Academic Press, pp 220–257, 1989.
18. Lam TJ: Environmental influences on gonadal activity of fish. *In* Hoar WS, Randall DJ, Donaldson EM (eds): Fish Physiology, Vol IX Reproduction, Part B, Behavior and Fertility Control. New York, NY, Academic Press, pp 65–116, 1983.
19. Lewbart GA: Preventive medicine for freshwater and marine aquarium fishes. Proceedings of the American Association of Zoo Veterinarians, St. Louis, MO, pp 75–80, 1993.
20. Lovell T: Nutrition and Feeding of Fish. New York, Van Nostrand Reinhold, 1989.
21. Moyle PB, Cech JJ: Fishes: An Introduction to Ichthyology. Englewood Cliffs, NJ, Prentice-Hall, 1982.
22. Navarre O, Halver JE: Disease resistance and humoral antibody production in rainbow trout fed high levels of vitamin C. Aquaculture 79(1–4):207–221, 1989.
23. Nelson JS: Fishes of the World, 2nd ed. New York, John Wiley and Sons, 1984.
24. Newman SG: Bacterial vaccines for fish. Annu Rev Fish Dis 3:145–185, 1993.
25. Noga EJ: Fish Disease. New York, Mosby–Year Book, pp 282–283, 1996.
26. Post GW: Nutrition and nutritional diseases of salmonids. *In* Stoskopf MK (ed): Fish Medicine. Philadelphia, WB Saunders, pp 343–358, 1993.
27. Sargent J, Henderson RJ, Tocher DR: The lipids. *In* Halver JE (ed): Fish Nutrition. New York, Academic Press, pp 154–218, 1989.
28. Smith LS: Introduction to Fish Physiology. Neptune City, NJ, TFH Publications, 1982.
29. Stoskopf MK: Fish Medicine. Philadelphia, WB Saunders, 1993.
30. Stoskopf MK: Shark pharmacology and toxicology. *In* Stoskopf MK (ed): Fish Medicine. Philadelphia, WB Saunders, pp 809–816, 1993.
31. Wedemeyer GA, Barton BA, McLeay DJ: Stress and acclimation. *In* Schreck CB, Moyle PB (eds): Methods for Fish Biology. Bethesda, MD, American Fisheries Society, pp 451–489, 1990.
32. Whitaker BR: Establishing a quarantine procedure for marine fish. Eastern States Veterinary Conference Proceedings, Orlando, FL, pp 552–554, 1991.
33. Whitaker BR: Common disorders of marine fish. Comp Cont Educ Sm Anim 13(6):960–967, 1991.
34. Whitaker BR: Quarantine and post mortem examination. Proceedings of the North American Veterinary Conference, Orlando, FL, pp 635–637, 1992.
35. Whitaker BR, Hecker B, Andrews C: Establishing a quarantine program for fishes. American Zoo and Aquarium Association Conference Proceedings, Atlanta, pp 282–287, 1994.

CHAPTER 25

Fish Pharmacotherapeutics

MICHAEL K. STOSKOPF

The decade of the 1990s has seen a major increase in understanding of drug kinetics in fish. Most research continues to be conducted on food fish species because of the need to establish therapies for infectious diseases occurring in the high-density rearing conditions of food production aquaculture. Nevertheless, this new information is useful to veterinarians managing the health of any fish species.

Many of the empiric drug doses found in the older literature are being supplanted by doses based on pharmacokinetic studies, and the principles of drug dose establishment, which function well for terrestrial species, appear to also apply to fish. The axiom that all fish are not the same is clearly being supported by the modern drug studies. Extrapolation between species has some risk, particularly for drugs with low therapeutic indices, and individual variation should be expected. Furthermore, drug kinetics can be quite different in multidose applications than in a single dose. Most commonly, elimination parameters become slower in multiple administrations. When this occurs, the duration and mean drug level in the animal is elevated over predicted values. Therefore, clinicians should be cautious when a multidose regimen is based only on single-dose kinetic studies.

The three basic rules of zoological clinical pharmacology apply to fish. When a clinician intends to treat an ailment in a species with a drug that he or she has never used in that species, the clinician should:

1. Learn everything possible about the known pharmacology of the drug including mechanisms of action and mechanisms of known untoward effects.

2. Try to locate someone who has used the drug in the intended species previously and learn from that person's experience.

3. Never use a drug in a new species for the first time in more animals than can be lost as a result of drug reactions or toxicity. This rule applies even after gaining information from someone with experience.

Additional factors that are not major considerations in terrestrial mammals and birds can become important when giving drugs to fish. These include the impact of water temperature, pH, hardness or salinity, and specific ion content on drug pharmacokinetics and pharmacodynamics. The effect of any of these factors can be different for different routes of administration for the same drug. Even though environmental factors complicate

the process of establishing dosage regimens through pharmacokinetic studies, the empiric approach (i.e., establishing dosage regimens based on observed therapeutic benefit without unacceptable complications) remains as valid for fish medicine as it is in terrestrial animal medicine.

ESTABLISHING A DOSAGE REGIMEN (Chart 25–1)

Selecting which pharmacokinetic parameters are most appropriate to use when establishing a dosage regimen can be challenging. Pharmacokinetic studies are not conducted under a set of standard conditions, nor is the handling of data (model fitting) standardized. This does not reflect a desire on the part of investigators to make life difficult for clinicians, rather it reflects the complexity of relating pharmacokinetics to both environmental conditions and the pharmacodynamics of the drug. Empiric experience has shown that some drugs are more efficacious when low, but effective, tissue concentrations can be maintained continually. These drugs include many that inhibit cell wall synthesis or function. They are generally drugs with little or no postantibiotic effect on bacterial growth such as the beta-lactams or erythromycin. For these drugs, the critical determinant of efficacy is the time that serum concentrations exceed the mean inhibitory concentration (MIC) required to inhibit bacterial growth. The elimination half-life ($T_{1/2}$-beta) is a very important tool for calculating their theoretic dosage regimens. Drugs with significant postantibiotic effects on bacteria include many antibiotics that inhibit protein or nucleic acid synthesis. For these drugs, efficacy is much more dependent on the peak tissue concentration reached in relation to the MIC than on the percentage of time that serum levels remain above a minimum effective concentration. Drugs of this type include the aminoglycosides and fluoroquinolones. Determination of appropriate dose intervals for these drugs often relies on peak serum drug concentrations and noncompartmental modeling parameters such as the integrated area under the curve (AUC) above MIC.

ENVIRONMENTAL PHARMACOLOGY

The application of drugs to fish can cause important environmental impacts. Several drugs commonly used

CHART 25–1:   Dosage Regimens

Drug	Route	Dose	Comments
Antibacterial Drugs			
Amoxicillin	PO	25 mg/kg BID	
Chloramphenicol	IM, PO	50 mg/kg once followed by 25 mg/kg OID	Avoid use in food fish
Enrofloxacin	IM, PO, IP	5 mg/kg OID	
Erythromycin	IM, PO	100 mg/kg OID	For bacterial kidney disease
Florfenicol	IM, PO, IP	40–50 mg/kg OID	
Gentamicin	IM	2.5 mg/kg every 72 hours	Nephrotoxicity
Naladixic acid	IM, PO	5 mg/kg OID	
Oxolinic acid	PO	5–25 mg/kg OID	Residues persist for 21 days in trout
Oxytetracycline	IM	10 mg/kg OID	Can immunosuppress fish
	PO	20 mg/kg TID	
	Bath	1 hour 100 mg/L	Freshwater fish
		1 hour 400 mg/L	Marine fish
Sarafloxacin	PO	10–14 mg/kg OID	Treat full 10 days
Sulfadimethoxine/ ormetoprim (Romet 30)	IM, PO	42 mg/kg sulfadimethoxine and 8 mg/kg ormetoprim OID	6-Wk withdrawal for salmonids; 3 days for catfish
Antifungal Drugs			
Miconazole	IM, PO, IP	10–20 mg/kg	
Ketoconazole	IM, PO, IP	2.5–10 mg/kg	
Itraconazole	PO	1–5 mg/kg	
Antiprotozoal Drugs			
Metronidazole	PO	25 to 30 mg/kg daily	
	PO	50 mg/kg	
Antihelminthics			
Albendazole	PO		Systemically absorbed
Ivermectin	PO		Low margin of safety
Mebendazole	PO	20 mg/kg 3 times weekly	
Niclosamide	PO	200 mg/kg 2 times 10 days apart	Metabolites toxic to sharks
	PO	5 g/kg feed 2 times 10 days apart	
Praziquantel	PO	5 mg/kg body weight	Repeat weekly up to 3 times
	Bath	3 to 6 hour 10 mg/L	Toxic to Coryodoras
Pyrantel pamoate	PO	10 mg/kg once	
Thiabendazole	PO	10–25 mg/kg 2 times 10 days apart	
	PO	66 mg/kg once	

Chart continued on following page

◆ **CHART 25–1: Dosage Regimens** *Continued*

Drug	Route	Dose	Comments
Other Therapeutics			
Butorphanol	IM	0.05–0.1 mg/kg	
Carp pituitary extract (P)	IM	5 mg/kg at 6-hr intervals	Combined with 20 IU human chorionic gonadotropin (HCG)
Dexamethasone	IM, IP	1–2 mg/kg	
Furosemide	IM	2–5 mg/kg PRN	Not effective in alkalosis
Haloperidol	IM	0.5 mg/kg	Combined with 1st luteinizing hormone analog (LRH-A) (see text)
HCG	IM	30 IU/kg at 6-hr intervals	
	IM	20 IU/kg at 6-hr intervals	Combined with 5 mg/kg CP
Hydrocortisone	IM, IP	1–4 mg/kg	
LRH-A	IM	2 µg/kg followed in 6 hour 8 µg/kg	
Reserpine	IM	50 mg/kg	Combined with 1st LRH-A (see text)

IM, intramuscularly; IP, intraperitoneally; PO, per os.
Tabular compilation of doses, although quickly accessible to the clinician, cannot substitute for a solid background in clinical pharmacology and careful review of the text.

for treatment in fish (e.g., sulfadimethoxine, oxytetracycline) persist for a prolonged time (years) in water or sediments. Care should always be taken to evaluate the disposition of water when drugs are given to fish. This becomes more of a concern as the drug delivery route becomes less precise. Bath or dip treatments, or per os (PO) administrations in feed of drugs excreted unchanged or as active metabolites pose high potential environmental risks. Options for mitigation include filtration of the treatment water, (activated carbon), with proper disposal of the extracted drug and filter media, or chemical treatment of the water before discharge. For example, some drugs are unstable in extreme pH and can be broken down to less active forms through proper manipulation of water pH. Other drugs can be oxidized into inactive components when subjected to ozone treatments, or photodegraded by intense light or solar exposure. It is important to take whatever steps are available to reduce environmental contamination with therapeutic drugs when planning treatments for fish.

ANTIBACTERIAL DRUGS

Three antibacterial drug preparations are approved by the Food and Drug Administration (FDA) for use in specific species of food fish for specific diseases. They are Terramycin, Romet, and Sulfamerazine. All other

use of antibacterials in fish is extralabel, and appropriate care should be taken to avoid drugs entering the human food supply. Culture and MIC determination are important tools for selecting and appropriately dosing antibacterial drugs in fish and should be used whenever possible. Recent reviews[1, 5–7] of antibiotic research in fish provide extensive summaries of MIC and pharmacokinetic data from individual studies.

When fish are still eating, oral administration of drug in feed is a preferred route because of the reduction of stress for the fish and labor for the clinician. Commercial gel diets make good vehicles for many drugs. The establishment of the veterinary drug order process by the FDA has also made the milling of drugs into pelleted feed more practical for larger scale applications. Palatability is a major issue in delivery of antibacterials in the food. Some drugs, such as erythromycin and potentiated sulfonamides, have significant palatability problems for many species of fish and can require addition of large amounts of fish oils or other attractants to induce the fish to eat them. Some antibiotics, such as erythromycin, are very susceptible to effects from the food they are combined with. The preparation base for the drugs should be assessed for any effects on drug efficacy.

When relatively few or particularly valuable fish are affected, parenteral administration may be the most appropriate route of delivery. Injection ensures more accurate delivery of the intended dose than oral or topical administrations. Intravenous (IV) administration is not commonly used because it can increase the time that the fish is manipulated, and perivascular injection is common when using the caudal tail vein. For relatively nonirritating drugs, intracoelomic (IP) injection is used if rapid drug absorption is important. Suspensions (e.g., sulfadimethoxine/ormetoprim) injected IP are not absorbed as quickly as expected, presumably because the drugs are not in solution. Intramuscular (IM) injection is commonly used, and, although some drugs are readily absorbed (aminoglycosides), bioavailability of others after IM injection (tetracyclines) can be fairly low. Some drugs cause local irritation and tissue necrosis at the injection site (tetracyclines, enrofloxacin), which should be considered before implementing prolonged, multiple-injection therapy regimens.

Amoxicillin

Amoxicillin is approved for use in food fish in the United Kingdom and has been used in Atlantic salmon infected with *Aeromonas salmonicida.* Oral doses of 120 mg/kg based on pharmacokinetic studies of young parr in fresh water at 16°C were not effective in clinical trials conducted on infected fish in salt water at lower temperatures. It is possible that palatability problems were a large factor in the inability to achieve useful serum drug concentrations. In treatment of display fish, amoxicillin has generally been used empirically in combination therapies at much lower doses (25 mg/kg PO BID).

Chloramphenicol

Chloramphenicol has long been associated with the rare human complication of aplastic anemia known as Gray's syndrome, making it an unlikely candidate for use in food fish. It has, however, been used extensively for treatment in ornamental fish species. Kinetic studies are available for the drug given PO by gavage to rainbow trout in fresh water at 17°C, but no careful studies have been published using the drug in tropical fish. Empirically, chloramphenicol appears more efficacious when delivered in dosage regimens closely patterned from terrestrial mammalian therapies (50 mg/kg initial dose followed by 25 mg/kg BID).

Enrofloxacin

One of the newest fluoroquinolones to become available, enrofloxacin is a DNA gyrase inhibitor with a broad spectrum of activity against gram-negative rods. It has been studied in trout, Atlantic salmon, and hybrid striped bass for efficacy against a wide range of bacterial pathogens. In vitro studies have shown that the MIC for enrofloxacin is higher at lower temperatures, which should be expected considering the mechanism of action of the drug and the general impact of temperature on bacterial reproduction. A number of kinetic studies have been performed, primarily on salmonids kept at various temperatures and given various doses.

One study showed bioavailability of orally administered enrofloxacin to vary from 42% at 15°C to 24% at 10°C. Field trials have shown good efficacy, with 5 mg/kg PO in feed daily for up to 10 days being the most common dosage regimen tested. The drug is used at the same dose when delivered IM. From studies using pacu under strict laboratory conditions, it is apparent that a considerable proportion of enrofloxacin is excreted unchanged into the water and that undosed control fish readily absorb and bioaccumulate enrofloxacin from the water.

Erythromycin

Erythromycin has received considerable investigative attention because of its potential for efficacy against bacterial kidney disease of salmonids (*Renibacterium salmoninarum*). A macrolide antibiotic, it is a bacteriostat that functions through inhibition of mRNA translation and protein synthesis. Palatability problems are common with this drug, especially at high doses (200 mg/kg). For the specific problem in salmonids, attention is focused on IM injection of erythromycin in brood fish within a month of spawning to produce protective drug concentrations in the yolk of eggs. This strategy is designed for breaking vertical transmission of the disease. Applications in display fish have been extremely limited. Oral medication in the feed delivered at 100 mg/kg body weight per day for 7 to 10 days is the most commonly used regimen.

Florfenicol

Florfenicol, an analog of thiamphenicol, which is itself a derivative of chloramphenicol, does not appear to cause Gray's syndrome in humans. It is, therefore, being evaluated for potential use in a variety of food species, including Atlantic salmon. Florfenicol appears to be rapidly absorbed from the intestine in salmon (bioavailability of 96%), with rapid distribution and metabolism. It is excreted primarily as an aminated derivative. In vitro florfenicol is approximately one to two times less active than chloramphenicol, but clinical trials in Atlantic salmon parr challenged with *Aeromonas salmonicida* showed excellent efficacy at a dose of 20 mg/kg. Most empiric use in display fish is centered on a dosage regimen of 40 to 50 mg/kg given daily or BID, usually PO.

Gentamicin

The building case for gentamicin as a nephrotoxic agent in fish has dramatically reduced use of the drug in clinical settings. In general, the kinetics of aminoglycosides tend to be similar in a given species, and extrapolation from single dose gentamicin and tobramicin studies conducted in sharks has resulted in a dosage regimen of 2.5 mg/kg every 3 days IM for any aminoglycoside being used clinically in a wide range of fish species. This practice may hold some risk. Aminoglycosides are excreted essentially unchanged in the urine, making consideration of the normal environment (salinity) and renal physiology of the fish very important elements in arriving at nontoxic dosage regimens. Dosages as low as 1 mg/kg every 33 hours have caused extensive renal tubular necrosis in freshwater species (channel catfish). This, and the probable need to deliver the drug parenterally because of its low lipid solubility, make gentamicin unattractive for treatment of fish. Attempts to achieve useful plasma concentrations through bath administration have been thwarted by the tendency of gentamicin to plate to glass surfaces of treatment tanks and by the lipophobic nature of the drug.

Naladixic Acid

Naladixic acid, one of the original quinolone antibiotics discovered more than 20 years ago, has been used in the pet trade for the treatment of undiagnosed bacterial infections in fish. It is used in food fish (Ayu) in Japan with a 7-day withdrawal time. Pharmacokinetic studies in rainbow trout and amago salmon held at the same temperature showed little species variation in kinetic parameters. Bioavailability after oral administration appears to approach 100% and distribution is rapid. The drug accumulates in bile and does not distribute well into fat. The current empiric dose most commonly used is 5 mg/kg PO given daily.

Oxolinic Acid

Oxolinic acid is another of the original quinolone antibiotics. It is a registered fish therapeutant in Japan and is used extensively there. Oxolinic acid MICs for fish pathogens are generally in the range of 0.075 to 0.3 μg/ml; however, the MIC against some *Vibrio* species and *Pseudomonas fluorescens* can exceed 3 μg/ml. The pharmacokinetics of this drug vary with temperature and with the species being treated. Elimination is slower in marine fish and elimination half-lives are prolonged at lower temperatures. Bioavailabilty through the oral route is relatively poor (20% at 7.5°C in Atlantic salmon in sea water), increasing environmental risks of using the drug. Although the drug is used extensively in the hobby trade, no published pharmacokinetic data or clinical challenge trials are available to evaluate the commonly used dosage regimens (5 to 25 mg/kg PO daily).

Oxytetracycline

The tetracyclines are broad-spectrum bacteriostatic protein synthesis inhibitors that are used extensively in the treatment of bacterial, mycoplasmal, chlamydial, rickettsial, and protozoal infections in fish and other animals. Oxytetracycline is FDA approved for specific uses in food fish and is widely used in food fish production. It is also used extensively in the treatment of display fish and is administered by a variety of routes, including parenteral injection and immersion baths. Good or moderate activity (MIC < 4 μg/ml) can be achieved against selected gram-positive aerobes and a wide spectrum of gram-negative organisms. Oxytetracy-

cline is less lipid soluble than minocycline or doxycycline but less highly bound to plasma proteins. Oxytetracycline is excreted essentially unchanged in the urine and, to some degree, in the bile where enterohepatic circulation can occur. The drug is remarkably stable in cold marine habitats and poses an important environmental concern. Oxytetracycline pharmacokinetics in fish have been more extensively studied and reported than for any other antibiotic. Bioavailabilty of oxytetracycline varies dramatically with experimental conditions and the species of fish used, leaving room for considerable controversy over the effectiveness of oral and bath administrations. High bioavailability through the oral route has been documented in trout (>80%), but, in the goldfish, bioavailability of less than 1% may be due to the lack of a true stomach or a highly acidic region of the gut to ionize the drug and facilitate absorption. The issue of bioavailability from IM injection is also murky, with studies showing bioavailability to be high in African catfish (>80%) and low in hybrid striped bass. Empiric experience with the drug depends greatly on the susceptibility of the pathogen being treated. Immunosuppression of treated fish through alteration of macrophage function and the possibility of hepatic damage from excessively high doses and hepatic recirculation should be kept in mind when administering this drug. The most commonly applied dosage regimens are 10 mg/kg IM, 20 mg/kg TID in feed, or 1 hour baths at 100 mg/L in fresh water, 400 mg/L in marine water.

Sarafloxacin

Sarafloxacin has received extensive investigation and is a very strong candidate for use in food fish. This modern generation fluoroquinolone has been very effective in field trials against enteric septicemia of channel catfish. The salmonid industry hopes that the relatively rapid metabolism of the drug will result in shorter withdrawal times than currently approved antibiotics. FDA concerns about the use of fluoroquinolones in food species and environmental impact questions have put approval of Sarafloxacin on hold, and the drug has not been available for extensive testing in other species of fish. It does, however, hold promise in nonfood fish in the future. Dosage regimens of 10 to 14 mg/kg PO for 10 days are usually effective.

Sulfadimethoxine/Ormetoprim (Romet 30)

Sulfadimethoxine/ormetoprim combination therapy is one of the three FDA approved medications for systemic treatment of bacterial diseases in food fish. Both of these drugs have high bioavailability when administered orally or parenterally, and they distribute broadly in the tissues. Their spectrum of efficacy is wide and they are routinely used in extralabel applications. Caution interpreting the kinetic parameters of these drugs is advised because replication of the dissolution of either drug into an acceptable IV formulation has not been successful in the author's laboratory. Nevertheless, administered orally, the combination is empirically efficacious against a fairly broad range of bacterial infections in fish and can be used successfully to treat bacterial septicemias in ornamental species. A routine oral dose is 42 mg/kg of sulfadimethoxine and 8 mg/kg of ormetoprim in the feed. Both drugs are stable in water and pose the environmental risk of persistence in sediments and the water column.

ANTIFUNGAL DRUGS

Advances in antifungal pharmacology in fish have not been as rapid as those in antibacterial therapy. This is probably due in part to the lack of sophistication in specific antemortem diagnosis of systemic fungal diseases in fish. There are currently no antifungal drugs approved for parenteral use in food fish in the United States. Any use of systemic antifungal drugs in fish is extralabel and the clinician should ensure that the fish will not enter the human food supply.

One of the challenges in determining doses for an antimycotic drug is the lack of accepted and validated methods for determining in vitro the drug concentration that will inhibit a given fungal organism. This has made drug selection for treating fungi pathogenic to fish somewhat arbitrary, particularly when the taxonomic relationship to fungi infecting mammals is unclear. In these situations, clinicians have had to rely on absorption and elimination data derived from mammalian studies.

Amphotericin B has not been used extensively in fish. In mammals, the drug is essentially not absorbed from the gastrointestinal (GI) tract, much like the related nystatin, and there is little reason to expect this to be different for fish. When the large number of untoward side effects in mammals are considered, clinicians have generally chosen other drugs. Flucytosine, on the other hand, is well absorbed from the mammalian GI tract, but is essentially excreted entirely by the renal route in mammals. Dosing drugs with obligate renal excretion has been shown to be complex in fish, and concerns about potential toxicity have encouraged clinicians to gravitate toward the imidazoles and triazoles. Miconazole (10 to 20 mg/kg IP, PO, IM) and ketoconazole (2.5 to 10 mg/kg PO, IP) were used in a variety of individual cases of systemic fungal disease with variable success, primarily in marine tropical fishes, early in the past decade, but their use has been largely supplanted by the selection of newer drugs. Itraconazole is probably less well absorbed from the gut than ketoconazole, and, in mammals, serum concentrations are much lower for the same dose. However, the potential for therapeutic effectiveness against a wider range of filamentous fungi and the lack of renal excretion has made it an attractive choice for use in fish. Itraconazole has been used with variable success in isolated cases in marine tropical reef teleosts. I am only aware of administrations in the food, and doses have ranged from 1 to 5 mg/kg body weight given daily to weekly.

Fluconazole promises to supplant the other triazoles in mammals because of its improved bioavailability, which is not altered by food or gastric pH. The challenge of finding an effective and safe dose empirically for this drug in fishes is complicated by the probability that fish, like mammals, excrete about 90% of the administered dose through renal mechanisms. The complex interaction between gill and kidney in teleosts adapted to different waters makes it unlikely that a single empiric dose for fluconazole will serve all fish species equally well.

ANTIPROTOZOAL DRUGS

Development of effective systemic drugs for the treatment of protozoal infections has not progressed far in the past decade. The situation for human therapy is not advanced over the animal drug market in this arena and offers little in the way of potential new treatments. This is a particularly difficult issue for veterinarians treating illness in fish because protozoal infections make up a large part of the disease spectrum seen in aquarium and aquacultural fishes. There are currently no antiprotozoal drugs approved for parenteral use in food fish in the United States and any systemic application to fish is extralabel. Therefore, treated fish should not enter the human food supply. Many of the protozoal infections of fish are treated as ectoparasites and the use of formalin as a bath is approved by the FDA for use in salmonids and catfish. Other approaches focus on alteration of the water pH, hardness or salinity, temperature, or even dilutional impacts of massive water changes.

Much of the human drug development efforts for antiprotozoal drugs is aimed at trypanosomes, schistosomes, and amebae. These organisms are not generally recognized as major problems for most fish and most of these drugs pose environmental, toxic, or oncogenic risks that make them of questionable application in fish. One drug that has found application is metronidazole. It has good efficacy against many flagellates, amebae, and anaerobic bacteria. Metronidazole is essentially insoluble in water, so baths are not very effective against systemic infections. Oral administration in gel foods is the preferred route of administration. Metronidazole distributes well in mammals, getting into all secretions and cerebrospinal fluid. Although renal excretion occurs, hepatic metabolism is the major route of excretion in mammals and probably fish. Kinetic and metabolism studies in fish are needed. Older, empiric doses of 50 mg/kg body weight daily have been efficacious in many cases, but the need for these high doses is probably related to delivery problems. Delivered well in gel foods, lower doses of metronidazole (25 to 30 mg/kg body weight/day) should effectively reach the serum levels necessary to kill most susceptible protozoa (8 µg/ml mean effective concentration [MEC]). Very little is known about the efficacy or pharmacokinetic dosing of older antimalarial or antiameba drugs for fish.

ANTIHELMINTHICS

There are no antihelminthic drugs approved for systemic use in food fishes in the United States and any use is extralabel. The clinician should prevent treated fish from entering the human food supply. Dichlorvos and related drugs have found acceptance in foreign aquaculture production but not in the United States. Many helminthic infections of fish have complex life cycles with one or more intermediate hosts involved. Direct treatment of the fish is only a partial and temporary solution in these cases.

Albendazole

Like mebendazole, albendazole is a derivative of the benzimidazole carbamate, but unlike mebendazole, albendazole is very well absorbed from the GI tract. This makes the drug useful for treatment of extraluminal helminth infections. The drug is metabolized in the liver and excreted as metabolites, primarily by the kidneys, although the contribution of the gills has not been studied. The drug should not be used with brood fish because teratogenic effects are well documented.

Ivermectin

An avermectin or macrocyclic lactone, ivermectin is primarily excreted unchanged in the feces by mammals and renal excretion is minimal. As a nemacide, the drug is notably more effective against certain nematode families than others. In fish, it has been examined primarily for use against crustacean parasites (copepods), primarily in marine species. High doses appear to be required for this application. The margin of safety for this drug is small, and environmental impacts on beneficial crustaceans are a major concern. Toxicity is observed clinically, usually by the appearance of neurologic signs manifest as abnormal swimming and behavior. Cardiovascular effects should also be expected but are not routinely looked for in fish. The central nervous system effects of ivermectin toxicity appear to be reversible with removal of the drug.

Mebendazole

Mebendazole is closely related to albendazole, but has extremely poor absorption from the GI tract (10% to 20%). The drug is rapidly metabolized and an extensive first-pass metabolism affects pharmacokinetics of the drug significantly. It is generally administered at a dose of 20 mg/kg body weight once a week for three treatments, given orally in food for the treatment of GI nematodes. There is little or no renal metabolism of the drug, which is conjugated in the liver of mammals. Mebendazole is embryotoxic to fish and is also teratogenic, causing a high prevalence of deformed fry if administered to brood fish preparing to spawn.

Niclosamide

Niclosamide has been supplanted by the use of praziquantel for the treatment of cestodiasis in fish. The traditional treatments have been 200 mg/kg body weight given orally in feed twice, 10 days apart. Alternatively, 5 g/kg feed can be delivered ad lib for 2 days, 10 days apart. Although the use of niclosamide represented a major advance over the use of arsenicals, which were used extensively for the treatment of cestodes in fish historically, it still represents some risk of toxicity. Elasmobranchs appear to be particularly sensitive. The timing of niclosamide toxicity in sharks relative to dose administration suggests that the drug may be excreted as a toxic metabolite capable of efficient enough absorption across the gills to rapidly reach toxic serum levels.

Praziquantel

Praziquantel is rapidly absorbed orally with extensive first-pass clearance as metabolites in the urine in mammals. This results in transient and low serum concentrations, which appears to also occur in fish. Furthermore, based on clinical observations of therapeutic effects on fish sharing water systems with treated fish, it appears that the drug may be rapidly absorbed by the gills; however, controlled studies have not been performed. Praziquantel is effective against many trematodes and cestodes. At lower doses, the drug causes the worms to lose attachment to their host. At higher doses, praziquantel affects tegument integrity, allowing host defense mechanisms to kill the parasite. This mode of action poses a problem for in vitro testing of efficacy against trematode genera because death of the worm is not a reasonable end point, but rather vacuolization and vesiculation of tegument are. Even then, the quality of the host reaction has a major impact on the success of therapy. Praziquantel is empirically administered at doses of 5 mg/kg body weight in food or as a 3- to 6-hour bath at 10 mg/L.

Pyrantel Pamoate

Pyrantel pamoate is a depolarizing neuromuscular blocking agent that functions as a nicotinic activator and a weak cholinesterase inhibitor. It has been used in fish for the treatment of gastric nematodes. The drug is poorly absorbed from the GI tract and has little or no value in treating extraluminal infections. Pyrantel pamoate is mostly excreted unchanged in the feces and poses an environmental risk. It is routinely administered in food at a dose of 10 mg/kg body weight.

Thiabendazole

Thiabendazole has been used at a dose of 10 to 25 mg/kg given orally in the feed twice, 10 days apart, for the treatment of gastric nematodes in several species of fish. Higher doses (66 mg/kg) have also been advocated. The drug is rapidly absorbed from the GI tract and excreted primarily as active metabolites by the kidney. Clinically, it is common for fish to go off feed after thiabendazole therapy, presumably from GI upset. This anorexia generally resolves within 2 to 4 days of drug administration and is more severe when higher doses are administered.

STEROIDS

The use of steroids in the management of fish health is a relatively recent development. All use of systemic steroids in fish is extralabel. This limits the application of steroid therapy for food fish; however, for display and pet fish, the judicious application of systemic steroid therapy can be a valuable adjunct to the treatment of shock, trauma, or chronic stress syndromes. All steroid doses in fish have been developed on an empiric basis, for the most part in uncontrolled clinical applications. I know of no pharmacokinetic data or controlled clinical trials testing these drugs in fish. Apparent clinical benefit can be derived from the parenteral administration of dexamethasone at 1 to 2 mg/kg body weight. Empirically, the duration of effect appears to be less than 6 hours in koi and goldfish, requiring multiple treatments daily to maintain critically ill patients. Hydrocortisone has also been used effectively as an emergency drug in fish. Doses have ranged between 1 and 4 mg/kg, usually administered IP for shock. Considerably more clinical experience needs to be gained with these drugs before definitive dosage regimens can be established, but they appear to be useful adjuncts to fluid therapy when treating severely traumatized animals.

DIURETICS

The only diuretic to have received appreciable clinical use in fish to date has been furosemide. This drug has been administered IP or IM in cases of ascites or general edema at levels of 2.5 to 5 mg/kg. Dose intervals have ranged from 12 to 72 hours. The degree of impact on the disease process varies with the cause of the excessive fluid accumulation, the species of fish being treated, and the salinity of the fish's environment. Furosemide is a high-ceiling diuretic, which, in mammals, exerts its effects on the loop of Henle, inhibiting electrolyte reabsorbtion (Na^+, Cl, Mg^{2+}, Ca^{2+}) in the ascending limb. It is also a weak carbonic anhydrase inhibitor and enhances renal blood flow in mammals. These effects are not limited to the kidney in mammals and the impact of furosemide on gill physiology in fish should be investigated. I know of no pharmacokinetic or physiologic studies of this drug in fish, but the relatively common appearance of dropsy or tissue edema in diseased fish suggests that it might bear further investigation.

ANALGESICS

With the advent of new procedures using established fish anesthetics, the question of postoperative analgesia is being explored. For a more complete synopsis of recent developments in anesthetic pharmacology in fish, refer to Chapter 24. Briefly, however, the most significant advances in fish anesthesia in the past 5 years have not been due to the introduction of new drugs, but rather to the accumulation of evidence that careful measured delivery of the established fish anesthetics such as tricaine methane sulfonate (MS-222) reduces recovery time and increases the safe duration of anesthesia that can be achieved. This has increased the success of more extensive and prolonged surgical interventions in fish.

Butorphanol administered IM (0.1 mg/kg) to a koi 24 hours after an extensive celiotomy for removal of an abdominal mass empirically appeared to reduce discomfort significantly and allowed rapid return to normal mobility and appetite with no observed untoward effects. Administration to other postsurgical fish at doses of 0.05 to 0.1 mg/kg have not been deleterious and appear to have facilitated recovery. The application of analgesics in fish warrants further attention by clinicians and investigators.

REPRODUCTIVE HORMONES

The use of hormone induction to spawn brood fish is an important aspect of economic production for several species of aquaculture fish. The technique is less commonly applied to display fish production, but has excellent potential for spawning species difficult to breed in captivity. The use of hormones in fish is extralabel in the United States and treated brood fish should not enter the human food supply. The use of hormones to induce spawn merely stimulates the release of eggs. It does not cause eggs to mature and should not be administered unless the eggs are mature. The optimal doses for the various hormones used to induce spawning in fish vary across species and in the hands of different investigators. Human chorionic gonadotropin (HCG) is used extensively in spawning of a variety of fish species. It is commonly administered in two IM injections separated by about 6 hours. The total dose for most species of ornamental fish is 60 IU/kg. HCG is sometimes used in conjunction with carp pituitary extract (CP), giving two injections of 20 IU/kg HCG and 5 mg/kg of CP. Fish also release eggs in response to administration of the synthetic luteinizing hormone analog LRH-A, given alone or in conjunction with dopamine blocking agents such as reserpine or haloperidol. The first injection of LRH-A is usually 2 μg/kg IM followed 6 hours later by 8 μg/kg IM. In species that do not respond to LRH-A alone, reserpine at 50 mg/kg or haloperidol at 0.5 mg/kg can be administered with the first injection of LRH-A.

REFERENCES

1. Bowser PR, Babish JG: Clinical pharmacology and efficacy of fluoroquinolones in fish. Annu Rev Fish Dis 1:63–66, 1991.
2. Munday BL: Fish. *In* Cooper BS (ed): Antimicrobial Prescribing Guidelines for Veterinarians. Sydney, Australia, Post Graduate Foundation, University of Sydney, pp 305–325, 1995.
3. Prescott JF, Baggot JD: Antimicrobial Therapy in Veterinary Medicine, 2nd ed. Ames, IA, Iowa State University Press, 1993.
4. Smith P, Hiney MP, Samuelsen OB: Bacterial resistance to antimicrobial agents used in fish farming: a critical evaluation of method and meaning. Annu Rev Fish Dis 4:273–313, 1994.
5. Stoffregen DA, Bowser PR, Babish JG: Antibacterial chemotherapeutants for finfish aquaculture: a synopsis of laboratory and field efficacy and safety studies. J Aquatic Anim Health 8(3):181–207, 1996.
6. Stoskopf MK: Fish Medicine. Philadelphia, WB Saunders, 1993.
7. Sundlof SF, Riviere JE, Craigmill AL: A comprehensive compendium of minor species drugs. *In* FARAD: The Food Animal Residue Avoidance Databank. Gainesville, FL, University of Florida, pp 167–169, 1992.

REPTILES

CHAPTER 26

Use of Antimicrobial Drugs in Reptiles

ELLIOTT R. JACOBSON

Reptiles are a diverse group of vertebrates, consisting of approximately 6400 species. They vary in size from small geckos weighing only a few grams up to large marine turtles and crocodilians which approach 900 kg. Reptiles are popular as pets, as display animals in zoological collections, and as research animals both in the laboratory and the field. Infectious diseases are known to cause illness and death in captive reptiles,[1, 12, 14, 16, 26, 48] and recently several diseases have surfaced as health problems of wild reptiles. For some unexplained reason, more diseases are reported in chelonians than in other groups of reptiles (see Chapter 30). A variety of bacteria have been incriminated as either primary or secondary pathogens, and infections caused by gram-negative bacteria are more common than those caused by gram-positive bacteria. Of the aerobes, *Pseudomonas aeruginosa, Aeromonas hydrophila, Providencia rettgeri, Morganella morganii, Salmonella arizonae,* and *Klebsiella oxytoca* have frequently been isolated from healthy and ill captive reptiles, becoming invasive when conditions either change the resistance of the host or select for pathogenic organisms.[14, 27] These organisms may also become invasive following a primary viral disease such as gram-negative infections in ophidian paramyxovirus pneumonia.[31] Compared to clinically healthy desert tortoises, *Pasteurella testudiniis* is more commonly isolated from the nasal cavity of animals

with mycoplasmosis.[35, 36] Some groups of reptiles seem particularly susceptible to infection with specific types of bacteria. For instance, the American alligator (*Alligator mississippiensis*)[18] and aquatic chelonians[38] are susceptible to *A. hydrophila* infections. In the green iguana (*Iguana iguana*), an unusual *Neisseria* species has been commonly isolated from the oral cavity and bite wounds.[57]

Mycotic infections are also commonly seen in all major groups of captive reptiles, with the integumentary and respiratory systems most often being involved.[1, 50] The dermatomycoses of mammals caused by *Microsporum* and *Trichophyton* are rarely reported in reptiles. However, fusariosis, geotrichosis, phycomycosis, and chromomycosis appear to be relatively common. Predisposing factors such as suboptimal cage temperatures and filthy environmental conditions are often involved. Most cases of mycotic disease in reptiles are diagnosed at necropsy. As a result, there are relatively few reports that discuss medical management.[24, 28, 33]

This chapter focuses on the use of antimicrobial drugs as an important part of medically managing reptiles ill with bacterial and mycotic disease. Selection of specific antimicrobials is more difficult in reptiles than in mammals and birds because of the broad range of behavioral, anatomic, and physiologic peculiarities of the various species within the class Reptilia. Furthermore, only 20 pharmacokinetic studies have been performed in 34 of the 6400 species of reptiles (only one pharmacokinetic study has been done in a lizard). Thus, at times, the selection of an appropriate antimicrobial is often more of an art than a science. Extrapolation from one species to the next is often used when determining drug dosages in a species for which no pharmacokinetic data are available. Metabolic scaling of antimicrobial drugs has been used to circumvent this problem[66] but there are no data to validate this approach in dosing a reptile with an antimicrobial drug.

ANTIMICROBIAL DRUGS USED FOR MICROBIAL INFECTIONS: SCIENTIFICALLY DERIVED DOSES

This section addresses scientifically derived doses based on plasma and serum concentrations and pharmacokinetic studies by order of Reptilia, starting with Chelonia (Tables 26–1, 26–2), and discusses empirically derived dosages that have been recommended in veterinary medical literature.

Chelonia: Turtles and Tortoises

PENICILLINS

A study of carbenicillin in the Greek (spur-thigh) tortoise (*Testudo graeca*) and Hermann's tortoise (*Testudo hermanni*) indicated a biphasic increase in serum levels of carbenicillin after intramuscular (IM) administration of 400 mg/kg of body weight.[45] Because tortoises have an extremely large bladder, it was hypothesized that the bladder may act as a reservoir for certain antibiotics, making them available for recycling. Even so, carbenicillin proved to be safe and effective when administered at a dosage of up to 400 mg/kg every 48 hours. A

preliminary serum concentration study has been conducted on ampicillin in Hermann's tortoises.[67] While *P. aeruginosa*, and most strains of *Salmonella* species and *Klebsiella* species were resistant to this antibiotic, an average minimum inhibitory concentration (MIC) of 2.85 μg/ml was found to be sufficient against *Staphylococcus* species. Administration of ampicillin at 50 mg/kg IM every 12 hours resulted in blood levels considered therapeutic against this organism.

TETRACYCLINES

Blood concentrations for a tetracycline in reptiles is only available for doxycycline in Hermann's tortoise.[67] In this study, MICs for *Staphylococcus* species and *Klebsiella* species were found to be 8.9 μg/ml and 5.6 μg/ml, respectively. *P. aeruginosa* and *Salmonella* species were found to be resistant. For doxycycline, a loading dose of 50 mg/kg and then 25 mg/kg, administered IM every 3 days, was considered a therapeutic regimen for *Staphylococcus* and *Klebsiella* infections. For the most part, there are few instances in which tetracycline administration would be recommended in reptiles. Chlamydiosis has been reported in green turtles (*Chelonia mydas*)[23] and tetracycline would be indicated for treatment of chelonians suspected of having this disease.

AMINOGLYCOSIDES

Historically, the aminoglycoside antibiotics gentamicin and amikacin have been two of the most commonly used antibiotics in treating reptiles ill with gram-negative microbial infections. Gentamicin, however, has a narrow safe therapeutic range and cases of nephrotoxicity have been reported in reptiles.[24, 53] There are no reports in the reptile literature of amikacin induced nephrotoxicity. Because of this, gentamicin is no longer used as commonly as amikacin. However, sensitivity patterns of various gram-negative bacteria are not al-

TABLE 26–1. Antimicrobial Drug Doses in Chelonians (Turtles and Tortoises) and Crocodilians (Alligators, Crocodiles)

Order	Drug	Species	Dose (mg/kg)	Dose Interval (hours)	Route of Administration	Reference
Chelonia	Carbenicillin	Greek tortoise	400	48	IM	45
	Ampicillin	Hermann's tortoise	50	12	IM	67
	Doxycycline	Hermann's tortoise	50	Loading dose	IM	67
			25	72		
	Gentamicin	Painted turtle	10	48	IM	9
		Red-eared slider	6	72–96	IM	60
		Gopher tortoise	5	48	IM	10
	Enrofloxacin	Box turtle	2.5	96–120	IM	Aucoin, personal communication
		Hermann's tortoise	10	24	IM	67
		Gopher tortoise	5	24–48	IM	59
		Indian star tortoise	10	12–24	IM	61
	Ketoconazole	Gopher tortoise	15–30	24	PO	56
Crocodilia	Gentamicin	American alligator	1.75	72–96	IM	34
	Amikacin	American alligator	2.25	72–96	IM	34

TABLE 26–2. Antimicrobial Drug Doses in Squamates (Lizards and Snakes)

Suborder	Drug	Species	Dose (mg/kg)	Dose Interval (hours)	Route of Administration	Reference
Lacertilia (lizards)	Cefoperazone	Tegu	125	24	IM	41
Ophidia	Carbenicillin	Mangrove snake King snake Reticulated python Great Plains rat snake Yellow rat snake Black rat snake	400	24	IM	44
	Piperacillin	Blood python	100	48	IM	20
	Cefoperazone	False water cobra	100	96	IM	41
	Ceftazidime	Mangrove snake Boa constrictor Reticulated python Burmese python Yellow rat snake	20	72	IM	43
	Chloramphenicol	Bull snake	40	24	SQ	7
		Red-bellied water snake Midland water snake Gray rat snake Corn snake Eastern king snake Eastern indigo snake Black racer Hog-nose snake Copperhead Cottonmouth Timber rattlesnake Eastern diamondback rattlesnake Reticulated python Indian rock python Burmese python Boa constrictor	50	12–72	SQ	11
	Gentamicin	Bull snake	2.5	24	SQ	8
		Blood python	2.5 1.5	Loading dose 96	IM	20
	Amikacin	Bull snake	5 2.5	Loading dose 72	IM	49
	Ciprofloxacin	Reticulated python	2.5	48–72	Oral	40
	Enrofloxacin	Burmese python	10 5	Loading dose 48	IM IM	70

ways equivalent when comparing these two drugs; the author has seen isolates obtained from reptiles that are sensitive to gentamicin and not amikacin. Thus, with certain gram-negative bacterial infections, gentamicin may be preferred over amikacin.

In the painted turtle (*Chrysemys picta*) maintained at 26°C, $T_{1/2}$ for gentamicin was 32 hours and the suggested dosage was 10 mg/kg IM every 48 hours.[9] In the red-eared slider (*Chrysemys scripta elegans*), 6 mg/kg IM produced therapeutic plasma concentrations for 2 to 5 days.[60]

In the gopher tortoise (*Gopherus polyphemus*), pharmacokinetic studies of amikacin were conducted in two groups of tortoises administered 5 mg/kg body weight (shell included) acclimated at either 20° or 30°C.[10] As part of this study, the effect of multiple dose administrations and effects of acclimation temperature on oxygen consumption were also studied. The mean residence time for amikacin in the 30°C tortoises (22.67 ± 0.50 hours) was significantly less than that of the 20°C group (41.83 ± 3.23 hours). The clearance rate of the warmer acclimated tortoises was approximately twice as fast as that of the cooler acclimated tortoises. Similarly, oxygen consumption was found to be approximately twice as great at the higher acclimation temperature. Results of this study indicated that, in gopher tortoises acclimated at 30°C, amikacin should be administered IM at 5 mg/kg every 48 hours.

FLUOROQUINOLONES

Although several fluoroquinolones have become popular antibiotics for treatment of reptiles ill with bacterial infections, few experimental studies have been performed to determine proper doses and frequency of administration.

In a study with IM administration of enrofloxacin in box turtles (*Terrapene carolina*), results indicated that this species should be dosed at 5 mg/kg of body weight every 4 to 5 days (D. Aucoin, personal communication). In Hermann's tortoise, the recommended dose for enrofloxacin administration was 10 mg/kg given IM every 24 hours.[67] This dose and frequency of administration was based on blood concentrations and MICs of several bacterial isolates including *P. aeruginosa*, *Klebsiella* species, and *Salmonella* species. The results of a pharmacokinetic study in adult gopher tortoises indicated that enrofloxacin should be administered at 5 mg/kg IM every 24 to 48 hours to maintain blood concentrations above the MIC of bacteria considered to be potential pathogens in this species.[59] In gopher tortoises, administration of enrofloxacin daily for 5 days resulted in increased mean trough and peak plasma concentrations of enrofloxacin. In Indian star tortoises (*Geochelone elegans*), a pharmacokinetic study indicated that enrofloxacin should be administered at 10 mg/kg IM every 12 hours for treatment of *Pseudomonas* species and *Citrobacter* species infections and every 24 hours for other bacterial infections.[61]

The aforementioned studies indicate that, even with taxonomically related species, there is considerable variation in pharmacokinetic parameters of certain antibiotics.

KETOCONAZOLE

There has been only one study concerning blood concentrations and pharmacokinetics of the antifungal drug ketoconazole in a reptile. In a multiple dose study in gopher tortoises, the administration of ketoconazole, given orally every 24 hours at 15 and 30 mg/kg of body weight, resulted in concentrations of drug in plasma that were considered therapeutic.[56]

Crocodilia: Alligators, Caiman, Crocodiles, Gharial

AMINOGLYCOSIDES

In crocodilians, scientifically derived antimicrobial drug doses are only available for gentamicin and amikacin in American alligators (*A. mississippiensis*). In juvenile American alligators maintained at a water temperature of 22°C, gentamicin was absorbed rapidly after IM administration, with a biphasic distribution having both rapid and slow phases for both dosages administered.[34] The $T_{1/2}$ values for the 1.25 mg/kg and 1.75 mg/kg dosages were 37.8 hours and 75.4 hours, respectively. The recommended dosage of gentamicin in American alligators was 1.75 mg/kg every 72 to 96 hours.

In juvenile American alligators maintained at a water temperature of 22°C, amikacin was absorbed rapidly after IM administration, with a biphasic disposition having both rapid and slow phases.[34] The $T_{1/2}$ values for alligators administered 1.75 mg/kg and 2.25 mg/kg were 49.4 and 52.8 hours, respectively. The peak concentrations following administration of a second dose

at 96 hours were greater than those achieved following the first injection. The recommended dosage was 2.25 mg/kg IM every 72 to 96 hours.

Squamata: Lizards and Snakes

Lizards (suborder Lacertilia) and snakes (suborder Ophidia) comprise the majority of extant reptiles. Therefore, it is surprising that, whereas several pharmacokinetic drug studies have been conducted in snakes, there has been only one study in a lizard. Antimicrobial doses in lizards are generally extrapolated from those determined in other reptiles or calculated by metabolic scaling.[58, 65]

PENICILLINS

There are few pharmacokinetic studies involving penicillins in snakes. A study was conducted with carbenicillin in nine snakes of five different species, including a mangrove snake (*Boiga dendrophila*), two king snakes (*Lampropeltis getulus*), a reticulated python (*Python reticulatus*), a Great Plains rat snake (*Elaphe guttata emoryi*), a yellow rat snake (*Elaphe obsoleta quadrivittata*), and three black rat snakes (*Elaphe obsoleta obsoleta*); all snakes were ill with a variety of pathologic conditions.[44] In snakes receiving carbenicillin at 400 mg/kg of body weight IM, peak plasma concentrations of 177 and 270 μg/ml were reached 1 hour after the initial injection, and therapeutic levels greater than 50 to 60 μg/ml were maintained for at least 12 hours. This dose was significantly higher than doses previously recommended in the literature for mammals. No recommendations were given concerning frequency of administration.

Piperacillin, which is highly active against many aerobic gram-negative organisms, including *P. aeruginosa*, has been evaluated in blood pythons (*Python curtis*).[20] MICs of piperacillin were determined for several species of gram-negative bacilli isolated from the upper respiratory tract of snakes ill with pneumonia. Piperacillin at 100 mg/kg of body weight IM resulted in blood levels that far exceeded the MIC of all bacteria evaluated. The serum $T_{1/2}$ was 12.3 to 17 hours and the recommended dosing interval was every 48 hours.

CEPHALOSPORINS

There is only one pharmacokinetic study for an antimicrobial in a lizard. Cefoperazone, a third-generation beta-lactam antibiotic, was administered as a single IM dose of 200 mg/kg to tegus (*Tupinambis teguixin*)[41] maintained at 24°C. Peak serum levels were reached at 4 hours following injection and at 24 hours had declined to subtherapeutic levels. The recommended dosage was 125 mg/kg every 24 hours. For other antibiotics in lizards, clinicians either extrapolate from doses determined for other reptiles or use metabolic scaling.[58, 65]

Serum concentrations also have been determined for cefoperazone in the colubrid snake (*Hydrodynastes gigas*).[41] Following IM administration of 100 mg/kg cefoperazone, serum levels peaked at 8 hours and therapeutic levels were maintained for more than 96 hours. The recommended dosage was 100 mg/kg every 96 hours.

Another third-generation beta-lactam antibiotic is ceftazidime. Because of its enhanced antipseudomonal activity, its minimal nephrotoxic effects, and the ability to deliver a large dose in a relatively small volume, ceftazidime is often selected for use in reptiles. However, pharmacokinetic studies are limited to snakes. In a study involving several species of snakes, ceftazidime showed a high level of in vitro activity against Enterobacteriaceae and other gram-negative bacilli, with only 9 of 32 strains tested by disc diffusion being resistant.[43] The five following species of snakes were used and maintained at 30°C: mangrove snake, boa constrictor (*Boa constrictor*), reticulated python, Burmese python, and yellow rat snake. Peak plasma antibiotic levels after a single IM injection of 20 mg/kg were reached 1 to 8 hours after the initial injection, and therapeutic levels were maintained for at least 96 hours. No obvious side effects were noted. A dosage of 20 mg/kg every 72 hours was recommended.

CHLORAMPHENICOL

In bull snakes (*Pituophis melanoleucus catenifer*) administered Chloromycetin succinate subcutaneously (SQ) at 40 mg/kg body weight, $T_{1/2}$ was 5.2 hours, in comparison with 1.5 to 3 hours for mammals.[7] On the basis of this study, the author recommended that this dose be administered every 24 hours for 5 to 14 days, depending on the clinical situation and clinical response. Two snakes in this study that were maintained at 24°C were administered 12 mg/kg Chloromycetin palmitate per os (PO); absorption was slow and therapeutic levels were not reached. In another study, the following 16 species were used: (1) red-bellied water snake (*Nerodia erythrogaster*), (2) midland water snake (*Nerodia sipedon*), (3) gray rat snake (*Elaphe obsoleta spiloides*), (4) corn snake (*Elaphe guttata guttata*), (5) eastern king snake (*Lampropeltis getulus getulus*), (6) eastern indigo snake (*Drymarchon corais couperi*), (7) black racer (*Coluber constrictor*), (8) hog nose snake (*Heterodon platyrhinos*), (9) copperhead (*Agkistrodon contortrix*), (10) cottonmouth (*Agkistrodon piscivorus*), (11) timber rattlesnake (*Crotalus horridus horridus*), (12) eastern diamond-back rattlesnake (*Crotalus adamanteus*), (13) reticulated python, (14) Indian rock python (*Python molurus molurus*), (15) Burmese python, and (16) boa constrictor. The $T_{1/2}$ was quite different between these species, varying from 3.3 hours in the eastern indigo snake to 22.1 hours in the midland water snake.[11] The recommended dose was 50 mg/kg, but the frequency of administration varied from every 12 hours to every 72 hours.

AMINOGLYCOSIDES

Gentamicin was the first aminoglycoside to be used in treating reptiles with severe gram-negative bacterial infections. Gentamicin, however, has a narrow safe therapeutic range and cases of nephrotoxicity have been reported in reptiles, particularly snakes administered

mammalian dosages.[24, 53] In one of the first antimicrobial drug studies in a reptile, it was demonstrated that, in bull snakes kept at 24°C, the $T_{1/2}$ for gentamicin was 82 hours.[8] It was clear from this work that gentamicin was eliminated much more slowly than in mammals and this accounted for toxicities seen when snakes were administered a mammalian dosing regimen. On the basis of these findings, an IM dose of 2.5 mg/kg every 72 hours was recommended. In another study in blood pythons, a loading dose of 2.5 mg/kg followed by a maintenance dose of 1.5 mg/kg every 96 hours was recommended.[19]

There is only a single pharmacokinetic study of amikacin in snakes. In gopher snakes (*Pituophis melanoleucus*) maintained at 37°C, although the half-life was not significantly different from those maintained at 25°C, there was a larger volume of distribution and a more rapid body clearance at 37°C than at 25°C.[49] The authors recommended that amikacin be administered IM at 5 mg/kg (loading dose) followed by 2.5 mg/kg every 72 hours.

FLUOROQUINOLONES

Results of a study involving the oral administration of ciprofloxacin in reticulated pythons indicated that this drug should be administered at 2.5 mg/kg every 48 to 72 hours.[40] In juvenile Burmese pythons (*Python molurus bivittatus*) that received an IM injection of enrofloxacin at 5 mg/kg of body weight, the mean maximal plasma concentration was reached at 5.75 hours after injection.[70] Multiple dose studies indicated that, over a 5-day period of sampling, even though there was a stepwise increase in mean trough plasma concentrations of enrofloxacin, peak plasma concentrations did not significantly increase during the sampling period. These results indicated that, when treating young Burmese pythons for *Pseudomonas* infections, enrofloxacin should be administered at an initial dose of 10 mg/kg followed by 5 mg/kg every 48 hours.

COMBINATION DOSING

The aminoglycosides gentamicin and amikacin are often used in combination with penicillins and cephalosporins for treatment of severe gram-negative infections in reptiles, such as those caused by *Pseudomonas* and *Proteus*. Aminoglycosides are often combined with either carbenicillin or piperacillin. Because clinical studies have demonstrated antagonisms between gentamicin and carbenicillin, these drugs should not be mixed before injection because chemical interaction will result in complex formation and inactivation of these antibiotics.[62] One dosing regimen begins with the administration of gentamicin or amikacin on day one, followed by carbenicillin or piperacillin on day 3 (48 hours later). Both drugs are then administered every 3 days for a total of 7 to 9 treatments for each antibiotic.

Another combination that is routinely used is gentamicin or amikacin in combination with ceftazidime. No antagonisms have been reported between these antibiotics. The aminoglycoside is administered on day 1, followed by ceftazidime on day 2. Both drugs are then administered every 3 days, with a total of 7 to 9 treatments for the aminoglycoside and up to 21 treatments with ceftazidime. The author has never observed negative side effects of ceftazidime in reptiles.

Bacteroides, Fusobacterium, Clostridium, and *Peptostreptococcus* have been cultured from a variety of lesions in reptiles including subcutaneous and hepatic abscesses.[68] Because aminoglycosides are uniformly ineffective against anaerobes, the author recommended that antibiotics effective against anaerobes such as carbenicillin, ceftazidime, and metronidazole be used in treating infections with these organisms in reptiles. In most cases, when anaerobes were isolated, aerobes were also cultured, so combined antibiotic therapy with an aminoglycoside and one of the aforementioned antibiotics efficacious against anaerobes was indicated.

ANTIMICROBIAL DRUGS USED FOR MICROBIAL INFECTIONS: EMPIRICALLY DERIVED DOSES

Trimethoprim/Sulfonamides

Even though the author has used trimethoprim/sulfonamides in reptiles, there are no pharmacokinetic studies for determining appropriate doses. The author has used injectable trimethoprim/sulfadiazine at 30 mg/kg, the first two doses administered 24 hours apart and then every 48 hours. No toxic effects have been seen in any of a wide variety of reptile species medicated. The veterinary injectable form is not readily available in the United States.

Tylosin

The author is not aware of any pharmacokinetic studies of tylosin in reptiles. Still, this antimicrobial has been administered IM to reptiles, particularly those with respiratory disease, at 5 mg/kg every 24 hours.[37]

Metronidazole

Infections with anaerobic bacteria are seen in ill reptiles. In one study of 39 specimens collected from reptiles, 21 yielded the following anaerobic bacteria: *Bacteroides, Fusobacterium, Clostridium,* and *Peptostreptococcus.*[68] In vitro sensitivity testing indicated that all isolates that were tested were sensitive to metronidazole. Although no pharmacokinetic studies have been reported with metronidazole in reptiles, this drug is often used in reptiles with amebiasis and trichomoniasis. In general, the dose used for treating reptiles with amebic and trichomonad infections is generally 100 mg/kg PO given as a single dose and repeated in 2 weeks, but, for bacterial infections, the recommended dosage is 20 mg/kg once per day for a minimum of 1 week.

Nystatin

Although there are no pharmacokinetic studies of nystatin in the literature, this drug has been administered orally to reptiles with *Candida* infections of the oral cavity and gastrointestinal tract. The recommended dosage was 100,000 IU/kg every 24 hours.[25]

SOAKS AND DIPS FOR AQUATIC CHELONIANS

Necrotizing or proliferative skin lesions commonly develop in captive hatchling marine turtles, especially when they are raised under crowded conditions. To evaluate the effect of several different dips on loggerhead sea turtles (*Caretta caretta*), hatchlings were soaked in various concentrations of several chemicals.[46] No external injuries were observed in hatchlings that were bathed for 10 days in seawater containing one of the following chemicals: (1) 0.1 to 0.4 ppm potassium permanganate, (2) 25 to 400 ppm formalin, and (3) 0.1 to 0.4 ppm malachite green. The following concentrations produced either irritating or toxic effects: (1) 0.8 ppm potassium permanganate, (2) 800 ppm formalin, and (3) 0.8 ppm and 1.6 ppm malachite green. In Florida soft-shell turtles (*Trionyx ferox*) with cutaneous mucormycosis, affected turtles were immersed for 15 minutes in a solution of 0.15 mg/L malachite green three times daily for 1 week.[33] Turtles were thoroughly rinsed with fresh water following the immersions to reduce eye irritation. There was a regression in lesions in treated turtles, with mild conjunctivitis being an adverse side effect.

SELECTION OF ANTIMICROBIAL DRUGS

The selection of an antimicrobial drug involves multiple host-, drug-, and bacteria-specific factors, which should be taken into account before administration. A primary consideration is identification of the causative agent. If a lesion is present, in addition to collecting a swab specimen for culture, a biopsy specimen should be collected for cytologic and histologic evaluation. This is essential when interpreting the significance of cultured microbes. In reptiles suspected of being septic, blood samples should be obtained for culture. Techniques for collecting specimens from reptiles are discussed elsewhere.[29]

Bacterial infections are commonly encountered in captive reptiles, either as primary or secondary invaders. Mixed bacterial infections are routinely seen. Although infections with gram-positive microbes have been reported in reptiles, as discussed earlier, gram-negative infections are more commonly seen. In one study, *Pseudomonas, Providencia, Proteus,* and *Morganella* accounted for 44% of isolates from ill reptiles.[28] A variety of fungal diseases has also been reported in reptiles.[50] *Aspergillus, Fusarium, Geotrichum, Paecilomyces, Candida,* and a variety of Phycomycetes have been identified as causative agents of fungal disease in reptiles.

Following isolation and identification of the causative bacterial agent, MICs of antibiotics should be determined. Once MICs are known, selection of the most appropriate antibiotic depends on the following: (1) system affected and type of lesion, (2) antibiotic pharmacodynamics and pharmacokinetics, and (3) size, clinical condition, temperament, and immune status of the host.

In selecting an antibiotic, the clinician should choose a drug that will reach therapeutic concentrations in the affected tissue. There are several special biologic features of reptiles that influence treatment. First, reptiles often produce granulomatous inflammation in response to a variety of pathogens.[52] Because most antibiotics do not readily penetrate well-developed granulomas, the list of affective drugs may be short. Where mature granulomas are located subcutaneously, concurrently with use of appropriate antimicrobials, most of these lesions should be removed surgically.

Pharmacologic properties of antibiotics need to be considered, and, as discussed, the clinician must select a drug that will penetrate the affected tissue and lesion. Furthermore, potential side effects and toxicities of the drugs must be considered. For instance, gentamicin-associated visceral gout has been reported in reptiles when this antibiotic was administered at mammalian therapeutic dosages.[24, 53]

Selecting a bacteriostatic drug versus a bactericidal drug is an important consideration. Even when the ill reptile is maintained under ideal environmental conditions, the immune status of the animal may be suboptimal. Because many ill reptiles, especially those with chronic infections, appear to be immunocompromised, bactericidal antibiotics rather than bacteriostatic drugs are generally recommended.[28]

Size and temperament of the animal may also influence the drug being selected, including the route of administration. Most species of reptiles weigh less than 100 g and many weigh less than 30 g. In some species of lizards, adults weigh only a few grams. Administering drugs to these animals can be extremely difficult. The clinician may be limited to those antibiotics that can easily be diluted to a concentration that can be precisely and safely injected. At the other end of the spectrum are the very large, dangerous reptiles. In these animals, the clinician may choose to administer a drug that can be given in a relatively small volume via an injection dart. In dangerous reptiles such as venomous snakes, a drug that can be administered every few days rather than daily is preferred. Some reptiles are extremely timid and nervous, and may not be suitable for injection. In such cases, the antibiotic must be administered orally, preferably in food if the animal is still feeding. Thus, the route of administration also influences the choice of antibiotics to be administered.

ENVIRONMENTAL AND PHYSIOLOGIC CONSIDERATIONS

Because reptiles are ectotherms, their physiology and behavior are markedly affected by environmental temperature. Most species show varying degrees of thermoregulation during the course of daily activity and, with temperate species, seasonal changes. Daily activity is conducted within a thermal optimal temperature zone, which may show both age-related and seasonal changes. The range of this zone varies among species, especially among those adapted to widely different habitats. Nocturnal reptiles, diurnal desert reptiles, diurnal temperate forest reptiles, tropical reptiles, montane reptiles, and aquatic reptiles may all have markedly different thermal requirements. When calculating drug doses and in treatment of ill reptiles, it is important to consider that environmental temperature has profound effects on physiologic processes of reptiles. A review of activity temperatures of reptiles can be found elsewhere.[2]

Health status may affect temperature preferences of reptiles, thereby affecting metabolism. Behavioral fever has been described in reptiles in which a behavioral temperature of 2°C developed in desert iguanas (*Dipsosaurus dorsalis*) when injected with a killed bacteria (*A. hydrophila*).[69] That is, when placed in a temperature gradient, lizards injected with bacteria thermoregulated at body temperatures 2°C above controls. Furthermore, when desert iguanas were injected with live *A. hydrophila*, those maintained at an elevated ambient temperature had a significant increase in survival rate compared to those maintained at lower temperatures.[42] Some clinicians[49] have used this information by recommending that reptiles ill with microbial infection should be treated and maintained at the upper limits of their optimal temperature zone. Other clinicians[63] have successfully treated illness in pythons using a method termed *thermotherapy*. Pythons with signs of respiratory disease showed clinical improvement after being maintained at a temperature range of 92° to 97°C. The basis for this more than likely includes the direct effect of temperature on immune function in reptiles.

Several studies have demonstrated that the humoral response and graft rejection in reptiles is temperature dependent.[13] Whereas a maximum humoral response is seen at temperatures within the thermal optimal temperature zone, suboptimal temperatures resulted in a slower response to injected antigens and a longer period before allografts were rejected. At 10°C, snapping turtles (*Chelydra serpentina*) do not react to allografts at all.[6] The author of this paper has made several observations in which bacterial sepsis developed in reptiles subjected to transient temperatures approaching the critical thermal maximum following a reduction of ambient temperature to optimal levels. Other physiologic changes may occur if a reptile is maintained continuously at the warm body temperatures that they preferentially select for shorter periods of time during normal daily activity. In studies with the lizards *Urosaurus ornatus, Sceloporus virgatus,* and *Sceloporus graciosus* when exposed 10 hours per day for 3 weeks to temperatures 1° to 2°C above their respective preferred ranges suffered marked spermatogenic damage and a decline in appetite and body weight.[47]

Maintaining reptiles at the upper limits of their optimal temperature zone has additional complications. In Benedict's 1932 study[4] of water loss in pythons, the three average values for insensible perspiration during a 24-hour period were 0.4, 4.0, and 7.3 g/kg in snakes maintained at 20°, 26°, and 33°C, respectively. In another study with the snakes *Coluber ravergieri, Spalerosophis cliffordi, Vipera palaestinae,* and *Aspis cerastes,* total evaporative water loss in resting and active snakes increased with temperature, with the values at 35°C being twice as high as those maintained at 22°C.[15] At higher environmental temperatures, more fluids are lost, and with an ill reptile, especially one with respiratory, gastrointestinal, or integumentary system disease, excessive fluid loss may occur, thus further compromising the health status of the animal. Evaluating the hydration status of these animals becomes critical if thermotherapy is used.

Whereas metabolism is increased at elevated temperature, thereby "helping" to control or kill the infectious agent, the pharmacokinetics of the administered drug also may be affected. In gopher snakes administered amikacin and housed at 37°C, the volume of distribution of the antibiotic was larger and it was more rapidly cleared than in those housed at 25°C.[49] In a study in gopher tortoises acclimated at 20° and 30°C and administered amikacin at 5 mg/kg body weight (shell included),[10] the half-life was significantly less at 30°C than in the group maintained at 20°C. The clearance rate of amikacin in the warmer acclimated tortoises was approximately twice as fast as that of the cooler acclimated tortoises. Change in clearance rates may influence potential toxic effects of certain drugs. In a study with gentamicin in water snakes (*Nerodia fasciata*), toxic effects on the kidney were more severe at 30°C than at 20°C.[21] This effect of ambient temperature on metabolism and drug toxicity must be considered when determining the most appropriate dosage and administration interval. Even though a temperature range of 30° to 35°C may be ideal for many reptiles, some species have a lower thermal optimal range and others have a higher range.

The half-lives of a number of antibiotics appear to be considerably longer in reptiles than in mammals. However, the proper dosing has only been determined in a few species. Because reptiles are a highly diverse group, both anatomically and physiologically, it may not be scientifically correct to extrapolate from one species to the next. For instance, even though enrofloxacin was found to have prolonged blood concentrations following an IM injection of 5 mg/kg of body weight in box turtles (D. Aucoin, personal communication, 1993), in Hermann's tortoise, the therapeutic blood concentrations lasted only 24 hours following an IM injection of 10 mg/kg.[67] Differences more than likely also exist within a species, varying with age and size.

ADMINISTRATION OF ANTIMICROBIALS

In most cases, antimicrobials are given by injection, either SQ or IM. The author generally administers oral antimicrobials only when there is primary infection of the gastrointestinal tract, when an animal does not tolerate injections and has to be medicated in its feed, and when the required drug is only available in an oral form. In farming operations of reptiles such as with crocodilians and sea turtles, when large numbers of reptiles are ill and have to be treated, it may not be practical to administer drugs by injection. In such cases, oral medication is generally the preferred route of administration.

Several problems exist with oral medication of reptiles. First, very few pharmacokinetic studies have been performed on drugs administered orally to reptiles. Thus, for most antimicrobials, the dose selected is not based on science. The gastrointestinal transit time varies greatly between the various groups and species of reptiles, being the slowest in the large herbivorous reptiles. Even in some carnivorous reptiles, the transit time may be quite prolonged. Thus, in these animals it may be difficult to achieve optimal therapeutic concentrations of antimicrobials in blood following administration of oral medicants.

Even though many oral medicants can be administered in the food of ill reptiles that are feeding, orally medicating reptiles that are not feeding may not be a simple task. Venomous snakes and large crocodilians are dangerous to handle and manipulate for administration of oral drugs. It may be impossible to extricate the head beyond the shell margins and force open the mouths of many species of turtles and tortoises. The keratinized epidermal hard parts over the mandibles and dentary bones are easily traumatized, and extreme care must be taken in trying to force the mouth open. The giant tortoises are particularly difficult to give oral medicants. These reptiles must be anesthetized and a pharyngostomy tube inserted for oral medication to be given.[54]

As a generalization, snakes are the easiest group of reptiles to orally medicate. The mouths of most snakes are simple to open and, because the glottis is in an extremely cranial position, is easily avoided. A lubricated French catheter or nasogastric tube can be passed down the esophagus of the snake with minimal resistance. Catheters that are very rigid should be avoided. It is important to have the snake relatively straight when passing the catheter. Because the cranial esophagus is extremely thin in most species, the end of the catheter should be round and smooth. The stomach of most snakes is from one third to one half of the way down the distance from the head to cloaca, but it is not necessary to pass a catheter as far as this organ. In most situations, passing the catheter halfway between the stomach and oral cavity is satisfactory.

Most of the antibiotics commonly used in reptile medicine are administered either IM or SQ. The problem with intravenous administration of antibiotics is that, except in tortoises, peripheral vessels cannot be visualized.[32] Even though blood can be collected from a number of sites in different species of reptiles,[55, 64] most of this sampling is "blind" and may not be suitable for repetitive infusions. With SQ and IM drug administrations, the author avoids administering drugs that require large volumes per kilogram of body weight, especially if the drug is irritating to surrounding tissues. For instance, necrotizing skin lesions developed in several snakes following injection of more than 1 ml of enrofloxacin at a single site.

Because most species of reptiles have a well-developed renal portal system, with blood from the caudal half of the body going to the kidneys before reaching systemic circulation, SQ and IM injections often are administered in the cranial half of the body. This is particularly important when injecting drugs that are potentially nephrotoxic and those that are eliminated primarily through the renal system. However, few studies have looked at this potential problem scientifically (see Chapter 32). In a recent study, red-eared sliders received either gentamicin (10 mg/kg) or carbenicillin (200 mg/kg) in a forelimb or hindlimb.[22] No significant differences were found in any of the pharmacokinetic determinants in turtles given gentamicin. With carbenicillin, those that received the drug in a hindlimb had significantly lower blood levels for the first 12 hours after injection than those that received it in a forelimb. However, because blood levels for both injection sites were still well above the MIC for organisms generally treated with carbenicillin, this difference was not considered clinically significant. Still, the renal portal system varies in development between various groups of reptiles and further work is needed before broad generalizations can be made.

Snakes are the easiest reptiles to inject because of the large dorsal muscle masses associated with the ribs and vertebrae. In lizards, the muscle masses associated with the forelimbs are not substantial and small volumes of drug are needed in these animals. Tortoises, especially the large tortoises, have extremely thick epidermal hard parts on the cranial aspect of their forelimbs, therefore injections are generally made through the thinner skin on the caudal (posterior) aspect of the forelimbs.

A special feature of all snakes (those with eyes) and some lizards is the spectacle. The spectacle embryologically represents a fusion of the upper and lower eyelids, which have become transparent. It is present as a permanent structure over the cornea and is shed with skin during ecdysis. Infections of the subspectacular space have been reported[51] and topical antibiotics do not appear to move across this structure. In treating such infections in reptiles, a wedge needs to be removed from the spectacle and then appropriate topicals applied directly onto the globe and within the space.

METABOLIC SCALING

The allometric equation $y = a \cdot x^b$ has been used to scale many morphologic and physiologic attributes relative to body mass. For instance, in eutherian mammals, the equation $P_{met} = 70M_b^{0.75}$ has been used to describe the relationship between metabolic rate (P_{met}) and body mass (M_b).[39] This relationship between metabolic rate and body mass has been used in determining appropriate dosages and dosing intervals of antibiotics both intraspecifically for different sized reptiles and interspecifically for those reptiles in which antibiotic pharmacokinetic studies have not been performed using a similar allometric equation (MEC = 10[kg]$^{0.75}$).[58, 64, 65] However, in a recent review of the subject, no single equation was considered appropriate for all reptiles because the mass constant varies from 1 to 5 for snakes

and 6 to 10 for lizards; no values for chelonians or crocodilians are available.[29]

Even though metabolic scaling of antibiotics is a simple mathematical process, a number of problems surface when this approach is examined more closely. First, unless the mass constant for the unknown species approximates that of the known species, inappropriate dosages and intervals of administration are calculated. When metabolic allometric equations are compared among different reptiles, there appears to be significant variability in these data between different studies. For instance, Bartholomew and Tucker,[3] in looking at metabolic data on lizards ranging in size from 2 g to 4.4 kg, calculated the allometric equation to be $P_{met} = 6.84M_b^{0.62}$. This is different than findings by Bennet and Dawson[5] for 24 species of lizards ranging in weight from 0.01 to 7 kg, for which the equation $P_{met} = 7.81M_b^{0.83}$ was determined. Furthermore, still different equations have been calculated for snakes.[17] In determining resting metabolic rate of 34 species from genera of boas and pythons, the mass exponents of different species showed considerable variation.[10a] Second, the variable body temperature of ectotherms compounds the ability to derive a universal equation, even for a single species. It is well known that metabolism of ectotherms varies directly with body temperature.[5] As body temperature increases, so does metabolism. Thus a reptile at 20°C consumes less oxygen per unit time than the same animal maintained at 30°C.[10a, 30] This is reflected by changes in mass constant with changes in environmental temperature.[10a]

Pharmacokinetic differences may exist between species within the same family, independent of metabolic rate. For instance, the $T_{1/2}$ of enrofloxacin in the Indian star tortoise was 5.1 hours,[61] whereas for the gopher tortoise it was 23.1 hours.[59] In a study involving the administration of chloramphenicol in 87 snakes of 16 different species, the biologic half-life varied from 3.3 hours in the indigo snake to 22.1 hours in the midland water snake.[11]

All available pharmacokinetic studies and metabolic allometric equations are derived from clinically healthy reptiles. Differences more than likely exist between healthy and ill reptiles in regard to uptake, distribution, and elimination of drugs and overall metabolism.

Even though metabolic scaling of antibiotics is a potentially useful and practical tool in drug dosing, the aforementioned limitations must be considered when dosing an ill reptile. Until more scientifically derived information is available for demonstrating the accuracy of metabolic scaling of antibiotics in reptiles, the clinician must be aware of the limitations of this approach. On the surface this appears to be better than extrapolation, but developing a single equation for all reptiles may not be valid. Metabolic scaling is most useful when calculating doses in a species for which a specific equation has been determined under specific environmental conditions. A validation study using enrofloxacin in the green iguana is being conducted (L. Maxwell, personal communication, February 1988) and should provide valuable information on this approach in dosing drugs in reptiles.

Acknowledgments

Portions of this chapter were borrowed from Jacobson ER: Use of antimicrobial therapy in reptiles, *in* Antimicrobial Therapy in Caged Birds and Exotic Pets, An International Symposium, Trenton, NJ, Veterinary Learning Systems, 1995; and from Jacobson ER: Metabolic scaling of antibiotics in reptiles: basis and limitations, Zoo Biology 15:329–339, 1996.

REFERENCES

1. Austwick PKC, Keymer IF: Fungi and actinomycetes. *In* Cooper JE, Jackson OF (eds): Diseases of the Reptilia, vol I. London, Academic Press, pp 192–231, 1981.
2. Avery RA: Field studies of reptilian thermoregulation. *In* Gans C, Pough FM (eds): Biology of the Reptilia, vol 12C. London, Academic Press, pp 93–166, 1980.
3. Bartholomew GA, Tucker VA: Size, body temperature, thermal conductance, oxygen consumption, and heart rate in Australian varanid lizards. Physiol Zoo 37:341–354, 1964.
4. Benedict FG: The Physiology of Large Reptiles. Washington, DC, Carnegie Institution of Washington, 1932.
5. Bennet AF, Dawson WR: Metabolism. *In* Gans C, Dawson WR (eds): Biology of the Reptilia, Physiology A, vol 5. New York, Academic Press, pp 127–223, 1976.
6. Borysenko M: Skin allograft and xenograft rejection in the snapping turtle, *Chelydra serpentina*. J Exp Zool 170:341–358, 1969.
7. Bush M, Smeller JM, Charache P, et al: Preliminary study of antibiotics in snakes. Proceedings of the Annual Meeting of the American Association of Zoo Veterinarians, St. Louis, pp 50–54, 1976.
8. Bush M, Smeller JM, Charache P, et al: Biological half-life of gentamicin in gopher snakes. Am J Vet Res 39:171–173, 1976.
9. Bush M, Custer R, Smeller JM, et al: Preliminary study of gentamicin in turtles. Proceedings of the Annual Meeting of the American Association of Zoo Veterinarians, Honolulu, pp 71–73, 1977.
10. Caligiuri RL, Kollias GV, Jacobson ER, et al: The effects of ambient temperature on amikacin pharmacokinetics in gopher tortoises. Vet Pharmacol Ther 13:287–291, 1990.
10a. Chappell MA, Ellis TM: Resting metabolic rates in boid snakes: allometric relationships and temperature effects. J Comp Physiol [B] 157:227–235, 1987.
11. Clark CH, Rogers ED, Milton SL: Plasma concentrations of chloramphenicol in snakes. Am J Vet Res 46:2654–2657, 1985.
12. Clark HF, Lunger PD: Viruses. *In* Cooper JE, Jackson OF (eds): Diseases of the Reptilia, vol I. London, Academic Press, pp 135–164, 1981.
13. Cooper EL, Klempau AE, Zapata AG: Reptilian immunity. *In* Gans C, Billet F, Maderson PFA (eds): Biology of the Reptilia, vol 14C. New York, Wiley, pp 599–678, 1985.
14. Cooper JE: Bacteria. *In* Cooper JE, Jackson OF (eds): Diseases of the Reptilia, vol I. Academic Press, London, pp 165–191, 1981.
15. Dmi'el R: Relation of metabolism to body weight in snakes. Copeia 1972:179–181, 1972.
16. Frye FL: Reptile Care, vols I and II. Neptune City, NJ, TFH, 1991.
17. Galvao PE, Tarasantchi J, Guertzenstein P: Heat production of tropical snakes in relation to body weight and body surface. Am J Physiol 209:501–506, 1965.
18. Gorden RW, Hazen TC, Esch GW, Fliemans CB: Isolation of *Aeromonas hydrophila* from the American alligator (*Alligator mississippiensis*). J Wildl Dis 15:239–243, 1979.
19. Hilf M, Swanson D, Wagner R, et al: Pharmacokinetics of gentamicin and piperacillin in blood pythons: new dosing regimen. Proceedings of the 13th International Symposium for the Propagation and Husbandry of Reptiles, Phoenix, pp 87–90, 1989.
20. Hilf M, Swanson D, Wagner R, et al: Pharmacokinetics of piperacillin in blood pythons (*Python curtis*) and in vitro evaluation of efficacy against aerobic gram-negative bacteria. J Zoo Wildl Med 22:199–203, 1991.
21. Hodge MK: The effect of acclimation temperature on gentamicin nephrotoxicity in the Florida banded water snake (*Natrix fasciata*). Proceedings of the Annual Meeting of the American Association of Zoo Veterinarians, Knoxville, TN, pp 226–237, 1978.
22. Holz P, Conlon PD, Crawshaw GJ, Burger J: The reptilian renal portal system and its effect on drug kinetics. Proceedings of the

Annual Meeting of the Association of Reptile and Amphibian Veterinarians and American Association of Zoo Veterinarians, Pittsburgh, pp 95–96, 1994.
23. Homer BL, Jacobson ER, Schumacher J, Scherba G: Chlamydiosis in green sea turtles. Vet Pathol 31:1–7, 1994.
24. Jacobson ER: Gentamicin-related visceral gout in 2 boid snakes. Vet Med Small Anim Clin 71:361–363, 1976.
25. Jacobson ER: Necrotizing mycotic dermatitis in snakes: clinical and pathologic features. J Am Vet Med Assoc 177:838–841, 1980.
26. Jacobson ER: Infectious diseases of reptiles. *In* Kirk RW (ed): Current Therapy, vol 7. Philadelphia, WB Saunders, pp 625–633, 1980.
27. Jacobson ER: Reptiles. *In* Harkness J (ed): The Veterinary Clinics of North America. Philadelphia, WB Saunders, pp 1203–1225, 1987.
28. Jacobson ER: Laboratory investigations. *In* Beynon PH, Lawton MPC, Cooper JE (eds): Manual of Reptiles. Gloucestershire, England, British Small Animal Veterinary Association, pp 50–62, 1992.
29. Jacobson ER: Metabolic scaling of antibiotics in reptiles: basis and limitations. Zoo Biol 15:329–339, 1996.
30. Jacobson ER, Whitford WG: The effect of acclimation on physiological response to temperature in the snakes, *Thamnophis proximus* and *Natrix rhombifera*. Comp Biochem Physiol 35:439–449, 1970.
31. Jacobson ER, Gaskin JM: Paramyxovirus infection of viperid snakes. *In* Biology of Pit Vipers. Tyler, TX, Selva, pp 415–419, 1992.
32. Jacobson ER, Schumacher J, Green ME: Techniques for sampling and handling blood for hematologic and plasma biochemical determinations in the desert tortoise, *Xerobates agassizii*. Copeia 1:237–241, 1992.
33. Jacobson ER, Calderwood MB, Clubb SL: Mucormycosis in hatchling Florida softshell turtles. J Am Vet Med Assoc 177:835–837, 1980.
34. Jacobson ER, Brown MP, Chung M, et al: Serum concentration and disposition kinetics of gentamicin and amikacin in juvenile American alligators. J Zoo Anim Med 19:188–194, 1988.
35. Jacobson ER, Gaskin JM, Brown MB, et al: Chronic upper respiratory tract disease of free-ranging desert tortoises (*Xerobates agassizii*). J Wildl Dis 27:296–316, 1991.
36. Jacobson ER, Brown MB, Schumacher IM, et al: Subclinical mycoplasmosis and the desert tortoise, *Gopherus agassizii*, in Las Vegas Valley, Nevada. Chelon Conserv Biol 1:279–284, 1995.
37. Jenkins JR: Medical management of reptiles. Compendium on Continuing Education 13:980–988, 1991.
38. Keymer IF: Diseases of chelonians: (2) necropsy survey of terrapins and turtles. Vet Rec 103:577–582, 1978.
39. Kleiber M: The Fire of Life: An Introduction to Animal Energetics. New York, Wiley, 1961.
40. Klingenberg RJ, Backner B: The use of ciprofloxacin, a new antibiotic, in snakes. Proceedings of the 15th International Symposium on Captive Propagation and Husbandry of Reptiles and Amphibians, Seattle, pp 127–140, 1991.
41. Klingenberg RJ: Therapeutics. *In* Mader DR (ed): Reptile Medicine and Surgery. Philadelphia, WB Saunders, pp 299–321, 1996.
42. Kluger MJ, Ringler DH, Anver MR: Fever and survival. Science 188:166–168, 1975.
43. Lawrence K: Preliminary study on the use of ceftazidime, a broad spectrum cephalosporin antibiotic, in snakes. Res Vet Sci 36:16–20, 1984.
44. Lawrence K, Needham JR, Palmer GH, et al: A preliminary study on the use of carbenicillin in snakes. J Vet Pharmacol Ther 7:119–124, 1984.
45. Lawrence K, Palmer GH, Needham JR: Use of carbenicillin in 2 species of tortoise (*Testudo graeca* and *T hermanni*). Res Vet Sci 40:413–415, 1986.
46. Leong JK, Wheeler RS, Lansford LM: Tolerance and responses of normal and diseased loggerhead turtles (*Caretta caretta*) to some chemotherapeutics. Proceedings of the 11th Annual Meeting of World Mariculture Society, New Orleans, 1980.
47. Licht P: The relation between preferred temperature and testicular heat sensitivity in lizards. Copeia 1965:428–436, 1965.
48. Mader DR: Reptile Medicine and Surgery. Philadelphia, WB Saunders, 1996.
49. Mader DR, Conzelman GM, Baggot JD: Effects of ambient temperature on the half-life and dosage regimen of amikacin in the gopher snake. J Am Vet Med Assoc 187:1134–1136, 1985.
50. Migaki G, Jacobson ER, Casey HW: Fungal diseases of reptiles. *In* Hoff GL, Frye FL, Jacobson ER (eds): Diseases of Amphibians and Reptiles, New York, Plenum Press, pp 183–204, 1984.

51. Millichamp N, Jacobson ER, Wolf E: Diseases of the eye and ocular adnexae in reptiles. J Am Vet Med Assoc 183:1205–1212, 1983.

52. Montali R: Comparative pathology of inflammation in the higher vertebrates (reptile, birds and mammals). J Comp Pathol 99:1–26, 1988.

53. Montali RJ, Bush M, Smeller JM: The pathology of nephrotoxicity of gentamicin in snakes: a model for reptilian gout. Vet Pathol 16:108–115, 1979.

54. Norton TM, Jacobson ER, Caligiuri R, Kollias GV: Medical management of a Galapagos tortoise (*Geochelone elephantopus*) with hypothyroidism. J Zoo Wildl Med 20:212–216, 1989.

55. Olson GA, Hessler JR, Faith FE: Techniques for blood collection and intravascular infusions of reptiles. Lab Anim Sci 25:783–786, 1975.

56. Page CD, Mautino M, Derendorf H, et al: Multiple dose pharmacokinetics of ketoconazole administered to gopher tortoises (*Gopherus polyphemus*). J Zoo Wildl Med 22:191–198, 1991.

57. Plowman CA, Montali RJ, Phillips LG, et al: Septicemia and chronic abscesses in iguanas (*Cyclura cornuta* and *Iguana iguana*) associated with a *Neisseria* species. J Zoo Anim Med 18:86–93, 1987.

58. Pokras MA, Sedgwick CJ, Kaufman E: Therapeutics. *In* Beynon PH, Lawton MPC, Cooper JE (eds): Manual of Reptiles. Gloucestershire, England, British Small Animal Veterinary Association, pp 194–213, 1992.

59. Prezant RM, Isaza I, Jacobson ER: Plasma concentrations and disposition kinetics of enrofloxacin in gopher tortoises (*Gopherus polyphemus*). J Zoo Wildl Med 25:82–87, 1994.

60. Raphael BL, Clark CH, Hudson R: Plasma concentrations of gentamicin in turtles. J Zoo Anim Med 16:138–139, 1985.

61. Raphael BL, Papich M, Cook RA: Pharmacokinetics of enrofloxacin after a single intramuscular injection in Indian star tortoises. 25:88–94, 1994.

62. Riff LJ, Jackson GG: Laboratory and clinical conditions for gentamicin inactivation by carbenicillin. Arch Intern Med 130:887–890, 1972.

63. Ross RA: The Bacterial Diseases of Reptiles. Stanford, CA, Institute for Herpetological Research, 1984.

64. Samour HJ, Rishey D, March T, et al: Blood sampling techniques in reptiles. Vet Rec 12:472–478, 1984.

65. Sedgwick CJ, Borkowski R: Allometric scaling: extrapolating treatment regimens for reptiles. *In* Mader DR (ed): Reptile Medicine and Surgery. Philadelphia, WB Saunders, pp 235–241, 1996.

66. Sedgwick CJ, Moffat S, Kollias GV: Scaling antimicrobial drug dosage regimens to minimum energy cost rather than body weight. Proceedings of the Annual Meeting of the American Association of Zoo Veterinarians, Louisville, KY, pp 15–20, 1984.

67. Spörle H, Göbel T, Schildger, B: Blood-levels of some anti-infectives in the Hermann's tortoise (*Testudo hermanni*) [Abstract]. *In* 4th International Colloquium on Pathology and Medicine of Reptiles and Amphibians, Bad Nauheim, Germany, 1991.

68. Stewart JS: Anaerobic bacterial infections in reptiles. J Zoo Wildl Med 21:180–184, 1990.

69. Vaughn LK, Bernheim HA, Kluger MJ: Fever in the lizard *Dipsosaurus dorsalis*. Nature 252: 473–474, 1974.

70. Young LA, Schumacher J, Papich MG, Jacobson ER: Disposition of enrofloxacin and its metabolite ciprofloxacin after intramuscular injection in juvenile Burmese pythons (*Python molurus bivittatus*). J Zoo Wildl Med 28:71–79, 1997.

CHAPTER 27

Chameleon Medicine

MICHAEL T. BARRIE

Chameleons are highly specialized arboreal reptiles. Most species are found in sub-Saharan Africa and Madagascar. In captivity, chameleons are well known as being delicate, requiring close individual attention to nutritional, environmental, and social needs. The family Chamaeleonidae has two subfamilies, Chamaeleoninae and Brookesinae. The subfamily Chamaeleoninae contains two genuses, *Chameleo* and *Bradypodion*. *Chameleo* species are those most frequently seen in herpetologic collections. *Bradypodion* species are also known as dwarf chameleons. The subfamily Brookesinae consists of the genuses *Brookesia* and *Rampholeon*.

BIOLOGIC DATA

Most species of chameleons have a laterally flattened body. Opposing toes on their feet and a prehensile tail are adapted to walking on branches. Turret-like eyes that move independently allow observation of two objects at once or provide binocular vision when focusing on prey. Chameleons use stealth to catch prey, walking in a slow halting gait that has been described as resembling leaves moving in a breeze. Their coloration provides excellent camouflage to foil prey and predators alike. An elastic tongue, connected to a long hyoid apparatus, can catch prey several body lengths away. Chameleons change color according to mood, reproductive status, and for thermal regulation, and not, as is widely believed, to match their surroundings. They are not fast runners but some species will jump off a branch and drop to the ground if threatened. Species of the subfamily Brookesinae differ from this general description in that they are more terrestrial, have non-prehensile or weakly prehensile tails, and have little ability to change colors. The chameleon ear is simple, lacking an external aperture or tympanic membrane. The lungs are also very simple in structure, and, in many species,

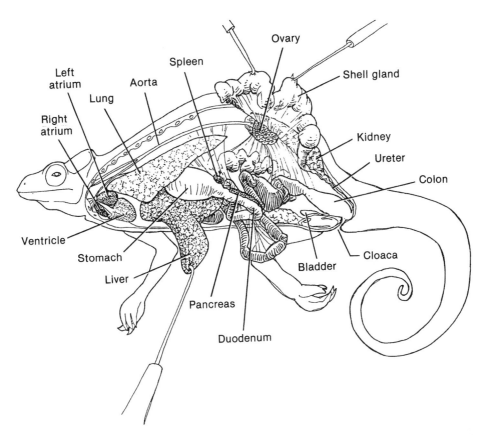

FIGURE 27–1. Lateral, midsagittal view of a female chameleon. (From Barten SL: Lizards. *In* Mader DR [ed]: Reptile Medicine and Surgery. Philadelphia, WB Saunders, p 50, 1996.)

there are finger-like sacculations that have been used as a means of classification. The intestines are often pigmented black. Figures 27–1 and 27–2 show basic anatomy of a chameleon.

As a group, chameleons have diversified into a variety of preferred natural habitats, many species having very specialized environmental needs. The panther chameleon (*Furcifer pardalis*), which tends to thrive in degraded forests, is hardier in captivity, being more tolerant to varying environmental conditions. Husbandry requirements differ dramatically among species and thorough research of specific environmental and nutritional needs is paramount. Several excellent reviews of husbandry that address the needs of individual species have been published.[5, 9–13, 17, 21, 28, 31] The life expectancy of chameleons in nature may be short. Species that come from environments with heavy predatory pressures may only live one season and, as a result, reproduce at a young age. Jackson's chameleon (*Chamaeleo jacksonii*) and Parson's chameleon, *Chamaeleo parsonii (Calumma parsonii),* have been reported to live as long as 9 and 7 years, respectively, in captivity.[28]

Blood can be taken from the tail vein in large species and via cardiac puncture from the right or left axilla in smaller species. The hemogram of reptilian blood can be quite variable and dependent on external factors. Normal parameters are not well established for chame-

leon species but examination of blood smears and plasma chemical values can be a useful adjunct to a thorough physical examination. The hemogram may be useful in assessing inflammation, parasitemia, and anemia. Techniques for evaluating blood have been described.[6, 24]

HUSBANDRY

Providing an optimal environment for chameleons is especially important to this delicate group of animals. Proper chameleon care is specialized and intensive. Subtle environmental deficiencies can result in failure to thrive. Enclosure size, perching, lighting quality and intensity, thermal gradients, natural climatic cycles, nutrition, and social interaction are a few of the factors to consider when trying to understand the needs of a chameleon. Adequate housing should generally provide for a spacious, buoyant environment. Chameleons do not do well in glass-sided aquariums. Nonabrasive screen or plastic-coated wire with covered edges is needed to protect the animal's feet. Chameleons must be carefully observed on a daily basis to ensure they are eating and drinking.

Chameleons need a nighttime temperature decrease of 5° to 10° F. Daytime highs depend on the species.

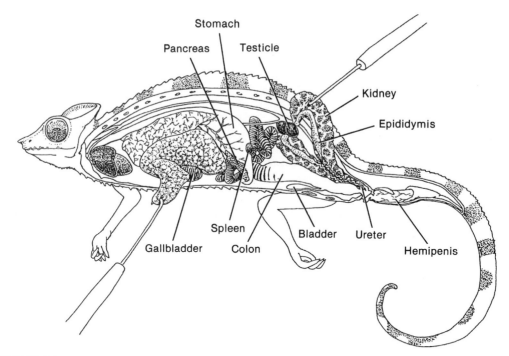

FIGURE 27–2. Lateral, midsagittal view of a male chameleon. (From Barten SL: Lizards. *In* Mader DR [ed]: Reptile Medicine and Surgery. Philadelphia, WB Saunders, p 50, 1996.)

Montane species such as *C. jacksonii, Chamaeleo fisheri,* and *Chamaeleo montium* do best at 70° to 80°F, whereas tropical lowland species need highs of 80° to 90°F. Basking site temperatures should be in the range of 82° to 85°F for montane species and 90° to 95°F for lowland species. Any enclosure should always provide a thermocline.[9] Providing suitable gradients that allow thermal choices within the chameleon's space reduces stress and resultant negative effects on metabolic status.

Because most chameleons do not drink from standing water, they must be watered with a hand sprayer or provided with a drip system. Humidity needs differ depending on the species and their natural habitat, with 50% to 60% humidity generally being adequate. Because chameleons are solitary and territorial, it is stressful for individuals, particularly males, to be placed within sight of each other.

FEEDING AND NUTRITION

Crickets and mealworms provide the basic diet for chameleons, but a broad range of insects, spiders, and snails, including field sweepings if possible, are recommended. Cockroaches are becoming increasingly popular as a supplement. *Blaberus* species or juvenile Madagascan hissing cockroaches (adults are too chitinous) can be grown in culture and provide excellent nourishment.

If natural sunlight is not available, a vitamin supplement containing calcium and vitamin D_3 should be provided by dusting food items or "gut loading" crickets a diet high in calcium and vitamin D_3 for several days before feeding out.[1, 28] Ferguson and colleagues[19] determined that an ultraviolet-B (UV-B, 290–320 nm) light source is needed for chameleons kept exclusively indoors. The intensity of UV-B from a "full spectrum" fluorescent lamp is not sufficient and should be supplemented 1 hour per day, 5 days per week with a UV-B sun lamp. It is important that chameleons have the choice to shelter themselves from this light if they desire.[19]

Very large chameleons, such as Parson's chameleon, eat pinky or fuzzy mice, geckos, or other small lizards on occasion. Vegetable debris has been found in the stomachs of panther chameleons and this and other species have been observed occasionally eating leaves and flowers.[4, 28] Hatchling chameleons have voracious appetites and tend to grow rapidly. They must be fed at least daily.

REPRODUCTION

Chameleon species are either viviparous or ovoviviparous and most breed readily in captivity. Females of various species signal their receptivity with distinctive color patterns. When they become gravid, they display a distinctive color change. Nonreceptive females react aggressively to advances by males. Viviparous *Chamaeleo* species lay large numbers of eggs and require appropriate soil substrate for oviposition, a proper nest site being fundamentally important in this phase. Moistened top soil or potting soil in a bucket or tub placed in the female's enclosure well in advance of oviposition has been successful for some herpetoculturists. It is important that the size of the container be wide enough and deep enough to fully accommodate the female. Depending on species and size of the animal, the depth may need to be up to 12 inches. *Brookesia* species lay only two to four eggs. Females need privacy (no handling) during this time. Lack of an acceptable nest site causes the female to postpone laying, resulting in dystocia.

Dystocia is too frequent in captive chameleons and commonly results in death. Causes include a stressful environment, inappropriate nesting conditions, which cause the female to delay laying, and poor nutritional status. Female chameleons should be in robust condition and with good energy stores before breeding. Individuals with marginal energy stores are candidates for dystocia. Therefore, close attention to keeping breeding females well fed is imperative. It is thought that female panther chameleons, and probably males as well, do not survive to a second breeding season in the wild.[18] With individuals that die near the time of oviposition, it is possible to recover viable eggs at the time of death via a postmortem cesarean.[8] Female chameleons possess the capability of storing spermatozoa and fertilizing subsequent clutches even in the absence of a male. A correlation has been observed with survivability of clutches and females that were not allowed to regain condition before breeding again. The vitality of these hatchlings worsened with each subsequent clutch.[9]

INFECTIOUS DISEASES

Viruses may play an important role in some diseases of chameleons, but relatively few are reported. This is probably because viruses are more difficult to investigate and are easy to overlook. An adeno-like virus was described by Jacobson and Gardiner[22] from the trachea and esophagus of a Jackson's chameleon. Opisthotonos developed in this animal before its death. A Meller's chameleon was seen to exhibit similar signs, which had inclusion bodies in the brain, suggesting a viral origin. A flap-necked chameleon was reported to have a concurrent pox and chlamydia infection in circulating monocytes.[23]

Bacterial infections are common and are often a direct result of shipping stress or improper housing conditions. Such infections can be difficult to successfully treat once they are established. Abscesses should be debrided and cultured if possible. Foot abscesses may be caused by rough wire enclosures and occasionally progress to generalized cellulitis of the limb. Stomatitis and osteomyelitis of the mandible are frequently observed and should be treated with systemic antibiotics and topical debridement, the choice of antibiotic depending on culture and sensitivity. Septic arthritis, affecting the elbow or stifle joints, is often evident by swelling of the affected joint, with radiographs confirming the severity of the infection. Ophthalmic infections can be challenging to treat in chameleons because of their narrow palpebral fissure, limiting exposure. In one zoological collection, bacterial infections were responsible for roughly half of the deaths that showed histopathologic change. *Pseudomonas, Proteus,* and *Salmonella* were the most common organisms cultured from these lesions.[3] Intussusceptions of the small intestine have been observed, usually associated with enteritis or parasitism. Many bacterial infections of the visceral organs could be secondary to parasitic or viral infections but may be difficult to identify once the animal shows signs of illness.

Fungal diseases affecting the liver, intestines, and skin have also been reported.[2, 29, 30]

PARASITIC DISEASES

Chameleons frequently carry large numbers of parasites. Parasitic infections can be self-limiting or perpetual depending on several factors, including the life cycle of the parasite. Strict hygienic husbandry habits that include expedient removal of excrement and measures that prevent food items from becoming contaminated with feces help limit reinfections of those parasites that require an intermediate host. Not all infections result in disease and some caution should be exercised when medicating animals with heavy worm burdens. Illness or death of the host may occur as a result of the large number of dead parasites that must be reabsorbed.[25, 27] Parasite burdens from wild-caught individuals may vary depending on the time of year the animal was collected.[18]

Ascarids and strongyle ova are common findings in fecal samples from newly purchased individuals. Coccidia species infect the intestines or the biliary system and may result in enteritis or cholecystitis. Cryptosporidia have been observed infrequently by myself and have been described by Dillehay and colleagues[14] Microfilaremia is common, especially in *C. pardalis, Chamaeleo ousteleti,* and *Chamaeleo verrucocus.* Adult *Foleyella* species are found outside the vascular system in subcutaneous, buccal, perirenal, and air sac surfaces as well.[20, 34] Transmission occurs through blood-sucking arthropods. Adult filarid worms living in the coelomic cavity or under the skin are resistant to treatment. I have frequently found apparently healthy worms during necropsy examinations of chameleons that had several anthelmintic treatments. Protozoan hemoparasites (*Leishmania, Trypanosoma, Pirhemocyton*) can be observed in blood smears of wild-caught animals and in most cases occur in low numbers, not apparently causing illness.[33]

THERAPEUTICS

Differentiating the cause of illness can be challenging because, typically, chameleons appear depressed without specific signs. Chameleons showing even early signs of systemic illness should prompt a poor prognosis. A sunken appearance to the eyes and a pale dull appearance may be the first sign of a problem. Ill chameleons quickly stop eating and drinking. Individual and timely attention to a sick chameleon is important for successful treatment. Careful attention to husbandry and correction of any deficiencies in temperature, light exposure, or social conditions are fundamental. Supportive care, with oral administration of electrolytes and hand feeding of food items, baby food formulas, or commercial enteral diets, is often necessary. Guidelines for nutrition support in the sick reptile is addressed by Donoghue and Langenberg.[15, 16] Chameleons respond to appropriate antibiotic therapy if their condition is not too severe. Antimicrobials should be selected according to culture and sensitivities when possible. Excellent formularies for reptiles provide guidelines that can be used to medicate chameleons.[7, 32] Darkening of the skin and irritation at injection sites have been reported by persons who recommend avoiding injectable modalities of treatment in chameleons.[26] These occasional reactions from injectable therapeutics (IM or SQ) have not been a significant problem in my experience. Some chameleons have been on long-term injectable enrofloxacin and amikacin for intractable infections without toxicity.

MISCELLANEOUS DISEASES

A relatively high percentage of chameleons die without discernible pathology.[3] Metabolic bone disease occurs in chameleons as it does in other reptiles. Inappropriate amounts of calcium, phosphorus, and vitamin D_3 and a lack of UV-B exposure result in the classic signs of tremors, folding fractures, or jaw swelling. Treatment should address correcting the diet and administering a calcium supplement (calcium gluconate). Gular edema has been attributed to renal disease associated with hypervitaminosis D_3. Excessive vitamin A is also thought to be a cause of gular edema.[31]

RESTRAINT AND ANESTHESIA

Physical restraint of chameleons is easy for minor procedures. Care should be taken not to damage the chameleon's feet when pulling it off its perch. Chameleons feel less threatened if allowed to grip a branch or hand during examination.[25] Grasping a chameleon by the sides usually provokes an aggressive gaping response allowing examination or treatment of the oral cavity. Care must be taken not to injure chameleons that refuse to open their mouth voluntarily. Isoflurane via mask is an effective anesthetic for surgical procedures, with induction taking 45 minutes or longer. To reduce stress during induction, the animal can be sealed in a chamber or a zippered plastic bag insufflated with oxygen and 4% isoflurane. Ketamine (15 mg/kg) can be used to speed induction but greatly prolongs recovery.

SURGERY

Intracoelomic surgery should be done with a paramedian approach to avoid the ventral abdominal vein. Long cartilaginous ribs, which often extend over much of the abdomen, can be avoided by incising longitudinally between them. In cesarean sections, eggs can be removed from the normally thin, friable uterus with a single uterine incision. This is done by infusing the uterus with sterile saline and floating the eggs out. Closure of the body wall is done in two layers.

REFERENCES

1. Allen ME, Oftedal OT: Dietary manipulation of the calcium content of feed crickets. J Zoo Wldl Med 20(1):26–33, 1989.
2. Austwick PKC, Keymer IF: Fungi and actinomycetes. *In* Cooper JE, Jackson OF (eds): Diseases of the Reptilia. New York, Academic Press, p 213, 1981.
3. Barrie MT, Castle E, Grow D: Diseases of chameleons at the Oklahoma City Zoological Park. Proceedings of the Annual Meeting of the American Association of Zoo Veterinarians, St. Louis, MO, p 1, 1993.
4. Bartlett RD, Bartlett PP: Chameleons: A Complete Pet Owners Manual. Hauppauge, NY, Barron's Educational Series, p 29, 1995.
5. Bustard R: Keeping and breeding oviparous chameleons. Br Herp Soc Bull 27:1–16, 1989.
6. Campbell TW: Clinical pathology. *In* Mader DR (ed): Reptile Medicine and Surgery. Philadelphia, WB Saunders, pp 248–257, 1996.
7. Carpenter JW: Exotic Animal Formulary. Manhattan, KS, Greystone Publications, 1996.
8. Castle E: Husbandry and breeding of chamaeleons *Chamaeleo spp* at Oklahoma City Zoo. Int Zoo Yearbook 29:74–84, 1990.
9. Castle E: Proceedings of the 1st Annual Canadian Herpetological Symposium on Captive Propagation and Husbandry, Druinheller, Alberta, Canada, 1994.
10. de Vosjoli P: The General Care and Maintenance of True Chameleons, Part I: Husbandry. Lakeside, CA, Advanced Vivarium Systems, 1990.
11. de Vosjoli P: True Chameleons, Part II: Notes on Popular Species, Diseases and Disorders. Lakeside, CA, Advanced Vivarium Systems, 1990.
12. de Vosjoli P: The Lizard Keepers Handbook. The Herpetological Library. Lakeside, CA, Advanced Vivarium Systems, 1994.
13. de Vosjoli P, Ferguson GW (eds): Care and Breeding of Panther, Jackson's, Veiled and Parson's Chameleons. The Herpetological Library. Lakeside, CA, Advanced Vivarium Systems, 1995.
14. Dillehay DL, Boosinger TR, MacKenzie S: Gastric cryptosporidiosis in a chameleon. J Am Vet Med Assoc 189(9):1139–1140, 1986.
15. Donoghue S: Veterinary nutrition management of amphibians and reptiles. J Am Vet Med Assoc 208(11):1861–1920, 1996.
16. Donoghue S, Langenberg J: Nutrition. *In* Mader DR (ed): Reptile Medicine and Surgery. Philadelphia, WB Saunders, p 148, 1996.
17. Ferguson GW: Old-World chameleons in captivity: growth, maturity, and reproduction of Malagasy panther chameleons (*Chamaeleo pardalis*). *In* Murphy JB, Adler K, Collins JT (eds): Captive Management and Conservation of Amphibians and Reptiles. Contributions to Herpetology, vol 11. Ithaca, NY, Society for the Study of Reptiles and Amphibians, pp 323–331, 1994.
18. Ferguson GW: Taxon management account, panther chameleon *Chamaeleo furcifer pardalis*. *In* Hammack S (ed): Lizard Advisory Group Taxon Management Accounts. American Zoo and Aquariums Association, Wheeling, WV, 1995.
19. Ferguson GW, Jones JR, Gehrmann WH, et al: Indoor husbandry of the panther chameleon *Chamaeleo [Furcifer] pardalis*: effects of dietary vitamins A and D and ultraviolet irradiation on pathology and life-history traits. Zoo Biol 15:279–299, 1996.
20. Frank W: Endoparasites. *In* Cooper JE, Jackson OF (eds): Diseases of the Reptilia. New York, Academic Press, p 337, 1981.
21. Grow D: Management of Chamaeleonidae at the Oklahoma City Zoo. *In* Staub R (ed): Captive Propagation of Reptiles and Amphibians. Northern California Herpetology Society, Davis, CA, pp 67–75, 1991.
22. Jacobson ER, Gardiner CH: Adeno-like virus in esophageal and tracheal mucosa of a Jackson's chameleon (*Chamaeleo jacksoni*). Vet Pathol 27:210–212, 1990.
23. Jacobson ER, Telford SR: Chlamydial and poxvirus infections of circulating monocytes of a flap-necked chameleon (*Chamaeleo delpis*). J Wldl Dis 26(4):572–577, 1990.
24. Jacobson ER: Blood collection techniques in reptiles: laboratory investigations. *In* Fowler ME (ed): Zoo and Wild Animal Medicine: Current Therapy 3. Philadelphia, WB Saunders, 1993.

25. Jenkins JR: Husbandry and diseases of Old World chameleons. J Small Exotic Anim Med 1(4):166, 1992.
26. Klingenberg RJ: Therapeutics. *In* Mader DR (ed): Reptile Medicine and Surgery. Philadelphia, WB Saunders, p 308, 1996.
27. Lane TJ, Mader DR: Parasitology. *In* Mader DR (ed): Reptile Medicine and Surgery. Philadelphia, WB Saunders, pp 185–203, 1996.
28. Le Berre F: The New Chameleon Handbook. Hauppauge, NY, Barron's Educational Series, 1995.
29. Migaki G, Jacobson ER, Casey HW: Fungal diseases in reptiles. *In* Hoff GL, Frye FL, Jacobson ER (eds): Diseases of Amphibians and Reptiles. New York, Plenum Press, p 185, 1984.
30. Shalev M, Murphy JC: Mycotic enteritis in a chameleon and a brief review of phycomycoses of animals. J Am Vet Med Assoc 171:872–875, 1977.
31. Stahl SJ: Veterinary Management of Old World Chameleons. *In* Striple PO (ed): Advances in Herpetoculture—International Symposium, Inc., Palo Alto, CA, Number 1, pp 151–160, 1996.
32. Stein G: Reptile and amphibian formulary. *In* Mader DR (ed): Reptile Medicine and Surgery. Philadelphia, WB Saunders, p 465, 1996.
33. Telford SR: Hemoparasites of reptiles. *In* Hoff GL, Frye FL, Jacobson ER (eds): Diseases of Amphibians and Reptiles. New York, Plenum Press, p 385, 1984.
34. Thomas CL, Artwohl JE, Pearl RK, et al: Swollen eyelid associated with *Foleyella sp* infection in a chameleon. J Am Vet Med Assoc 209(5):972–973, 1996.

CHAPTER 28

Crocodilian Anesthesia

MARK LYNN LLOYD

This chapter is a concise, complete clinician's reference to modern drugs for crocodilian anesthesia and immobilization. Using the data herein, a veterinarian can confidently perform crocodilian immobilizations for a variety of procedures. The clinician can control the anesthetic event by anticipating the potential side effects, duration of the drugs, and limitations of each choice.

The emphasis of this chapter is limited to the best available and new experimental agents for crocodilians. Other chemical immobilizing agents are also discussed for comparison. This is not a comprehensive listing of every published crocodilian immobilization drug and its use. Several other excellent review publications are available. The most useful current references are also provided for a complete review if further investigation is required.

IMMOBILIZATION CRITERIA

The strength, size, and location of crocodilians often necessitate special immobilization considerations. Immobilization drug choice must be made on evaluation of the specific needs of the individual specimen, the working environment, and the planned procedure. In addition to choosing the optimal agent for the specimen's well-being, the safety of the personnel and the expense of the agent used, which becomes significant in massive individuals or large groups of specimens, must also be considered.

Individual Specimen Considerations

There are many factors involved in selection of the best immobilization agent for the individual specimen. In crocodilians small enough to be manually restrained with or without mechanical devices, local anesthetic procedures, gas induction, or intravenous (IV) immobilization may be used. IV administration of anesthetics offers several advantages, including a rapid induction and potentially a rapid drug clearance and recovery. In addition, a lower dosage by IV bolus may provide an equivalent anesthetic depth to higher doses administered subcutaneously (SQ), intramuscularly (IM), or by intracoelomic (ICe) means. Finally, a wider range of drug choices may be used intravenously, including more recently introduced drugs such as propofol.[3] This route is severely limited in many specimens because of their size. Primary venous access in crocodilians is via the ventral caudal vein, located in the powerful tail, and the dorsal jugular vein (dorsal vertebral sinus), located between cervical vertebrae dorsal to the spinal cord (and in close proximity to the jaws and sharp teeth).[9, 12] Neither area is readily accessible in large, uncooperative animals.

Massive specimens are also predisposed to increased cardiopulmonary depression. Respiratory compromise is most significant in large, obese, long-term captive crocodilians. All immobilizing agents cause dose-dependent respiratory compromise. Paralytics, barbiturates, and alpha$_2$ agonists cause severe pulmonary depression in crocodilians.[1, 2, 6, 9, 13, 15] Death has occurred

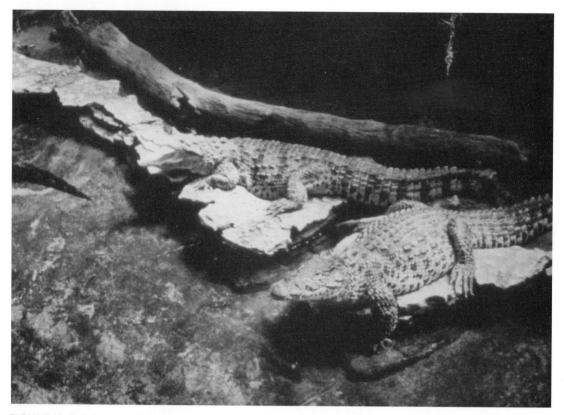

FIGURE 28–1. Cuban crocodiles (*Crocodylus rhombifer*). Note the mouth gaping, typical of crocodilians at rest and an initial sign of anesthetic induction as the muscles relax. This large enclosure and deep pool is unsuitable for safe immobilization, Toledo Zoo Exhibit.

resulting from respiratory insufficiency in very large long-term captive American alligators (*Alligator mississippiensis*) and false gharials (*Tomistoma schlegelii*). Dissociatives and gas anesthetics cause less respiratory compromise.[1, 2, 15, 16] Doxapram can centrally antagonize the respiratory depressive effects of most anesthetics as an adjunct agent and specific reversal agents may also be used.[6] Recovering animals that are quiet and unmonitored are at most risk because they lack external stimulation.

Some species appear more sensitive to specific drugs. For example, in at least 10 species of crocodilians, including the American alligator and false gharials, noncompetitive (depolarizing) neuromuscular blocking agents such as succinylcholine appear to have a wide margin of safety.[1, 2, 9, 13] According to some authors, competitive (non-depolarizing) agents, such as gallamine, however, have been associated with unacceptable morbidity and mortality rates in large American alligators.[9, 11] They may require a lower dose than other crocodilians or gallamine may be unsafe in that species altogether. Bonnie Raphael, (Wildlife Conservation Society, Bronx Zoo, New York, personal communication, October 1996) reported deaths in two very large false gharials during overnight recovery from gallamine, despite the use of neostigmine reversal. Years previously when they were considerably smaller, these same animals had been immobilized uneventfully several times

with gallamine. The animals did require repeated doses of neostigmine on occasion. The unmonitored, unstimulated, prolonged recovery may have allowed severe cardiopulmonary depression to occur in these massive animals.

The temperament of the species or specimen may warrant chemical restraint even in smaller individuals. Highly aggressive, documented human attackers, such as saltwater crocodiles (*Crocodylus porosus*), Nile crocodiles (*Crocodylus niloticus*), and Cuban crocodiles (*Crocodylus rhombifer*), should routinely be chemically immobilized for the safety of the personnel. More docile species such as the alligators and long-term captive crocodilians may be manually restrained or "coaxed" into cooperation or restrained with low-dose sedation.

Wild-caught or agitated individuals may injure themselves under manual restraint alone. Even without gross trauma, negative sequelae can occur without chemical restraint. Three of five unsedated wild adult Nile crocodiles died of undocumented causes when captured and moved. A mugger crocodile (*Crocodylus palustris*) was anorexic for 18 months after transport within the Philadelphia Zoo.[13]

Gavialinae (gharials, or *Gavialis gangeticus*) and Tomistominae (false gharials) have elongated, relatively fragile rostra and cannot feed normally if either the mandibular or maxillary rostrum is fractured or amputated. The risk of anesthesia may be greatly outweighed by the risk of potential rostral trauma during unsedated manual restraint. Although these subfamilies are often more timid and docile to work with than their relatives, light anesthesia may be advantageous.[11]

Exotic animal veterinarians have long been convinced of the advantages of "better living through chemistry" in many species. Physical restraint is seldom safer than carefully chosen modern immobilization agents. Crocodilians restrained with ropes, noose poles, and mechanical devices tend to spin violently, potentially strangulating and injuring the animal. Manual restraint techniques and equipment *can* be used effectively and safely to achieve control of the animal and may complement chemical immobilization.[5, 10, 20]

Environmental Considerations

Immobilization and recovery are best accomplished in a small enclosure that allows limited subject mobility. Water in the enclosure should not be deeper than the animal's maxilla (Fig. 28–1). Drowning has been observed in animals after administration of immobilization agents when the specimens retreated into deep water.[13] Dissociative agents, such as ketamine and tiletamine, may offer some benefit by maintaining pharyngeal reflexes better than other agents in an area with drowning potential.[1, 2, 15, 19]

Individuals to be immobilized should be sequestered. Cohabitant animals pose a threat to the subject and staff as potential attackers; furthermore, they have been responsible for suffocating recovering specimens by simply laying on top of them.[12, 13] Field conditions may not allow for environmental manipulations, but selection of appropriate drugs and innovative capture devices can assist in safe immobilization. Take advantage of shade or sun to facilitate thermoregulation during recovery. Recovering animals far enough from water that they must be able to ambulate to reach it can also make the procedure as safe as possible.[4, 5, 10, 20]

Many authors emphasize the importance of maintaining reptilian patients at preferred body temperature for optimal immobilization and recovery.[1, 6, 13] All species, especially mammals, cannot recover appropriately if hypothermic. It is equally important in crocodilians even though they can function at a wider range of body temperatures. Metabolism and excretion of immobilization agents can be significantly altered by changes in body temperature. The large body mass of crocodilians confers large thermal mass, which allows an increased measure of safety for short procedures, but it can also prolong rewarming in case large specimens become hypothermic.

Procedure

Crocodilia are most often immobilized for translocation, biometric evaluation, and minor medical procedures such as physical examination (Figs. 28–2 to 28–4), gastric lavage (Fig. 28–5), phlebotomy (Figs. 28–6, 28–7), and radiography (Figs. 28–8, 28–9). Surgical procedures are infrequent. They are usually conducted for traumatic injury and occasionally for foreign body enterotomy. Most procedures are not painfully invasive, beyond venipuncture. Therefore, selection of an appropriate immobilizing agent can be based on the other considerations.

Choice of immobilization agent should also be based on the type of procedure planned. Only anesthetic agents that block nociperception and provide analgesia should be used for painful procedures. Paralytic agents do not provide any analgesia. Moreover, they also do not provide even loss of proprioception or consciousness. Even noninvasive procedures should include visual and auditory barriers such as blindfolds and towels

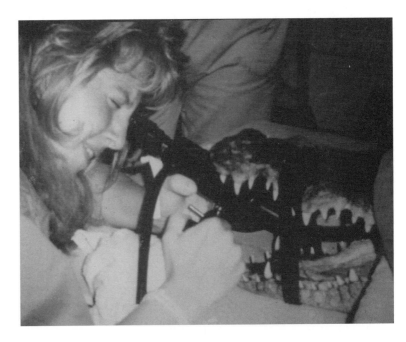

FIGURE 28–2. Wynona Shellabarger, Toledo Zoo, performs gastric endoscopy in a Cuban crocodile (*Crocodylus rhombifer*) under gallamine immobilization with a 2 × 6 × 12 inch wooden oral speculum.

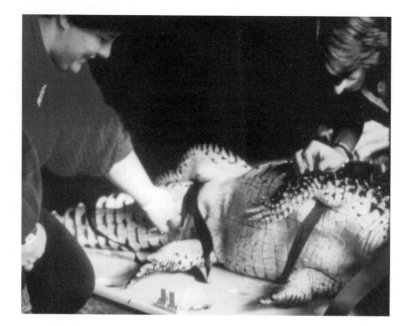

FIGURE 28–3. Ann Manharth, Toledo Zoo, performs a digital cloacal examination on a crocodile for sexing.

to minimize stress.[6, 13] Heart and respiratory rates may even escalate with paralytics during the procedure, at least in part because of external stimulation in a conscious state while paralyzed. This can be advantageous. Acute fatal anesthetic complications are usually due to depression of cardiovascular or respiratory systems. As discussed, after the procedure is complete, life-threatening cardiopulmonary depression can occur in the absence of external stimulation.

Potent analgesics for painful procedures include alpha$_2$ agonists and narcotics, but these are also potent cardiopulmonary depressants.[1, 2, 7, 13, 15] Dissociatives combined with benzodiazepines are less depressive and provide good analgesia, but they may also prolong recovery.[1, 6, 15] Volatile gas anesthetics provide excellent analgesia with minimal cardiopulmonary depression, but they must be used after induction with an injectable agent except in very small specimens, which can be masked or intubated while unsedated.[1, 2, 15, 16]

PARALYTIC IMMOBILIZATION DRUGS

Paralytic agents are historically one of the most commonly used crocodilian immobilization drugs. They re-

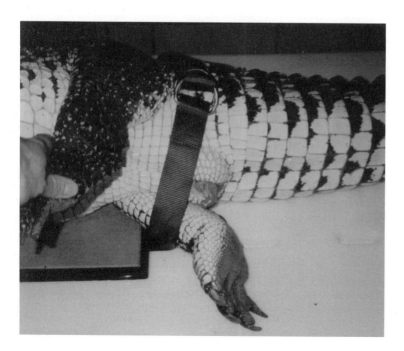

FIGURE 28–4. Penile eversion in a crocodile immobilized with gallamine undergoing radiography.

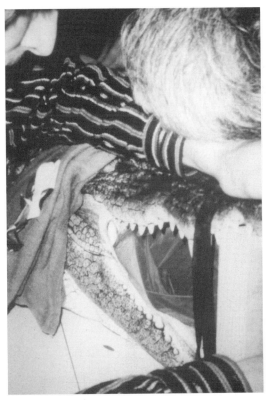

FIGURE 28–5. Manual removal of gastric foreign body in an immobilized crocodile. The clinician wears a rectal sleeve and uses a 2 × 6 inch wooden oral speculum; a rubber inner tube band is placed on the animal's mandible.

main an excellent choice for safety and efficacy in most crocodilian species and procedures. They must be used judiciously, only for procedures of minimal discomfort, unless combined with analgesics or anesthetics.[4, 6, 9, 12, 13, 14, 17, 21]

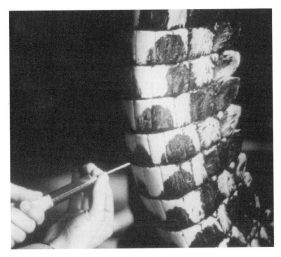

FIGURE 28–6. Caudal venipuncture of a crocodile, using an 18-gauge, 3½-inch spinal needle and a 12-ml syringe.

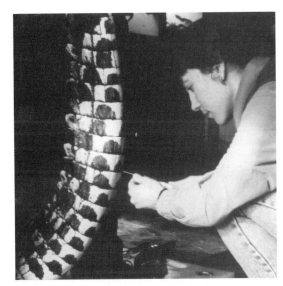

FIGURE 28–7. Joanne Desanto performs caudal venipuncture in a Cuban crocodile (*Crocodylus rhombifer*).

Flaccid paralysis also requires special considerations for the musculoskeletal support. A "back board" or some form of "stretcher" to support the vertebral column is essential (Fig. 28–10). When rolling or manipulating a large paralyzed crocodilian, spinal or articular luxation can occur.[4, 12]

Gallamine Triethiodide

Gallamine triethiodide is a non-depolarizing competitive neuromuscular blocking agent that can be reversed with neostigmine. It is the most commonly used immobilizing agent in South African crocodile farms and

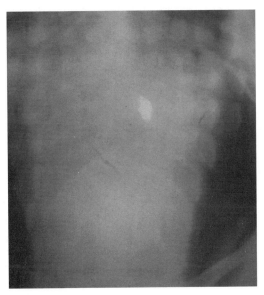

FIGURE 28–8. Dorsoventral radiograph of a metallic dense gastric foreign body in a crocodile (coin).

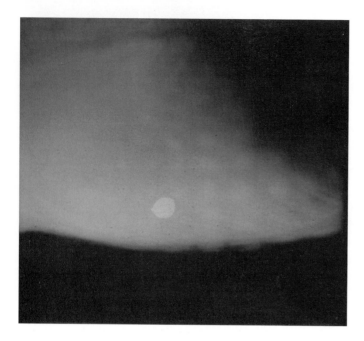

FIGURE 28–9. Lateral radiograph of a metal dense gastric foreign body in a crocodile (coin).

field research.[4] Recovery can be prolonged from hours to days without reversal.[1, 6, 12, 13, 15, 21] Respiratory and heart rate increase under gallamine immobilization during a procedure. This may be due to either the direct effect of the drug or to visual, auditory, and tactile stimulation while the animal is completely conscious but paralyzed.[13]

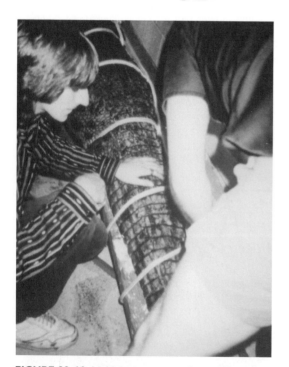

FIGURE 28–10. Multiple straps are used to stabilize an immobilized crocodile on a wooden 2 × 12 inch backboard.

The muscarinic effects of neostigmine (e.g., salivation, emesis) can be prevented by premedication with atropine or glycopyrrolate. Fasting the animal for at least 72 hours minimizes the chance for aspiration with any crocodilian immobilization. In 265 trials in several species of crocodilians, only three deaths were recorded. Those deaths were attributed to post-immobilization mismanagement. Drowning in deep water and asphyxiation from the weight of a conspecific that climbed onto the dorsum of the recovering specimen were cited as causes. Repeated immobilizations with gallamine, eight times over a 6-year period in one Nile crocodile, resulted in no observable cumulative effects. Redosing with neostigmine is commonly necessary to ensure complete reversal.[12, 13]

Elliot Jacobson (personal communication, October 1996) of the University of Florida claims that gallamine is unsafe in American alligators (*Alligator mississippiensis*). The immobilization dose was approximately 1 mg/kg and the animals were not given neostigmine reversal. The specimens were very large, and two of five animals died. Although no comparable reports were found, gallamine should be used with caution, if at all, in either American or Chinese alligators (*Alligator sinensis*). As discussed, Bonnie Raphael has also observed fatal immobilization sequelae in overnight recoveries of large adult false gharials.

Succinylcholine Chloride

Succinylcholine chloride is a depolarizing neuromuscular blocking agent. It has been used in numerous species of crocodilians with success. The major disadvantage is the inability to reverse this noncompetitive paralytic. Recovery is sometimes prolonged, up to 12 hours.[6, 13, 15, 21]

DISSOCIATIVE ANESTHETICS

Although reptiles are highly resistant to the effects of dissociative anesthetics, compared to mammals, this group of drugs continues to be one of the safest overall choices in all reptiles. One author reported more than 1000 anesthetic episodes without a single associated death.[6] Pharyngeal reflexes tend to be maintained, cardiopulmonary function is minimally depressed, and low doses can be safely combined with other anesthetics to produce the desired effect. The greatest disadvantage is the often prolonged recovery, taking up to 24 hours.[1, 2, 6, 9, 13, 19] IV administration may accelerate induction and recovery. Yohimbine is reported to partially reverse the effects of dissociates.[6] Isotonic fluids and diuretics may also increase the renal clearance.[1, 2, 6, 9, 15, 19]

Ketamine Hydrochloride

Ketamine hydrochloride provides minimal muscle relaxation and questionable analgesia when used alone. It can be combined with benzodiazepines or alpha$_2$ agonists to provide relaxation. Ketamine, as commercially supplied in a 100-mg/ml solution, may require a volume that can be prohibitive to administer in large specimens. For example, a 75-kg animal may require 25 to 50 ml to immobilize. Lyophilized ketamine can be used to decrease the drug volume. Doses over 100 mg/ml usually require intermittent positive pressure ventilation in crocodilians.[1, 2, 6, 9, 13, 15, 19]

Tiletamine

Tiletamine, the dissociative component of telazol, is more potent than ketamine, and, in combination with zolazepam, a benzodiazepine, it provides good analgesia and relaxation. Recovery may still take several hours.[6, 13] It is commercially available as a lyophilized powder and can be reconstituted up to 500 mg/ml, thus making it more suitable for large specimens. It does lose potency rapidly after reconstitution but it lasts 5 days if refrigerated, according to the manufacturer. The author of this chapter has used reconstituted telazol kept frozen in a "home" refrigerator freezer (~15° to 32°F [−10° to 0°C]) for up to 1 month with no apparent clinical loss in potency, although this is not recommended by the manufacturer.[6, 15]

NARCOTICS

Etorphine

Etorphine has been used with excellent success in crocodilians since the 1960s.[1, 6, 13, 15] It provides rapid induction and excellent analgesia. Even without reversal, spontaneous recovery occurs within 1 to 3 hours. There is a wide species variability in effective drug dosage, with some species being extremely resistant to etorphine even at very high doses.[9, 13] Etorphine is expensive to use in large animals or groups of specimens, potentially hundreds of dollars. Etorphine is extremely dangerous

to personnel. It should never be used without the human antagonist naloxone on hand. Staff should be prepared to administer the antidote IV immediately and perform cardiopulmonary resuscitation in case of accidental human exposure. Although etorphine is an excellent choice for safety and efficacy for the crocodilian, it poses an unacceptable risk for the human immobilization team. With the availability of agents that are safer for humans, there is little need to rely on etorphine for crocodilian immobilization.[1, 2, 9, 13, 15]

Oxymorphone

Oxymorphone is much safer than etorphine for personnel and is an excellent analgesic and muscle relaxant. It causes less cardiopulmonary depression than etorphine and can be reversed as well. Tachypnea has been observed in some species. Oxymorphone is 100 to 1000 times less potent than etorphine; therefore, the volume required may be excessive except in small specimens. Published dosages in other reptiles range from 0.1 to 1.5 mg/kg.[6] The author has administered as much as 30 mg/kg IM in radiated tortoises (*Geochelone radiata*) with little or no clinical effect. No published data are available on its use in crocodilians. Despite the safety advantages over etorphine, oxymorphone needs further investigation in crocodilians.

ALPHA$_2$ AGONISTS

Alpha$_2$ agonists provide variable muscle relaxation and fair analgesia. They are variably reversible with several antagonists, which is the biggest advantage of this class of drugs. Newer, more potent alpha$_2$ agonists and reversal agents are being investigated in crocodilians.[6, 7] The disadvantages of these agents include severe cardiopulmonary depression and prolonged recovery without reversal of more than 12 hours. Cardiopulmonary side effects may be anticipated and controlled by administration of parasympatholytics and doxapram. Alpha$_2$ agonists are at their best when combined with premedications or dissociative anesthetics to lower the dose of both via synergism.[1, 2, 6, 18]

Xylazine

Xylazine is readily available and may be reversed. It is best used in combination with ketamine.[1, 2, 6, 15, 18] It can also be combined with inhalant gas anesthetics.[2] Its effects can be variable in crocodilians as can be the efficacy of yohimbine reversal. Without reversal, xylazine may last up to 12 hours.[6] It is a reasonable choice for crocodilian immobilization but the side effects make it less than the ideal crocodilian anesthetic.

Detomidine

Detomidine is approximately 10 times more potent than xylazine. The reversal agent atipamezole may be more effective than yohimbine for detomidine. Detomidine can be reversed with yohimbine, but it may require a higher dose than the dose for xylazine reversal. Detomidine is commercially available in the United States, approved for use in equids.

Medetomidine

Medetomidine is experimentally available in the United States. It is more potent than either xylazine or detomidine. Research is currently under way on its use in crocodilians and reversal with atipamezole. According to the research, this alpha$_2$ agonist shows the most promise in safety and efficacy for crocodilians.[7, 15]

OTHER INJECTABLE AGENTS FOR CHEMICAL RESTRAINT

Propofol

Propofol is a potentially exceptional new immobilization drug in crocodilians. It is currently available in the United Kingdom as a veterinary product but in the United States it is only available as a human product. It is moderately expensive, contains no preservative, and is currently only available in a 200-mg glass ampule (enough for a 15- to 20-kg animal). It is recommended that the unused portion of the ampule be discarded after 24 hours.

Some authors consider propofol to be the induction agent of choice. It is most effective when administered IV, limiting its use in large crocodilians. In reptiles, propofol is ineffective in providing rapid induction and deep anesthesia when equivalent dosages are administered IM without adjunct drugs to accelerate absorption.[3] The author of this chapter is currently researching the effect of combination of propofol and hyaluronidase injected IM to enhance absorption and accelerate induction in reptiles.

Propofol has a short duration when administered IV in reptiles; its effects last only 45 to 90 minutes. It provides excellent relaxation and can be readily combined with gas anesthetics for maintenance. When IV administration is possible, some authors recommend propofol induction via IV bolus and anesthetic maintenance with isoflurane via endotracheal tube as the drug combination of choice.[3] It has not been used extensively in crocodilians but results in other reptiles have been exceptional.

Tricaine Methanesulphonate

Tricaine methanesulphonate causes rapid induction when administered IM or ICe. Recovery can be prolonged, sometimes taking up to 30 hours. This is usually unacceptable for most procedures. Other anesthetic choices allow quicker recovery and better depth control.[6, 13]

Barbiturates

Barbiturates have severe cardiopulmonary depressive effects at doses high enough to induce stage three anes-thesia in reptiles. Even short-acting and ultra short-acting preparations cause prolonged recovery in reptiles. Induction is slow, unless the drug is administered IV, and recovery may take days. *Flumazenil* is used to antagonize barbiturate overdoses in humans but its use is undocumented as a reversal agent in crocodilians. Barbiturates provide a narrow margin of safety and usually require premedication or parasympatholytic agents to compensate for the untoward side effects. Barbiturates should not be routinely used for crocodilian anesthesia because too many safer drug choices are available.[1, 2, 6, 9, 13, 18]

VOLATILE GAS ANESTHETICS

Gas anesthetics can be used for induction in small specimens, but reptiles often use controlled apnea and resist face mask or chamber induction for as long as 20 minutes. Intubation is often difficult or impossible in an awake animal. Therefore, all gas anesthetics are best used for maintenance after induction with a short-acting injectable agent. Intubation with a cuffed endotracheal tube can take advantage of the complete tracheal rings in crocodilians to seal the trachea well.

The glottis of reptiles is closed between respirations. Furthermore, crocodilians have an extended rigid soft palate that works in conjunction with the gular fold at the base of the tongue to occlude the oropharynx from the oral cavity. This allows the mouth to be open under water without compromising nasal respiration. It also requires the clinician to manually separate the tissues to gain sight and access to the glottis. Usually, at least two individuals are needed to accomplish this task.[2, 6, 13, 16]

Isoflurane

Isoflurane is the anesthetic maintenance drug of choice. It provides analgesia, muscle relaxation, and rapid recovery with spontaneous or manual ventilation. The rapid recovery may even be a disadvantage if a large specimen must be transported some distance back to an enclosure. After the isoflurane is discontinued, rapid recovery may place personnel at risk. Applying a constricting band around the animal's mandible may be prudent until all staff have left the recovery enclosure. Isoflurane usually provides recovery within minutes with either spontaneous or intermittent positive pressure ventilation.[1, 6, 13, 16, 18]

Halothane

Even though isoflurane is superior, many clinicians still have only halothane vaporizers available. Halothane is more hepatotoxic and cardiotoxic to both the patient and the staff. Induction and recovery are slightly prolonged and may partially depend on hepatic metabolism of the anesthetic as well as expiratory clearance.[2, 6, 13, 16]

ADJUNCT THERAPEUTIC AGENTS (Table 28–1)

Hyaluronidase

Hyaluronidase is a proteolytic enzyme shown to enhance and accelerate the absorption of both SQ and IM drugs injected simultaneously. It is approved for use in the SQ administration of renal contrast media or iso-

tonic fluids in humans.[12] The author of this chapter has combined hyaluronidase with various drugs administered SQ or IM in numerous species. Renografin, lactated Ringers solution, 0.9% saline solution, telazol, ketamine, xylazine, etorphine, carfentanil, diprenorphine, yohimbine, gallamine, neostigmine, and doxapram were successfully combined and drug effects were accelerated in all cases. No gross adverse effects were observed.

The most critical phases of immobilization are induction and recovery in which most anesthetic compli-

TABLE 28–1. Crocodilian Immobilization Drugs and Adjunct Therapeutic Agents

Drug	Dose (mg/kg)	Comments and Precautions	Source (Mfg)	Ref.
Dissociatives				
Ketamine hydrochloride	20–40 sedative 40–80 anesthetic IM, SC, ICe	>100 mg/kg may require IPPV LD50 150 mg/kg Prolonged recovery: 6–24 hours Voluminous unless lyophilized	Ketaset, Aveco Co., Inc.	1, 6, 9, 11, 13, 15, 19
Telazol (tiletamine zolazepam)	5–10 sedative 10–40 anesthetic IM, SC, ICe IM, SC, ICe	Better analgesia and relaxation than ketamine Supplied lyophilized, allowing small volumes of concentrate Recovery less prolonged, 1–4 hours	Telazol, AH Robins Co.	1, 6, 11, 13, 15
Paralytics				
Gallamine (not anesthetic)	0.05–0.5 sedative 0.5–1.25 immobilization IM, SC, ICe	Prolonged recovery without reversal Reversable with neostigmine Deaths recorded in *A. mississippiensis*, without reversal and *T. schlegelii* after reversal, overnight	Flaxedil, American Cyanamid Co.	1, 4, 6, 9, 13, 21
Succinylcholine (no antagonist; not anesthetic)	0.25 w/diazepam 0.5–2.0 sedative 3–5 immobilization IM, SC, ICe	0.4 mg/kg diazepam, 20 minutes before premedication Recovery 3–4 hours Recovery: 2–4 hours at low dose Recovery: 6–12 hours at high dose Apnea and arrhythmias at high dose	Anectine, Burroughs Wellcome Co.	1, 6, 9, 13, 15, 17, 21
Volatile Gases				
Isoflurane	3%–5% induction 1%–2% maintenance	Drug of choice for safety, analgesia, and recovery Moderately expensive Usually requires injectable induction for large animals Rapid recovery	AErrane, Anaquest	1, 15, 16
Halothane	3%–5% induction 2%–3% maintenance	Secondary choice to isoflurane Less expensive Recovery slightly longer than for isoflurane	Halothane, Fort Dodge	1, 6, 15, 16
Narcotics				
Etorphine (M99)	0.05–20 SQ, ICe, IM	Short recovery 1–2 hours, also reversible Wide range of susceptibility May be prohibitively expensive Significant safety concerns with staff	M99, American Cyanamid Co. & Lemmon Co.	1, 6, 13, 15
Alpha₂ Agonists				
Xylazine	1.0–2.0 IM, SQ	Follow with 20 mg/kg ketamine Recovery in 6–12 hours Yohimbine reversal Depresses cardiopulmonary function	Xyla-Ject, Phoenix Pharmaceutical, Inc.	1, 2, 6, 15
Medetomidine	0.04–0.16 IM, SQ	Reverse with atipamezole Experimental	Medetomidine Wildlife Pharmaceutical	7, 15

Table continued on following page

TABLE 28–1. **Crocodilian Immobilization Drugs and Adjunct Therapeutic Agents** *Continued*

Drug	Dose (mg/kg)	Comments and Precautions	Source (Mfg)	Ref.
Alpha₂ Agonists *Continued*				
Detomidine	1.0 IM, SQ	Reversal with yohimbine or atipamezole Experimental	Domesedan, Ciba Geigy, Ltd.	7
Propofol	10–15 IV	Short duration: 0.5–1.5 hours IV preferred in reptiles Maintain on gas anesthetics Experimental IM w/hyaluronidase	Diprivan, Zeneca Pharmaceutical	3
Tricaine	70–110 IM, ICe	Recovery unacceptably prolonged: 10 hours	MS-222, Sandoz	1, 6, 13
Premedication				
Atropine	0.01–0.04 IM, SQ, IV, ICe	Sympatholytic Antagonizes cardiac depression from most anesthetics and muscarinic effects from neostigmine (emesis, salivation, respiratory secretions)	Atropine SA, Butler	1, 6, 12, 15
Glycopyrrolate	0.01–0.05 IM, SQ, IV	Sympatholytic, effects similar to atropine but more prolonged and less gastrointestinal ileus	Robinul-V, Aveco	16
Diazepam	0.25 0.2–0.6	20 minutes before succinylcholine Recovery in 3 hours With dissociatives	Diazepam, LyphoMed, Inc.	1, 6, 15, 17
Medazolam	2.0	Premedication for dissociatives Use in crocodilians poorly documented	Versed, Roche	18
Doxapram	5–10	Direct respiratory stimulant Use with any respiratory depressant Reported to (partially) reverse dissociatives Voluminous in large specimens	Dopram-V, Fort Dodge	6
Hyaluronidase	150 IU/L 25 IU/dose	SQ fluid absorption/distribution acceleration Mixed in syringe with anesthetic, premedication emergency, reversal drugs Caution with non-IV drugs	Wydase, Wyeth Labs, Inc.	12
Yohimbine	0.1	Alpha₂ agonist reversal, commercially available Variable results	Yobine, Lloyd Laboratories	6
Atipamezole	0.05–1.0	Available for experimental use More effective reversal than yohimbine May soon be commercially available	Atipamezole, Wildlife Pharmaceutical	7
Flumazenil	1 mg/20 mg of zolazepam	Reversal agent for barbiturates and benzodiazepines, experimental in crocodilians	Romazicon, Roche	
Neostigmine	0.25	Reversal for non-depolarizing/competitive neuromuscular paralytics (gallamine) Atropine or glycopyrrolate may prevent muscarinic side effects	Neostigmine, Bristol-Myers Squibb Co.	1, 4, 6, 9, 12, 13

cations occur. Early attempts at physical restraint before induction is complete may result in thrashing, aggressive, erratic, and traumatic behaviors. The more rapid the induction, the sooner the veterinary staff can monitor, examine, and stabilize the patient. The sooner the planned procedure is initiated, the sooner it is completed, minimizing necessary anesthetic time.

A prolonged recovery increases the risk of anesthetic complications beyond the minimum required time. Hypothermia, aspiration, drowning, or from cohabitant conspecifics injury may occur during recovery. Cardiopulmonary depression may become severe without stimulation. Because of the prolonged recovery with most crocodilian anesthetics, crocodilians are often left unmonitored overnight to recover, after the staff has left for the day.[13] If cardiopulmonary depression occurs, it may be unnoticed until the following day. To minimize induction and recovery time, the author uses hyaluronidase with both immobilizing and reversal agents.

Premedications and emergency drugs have a more

rapid onset if combined with hyaluronidase as well. In a group of Cuban crocodiles immobilized with gallamine, recovery was more rapid in specimens reversed with neostigmine and hyaluronidase compared to those reversed with neostigmine alone. Repeat doses of neostigmine were also required in some animals not receiving hyaluronidase with neostigmine.[12]

Caution should be exerted with drugs that are potentially toxic if given IV. Because of accelerated absorption, these drugs should *not* be used with hyaluronidase IM or SQ. Potassium chloride and potassium penicillin, for example, may be cardiotoxic if absorbed too rapidly.

Parasympatholytic Drugs

Parasympatholytic drugs such as atropine and glycopyrrolate can be used in crocodilians to counteract anesthetic side effects such as salivation, respiratory secretion, emesis, cardiac arrhythmias, and bradycardia.[1, 6, 13, 18] They are particularly useful to block the undesirable muscarinic effects of neostigmine reversal.[6, 13] The profound cardiac depression of alpha$_2$ agonist anesthetics can be minimized with parasympatholytics as well.

Doxapram

Doxapram directly stimulates the central nervous system respiratory center to counteract the depressive effects of many anesthetics such as dissociatives, alpha$_2$ agonists, narcotics, and volatile gases. Because it is centrally active, it is effective against almost any respiratory depressant. Even if the respiration has been adequate during manipulation, it may be prudent to administer a dose of doxapram routinely at the end of each procedure to stimulate breathing through the recovery.[6]

Benzodiazepine Tranquilizers

Diazepam and *midazolam* potentiate the effects of dissociative anesthetics and paralytics but they may also extend the recovery time.[1, 17] Either drug may be used as a premedication or given simultaneously with most anesthetics. Even at high doses, it is difficult to induce anesthesia with benzodiazepines alone. Diazepam is approximately 10 times more potent than midazolam. Premedication with diazepam has been shown to decrease the dose of succinylcholine induction by 10-fold, in order to eliminate the righting reflex in 23 of 26 American alligators. Respiration was spontaneously maintained in all of the animals and most animals recovered within 3 hours with no ill effects. In fact, 23 animals produced fertile eggs the following year.[17] Ketamine and diazepam combination anesthesia without reversal may have a recovery of more than 6 hours in crocodilians, approximately the same as ketamine alone.[6]

Zolazepam is not available alone but is synergistic with the dissociative anesthetic tiletamine in telazol. It provides excellent relaxation and smooths recovery. Without reversal, recovery may take up to 4 hours.[1, 6, 18] Bonnie Raphael (personal communication, October 1996) has used flumazenil to antagonize zolazepam in crocodilians with good results.

REVERSAL AGENTS

Neostigmine

Neostigmine reverses the effects of competitive neuromuscular blocking agents such as gallamine but its muscarinic side effects such as vomiting, regurgitation, and purgation may predispose specimens to aspiration pneumonia. Parasympatholytics can block these side effects. Withholding food for at least 72 hours before neostigmine administration is prudent as well.[6, 13]

Atipamezole

Atipamezole is a reversal agent to the newer, more potent, experimental alpha$_2$ agonists such as detomidine and medetomidine. It is currently under investigation and appears to be more effective than yohimbine and xylazine combination.[7]

Yohimbine

Yohimbine is antagonistic to alpha$_2$ agonists commonly used to reverse xylazine and may partially reverse dissociatives such as ketamine.[6] Yohimbine is less effective than atipamezole, and, in the author's experience, the reversal is less dependable, even among various species of mammals.

Flumazenil

Flumazenil can be used to reverse benzodiazepines and barbiturates. It has not been used extensively in reptiles but has been used to reverse zolazepam in some crocodilians. It is available currently as a human pharmaceutical.

RECOMMENDATIONS

Immobilization duration is the greatest obstacle in crocodilian immobilization. Many drugs provide rapid induction, a wide margin of safety for the animal, and adequate analgesia, but recovery times may last several hours. Selection of an agent that can be reversed or has a short duration is preferable for most procedures. Hyaluronidase can be used to accelerate induction as well as recovery if an antagonist is available.

Injection sites are limited in crocodilians because of their dorsal osteoderms and thick caudal scutes. Femoral and brachial musculature are excellent IM injection sites. The lateral surfaces of the tail base can also be used for IM injection. Intracoelomic space can most easily be accessed through the paralumbar fossae.[13]

Monitoring anesthetic depth can be accomplished in several ways. The anesthetic generally affects the patient cranially to caudally, affecting the tail last.[6] Loss of righting reflex can be ambiguous because small crocodilians gently placed in dorsal recumbency may be temporarily immobile even when completely awake. Any disturbance or rough handling immediately elicits a response. If an anesthetized animal fails to respond to disturbance, prodding, or rough handling, it is at least heavily sedated.[17] Mouth gaping is often seen as the muscles relax with neuromuscular blocking agents. Reluctance to close the mouth when touched with a long tool is good evidence of immobilization induction (see Fig. 28–1). The digits may be elevated off the ground as the extremities relax.[4]

Respiratory rates in minimally stimulated unsedated American alligators and caiman (*Caiman crocodilus*) were an average of one to three breaths per minute. Heart rates in those same individuals were 11 to 17 beats per minute. These rates can be used for comparison to the heart and respiratory rates of immobilized crocodilians.[8]

The final choice of an appropriate immobilizing agent should be made based on the requirements of the specimen, procedure, and the environment compared to the available drugs and their individual advantages and limitations. An informed clinician can choose an appropriate drug, anticipate side effects, and prepare for potential outcomes.

Acknowledgments

Special thanks to the veterinary and reptile departments of the Toledo Zoo, Toledo, Ohio. Their mentorship and support allowed the author to enhance his skills and instilled confidence in crocodilian medicine and husbandry. Thanks are also extended to Dr. Kevin Wright of the Philadelphia Zoo for his assistance in crocodilian anesthesia literature procurement.

REFERENCES

1. Bennet RA: Anesthesia. *In* Mader DR (ed): Reptile Medicine and Surgery. Philadelphia, WB Saunders, pp 241–247, 1996.
2. Burke TJ: Reptile anesthesia. *In* Fowler ME (ed): Zoo and Wild Animal Medicine, 2nd ed. Philadelphia, WB Saunders, pp 153–155, 1986.
3. Divers SJ: The use of propofol in reptile anesthesia. Proceedings of the Annual Conference of the Association of Reptilian and Amphibian Veterinarians, Sacramento, CA, pp 57–59, 1996.
4. Fleming GJ: Capture and chemical immobilization of the Nile crocodile (*Crocodylus niloticus*) in South Africa. Proceedings of the Annual Conference of the Association of Reptilian and Amphibian Veterinarians, Sacramento, CA, pp 63–66, 1996.
5. Fowler ME: Restraint and Handling of Wild and Domestic Animals. Ames, IA, Iowa State University Press, pp 286–310, 1985.
6. Frye FL: Biomedical and Surgical Aspects of Captive Reptile Husbandry, 2nd ed. Malabar, Krieger Publishing Company, 1991.
7. Heaton-Jones TJ: Development of anesthesia in crocodilians. Proceedings of the Annual Conference of the Association of Reptilian and Amphibian Veterinarians, Sacramento, CA, p 61, 1996.
8. Huggins SE, Hoff HE, Pena RV: Heart and respiratory rates in crocodilian reptiles under conditions of minimal stimulation. Physiol Zool 42:320–333, 1969.
9. Jacobson ER: Immobilization, blood sampling, necropsy techniques and diseases of crocodilians: a review. J Zoo Anim Med 15:38–45, 1984.
10. Jones D, Hayes-Odum L: A method for the restraint and transport of crocodilians. Herpetol Rev 25:14–15, 1994.
11. Lane TJ: Crocodilians. *In* Mader DR (ed): Reptile Medicine and Surgery. Philadelphia, WB Saunders, pp 78–94, 1996.
12. Lloyd ML, Reichard T, Odum A: Gallamine reversal in Cuban crocodiles (*Crocodylus rhombifer*) using neostigmine alone versus neostigmine with hyaluronidase. Proceedings of the Joint Conference of the American Association of Zoo Veterinarians and the Association of Reptilian and Amphibian Veterinarians, Pittsburgh, PA, 1994.
13. Loveridge JP: The immobilisation and anaesthesia of crocodilians. Int Zoo Yearbook 19:103–112, 1979.
14. Messel H, Stephens DR: Drug immobilization of crocodiles. J Wildl Management 44:295–296, 1980.
15. Page CD: Current reptilian anesthesia procedures. *In* Fowler ME (ed): Zoo and Wild Animal Medicine, 3rd ed. Philadelphia, WB Saunders, pp 140–143, 1986.
16. Sedgewick CJ: Inhalation anesthesia for captive wild mammals, birds, and reptiles. *In* Fowler ME (ed): Zoo and Wild Animal Medicine, 2nd ed. Philadelphia, WB Saunders, pp 51–56, 1986.
17. Spiegel RA, Lane TJ, Larsen RE, et al: Diazepam and succinylcholine chloride for restraint of the American alligator. J Am Vet Med Assoc 185:1335–1336, 1984.
18. Stein G: Reptile and amphibian formulary. *In* Mader DR (ed): Reptile Medicine and Surgery. Philadelphia, WB Saunders, pp 465–472, 1996.
19. Terpin KM, Dodson P: Observations on ketamine hydrochloride as an anaesthetic for alligators. Copeia 1:147–148, 1978.
20. Webb GJW, Messel H: Crocodile capture techniques. J Wildl Management 41:572–575, 1977.
21. Woodford MH: The use of gallamine triethiodide as a chemical immobilizing agent for the Nile Crocodile (*Crocodilus niloticus*). E Afr Wildl J 10:67–70, 1972.

CHAPTER 29

Medical Management of Sea Turtles in Aquaria

BRENT R. WHITAKER

HOWARD KRUM

Sea turtles have long been popular exhibit animals in public aquaria. Their gentle yet curious temperament, ability to cohabitate with many other species, longevity, large size, and readily adaptable nature have contributed to their popularity among both visitors and husbandry staff. Of the world's seven species of sea turtles, those most commonly displayed by aquaria include the loggerhead (*Caretta caretta*), hawksbill (*Eretmochelys imbricata*), green (*Chelonia mydas*), and Kemp's ridley (*Lepidochelys kempii*) (Table 29–1). The leatherback (*Dermochelys coriacea*) is the largest and most unusual of sea turtles with enormous front flippers and a shell that is covered with a dark, firm skin. It is rarely displayed, however, because it requires a large amount of space and a specialized diet, which includes cnidarians (e.g., medusa, siphonophores), tunicates (e.g., salps, pyrosomas), and jellyfish, all of which are difficult for most aquaria to provide in sufficient quantity.

In the wild, sea turtles face many dangers that threaten their populations with extinction. Predation of adult turtles by humans and sharks, destruction of nesting beaches, consumption of eggs by humans and other animals, pollutants including petroleum products and plastic debris, and accidental injury from trawlers and

TABLE 29–1. Characteristics of Sea Turtle Species Commonly Kept in Aquaria

Sea Turtle	Identifying Characteristics	Estimated Age of Maturity (Years)	Size Hatchling/Adult (SCL)	Weight	Natural Diet
Loggerhead *Caretta caretta*	5 Vertebral scutes 5 Costal scutes 11–12 Marginal scutes Nuchal scute in contact with first costal on each side	12–35	Adult approx. 92 cm Hatchling 45 mm	113–115 kg Approx. 20 g	Primarily carnivorous; crabs, shrimp, jellyfish; a variety of mollusks; may scavenge fish
Green *Chelonia mydas*	4 Pairs lateral scutes Elongated prefrontal scales	20–50	Adult 88–117 cm Hatchling approx. 50 mm	65–160 kg Approx. 25 g	Primarily herbivorous; sea grasses and algae; jellyfish, shellfish, and other marine animals
Hawksbill *Eretmochelys imbricata*	4 Pairs costal scutes 2 Claws on each flipper posteriorly overlapping scutes	Unknown	Adult 63–91 cm Yearling 20 cm	Approx. 80 kg	Variety of foods; sponges, algae, variety of invertebrates
Kemp's ridley *Lepidochelys kempii*	5 Pairs vertebral scutes 5 Pairs costal scutes 12 Pairs marginal scutes on carapace; bridge joining carapace and plastron has 4 scutes, each with a pore	6–7	Adult approx. 65 cm Hatchling 42–48 mm	<45 kg 15–20 g	Crustaceans, jellyfish, and mollusks

(Data from references 9, 34–38.)

powerboats have been implicated in the decline of sea turtle populations. Within the United States, all sea turtles are protected by the Endangered Species Act of 1973, thus aquaria must obtain special permits from the U.S. Fish and Wildlife Service in order to have them. Five species of sea turtles frequent United States coastal waters. Of these, the hawksbill, Kemp's ridley, and leatherback are currently listed as endangered, whereas the loggerhead is considered threatened. Floridian and east pacific breeding populations of the green sea turtle are listed as endangered, whereas the remainder of this species is labeled as threatened.[34] The status of each species is reviewed every 5 years to determine whether a change in listing is warranted.

Health problems in captive sea turtles may be minimized through the development of proper husbandry practices and a sound preventive medicine program. Modern aquaria are committed to sea turtle conservation, research, and education, and much of what has been learned about the medical care of these animals is the result of years of working with both stranded and collection sea turtles. Providing an appropriate environment, nutritional plan, and program of medical care is essential to maintaining good health among sea turtles in aquaria.

ENVIRONMENTAL CONSIDERATIONS

As with most other species kept in zoos or aquaria, proper environmental conditions contribute significantly to maintaining good health in sea turtles.[52] The information obtained during the collection of an accurate environmental history and performance of the environmental examination can yield valuable diagnostic and prognostic data. Sea turtle health problems may take many months to manifest in overt disease. An animal's history should therefore include a thorough evaluation of the environmental data accumulated over the past several months. The most important environmental considerations for sea turtles in captivity include water quality (temperature, salinity, pH, chlorine, ozone, ammonia, nitrite, nitrate concentrations, and total coliform bacteria counts), lighting (intensity, duration, wavelength, photoperiod), enclosure construction (shape, materials, substrate, decor), water depth and current flow pattern, and ambient sound levels. These parameters should be monitored and recorded on a regular basis. In addition, the interactions between the sea turtle and its tank mates should be examined.

Sea turtles should be housed in an appropriately designed enclosure. Although these animals are adapted to living in bays and the open ocean, they can successfully adjust to captivity, as long as tank parameters (e.g., overall shape, volume, materials used, decor obstacles, and water depth) and current patterns are considered. Hatchlings, which spend much of their time floating at the surface, are given buoyant sargasm or artificial seaweed on which they can rest and feed. Larger turtles must be given significantly more room to dive, swim, and surface. Tank shape, water depth, and

decor selection and placement become more important as the overall tank volume is reduced. Sea turtles can negotiate most obstacles as long as they have the opportunity to visualize an object and react. This is important because injuries have resulted from collision with obstacles when excited sea turtles are returned to both novel and known enclosures. In general, we have found that, as tank volume is reduced, the enclosure should become more cylindrical with few or no obstructions. We have successfully rehabilitated or maintained stranded Kemp's ridleys (25- to 60-cm straight carapace length) in cylindrical "flexible" fiberglass tanks (Solar Components Inc., Manchester, NH) as small as 54 inches in diameter by 50 inches deep for 3 to 5 months. Larger sea turtles should not be kept in shallow enclosures (i.e., less than 2 to 3 feet in depth) unless they are ill, because abrasions and pressure sores are likely to develop on their plastron. In addition, a pattern of water flow and current strength should be provided to allow the turtle several resting or sleeping spots.

Sea turtles may be destructive, biting both decor and divers. Sturdy, nonabrasive materials must therefore be used when creating underwater exhibits. Turtles also dig in the substrate, destroying portions of the biologic filter if encountered. All materials acquired by a curious turtle are subject to consumption, which can cause gastrointestinal (GI) upset, ulceration, obstruction, or perforation. Toxicity may also occur. Young turtles commonly ingest large amounts of gravel or crushed coral, resulting in impaction (Fig. 29–1). Healthy adult sea turtles, which are capable of remaining underwater without oxygen for up to 2 hours, are unlikely to become trapped and drown in a well-designed enclosure.

Some water quality parameters, such as temperature and chlorine or ozone concentrations, may directly and rapidly affect sea turtle health. Others parameters including pH and ammonia concentration are of less immediate concern, but are indicative of problems with water filtration that must be addressed. The most com-

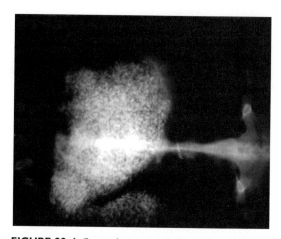

FIGURE 29–1. Sea turtles commonly ingest foreign bodies. This 10-kg loggerhead sea turtle consumed a large amount of gravel from its exhibit, which resulted in the animal's death. (Courtesy of Dr. Bob George, Virginia Marine Science Museum.)

monly maintained sea turtles in North America generally do well in seawater maintained between 25° and 28°C. Although healthy adult turtles can tolerate sustained water temperatures slightly higher or lower than this range, significant and persistent deviation will likely result in ill health.[19, 25, 57] Like in other reptiles, persistently low body temperatures influence the turtle's metabolism, resulting in decreased immunologic function[52, 57] and altered drug pharmacokinetics.[23] In addition, GI peristalsis may be inhibited enough so that overgrowth of the resident bacterial flora compromises health.[29] Low water temperatures can induce a state of inactivity or torpor commonly called cold stunning. Although hundreds of wild sea turtles succumb to prolonged hypothermia annually in the United States,[13, 29, 32] it is rarely seen in aquaria where carefully controlled environments are provided.

Outdoor enclosures with direct sunlight may provide certain benefits not available to sea turtles housed indoors with artificial lighting. It has been widely reported that sea turtles bask or float quietly at the water surface in the wild. Sapsford and Van der Riet[44] recorded a core body temperature of a basking loggerhead that was 3° to 4°C above ambient water temperature. Although the importance and function of sea turtle basking behavior are unknown, it seems plausible that this allows the animal to thermoregulate and carry out vitamin D conversion as observed in other reptile species.[15]

Full-spectrum artificial lighting that provides ultraviolet (UV) A, UV B, and infrared light may benefit sea turtles when natural sunlight is unavailable. Although artificial basking lights are not typically used in indoor sea turtle enclosures, they are recommended for turtles fighting disease or recovering from injury. In addition, a consistent photoperiod should be provided. A lighting duration of 12 to 18 hours per 24 hours is adequate to balance the needs of the display facility and those of the animal. For example, conditions of near constant light are unnatural for turtles and likely to be low-level, chronic stressors.

Large filtration systems typically use either chlorine or ozone injection to oxidize the organic material produced during animal metabolism and waste breakdown, as well as to reduce bacterial loads. Both methods may effectively aid in water quality maintenance; however, their oxidative potential can irritate the mucous membranes and eyes. Sea turtles have been successfully maintained in water with total chlorine concentrations of 1 ppm or less. As with any aquatic species, it is recommended that there be no residual ozone in the actual enclosure water.

Because most sea turtle enclosures in public aquaria are mixed species exhibits, there is potential for trauma to be inflicted by tank mates. Large sharks are known to injure slower moving sea turtles. Even smaller fish species such as queen angel fish *(Holancathus ciliaris)* have been seen to pick at and traumatize a sea turtle's eyes and exposed lesions while the animal is resting. The potential for disease transmission among tank mates does exist, but can be minimized by maintaining excellent water quality and establishing a quarantine program for new arrivals.

NUTRITION

Depending on the supply of local foodstuffs, providing captive sea turtles with their natural diet (see Table 29–1) in sufficient quantity may present a significant challenge. Adult green sea turtles are considered to be primarily herbivorous although they are known to consume marine animals in the wild.[56] In captivity, they do well offered a diet of leafy vegetables, such as romaine lettuce,[9] mixed with small amounts of fish and invertebrates. Hatchling green turtles and other adult sea turtles are carnivorous and are often fed a diet consisting of fish, crabs, squid, and shellfish. Commercial pelleted turtle feed, modified trout chow, and gelatin-based diets have also been used with varied levels of success.

A balanced diet of high quality foods providing protein, fats, moisture, carbohydrates, vitamins, and minerals is required by captive sea turtles. The protein content of most food fishes ranges from 12% to 22%; these provide a variety of amino acids and are highly digestible. Pelleted diets contain up to 25% to 45% protein to obtain rapid growth. When formulating a dietary plan, the source of protein and the species to be fed must be considered. For example, loggerhead sea turtles, which are primarily carnivorous, fed a floating trout chow presumably containing a significant amount of vegetable matter did not grow nearly as well as green sea turtles, which are primarily herbivorous, given the same diet. The loggerhead turtles' growth rate increased substantially when their diet of pellets was supplemented with fish.[49] Pelleted foods contain much less fresh water as compared to that found in fish and invertebrates of equal mass. The water content of fish is inversely proportional to the amount of fat present. Food fishes such as mackerel and herring have more fat and less water than do the leaner smelt and capelin. Those prey items with more fat are higher in calories. Squid, shrimp, and other invertebrates are rich in water and carbohydrates, but low in fat, necessitating a larger consumption of these items to provide sufficient caloric intake.

The energy requirements of most captive sea turtles are commonly provided by feeding a mixture of fish and invertebrates such as smelt, herring, capelin, mackerel, squid, crabs, and shrimp. Only high quality food fit for human consumption should be fed. Commercially prepared fish that have been rapidly frozen following capture, glazed, and packed in containers impervious to air and moisture have the longest shelf life. Most frozen fish should be maintained at −25° to −30°C for no longer than 6 to 8 months; invertebrates and fish containing little fat may be kept longer. Dark muscled species of fish, such as mackerel, should be stored no longer than 4 months because their high levels of unsaturated fats and the presence of oxygen-binding myoglobin hasten rancidity. Frozen items to be thawed are first placed in a refrigerator (4° to 6°C) for up to 24 hours before placing them into cold water (<8°C). Soaking fish in water for extended periods of time promotes the loss of nutrients and should be avoided.[18] When preparing the diet for the day each food item should be examined for freshness. If the fish or invertebrate needs to be cut into pieces, this should be done just before feeding to retain the moisture in the food. All food should be refrigerated or placed on ice until used. Any remaining food should be discarded at the end of the day.

The loss of vitamins from foodstuffs begins soon after manufacture or processing. Providing a multivitamin twice a week is therefore recommended. Additional supplements of thiamine and vitamin E are often added to the diets of fish-eating animals. Thiamine deficiency occurs in marine animals that consume large quantities of food fish such as herring, smelts, and capelin, which contain thiaminase in their tissues. Because most fish tissue contains a large proportion of unsaturated fats, the addition of antioxidants such as vitamin E should also be considered. A safe and effective dosage for the supplementation of fish diets is thiamine at 25 mg/kg and vitamin E at 100 IU/kg of fish fed.[18]

Daily energy requirements depend on a sea turtle's reproductive status, level of activity, water temperature, and individual needs. Young, growing animals as well as those fighting illness or repairing an injury have a greater caloric need. Because reptiles are ectotherms, their body temperature closely follows that of their environment. In warmer waters, increased metabolic function enables the turtle to fully use food products that are consumed, resulting in optimal growth. Cooler waters may lead to diminished metabolic activity, resulting in the maldigestion of food products or even the inability to capture prey.

Both underfed animals and those that refuse to feed begin to lose weight.[12] The clinician must therefore take into account the animal's physiologic state congruent with environmental parameters when assessing a turtle reported with anorexia or weight loss. A general rule of thumb is to feed hatchling turtles 5% of their body weight, yearling turtles 3% of their body weight, and 2 year olds 1.5% of their body weight daily. By 1 to 2 years of age, turtles may be weaned from gelatin diets that foul the water more so than from other foods.[16] A daily growth rate of 1.87% has been reported for loggerhead sea turtles maintained in 20°C water and fed a diet of horse mackerel (*Trachurus japonicus*).[40] Because a

number of variables influence caloric needs, it is recommended that turtles younger than 1 year of age be weighed at least weekly initially, and then monthly as weight gains become evident.

Few nutritional diseases have been observed in captive sea turtles. Cachectic myopathy in oceanarium-reared turtles has been associated with ulcerative stomatitis and endocarditis,[19] although any chronic disease process resulting in an animal's inability to assimilate nutrients causes wasting. GI obstruction may occur, especially in hatchlings, if fed inappropriately sized or selected food items.[17] Anemia, hypoproteinemia, and hypoglycemia are commonly observed changes in malnourished turtles. We have observed dramatic abnormalities in blood, growth (Fig. 29–2), and skeleton indicative of malnutrition in 1-year-old captive-reared loggerhead sea turtles fed freeze-dried krill without vitamin or mineral supplementation. Cortical thinning, bowed femurs, and healed pathologic fractures were seen in these turtles whose average straight carapace length was 12.96 cm and weight was only 0.344 kg. In comparison, clutch mates provided a diet of cut fish, shrimp, and krill rolled in a balanced calcium phosphorus supplement had a notable inverse in their calcium:phosphorus ratio, although radiographs showed no bony abnormalities. These turtles were also significantly larger than their clutch mates with an average straight carapace length of 22.0 cm and weight of 1.8 kg.[47] After changing both groups of animals to a gelatin diet (Table 29–2), an improvement in the calcium:phosphorus ratio, serum calcium, and albumin occurred. Subsequent clutches fed the gelatin diet developed normally and in good health. Life-threatening anemias have also been observed in juvenile loggerhead and Kemp's ridley turtles fed only squid and shrimp. These animals are found listless, floating, and hyperventilating with packed cell volumes one half to one third the normal values. Evidence of malnutrition in these turtles include muscular atrophy, a concave plastron, and sunken eyes. If intervention is undertaken early enough, these animals respond well to an improved diet and supplementation with iron.[17]

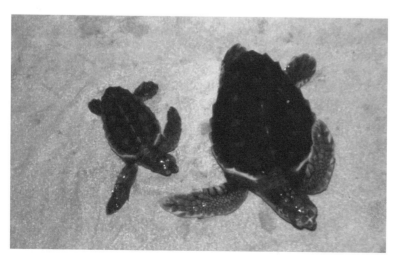

FIGURE 29–2. Dietary deficiencies may lead to poor growth as well as other physiologic changes, as seen in the smaller of these clutch mates, which was fed only freeze-dried krill. The larger of these loggerhead sea turtles received cut fish, shrimp, and krill coated with a calcium-phosphorus supplement. (Courtesy of Dr. Andy Stamper, National Aquarium, Baltimore.)

TABLE 29–2. Sea Turtle Gelatin Diet

Ingredient	Weight (g)	% of Diet
Trout Chow	425	8.0
Fish (various species)	565	10.6
Squid (viscera removed)	282	5.3
Peeled shrimp	282	5.3
Spinach (fresh or frozen)	142	2.8
Carrots (fresh)	142	2.7
Gelatin (unflavored)	450	8.5
Water 2800 ml	2800	53.0
Supplements:		
Sea Tabs (Pacific Research Lab, Inc., El Cajon, CA)	#4 500-mg tablets	0.04
Amino Acid Complex 1000	#4 500-mg tablets	0.04
Spirolina (Lightforce, Santa Cruz, CA)	50 ml powder (28 g)	0.50
Rep-Cal (Rep-Cal Research Labs, Los Gatos, CA)	200 ml powder (180 g)	3.4

Modified from Stamper MA, Whitaker BR: Medical observations and implications on "healthy" sea turtles prior to release into the wild. Proceedings of the Annual Meeting of the American Association of Zoo Veterinarians, Pittsburgh, PA, pp 182–185, 1994.

COLLECTION AND RESTRAINT

Capture and Physical Restraint

Many examination and treatment procedures are preferably accomplished without the use of sedatives or general anesthetics because these animals are usually slow to recover from the effects of these drugs. Hatchling and young sea turtles weighing less than 10 kg are easily collected and restrained without special equipment. This is done by gently grasping the lateral margins of the turtle's shell with one or both hands. Care must be taken not to compromise respiration by exerting excessive pressure on the flexible shell. Larger turtles are best handled by firmly grasping the carapace just caudal to the head with one hand and grasping between the hind flippers with the other. Heavier animals may require strong and able assistants to lift each side of the shell. Very large sea turtles may require additional equipment such as a mechanical hoist and padded carrier from which water can freely drain as it is lifted from the surface. Healthy sea turtles resist restraint by attempting to bite and vigorously slapping their flippers, which may have sharp claws. Handlers must be wary of the animal's beak; even small sea turtles can inflict a painful bite if given the opportunity.

Once collected, large turtles are placed onto a thick piece of foam for examination and collection of samples. The flippers may be held at the animal's side and the head secured. Many turtles become calm if they are placed on their back, allowing for procedures such as an ultrasound examination or the administration of fluids to be conducted without additional restraint. Pieces of foam or rolled towels can be used to support and stabilize the carapace. To place a larger turtle on its back, the flipper closest to the ground is tucked against the animal's body and the turtle is gently rolled onto its back.

Seriously ill sea turtles that are unable to swim will drown if placed in more than a few inches of water. A sling may be fashioned that allows the turtle to float with its head above water while reducing pressure on the plastron, which otherwise may result in respiratory compromise.

Chemical Restraint

Sedation and the induction and maintenance of general anesthesia may be safely accomplished in sea turtles.[30, 45, 54] As with any other patient, a thorough preoperative health evaluation with complete blood count (CBC), blood chemistry profiles, blood gases, coagulation evaluation, and survey radiography is recommended. Baseline information including body temperature, pulse, and respiration rates should also be obtained as part of the preanesthetic assessment. When possible, dehydrated turtles should receive fluid therapy in advance of planned procedures. Depending on the specific procedure and the animal's condition, fluids may be administered by intracoelom (ICe), subcutaneous (SQ), intraosseous (IO), or intravenous (IV) routes. Fluid administration by gastric lavage or per os (PO) is usually less efficacious because of the propensity for passive fluid regurgitation in sea turtles.

Injectable anesthetics have been used extensively and safely in reptile medicine, both as induction agents and for general anesthesia.[5, 6] The main drawbacks of the most commonly used injectable drugs center around their lengthy and sometimes unpredictable half-lives and an inability to reverse their effects rapidly. In addition, most have not been thoroughly tested in sea turtle species. For example, IV sodium pentobarbital has been shown to produce unacceptably high morbidity and mortality rates in Kemp's ridleys as compared with its use in green sea turtles.[54] For these reasons and because all sea turtle species are threatened or endangered, we recommend only the use of ketamine, which we have used safely and effectively. As injectable drugs with reversal agents become available, their use should be evaluated.

Ketamine (25 mg/kg IV[7] or IM) is most useful as an induction agent or for providing a light sedative effect for short-term procedures. Used at higher doses (50 to 70 mg/kg IM),[48] recovery times may be excessively long and unpredictable. A combination of ketamine (10 ml) and acepromazine (1 ml) administered IV gives a more rapid induction and recovery. Doses as small as 8–12 mg/kg IV provide excellent sedation and allow the clinician to readily intubate the turtle. Table 29–3 provides allometrically scaled doses for administering this mixture to larger sea turtles. Leatherback sea turtles require approximately 15% more than the calculated doses.[16] General anesthesia may also be induced with the use of inhalant agents via a mask or direct intubation with subsequent forced ventilation. Moon and Stabenau[30] report that unsedated direct orotracheal intubation and ventilation with 2% to 5%

TABLE 29–3. Allometrically Scaled Dosages for a Mixture of Ketamine (10 ml) and Acepromazine (1 ml) Administered to Larger Sea Turtles

Weight (kg)	Dosage (mg/kg)*
10	30
15	26.8
20	25
50	19.9
100	16.7
150	15.2
200	14.1
250	13.3
300	12.7
350	12.3
400	11.8
450	11.5

*Leatherback sea turtles require up to 15% more drug than the calculated dose.

Printed with permission of Dr. Bob George, personal communication, 1996.

isoflurane produced anesthesia in approximately 7 minutes in Kemp's ridleys. Isoflurane appears to be safe and effective for use in Kemp's ridley, green, and loggerhead sea turtles.[45] Orotracheal intubation is fairly simple because the glottis is easily visualized just caudal to the base of the tongue. As in some other marine species, the tracheal rings of sea turtles are complete and care should be taken not to overinflate the endotracheal cuff. New anesthetics and the appropriate choice of an anesthetic carrier gas are being investigated with the goal of reducing the duration of recovery. Procedures have been attempted with various combinations of O_2, CO_2, NO, and room air. Currently, only the use of either 100% O_2 or a mixture of O_2 with up to 50% NO can be recommended.

At surgical planes of anesthesia, assisted ventilation is necessary. Tidal volumes can be estimated at approximately 50 ml/kg,[14] but may be significantly reduced with lung compromise. Ventilation pressures should not exceed 15 cm H_2O and rates should be between 2 and 8 ventilations/minute.[30] Intraoperative blood gas analysis may provide valuable information on the animal's respiratory and metabolic status, allowing adjustments in ventilation technique to be made.

Monitoring the patient closely is imperative during the use of anesthetics. Limb withdrawal and ocular reflexes diminish as the depth of anesthesia increases. As with any anesthetized patient, core body temperature and heart rate should be continuously monitored. Temperature should be monitored by using a flexible rectal probe. Correct placement is best accomplished by advancing the lubricated probe into the cloaca while directing it craniodorsally and slightly toward the left side of the turtle. This directs the probe away from the opening of the urinary bladder. The descending colon curves sharply and transversely to the right side of the animal at approximately the level of the mid-plastron.

Passing the probe further than the flexure may be difficult and is potentially dangerous.

Heart rate and pulse rate may be monitored and evaluated through the use of a variety of equipment including an electrocardiogram (ECG), direct cardiac ultrasound (echocardiography), pulse oximetry, and a Doppler blood flow meter. Adhesive ECG pads (Trauma Trode, LMI Medical, Grand Rapids, MI) adhere well to the dry shell and can be placed on either the plastron, carapace, or skin. On the plastron, one lead can be placed on each of the pectoral scutes and one on the left femoral scute (Fig. 29–3). This lead placement can be used for obtaining a "lead II" ECG tracing. Echocardiography provides information about heart rate and is a means for evaluating cardiac contractility. A pulse oximeter with a rectal reflectance probe may provide heart rate information and relative values for blood oxygen saturation[33] but should only be used as an adjunct to other more reliable means of pulse monitoring. The Doppler blood flow meter provides reliable and valuable information. The velocity of blood flow in hypothermic patients, however, may be too slow to be reliably detected through this method. Alternatively, some anesthetic agents may induce a significant bradycardia and reduce systemic blood pressure, both of which may potentially be ameliorated by the administration of atropine IV[30] or intratracheally if detected early enough. The best sites to position the Doppler probe are at the mediastinal and inguinal acoustic windows,

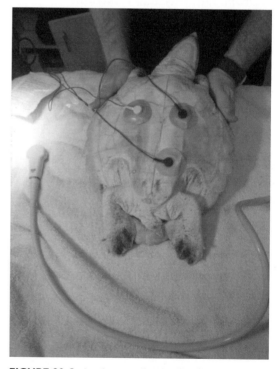

FIGURE 29–3. An electrocardiogram (ECG) can be obtained through the use of a standard ECG machine and three leads (LL, RA, LA) attached to the dry plastron with Trauma Trode ECG pads. A similar attachment of the leads to the carapace produces similar results.

aiming the transducer at the cardiac and the renal vasculature, respectively. It may be useful to image the vessels with ultrasound before the Doppler blood flow meter is used.

Support during recovery from anesthesia should include precise control of body temperature and fluid therapy. The latter is particularly important if significant blood loss occurred during the procedure. Recovery from general anesthesia may take from 2 to 6 hours [45] up to 24 hours. Ventilation and perfusion mismatches and intracardiac shunting are suspected to contribute to the variability in recovery period duration.[30] When possible, surgical procedures should be planned for the early morning to facilitate close monitoring during the recovery phase. Assisted ventilation should be continued until the animal rejects the endotracheal tube. Usually, arousal from anesthesia is immediately preceded by a rapid increase in heart and respiratory rate.[30]

PHYSICAL EXAMINATION AND CLINICAL TECHNIQUES

Physical Examination

Annual or even semiannual physical examinations should be performed on all sea turtles maintained in captivity. The extent of examination is likely dictated by patient size, expertise of staff members, and availability of equipment. The examination of the sea turtle should begin by collecting weight and measurements. Measurements commonly include straight and curved carapace lengths, straight and curved carapace widths, and straight plastron length (Fig. 29–4). These measurements help the clinician evaluate and quantify nutritional problems such as obesity, cachexia, and metabolic bone problems. Sunken eyes, depressed pectoral muscles, and a convex plastron are signs of weight loss and dehydration. The bony carapace and plastron provide a challenge to the clinician by limiting auscultation,

palpation, and ultrasonographic examinations. The animal's entire integument should be examined to note any abnormalities such as discolorations, lacerations, or ulcerations. Captive sea turtles may succumb to an ulcerative dermatitis caused by any of a variety of bacteria or fungi. In addition, the clinician should look for any shape defects and ectoparasites such as leeches or barnacles. All growths should be examined grossly and biopsied, especially when significant changes in size, shape, or consistency are noted over a short period of time. Fibromas, cutaneous papillomas, and fibropapillomas are three lesions associated with the disease syndrome known as green sea turtle fibropapillomatosis, which also affects loggerhead, olive ridley, and hawksbill sea turtles.[17, 21] This disease should be ruled out for any animal with aberrant skin growths.[3, 21]

Examination of the oral cavity is possible without sedation. Once the animal is quieted, the mouth may be opened with constant, gentle pressure on the lower jaw. Rolled cloth strips are then looped around the lower and upper beak and gently retracted, enabling an unobstructed view of the oral cavity. Care should be taken when a bite block is used so as not to fracture or chip the beak when the animal bites down. The animal's powerful jaws can easily sever a finger. Despite the extra effort required, oropharyngeal examination may be useful to detect ulcerative stomatitis or obstructive rhinitis syndromes.[17] The eyes are easily and thoroughly evaluated with standard ophthalmologic tools to note any corneal, iridal, or lenticular problems. Suspected corneal ulcers may be confirmed with fluorescein dye and a cobalt light. Pupillary light reflexes are not of diagnostic value in sea turtles. Uveitis may be indicative of systemic disease or localized infection. Cataracts have been noted on rare occasion and may be removed surgically, but they are unlikely to seriously debilitate captive sea turtles. The structure of the sea turtle ear is such that anything other than external evaluation of the tympanic membrane is precluded. Abdominal palpation should be attempted through the inguinal "windows."

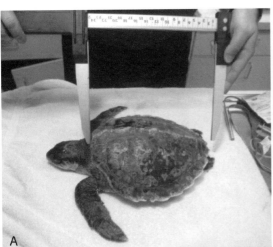 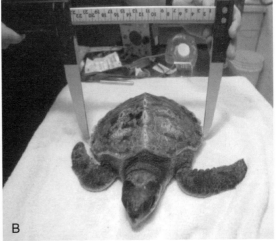

A B

FIGURE 29–4. Calipers are used to measure straight carapace length *(A)* and straight carapace width *(B)*. A flexible tape measure placed directly on the shell measures curved carapace length and curved carapace width.

With practice, it may be possible to appreciate distended or impacted loops of intestine, abdominal masses, and the presence of eggs. A visual examination of the cloaca should be performed as well.

Respiratory rate and effort should be noted before handling the sea turtle. Auscultation of the lung fields should be attempted; however, plain film radiography and even the animal's attitude in the water column are likely to be more sensitive indicators of respiratory diseases such as bacterial and fungal pneumonias. Core body and ambient water temperatures as well as pulse rate should recorded. At any time during the physical examination it is likely that the animal will urinate or defecate, and containers should be on hand for collection of these samples. Fecal examination should be performed looking for signs of nematode, trematode, and coccidial parasitic infection.[11, 19, 20, 50] Survey radiographs and ultrasonography, as well as blood collection, should be attempted during the annual or semiannual physical examination. The data collected during the physical examination provide invaluable individual animal references if future health problems arise.

Blood Collection and Analysis

The routine analysis of blood including hematology and blood chemistries is an important component of monitoring the health status of collection turtles. Age,

sex, size, health, habitat, and diet all influence hematologic and serologic parameters. For these reasons, it is difficult to compare values obtained for captive animals to those published for wild sea turtle populations.[7, 9, 17, 28, 55] Normal values must therefore be established for each individual, taking care to minimize any variability in acquisition, handling, or analysis of samples. Table 29–4 provides blood data collected from rehabilitated Kemp's ridley turtles and captive juvenile loggerhead sea turtles.

Blood may be collected from several sites including the dorsal cervical sinus, the jugular vein, and metatarsal vessels (Fig. 29–5). The use of cardiac puncture is commonly described in earlier literature, but is no longer used because it is potentially dangerous and unnecessary.[41] The dorsal cervical sinus is most commonly used because sufficient quantities of blood may be safely and rapidly collected. Vaccutainers or syringes with 20- to 22-gauge 1-inch or 1½-inch needles are used in larger turtles, whereas insulin syringes (26-gauge needles) work well for hatchlings weighing as little as 20 g,[4] although the distortion of cells is more likely when smaller bore needles are used. Proper positioning of the head and neck is necessary to ensure a successful collection. This is done by placing the turtle on the edge of a table or a foam pad, firmly grasping the head, and extending it slightly downward. The site is prepared with a disinfectant for venipuncture and the

TABLE 29–4. Hematology and Blood Chemistry Values for Healthy Rehabilitated Kemp's Ridley and Captive Loggerhead Sea Turtles

	Rehabilitated Kemp's Ridley Turtles Before Release from the New England Aquarium			Captive Loggerhead Turtles Weighing less than 2 Kg Housed at the National Aquarium in Baltimore		
	Serum Chemistry	SD	n	Plasma Chemistry	SD	n
Glucose	118.7	16.7	15	131.4	10.2	9
Urea nitrogen (mg/dl)	161.7	28	15	101.7	17.8	6
Uric acid (mg/dl)	—	—	—	0.7	0.3	7
Sodium (mEq/L)	150.0	4	15	157	1	3
Potassium (mEq/L)	4.1	0.8	15	4.6	0.4	3
Chloride (mEq/L)	115.5	3.9	15	121	9.8	3
Calcium (mg/dl)	6.3	1.3	15	7.1	0.8	8
Phosphorus (mg/dl)	9.0	1.8	15	5.3	3.5	8
Magnesium (mg/dl)	—	—	—	2.42	0.8	6
Aspartate aminotransferase (IU/L)	160.7	42.6	15	122.5	37.8	9
Alkaline phosphatase (IU/L)	465.3	306.4	15	73.9	36.9	9
Lactic dehydrogenase (IU/L)	6297.7	5284.8	14	108.8	63.5	9
Creatine kinase (IU/L)	2832	1698.6	15	1614.5	1677.0	4
Total protein (g/dl)	3.2	0.6	15	2.0	0.8	9
Albumin (g/dl)	1.6	0.3	15	1.0	0.26	9
Globulin (g/dl)	1.6	0.4	15	0.95	0.65	8
Hematology						
Hematocrit (%)	30.1	3.0	15	22.0	5.33	11
RBC × 10⁶/UL	—	—	—	0.39	0.08	10
WBC (Nat Herricks) × 10³/UI	—	—	—	14.67	5.8	12

RBC, red blood cells; WBC, white blood cells.

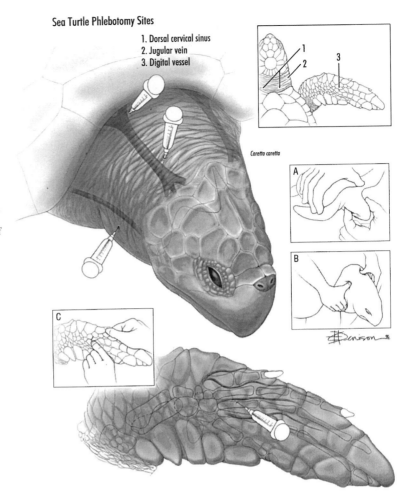

Sea Turtle Phlebotomy Sites

1. Dorsal cervical sinus
2. Jugular vein
3. Digital vessel

Caretta caretta

FIGURE 29–5. The dorsal cervical sinus and jugular vein provide excellent routes for the collection of blood from sea turtles weighing as little as 20 g. Intravenous catheters may also be placed in these vessels for the administration of drugs or fluids. The metatarsal vessels can also be used to collect blood from larger sea turtles.

needle is inserted paramidline, angled slightly toward the shell. If unsuccessful, the needle should be fully removed and repositioned to locate the sinus. There are many possible approaches to this sinus as can be seen by studying the turtle's anatomy. The exact location of these vessels often changes in ill and emaciated sea turtles as compared to healthy ones. This is probably due to a lack of supporting fat bodies and musculature, allowing the vessels to deviate laterally from where they would be expected to be found in a healthy animal (Walsh M, personal communication, 1996).[51] Ultrasound should be used to locate these vessels when blood collection is difficult or to locate the best site for catheter placement (Fig. 29–6).

Sodium or lithium heparin is the anticoagulant of choice. Hemolysis occurs if blood is placed in EDTA because of the chelation of calcium and other ions.[8] Immediately after collection and mixing of the blood, smears are made and air dried. Either plasma or serum may be used for chemistry analysis; however, data from plasma provide more consistent results. This has been attributed in part to the variability in time required for clot formation to occur, allowing chemical composition of the sample to change.[8]

For comparison of diagnostic samples, it is extremely important that the same analytic methods be used. For example, drastic differences in total white blood cell (WBC) count have been noted in two commonly used analytic methods: Nat-Herrick method and the Eosinophil Unopette.[2] Because the Eosinophil Unopette method requires the WBC differential for calculation of the total WBC count,[10] it is also important that the same staining methods for blood smears be used when comparing data. Dif-Quik stain, for example, poorly differentiates basophils, potentially altering the overall percentages of cell types reported, resulting in an inaccurate calculation of total WBC. We have found the May-Grunwald, Wright's-Giemsa stains excellent for preparing blood smears collected from sea turtles.[1] In general, the total WBC counts obtained with the Nat-Herrick method are greater than those acquired with the use of the Unopette stain. In one study of 32 blood samples collected from loggerhead sea turtles, counts determined through the Nat-Herrick method exceeded those obtained through the Unopette method by 2% to 68%, with an average of 38.5%.[2] The reason for this discrepancy of WBC is not fully understood but its potential impact upon diagnostic interpretation is clear.

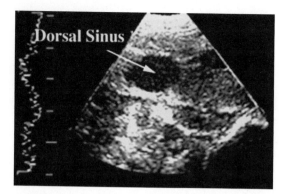

FIGURE 29–6. Ultrasonography can be used to locate the dorsal sinus for blood collection or intravenous catheterization. The dorsal sinus in this 25-kg turtle is approximately 1 × 2 cm, as seen in this transverse section obtained with a 5.0-MHz probe placed dorsally in the mid-neck region. (Courtesy of Dr. Roger Williams, National Aquarium, Baltimore.)

Diagnostic Imaging

Radiologic and ultrasonographic examinations are readily carried out in all but the largest of turtles, providing the clinician with valuable diagnostic information. In general, sea turtles need not be sedated for radiographic or ultrasound examinations. These animals usually struggle for a period of time but then become quiet and manageable, especially when placed in ventrodorsal recumbency.

Survey radiographs should be taken of each sea turtle in the collection as part of its periodic wellness examination. Diagnostically, radiology is useful for evaluating the extent of external trauma in the chelonian patient, determining mineralization of soft tissues, detecting foreign bodies, monitoring the development of bones, and assessing the health of the respiratory tract.[27] We recommend that at least three views be obtained at each examination including ventrodorsal, cranial-caudal, and lateral exposures. The mAs and kvp settings used for whole body radiography are usually inappropriate for the extremities. Radiograph machines with high mA (200 to 300 mA) capabilities and small focal spots are ideal. High-detail, rare earth intensifying screens and compatible film combinations have been recommended for reptilian subjects.[46]

It is important when attempting to image the respiratory tract that the turtle be allowed to take a deep breath just before exposure. This allows for the fullest expansion of the lung field and a more thorough evaluation. Lateral and cranial-caudal views are usually taken with the animal in dorsoventral recumbency, with the use of a horizontal beam.[31] These views maximize evaluation of the respiratory track while screening for bony abnormalities and foreign bodies. Radiographic contrast studies (air and barium) of the GI tract have been used in chelonians, but interpretation is sometimes difficult because of the relatively long GI transport times.[22]

The use of ultrasound as a diagnostic tool is particularly well suited to the evaluation of soft tissues such as the intestine, liver, and kidneys. Many of the more superficial tissues in smaller turtles may be imaged with a 7.5-MHz transducer. Linear array transducers generally produce an image that is easier to interpret, but the relatively large footprint of the transducer reduces its usefulness in smaller turtles. A 3.5- or 5-MHz curvilinear transducer is more useful for imaging the deeper tissues of larger turtles. Active animals are generally easier to image out of water, but require liberal amounts of coupling gel. Debilitated turtles, however, are best kept partially submerged in water enhancing image quality. Probes not designed for immersion in water should be protected by placing them in a water-tight plastic sleeve. Three acoustic windows for visceral examination exist in the sea turtle: the mediastinal, the axillary, and the inguinal. These are similar to those described by Penninck et al.[42] for the gopher tortoise (*Xerobates agassizi*). Working craniocaudally, a 7.5 linear array transducer may be used to visualize the vasculature of the head and neck. This method may be used to aid phlebotomy or catheterization attempts in severely dehydrated patients. Cardiac imaging is best attempted via the mediastinal acoustic window. A three-chamber, frontal-coronal section can be accomplished by placing a 3.5- or 5-MHz curvilinear transducer near the gular scute and aiming toward the center of the plastron (Fig. 29–7A). The axillary windows may be used to image the liver, pectoral muscles, and heart as well as the associated vasculature. Ultrasound-guided biopsy of the liver can be accomplished via the right axillary window (see Fig. 29–7B). The inguinal windows provide excellent access to image the kidneys, urinary bladder, stomach, intestines, right liver lobe, and gallbladder (see Fig. 29–7C).

Further diagnostic imaging techniques including the use of magnetic resonance imaging and computed tomography should be considered. Universities and research hospitals are most likely to have machines as well as interested diagnosticians who are often willing to work with the veterinarian to aid these threatened and endangered animals.

Abdominocentesis

The accumulation of fluid within the coelomic cavity often accompanies disease processes affecting the hepatic, renal, or cardiovascular system. Samples of fluid are acquired by placing the turtle in ventrodorsal recumbency, extending a rear flipper caudally, and inserting a needle anterior to the femur in a craniomedial direction. Length and diameter of the needle depend on the size of the animal. Ultrasonography may help the clinician avoid distended loops of intestine and locate pockets of fluid more efficiently. A complete analysis of the fluid should include anaerobic and aerobic bacterial culture, cytology, and assessment of protein content. The same technique may also be used to withdraw accumulated gas in the coelomic cavity, which can occur as a result of a tear in lung tissue.

Laparoscopy and Endoscopy

Laparoscopy enables the clinician to perform an internal examination and collect biopsies in sea turtles without

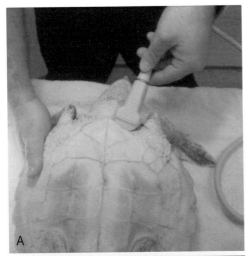

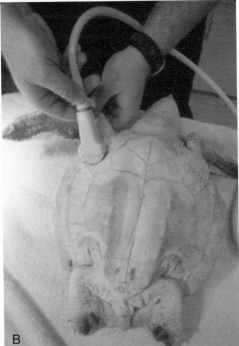

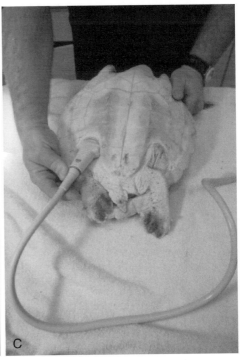

FIGURE 29–7. Ultrasonography can be used to locate blood vessels, assess cardiac function, perform biopsies, and examine soft tissues. *A,* The mediastinal acoustic window allows imaging of the heart. *B,* The right axillary acoustic window enables ultrasound-guided biopsies of the liver to be performed. *C,* The inguinal acoustic windows can be used to image the kidneys, urinary bladder, stomach, intestines, right liver lobe, and gallbladder.

major surgery. Rigid laparoscopes are available in a variety of sizes. Larger scopes provide better optics and a larger field of view; however, selection is often based on animal size and availability of equipment. The turtle should be placed on its back with its cranial carapace tipped slightly downward so that the intestines fall away from the site of entry just anterior to the right or left rear flipper. Insufflation with CO_2 is often necessary to carry out a complete examination. Changing the turtle's position during the examination helps the clinician by shifting tissues, allowing additional structures to be viewed.

Endoscopy provides a nonsurgical alternative for foreign body removal and examination of the stomach. Protection of the flexible endoscope is provided by passing it through a wooden bite block or short padded PVC pipe wedged in the oral cavity (Fig. 29–8). Heavy sedation is often required to carry out a complete and successful examination. In our experience, it may be hard to pass any tube, even an endoscope, down the distal esophagus, which turns sharply to the animal's left under the heart before passing through the muscular esophageal sphincter and into the stomach. Rotating the turtle may assist the entry of the endoscope as well as provide a more thorough examination of the chamber. While biopsy samples are easily taken, retrieving foreign bodies through an endoscope may be challenging because of the presence of the sharply pointed papillae that line the esophagus (Fig. 29–9). Designed to prevent the loss of ingested items while extruding unwanted

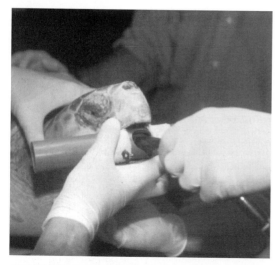

FIGURE 29–8. An endoscope is passed through a small padded PVC pipe, protecting it from the powerful bite of a loggerhead sea turtle. (Courtesy of George Grall, National Aquarium, Baltimore.)

seawater, the papillae tend to impale or catch items as they are withdrawn.

Cerebrospinal Fluid

Cerebrospinal fluid (CSF) may be obtained for cytology and culture from adult sea turtles showing signs of neurologic disease. For animals weighing 20 to 40 kg, a 2- to 3-inch, 22- to 25-gauge needle is directed cranioventrally into the neck, on the midline and just caudal to the supraoccipital protrusion.[41] The head must be fully extended downward, allowing the needle to miss the atlas, pass through the foramen magnum, and enter the subcranial space. Resistance in the form of a cartilaginous-like material may be encountered immediately before entering the CSF. This material is differentiated from bone in that gentle but constant and even pressure results in forward progress of the needle. If the sample is contaminated with blood after drawing a small amount of fluid, a second clean syringe is used. Up to 2 to 3 ml of CSF may be withdrawn safely from sea turtles weighing 20 to 40 kg.[41]

QUARANTINE

All sea turtles new to a collection should be quarantined for a minimum of 60 days. This provides the caregiver time to assess the overall behavior and health of the animal before introduction into the colony. Diseases such as spirochidiasis, a potentially deadly infection caused by intravascular trematodes, have been found in several species of sea turtle with greater than a 30% infection rate of the wild-caught loggerhead *Caretta caretta*. Although the life cycle of this trematode, ap-

proximately 30 to 60 days, is not completely understood, this parasite causes illness and mortality as a result of egg migration, the presence of adult worms, and secondary infection.[53] Additionally, fibropapillomas, which are thought to be caused by a papillomavirus, have been found to infect multiple species of sea turtles. Other than the surgical removal of the masses, no other treatment is available for this disease, making it imperative that new arrivals be quarantined.

A complete physical examination including the collection of blood for a CBC and chemistries should be executed shortly after the turtle's arrival and just before its exit from quarantine. Radiographs should be obtained and scrutinized for evidence of respiratory disease, bony abnormalities, ingestion of foreign objects, or other signs of potential illness.

Quarantined turtles should be housed in isolated tanks, each with its own filtration system. When possible, separate and dedicated equipment (e.g., nets, siphons, feeding tubes) should be provided for each quarantine system to minimize the spread of contagious diseases between animals. After use, all organic debris should be washed from the tools before placing them in a disinfectant bath (see Chapter 7). Staff must be encouraged to wash their hands with a disinfectant soap after handling quarantined turtles or working in their tanks.

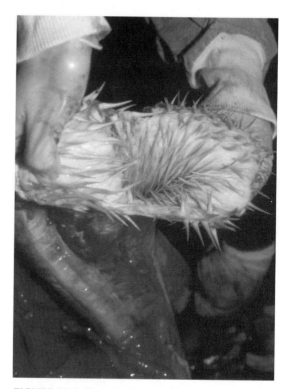

FIGURE 29–9. Sharply pointed papillae line the sea turtle's esophagus, making the removal of foreign bodies from the stomach through an endoscope a challenge. All tubes passed into the stomach should be smooth, without a side portal that may be caught by the papillae upon withdrawal.

THERAPEUTIC CONSIDERATIONS

Emergency Situations

The incidence of "emergency" medical situations encountered with sea turtles maintained in captivity is low. Most medical problems are of a chronic, insidious nature precipitated or induced by nutritional inadequacies or suboptimal environmental conditions. Emergency situations most likely to occur include traumatic injury by tank mates, prolonged forced submergence ("drowning"), and hypothermia resulting from life support system failure.

Regardless of the cause, if a turtle is nonresponsive and not respiring, resuscitation attempts should be initiated. Establishment of a patent airway via orotracheal intubation and subsequent forced ventilation (2 to 8 breaths per minute) with 100% oxygen should be the first priority. Second, an evaluation of cardiac activity should be attempted with the use of an ECG, Doppler blood flow meter, or direct cardiac ultrasound examination. Weak, depressed, or irregular cardiac activity has been improved with epinephrine and atropine therapies administered via IV, IP, IM, intratracheal, and intracardiac routes. In a true emergency, direct access to the vascular system is desired. Before attempting catheterization, blood should be collected for fast evaluation of blood gases, pH, lactate, hematocrit, total protein, osmolality, glucose, sodium, potassium, chloride, and blood urea nitrogen. Core body temperature should be continuously monitored and regulated.

Intravenous catheterization can be attempted at the sites used for blood collection. In severely dehydrated patients or those in shock, a cut-down may be necessary to visualize the vessel and ensure accurate catheter placement. Maintaining patency of the IV catheter may be difficult, especially in turtles displaying any level of activity. More rapid and reliable vascular access can be obtained via an intraosseous catheter placed in the distal humerus (Fig. 29–10). A standard spinal needle appropriately sized to the animal works well. The stylet prevents bone "coring" and subsequent blockage of the needle. Catheter insertion is accomplished by positioning the animal in dorsoventral recumbency, facing the examiner. Right-handed veterinarians can stabilize the left foreflipper with the left hand and insert the needle in the distal one fourth of the medial aspect of the humerus at an angle of approximately 30 to 45 degrees from parallel. Care should be taken to insert the needle as distal as possible without entering the joint capsule. This placement helps avoid the major nutrient foramen. Positioning of the needle should be confirmed with radiography. The catheterized limb can be folded and secured with tape to the carapace. Other routes for fluid administration include PO, SQ, and ICe, all of which are less efficacious in an emergency.

Fluid selection should be based on initial blood results. Hypoglycemia, for example, is commonly observed in dehydrated turtles and should be addressed by administering a 5% dextrose solution intracoelomically.[52] Fluid types and routes of administration[29] are found in Table 29–5. Rates of administration usually

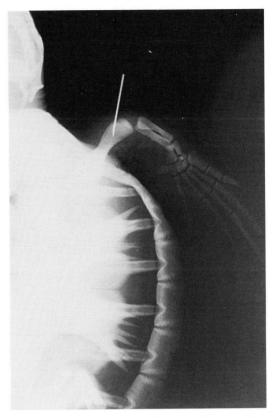

FIGURE 29–10. Intraosseous catheters provide an excellent route for the administration of fluids to sea turtles. Proper placement of the needle into the humerus should be confirmed through radiography.

range from 1% to 3% body weight per 24 hours as directed by blood parameters and clinical response. In addition, turtles that can swim may be placed in pools with fresh water, which can aid rehydration attempts.

Hydration status may be estimated by concurrent evaluation of hematocrit, plasma osmolality, total protein, sodium, and chloride concentrations and tear and urine osmolality [39, 43] as compared with individual baseline values. In addition, subjective indicators such as skin turgor, degree of enophthalmos, presence of tearing and urine production, and plastron or carapace wrinkling can be valuable indicators of hydration status.

Therapeutics

Relatively little is known about safe and efficacious drug dosing regimens for reptiles as compared with traditional domestic species. Only a few pharmacokinetic studies have been performed on a small number of reptilian species with the most commonly used therapeutics.[24] We are unaware of any published pharmacokinetic studies for sea turtles. Decisions regarding drug dose and dosing frequency in reptile medicine are complicated by the animals' largely ectothermic nature and, thus, widely varying metabolic states. The health state of the individual animal is also likely to affect uptake,

TABLE 29–5. Therapeutics

Type	Therapeutic	Dosage	Route	Frequency	Duration*	Reference
Antibacterial	Amikacin	2.5–3.0 mg/kg	IM†	q 72 hour	5 Txs	9
	Chloramphenicol	30–50 mg/kg	IM	q 24 hour	7–10 Txs	9
	Chloramphenicol	50 mg/kg	PO	q 24 hour	7–10 Txs	9
	Enrofloxacin	5 mg/kg	IM	q 48 hour	10–30 Txs	26
	Triple antibiotic ointment	prn	TOP	q 24 hour	prn	
Antifungal	Fluconazole		IM	q 48 hour	30–40 Txs	26
Parasiticide	Fenbendazole	50–100 mg/kg	PO	q 10–14 days	2 Txs	9
Antiseptic‡	Chlorhexidine	1:40 dil	TOP	prn	5 minute contact time	
	Povidine iodine	1:10 dil	TOP	prn	5 minute contact time	
Emergency (cardiac)	Atropine sulfate	0.04 mg/kg	IM, IV, ICe-diluted with 10 ml 0.9% saline, intratracheally, intracardiac			30
Fluid therapy	Lactated Ringer's solution (LRS)	1–3% TBW	ICe, PO, SQ, IV	q 24–48 hour	prn	
	LRS: 2.5% dextrose solution	1:1 solution 1–3% TBW	ICe, PO, IV	q 24–48 hour	prn	
	2.5% Dextrose: 0.45% saline	2:1 solution 1–3% TBW	ICe, IO, PO, IV	q 24–48 hour	prn	
	0.9% saline	1–3% TBW	PO	q 24–48 hour	prn	
	Fresh water	1–3% TBW	PO	q 24–48 hour	prn	

ICe, intracoelomically; TOP, topically; TBW, total body weight; dil, dilution; Txs, treatments.
*Duration of treatment should be determined by clinical response to therapy and periodic evaluation of blood work.
†Most IM therapeutics should be administered in pectoral muscles to avoid direct renal transport.
‡Solutions should be thoroughly removed by rinsing after appropriate contact time.

distribution, elimination, and metabolism of drugs that are administered. For these reasons, it has been suggested that the principles of allometric scaling may not be applicable to reptiles.[23, 24] We have used both "traditional" dosing and allometric scaling regimens of antimicrobial agents for sea turtles and have attempted to measure blood levels for two agents with inconclusive results.[26] We recommend that, in light of the lack of substantive evidence of drug safety and efficacy, medications be used conservatively. Selection of the antimicrobial agent should be based on microbial culture and sensitivity results. Periodic hematology and blood chemistry evaluation helps the clinician monitor the animal's response to therapy. In addition, the concentration of some drugs may be determined in serum, allowing modification of the dosage as necessary.

Table 29–5 lists therapeutic agents and dosing regimens that have been used with success in sea turtles. In general, therapies should be extended well beyond (2 to 3 weeks) the resolution of clinical signs of disease whenever possible. We have used the combined antibacterial and antifungal therapies of enrofloxacin and fluconazole for periods of 2 to 3 months with apparent safety and efficacy.

Shell lesions should be assessed and treated as soon as they are noticed. The likelihood of infection with waterborne opportunistic pathogens can be minimized by maintaining the animal in a clean environment. Deep wounds should be debrided, cleansed, and coated with a petroleum-based antibiotic ointment over which a transparent Tegaderm (3M Health Care, St. Paul, MN) patch is applied. Best results are achieved by using Super Glue to secure the margin of the patch to dry shell.[52]

Acknowledgments

We wish to thank Dr. Bob George, Dr. Roger Williams, Ms. Jill Arnold, Ms. Pam Lyons, and Dr. Chris Andrews for taking the time and effort to thoroughly review this chapter. Furthermore, we wish to thank Ms. Susie Ridenour who conducted a thorough literature search and provided us with many useful references, as well as Ms. Cynthia Smith who compiled the blood data for rehabilitated Kemp's ridley turtles. The illustration was created by Erica Denison, a student of the Johns Hopkins School of Art as Applied to Medicine. Finally, we acknowledge Ms. Jill Arnold, Ms. Christine Steinert, Mr. David Schofield, Ms. Pam Lyons, Ms. Connie Merigo, and the animal care staff at the New England Aquarium whose interest and dedication has helped us to better understand the medical management of sea turtles in aquaria.

REFERENCES

1. Arnold J: Personal communication, 1996.
2. Arnold J: White blood cell count discrepancies in Atlantic loggerhead sea turtles: Natt-Herrick vs. Eosinophil Unopette. Proceedings of the Annual Meeting of the Association of Zoo Veterinarian Technicians, Cleveland, OH, pp 15–22, 1994.
3. Balazs GH: Fibropapillomas in Hawaiian green turtles. Mar Tur News Letter 39:1, 1986.
4. Bennett JM: A method for sampling blood from hatchling loggerhead turtles. Herp Rev 17(2):43, 1986.
5. Bennett RA: Anesthesia. *In* Mader D (ed): Reptile Medicine and Surgery. Philadelphia, WB Saunders, pp 241–247, 1996.
6. Bennett RA: A review of anesthesia and chemical restraint in reptiles. J Zoo Wildl Med 22:282–303, 1991.
7. Bolten AB, Bjorndal KA: Blood profiles for a wild population of green turtles (*Chelonia mydas*) in the southern Bahamas: Size-

specific and sex-specific relationships. J Wildl Dis 28(3):407–413, 1992.

8. Bolten AB, Jacobson ER, Bjorndal KA: Effects of anticoagulant and auto analyzer on blood biochemical values of loggerhead sea turtles (*Caretta caretta*). Am J Vet Res 53(12):2224–2227, 1992.

9. Campbell TW: Sea turtle rehabilitation. *In* Mader D (ed): Reptile Medicine and Surgery. Philadelphia, WB Saunders, pp 427–436, 1996.

10. Campbell TW: Avian Hematology and Cytology. Ames, IA, Iowa State University Press, 1988.

11. Dailey MD, Fast ML, Balazs GH: *Carettacola hawaiiensis* n. sp. (Trematoda: Spirorchidae) from the green turtle, *Chelonia mydas*. Hawaii J Parasitol 77(6):906–909, 1991.

12. Donoghue S, Langenberg J: Nutrition. *In* Mader DR (ed): Reptile Medicine and Surgery. Philadelphia, WB Saunders, p 149, 1996.

13. Ehrhart LM, Witherington BE: Hypothermic stunning and mortality of marine turtles in the Indian River Lagoon System, Florida. Copeia 3:696–703, 1989.

14. Gatz RN, Glass ML, Wood SC: Pulmonary function of the green sea turtle, *Chelonia mydas*. J Appl Physiol 62:2:459–463, 1987.

15. Gehrmenn WH: Evaluation of artificial lighting. *In* Mader D (ed): Reptile Medicine and Surgery. Philadelphia, WB Saunders, pp 463–465, 1996.

16. George R: Personal communication, 1997.

17. George R: Health problems and diseases of sea turtles. *In* Lutz PL, Musick J (eds): The biology of sea turtles. Boca Raton, FL, CRC Press, pp 363–382, 1996.

18. Geraci JR: Nutrition and nutritional disorders. *In* Fowler ME (ed): Zoo and Wild Animal Medicine, 2nd ed. Philadelphia, WB Saunders, p 761, 1986.

19. Glazebrook JS, Campbell RSF: A survey of the diseases of marine turtles in northern Australia. II. Oceanarium-reared and wild turtles. Dis Aquat Org 9:97–104, 1990.

20. Grodon AN, Kelly WR, Lester JG: Epizootic mortality of free-living green turtles, *Chelonia mydas,* due to coccidiosis. J Wildl Dis 29(3):490, 1993.

21. Herbst LH: Fibropapillomatosis of marine turtles. Annu Rev Fish Dis 4:389, 1994.

22. Holt PE: Radiological studies of the alimentary tract in two Greek tortoises (*Testudo graeca*). Vet Rec 103:198–200, 1978.

23. Jacobson ER: Metabolic scaling of antibiotics in reptiles: basis and limitations. Zoo Biol 15:329–339, 1996.

24. Klingenberg RJ: Therapeutics. *In* Mader D (ed): Reptile Medicine and Surgery. Philadelphia, WB Saunders, pp 299–321, 1996.

25. Krum NH, Whitaker BR: Unpublished observations, 1996.

26. Krum HN, Spina S, Cooper R, Merigo C: Aerobic and anaerobic bacterial culture and in vitro antimicrobial sensitivity results for cold-stunned Kemp's ridley and loggerhead sea turtles; preliminary in vitro pharmacokinetic results of two antimicrobials. Proceedings of the Annual Symposium on Sea Turtle Biology and Conservation, Hilton Head, SC, in press.

27. Krum HN, Spina S, Cooper R, Merigo C: The use of plain radiography as a diagnostic and prognostic tool for debilitated Kemp's ridley turtles. Proceedings of the Annual Symposium on Sea Turtle Biology and Conservation, Hilton Head, SC, in press.

28. Lutz PL, Dunbar-Cooper A: Variations in the blood chemistry of the loggerhead sea turtle, *Caretta caretta*. Fisheries Bulletin 85(1):37–43, 1987.

29. Merigo C, Krum HN: A summary of the 1995 live sea turtle strandings on Cape Cod, MA, USA; associated critical care techniques. Proceedings of the Annual Symposium on Sea Turtle Biology and Conservation, Hilton Head, SC, in press.

30. Moon PF, Stabenau EK: Anesthetic and postanesthetic management of sea turtles. J Am Vet Med Assoc 208(5):720–726, 1996.

31. Morgan JP: Reptiles and amphibians. *In* Morgan JP (ed): Techniques of Veterinary Radiography, 5th ed. Ames, IA, Iowa State University Press, pp 448–453, 1993.

32. Morreale SJ, Meylan AB, Sadove SS, Standora EE: Annual occurrence and winter mortality of marine turtles in New York waters. J Herp 26:301, 1993.

33. Murray M: Cardiology and circulation. *In* Mader D (ed): Reptile

Medicine and Surgery. Philadelphia, WB Saunders, pp 95–104, 1996.

34. National Marine Fisheries Service and U.S. Fish and Wildlife Service: Recovery Plan for U.S. Population of Atlantic Green Turtle *Chelonia mydas*. Washington, DC, National Marine Fisheries Service, 1991.

35. National Marine Fisheries Service and U.S. Fish and Wildlife Service: Recovery Plan for U.S. Population of Loggerhead Turtle *Caretta caretta*. Washington, DC, National Marine Fisheries Service, 1991.

36. National Marine Fisheries Service and U.S. Fish and Wildlife Service: Recovery Plan for U.S. Population of Kemp's Ridley Sea Turtle *Lepidochelys kempii*. Washington, DC, National Marine Fisheries Service, 1991.

37. National Marine Fisheries Service and U.S. Fish and Wildlife Service: Recovery Plan for U.S. Population of Leatherback Turtles *Dermochelys coriacea* in the U.S. Caribbean, Atlantic, and Gulf of Mexico. Washington, DC, National Marine Fisheries Service, 1991.

38. National Research Council: Decline of the sea turtles. Washington, DC, National Academy Press, 1990.

39. Nicolson SW, Lutz P: Salt gland function in the green sea turtle *Chelonia mydas*. J Exp Biol 144:171–184, 1989.

40. Nuitja INS, Uchida I: Preliminary studies on the growth and food consumption of the juvenile loggerhead turtle (*Caretta caretta* L.) in captivity. Aquaculture 27:157–160, 1982.

41. Owens DW, Rutz GJ: New methods of obtaining blood and cerebrospinal fluid from marine turtles. Herpetologica 36(1):17–20, 1980.

42. Penninck DG, Stewart JS, Murphy JP, Pion P: Ultrasonography of the California desert tortoise (*Xerobates agassizi*): anatomy and application. Vet Rad 32(3):112–116, 1991.

43. Prange HD, Greenwald L: Effects of dehydration on the urine concentration and salt gland secretion of the green sea turtle. Comp Biochem Physiol 66A:133–136, 1980.

44. Sapsford CW, Van der Riet M: Uptake of solar radiation by the sea turtle, *Caretta caretta*, during voluntary surface basking. Comp Biochem Physiol 63A:471–474, 1979.

45. Shaw S, Kabler S, Lutz P: Isoflurane—a safe and effective anesthetic for marine and freshwater turtles. Proceedings of the International Wildlife Rehabilitation, Naples, FL, pp 112–119, 1992.

46. Silverman S, Janssen DL: Diagnostic imaging. *In* Mader D (ed): Reptile Medicine and Surgery. Philadelphia, WB Saunders, pp 258–264, 1996.

47. Stamper MA, Whitaker BR: Medical observations and implications on "healthy" sea turtles prior to release into the wild. Proceedings of the Annual Meeting of the American Association of Zoo Veterinarians, Pittsburgh, PA, pp 182–185, 1994.

48. Stein G: Reptile and amphibian formulary. *In* Mader D (ed): Reptile Medicine and Surgery. Philadelphia, WB Saunders, pp 465–472, 1996.

49. Stickney S, White DB, Perlmutter D: Growth of green and loggerhead sea turtles in Georgia on natural and artificial diets. Bull Georgia Acad Sci 31:37–44, 1973.

50. Upton SJ, Odell DK, Walsh MT: *Eimeria caretta* sp. nov. (Apicomplexa: Eimeriidae) from the loggerhead sea turtle, *Caretta caretta* (Testudines). Can J Zool 68:1268–1269, 1989.

51. Walsh M: Personal communication, 1996.

52. Wiles M, Rand TG: Integumental ulcerative disease in a loggerhead turtle *Caretta caretta* at the Bermuda Aquarium: microbiology and histopathology. Dis Ag Org 3:85, 1987.

53. Wolke RE, Brooks DR, George A: Spirorchidiasis in loggerhead sea turtles (*Caretta caretta*). Pathol J Wildl Dis 18(2):175–185, 1985.

54. Wood FE, Critchley KH, Wood JR: Anesthesia in the green sea turtle, *Chelonia mydas*. Am J Vet Res 43:1882–1883, 1982.

55. Wood FE, Ebanks GK: Blood cytology and hematology of the green sea turtle *Chelonia mydas*. Herpetologica 40(3):331–336, 1986.

56. Wood JR, Wood FE: Growth and digestibility for the green turtle (*Chelonia mydas*) fed diets containing varying protein levels. Aquaculture 25:269–274, 1981.

57. Zapata AG, Varas A, Torroba M: Seasonal variations in the immune system of lower vertebrates. Immunol Today 13:142, 1992.

CHAPTER 30

Health Assessment of Chelonians and Release into the Wild

ELLIOTT R. JACOBSON

JOHN L. BEHLER

JAMES L. JARCHOW

The status of living turtles and tortoises is in perilous decline. Chelonian specialists believe that 50% of taxa are facing serious challenges. Causes for decline in status range from elevated subsistence hunting, unbridled commercial collection for food and exotic pet markets, debilitating diseases, increased predation, alien plant introductions and diminished forage quality, dramatic mortality rates as a consequence of highway construction, human-set fires, protracted droughts, and poor wildlife management and land-use practices. Most seriously affected are the tortoises, large river turtles, marine turtles, and the small special rarities sought by the hobbyists. The burgeoning human population in southern Asia and elsewhere in developing countries in tropical and subtropical regions is consuming tons of turtles and tortoises daily,[36, 44] and some species will be lost before they are even acknowledged as such. Of 42 tortoise species, one is considered critically endangered, four are considered endangered, and 18 are listed as vulnerable in the 1996 International Union for Conservation of Nature (IUCN) Red List of Threatened Animals. The leatherback and six other marine turtles are listed as critically endangered (2), endangered (3), or vulnerable (1). Among freshwater turtles, 51 are considered threatened, with five being listed as critically endangered, 17 as endangered, and 29 as vulnerable.

Herpetologists, veterinarians, and wildlife managers must minister to vanishing chelonian resources and their fragmented habitats. Herpetologists are scrambling to classify new species, document their status and natural histories, and provide assistance to wildlife managers. Veterinarians are faced with health crises at the individual and population levels and increasingly are asked to guide the actions of conservation biologists who plan turtle rescue efforts. The exotic pet trade preys heavily on wild populations where habitat remains intact. Harvesting of turtles and tortoises continues at a given location until it is no longer profitable. Results of several studies[7, 8, 13] indicated that the removal of modest numbers of adult and older juvenile turtles has deleteri-

ous effects on the populations, which cannot easily be offset, and strongly suggest that long-lived chelonians cannot tolerate commercial collection. As stated by Congdon,[7] "The concept of sustainable harvest of already-reduced populations of long-lived organisms appears to be an oxymoron."

Chelonian recovery stations or conservation centers have developed in response to dramatic decline of native turtle stocks and the huge number of displaced animals, unwanted pets, and confiscations. Centers have developed for tortoises and/or freshwater turtles in southern Europe, Africa, northwestern Madagascar, India, and western North America. Other such stations for marine turtles have been established in scattered locations circumtropically. Often, these centers, despite meager funds, have impressive educational programs. "Shortcuts," however, are often taken in the captive management and repatriation elements of such conservation programs. Many centers lack special veterinary and herpetologic expertise, and they cannot afford the expense of securing such support. In such situations, health screens and genetic assessments are often lacking, and rigid quarantine facilities are inadequate or absent. Repatriation protocols are generally developed without wildlife and veterinary science expert review. When a recovery center includes relocation, repatriation, or translocation exercises among its programs, the motives for advocating these strategies must be carefully examined through peer review before the release and recommended pre- and post-release biologic and management criteria are followed.[5, 11, 55] It is imperative that projects be carefully monitored so that accurate results, either positive or negative, can be published.

In this chapter, guidelines for release of captive and confiscated chelonians are developed. The guidelines are likely to need modification or revision to meet the needs of specific programs. Understanding infectious diseases of chelonians and how to perform health evaluations of chelonians are essential to any release program; these topics are also discussed.

PHYSICAL AND CLINICAL EVALUATION

For captive and wild chelonians, history becomes essential when interpreting findings and understanding the basis for many medical problems.[21] Collecting information on the diet of the captive chelonian is important when trying to assess the health status of the animal. Similarly, quality of forage in the field needs to be assessed when determining the status of individual wild tortoises or populations. For aquatic chelonians, assessment of water quality is essential. Chemical spills and chemical run-offs from agricultural lands have deleterious effects on the habitat of these animals. Developing a good database on environmental conditions for both captive and wild animals is necessary when trying to assess health of these animals.

The following questions are routinely asked before chelonians are examined at the Veterinary Medical Teaching Hospital (VMTH), University of Florida:

1. What is the species being evaluated? Common and scientific names should be recorded.

2. What is the origin of the animal? Is it wild caught or captive bred?

3. How long has the chelonian been in captivity?

4. What is the enclosure or cage design? Is the chelonian kept outdoors or indoors? Has it been exposed to other species of chelonians or other reptiles?

5. What is the thermal environment of the chelonian?

6. What is the humidity and photoperiod?

7. What is the nutrition of the chelonian? How often is it fed? How is the food stored?

8. For terrestrial species, how is water offered and how often is it changed?

9. How often does the chelonian defecate and what is the consistency of the feces?

10. Does the owner have a quarantine program and, if so, how long are animals quarantined?

11. Have there been previous disease problems with this animal or others in the collection?

12. What is the attitude and behavior of the chelonian? Have there been recent behavioral changes?

13. What is the chief complaint?

As a group, chelonians are difficult animals to evaluate clinically. Many species are capable of withdrawing into the margins of their shell when threatened, becoming "bony boxes." Clinicians experienced in evaluating chelonians have devised methods for coaxing them out of their shells. For medium to small-sized chelonians, one method is to push in or gently touch the hindlimbs, which often results in head extension. Slow, deliberate movements reduce fearful responses and retraction into the shell. Many tortoises extend their forelimbs and head if tilted slightly downward, perhaps in an effort to avoid falling. Above all, examination of a frightened chelonian requires patience.

At times, sedation or anesthesia is required. Drugs such as ketamine, telazol, and succinylcholine have been used to allow a detailed physical examination, particularly with large and giant tortoises.[21, 49] Even for those species that move about freely despite manipula-tions by the clinician, judging their health status is no simple matter. Difficulties are compounded in the field where the investigator may only be able to judge the animal at a distance or when the animal is collected under conditions in which there is limited equipment and limited time to conduct a thorough evaluation. Health assessment in the field may require a different approach from health assessment in a clinical practice, university teaching hospital, research laboratory, or well-equipped conservation center.

A thorough physical examination is the starting point for assessing chelonian health. First, however, the chelonian should be observed in water if aquatic and on land if terrestrial. The alertness of the animal and its ability to ambulate should be noted. Weight (W) and carapace length in the midline (MCL) are easy to obtain (except in giant tortoises and large marine turtles) and may provide valuable information. These data should be collected whenever a chelonian is handled for health assessment. Clinical condition has been assessed using W in relation to MCL in captive spur-thighed tortoises and Hermann's tortoises.[40] To determine whether the relationship between W and MCL could be used to discriminate between healthy desert tortoises and desert tortoises with signs of upper respiratory tract disease, the logarithm of MCL was regressed on the logarithm of W for both groups.[35] A significant difference was found between the regression lines for the two groups, with tortoises with clinical signs weighing about 7% less than clinically healthy tortoises, but several ill tortoises weighed the same as healthy tortoises. The presence of uroliths, a large volume of coelomic exudate, and intestinal gravel accumulations elevate body weight of ill tortoises. In clinical practice, James L. Jarchow has used weight loss during hibernation as an early indicator of disease in captive desert tortoises. Tortoises exhibiting a winter weight loss of 8% or more are often found, when clinically evaluated, to be affected by a disease process.

The shell should be examined for the quality of its scutes. Any lesions seen should be recorded. Seams between adjacent scutes can be examined for evidence of new growth. In captive tortoises, excessive pyramiding of carapacial scutes is commonly seen and is thought to have a dietary basis. The soft integument should also be examined. Special attention should be given to evidence of abnormal patterns of keratinization, desquamation, ulceration, erythema, cutaneous discharges, and swelling.

Legs should be gently extended to look for any lesions in the areas around the distal end of the limbs. Asymmetric patterns of toenail wear may be associated with lameness in terrestrial species. Limbs should be examined for soft tissue swelling, muscle atrophy, and painful responses to manipulation. The joints of opposite limbs should be compared to identify swelling and evaluate range of motion.

Relative position of each globe in its orbit should be noted. Unilateral enophthalmos may result from phthisis or orbital injury. Bilateral enophthalmos may result from dehydration, inanition, or microphthalmia. Unilateral exophthalmos may be the result of a retrobulbar abscess, tumor, or injury. Bilateral exophthalmos may result from vascular obstruction or generalized edema.

The chelonian cornea and lens should be clear as in other vertebrate species. Corneal ulcers are often covered by tenacious, caseous plaques that may protect healing tissue. The anterior chamber of the eye should be free of blood or exudate. The color of each iris and pupil shape and size should be compared. Magnification and adequate illumination of the eye are critical to effective examination.

The beak should be examined for fractures and mal-occlusion, which may predispose tortoises to dehydration. The presence of moisture or dried mucus on the beak may indicate oral infection, ulceration, or irritation from a foreign body. Many species of aquatic chelonians open their mouth in a defensive gape when held, allowing examination of the oral cavity. Small and medium-sized tortoises require extension of the neck and manual restraint of the head; care should be taken to hold the head from the base of the skull, avoiding pressure on tympanic membranes and mandibular joints. If the tortoise vigorously resists restraint, chemical restraint should be provided to avoid injury to retractor muscles of the neck. The mouth is then opened by pushing the mandible downward with a fingertip on the front of the lower beak. If there is too much resistance, a dull curved dental scaler may be placed over the tip of the lower beak and the jaws gently pried open. Larger tortoises may be placed on a table at eye level and with illumination directed at the head and with slow, deliberate movements, the dental scaler is hooked over the lower beak. The tortoise usually attempts to dislodge the instrument by opening its mouth. If the scaler is then pushed gently downward, the tortoise opens its mouth widely, allowing examination without head restraint. Giant tortoises generally require either chemical restraint or "teasing" with a favorite food item to allow examination of the oral cavity.

Color of oral mucous membranes should be noted. Cyanosis, pallor, and congestion are significant as in other vertebrate species. Petechiation, ulceration, and the presence of mucoid or caseous exudates, often accumulating in the choanae, should be noted. If the head is restrained, the glottis may be examined by elevating the base of the tongue with a finger under the mandible. Blood in the oral cavity, mandibular instability, and/or asymmetry of oral structures may indicate cephalic trauma.

The nares should be patent and free of discharges or dried mucus. Cutaneous erosion or depigmentation around or below the nares may indicate a history of chronic nasal discharge. Even if the nares are dry, the presence and character of nasal exudate may be evaluated by pressing on the intermandibular tissue, pushing the tongue dorsally into the choanae, thus expelling any free exudate in the nasal cavity out through the external nares. Any mucous discharge should be considered abnormal.

Temporal muscles should appear plump and full. A sunken appearance over temporal areas may indicate cachexia or severe dehydration. Areas of discoloration, swelling, or asymmetry may indicate localized infection

or trauma. Tympanic membranes should be included in the examination process.

The lung fields of chelonians may be effectively percussed through the carapace. The technique consists of resting the animal on the palm of one hand or similar platform and then tapping the carapace with the index finger of the other hand. The tone of the sound produced over each costal scute on one side should be the same as that from the corresponding site of the other side. A dull sound denotes fluid or increased soft tissue mass below the point of percussion. Undermined, superficial lesions of carapacial scutes or dermal bone plates produce a "tinny" sound. A useful diagnostic screen for pneumonia in aquatic species consists of placing the turtle in water and noting changes in buoyancy; turtles with pulmonary disease may float with one side up or be incapable of diving.

In small chelonians, the caudal part of the coelomic cavity may be palpated by placing a finger cranial to each relaxed hindlimb, in the soft tissue axillary region (femoral fossa). Shelled eggs and cystic calculi may be detected by tilting the cranial region of the shell upward and rocking it from side to side. Hard structures such as eggs and calculi can be palpated as they bounce off the fingertips.

Specific diagnostic procedures are useful in determining the cause of some diseases that have epizootic potential. Tortoises exhibiting stomatitis with or without a caseous exudate may be lightly anesthetized and swabs or scrapings of oral epithelium submitted for cytologic examination to identify intranuclear herpesvirus inclusions. Transtracheal washes may provide adequate samples for bacterial culture and cytology for herpesvirus and iridovirus inclusion identification. Inflammatory exudates and ulcerative lesions should be cultured routinely and submitted for cytologic examination. Tortoises with signs of rhinitis should be tested for mycoplasma using enzyme-linked immunosorbent assay and polymerase chain reaction methods.[4] Wet mounts of fecal smears as well as fecal flotation should be used in examinations for enteric parasites. *Hexamita* trophozoites are most readily detected in a wet mount consisting of a mixture of urine and feces. Most chelonians are colonized by a variety of innocuous oxyurids and ciliates. Those parasites that are potentially harmful or are atypical for a given host should be identified and the chelonian treated with appropriate parasiticides.

In a veterinary hospital, radiography can be used to evaluate a variety of internal structures such as lungs, gastrointestinal system, reproductive tract, and bladder. Magnetic resonance imaging may be used to determine lesions in pulmonary and visceral organs. Ultrasound imaging of the reproductive tract, can be done both in a clinic and in the field. Endoscopy can be used to examine and collect biopsy specimens from the gastrointestinal tract, reproductive organs, and other visceral structures. Blood, urine, biopsy specimens, and exudates should be collected for a variety of clinical evaluations. Various collection sites can be used for obtaining blood from chelonians, each having advantages and disadvantages.[22, 33, 59] Blood values have been reported for several species of chelonians, including the desert tortoise,[57] gopher tortoise,[61] Mediterranean tortoises,[43] radiated tortoise,[47] and loggerhead turtles.[2] However, values between captive and wild tortoises vary with season, age, and sex differences, making interpretation extremely difficult.

Continued data collection for free-ranging chelonians is needed to assess health, both in the field and in captivity. Correlative studies need to be performed because data become meaningful only in the context of the whole animal. As more and more data accumulate and new methods and technologies become available, health assessment will become more of a science than an art.

DEVELOPMENT OF A DECISION TREE FOR MANAGEMENT OF CAPTIVE, TRANSLOCATED, AND SEIZED CHELONIANS

Turtles and tortoises are popular pets. In 1992 there were approximately 2.4 million turtles in U.S. households.[58] Many captive chelonians are purchased as wild-caught animals; others, such as the desert tortoise, are offered through adoption programs in response to land development. More than 230,000 desert tortoises are kept in captive or semicaptive conditions in California and Las Vegas Valley, Nevada.[24]

As with other trades in animals, the pet trade has resulted in large numbers of chelonians being confiscated. How to manage those animals and what to do with them have surfaced as major issues in chelonian conservation. Furthermore, injured chelonians are brought into rehabilitation facilities for treatment and eventual return to the wild, and other chelonians are made homeless by loss of habitat to development and agriculture. Even though returning captive chelonians to the wild, through repatriation, re-introduction, or translocation programs, is often perceived by the public as the proper or humane thing to do, it may result in more harm than good. Stringent guidelines need to be developed to ensure that there is merit in releases back to the wild, but realistic, unambiguous guidelines are not easy to develop. In response to confiscation of live animals by governmental authorities, the 1994 Convention on International Trade in Endangered Species of Wild Fauna and Flora (CITES) developed guidelines for the disposal of confiscated animals.[6] In the CITES guidelines, the ultimate decision on the disposition of animals must achieve the following goals:

1. Maximize conservation value of the specimens without in any way endangering the health, behavioral repertoire, or conservation status of wild or captive populations of the species
2. Discourage further illegal or irregular trade in the species
3. Provide a humane solution, whether that involves maintaining the animals in captivity, returning them to the wild, or using euthanasia to destroy them

Ultimately, for both captive chelonians being considered for return to the wild or wild chelonians being considered for translocation or reinforcement and supplementation programs, the welfare and health of the recipient population is paramount.

In the 1994 CITES guidelines for the disposition of confiscated live animals, decision trees were developed for both "captive" (Fig. 30–1) and "return to the wild" (Fig. 30–2) options. The decision trees are useful in facilitating consideration of what option to follow. These trees have been slightly modified to be used as guidelines in making recommendations on disposition of confiscated, injured, and otherwise displaced chelonians. As in the CITES guidelines, a question and answer format is used. Philosophical and moral issues are excluded from such a format of decision making and are discussed later.

DECISION TREE ANALYSIS

The following questions should be asked when determining whether a captive chelonian should be maintained in captivity, returned to the wild, or euthanized. Captive chelonians are considered to be donors and the free-ranging population are recipients. For re-introduction programs, recipients are no longer present and reference is made only to donors. The various categories of captive chelonians that may be returned to the wild include (1) confiscated chelonians, (2) those propagated in captivity, (3) those displaced from wild habitat, and (4) those found in the wild ill or injured and receiving treatment in a veterinary clinic or wildlife rehabilitation facility.

◆ **Question 1: Will returning the chelonian to the wild make a significant contribution to the conservation of the species, either through education or other means?**

There are several considerations that need to be addressed when answering this question. First, information is needed on the taxonomic status of the species, subspecies, or local population receiving donors. Are donors and recipients of the similar genetic background? If populations are stable, there may be limited or no biological value in returning the animal to the wild. Major problems in returning animals to the wild center around (1) possibility of disease introduction by donor into recipient population, (2) displacement of recipients by donors, and (3) failure of donor to be incorporated into population or survive in the recipient's habitat. Because of such problems, it is essential that the potential conservation merit of the release be determined. Sometimes, even in a stable population, return of certain individuals may be deemed useful if there is educational merit. Education is useful in publicizing the plight of many species, and release programs often attract the attention of the public. However, it is imperative that the public be educated properly about the inherent difficulties and problems with such programs.

◆ **Answer:** Yes: Go to "Return to Wild Decision Tree"

No: Investigate captivity options

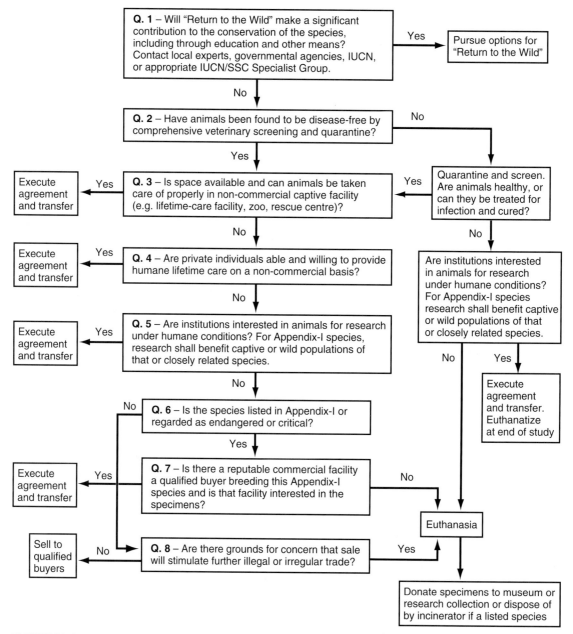

FIGURE 30–1. Decision tree for captive options. (From CITES: Appendix I Resolution Conf.9.11. Disposal of Confiscated Live Animals of Species Included in the Appendices. Adopted at the Ninth Meeting of the Conference of the Parties to CITES, the Convention on International Trade in Endangered Species of Wild Fauna and Flora, November 7–18, 1994.)

DECISION TREE ANALYSIS: CAPTIVITY

The decision to maintain turtles in captivity is based on less complicated considerations than the decision of whether to return them to the wild. However, the large numbers of captive chelonians—including confiscated, captive-bred, displaced, unwanted pets, and injured animals—often drive decisions on whether to return them to the wild, especially when euthanasia is the only

alternative. As stated, return to the wild should be based on conservation merit alone; using any other basis is irresponsible.

◆ **Question 2: Have chelonians been found to be disease-free and in proper condition by comprehensive veterinary screening and quarantine?**

As discussed previously in this chapter, a wide variety of infectious diseases have been identified in chelo-

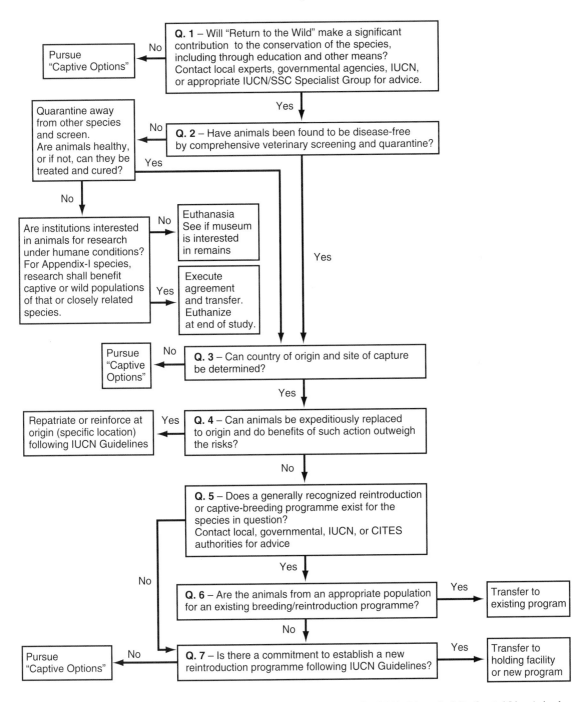

FIGURE 30–2. Decision tree for return to the wild. (From CITES: Resolution Conf.9.11. Disposal of Confiscated Live Animals of Species Included in the Appendices. Adopted at the Ninth Meeting of the Conference of the Parties to CITES, the Convention on International Trade in Endangered Species of Wild Fauna and Flora, November 7–18, 1994.)

nians. The infectious diseases discussed probably represent only a small number of diseases that turtles may harbor and with which they can become infected. Many noninfectious diseases also have been described.[20] Chelonians in captivity may not be in proper condition or have the proper behavioral repertoire to survive in the wild. It is essential that animals designated for return to the wild be evaluated as thoroughly as possible. A veterinarian should be involved in the process. It is important to determine whether the chelonian has been isolated from nonnative species or whether it is possible that there has been exposure to exotic pathogens. Aquatic species fed mollusks, arthropods, and fish may be exposed to immature stages of parasites with complex life cycles that later may be introduced into naive populations. If the chelonian being considered for release was reared or maintained in the vicinity of exotic species, it is possible that it has become infected with a foreign pathogen. A catastrophe could happen if an exotic pathogen is introduced into a naive population. In general, no ill turtles should be returned to the wild. The exception is when the donor was derived from a host population that is affected with the pathogen or disease and will be returned to that population. For example, because more than 50% of green turtles in certain populations are affected with fibropapillomatosis, returning affected turtles to those populations has little impact on the spread of disease. However, turtles with tumors should never be added to a population that is tumor free.

♦ **Answer:** Yes: Proceed to Question 3.
　　　　　　No: Quarantine or maintain isolated from other species, especially nonnative species. If the chelonian has a chronic and incurable disease, it should be euthanized or considered for research studies involving the particular disease process, including biologic effects.

♦ **Question 3: Is space available in noncommercial captive facility (e.g., lifetime-care facility, zoo, or rescue center) and will proper care be given?**

Although a variety of noncommercial facilities may be available for captive chelonians, a facility capable of providing proper housing, husbandry, and long-term care must be found. It is far easier to accept captive turtles of various kinds than to take care of them properly. If other animals in the collection would be at risk from diseases or potential diseases from the donor, the turtles should not be accepted. A formal agreement should be established between the parties involved ensuring that there is (1) commitment to lifetime care, (2) exclusion from sale of the chelonians involved, or (3) euthanasia when space is no longer available or transfer to another appropriate facility is not possible. In many countries, no facilities are available, and help and recommendations are needed from international organizations. Governmental approval and involvement are necessary for nationally and internationally protected species.

♦ **Answer:** Yes: Execute agreement and transfer.
　　　　　　No: Proceed to Question 4.

♦ **Question 4: Are private individuals able and willing to provide humane lifetime care?**

There are many private individuals in the United States and overseas who breed turtles and tortoises. For most of these individuals, offspring are sold through the pet trade, primarily overseas, because, in the United States, it is illegal to sell chelonians as pets with a carapace length in the midline less than 4 inches. Furthermore, as with many breeders, chelonian breeders often specialize in certain species, families, or groups of chelonians. Some breeders specialize in tortoises and others in certain aquatic turtles. Some have developed home pages on the World Wide Web, listing stock and

prices. Lists of reputable breeders interested in acquiring confiscated animals and other captives need to be developed. State herpetologic organizations can generally provide information on breeders within their own state. Formal agreements need to be developed concerning the responsibilities of the private individual and disposition of any offspring produced. In California and Nevada, formal adoption programs have been established for displaced desert tortoises, with information provided to private individuals on husbandry and health problems. An upper respiratory tract disease has been described in captive and wild desert tortoises (see Infectious Disease), and ill captives have been released to the wild. It is essential that recipients of chelonians understand the consequences of such releases and guard against their occurrence.

♦ **Answer:** Yes: Execute agreement and transfer.
　　　　　　No: Proceed to Question 5.

♦ **Question 5: Are institutions interested in chelonians for research conducted under humane conditions?**

The confiscated or otherwise permanent captive chelonian may be valuable in research projects. If the chelonian has a chronic illness, there may be researchers interested in studies on the particular disease. However, for most biologic studies, ill animals should not be used in research projects. Biologic data collected from ill animals may not be relevant in answering questions concerning "normal" animals.

♦ **Answer:** Yes: Execute agreement and transfer.
　　　　　　No: Proceed to Question 6.

♦ **Question 6: Is the species listed in CITES Appendix I or regarded as endangered or critical?**

Commercial sale of tortoises and turtles listed in CITES Appendix I should not be permitted unless the activity is carefully regulated through governmental permitting and identification documentation programs. Any action that may stimulate trade in CITES Appendix I species is ill advised. This policy should be applied to all species recognized as threatened or endangered by CITES or Endangered Species Act (ESA) of the United States, or by wildlife laws of foreign countries.

♦ **Answer:** Yes: Proceed to Question 8.
　　　　　　No: Proceed to Question 7.

♦ **Question 7: Is there a commercial facility or qualified buyer breeding this species and is that facility or person interested in the chelonians?**

There are recognized facilities and individuals breeding endangered species. Where breeding facilities are in the country of origin, at the site within the geographic range of the species, care must be taken when importing confiscated and otherwise captive maintained chelonians from other locations or countries. There is always the risk of introducing foreign pathogens with the donated animals. When the breeding facility is in the same country where the donated chelonians are located, certain risks are reduced, but chances of introducing a pathogen into a stable collection still exist. When considering placing such donors in breeding programs, one outcome may be stimulation of trade in the particular species, especially when hatchlings are produced. Encouraging trade in listed species should be avoided.

◆ **Answer:** Yes: Execute agreement and transfer.
　　　　　No: Euthanize and dispose of carcass.

◆ **Question 8: Are there grounds for concern that sale will stimulate further illegal or irregular trade?**

The sale of chelonians for the pet trade has been a large international business for many years. Certain rare and unusually patterned species are particularly attractive. In 1996 a large group of ploughshare tortoises (*Geochelone yniphora*) were stolen from a noncommercial, conservation breeding program facility in northwest Madagascar, with some tortoises eventually being offered for sale in a published dealer's list from the Czech Republic. There is significant trade in blackmarketed listed species, and confiscated and otherwise captive chelonians should not be offered to a breeding program if ultimately the offspring or donated animals are to be sold, thereby encouraging trade in this species. The worldwide exploitation of endangered species for sale in the pet trade needs to be tightly regulated. However, it also must be realized that captive-bred animals usually make healthier pets, thereby reducing pressures on collecting wild animals for trade.

◆ **Answer:** Yes: Euthanize and dispose of carcass.
　　　　　No: Go to Question 7.

DECISION TREE ANALYSIS: RETURN TO THE WILD

◆ **Question 2: Have chelonians been found to be disease free by comprehensive veterinary screening and quarantine?**

Chelonians intended for release to the wild need to be thoroughly evaluated to ensure that they are free of known infectious diseases and are healthy. This is with the realization that only a small number of specific health problems that occur in these animals are recognized and that there is limited ability in diagnosing disease problems. A veterinarian should be involved in the process. Doing a thorough physical examination on one or a few chelonians is achievable, but doing such evaluations on large numbers of animals may not be practical or cost effective. Minimally, the animal needs to be given a physical examination and samples should be collected for tests designed to screen for exposure to pathogens known to cause problems in the species being released. For instance, desert and gopher tortoises are known to be susceptible to mycoplasmosis and those species should be tested for exposure to the causative agent before their release. If examination determines that the chelonian is not healthy, it should be quarantined. If the chelonian cannot be successfully cured, it

should be euthanized. As discussed previously in this chapter, herpesvirus infections are responsible for significant mortality rates in certain species and groups of chelonians. Chelonians originating from facilities where herpesvirus infection has been identified should be stringently evaluated before their release. The prevalence of herpesviruses in wild populations of any chelonians is unknown and more information is needed before recommendations can be made on what to do with chelonians originating from a facility where this virus has been identified.

◆ **Answer:** Yes: Proceed to Question 3.
　　　　　No: Quarantine minimally for 90 days; reassess Question 2 after quarantine. If the animal has a chronic and incurable infection or condition, first offer the animal to research institutions. If it is impossible to place the animal in such an institution, it should be euthanized.

◆ **Question 3: Can country of origin and site of capture be determined?**

The origin of the confiscated or otherwise captive chelonian should be determined before its release. It is inappropriate to mix chelonians that differ genetically. This may require genetic analysis such as determining sequences for mitochondrial DNA.

◆ **Answer:** Yes: Proceed to Question 4.
　　　　　No: Pursue "captive" options.

◆ **Question 4: Can chelonians be expeditiously replaced to origin and do benefits of such action outweigh risks?**

The various threats to the recipient wild chelonian population should be addressed by herpetologists with special expertise with the taxon in question.

◆ **Answer:** Yes: Repatriate and reinforce at origin (specific location) following IUCN guidelines.[19]
　　　　　No: Proceed to Question 5.

◆ **Question 5: Does an officially recognized captive-breeding or reintroduction program exist for the species in question?**

If a captive breeding program or reintroduction program involving confiscated and permanent captive chelonians exists, contact should be made with coordinators of the program and animals should be offered to the program.

◆ **Answer:** Yes: Proceed to Question 6.
　　　　　No: Proceed to Question 7.

◆ **Question 6: Are the animals from an appropriate population for an existing breeding or reintroduction program?**

Chelonians to be returned to the wild should be reintroduced or reinforcement should occur only into populations of the same genetic background. In most situations, there is limited conservation value in introducing animals of different genetic background into a wild population. If the population being reinforced does not have enough individuals to sustain the population, chelonians of a closely related genotype may be suitable.

◆ **Answer:** Yes: Transfer to existing program.
No: Proceed to Question 7.

◆ **Question 7: Is there a commitment to establish a new reintroduction program following IUCN guidelines?**

When chelonians cannot be transferred to an existing reintroduction program, return to the wild is recommended only when (1) appropriate habitat has been identified, (2) sufficient funds are available to support the program over many years, (3) sufficient numbers of animals are available for reintroduction or reinforcement. In most situations, habitat or money is not available to carry out these programs.

◆ **Answer:** Yes: Transfer to holding facility or new program.
No: Pursue "captive" options.

PHILOSOPHICAL ISSUES IN RETURNING CHELONIANS TO THE WILD

Many individuals who are involved in chelonian conservation issues develop strong emotional ties with the animals. Large numbers of chelonians are continuously confiscated in the pet trade or are brought into care facilities because (1) there is failure to meet either export or import requirements, (2) the animals have injuries, (3) the animals are displaced because of habitat destruction, or (4) the animals were pets that have become unwanted. For persons concerned about these animals, it is not easy to decide what to do with them. Even when a decision tree is used to determine disposition, emotions may still override the original goals. Emotions are not considered in the decision tree. At the Veterinary Medical Teaching Hospital, University of Florida, many injured gopher tortoises, box turtles, fresh water aquatic emydine turtles, and marine turtles are seen and there is an attempt to return these originally

TABLE 30–1. Infectious Diseases and Pathogens of Chelonians

Pathogen	Species	Lesion	Reference
Virus			
Herpesvirus	Green turtle	Skin necrosis	54
Herpesvirus	Green turtle	Pneumonia, tracheitis, conjunctivitis	30
Herpesvirus	Green turtle	Fibropapilloma	25
Herpesvirus	Freshwater turtles	Hepatic necrosis	10, 12, 32
Herpesvirus	Tortoises	Stomatitis, pharyngitis, pneumonia, encephalitis	9, 16, 26, 52, 53
Iridovirus	Hermann's tortoise	Hepatic necrosis	17
	Gopher tortoise	Tracheitis, pneumonia	62
Bacteria			
Gram-negatives	Freshwater turtles	Septicemia	28, 37, 38
Salmonella	Turtles and tortoises	None; carriers	3, 39, 41, 51
Mycoplasma	Desert tortoise	Rhinitis	9, 29
	Gopher tortoise	Rhinitis	50
Chlamydia	Green turtle	Myocarditis, hepatitis, splenitis	18
Dermatophilus	Tortoises and turtles	Epidermal necrosis	48
Fungi			
Aspergillus	Aldabra and Galapagos tortoises; green turtles	Pneumonia	1, 14, 31
Geotrichum			
Paecilomyces			
Beauvaria			
Protozoa			
Entamoeba invadens	Tortoises and turtles	Enteritis, hepatic necrosis	27
Caryospora cheloniae	Green turtles	Enteritis	45
Intranuclear coccidia	Radiated tortoise	Nephritis, enteritis, pancreatitis	34
Hexamita parva	Tortoises and turtles	Nephritis	64
Trematoda			
Spirorchid trematodes	Freshwater and marine turtles	Vascular disease	15, 42, 63
Nematoda			
Proatractis	Tortoises	Colitis	56
Diptera			
Cistudinomyia cistudinis	Box turtle, gopher tortoise, Aldabra tortoise	Dermatitis	40, 60

wild turtles back to the wild as soon as possible. However, some of these chelonians, especially injured gopher tortoises, may be under care for up to 6 months. The longer an animal is in care and receiving treatment, the more difficult it is to euthanize it. When dozens, hundreds, and even thousands of chelonians are confiscated by government authorities, who generally have extremely limited budgets for such operations, the pressures are particularly great to determine the disposition of the animals as soon as possible. By far, euthanasia is the most expedient solution to this dilemma. The more common the species, both in the wild and captivity, the greater the probability of euthanasia. Justification is easy when the animals are obviously ill and suffering. Justification becomes less defensible, however, when animals are apparently healthy. Large numbers of domestic animals such as dogs, cats, and horses are euthanized every day in the United States because there are not enough homes in which to place these animals and not enough facilities to maintain them until placement is possible. Does quality of life matter? Should that be considered in the equation when coming to a resolution? Certainly, it is hard to justify maintaining animals if certain minimal needs are not being met. When they are not, euthanasia needs to be performed.

INFECTIOUS DISEASES

Captive chelonians, including marine, freshwater aquatic, and terrestrial species, are susceptible to a wide variety of infectious diseases. Regarding wild chelonians, several diseases have emerged as major health problems. More diseases have been reported in wild chelonians compared to other major groups of reptiles.[23] Whether this is an indication of a greater prevalence of disease in this order compared to other reptiles or simply a reflection of the number of worldwide studies involving chelonians remains to be determined. When chelonians die, the shells are left behind as monuments to the loss of the individuals from the population, favoring the discovery of epizootics. Additionally, because of their benign nature, chelonians are often observed in the field by the lay public, which also favors the reporting of disease problems in ill populations.

Of viral diseases, herpesviruses have surfaced as important pathogens in turtles and tortoises. Various gram-negative bacteria have been implicated as causes of septicemias in wild and captive aquatic turtles. There are numerous reports of pulmonary fungal disease in tortoises and fungal shell disease in aquatic species. Although few parasites have been implicated as significant pathogens in chelonians, the spirorchid trematodes are problematic in freshwater and marine turtles. Table 30–1 lists the most significant infectious diseases of chelonians.

REFERENCES

1. Andersen S, Eriksen E: Aspergillose bei einer Elephantenschildkrote (*Testudo gigantea elephantina*). X Internationalen Symposiums uber die Erkrankungen der Zootiere. Berlin, Akademie der Wissenschaften der DDR, pp 65–67, 1968.
2. Bolten AB, Jacobson ER, Bjorndal KA: Effects of anticoagulant and autoanalyzer on blood chemistry values of loggerhead sea turtles (*Caretta caretta*). Am J Vet Res 52:2224–2227, 1992.
3. Boycott JA, Taylor J, Douglas SH: Salmonella in tortoises. J Pathol Bact 65:401–411, 1953.
4. Brown MB, Schumacher IM, Klein PA, Harris RK, Correll T, Jacobson ER: *Mycoplasma agassizii* causes upper respiratory tract disease in the desert tortoise. Infect Immun 62:4580–4586, 1994.
5. Burke R: Relocations, repatriations, and translocations of amphibians and reptiles: taking a broader view. Herpetologica 47:350–357, 1991.
6. CITES: Resolution Conf.9.11. Disposal of Confiscated Live Animals of Species Included in the Appendices. Adopted at the Ninth Meeting of the Conference of the Parties to CITES, the Convention on International Trade in Endangered Species of Wild Fauna and Flora, Fort Lauderdale, FL, 1994.
7. Congdon JD, Durham AE, van Loben Sels RC: Delayed sexual maturity and demographics of Blanding's turtles (*Emydoidea blandingii*): implications for conservation and management of long-lived organisms. Conservation Biology 7:826–833, 1993.
8. Congdon JD, Durham AE, van Loben Sels RC: Demographics of common snapping turtles (*Chelydra serpentina*): implications for conservation and management of long-lived organisms. Am Zool 34:397–408, 1994.
9. Cooper JE, Gschmeissner S, Bone RD: Herpes-like virus particles in necrotic stomatitis of tortoises. Vet Rec 123:554, 1988.
10. Cox WR, Rapley A, Barker IK: Herpesvirus-like infection in a painted turtle (*Chrysemys picta*). J Wildlf Dis 16:445–449, 1980.
11. Dodd CK: Disease and population declines in the flattened musk turtle *Sternotherus depressus*. Am Midl Natur 119:394–401, 1988.
12. Frye FL, Oshiro LS, Dutra FR, et al: Herpesvirus-like infection in two Pacific pond turtles. J Am Vet Med Assoc 171:882–884, 1977.
13. Garber SD, Burger J: A 20-year study documenting the relationship between turtle decline and human recreation. Ecological Applications 5:1151–1162, 1995.
14. Georg LE, Williamson WM, Tilden EB, Getty RE: Mycotic pulmonary disease of captive giant tortoises due to *Beauvaria bassiana* and *Paecilomyces fumoso-roseus*. Sabouraudia 2:80–86, 1962.
15. Glazebrook JS, Campbell RSF: A survey of the diseases of marine turtles in northern Australia. II. Oceanarium-reared and wild turtles. Dis Aquat Org 9:97–104, 1990.
16. Harper PAW, Hammond DC, Heuschele WP: A herpesvirus-like agent associated with a pharyngeal abscess in a desert tortoise. J Wildl Dis 18:491–494, 1982.
17. Heldstab A, Bestetti G: Spontaneous viral hepatitis in a spur-tailed Mediterranean land tortoise (*Testudo hermanni*). J Zoo Anim Med 13:113–120, 1982.
18. Homer BL, Jacobson ER, Schumacher J, Scherba, G: Chlamydiosis in mariculture-reared green turtles (*Chelonia mydas*). Vet Pathol 31:1–7, 1994.
19. IUCN: Re-Introduction Specialist Group, Species Survival Commission. Guidelines for Re-Introductions, as approved by 41st Meeting of Council, International Union for Conservation of Nature, May 1995.
20. Jackson OF, Cooper JE: Nutritional diseases. *In* Cooper JE, Jackson OF (eds): Diseases of the Reptilia, vol 2. London, Academic Press, pp 409–428, 1981.
21. Jacobson ER: Reptiles. *In* Harkness JE (ed): Veterinary Clinics of North America: Small Animal Practice. Philadelphia, WB Saunders, pp 1203–1225, 1987.
22. Jacobson ER: Blood collection techniques in reptiles: laboratory investigations. *In* Fowler ME (ed): Zoo and Wild Animal Medicine: Current Therapy 3. Philadelphia, WB Saunders, pp 144–152, 1993.
23. Jacobson ER: Diseases in turtles and tortoises: the chelonian charisma vs coincidence conundrum. *In* J. van Abemma (ed): Proceedings, Conservation, Restoration, and Management of Tortoises and Turtles. An International Conference. State University of New York, Purchase, New York, Turtle and Tortoise Society, pp 89–90, 1992.
24. Jacobson ER, Brown MB, Schumacher IM, Collins BR, Harris RK, Klein PA: Mycoplasmosis and the desert tortoise (*Gopherus agassizii*) in Las Vegas Valley Nevada. Chelon Conserv Biol 1:279–284, 1995.
25. Jacobson ER, Buergelt C, Williams B, Harris, RK: Herpesvirus in cutaneous fibropapillomas of the green turtle *Chelonia mydas*. Dis Aquatic Org 12:1–6, 1991.
26. Jacobson ER, Clubb S, Gaskin JM, Gardiner, C: Herpesvirus-like infection in Argentine tortoises. J Am Vet Med Assoc 187:1227–1229, 1985.

27. Jacobson ER, Clubb S, Greiner EC: Amebiasis in red-footed tortoises. J Am Vet Med Assoc 183:1192–1194, 1983.
28. Jacobson ER, Gardiner CH, Barten SL, Burr DH, Bourgeois AL: *Flavobacterium meningosepticum* infection of a Barbour's map turtle (*Graptemys barbouri*). J Zoo Wildl Med 20:474–477, 1989.
29. Jacobson ER, Gaskin JM, Brown MB, et al: Chronic upper respiratory tract disease of free-ranging desert tortoises, *Xerobates agassizii*. J Wildl Dis 27:296–316, 1991.
30. Jacobson ER, Gaskin JM, Roelke M, et al: Conjunctivitis, tracheitis, and pneumonia associated with herpesvirus infection in green sea turtles. J Am Vet Med Assoc 189:1020–1023, 1986.
31. Jacobson ER, Gaskin JM, Shields RP, White FH: Mycotic pneumonia in mariculture reared green sea turtles. J Am Vet Med Assoc 175:929–933, 1979.
32. Jacobson ER, Gaskin JM, Wahlquist H: Herpes-like virus infection in map turtles. J Am Vet Med Assoc 181:1322–1324, 1982.
33. Jacobson ER, Schumacher J, Green ME: Field and clinical techniques for sampling and handling blood for hematological and plasma biochemical determinations in the desert tortoise, *Xerobates agassizii*. Copeia 1992:237–241, 1992.
34. Jacobson ER, Schumacher J, Telford SR, et al: Intranuclear coccidiosis in radiated tortoises (*Geochelone radiata*). J Zoo Wildl Med 25:95–102, 1994.
35. Jacobson ER, Weinstein M, Berry K, et al: Problems with using weight vs length relationships to assess tortoise health. Vet Rec 132:222–223, 1993.
36. Jenkins MD: Tortoises and freshwater turtles: the trade in Southeast Asia. TRAFFIC International, United Kingdom, 1995.
37. Kaplan HM: Septicemic ulcerative cutaneous disease of turtles. Lab Anim Care 7:273–277, 1957.
38. Keymer IF: Diseases of chelonians: (2) necropsy survey of terrapins and turtles. Vet Rec 103:577–582, 1978.
39. Klemens MW: Repatriation of confiscated tortoises: conscience-clearing expediency or sound wildlife management? Re-Introduction News 10:5–6, 1995.
40. Knipling EF: The biology of *Sarcophaga cistudinis* Aldrich (Diptera), a species of Sarcophagidae parasitic on turtles and tortoises. Entomol Soc, Washington 39:91–101, 1937.
41. Lamm SH, Taylor A, Gangarosa EJ, et al: Turtle-associated salmonelloses I. An estimation of the magnitude of the problem in the United States. Am J Epidemiol 95:511–517, 1972.
42. Lauckner G: Diseases of reptilia. *In* Kinne O (ed): Diseases of Marine Animals. Hamburg, FRG, Biologische Anstalt Helgoland, pp 443–626, 1985.
43. Lawrence K: Seasonal variation in blood chemistry of long term captive Mediterranean tortoises (*Testudo graeca* and *T. Hermanni*). Res Vet Sci 43:379–383, 1987.
44. Le Dien D, Broad S: Investigations into Tortoise and Freshwater Turtle Trade in Vietnam. IUCN Species Survival Commission. Gland, Switzerland and Cambridge, UK, IUCN, pp 34, 1995.
45. Leibovitz L, Rebell G, Boucher GC: *Caryospora cheloniae* sp nov: a coccidial pathogen of mariculture-reared green sea turtles (*Chelonia mydas mydas*). J Wildl Dis 14:269–275, 1978.
46. Leong JK, Smith DL, Revera DB, et al: Health care and diseases of captive-reared loggerhead and Kemp's ridley sea turtles. *In* Caillouet CW, Landry AM (eds): Proceedings of the First International Symposium on Kemp's Ridley Sea Turtle Biology, Conservation, and Management, Galveston, TX, pp 178–201, 1989.
47. Marks S, Citino SB: Hematology and serum chemistry of the radiated tortoise (*Testudo radiata*). J Zoo Wildl Med 21:342–344, 1990.
48. Masters AM, Ellis TM, Carson JM, et al: *Dermatophilus chelonae* sp. nov., isolated from chelonids in Australia. Int J Syst Bacteriol 45:50–56, 1995.
49. Mautino M, Page CD: Biology and medicine of turtles and tortoises. *In* Quesenberry E, Hillyer EV (eds): Veterinary Clinics of North America, Small Animal Practice, Exotic Pet Medicine I. Philadelphia, WB Saunders, pp 1251–1270, 1993.
50. McLaughlin GS: Upper respiratory tract disease in gopher tortoises, *Gopherus polyphemus*: pathology, immune responses, transmission, and implications for conservation and management. Ph.D. dissertation, University of Florida, 1997.
51. McNeil E, Hinshaw WR: Salmonella from Galapagos turtles, a gila monster, and an iguana. J Vet Res 7:62–63, 1946.
52. Muller M, Sachsse W, Zangger N: Herpesvirus-Epidemie beider griechischen (*Testudo hermanni*) und der maurischen Landschildkrote (*Testudo graeca*) in der Schweiz. Schweiz Arch Tierhelk 132:199–203, 1990.
53. Pettan-Brewer KCB, Drew ML, Ramsay E, et al: Herpesvirus particles associated with oral and respiratory lesions in a California desert tortoise (*Gopherus agassizii*). J Wildl Dis 32:521–526, 1996.
54. Rebell H, Rywlin A, Haines HA: Herpesvirus-type agent associated with skin lesions of green turtles in aquaculture. Amer J Vet Res 36:1221–1224, 1975.
55. Reinert HK: Translocation as a conservation strategy for amphibians and reptiles: some comments, concerns, and observations. Herpetologica 47:357–363, 1991.
56. Rideout BA, Montali RJ, Phillips LG, Gardiner CH: Mortality of captive tortoises due to viviparous nematodes of the genua *Proatractis* (Family Atractidae). J Wildl Dis 23:103–108, 1987.
57. Rosskopf WJ: Normal hemogram and blood chemistry values for California desert tortoises. VM/SAC 77:85–87, 1982.
58. Salzberg A: Report on import/export turtle trade in the United States. Proceedings of the International Congress of Chelonian Conservation, Gonfaron, France, pp 314–322, 1995.
59. Samour HJ, Risley D, March T, et al: Blood sampling techniques in reptiles. Vet Rec 12:472–477, 1984.
60. Stover J, Norton T, Jacobson ER, Rider PJ: *Cistudinomyia cistudinis* infestation in Aldabra tortoises (*Testudo gigantea*). Third International Colloquium on the Pathology of Reptiles and Amphibians, Orlando, FL, pp 109–110, 1989.
61. Taylor RW, Jacobson ER: Hematology and serum chemistry of the gopher tortoise, *Gopherus polyphemus*. Comp Biochem Physiol 2A:425–428, 1981.
62. Westhouse RA, Jacobson ER, Harris RK, et al: Respiratory and pharyngo-esophageal iridovirus infection in a gopher tortoise (*Gopherus polyphemus*). J Wildl Dis 32:682–686, 1996.
63. Yamaguti Y: Synopsis of the Digenetic Trematodes of Vertebrates, Vol 1. Keugaku, Tokyo, Japan, 1971.
64. Zwart P, Truyens EHA: Hexamitiasis in tortoises. Vet Parasitol 1:175–183, 1975.

CHAPTER 31

Organ Location in Snakes for Diagnostic and Surgical Evaluation

HELEN E. McCRACKEN

The internal organs of a snake are elongated, attenuated, and arranged sequentially, with some overlap, along the length of the narrow body cavity (Fig. 31–1). The organ sequence, with the exception of the lungs, is constant for all species, but the relative position and size of viscera, as a function of body length, vary significantly both between and within taxonomic families.[2, 3, 5, 7, 8, 10, 16] Knowledge of these anatomic details and their interspecies variations is helpful in the diagnosis and treatment of many disease conditions in snakes. There are records in the literature of this information for numerous species,[2–11, 13, 16] but such data are not available for many snakes.

METHODS

A study was made of the internal anatomy of 81 adult snakes of 24 species belonging to the families Boidae, Colubridae, Elapidae, and Crotalidae (Table 31–1). Each cadaver was opened along its full length by mid-ventral incision and straightened, and measurements were made (to the nearest millimeter) of the distance from the snout to the anterior and posterior poles of each major internal organ. The ratio of each of these measurements to the snout-cloaca length of the snake was then calculated to determine the position of each organ in relation to body length. An alternative method used in other studies[2, 3] was to record the number of ventral scutes between the snout or cloaca and the various organs. A comparison of the two methods revealed the former to be more precise because of individual variation in the total number of ventral scutes.[16] These data were obtained for two purposes: to assist in the location of specific organs in a snake so that certain procedures (e.g., radiography, surgical biopsy) may be executed and to aid in the diagnostic approach to palpable and visible internal masses in snakes.

RESULTS

The species mean plus or minus standard deviation ($\bar{x} \pm$ s.d.) of the relative position of the poles of each organ were computed for the three species with the greatest sample size: *Morelia spilota* (both subspecies; $n = 22$), *Liasis childreni* ($n = 11$), and *Morelia amethistina* ($n = 7$). This statistic of the data was similarly calculated for each family, with measurements from all specimens examined; the results are presented in Figures 31–2 and 31–3. Gallbladder, spleen, pancreas, oviducts, thyroid, and adrenal glands are not represented in these graphs because they were uniformly found in the same organ associations in all species examined (see Sequence of Internal Organs section next). Therefore, data presented for other organs may be used to locate them.

The relative positions and lengths of viscera were found to be reasonably constant for each species, regardless of individual body length. Distinct differences were observed between species, with greater differences between, than within, snake families. It was concluded that the most accurate data to use for diagnostic purposes would be those collected for the species in question. If these are unavailable, the mean values computed for each family are used. The greater variation present in the family mean data decreased the accuracy of prediction of organ position, but in most cases this is of little consequence because of the relatively long lengths of most snake viscera.

SEQUENCE OF INTERNAL ORGANS

The sequence of positioning of viscera, for all organs except the lungs, was constant for all species examined. The following organ associations were observed in all specimens examined:

- The heart is positioned immediately cranioventral to the point of termination of the trachea and is quite mobile, perhaps as an adaptation to facilitate the passage of relatively large prey items past it.[12]
- The thyroid gland is situated immediately anterior to the heart, with the thymus and paired parathyroid glands immediately cranial to it, lying within aggregations of adipose tissue in well-conditioned snakes. The thymus does not involute with maturity as it does in higher vertebrates.[12]

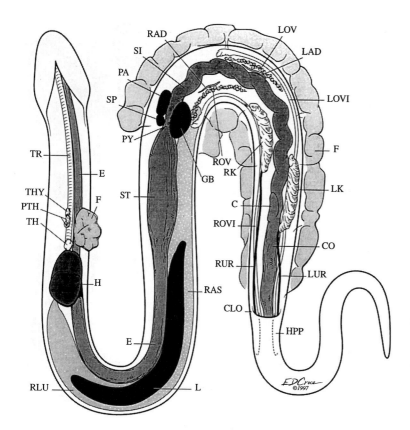

FIGURE 31–1. Internal anatomy of a female snake, ventral aspect; celomic fat bodies reflected laterally.

TR trachea	PY pylorus	RK right kidney
E esophagus	SI small intestine	LK left kidney
THY thymus	GB gall bladder	RUR right ureter
PTH parathyroid gland	SP spleen	LUR left ureter
TH thyroid gland	PA pancreas	C cecum
F fat body	RAD right adrenal gland	CO colon
H heart	LAD left adrenal gland	CLO cloaca
RLU right lung	ROV right ovary	HPP postion of hemipenal
RAS right air sac	LOV left ovary	pocket in male
L liver	ROVI right oviduct	
ST stomach	LOVI left oviduct	

- The gallbladder is positioned adjacent to the gastric pylorus, some distance caudal to the posterior pole of the elongated, spindle-shaped liver. The pancreas and spleen, fused in some species as a splenopancreas,[12] are generally very close to the gallbladder, forming a clustered organ triad. The cranial pole of the right ovary is situated at the level of this triad, or at a short distance caudal to it. In many boids, the right testis is similarly positioned, but in other species, in which the testes are shorter than the ovaries, the anterior pole of the right testis is further caudal.
- The right gonad, left gonad, right kidney, and left kidney are arranged sequentially in that order, with a variable degree of overlap. Gonadal size varies seasonally.[12] The oviducal infundibula open immediately craniolateral to the anterior poles of their respective ovaries. The pink, filiform adrenal glands lie immediately mesial to their respective gonads, incorporated in the gonadal mesentery.

- The gastrointestinal tract is essentially linear with a slight degree of concertina-like folding of the small intestine. In boids and some other species, a small cecum is present at the junction of small intestine and colon, situated at approximately 50% to 75% of the distance from pylorus to cloaca.
- Celomic fat is distributed in distinct bodies arranged in adjacent chains in mesentery lying ventral to all other viscera. In most species, these chains commence between the posterior pole of the liver and the gallbladder and continue to the level of the cloaca. In well-conditioned and obese snakes, small fat aggregations are also present immediately cranial to the heart.

Trachea and lung positioning and morphology vary greatly between species. In all species, the trachea is supported by incomplete cartilaginous rings. Boids have a simple trachea that bifurcates at the level of the heart; the short bronchi open into two saccular lungs, and the

TABLE 31–1. Specimens Used in Study

Family	Scientific Name	Common Name	Sample Size
Boidae	*Aspidites melanocephalus*	Black-headed python	3
	Boa constrictor	Boa constrictor	1
	Corallus caninus	Emerald tree boa	2
	Liasis childreni	Children's python	11
	Liasis olivaceus	Olive python	4
	Morelia amethistina	Amethystine python	7
	Morelia spilota spilota	Diamond python	12
	Morelia spilota variegata	Carpet python	10
Colubridae	*Boiga irregularis*	Brown tree snake	2
	Elaphe guttata	Cornsnake	4
	Stegonotus cucullatus	Slate-grey snake	1
	Dendrelaphis punctulatus	Green tree snake	1
	Elaphe taeniura freesei	Taiwan beauty snake	1
Elapidae	*Acanthophis antarcticus*	Death adder	5
	Austrelaps superbus	Copperhead	3
	Notechis ater	Black tiger snake	1
	Notechis scutatus	Eastern tiger snake	3
	Oxyuranus scutellatus	Taipan	1
	Pseudechis porphyriacus	Red-bellied black snake	1
	Pseudonaja textilis	Eastern brown snake	2
Crotalidae	*Agkistrodon bilineatus*	Cantil	2
	Bothrops schlegeli	Eyelash viper	1
	Crotalus atrox	Western diamondback rattlesnake	1
	Sistrurus catenatus tergeminus	Western massasauga	2

right lung is slightly longer in most species. The lungs extend a short distance past the commencement of the liver and then continue caudally as membranous air sacs that terminate close to the gallbladder. The point of junction of lung and air sac cannot be accurately measured because the vascularized lung parenchyma gradually decreases in density and disappears over a transitional area.[16] In colubrids and elapids, the left lung is extremely reduced or absent. The trachea bifurcates or opens into the single lung at the level of the heart. In some species (e.g., *Elaphe guttata* and *Pseudechis porphyriacus*), there is a simple trachea; in others, the cartilaginous rings of the trachea open dorsally into a membranous sac for the full length (e.g., *Notechis* species) or caudal half (e.g., *Boiga irregularis* and *Stegonotus cucullatus*) of the trachea. Some elapids (e.g., *Pseudonaja* species and *Acanthophis antarcticus*) have a short tracheal lung in which the lung commences 3 to 4 cm anterior to the heart as a saccular extension off open tracheal rings. After the termination of the trachea at the level of the heart, the lung continues as a saclike structure. Lung and air sac lengths of most colubrids and elapids are similar to those of boids, but they are longer in some species. In *Oxyuranus scutellatus,* the lung extends a short distance past the posterior pole of the liver and continues as an air sac to just anterior to the cloaca. Crotalids have a single tracheal lung (the left lung is absent) that commences a short distance caudal to the base of the skull and extends the full length of the trachea. Posterior to the termination of the trachea, the lung continues for a short distance before becoming contiguous with an air sac of variable length.

CLINICAL APPLICATION OF DATA

Location of Specific Organs for Clinical Examination

Unless the examiner is very familiar with snake anatomy, it is difficult to determine the site of most internal organs by simple visual examination or palpation, because there are few landmarks to guide the clinician. The data collected in this study may be used to locate organs for specific diagnostic and therapeutic procedures such as radiography, ultrasonography, magnetic resonance imaging, computed tomographic (CT) scans, endoscopy, biopsy, and surgery. It may also be used to locate the heart for monitoring or cardiocentesis in large, well-muscled snakes and in moribund animals in which the beat is not easily visualized and the heart is not readily palpable.[15] In these situations, the snout-cloaca length of the snake is measured, and the positional data from Figure 31–2 or 31–3 are used to calculate the approximate locations of the target organs.

Diagnosis of Internal Masses

Visible or palpable intracelomic masses are common clinical findings in snakes, either as presenting signs or as observations made during examination. The most common causes are intestinal impaction, retained eggs or fetuses, and abscesses or granulomas within organs or external to them. Differential diagnoses also include neoplasia; ingested foreign bodies; intestinal intussus-

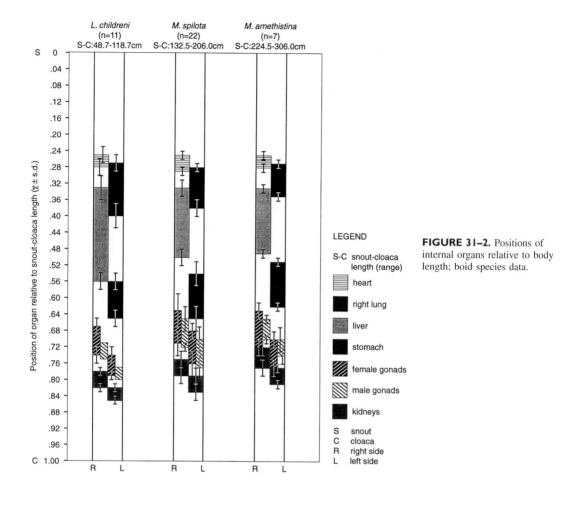

FIGURE 31–2. Positions of internal organs relative to body length; boid species data.

LEGEND

S-C   snout-cloaca length (range)

heart

right lung

liver

stomach

female gonads

male gonads

kidneys

S   snout
C   cloaca
R   right side
L   left side

ception; uric acid colonoliths; cardiomyopathy; pericardial effusion; goiter; renal and visceral gout; cholecystomegaly resulting from bile duct obstruction or coccidiosis; ripe or atretic follicles; inflammation of any organ, including omphalitis, steatis, gastritis caused by *Cryptosporidium* and *Monocercomonas*, and colitis resulting from *Entamoeba* infection.[1, 15] A knowledge of the organs located at the sites of such masses is integral to their diagnosis. The anatomic data collected in this study have proved very successful diagnostic aids in this regard. In addition to history taking, complete physical examination, plain radiography, and palpation of the mass to assess its hardness, texture, discreteness, and movability, the distances from snout to cloaca and snout to anterior pole of mass and the dimensions of the mass are measured. The ratio of snout-mass length to snout-cloaca length is then calculated and compared with the anatomic positional values obtained for the species concerned, if available, or, alternatively, with the family values. The calculated ratio is used to determine (1) whether the mass would be in the esophagus, stomach, or intestine, if it were intraintestinal, or (2) which organ the mass would be associated with, if it were extraintestinal. A differential diagnosis for the mass can then be established. Intra-intestinal and extra-intestinal masses can generally be distinguished reliably

by plain radiography, the former being typically irregularly shaped and of heterogeneous density, including bony spicules. Abscesses, granulomas, neoplasms, and swollen organs are generally discrete masses of homogeneous soft tissue density. Contrast radiography or endoscopic examination may be used in addition.

◆ CASE REPORTS

Case I

An adult female *Vipera ammodytes* had a large visible swelling (approximately 4 cm long, 2.5 cm in diameter) in the caudal body cavity. The snout-mass distance was 35 cm, and the snout-cloaca length, 45 cm; the ratio of these values was 0.78. Because no positional data were available for this species, the mean values for the Crotalidae were used. This ratio (0.78) corresponds with the positions of the intestine, left ovary, and oviduct (see Fig. 31–3). On palpation, the mass was firm, smooth, and discrete and could not be advanced. Plain radiographs demonstrated a discrete mass of homogeneous soft tissue density. The preliminary diagnosis was an abscess or a tumor involving the left ovary or oviduct. A celiotomy at the site revealed a discrete, cream,

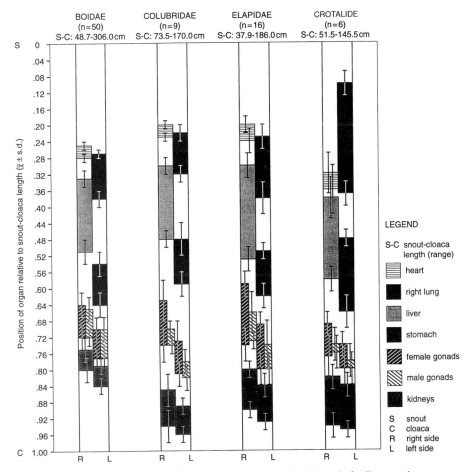

FIGURE 31–3. Positions of internal organs relative to body length; family mean data.

fleshy mass lying ventrolateral (left side) to the intestine and occupying almost the entire width of the body cavity. A duct (approximately 3 mm wide) resembling the oviduct protruded from its caudal pole. A similar duct ran longitudinally in the mesentery on the right side of the mass. The mass was presumed to represent neoplastic change of the left ovary, inasmuch as there was no trace of normal gonad at the site. The lesion was removed by blunt dissection and surgical ligation of the presumptive left oviduct. The presumptive right oviduct was preserved. Histopathology revealed the mass to be an adenocarcinoma involving the ovary, probably of oviduct origin.

Two weeks after surgery, a decision was made to surgically examine the right ovary for evidence of neoplasia, because recent radiographs had revealed a small indistinct mass of similar density to the original tumor, at a site just cranial to it. The incision was elected to commence 31.0 cm from the snout, on the basis of the mean value for the position of the anterior pole of the right ovary in the other crotalids (0.69, because 0.69 × 45 cm = 31.0 cm; see Fig. 31–3). This incision (3 cm in length) was in the exact position desired, and the right ovary and

oviduct and all other organs visualized were found to be normal. Nothing was seen to explain the radiographic finding. The snake had no further problems until it died 3 years later of an unrelated condition and was found at autopsy to have no evidence of neoplasia.

Case 2

An adult female *M. amethistina* had several large palpable internal masses and a history of anorexia for 8 months. The snout-cloaca length was 288 cm. The largest mass (approximately 6 cm long, 3 cm in diameter) was 141 cm from the snout (positional ratio of 0.49). The other masses (each 2 to 3 cm in diameter) lay in a chain 31 cm long, commencing 179 cm from the snout (positional ratio of 0.62). These ratios were compared with positional data for *M. amethistina* (see Fig. 31–2). The value of 0.49 corresponds with the positions of the posterior pole of liver, esophagus, and air sac, and 0.62 corresponds with the location of pylorus, and hence the organ triad of gallbladder, spleen, and pancreas, and with the anterior pole of the right ovary and oviduct. On palpation, all masses were firm, discrete, and immobile. Plain radiographs of both areas revealed discrete masses of homogeneous soft tissue density. The preliminary diagnosis was an abscess or tumor on the caudal liver pole and either large follicles on one or both ovaries or unfertilized eggs in the oviducts. An exploratory celiotomy over the site of the first mass revealed a large encapsulated abscess under the liver capsule at the caudal pole. The abscess was removed, but a poor prognosis was given because adjacent liver tissue was pale, mottled, and very friable with several pinpoint white masses on the surface. The snake recovered from anesthesia but died overnight. Necropsy revealed focal chronic hepatic abscessation with locally extensive hepatitis and multiple large degenerate follicles on both ovaries.

DISCUSSION

Of the snakes examined in this study, only *M. spilota* and the elapid species have been previously similarly described.[2, 16] These earlier studies, however, did not include measurements of all major viscera. It was determined, by examining the distribution of range from the unit normal,[14] that a sample size of at least 12 is required for a reasonable estimate of the range of values in a population. Because of the opportunistic nature of specimen acquisition, this minimum sample size was achieved only for *M. spilota* ($n = 22$) and the Boidae ($n = 50$) and Elapidae ($n = 16$). The smaller data sets presented for the other species and families are therefore less reliable statistically but have nevertheless proved useful diagnostically, as demonstrated in the cases just described.

REFERENCES

1. Barten SL, Davis K, Harris RK, Jacobson ER: Renal cell carcinoma with metastases in a corn snake (*Elaphe guttata*). J Zoo Wildl Med 25(1):123–127, 1994.
2. Bragdon DE: A contribution to the surgical anatomy of the water snake, *Natrix sipedon sipedon*; the location of the visceral endocrine organs with reference to ventral scutellation. Anat Rec 117:145–161, 1953.
3. Brongersma LD: Notes on *Maticora bivirgata* (Boie) and on *Bungarus flaviceps* Reinh. Zoologische Mededelingen, Rijksmuseum Van Natuurlijke Historie Te Leiden 30(1):1–29, 1948.
4. Brongersma LD: Notes on *Pseudoxenodon inornatus* (Boie) and *Pseudoxenodon jacobsonii* Lidth. Proc Kon Ned Akad Wet 53(9):3–10, 1950.
5. Brongersma LD: Some notes upon the anatomy of *Tropidophis* and *Trachyboa* (Serpentes). Zoologische Mededelingen, Rijksmuseum Van Natuurlijke Historie Te Leiden 31(11):107–124, 1951.
6. Brongersma LD: Notes on New Guinean reptiles and amphibians. V. Proc Kon Ned Akad Wet Series C 59(5):599–610, 1956.
7. Brongersma LD: Notes upon the trachea, the lungs, and the pulmonary artery in snakes III. Proc Kon Ned Akad Wet Series C 60(4):451–457, 1957.
8. Brongersma LD: Upon some features of the respiratory and circulatory systems in the Typhlopidae and some other snakes. Extrait Des Archives Neerlandaises De Zoologie. Tome XIII, I. Supplement:120–127, 1958.
9. Brongersma LD: Notes on *Liasis boeleni* Brongersma. Proc Kon Ned Akad Wet Series C 72(2):124–128, 1969.
10. Diani AR: A comparative study of the ophidian digestive tract. Ph.D. dissertation, St. Louis University, 1974.
11. Frenkel G, Kochva E: Visceral anatomy of *Vipera palestinae*: an illustrated presentation. Isr J Zool 3:145–163, 1970.
12. Funk RS: Snakes. *In* Mader DR (ed): Reptile Medicine and Surgery. Philadelphia, WB Saunders, pp 34–46, 1996.
13. Klauber LM: Rattlesnakes: Their Habits, Life Histories and Influence on Mankind. Los Angeles, University of California Press, 1968.
14. Pearson ES, Hartley HO (eds): Biometrika Tables for Statisticians, 2nd ed, vol 1. Cambridge, UK, Cambridge University Press, 1962.
15. Russo EA: Diagnosis and treatment of lumps and bumps in snakes. Compend Contin Educ Pract Vet 9(8):795–807, 1987.
16. Wallach V: A cladistic analysis of the terrestrial Australian Elapidae. *In* Grigg G, Shine R, Ehmann HE (eds): Biology of Australasian Frogs and Reptiles. Sydney, Australia, Royal Zoological Society of New South Wales, pp 223–253, 1985.

CHAPTER 32

The Reptilian Renal-Portal System: Influence on Therapy

PETER H. HOLZ

A renal-portal system is present in most fishes and in all amphibians, reptiles, and birds. It is absent in mammals, except embryonically.[5] The renal-portal system (Fig. 32–1) collects blood from the tail, hind limbs, and pelvic region and carries a portion of that blood to the kidneys. Blood within the kidneys percolates through capillaries that surround the proximal and distal convoluted tubules of the nephrons and then exits into the postcaval vein, which transports it back to the heart. Renal-portal blood perfuses only the tubules and not the glomeruli.[17] Consequently, the tubules receive mixed venous and arterial blood, the latter originating from the efferent arterioles.

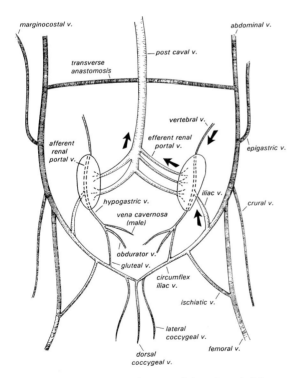

FIGURE 32–1. Renal portal system of the red-eared slider (dorsal view). Arrows indicate direction of blood flow. The oval stippled organs represent the kidneys.

marginocostal v.

abdominal v.

post caval v.

transverse anastomosis

vertebral v.

afferent renal portal v.

efferent renal portal v.

epigastric v.

hypogastric v.

iliac v.

crural v.

vena cavernosa (male)

obdurator v.

gluteal v.

circumflex iliac v.

ischiatic v.

lateral coccygeal v.

dorsal coccygeal v.

femoral v.

The function of the renal-portal system has been reviewed by Dantzler.[5] Fishes, amphibians, and reptiles cannot produce hypertonic urine because they lack a loop of Henle. Therefore, to decrease water loss, the glomerular filtration rate must decrease. This is accomplished through the action of arginine vasotocin, which causes constriction of the afferent glomerular arterioles.[21] Consequently, blood flow through the glomerulus ceases. The renal-portal system continues to supply blood to perfuse the tubule cells and prevent them from undergoing ischemic necrosis.

In all species examined, blood may be shunted through or around the kidneys, depending on the need of the individual. A valve that controls blood flow to the kidneys has been described in chickens.[1] A smaller but similar structure has been identified in the red-eared slider (*Trachemys scripta elegans*).[8] Radioangiographic studies in this species indicate that blood from the tail may be shunted through or around the kidneys (Figs. 32–2, 32–3), but much of the blood from the hindlimb bypasses the kidney and flows to the liver (Fig. 32–4).[8] The alteration in blood flow is likely a result of the action of the valve: when the valve is closed, blood enters the kidney; when the valve is open, blood bypasses the kidney. It is unknown, at this stage, what controls the valve. In poultry the valve opens in response to adrenaline and closes in response to acetylcholine.[20]

A number of authors[9, 14–16, 23] state that drugs should not be injected into the caudal portion of the body of reptiles because the renal-portal system will carry them to the kidneys, leading to rapid excretion and possible nephrotoxicity. However, these assertions are not based on any experimental data. One study suggests that the renal-portal system has no effect on drug kinetics.[8]

Two commonly used antibiotics, gentamicin and carbenicillin, were selected to determine the effect of the renal-portal system on drug kinetics in the red-eared slider. Location of the injection, whether in the forelimb or in the hindlimb, did not affect the pharmacokinetics of gentamicin. Intuitively, this is a logical result because gentamicin is excreted almost solely by glomerular filtration.[25] Because the renal-portal system provides blood only to the renal tubules,[17] gentamicin carried to the kidney is not excreted before gaining access to the systemic circulation.

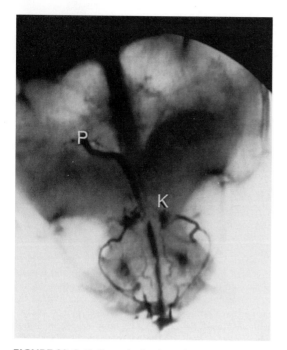

FIGURE 32–2. Radiograph of red-eared slider injected with radiopaque dye in the dorsal coccygeal vein. Note dye perfused the kidneys. K, kidney; P, post caval vein.

gentamicin in eastern box turtles (*Terrapene carolina carolina*), and by Jensen and Westerman,[10] who reported no site differences when amikacin was used in the ostrich (*Struthio camelus*). Evidence thus indicates that aminoglycosides, and other drugs that are excreted primarily by glomerular filtration, may be administered in either the forelimb or the hindlimb without a loss of therapeutic effect.

Drugs excreted by tubular secretion could potentially be affected by the renal-portal system. However, because only a small portion of the blood flow from the hindlimb is diverted through the kidney, any potential effect will be minor and unlikely to be clinically significant. This was demonstrated in the carbenicillin study. Studies on the kinetics of piperacillin[7] and ceftazidime,[13] in which recommended doses were used, also yielded blood levels greatly in excess of MIC. Up to 85% of the drug would have to be excreted during its first pass through the kidney to produce a significant effect on blood levels. A study in which radiolabeled macroaggregated albumin was injected in the femoral vein resulted in a maximum uptake by the kidney of approximately 20%.[8] Consequently, this high rate of drug elimination appears extremely unlikely.

Because the renal-portal system functions to protect tubules during periods of dehydration, it could be argued that clinically ill, potentially dehydrated reptiles may be more affected than the healthy ones examined, inasmuch as blood flow through the renal-portal system is increased. However, when the glomerulus is closed, the associated tubule collapses, because fluid no longer passes through it. Consequently, transport across the

Carbenicillin was selected because a significant portion of this drug is excreted by tubular secretion.[11] Because of the large volume of drug required in relation to the small muscle mass of the sliders' limbs, half the recommended carbenicillin dose was used.[12] Experimental results indicated a slightly lower blood level during the first 8 hours after injection for animals injected in the hindlimb. No difference was detected after this time period. For a drug to be effective, it should achieve a blood level four times above the minimum inhibitory concentration (MIC) of the pathogen being treated.[4] Lawrence and coworkers[13] calculated the MIC for a number of potential reptile pathogens. Despite the difference in kinetics and the lower dose used, carbenicillin blood levels were well in excess of this threshold, regardless of the injection site. Therefore, organisms would be treated effectively, regardless of whether the carbenicillin was administered in the forelimb or the hindlimb.

When the histologic appearances of red-eared slider kidneys receiving gentamicin, carbenicillin, and no antibiotics were compared, no significant difference could be detected. There was no evidence of nephrotoxicity, regardless of the drug received or the injection site.[8]

On the basis of the knowledge of renal-portal anatomy and physiology and the results of the antibiotic pharmacokinetic studies, several recommendations concerning reptile therapeutics can be made. Because all aminoglycosides have a mode of excretion similar to that of gentamicin,[25] it is likely that none of them are influenced by renal-portal perfusion. Support for this conclusion is provided by Beck and associates[2] who found no effect of injection site on the kinetics of

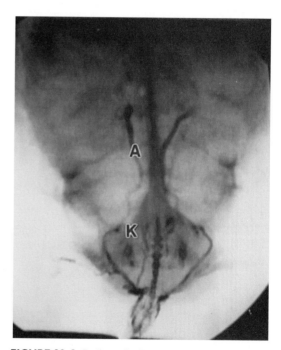

FIGURE 32–3. Radiograph of red-eared slider injected with radiopaque dye in the dorsal coccygeal vein. Note dye entered the abdominal vein and bypassed the kidneys. A, abdominal vein; K, kidney.

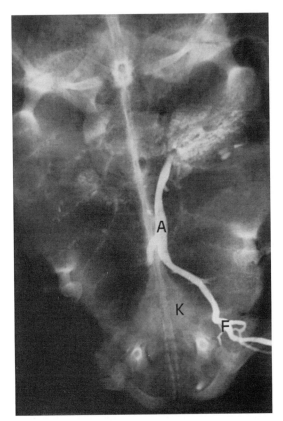

FIGURE 32–4. Radiograph of red-eared slider injected with radiopaque dye in the femoral vein. Note dye entered the abdominal vein and bypassed the kidney. A, abdominal vein; F, femoral vein; K, kidney.

epithelium ceases.[22] Therefore, even though more drug might be entering the kidney, more would not necessarily be excreted. As nephrons cease to filter, it is possible that less drug would be excreted and higher blood levels might occur.

Experimental work indicates that much of the blood from the hindlimb flows directly to the liver.[8] This has potential implications for drugs that are excreted predominantly through hepatic metabolism. Some of the fluoroquinolones, such as enrofloxacin,[24] are in this category. Drugs administered orally are also transported to the liver before entering the systemic circulation. For drugs with a high hepatic extraction ratio, such as propranolol, only a small portion of the oral dose reaches the systemic circulation, as a result of hepatic presystemic elimination.[6] However, a high hepatic extraction ratio is not characteristic of the fluoroquinolones, which achieve comparable blood levels whether administered orally or parenterally.[24] Consequently, their pharmacokinetics are unlikely to be influenced by injection site.

Aminoglycosides are unusual in that they are excreted almost solely by glomerular filtration. The majority of drugs have both a renal and a hepatic component to their excretion, further diluting the potential effect of the renal-portal system. It is more likely that blood levels are subtherapeutic because of species differences, as demonstrated for enrofloxacin[18, 19] and chloramphenicol,[3] than because of any perceived influence of injection site.

Extrapolation across drug groups can be difficult. All the components of a particular drug's metabolism must be taken into consideration to determine the most likely effect of the renal-portal system on the drug's kinetics. According to current research, it seems unlikely that injection site has any influence on the activity of a drug. Thus the caudal area of reptiles is available for drug administration, with the advantages of increased operator safety because of greater distance from the subject's mouth, a greater muscle mass in many species, and the flexibility of being able to rotate repeated injections through sites on four limbs, rather than two, in quadrupeds.

REFERENCES

1. Akester AR: Radiographic studies of the renal portal system in the domestic fowl (*Gallus domesticus*). J Anat 98:365–376, 1964.
2. Beck K, Loomis M, Lewbart G, et al: Preliminary comparison of plasma concentrations of gentamicin injected into the cranial and caudal limb musculature of the eastern box turtle (*Terrapene carolina carolina*). J Zoo Wildl Med 26:265, 1995.
3. Clark CH, Rogers ED, Milton JL: Plasma concentrations of chloramphenicol in snakes. Am J Vet Res 46:2654, 1985.
4. Conzelman GM: Pharmacotherapeutics of aminoglycoside antibiotics. J Am Vet Med Assoc 176:1078–1080, 1980.
5. Dantzler WH: Comparative aspects of renal function. *In* Seldin DW, Giebisch G (eds): The Kidney: Physiology and Pathophysiology. New York, Raven Press, pp 333–364, 1985.
6. Gibaldi M: Biopharmaceutics and Clinical Pharmacokinetics, 3rd ed. Philadelphia, Lea & Febiger, 1984.
7. Hilf M, Swanson D, Wagner R, Yu VL: Pharmacokinetics of piperacillin in blood pythons (*Python curtus*) and in vitro evaluation of efficacy against aerobic gram-negative bacteria. J Zoo Wildl Med 22:199, 1991.
8. Holz, P: The reptilian renal portal system and its effect on drug kinetics. D.V.Sc. dissertation, University of Guelph, 1994.
9. Jacobson ER: Use of chemotherapeutics in reptile medicine. *In* Jacobson ER, Kollias GV Jr (eds): Exotic Animals. New York, Churchill Livingstone, pp 35–48, 1988.
10. Jensen J, Westerman E: Amikacin pharmacokinetics in ostrich (*Struthio camelus*). Proceedings of the American Association of Zoo Veterinarians, South Padre Island, TX pp 238–242, 1990.
11. Kucers A, Bennett NM: The Use of Antibiotics, 3rd ed. London, William Heinemann Medical Books, 1979.
12. Lawrence K: Use of carbenicillin in two species of tortoise (*Testudo graeca* and *T. hermanni*). Res Vet Sci 40:413–415, 1986.
13. Lawrence K, Muggleton PW, Needham JR: Preliminary study on the use of ceftazidime, a broad spectrum cephalosporin antibiotic, in snakes. Res Vet Sci 36:16–20, 1984.
14. Mader DR: Antibiotic therapy. *In* Frye FL (ed): Biomedical and Surgical Aspects of Captive Reptile Husbandry, 2nd ed. Malabar, Krieger, pp 621–634, 1991.
15. Mautino M, Page CD: Biology and medicine of turtles and tortoises. Vet Clin North Am Sm Animal Pract 23:1251–1270, 1993.
16. McDonald HS: Methods for the physiological study of reptiles. *In* Gans C, Dawson WR (eds): Biology of the Reptilia, vol 5. London, Academic Press, pp 19–125, 1976.
17. Perschmann C: Über die Bedeutung der Nierenpfortader insbesondere für die Ausscheidung von Harnstoff und Harnsaure bei *Testudo hermanni* Gml und *Lacerta viridis* Laur. sowie über die Funktion der Harnblase bei *Lacerta viridis* Laur. Zool Beitr 2:447–480, 1956.
18. Prezant RM, Isaza R, Jacobson ER: Plasma concentrations and disposition kinetics of enrofloxacin in gopher tortoises (*Gopherus polyphemus*). J Zoo Wildl Med 25:82–87, 1994.
19. Raphael BL, Papich M, Cook RA: Pharmacokinetics of enrofloxacin after a single intramuscular injection in Indian star tortoises (*Geochelone elegans*). J Zoo Wildl Med 25:88–94, 1994.
20. Rennick BR, Gandia H: Pharmacology of smooth muscle valve in

renal portal circulation of birds. Proc Soc Exp Biol Med 85:234–236, 1954.
21. Sawyer WH: Effect of posterior pituitary extracts on urine formation and glomerular circulation in the frog. Am J Physiol 164:457–464, 1951.
22. Schmidt-Nielsen B, Davis LE: Fluid transport and tubular intercellular spaces in reptilian kidneys. Science 159:1105–1108, 1968.
23. Schmidt-Nielson B, Skadhauge E: Function of the excretory system

of the crocodile (*Crocodylus acutus*). Am J Physiol 212:973–980, 1967.
24. Vancutsem PM, Babish JG, Schwark WS: The fluoroquinolone antimicrobials: structure, antimicrobial activity, pharmacokinetics, clinical use in domestic animals and toxicity. Cornell Vet 80:173–186, 1990.
25. Whelton A, Neu HC (eds): The aminoglycosides: microbiology, clinical use, and toxicology. New York, Marcel Dekker, 1982.

CHAPTER 33

Periodontal Disease in Lizards

HELEN E. McCRACKEN

Periodontal disease is a significant cause of morbidity in captive lizards, occurring primarily in agamids and chameleons. This disorder was first described in 1994 in a review of 42 cases seen by the author during a 5-year period.[11] The species affected were all agamids and chameleons, including the common bearded dragon (*Pogona barbata*), inland bearded dragon (*Pogona vitticeps*), dwarf bearded dragon (*Pogona brevis*), eastern water dragon (*Physignathus lesueurii*), frilled lizard (*Chlamydosaurus kingii*), sail-finned water dragon (*Hydrosaurus pustulatus*), and Jackson's chameleon (*Chamaeleo jacksonii*).[11] Periodontal disease is also seen infrequently in lizards from other families, including the Eastern blue-tongue skink (*Tiliqua scincoides scincoides*) and the banded Fijian iguana (*Brachylophus fasciatus*) (Table 33–1).

The term *periodontal disease* refers to diseases of the periodontium, which in mammals comprises the gingiva, periodontal ligament, alveolar bone, and cemental surface of the tooth. Periodontal disease includes gingivitis, periodontitis, and periodontal abscessation.[6] Gingivitis is reversible inflammation of the marginal gingiva, caused by bacteria in plaque, an invisible material that accumulates on teeth and gums if they are not kept clean by mastication of a diet of suitable texture and consistency. Periodontitis is the extension of gingivitis to involve the periodontal ligament, causing irreversible loss of connective tissue attachment and bone.[2] The bacteria in plaque are initially predominantly non-motile, gram-positive aerobic cocci. As the plaque matures, however, there is a change to a predominantly anaerobic flora, including gram-negative motile rods and spirochetes.[2, 8] Clinical signs of periodontal disease in mammals include gingival erythema and swelling, supragingival and subgingival accumulation of dental calculus (mineralized plaque), periodontal pockets, and

gingival recession. Gingival hyperplasia may also occur.[6]

The dental and gingival anatomy of agamids and chameleons differs markedly from that of mammals. Agamids and chameleons are unique among lizards in that they have acrodont dentition. The only other reptile with this dentition type is the tuatara. Acrodont teeth are simple laterally compressed triangular structures that are ankylosed to the crests of the mandibles and maxillae. They are not continually replaced throughout life as are the teeth of other reptiles, but progressively wear with age. Other lizards have pleurodont teeth that are affixed to the lingual aspect of the jaws, in some cases resting on and attached to a bony shelf. These teeth are continually shed and replaced. Many agamids have a few pleurodont teeth rostrally.[4] A major difference between these dentition types is the position of the gingival margin (i.e., the visible gum line). In pleurodonts, as in mammals, this margin is immediately distal to the crests of the mandibles and maxillae, whereas in acrodonts it is at a faint longitudinal ridge of bone several millimeters from this point (Fig. 33–1). The exposed bone distal to the gingival margin has a slight sheen, distinguishing it from the bone to which soft tissue is attached. Therefore, the periodontium of acrodont lizards consists of the gingiva, the bone-gingiva interface, and the bone of the mandibles and maxillae. There is no periodontal ligament.

CLINICAL FINDINGS

Periodontal disease in lizards is a progressive condition. The earliest signs are mild erythema at the gingival margin and minimal calculus deposition on the teeth and exposed bone of the jaws. Both lingual and buccal aspects of the jaws are affected. Progressively heavier

TABLE 33–1. Lizard Periodontal Disease Cases, Melbourne Zoo, Australia, 1989–1996

Species	Mild to Moderate Periodontal Disease*		Severe Periodontal Disease Without Osteomyelitis†		Severe Periodontal Disease With Osteomyelitis‡	
	No. of Cases	No. Resolved	No. of Cases	No. Resolved	No. of Cases	No. Resolved
Pogona barbata	6	6	3	3	4	3
Pogona vitticeps	4	4	3	1	3	2
Pogona minor	2	2	2	2	1	—
Physignathus lesueurii lesueurii	4	4	—	—	—	—
Chlamydosaurus kingii	5	5	—	—	—	—
Hydrosaurus pustulatus	2	2	—	—	—	—
Chamaeleo jacksonii	—	—	—	—	3	1
Tiliqua scincoides	1	1	—	—	—	—
Brachylophus fasciatus	1	1	—	—	—	—
Total	25	25	8	6	11	6

*Cases with mild to moderate gingivitis, with or without mild to moderate gingival recession, with or without mild to moderate calculus deposition.

†Cases with moderate to heavy calculus deposition, extensive gingival recession, and inflammation with or without hyperplasia. Some lizards had localized subcutaneous abscesses over the mandible or maxilla.

‡Cases with associated osteomyelitis lesions in the maxilla or mandible. Most lizards had localized subcutaneous abscesses adjacent to bone lesion.

calculus deposition, more intense gingival erythema and swelling, and varying degrees of recession of gingiva from its point of normal attachment occur, exposing the underlying bone of the jaws. Gingival recession may progress until the entire lateral aspect of the mandibles and maxillae is exposed. In some cases, the ventral border of the mandibles is exposed, resulting in pocket formation ventral to the bone and creating the potential for food impaction. In advanced disease, gingival hyperplasia, suppurative gingivitis with pocket formation, and subcutaneous abscessation over mandibles or maxillae may also be present. Focal or multifocal osteomyelitis of the mandible or maxilla may also occur, in some cases precipitating pathologic fractures. Most cases of

osteomyelitis involve localized subcutaneous abscesses adjacent to the bone lesion. Some cases eventuate in fatal systemic infections, including septicemia and pneumonia.

HISTOPATHOLOGY

Histologic examination of the jaws of a healthy agamid (Figs. 33–2, 33–3) reveals the acrodont teeth to be composed of dentine in regular parallel dentinal tubules. With age, these structures are progressively worn until they no longer exist. The margins of the mandibles and maxillae then serve as the masticatory cutting edges.[4]

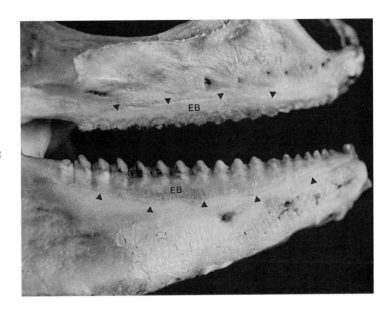

FIGURE 33–1. Skull of healthy *Physignathus lesueurii lesueurii* showing acrodont teeth, position of gingival margin *(arrows),* and exposed bone of mandible and maxilla (EB).

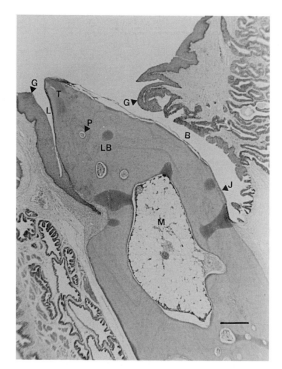

FIGURE 33–2. Cross section of mandible of healthy *Pogona barbata.* T, acrodont tooth; LB, lamellar bone; P, pulp tissue; M, bone marrow; B, buccal gingival sulci; L, lingual gingival sulci; J, junctional epithelium; G, gingival margin. (Hematoxylin and eosin; bar = 300 μm.)

Vital pulp tissue with an intact layer of odontoblasts is present distally, and the dentinal tubules emanate from these cells. The teeth are in continuity with vital lamellar bone that contains numerous osteocytes in lacunae. A gingival sulcus is present on both buccal and lingual aspects with thin (approximately three cell rows), flat, nonkeratinized stratified squamous epithelium attached to the bone. This junctional epithelium is in continuity with thicker, nonkeratinized stratified squamous epithelium of the gingival sulcus.

In specimens with clinical evidence of disease (Figs. 33–4, 33–5), dental calculus covered with bacteria is present on the tooth and bone surfaces both supragingivally and subgingivally, on both the buccal and lingual aspects of the jaws. In many cases, the bone adjacent to these calculus deposits lacks osteocytes and hence is considered to be nonvital. Numerous inflammatory cells (both mononuclear leukocytes and heterophils) may be present in the bone marrow. The junctional epithelium attachment migrates proximally, increasing the depth of the gingival sulcus, and adjacent bone is irregular and resorbed to varying degrees. In some cases, significant bone defects are present, filled with large clumps of dental calculus. Occasionally, multinucleated giant cells are present in the areas of bone resorption. Aggregations of inflammatory cells, predominately mononuclear leukocytes, are present in the underlying connective tissue of the gingival sulcus, and the junctional epithelium may be hyperplastic with a convoluted surface.

BACTERIOLOGY

A study was undertaken of the bacterial flora present at the bone-gingiva junction in healthy agamids and in those with periodontal disease.[11] The results are summarized in Table 33–2. The group of healthy lizards was composed of two *P. vitticeps* and three *P. minor;* the affected lizards were two *P. vitticeps,* three *P. barbata,* one *P. minor,* four *P. lesueurii lesueurii,* five *C. kingii,* and two *H. pustulatus.* Aerobic bacteria cultured from the healthy lizards included *Escherichia coli,* other coliforms, and *Corynebacterium* species. A wider range of aerobes was cultured from the affected lizards, including *Pseudomonas* species, *E. coli,* other coliforms, *Proteus* species, *Acinetobacter* species, *Aeromonas* species, *Staphylococcus* species, and *Streptococcus* species. Anaerobic bacteria from these animals were predominantly gram-negative bacilli, including *Bacteroides* species, and *Fusobacterium* species. Anaerobic streptococci and *Clostridium* species were also present.[11]

Pseudomonas species was demonstrated to be causally associated (Fischer's exact test, $p = 0.01$) with the presence of periodontal disease, and there was a trend for causal association with *Bacteroides* species. The findings of this study demonstrate a similarity to the microbiology of mammalian periodontal disease. In affected mammals, there is a change from the predominantly aerobic flora of the healthy mouth to a princi-

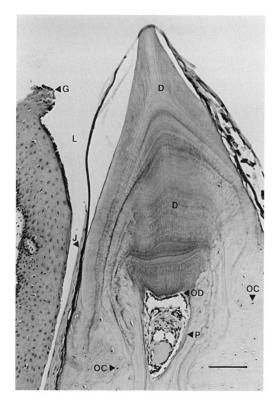

FIGURE 33–3. Mandible of healthy *Pogona barbata.* D, dentinal tubules; OD, odontoblasts; OC, osteocytes. (Hematoxylin and eosin; bar = 100 μm.)

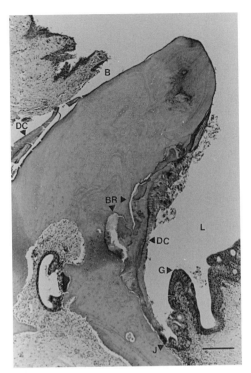

FIGURE 33–4. Maxilla of *Pogona vitticeps* with periodontal disease. DC, dental calculus; BR, bone resorption. (Hematoxylin and eosin; bar = 300 μm).

pally anaerobic flora, including spirochetes.[8] However, whereas the predominant aerobes in mammalian mouths are gram-positive cocci,[8] gram-negative bacilli predominated in the agamids, as has been reported for the oral flora of other reptiles.[3] Bacteria cultured from osteomyelitis lesions in seven agamids and two chameleons included *Pseudomonas aeruginosa* (n = 4), *Proteus* species (n = 1), *E. coli* (n = 1), *Corynebacterium* (n = 1), *Yersinia enterocolitica* (n = 1), and *Proteus mirabilis* (n = 1).[11]

EPIDEMIOLOGY AND POSSIBLE CAUSES

Periodontal disease has been seen only in captive lizards. Examination of alcohol-preserved museum speci-

TABLE 33–2. Bacteria Cultured from Bone-Gingiva Junction of Healthy and Affected Agamid Lizards

Culture Result*	Healthy Mouths (n = 5)	Affected Mouths (n = 17)
Aerobes only	5	2
Aerobes and anaerobes	—	8
Aerobes, anaerobes, and spirochetes	—	7

*Cultures performed aerobically at 28° and 35°C and anaerobically at 35°C.

mens of wild-caught adult and juvenile *P. vitticeps* (n = 8), *P. barbata* (n = 5), *P. lesueurii* (n = 8), and *C. kingii* (n = 5) detected no evidence of periodontal calculus, gingival swelling, recession, or bone loss.[11] In the reported cases of disease in captive lizards, there was no apparent gender predilection, and the age of affected animals ranged from 2 to more than 20 years (exact age unknown).

Inappropriate captive diet appears to be the major precipitating factor in this disease. The natural diet of most agamids and chameleons consists mainly of a wide range of insects and arachnids, including hard-bodied species such as beetles and cockroaches and relatively large species such as grasshoppers and locusts. Small vertebrates, mainly lizards, are eaten occasionally.[5, 10] Some species, including *Pogona* species and *P. lesueurii,* also eat a variety of fruits, flowers, and leaves.[5]

In the reported cases of periodontal disease (see Table 33–1), *Pogona* species, *P. lesueurii lesueurii,* and *H. pustulatus* lizards were fed a diet of live crickets and mealworms regularly supplemented with a diced vegetable and fruit mixture. Although ideally this mixture is predominantly distinct, firm, 7- to 10-mm³ vegetable pieces, it was sometimes finely diced, soft, and mainly fruit. Nine *P. barbata* and *P. vitticeps* lizards were examined after 2 to 3 years on the soft diet and were found to have moderate to severe periodontal disease. Six *P. lesueurii lesueurii* and *H. pustulatus*

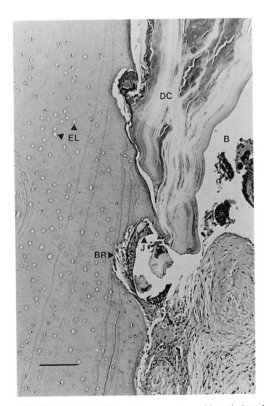

FIGURE 33–5. Mandible of *Pogona minor* with periodontal disease. EL, empty osteocyte lacunae. (Hematoxylin and eosin; bar = 100 μm).

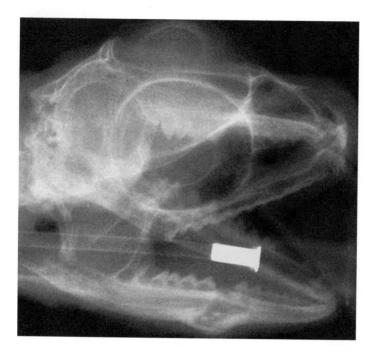

FIGURE 33–6. Radiograph of *Hydrosaurus pustulatus* with osteomyelitis of the mandible. Focal lucency, bone sequestra, peripheral bone sclerosis, and periosteal new bone can be seen.

lizards had mild disease after at least 4 years on the firm diet. Affected *C. jacksonii* and *C. kingii* lizards were fed only live insects, mostly crickets and mealworms; disease developed after periods of 2 to 4 years. It was concluded that all diets were inappropriately soft, precipitating excessive plaque accumulation.[11] Crickets and mealworms are soft-bodied insects that require minimal mastication compared with many of the natural prey items. The diets of *C. jacksonii* and *C. kingii* lizards were therefore modified to include harder and larger invertebrates such as grasshoppers, beetles, cockroaches, moths, and snails, which require longer periods of mastication. The diet of the omnivorous species is now composed of an increased proportion of insects, including the hard-bodied species, with less frequent firm fruit and vegetable supplementation. Dandelions, clover, and other flowers and leaves have been added as regular, more natural food items. No new cases of periodontal disease were diagnosed in the 2 to 3 years after these changes were implemented.

Systemic factors, including nutritional disorders and immunocompromise due to concurrent disease or environmental stress, may contribute to periodontal disease development in mammals by altering periodontal health and decreasing resistance to infection.[7] These may also be precipitating factors in lizards. Chameleons and some agamid species, including *C. kingii,* and *P. minor,* appear to be highly sensitive to captive environmental stress.[9]

DIAGNOSIS

Periodontal disease in lizards is an insidious condition in that it generally does not manifest with overt signs until it is well advanced. Earlier stages frequently go unnoticed because they are detectable only on examina-

tion of the oral cavity. Furthermore, these early changes are frequently not recognized as disease because many observers are unfamiliar with normal periodontal anatomy. Overt signs of the disease include severe gingival erythema and hyperplasia, focal facial subcutaneous swellings, and intermittent mouth gaping. Diagnosis of most cases is by clinical examination of a conscious patient, with the periodontal tissues revealed by dorsal and ventral reflection of the lips while the mouth is held closed. All lizards with subcutaneous facial abscesses are investigated for the presence of osteomyelitis. Most osteomyelitis lesions manifest as focal deficits or areas of soft bone in the surface of the jaws exposed by receded gingiva. These either are readily visible or are detected by exploration with a curet. Radiography is used to determine the extent and severity of these lesions. Other lesions occur within the bone and are detectable by radiography. Radiographic changes include bone lysis, presence of sequestra, adjacent areas of increased bone density, and periosteal new bone (Fig. 33–6). Material from abscesses and osteomyelitis lesions is submitted for aerobic and anaerobic culture and antibiotic sensitivity testing at 28° and 35°C. Gingival cultures are generally not helpful in guiding therapy because of the wide range of organisms present.

TREATMENT

Treatment of periodontal disease involves anesthesia to permit thorough removal of calculus by means of both hand instruments and ultrasonic scaling. Supragingival and subgingival scaling is performed on both buccal and lingual aspects. Gingival pockets are treated with curettage and irrigated liberally with 0.2% chlorhexidine mouthwash (Nolvosan, Fort Dodge, US; Chlorohex, Colgate-Orapharm, Australia). Chlorhexidine is the antiseptic of choice for the treatment of mammalian periodontal disease because it has a wide range of efficacy and binds electrostatically to bacterial and oral surfaces, thereby inhibiting bacterial adhesion.[2] After application, it produces an immediate bactericidal effect, followed by prolonged bacteriostatic action, reducing dental plaque formation and associated gingivitis.[1] Abscesses are incised, drained, curetted, flushed with sterile saline, and left open. Osteomyelitis lesions are treated by curettage, saucerization to prevent food entrapment, and thorough saline irrigation. Parenteral antibiotics are given in all cases, the drugs of choice being ceftazidime, 20 mg/kg IM every 72 hours, or a combination of amikacin, initially 5 mg/kg IM then 2.5 mg/kg every 72 hours, and piperacillin, 100 mg/kg IM every 48 hours. These drugs are all well distributed to bone and are generally effective against the range of organisms involved.[1] Antibiotics are later changed if indicated by culture and sensitivity results in patients with abscesses or osteomyelitis. Antibiotic course duration ranges from 2 to 4 weeks for mild to moderate cases to 6 to 10 weeks for cases involving osteomyelitis. In addition to undergoing parenteral therapy, the periodontal tissues and any open soft tissue or bone lesions are irrigated daily with 0.2% chlorhexidine or less frequently in lizards overly stressed by frequent handling. In osteomyelitis cases, anesthesia is repeated at 2- to 3-week intervals for thorough cleaning of lesions, including further curettage if necessary. If the lesions are progressive, repeated cultures are taken and antibiotics are changed if indicated. Radiographs are taken at the completion of therapy to confirm resolution of lesions. After cessation of treatment, oral bone deficits are checked frequently for food impaction and signs of infection. In most cases, these deficits eventually fill with bone or fibrous tissue. Prognosis is guarded for osteomyelitis in chameleons[9] and other sensitive species

because they may be chronically stressed by the intense and prolonged treatment required for resolution of this problem, and death may result. If the treatment intensity is decreased to reduce stress, lesions may fail to resolve, necessitating euthanasia. Treatment success is indicated in Table 33–1. Gingival recession is irreversible, and affected animals are prone to recurrent calculus deposition and gingivitis despite dietary modification. To prevent further progression of disease, affected animals are anesthetized for oral prophylaxis every 6 months.

REFERENCES

1. Badewitz-Dodd LH: Mims Annual, 17th ed. Sydney, Australia, IMS Publishing, 1993.
2. Coles S: The use of antimicrobial agents as an adjunct in the treatment of canine periodontal disease. Post-Graduate Committee of Veterinary Science, Control and Therapy 168, Supplement, University of Sydney, Sydney, Australia, 1992.
3. Cooper JE: Bacteria. *In* Cooper JE, Jackson OF (eds): Diseases of the Reptilia, vol 1. London, Academic Press, pp 165–191, 1981.
4. Edmund AG: Dentition. *In* Gans C, Bellairs Ad'A, Parsons TS (eds): Biology of the Reptilia, vol 1. London, Academic Press, pp 117–200, 1969.
5. Ehmann H: Encyclopaedia of Australian Animals. Sydney, Australia, Angus & Robertson, 1992.
6. Harvey CE, O'Brien JA, Rossman LE, et al: Oral, dental, pharyngeal and salivary gland disorders. *In* Ettinger SJ (ed): Textbook of Veterinary Internal Medicine, 2nd ed. Philadelphia, WB Saunders, pp 1126–1191, 1983.
7. Hennet PR: Periodontal disease and oral microbiology. *In* Crossley DA, Penman S (eds): Manual of Small Animal Dentistry, 2nd ed. Cheltenham, UK, BSAVA, pp 105–113, 1995.
8. Hennet PR, Harvey CE: Aerobes in periodontal disease in the dog: a review. J Vet Dent 8:9–11, 1991.
9. Jenkins JR: Husbandry and diseases of Old World chameleons. J Sm Exot Anim Med 1:166–171, 1992.
10. Martin J: Chameleons, Nature's Masters of Disguise. London, Blandford, 1992.
11. McCracken HE, Birch CA: Periodontal disease in lizards: a review of numerous cases. Proceedings of the American Association of Zoo Veterinarians, Pittsburgh, 108–115, 1994.

PART III

AVIAN MEDICINE

CHAPTER 34

Iron Overload in the Animal Kingdom

LINDA J. LOWENSTINE

LINDA MUNSON

Iron is essential for all living things. It plays a pivotal role in oxidation and reduction reactions by virtue of its ability to exist as either a ferrous (Fe^{2+}) or ferric (Fe^{3+}) ion. This property allows iron to participate in oxygen delivery (e.g., hemoglobin and myoglobin), oxidative metabolism (e.g., cytochrome P450), and other enzymatic processes (e.g., ribonucleic acid reductase), but it also makes iron a potent toxin. To keep iron under control, all living organisms have evolved proteins especially designed for iron uptake, transport (transferrins), utilization (e.g., hemoglobin), and storage (ferritin and hemosiderin).[5]

Iron storage occurs when iron uptake exceeds utilization, excretion, or both. Because mechanisms for excretion are limited, regulation of uptake is essential. During prenatal development, mammals receive iron transplacentally, whereas birds and reptiles rely on iron laid down in the yolk and albumin. Neonates are usually replete with iron. Postnatally, regulation of absorption occurs at the level of the duodenal enterocytes.[21] Iron uptake is high in infants and juveniles to accommodate growth and development. Normally uptake is minimal in adult mammals (mucosal blockade) but may be enhanced by anemia, pregnancy, or iron complexed with heme or in the presence of ascorbate and citrate. Iron absorption is blocked by the presence of phytates, tan-

nins, and other chemicals found primarily in fruits, leaves, and other plant parts. Some controversy exists as to whether mucosal blockade is present equally in all species of mammals and birds.

Iron storage is a normal physiologic process that becomes pathologic when excessive. Iron is stored in either ferritin or hemosiderin moieties. Ferritin is dispersed free in the cytosol and is not readily visualized on routine histologic study or with special stains for iron. Hemosiderin is seen as golden brown granules on hematoxylin and eosin staining and has a blue-green (Prussian blue) reaction with stains for iron (e.g., Perl's stain).[20] Especially in hepatocytes, hemosiderin must be distinguished from other pigments, such as lipofuscin and bile. Koalas (*Phascolarctos cinereus*), howler monkeys (*Alouatta* species), and golden lion tamarins (*Leontopithecus rosalia*) have all been reported to have pigmentary hepatopathy due to noniron pigments.[41]

Iron accumulation or overload is termed *hemosiderosis* or *siderosis* when toxic effects of iron are not identified and *hemochromatosis* when there is functional or morphologic evidence of iron toxicity. Hemosiderosis and hemochromatosis may be primary (hereditary) or secondary (to diet, infections, intoxications, certain anemias, and other conditions).[5, 35] Iron overload syndromes have been best described in humans, but there is also an expanding literature on iron overload in birds and some species of mammals. Little is known about iron overload in amphibians and reptiles. This chapter presents data on iron overload syndromes recognized in zoo and wild animals. Criteria for diagnosis and possible treatments are also discussed. For more detailed information on basic iron metabolism, the reader is referred to current texts and review articles.[5, 11, 19, 35]

IRON OVERLOAD

Mechanisms and Consequences

Iron overload is most often diagnosed postmortem. When a pathologist uses the term *hemosiderosis* or *siderosis,* it means that there is excessive stainable iron in cells, either parenchymal or phagocytic. Stainable iron may result from an absolute increase in intracellular iron or from a shift from ferritin to hemosiderin that takes place when iron stores are excessive or when an iron-containing cell is injured. Hemosiderosis may be the result of primary iron overload due to a hereditary lack of mucosal blockage of iron uptake, or it may be secondary to dietary or parenteral iron overload or a variety of other diseases.[1, 5, 19, 20] Inflammatory processes decrease the release of iron from cells of the reticuloendothelial (RE) system, causing increased storage and hypoferremia. This is thought to be a defense mechanism, "sequestering" iron from invading microorganisms that require iron for replication. RE cell iron increases in aplastic anemias (the so-called iron-loading anemias) or when red blood cells cannot properly utilize iron (thalassemia in humans), especially with concurrent transfusions or parenteral iron administration. Extravascular hemolysis due to hemoparasitism or other causes also increases iron stores. Catabolism of body tissues during fasting or starvation may lead to apparent iron overload. Dietary iron overload (either relative or absolute), especially in the face of liver damage, increases iron stores over time. Both copper deficiency (through ceruloplasmin deficiency) and copper excess seem to block release of iron from RE cells and hepatocytes. Cobalt deficiency also causes iron overload in some species.[20] Conversely, testosterone, estrone, and dexamethasone have been shown to increase iron release from cultured macrophages into the medium. This effect has also been demonstrated in vivo in experiments in which exogenous corticosteroids caused an increase in serum iron available for uptake and storage by hepatocytes.[42]

In hemochromatosis, the presence of the excess iron has proved toxic to the cell, tissue, or organ. In humans, hemochromatosis may be primary, as the result of a hereditary defect causing excessive enteric absorption of iron, or secondary, usually because of dietary overload accompanied by hepatic injury (e.g., alcoholic siderosis), aplastic anemias, or conditions in which there is abnormal utilization of iron by red blood cells (e.g., thalassemia) with or without parenteral iron administration. There is a trend in human medicine to reserve the term *hemochromatosis* for hereditary primary iron storage disease and to use *hemosiderosis* for all other

iron storage problems even in the face of severe organ damage. For veterinary purposes, the authors think it is better to stick to the classic definitions given earlier.

The end result of hemochromatosis is often fibrosis and, in the liver, cirrhosis. Cirrhosis is one of the most serious consequences or iron overload and has been reported in birds and some nonhuman mammals as well. However, toxins and infections that damage the liver can also lead to iron accumulation, so care must be exercised in interpretation of cause and effect. Risk of liver neoplasia is heightened in humans with hemochromatosis, and liver tumors have also been seen in birds and lemurs with iron overload.[8, 43, 44] Other factors, such as hepadnavirus infections and exposure to aflatoxins, may increase this risk. Iron overload may also increase susceptibility to infections, especially when serum iron levels are elevated.[11, 47]

Diabetes is another consequence of hemochromatosis in humans and is thought to be the result of both acinar and islet cell damage by iron. Although both iron overload and diabetes are seen in some species of birds (i.e., Toco toucan [*Ramphastos toco*]), no causal association has been made. Heart failure, due to cardiac arrhythmias induced by interference with electrical conduction or through direct myocardial fiber degeneration, is a common, sometimes fatal, sequela in humans with hemochromatosis. Myocardial iron is seen in animals with iron overload, and heart failure has been suspected in birds with hemochromatosis and coelomic effusions.[24]

Diagnosis

Clinical signs associated with iron overload in animals are usually referable to the liver, although heart failure has been reported. Cutaneous pigmentation and "bronze diabetes," which is a sequela of hemochromatosis in humans, have not been recognized in animals. Chronic wasting is a common feature in both birds and mammals. In birds, abdominal distention secondary to hepatomegaly and coelomic effusion are common signs often accompanied by dyspnea.[17, 24, 28, 37, 40, 47] Radiography may be useful in demonstrating hepatomegaly. Other imaging techniques for visualizing the liver, especially nuclear magnetic resonance, have been proposed for use in the diagnosis of iron overload in humans but are of value only in advanced disease. To the authors' knowledge, this has not been used in animals.

Liver enzyme levels are often elevated if hemochromatosis is present. Hypoproteinemia and other evidence of hepatic insufficiency may be present. Specific tests to assess iron status should be performed, including serum iron, total iron-binding capacity (TIBC), and serum transferrin levels, as well as the percentage of saturation of transferrin (calculated as serum iron ÷ TIBC × 100).[35] The range of normal iron levels varies among species, but average expected mammalian values would be on the order of a serum iron level of 100 μg/dl (range, 55–185 μg/dl); TIBC of about 300 μg/dl (range, 250–425 μg/dl); and a saturation of about 33%. Birds may have a higher saturation than mammals (up to 80%). Published values for avian serum or plasma iron levels vary widely, with the mean serum iron level ranging from 137 to 177 µg/dl in wild starlings to less than 358 µg/dl in ramphastids.[16, 48]

When an animal is in relative iron overload, there is increased saturation of the TIBC. If TIBC saturation is persistently increased, iron overload, liver disease, or abnormal erythropoiesis should be suspected. An elevation of serum iron level may be a reflection of iron overload, but increases can occur from a variety of other factors, including corticosteroid administration (in the dog and horse).[42] Serum ferritin concentrations can also be measured, as can free erythrocyte protoporphyrin and serum haptoglobin. Serum ferritin is the best measurement of iron stores and has been shown to correlate well in humans, dogs, pigs, cats, and horses,[42] but the usual test is immunologic and species specific, limiting its usefulness. Human ferritin antibodies would be expected to be cross-reactive with ape and Old World nonhuman primate ferritin, and horse antiferritin cross-reacts with black rhinoceros ferritin.

Liver biopsy is a mandatory diagnostic adjunct and is generally considered to be more accurate than serologic tests. Exploratory laparotomy (or postmortem examination) often reveals an enlarged liver with a dark, rusty color. If the condition is chronic, gross evidence of fibrosis and even cirrhosis with nodular hyperplasia may be present. Abdominal effusion and fibrin deposition may also be seen. Histologically, iron is found in the liver and may or may not be present in other organs or tissues as well. Sites often affected include heart, pancreas, kidneys, and endocrine organs.[24] The location of iron within the liver and other organs may provide clues about the pathogenesis of the excess iron storage (Table 34–1).

Iron stores can be quantified in biopsy samples by chemical methods often using colorimetry, by atomic absorption spectrophotometry (AAS), by x-ray microanalysis using a scanning electron microscope, or by estimation from histologic sections stained with iron-specific stains using image analysis techniques.[7, 9, 46] Iron levels have been measured from as little as 0.1-mg biopsy specimens using colorimetric methods, although samples weighing more than 0.4 mg were more useful.[32] Iron levels can be measured from deparaffinized samples and from formalin-fixed samples. Samples stored in saline, however, can lose up to 50% of their iron. Dry transportation or freezing of biopsy samples for chemical or AAS analysis is probably best.[32]

Liver iron concentrations are reported variously as micromoles or millimoles per gram or micrograms or milligrams per gram (which equals parts per million) on a dry weight (dw) or wet weight (ww) basis. This variation makes comparisons difficult. One mole of iron equals 55.85 g (the atomic weight). Conversion of ww to dw equivalent is somewhat of a problem, but values of 3.3 and 3.5 g of wet tissue have been estimated as being equivalent to 1 g of dried liver.[9, 18] There is not complete agreement on what constitutes a toxic level of iron in all species, and a wide range of values has been reported in zoo and wild animals. In humans, a level of greater than 400 µmol/g or 22.3 mg/g dw (6371 µg/g ww) is associated with fibrosis and is therefore pathologic,[19] whereas normal human adults usually have less than 1.8 mg/g dw (or 51 µg/g ww).[18] Average values

in reindeer liver range from about 290 µg/g ww in autumn to 2910 µg/g during migration,[3] whereas domestic cattle with hemochromatosis have liver iron concentrations of 8700 µg/g ww.[18] In normal birds, average liver iron levels range from about 170 µg/g ww in galliforms to 1311 to 1672 µg/g in wild starlings.[16, 33] Turkey poults are normally 186.9 µg/g dw (53 µg/g ww) but increased to 697 µg/g dw (199 µg/g ww) when starved for 4 days.[39] In species in which iron overload has been reported, captive individuals had higher levels even in clinically normal birds.[12, 13] The level in a toucan with clinical liver disease was 450 µmol/g dw (25,132 µg/g dw = 7180.7 µg/g ww).[9]

Treatment and Prevention

Principal treatments for iron overload are directed toward removing iron from the erythron by phlebotomy or from the parenchymal organs and RE system by chelation. Treatment of iron overload is best described in humans, but there are reports of both successful and unsuccessful treatment of birds and domestic mammals.[9, 23, 28, 34]

Mobilization of iron by chelation occurs slowly. The most widely used iron chelator is desferoxamine (DFO) B, which is specific for iron. Because of this specificity, it is an excellent tool for reducing iron overload, but it must be given parenterally and has a short plasma half-life.[14, 35] DFO cannot chelate iron from hemoglobin or transferrin. Therefore, the iron available for chelation is that which is stored in cells as ferritin, labile iron, or hemosiderin. DFO can enter hepatocytes and remove labile iron for excretion through the bile and feces. DFO can also compete with transferrin for iron at the hepatocyte membrane and solubilize iron for excretion by the kidneys through glomerular filtration and tubular secretion.

DFO is potentially toxic, and adverse effects documented in humans include ocular, auditory, and cerebral neurotoxicity, all of which are somewhat reversible after cessation of therapy. Acute hypersensitivity-mediated alveolar damage resembling acute respiratory distress syndrome has been reported in patients receiving continuous intravenous DFO. Increased bacterial and fungal infections such as yersiniosis and mucormycosis have been reported in human patients during iron chelation.

In anemia of chronic disease with siderosis of RE cells of liver, spleen, and bone marrow, the stored iron is poorly mobilized by DFO.[14]

Successful treatment of a channel-billed toucan (*Ramphastos vitellinus*) by chelation therapy has been reported.[9] A dose of 100 mg/kg DFO was administered daily subcutaneously in the dorsal neck or chest areas for 110 days. No adverse effects of this treatment were reported. The bird was also maintained on a low-iron diet (<65 ppm). The success of therapy was monitored with monthly hemograms and liver biopsies, samples of which were examined chemically and histologically using image analysis. During treatment, bacterial rhinitis developed. Serum iron levels increased after treatment, as did TIBC, and the liver iron levels declined from 450 to 28 µmol/g dw.

The use of phlebotomy for management of hemochromatosis has also been reported for two toucans[48]

TABLE 34–1. Location and Interpretation of Stainable Iron Stores

Organ	Cell Type	Interpretation
Liver	Kupffer cells	Extravascular hemolysis
		Starvation
		Dietary iron overload (acute)
		Chronic enteric parasitism or red cell parasitism
		Bacterial infections and other inflammatory processes
	Hepatocytes	Increased total iron-binding capacity saturation
		Normal during fetal life and in some neonates
		Corticosteroid administration
		Viral hepatitis
		Other inflammatory processes in liver
		Dietary iron overload (chronic)
		Genetic errors in iron absorption
		Dietary reasons for increased uptake (e.g., ascorbic acid, decreased phytates in diet)
		Decreased iron utilization in some anemias
		Parenteral iron overload (e.g., transfusions)
		Hepatic intoxication (e.g., lead, copper, petroleum products)
		Copper deficiency
		Chronic parasitism
	Macrophages	Centrilobular nodular siderosis—chronic passive congestion
		Nodular siderosis, perioportal or intralobular—hepatocellular necrosis
Spleen	Reticuloendothelial cells	Common incidental aging change
		Starvation or other generalized catabolism
		Increased extravascular hemolysis
		Decreased hematopoietic potential (e.g., anemia of chronic disease
		Chronic passive congestion (right-sided heart failure, hepatic portal hypertension)
Bone marrow	Siderophages	Aging change
		Decreased production of erythrocytes
		Abnormal utilization of iron by erythrocyte precursors
		Copper deficiency
		Anemia of chronic disease
Kidney	Tubular epithelium	Normal in hens during oviposition
		Hemoglobinuria, myoglobinuria, hematuria
		Cobalt deficiency in goats
	Glomeruli	Glomerular hemorrhage
		Entrapment of sideroleukocytes
Leukocytes	Monocytes	Sideroleukocytes
	Neutrophils	Equine infectious anemia
Lungs	Alveolar macrophages	Chronic passive congestion (left-sided heart failure)
		Localized hemorrhage or inflammation
Uterus	Macrophages	Recent estrus (carnivores) or menses (primates)
		Past pregnancy (all eutherian mammals)
Brain	Vessels and neurons	Incidental aging change
	Macrophages	Localized hemorrhage
Intestines	Lamina propria	Dietary iron overload
		Localized hemorrhage
		Incidental finding in horses, guinea pigs, and rabbits
		Necrosis of enterocytes, enteritis
		Starvation
Endocrines	Parenchyma	Generalized iron overload, primary hemochromatosis

and a mynah.[28] Phlebotomy in the toucans was at a rate of 1 ml/week until normal serum iron levels were reached in 4 weeks in one bird and 1 to 2 ml/week for more than 8 weeks in the second bird. On the basis of the experience with the mynah, a proposed treatment regimen included phlebotomy of a volume of 1 to 2 ml/day until clinical improvement or borderline anemia (whichever comes first) followed by weekly phlebotomy until serum iron level is less than 200 μg/ml. It was suggested that serum iron level, TIBC, aspartate aminotransferase level, albumin level, and packed cell volume be monitored; and a low-iron diet was also recommended. Phlebotomy has also been used to treat iron overload in domestic equids.[34]

Thus, success of either phlebotomy or chelation can be measured indirectly by changes in clinical parameters of iron status or by repeated liver biopsies evaluated by the methods described earlier.

Prevention of iron overload in susceptible species (see later discussion) is directed mainly at eliminating factors that exacerbate or contribute to the problem. Dietary modifications include feeding low-iron diets to susceptible birds (<65 ppm) and lemurs, providing more natural diet items or iron chelators such as tree gum for marmosets or tamarind juice and high-fiber biscuits for lemurs and leafy browse for follivores, and limiting dietary items like citrus fruits, which enhance iron abortion.[12, 43] Tap water, especially when it is carried in iron pipes, can also be a source of excess iron. Prevention of infectious diseases such as viral or bacterial hepatitides and hemoprotozoanoses is obviously warranted. For the many species in which the cause of iron overload is unknown, there are no specific prophylactic measures.

IRON OVERLOAD SYNDROMES

Amphibians and Reptiles

The literature on normal iron metabolism and derangements in amphibians and reptiles is not extensive. According to review of pathology records from two zoological collections, stainable hepatocellular iron is not uncommon in anuran amphibians and reptiles of all orders. It usually occurs in the presence of infections, chronic inanition, hepatic lipidosis, or other hepatocellular degeneration. Renal tubular hemosiderosis was also seen in a toad and in snakes and lizards with gram-negative sepsis, possibly secondary to hemolysis. On the basis of this limited study, reptilian iron overload appears to be indicative of an underlying disease problem rather than a primary cause of disease.

Birds

Since the 1970s, literature on iron overload syndromes in birds has been expanding, but there is still much confusion about the significance and pathogenesis. Part of the confusion arises from the indiscriminate use of the term *hemochromatosis* and the failure to distinguish between hemosiderosis and hemochromatosis and between primary and secondary hemochromatosis, especially in case reports. Also confounding is the fact that damage to the liver (e.g., toxins, chlamydial and other infections) may cause iron storage in hepatocytes. The presence of stainable iron does not necessarily mean that the iron caused the liver damage, although when the two are found together it is often tempting to evoke iron toxicity rather than to search extensively for an alternate explanation. It is clear, however, that in some species iron overload is a significant issue in successful captive propagation. It is also clear from the expanding literature on avian iron metabolism that birds may exhibit wide variation in iron storage at various stages of the life cycle, both in terms of age and seasonal events such as migration and molting, which are often accompanied by periods of fasting.

Both pigeons (*Columba livia*) and starlings (*Sturnus vulgaris*) are strong fliers and have larger hearts (relative to body weight), higher hematocrit and hemoglobin concentrations, and higher liver iron content than do relatively sedentary species such as chickens and quail.[16, 36] Seasonal variation in liver iron concentration has been noted in migratory common starlings, with the highest concentration corresponding to the end of moult before fall migration and in wintering birds and the lowest concentrations after breeding in the spring and summer months.[16, 33] Seasonal siderosis has also been reported in female eider ducks, which fast completely during egg laying and brooding (incubation and post-hatch).[2] Suggested pathogeneses for this increase include increased iron absorption before egg production, loss of liver parenchyma during fasting with relative increase in concentration of metals, and increased catabolism of body tissues and the erythron as the result of fasting during the reproductive period. Similar increase in stainable iron has been documented in mallard ducks (*Anas platyrhynchos*) in the postbreeding moult period.[7]

The effect of starvation and subsequent refeeding has been investigated in turkey poults.[39] Effects of starvation are thought to be mediated through corticosterone and glucagon, which cause catabolism of muscle in immature chickens. Increased storage of iron may be a way to conserve iron for reuse by the muscles after refeeding. Repeated starvation and refeeding can produce siderosis in other animal model systems especially if high-iron diets are fed. Starvation increases iron absorption and may cause a more efficient utilization of dietary iron.

Lead poisoning in a variety of water fowl has been associated with the presence of stainable iron in hepatocytes. The causal association with lead has been shown experimentally in cockatiels.[26] Sea birds (Cassin's auklets [*Ptychoramphus aleuticus*] and common murres [*Uria aalge*]) exposed experimentally or accidentally to oil also demonstrate hepatocellular and Kupffer cell iron development.[15] The stress of capture and captivity for as short as 7 days also increased stainable iron in control birds, although not to the extent seen in oil-covered birds. A combination of stress-induced increase in corticosteroids, damage to the erythron, and direct hepatotoxicity may be involved in both lead and oil intoxication.

Experimental iron overload has been produced by both parenteral and enteral (dietary) routes. Administration of intravenous iron dextran to chickens resulted in increased stainable iron in Kupffer cells after 24 hours and in hepatocytes after 48 hours. After 6 to 10 days, the iron was redistributed mainly to the hepatocytes with little stainable iron in the spleen, bone marrow, or intestinal tract. Pigeons and doves given iron in doses of 100 mg/kg body weight daily in their diet accumulated iron.[13] Oral vitamin C supplementation did not seem to have an effect on the mean level of iron in the liver. In another study, iron overload could also be produced in doves given iron doses of 50 mg/kg orally.[13] Liver iron levels became elevated in as little as 2 weeks of treatment, and the concentration increased over time. Feeding trials in mynahs (*Gracula* species) suggested that mynahs more avidly absorbed (or retained) dietary iron than did either doves or rats.[13]

Hemosiderosis is a common postmortem finding in a wide variety of avian species, many but not all of which are frugivorous or insectivorous. According to published reviews of zoo bird pathology as well as reviews by the authors,[7, 12, 17, 24, 44, 46] the orders and families of birds most often involved are presented in Table 34–2. The data coupled with experimental results suggest that in some families, especially Ramphastidae, Sturnidae, and Paradisaeidae, the iron storage may be primary or may be due to a specific sensitivity to dietary overload rather than secondary to infection or inflammation. In these species, iron storage is often found in many organs and tissues, and hepatocellular damage suggestive of hemochromatosis is fairly common. Some other species seem prone to iron overload development in the face of infections (e.g., flamingos and waterfowl). In others such as galliforms, psittacines, and seed-eating passerines (e.g., the finches), hemosiderosis is uncommon. Secondary hemosiderosis, however, can potentially occur in any species of bird, and there are reports in the literature of privately owned psittacines with iron overload reported to have hemosiderosis or even hemochromatosis.[40]

Mammals

In general, the identification of iron overload as a postmortem finding is much less common in mammals than in birds.

TABLE 34–2. **Birds in Which Hepatic or Multisystemic Hemosiderosis Is Often Found on Postmortem Examination**

Passeriformes
    Sturnidae* (mynahs and starlings)
    Paradisaeidae* (birds of paradise)
    Contigadie* (contigas, capuchin bird, umbrella bird)
    Piperidae (manakins)
    Ptylonorhynchidae* (bowerbirds)
    Emberizidae (tanagers, euphonias)
    Corvidae (magpies, crows)
    Laniidae (shrikes)
Coriciiformes
    Alcedinidae (kingfishers)
    Coraciidae (rollers)
    Bucerotidae* (hornbills)
Columbiformes
    Columbidae (fruit doves and imperial pigeons)
Piciformes
    Ramphastidae* (toucans, toucanettes, aracari)
Anseriformes
    Anatidae (eider ducks and others)
Ciconiiformes
    Pheonicopteridae (flamingos)
Cuculiformes
    Muscophagidae (turacos and go-away birds)

---

*Hemochromatosis may be found in addition to hemosiderosis.

NONHUMAN PRIMATES

Hepatocellular iron accumulation has been reported in lemurs,[43] common marmosets, and other callitrichids.[4, 10] It is a common finding in captive lowland gorillas and less so in free-ranging mountain gorillas.

In lemurs, the cause of hepatocellular iron accumulation is suspected to be the feeding of fruits rich in ascorbic acid in the context of a diet lacking the normal tannins, which inhibit iron absorption.[43] In laboratory-housed common marmoset (*Callithrix jacchus*) fed commercial primate diets, stainable iron varied considerably in amount among examined livers but was always present.[10] Accumulation was not related to gender, blood sampling frequency, or age and was present in controls as well as in animals that were part of toxicity assessment trials. Because marmosets normally eat sap and gums in the wild, they too may be suffering from an overavailability of iron as a result of a relative lack of iron-binding substances in their diets. In another colony of common marmosets, however, hemosiderosis was most pronounced in animals with "marmoset wasting syndrome"—chronic tubulointerstitial nephritis and anemia. Increasing the protein in the diet resulted in no further cases of wasting, renal disease, or hemosiderosis.[4]

Although experimental dietary-induced iron overload has been created in baboons and macaques, naturally occurring parenchymal siderosis is uncommon in cercopithecines, and primary hemochromatosis has not been described.[19]

In the lesser apes, hemosiderosis has been described in a siamang gibbon (*Hylobates syndactylus*) with concurrent atypical mycobacteriosis, which suggested that the iron accumulation may have occurred secondary to sequestration of iron.[29] A review of additional siamang necropsies at the same institution, however, revealed hemosiderosis in five of nine additional siamangs but none of the other gibbons. The exact pathogenesis of the hemosiderosis was uncertain. One interesting feature of siderosis in these siamangs was the presence of laminated circular iron concretions.

Examination of pathology reports from gorillas in the North American Species Survival Plan (SSP) cohort revealed that hepatocellular and intestinal pigmentation compatible with or confirmed to be iron was present in all age classes, including some neonates and stillborns. After the neonatal period, hepatocellular iron appears to accumulate with age regardless of gender. In the wild, gorillas are largely folivorous, supplementing their diets with little fruit, whereas citrus and other fruits and vegetables often supplement a commercially prepared diet for gorillas in captivity. Thus, increased ascorbic acid and decreased dietary phytates and tannins may play a role in the hemosiderosis of gorillas. Cardiovascular disease with chronic passive congestion and deficiencies of trace minerals such as copper could also be contributory. Similarly, hepatocellular and intestinal (lamina proprial) hemosiderosis is often present in the folivorous colobine monkeys, including the African colobus and Asian langurs.

A review of necropsy reports from older orangutans in the SSP population suggested that hemosiderosis is a less common finding than in gorillas. Systemic hemosiderosis involving hepatocytes and RE cells was occasionally present in old animals, especially those with fibrosing cardiomyopathy, chronic interstitial nephritis, or chronic infections such as bronchopneumonia, air sacculitis, or, in one case, a pelvic abscess. Severe hepatocellular siderosis was present in one old female with cirrhosis. As in the other primates discussed, the iron accumulation in orangutans may be multifactorial.

PERISSODACTYLS

Hepatic, splenic, and intestinal hemosiderosis without accompanying fibrosis is a common finding in captive back rhinoceroses (*Diceros bicornis*).[22, 27, 42] Hemolytic anemia is a common disease in this species, and black rhinos that die of anemia invariably have hemosiderosis. However, hemosiderosis also occurs without clinically evident hemolysis.[27] In a study comparing tissue iron deposition in free-ranging and recently caught rhinoceroses with that in rhinos that were held captive during translocation or in permanent captivity, significant iron deposition was found only in animals held 2 or more weeks. All captive black rhinos examined had systemic hemosiderosis. Iron deposits were identified in spleen, liver, lung, intestinal lamina propria, kidney, lymph nodes, adrenal glands, and bone marrow. Rhinoceroses with hemosiderosis were in poor body condition, but there was no concrete evidence of hemolysis or infection.[22]

In a review of four necropsies of zoo-housed Sumatran rhinos (*Didermocerus sumatrensis*), a species in which hemolytic anemia has not been documented, systemic hemosiderosis was present in all animals. It was more marked in two animals with chronic renal disease and weight loss than in animals that died of acute large colon torsion while in good nutritional condition.

Hemosiderosis does not seem to be as common a finding in either tapirs or equids. A review of mortality in tapirs (family Tapiridae) revealed a diagnosis of hemosiderosis in only 4 of 108 individuals (see Chapter 82). Two of these animals had chronic wasting of undetermined cause and two had chronic inflammatory disease processes.

Intestinal lamina proprial hemosiderosis, most pronounced in the duodenum, was considered to be an incidental but striking lesion in horses and ponies from one geographic area.[31] Siderosis associated with severe liver disease, including fibrosis, suggesting a diagnosis of hemochromatosis, has also been reported in horses and a pony, but the etiology was undetermined.[23, 34] It is possible that severe liver disease caused the accumulation of iron and not vice versa. Among zoo-housed equids, notable hemosiderosis of the liver, spleen, and intestine has been seen in Persian onagers.

ARTIODACTYLS

Neonatal hepatocellular hemosiderosis is also fairly common and is a reflection of the role of the liver in hematopoiesis in fetal life and the shift from fetal to postnatal types of hemoglobin found in some species.[20, 21] Examples of species in which it has been seen include Thompson's and Soemmering's gazelles (*Gazella tompsoni* and *Gazella sommerringi*), Markhor (*Capra falconer; heptneri*), West Caucasian tur (*Capra ibex caucasica*), mouflon sheep (*Ovis musimon*), Nubian ibex (*Capra ibex*), Burmese Thamin (*Cervus eldi*) and Formosan sika (*Cervus nippon*) deer, North Indian muntjac (*Muntiacus* species), and dik-dik (*Madoqua* species). Neonatal hemosiderosis is usually considered to be an incidental finding. In one gazelle and two sheep, however, intracanalicular bile stasis was also present, suggesting neonatal isoerythrolysis.

Neonatal hemosiderosis progressing to hemochromatosis has been identified in bongos (*Boocercus euryceros*) from one collection. Most calves had marked hepatic hemosiderosis at birth with prominent iron deposition in hepatocytes and iron-laden macrophages in portal areas. During the first few weeks, however, many neonates became progressively anorectic and lethargic and progressed to prostration and death. A few 2- to 4-week-old calves have had hepatic fibrosis and bile duct hyperplasia accompanying the accumulation of iron in hepatocytes, in portal siderophages, in Kupffer cells, and occasionally in biliary epithelium. Bongos in this group that survived to adulthood had iron predominantly in Kupffer cells, and bridging fibrosis was seen in only one adult. As mentioned, the presence of parenchymal iron in neonates by itself is not pathologic. However, the progression to hemochromatosis suggests that true iron overload was present and that there may have been a defect in transplacental iron transport. The disease in the bongo calves somewhat resembles neonatal hemochromatosis in human infants, the cause of which is poorly understood but is hypothesized to be a primary transplacental hyperabsorption of iron.[21] It also resembles hereditary hemochromatosis of Saler's cattle in which a common male ancestor was detected but for which the mode of inheritance has not been determined.[18]

Seasonal iron overload has been documented in Svalbard reindeer (*Rangifer tarandus*) from Norway.[3] This iron accumulation was influenced by starvation during the late winter and was exacerbated by ingestion of marginal forage plants such as mosses that were high in iron. In cases of starvation alone, iron accumulation was primarily in RE cells, whereas reindeer ingesting high iron forage had iron deposited in the hepatocytes as well.

In other adult hoofstock, severe hemosiderosis involving RE cells but also hepatocytes and renal tubular epithelium has been seen in bay duikers (*Cephalophus dorsalis dorsalis*) and a dik-dik (*Madoqua* species). The cause of the iron overload was not determined but was probably of the secondary type because most of these animals had evidence of concurrent infections or hemorrhage.

Splenic hemosiderosis is a common finding in aging artiodactyls and other animals.[20]

CARNIVORES

Felids. Hepatic hemosiderosis is common in captive cheetahs. In a survey of 75 captive cheetahs, Kupffer cell hemosiderosis was found in 83% and hepatocellular iron in 52%. Hemosiderosis has not been identified in the livers of 21 wild cheetahs examined to date. The hematocrit of cheetahs decreases proportional to the time in captivity, possibly indicating that subclinical hemolysis or erythron regeneration failure may be the basis for hepatic iron accumulation. It also is possible that acquisition of infections in captivity leads to iron shunting to the liver. Hemosiderosis is not accompanied by fibrosis and is not statistically correlated with veno-occlusive disease.

In snow leopards, 30 of 46 livers (65%) had iron accumulations (siderosis) in Kupffer cells or hepatocytes, which was moderate to severe in 24. Hepatic siderosis was less prevalent in leopards less than 1 year old (3 of 10) than in leopards more than 1 year old, although there was no increase in prevalence with age in leopards older than 1 year. Of 30 snow leopards with siderosis, 28 (93%) had concurrent subintimal fibrosis of sinusoids, central veins, and sublobular veins, but 10 of 43 (23%) leopards with subintimal fibrosis had no evidence of siderosis. Also, the degree of siderosis was not associated necessarily with the severity of vascular fibrosis.[30]

Hemosiderosis is occasionally seen in other big cats but not as prominently as in snow leopards and cheetahs. True hemochromatosis has not been seen by either author in any species of Felidae. Given the nearly purely carnivorous nature of the feline diet, these species would be expected to have a highly effective mucosal blockade to prevent excessive iron absorption.

Other Carnivores. Among other carnivores, hepatic hemosiderosis is often found in procyonids, including red pandas (*Ailurus fulgens*) and coati (*Nasua* species). An inciting cause is not always evident.

MARINE MAMMALS

Neonatal hepatocellular hemosiderosis is common in Pacific harbor seal pups (*Phoca vitulina richardsi*) found dead on the rookeries or dying in rehabilitation centers. Some but not all of these pups have had concurrent infections, especially gastroenteritis or omphalitis. A shift from fetal to postnatal hemoglobin is suspected, and neonatal jaundice is common. In northern elephant seals (*Mirounga angustirostris*), hepatocellular, Kupffer cell, and splenic hemosiderosis are impressive and ubiquitous in weanlings that die during rehabilitation. These pups normally undergo a postweaning fast in which they return nearly to their birth weight from a nursing weight of nearly four times as much. It is assumed that starvation contributes to the increase in stainable iron in these pups. Parasitism may also play a role.

Fasting is probably responsible for the ubiquitous presence of massive amounts of stainable iron in hepatocytes and Kupffer cells of California grey whales (*Eschrichtius gibbosus*) that strand on the California coast during migration, despite the implication of pollution by the lay press.

MISCELLANEOUS MAMMALS

As in species described earlier, neonatal hepatocellular hemosiderosis is thought to have been an incidental finding in several macropod joeys.

Hemosiderosis and hemochromatosis have been reported in the Afghan pika (*Ochotona rufescens*), a species in which there is a high prevalence of autoimmune hemolytic anemia.[25] In decreasing order of prevalence, iron was increased in the liver, gastrointestinal tract, mesenteric lymph nodes, spleen, kidney, adrenal gland, and bone. In the liver, both hepatocytes and Kupffer cells were involved in all animals. Two thirds of the animals had mild to moderate fibrosis, but this did not always correlate with the degree of stainable iron. It was postulated that both hemolysis and intestinal absorption played a role in the iron overload.

The rock hyrax is another species in which iron overload is commonly seen.[38] In the early reports of hemochromatosis in this species, iron was prominent in RE cells in intestine, spleen, lymph nodes, and hepatocytes. Hepatic fibrosis was also seen in many animals, suggesting that iron-associated hepatic damage or true hemochromatosis was present, but the amount of stainable iron was not always correlated with the degree of fibrosis. Historically, hyraxes were often infected with *Grassinema procavia,* which causes ulcerative gastritis and gastric hemorrhage. However, cases of severe hemosiderosis have been seen in hyrax without parasitism, although other inflammatory processes such as metritis were present. It is likely that the iron overload seen in the hyrax is multifactorial.

In gerbils, hepatic cirrhosis was associated with repeated episodes of endotoxin-induced hepatic necrosis and hemorrhage with resultant hemosiderosis.[6] The accumulation of iron was thought to contribute to the degree of fibrosis. Endotoxin-induced hepatic necrosis apparently is a common spontaneous lesion in many rodents, including gerbils, guinea pigs, and rats.[45] Several other rodent species in the collections reviewed had hepatocellular siderosis. Individuals that also had cirrhosis suggestive of true hemochromatosis included prehensile-tailed porcupine, rock cavy, and a kangaroo rat.

Hepatic hemosiderosis was also common in insectivores examined post mortem at one of the collections but was often associated with infectious disease processes. In the house shrew (*Suncus murinus*), however, predisposing factors were not readily apparent, which suggests the possibility of a primary iron storage problem.

CONCLUSION

In summary, the presence of stainable iron and presumptive iron overload is not an uncommon pathologic finding in captive and free-ranging wild animals. Hemosiderosis is much more common than hemochromatosis, which is seen commonly only in birds, lemurs, bongos, hyraxes, and pikas. Iron overload may be a primary disease problem in these species. It is found in many different scenarios, however. Predisposing conditions such as inflammatory or other chronic disease processes, dietary deficiencies or excesses, and possibly prolonged stress can sometimes be identified. Captive management clearly plays a role in some of the cases. Frequently, however, the pathogenesis or cause is conjectural. Iron overload syndromes throughout the animal kingdom need further documentation and research.

REFERENCES

1. Bonkovsky HL, Banner BF, Lambrecht RW, Rubin RB: Iron in liver diseases other than hemochromatosis. Semin Liver Dis 16:65–82, 1996.
2. Borch-Iohnsen B, Holm H, Jorgensen A, Horheim G: Seasonal siderosis in female eider nesting in Svalbard. J Comp Pathol 104:7–15, 1991.
3. Borch-Iohnsen B, Nilssen KJ: Seasonal iron overload in Svalbard reindeer liver. J Nutr 117:2072–2078, 1987.
4. Brack M, Rothe H: Chronic tubulointerstitial nephritis and wasting disease in marmosets. Vet Pathol 18(Suppl 6):45–54, 1981.
5. Brock JH, Halliday JW, Pippard MJ, Powell LW: Iron Metabolism in Health and Disease. London, WB Saunders, 1994.
6. Carthew P, Edwards RE, Dorman BM: Hepatic fibrosis and iron accumulation due to endotoxin-induced haemorrhage in the gerbil. J Comp Pathol 104:301–311, 1991.
7. Cork SC, Alley MR, Stockdale PHG: A quantitative assessment of hemosiderosis in wild and captive birds using image analysis. Avian Pathol 24:239–254, 1995.
8. Cork SC, Stockdale PHG: Carcinoma with concurrent haemosiderosis in an Australian bittern (*Botaurus poiciloptilus*). Avian Pathol 24:207–213, 1995.
9. Cornelissen H, Ducatelle R, Roels S: Successful treatment of a channel-billed toucan (*Ramphastos vitellinus*) with iron storage disease by chelation therapy: Sequential monitoring of the iron content of the liver during the treatment period by quantitative chemical and image analyses. J Avian Med Surg 9:131–137, 1995.
10. Davy CW, Edmunds JG: Hepatic iron levels in the marmoset (*Callithrix jacchus*). In Tucker MJ, Wadsworth PF (eds): Symposium on Marmoset Pathology. Alderley Park, Macclesfield, UK, ICI PLC, Pharmaceuticals Division, pp 1–6, 1985.
11. deSousa M, Brock JH (eds): Iron in Immunity, Cancer and Inflammation. London, John Wiley & Sons, 1989.
12. Dierenfeld ES, Pini MT, Sheppard CD: Hemosiderosis and dietary iron in birds. J Nutr 124:2685S–2686S, 1994.
13. Dorrenstein GM, Grinwis GM, Dominguez L, et al: An induced iron storage disease syndrome in doves and pigeons: A model for hemochromatosis in mynah birds. In Proceedings of the Association of Avian Veterinarians, New Orleans, pp 108–112, 1992.
14. Feldman BF, Kaneko JJ, Farver TB: Anemia of inflammatory disease in the dog: Availability of storage iron in inflammatory disease. Am J Vet Res 42:586–589, 1981.
15. Fry DM, Lowenstine LJ: Pathology of common murres and Cassin's auklets exposed to oil. Arch Environ Contam Toxicol 14:725–737, 1985.
16. Garcia F, Ramis J, Planas J: Iron content in starlings, *Sturnus vulgaris*. Comp Biochem Physiol 77A:651–654, 1984.
17. Gosselin SJ, Kramer LW: Pathophysiology of excessive iron storage in mynah birds. J Am Vet Med Assoc 183:1238–1240, 1983.
18. House JK, Smith BP, Maas J, et al: Hemochromatosis in Salers cattle. J Vet Intern Med 8:105–111, 1994.
19. Iancu TC: Animal models in liver research: Iron overload. Adv Vet Sci Comp Med 37:379–401, 1993.
20. Kelly WR: The liver and biliary system. In Jubb KVF, Kennedy PC, Palmer N (eds): Pathology of Domestic Animals, 4th ed, vol 2. San Diego, Academic Press, pp 319–406, 1993.
21. Knisely AS: Iron and pediatric liver disease. Semin Liver Dis 14:229–235, 1994.
22. Kock N, Foggin C, Kock MD, Kock R: Hemosiderosis in the black rhinoceros (*Diceros bicornis*): A comparison of free-ranging and recently captured with translocated and captive animals. J Zoo Wildl Med 23:230–243, 1992.
23. Lavoie JP, Teuscher E: Massive iron overload and liver fibrosis resembling hemochromatosis in a racing pony. Equine Vet J 25:552–554, 1993.
24. Lowenstine LJ, Petrak ML: Iron pigment in the livers of birds. In Montali RJ, Migaki G (eds): Comparative Pathology of Zoo Animals. Washington, DC, Smithsonian Institute Press, pp 127–135, 1980.
25. Madarame H, Kumagai M, Suzuki J, et al: Pathology of excessive iron storage in the Afghan pika (*Ochotona rufescens rufescens*). J Comp Pathol 103:351–359, 1990.
26. McDonald SE, Lowenstine LJ: Lead toxicosis in psittacine birds. Proceedings of the 25th International Symposium on the Diseases of Zoo Animals, Vienna, pp 183–196, 1983.
27. Montali RJ, Citino SB: Pathologic findings in captive rhinoceros. In Ryder OA (ed): Rhinoceros Biology and Conservation. San Diego, Zoological Society of San Diego, pp 346–349, 1993.
28. Morris PJ, Avgeris SE, Baumgartner RE: Hemochromatosis in a greater Indian hill mynah (*Gracula religiosa*): case report and review of the literature. J Assoc Avian Vet 3:87–92, 1989.
29. Munson L, Luibel FJ, Van Kruningen HJ: Siderophilic bodies associated with hemosiderois and atypical mycobacterial infection in an island siamang (*Hylobates syndactylus*). J Med Primatol 20:265–270, 1991.
30. Munson L, Worley MB: Veno-occlusive disease in snow leopards (*Panthera uncia*) from zoological parks. Vet Pathol 28:37–45, 1991.
31. Ochoa R, Kolaja GJ, Klei TR: Hemosiderin deposits in the equine small intestine. Vet Pathol 20:641–643, 1983.
32. Olynk JK, O'Neill R, Britton RS, Bacon BR: Determination of hepatic iron concentration in fresh and paraffin-embedded tissue: diagnostic implications. Gasteroenterology 106:674–677, 1994.
33. Osborn D: Seasonal changes in the fat, protein and metal content of the liver of the starling *Sturnis vulgaris*. Environ Pollut 19:145–155, 1979.
34. Pearson EG, Hedstrom OR, Poppenga RH: Hepatic cirrhosis and hemochromatosis in three horses. J Am Vet Med Assoc 204:1053–1056, 1994.
35. Ponka P, Schulman HM, Woodworth RC (eds): Iron Transport and Storage. Boca Raton, FL, CRC Press, 1990.
36. Ramis J, Planas J: Iron metabolism in pigeons. Q J Exp Physiol 63:383–393, 1978.
37. Randell MG, Patnaik AK, Gould WJ: Hepatopathy associated with excessive iron storage in mynah birds. J Am Vet Med Assoc 179:1214–1217, 1981.
38. Rehg JE, Burek JD, Strandberg JD, Montali RJ: Hemochromatosis in the rock hyrax. In Montali RJ, Migaki G (eds): The Comparative Pathology of Zoo Animals. Washington, DC, Smithsonian Institution Press, pp 113–125, 1990.
39. Richards MP, Roebrough RW, Steel NC: Effects of starvation and refeeding on tissue zinc, copper and iron in turkey poults. J Nutr 117:481–489, 1987.
40. Rupiper DJ, Read DH: Hemochromatosis in a hawk-head parrot (*Deroptyus accipitrinus*). J Avian Med Surg 10:24–27, 1996.
41. Schulman FY, Montali RJ, Bush M, et al: Dubin-Johnson–like syndrome in golden lion tamarins (*Leontopithecus rosalia rosalia*). Vet Pathol 30:491–498, 1993.
42. Smith JE, Chavey PS, Miller RE: Iron metabolism in captive black (*Diceros bicornis*) and white (*Ceratotherium simum*) rhinoceroses. J Zoo Wildl Med 26:523–532, 1995.
43. Spelman LH, Osborn KG, Anderson MP: Pathogenesis of hemosiderosis in lemurs: role of dietary iron, tannin and ascorbic acid. Zoo Biol 8:239–251, 1989.
44. Wadsworth PF, Jones DM, Pugsley SL: Hepatic hemosiderosis in birds at the Zoological Society of London. Avian Pathol 12:321–330, 1983.
45. Wagner JE, Manning PJ: The Biology of the Guinea Pig. New York, Academic Press, 1976.
46. Ward RJ, Iancu TC, Henderson GM, et al: Hepatic iron overload in birds: analytical and morphological studies. Avian Pathol 17:451–464, 1988.
47. Wilson RB: Hepatic hemosiderosis and *Klebsiella* bacteremia in a green aracari (*Pteroglossus viridis*). Avian Dis 38:679–681, 1994.
48. Worell A: Serum iron levels in ramphastids. Proceedings of the Association of Avian Veterinarians, Chicago, pp 120–130, 1991.

CHAPTER 35

Comparative Nutrition and Feeding Considerations of Young Columbidae

CHARLOTTE KIRK BAER

Columbids have some of the most distinctive diet and feeding strategies among all avian orders. Attributes related to the type of diet consumed and feeding strategies of columbid species may have evolved by natural selection. Recognition of different taxonomic classes of columbids and factors affecting the evolution of columbid species—including their expansive global range in habitat; traditional uses in research, education, recreation, and conservation; and physiologic mechanisms associated with feeding—provide a basis for understanding special aspects of columbid nutrition.

The perception by the general public that the pigeon is a nuisance or pest generally limits interest for the bird. However, the greatest number of pigeon species reside in subtropical or tropical areas, where wholesale destruction of tropical forests—primary pigeon habitat—is occurring, which prompts public concern. Complete devastation of the tropical forests in which most pigeon species exist could occur by the year 2040[3] if habitat destruction continues at its current rapid pace. Pigeon fanciers, scientists, environmentalists, and policymakers encourage the preservation of the tropical habitats of the pigeon. Propagation of these species in captivity is also important. Despite efforts to maintain and breed columbids in captivity by aviaries and zoological parks, the number of columbids continues to decline. For many endangered species in captivity, the fledgling success rate is less than 10%. Even though some aviculturalists are able to breed and hatch exotic pigeons in captivity, the squabs often do not survive to fledgling age. Inadequate parenting and improper feeding are major factors in the failure of squabs to survive in captivity. Artificial rearing of the species often does not succeed because of the limited information available on the basic elements of columbid management, such as feeding behavior and diet. The problems encountered in raising exotic pigeons in captivity and the lack of information on pigeon nutrition demonstrate the need for more research on these species.

CLASSIFICATION OF COLUMBIDAE

Feeding columbids is especially challenging because of the large variation among species and the diversity in natural history and origin of these birds. Larger species of the Columbidae family are referred to as pigeons, and the smaller species are referred to as doves. The family Columbidae is classified by Goodwin into four subfamilies containing 43 genera made up of about 300 species with 716 geographical races and forms.[14] The largest subfamily, Columbinae, is composed of the widespread familiar pigeons and doves, including the rock dove, mourning dove, wood pigeon, and the quail doves. Exotic species of this subfamily include the pheasant pigeon of New Guinea and the Nicobar pigeon, which inhabits small islands between the eastern Indian Ocean and the Philippines. The subfamily Treroninae is made up of tropical fruit–eating pigeons. The three groups of pigeons in this subfamily include green pigeons of the genus *Treron,* fruit doves of the genus *Ptilinopus,* and the larger imperial pigeons of the genus *Ducula.* The third subfamily, Didunculinae, includes only one species, the tooth-billed pigeon of Samoa. The subfamily Gourinae includes only the three species of crowned pigeons of New Guinea and nearby islands.

AVIAN LACTATION

Lactation is defined by Webster as "the secretion or formation of milk, a liquid that serves for the nourishment of young," and it is one of several physiologic features that characterize the mammalian class of animals. A few avian species, such as pigeons, doves, and some species of flamingoes[27] and penguins,[34] share with mammals the ability to secrete a milk for their young, or *lactate,* making them unique among birds. In birds and mammals, the milk produced transfers food from parent to offspring in a form that is readily used by immature young.

Milk production in mammals and birds is prolactin mediated.[18] The crop responds to increased levels of prolactin, as does the mammary gland, but the method of milk secretion in birds differs from that in mammals. Crop milk is a holocrine secretion in birds, whereas mammalian milk is an exocrine secretion from the mammary gland. Both male and female birds lactate, but only the female is capable of lactation in mammals.

Lactation in mammals has been described as a

method of adaptation to environmental conditions, enabling mammals to live and propagate in essentially all parts of the earth, even if the environment is extreme. Fish, reptiles, amphibians, and most birds are limited to habitation in temperate environments. Pigeons, however, possess the same method of adaptation, whereby nutrients in the form of milk are transferred from parent to offspring, allowing them to inhabit and reproduce in nearly any environment throughout the world.

From birth to weaning, the mammalian neonate is totally dependent on milk for nutrients. Similarly, crop milk is the sole source of nutrients for the squab during the first few days of life and remains the primary food of the young pigeon for the first week to 10 days after hatching. Gradually, crop milk is mixed with the adult diet and fed to hatchlings by both adult parents. Just as mammalian milk is essential for neonatal growth, crop milk is crucial for survival of squabs because they hatch in a relatively undeveloped state. Squabs are unable to use food found in their environment, cannot digest adult birds' diet, hatch with eyes unopened, and do not possess feathering for thermoregulation after hatching. Because of their dependency on parental secretions for nourishment, pigeons are unlike other avian species (such as the chicken or quail) that hatch with eyes open and are capable of obtaining and digesting seeds or pelleted diets. As in many mammalian species that grow rapidly during the neonatal stage of life, the nutrient-rich milk supports the rapid growth that squabs undergo during their first weeks of life.

Histologic Changes of the Lactating Avian Crop

The unique mechanism of milk secretion in the pigeon crop can be demonstrated histologically.[21] In response to the stimulatory effects of the anterior pituitary hormone prolactin, the crop begins to thicken around the eighth day of brooding. The hyperplastic appearance of the crop mucosal epithelium increases throughout brooding (18 to 21 days). Lipid droplets are incorporated within the squamous epithelium, and successive distal detachment of cells into the crop lumen constitutes the holocrine secretion of crop milk. Histologic differences in lactating versus nonlactating crop tissue are dramatic. The mucosal epithelium shows exaggerated hyperplasia, which could be confused histologically with a diseased state, but the presence of lipid and luminal contents would be suggestive of normal milk secretion.

Photomicrographs depicting changes in crop tissue during crop milk secretion are presented in Figures 35–1 and 35–2. Figure 35–1 illustrates a comparison between nonlactating and lactating crop tissue. Extensive hyperplasia of the mucosal epithelium is evident in lactating tissue. Crop milk is present in the lumen of the lactating crop. Figure 35–2 illustrates intracellular lipid droplets of the mucosal epithelium and the desquamation and sloughing of lipid laden cells constituting crop milk into the lumen of the crop gland.

CROP MILK COMPOSITION

The similarities between pigeon and mammalian lactation extend to the nutrient composition of the milk. Pigeon crop milk contains the same major macronutrients as mammalian milk—water, fat, protein, and ash—with the exception of carbohydrate (Fig. 35–3).[10, 13, 20, 22–24, 36] Differences between pigeon milk and most mammalian milks are found primarily in the carbohydrate and protein fractions. Most placental mammalian milks contain a significant amount of carbohydrate, but fur seal and sea lion milks contain only trace amounts of milk carbohydrate (lactose). Pigeon milk is devoid of lactose.[22–24]

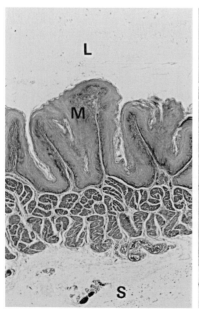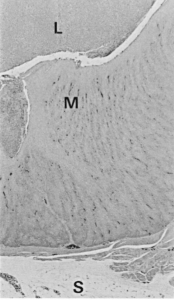

FIGURE 35–1. *Left,* Normal crop mucosal epithelium. *Right,* Lactating crop tissue from an adult male dove. L, lumen; M, mucosa; S, serosa. Hematoxylin and eosin stain; magnification, 40×. (From Kirk CL: Physiological hyperplasia associated with lactation in a dove. Comp Pathol Bull 25[4]:2–4, 1993. Reprinted with permission from the Registry of Comparative Pathology, Armed Forces Institute of Pathology, Washington, DC.)

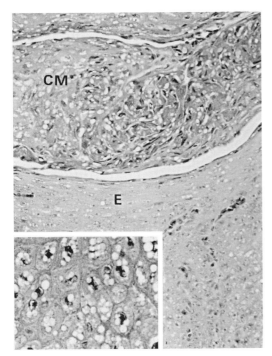

FIGURE 35–2. Hyperplastic mucosal epithelium (E) and intraluminal holocrine crop milk (CM). Hematoxylin and eosin stain; magnification, 400×. *Inset,* Intracellular lipid droplets in crop milk. Hematoxylin and eosin stain; magnification, 600×. (From Kirk CL: Physiological hyperplasia associated with lactation in a dove. Comp Pathol Bull 25[4]:2–4, 1993. Reprinted with permission from the Registry of Comparative Pathology, Armed Forces Institute of Pathology, Washington, DC.)

Milk Protein and Amino Acid Composition

High levels of crude protein (approximately 50% of dry matter) and fat (approximately 45% of dry matter) in pigeon crop milk support the assertion that crop milk is an energy-dense secretion that sustains the rapid growth of squabs.[10, 23, 24, 35] Altricial birds meet the demands for nestling growth by providing easily digested, nutrient-rich food to their young. Most altricial avian species provide insect or animal matter to their young, which is rich in protein and other readily available nutrients for growth. The pigeon, on the other hand, has evolved to meet the growth requirements of its young by secreting crop milk. In fruit-eating and vegetarian pigeon species, milk secretion is a logical form of feeding the young, because a fruit diet may not support rapid squab growth. Pigeon squabs require an energy-dense diet to support several physiologic mechanisms. Squabs are hatched in an undeveloped state, typically in clutches of two. Because the clutch size is small and squabs are immature in comparison with other avian species, squabs must huddle together to reduce the surface area exposed to air and to conserve the amount of energy expended to maintain stable body temperatures. Although energy expenditures are kept to a minimum

while squabs are completely ectothermic, a large amount of energy is devoted to rapid growth in addition to thermoregulation. To date, energy expenditures of the squab have not been partitioned, nor have they been quantitated. Observations on the physical state of pigeons at hatching and their rapid development, coupled with the nutrient composition of crop milk, suggest that squabs have significant energy requirements that are met by crop milk feeding.

The presence of high levels of protein in crop milk has prompted investigation into the amino acid content and composition of the milk protein. Amino acid composition of crop milk during early lactation is described in Table 35–1.[23, 24] Concentrations of most amino acids are higher in later lactation than they are during the first several days of lactation; this is especially true for methionine, lysine, and threonine. There appear to be significant changes in early crop milk amino acid concentrations; however, more research is needed to further substantiate apparent changes in amino acid concentrations.

Approximately 17% of the total nitrogen in crop milk is in the form of free amino acids. The amino acid content of crop milk suggests that it is a good source of animal protein and that nonessential amino acids may be important in squab development. Glutamic and aspartic acids are the prominent amino acids in crop milk.[23, 24] Because crop milk contains little carbohydrate, the energy required for metabolic processes in the squab may be partially supplied through glycogenesis of these amino acids.

Immunoglobulins are another important component of crop milk protein, similar to mammalian colostrum. Crop milk is a good source of immunoglobulin A (IgA), and it also contains some immunoglobulin C (IgC). Increased survival rates have been reported for squabs receiving crop milk during the first few days of life.[7, 15]

Fat and Fatty Acid Composition

Fatty acid composition of white Carneaux pigeon crop milk is presented in Table 35–2.[22, 24] Pigeon crop milk

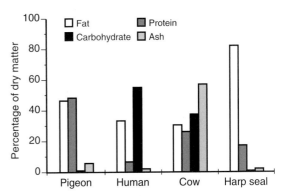

FIGURE 35–3. Comparison of pigeon milk with selected mammalian milks. (Data from reference 32; from Oftedal OT, Iverson SJ: Comparative analysis of nonhuman milks: A. Phylogenetic variation in the gross composition of milks. *In* Jensen RG [ed]: Handbook of Milk Composition. San Diego, Academic Press, pp 749–789, 1995.).

TABLE 35–1. Amino Acid Composition of White Carneaux Crop Milk (% As Is)

	Day 1		Day 2		Day 3	
Amino Acid	Mean	SEM*	Mean	SEM*	Mean	SEM*
Threonine†‡	0.571	0.025	0.552	0.021	0.694	0.025
Isoleucine†	0.523	0.022	0.484	0.019	0.571	0.023
Leucine†	1.022	0.051	0.962	0.042	1.157	0.051
Lysine†‡	0.946	0.028	0.886	0.023	1.059	0.028
Methionine†‡	0.318	0.015	0.311	0.012	0.377	0.015
Phenylalanine†	0.545	0.029	0.514	0.024	0.622	0.029
Tyrosine†	0.413	0.033	0.445	0.027	0.552	0.034
Valine†	0.629	0.029	0.589	0.024	0.700	0.029
Arginine†	0.836	0.038	0.786	0.031	0.954	0.038
Histidine	0.241	0.010	0.223	0.008	0.256	0.010
Alanine	0.642	0.041	0.629	0.033	0.739	0.041
Aspartic acid†	1.144	0.049	1.067	0.040	1.266	0.049
Glutamic acid	1.619	0.093	1.504	0.076	1.757	0.093
Glycine†	0.617	0.037	0.599	0.031	0.752	0.037
Proline	0.445	0.033	0.424	0.027	0.520	0.033
Serine†	0.609	0.035	0.571	0.028	0.727	0.035

*Standard error.
†Day 3 higher than day 2 ($P < 0.05$).
‡Day 3 higher than day 1 ($P < 0.05$).
From Kirk Baer CL, Thomas OP: Crop milk and squab growth in the Columbidae *(Columba livia)*. Proc Symp Comp Nutr Soc 1:75–77, 1996.

fat is primarily in the form of triglycerides (81.2%) and phospholipids (12.2%).[11] Cholesterol, cholesterol esters, monoglycerides, diglycerides, and free fatty acids comprise the remainder.

Crop milk is a good source of essential fatty acids. About half of the milk fatty acids are monoenes, and fatty acid profiles of columbid crop milk are similar across species.[11, 12, 24, 34, 35] Crop milk contains several fatty acids essential for growth in birds, specifically 18:2 (omega-6), 18:3 (omega-3), and 20:4 (omega-6).[22, 24, 30] Figure 35–4 illustrates the similarities between pigeon and mammalian milk fatty acids. As in mammalian milks, oleic acid (18:1) is the prominent fatty acid. Medium-chain fatty acids are relatively low in proportion to the total, similar to dog milk but unlike ruminant milks.[19] Although oleic and linoleic acids are present in similar proportions to mammalian milk, linoleic is pres-

ent in crop milk at higher levels than in dog, cow, bear, and elephant milks.[5, 19] High levels of oleic and linoleic acids may be important in the rapid development of the squab, because metabolites of these fatty acids are key components in the cell membranes of neural tissue and are also precursors of eicosanoids. Other fatty acids present in significant proportions are palmitic (16:0), stearic (18:0), and linoleic (18:2). The prominence of total unsaturated fatty acids is strikingly similar to that in the milk of fur seals.[35]

Fatty acid analysis can demonstrate the differences between pigeon crop milk secretion and adult pigeon pelleted feed, which could be stored in the adult pigeon crop.[22] The significantly different fatty acid profile of crop milk versus pigeon pelleted feed demonstrated that adult birds are not merely regurgitating their diet and feeding it to squabs, but instead are actually secreting

TABLE 35–2. Fatty Acid Composition (Weight %) of Pellet and White Carneaux Pigeon Crop Milk on Days 1 Through 3 After Hatching (Dry Matter Basis)

	Pellet		Day 1		Day 2		Day 3	
Fatty Acid	Mean	SEM*	Mean	SEM*	Mean	SEM*	Mean	SEM*
Oleic†	23.58	1.84	32.88	1.50	33.58	1.30	34.08	1.16
Linoleic†	2.14	1.58	23.77	1.29	23.57	1.12	22.51	1.00
Linolenic†	0.36	0.10	1.41	0.08	1.30	0.07	1.42	0.06
Total unsaturated	0.37	0.88	1.99	0.72	1.96	0.62	2.15	0.56
Total saturated	11.38	2.76	2.57	2.26	5.54	1.95	5.72	1.75
$>C_{18}$‡	9.02	2.99	7.23	2.44	7.23	2.11	7.23	1.89

*Standard error.
†Concentration of pellet lower than concentration of milk ($P < 0.001$).
From Kirk Baer CL, Thomas OP: Nutrient composition of crop milk and growth of squabs: new noninvasive techniques for milk collection and body composition determination in Columbidae *(Columba livia)*. Proceedings of the American Association of Zoo Veterinarians and Reptile and Avian Veterinarians. Pittsburgh, 1994, pp 302–304.
‡Other fatty acids greater than 18 carbons in length.

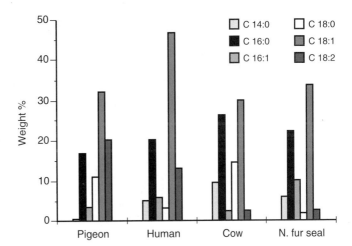

FIGURE 35–4. Fatty acid composition (weight percentage) of pigeon milk and other mammalian species. (Data from references 5, 19, 22, and 32.)

nutritive crop milk. However, milk samples obtained later in lactation, from squabs ingesting milk mixed with the adult diet, more closely reflect the fatty acid composition of the adult pelleted diet. [12, 22]

Milk Carbohydrate

The characteristic lack of significant levels of carbohydrate in crop milk is a reflection of the fact that the milk is a holocrine secretion, consisting primarily of sloughed epithelial cells (protein) and lipid droplets (fat). [9, 33] Determination of carbohydrate by difference as opposed to direct measurement may confound results and is entirely dependent on the accuracy of methodology used for determination of dry matter and other milk constituents.

Milk Mineral Composition

Mineral content of crop milk is presented in Table 35–3. [22, 24] Mineral concentration does not change during the first 3 days of lactation except for magnesium. Magnesium concentration appears to increase with time. Mineral analysis of crop milk indicates that it is similar to many mammalian milks and is uniquely comparable

to beaked whale milk (Table 35–4). [22, 37, 38] Both the beaked whale milk and pigeon crop milk are high in iron in comparison with milk of other mammalian species. High iron in marsupial milk, some rodent milks, and pigeon crop milk may be associated with the altricial status of the young.

Calcium and magnesium are important in squab growth. Crop milk contains notable amounts of both minerals, essential to normal bone growth and development. [10, 22] However, there has been one report of crop milk being devoid of calcium. [29] It is highly unlikely that parental crop milk fed to young squabs exclusively during the post-hatching stage of life contains no calcium, especially in view of the significant amount of calcium found in the carcasses of growing squabs. [22]

SQUAB GROWTH AND BODY COMPOSITION

Rapid growth rate of newly hatched columbids is an important consideration in the development of artificial formulas that are adequate to support this growth. The body weight of domestic white Carneaux and endangered Puerto Rican plain pigeons during the first 3 weeks after hatching is presented in Figure 35–5. A

TABLE 35–3. Mineral Composition of White Carneaux Pigeon Milk Days 1 Through 3 After Hatching (Dry Matter Basis)

Mineral	Day 1 Mean	Day 2 Mean	Day 3 Mean	SEM*
Calcium (%)	0.84	0.77	0.81	0.48
Potassium (%)	0.62	0.63	0.62	0.08
Magnesium (%)†	0.01	0.10	0.14	0.07
Sodium (%)	0.61	0.49	0.53	0.77
Iron (ppm)	445	417	425	38

*Standard error.
†Concentration higher on day 3 than days 1 and 3 (p <0.001).
From Kirk Baer CL, Thomas OP: Crop milk and squab growth in the Columbidae *(Columba livia)*. Proc Symp Comp Nutr Soc 1:75–77, 1996.

TABLE 35–4. Mineral Composition of Crop Milk and Other Mammalian Species

Milk	Sodium (mmol/L)	Potassium (mmol/L)	Calcium (mmol/L)	Magnesium (mmol/L)	Iron (µg/L)
Pigeon*†	29.60	19.90	25.20	5.92	54000
Human*	6.50	14.00	6.70	1.40	1000
Cow*	25.20	35.30	30.10	5.10	1100
Whale*‡	56.50	28.10	54.90	1.73	35000

*Data from reference 22.
†Data from reference 37.
‡Data from reference 38.

sigmoid curve is typical of body weight changes from birth to mature weight in most columbid species.

Body composition of many species changes during development. In general, the proportion of fat increases and the proportion of water decreases with age. The proportion of protein and ash is generally constant.[6, 26] During the development of domestic pigeons between days 1 and 7 after hatching, fat and water remain constant, carbohydrate content is lower, and crude protein content is higher immediately after hatching than later in development. The observed increase in carbohydrate in older squabs may be a consequence of more dietary carbohydrate in the gastrointestinal tracts of analyzed carcasses of older squabs consuming a mixture of milk and pelleted diet of the adults. The higher protein concentration of squabs immediately after hatching may represent a higher proportion of yolk that is quickly metabolized.

LIPOLYTIC ENZYMES

In all species examined to date, pancreatic lipase is unable to act on milk fat without previous initiation of lipolysis by preduodenal enzymes.[1, 16, 18, 25, 28] Facilitation of milk fat hydrolysis by pancreatic lipase is accomplished by the action of lingual or gastric lipase (or both) before dietary fat reaches the small intestine. In pigeons, it is unclear how pancreatic lipase is able to act on milk fat in the squab digestive tract without the presence of lingual or gastric lipase. Perhaps the answer lies in the difference between mammalian milk fat and avian milk fat. Mammalian milk fat is contained within fat globules. Triglycerides form the core, and the more polar phospholipids and cholesterol together with proteins make up the milk fat globule membrane, which is the barrier to pancreatic lipase. Conversely, avian milk fat is not "packaged" for transport as in mammalian milk secretion. The avian milk lipid is incorporated intracellularly and is passively sloughed into the crop lumen by epithelial desquamation of lipid-laden cells. Therefore, because there is not a fat globule membrane per se in avian crop milk, digestion of avian milk fat may be accomplished by pancreatic lipase. High levels of circulating lipoprotein lipase have been reported in the pigeon, and this enzyme plays a primary role in the incorporation of fat in crop milk.

FEEDING CONSIDERATIONS AND RECOMMENDATIONS

Natural History Considerations

Captive columbids require specialized diets, based on the species, feeding strategy, age, and reproductive status of the bird. Pigeons and doves fall naturally into three categories, with respect to diet: (1) seed-eating pigeons and doves; (2) fruit-eating pigeons of Africa, Australia, Asia, and the East Indies; and (3) fruit-eating crowned pigeons of New Guinea and surrounding coastal islands.

Although there might be differences between seed-eating and granivorous or fruit-eating columbids with regard to composition of the adult bird's diet and composition of crop milk produced, data are insufficient to make any conclusions. Several samples of crop milk produced by fruit-eating columbids (*Goura*) that were obtained opportunistically and analyzed suggest that crop milk in this species is not markedly different in composition from crop milk produced by seed-eating birds (C. Kirk Baer, unpublished data). More research is needed to elucidate any compositional differences

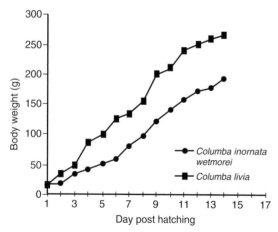

FIGURE 35–5. Growth rates of white Carneaux (*Columba livia*) and Puerto Rican plain (*Columba inornata*) pigeons. (Data from reference 22 and from Perez-Rivera: Optimal management of ring doves and giant runts to increase production of Puerto Rican plain pigeons [*Columba inornata wetmorei*] in captivity. Science 19[1]:22–28, 1991.)

between crop milk produced by seed-eating birds and milk produced by granivorous and fruit-eating species.

Importance of Sensory Contributions and Unique Feeding Behaviors

In addition to considering the natural history of the particular species being fed, special consideration also must be given to the unique feeding characteristics of columbids in general. Behavioral mechanisms play a key role in food intake of pigeons. Initiation of feeding by arousal and food recognition, followed by orientation and grasping food, and finally movement through the oral cavity and swallowing are well-defined stages of food intake in the pigeon. When the squab is fed, these stages are important considerations, especially as the bird grows older. Problems encountered in feeding squabs, such as refusal of the squab to accept food readily and inability of the squab to swallow, store, and digest artificial formulas, could be a result of abnormalities associated with the trigeminal sensory system, neural injury or disease, inappropriate presentation of food, inadequate sensory stimuli, or poor feeding techniques.[4]

Recognizing that specific senses are involved in each phase of feeding behavior, care should be taken to present the food in a manner that uses these senses. Pigeons possess taste buds, and it has been suggested that they perceive differences in flavors.[29, 31] Therefore, drastic or frequent changes in components of artificial milk replacers fed to orphaned squabs should be avoided. These changes should be avoided not only because they may result in differences in the palatability or taste of the diet, but also because any change in diet should be implemented gradually over a period of time (adaptation period). Similarly, odor might play a role in recognition and acceptance of artificial formulas and might be involved as a stimulus to eat. Vision is also a key component of feeding in the pigeon. Visual acuity of the pigeon's eye is excellent. Presentation of food to young, orphaned, sick, or injured pigeons might effect better results if provided in the two ranges of optimal visual acuity.

Food preference in older squabs and adult columbids is an additional consideration in developing diets for these birds. Seed selection or preference in birds, which is a common occurrence that often results in imbalances in nutrient intake or nutrient deficiencies, involves sensory processes that produce different responses to different seed types. The trigeminal sensorimotor system is one process involved in food preference; somatosensory input from the oral cavity is relayed to the central nervous system, resulting in positive response to particular types of food.

Production of Crop Milk

Crop milk production in Columbidae is an adaptation to environmental conditions that enable pigeons to live and propagate in a wide range of habitats throughout the world.[17] Male and female parent birds invest a

significant amount of physiologic resources into production of crop milk. Regulated by prolactin, this holocrine secretion is the primary source of nutrients for the parent-reared squab during the first 2 to 4 weeks after hatching. Similarly, a crop milk replacer should supply the primary source of nutrients for the hand-reared squab.

Simulating Characteristics of Natural Milk

Orphaned squabs should be fed in a manner that closely resembles natural feeding with regard to composition, quantity, and frequency of milk consumed by parent-raised birds. Providing the squab a nutrient-dense, readily digestible diet in appropriate quantities and at appropriate intervals for the first few days of life is crucial for survival.

Based on research available to date on domestic seed-eating columbids and several samples of crop milk from captive endangered fruit-eating pigeons, it has been determined that crop milk is rich in protein and fat and provides nutrients for rapid growth and development of young squabs. To simulate natural crop milk in early stages of lactation, protein and fat levels in artificial formulas should be approximately 45% to 55% and 38% to 48% of the dry matter, respectively. Artificial milk replacers should be formulated to contain 25% to 30% dry matter to simulate natural crop milk.

One of the most significant challenges in formulating an artificial milk replacer for any species, particularly for avian species, is determining the appropriate sources, not necessarily levels, of nutrients. Components and ingredients used to formulate milk replacers are extremely important considerations. Protein and fat can be provided from many different sources; however, the type and composition of fat and protein may be drastically different among available sources. The amino acid composition of crop milk protein appears (from limited data) to be most similar to avian muscle meat, possibly because the protein of natural crop milk is derived from hyperplastic, sloughed crop epithelial tissue. Therefore, a formula should be constituted to supply similar amounts and proportions of amino acids found in naturally produced crop milk. Glutamic acid, aspartic acid, and leucine are three amino acids found in significant quantities in crop milk and should be present in artificial milk replacers in similar levels and proportions. Sulfur-containing amino acids should not represent a large proportion of amino acids in milk replacers for columbids, because crop milk contains low levels of these nutrients. There is still debate over whether crop milk protein is a casein protein; however, crop milk is a good source of animal protein, containing all the essential amino acids required by birds in adequate proportions. The crop milk proteins and IgA and IgC might be important for immunity in young squabs.[7, 15] In general, breeders of pigeons have experienced increased successful rearing of squabs if the squabs have received crop milk during the first few days of life. There may be some benefit to acquiring natural crop milk and feeding it to squabs soon after hatching to provide a source of immunoglobulins and microflora that may be important for immunity and digestive function.

The fat source used in milk replacers should provide essential fatty acids. Oleic and linoleic acids are found in most mammalian milks and commercial milk replacers; they are the two primary fatty acids found in crop milk. These two fatty acids should be present in formulas at high levels (20% to 35% on a dry matter basis); crop milk contains higher levels of linoleic acid than most mammalian milks. A source of fat that contains half the milk fatty acids as monounsaturates and that is primarily in the form of triglycerides and phospholipids is recommended.

Carbohydrate should not constitute a significant portion of artificial milk replacers for young squabs. Because crop milk is almost devoid of carbohydrate during the first few days of life, an artificial formula for the young squab should contain no more than 0.5% on a dry matter basis. Apparently, squabs do not obtain energy for early rapid growth from milk carbohydrate, but rather they obtain caloric needs from high levels of milk fat and protein, and presumably from gluconeogenesis of the nonessential amino acids, glutamic and aspartic acids.

Four minerals most important to consider when developing a milk replacer for columbids are (1) calcium, (2) phosphorus, (3) magnesium, and (4) iron. High iron levels in crop milk, marsupial, and rodent milks are characteristic of the altricial status of the neonate, which is an important factor affecting survival when these species are artificially reared in captivity.

In general, crop milk composition does not appear to change during the first several days of lactation; therefore, daily changes in artificial diets fed to hand-reared squabs may not be required during the immediate period after hatching. However, the gross composition of crop milk changes significantly over time. The formulation of artificial milk replacers should be altered over time to reflect changes in composition of natural crop milk: dry matter, fat, and protein levels should remain relatively constant for the first week after hatching, and subsequently, carbohydrate levels and dry matter levels of the formula should increase. The increasing dry matter and carbohydrate content are a reflection of the increasing amounts of parent bird's diet that are gradually mixed with crop milk and are fed to the squab until 4 weeks of age.

Rapid Growth Considerations

Milk replacers should provide adequate energy and appropriate levels and proportions of nutrients to facilitate squab growth, which is rapid during the first 14 days of life and begins to slow after that period. Monitoring growth rate and body composition of columbids reared in captivity provides useful information for propagation of endangered and threatened species. Growth rates reflect the adequacy of milk replacers fed to squabs when compared with birds raised by parents. Body composition can be an indicator of normal physiologic development, and it should be monitored, if possible.

Digestive Capabilities of the Squab

Regardless of the adequacy and appropriateness of a formulated milk replacer, consideration must be given to the mechanisms for absorption and utilization of nutrients in the young columbid. Protein digestion occurs primarily in the proventriculus of the adult bird. Very young squabs possess lower levels of proteolytic enzymes than adult birds do, and it is not known what effect this difference may have on digestive capability.

Fat digestion appears to be unique in the pigeon when compared with other avian species. Pancreatic enzymes are most likely responsible for fat digestion in the pigeon, unlike other avian species that possess gastric lipase in the proventriculus. The mode of enzymatic action and lipolytic activity is not well defined for the pigeon.

Often, squabs reared on artificial formulas experience crop stasis, diarrhea, dehydration, and insufficient growth rates. These problems might be associated with the inability of the young bird to digest its food, as a result of underdeveloped or inadequate digestive enzyme function, or with inappropriate sources of nutrients for digestion. Because little digestion occurs in the crop of the very young bird, it is necessary to make certain that food passes from the crop to the proventriculus without extended delay. Overfeeding can hinder crop emptying and may exacerbate crop stasis or impaction. To simulate natural feeding behaviors observed in Columbidae, numerous small feedings spaced throughout the day and continued only in the presence of normal crop emptying are recommended.

REFERENCES

1. Abrams CK, Hamosh M, Lee TC, et al: Gastric lipase: localization in the human stomach. Gastroenterology 95:1460–1464, 1988.
2. Baer DJ, Rumpler WV, Barnes RE, et al: Measurement of body composition of live rats by electromagnetic conductance. Physiol Behav 53:1195–1199, 1993.
3. Barney GO (ed): The Global Report to the President. Washington, DC, U.S. Government Printing Office, 1980.
4. Berkhoudt H, Klein BG, Zeigler HP: Afferents to the trigeminal and facial motor nuclei in pigeon (*Columba livia*) central connections of jaw motor neurons. J Comp Neurol 209(3):301–312, 1980.
5. Bitman J, Wood DL, Hamosh M, et al: Comparison of the lipid composition of breast milk from mothers of term and preterm infants. Am J Clin Nutr 38:300–312, 1983.
6. Blaxter K: Reproduction and growth: postnatal growth. *In* Energy Metabolism in Animals and Man. New York, Cambridge University Press, pp 219–253, 1989.
7. Buhrows T, Bijker PGH, de Boer AM, et al: A study of the normal microflora in crop contents of neonatal domestic pigeons (*Columba livia domestica*). J Vet Nutr 2:17–21, 1993.
8. Castro G, Wunder BA, Knopf FL: Total body electrical conductivity (TOBEC) to estimate total body fat of free-living birds. Condor 92:496–499, 1990.
9. Chadwick A: Endocrinology of reproduction. *In* Abs M (ed): Physiology and Behavior of the Pigeon. New York, Academic Press, pp 55–72, 1983.
10. Davies WL: The composition of the crop milk of pigeons. Biochem J 33:898–901, 1939.
11. Desmeth M: Lipid composition of pigeon cropmilk: II. Fatty acids. Comp Biochem Physiol B Biochem Mol Biol 66:139–141, 1980.
12. Desmeth M, Vandeputte-Poma J: Lipid composition of pigeon cropmilk: I. Total lipids and lipid classes. Comp Biochem Physiol B Biochem Mol Biol 66:135–138, 1980.
13. Ferrando R, Wolter R, Fourlon C, et al: Le lait de pigeon. Ann Nutr Alim 25:241–251, 1971.

14. Goodwin D: Pigeons and Doves of the World, 2nd ed. London, British Museum (Natural History), 1977.

15. Goudswaard J, Noordzij A, van Dam RH, et al: Three immunoglobulin classes in the pigeon (*Columbia livia*). Int Arch Allergy Appl Immun 53:389–409, 1977.

16. Hamosh M: Lingual and Gastric Lipases: Their Role in Fat Digestion. Boca Raton, FL, CRC Press, 1990.

17. Hartwick RF, Kiepenheuer J, Schmidt-Koenig K: *In* Schmidt-Koenig K, Keeton WT (eds): Animal Migration, Navigation, and Homing: Proceedings in Life Sciences. New York, Springer Verlag, pp 107-118, 1978.

18. Horseman ND, Buntin JD: Regulation of pigeon cropmilk secretion and parental behaviors by prolactin. Annu Rev Nutr 15:213–238, 1995.

19. Iverson SJ, Kirk C, Hamosh M, et al: Milk lipid digestion in the neonatal dog: the combined actions of gastric and bile salt stimulated lipases. Biochim Biophys Acta 1083:109–119, 1991.

20. Kirk CL: The composition of crop milk in pigeons. Proceedings of the Ninth Doctor Scholl Conference on Nutrition of Captive Wild Animals, Chicago, in press.

21. Kirk CL: Physiological hyperplasia associated with lactation in a dove. Comp Pathol Bull 25(4):2–4, 1993.

22. Kirk Baer CL: Crop milk composition and squab growth in the Columbidae (*Columba livia*). M.S. thesis, University of Maryland, College Park, 1994.

23. Kirk Baer CL, Thomas OP: Nutrient composition of crop milk and growth of squabs: new noninvasive techniques for milk collection and body composition determination in Columbidae (*Columba livia*). Proceedings of the Association of Reptile and Amphibian Veterinarians and the American Association of Zoo Veterinarians, Pittsburgh, pp 302–304, 1994.

24. Kirk Baer CL and Thomas, OP: Crop milk and squab growth in the Columbidae (*Columba livia*). Proc Symp Comp Nutr Soc 1:75–77, 1996.

25. Kirk CL, Iverson SJ, Hamosh M: Lipase and pepsin activities in the stomach mucosa of the suckling dog. Biol Neonate 59:78–85, 1991.

26. Kleiber M: The Fire of Life: An Introduction to Animal Energetics. Huntington, NY, Robert E. Krieger, 1975.

27. Lang EM: Flamingos raise their young on a liquid containing blood. Experientia 19:532–533, 1963.

28. Liao TH, Hamosh P, Hamosh M: Gastric lipolysis in the developing rat: ontogeny of the lipases active in the stomach. Biochim Biophys Acta 754:1–9, 1983.

29. McLelland J: Digestive system. *In* McLelland J: Color Atlas of Avian Anatomy. Philadelphia, WB Saunders, 1991, p 52.

30. Mohrhauer H, Holman RT: The effect of dose level of essential fatty acids upon fatty acid composition of the rat liver. J Lipid Res 4:151–159, 1963.

31. Moore CA, Elliott R: Tastebuds on the pigeon tongue and mandible. J Comp Neurol 84:119–131, 1946.

32. Oftedal OT, Iverson SJ: Comparative analysis of nonhuman milks: A. Phylogenetic variation in the gross composition of milks. *In* Jensen RG (ed): Handbook of Milk Composition. San Diego, Academic Press, pp 749–789, 1995.

33. Patel MD: The physiology of the formation of "pigeon's milk." Physiol Zool 9(2):129–152, 1936.

34. Prevost J, Vitler V: Histologia de la sécrétion oesophagienne du manchot empereur. Proc Int Ornithol Cong 13:1085–1094, 1963.

35. Shetty S, Hedge SN: Changes in lipids of pigeon "milk" in the first week of its secretion. Lipids 26(11):930–933, 1991.

36. Sim JS, Hickman AR, Nwokolo E: Nutrient composition of squab crop contents during the first eight days post hatch. Poult Sci 65(Suppl 1):126, 1986.

37. Tormey K, Spaulding L, Studier EH, Kirk CL: Nitrogen and mineral composition of pigeon milk and nestlings. Michigan Academician: Papers of the Michigan Academy of Science, Arts, and Letters 27(3):381–382, 1995.

38. Ullrey DE, Schwartz CC, Whetter PA, et al: Blue-green color and composition of Stejneger's beaked whale (*Mesoplodon stejnegeri*) milk. Comp Biochem Physiol [B] 79:349–352, 1984.

CHAPTER 36

Medical Management of the California Condor

PHILIP K. ENSLEY

Veterinary participation in the conservation of the California condor *(Gymnogyps californianus)* evolved concurrently with the need by biologists for aggressive hands-on field studies in the 1980s. This was soon followed by the authorization of captive breeding programs at the Zoological Society of San Diego, Los Angeles Zoo, and, in 1993, the World Center for Birds of Prey in Boise, Idaho.[6] Together, these efforts resulted in the reintroduction of this species in California in 1992 and more recently in Arizona in 1996.

By 1980, there were estimated to be as few as 20 to 25 birds remaining in the wild, immediately north and west of Los Angeles, in addition to one captive specimen that had resided for several years at The Los Angeles Zoo. Thus, the clinical, surgical, and pathology experiences and data that have accumulated since 1980 originated from working with a relatively small population of birds.

Historical field population and biologic studies of the California condor by several reputable investigators[22, 32, 40, 42, 53, 54] have been nicely reviewed.[44] Decline of the wild population in this century is associated with habitat loss in the form of development and land use. Although difficult to quantify, one can add to this the direct disturbance by humans to include inadvertent poisoning through the use of dichlorodiphenyltrichloroethane (DDT), compound 1080, strychnine and cyanide use against agricultural pests and coyotes, and shooting. Lead poisoning by ingestion of lead bullet fragments in and from shot-contaminated carcasses was a probable factor in the death of condors but has been an only relatively recent documented finding involving three birds.[15] One additional factor in the species decline is its relatively slow reproduction rate. Efforts to salvage the California condor by public education of its endangered status and by setting aside recognized nesting habitat as restricted sanctuaries were critical steps, but they did not prove effective in reversing the downward population trend.[16]

In 1980, a modern research program was initiated, and the Condor Research Center in Ventura, California, was established. Authorized biologists were permitted to more vigorously study, identify, and monitor the remaining individual members of the wild population. These studies included capture, examination, diagnostic sampling, and release of radio-tagged birds and observation of active nest sites. These efforts produced significant information concerning the biology of the species. Perhaps the greatest single finding was that breeding pairs will lay a replacement for an egg lost early in the breeding season.[11, 41] This fact prompted the strategy for removal of eggs from nests for artificial incubation and hatching of chicks that would become part of the captive breeding population. Therefore, early veterinary clinical experiences consisted of examination of free flying birds, evaluation of chicks at nest sites removed for the captive breeding program, and monitoring the health of captive hatchlings and juveniles.[35]

During the winter of 1984–1985, there occurred an unexplained disappearance of several wild, non–radio-tagged birds. As a consequence, by early 1987, the remainder of the wild population was captured and placed in the captive breeding program.

In 1988–1989, 13 captive-bred female Andean condor (*Vultur gryphus*) chicks were released into the California condor's former range. These birds would act as a surrogate species, providing release technique experience and dispel doubts that reintroduction of the California condor was an achievable goal.[39] Before their recapture and subsequent release in Colombia, South America,[29] several of the Andean condors would overlap with the first reintroduced California condors in 1992. The Andean condor proved to be an invaluable model in learning captive condor husbandry[4, 8] and release technology.[49]

The goal of the California condor captive breeding program is to maintain a genetically diverse, long-lived, stable population of birds for the purpose of producing healthy chicks suitable for release to the wild. The goal of veterinary personnel is to provide health care to the captive population and advice and veterinary support to individuals managing the wild population.

BIOLOGIC DATA

The California condor is a New World, or Western hemisphere, vulture placed in the stork family, Ciconiidae, by the Committee on Classification and Nomencla-

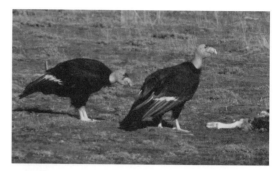

FIGURE 36–1. An adult pair of condors approach a calf carcass in the wild in 1983.

ture of the American Ornithologists' Union.[2] The condor is an obligate scavenger, or cathartid, eating the flesh of dead animals. It has the largest wingspread (8 to 9.5 feet) of any North American land bird; adults weigh 17 to 23 pounds.

Condors are soaring birds, riding thermals as they forage for food. Condors may consume 1 to 2 pounds per day, but they often go days without eating. Captive life expectancy in the case of one bird has been documented as reaching 45 years of age.[46]

Unlike the larger South American vulture, the Andean condor, to which it is often compared, the California condor is sexually monomorphic. Breeding maturity is reached at 5 to 7 years of age.

Juveniles have a grey-black color to their plumage, with the head and neck bare of feathers, revealing a greyish skin. As the bird matures, the head and neck change to a yellowish orange, reddish color. Between the external nares and the eyes, along the forehead, is a dark stubble of feather growth, giving the appearance of a black saddle. At maturity, the body plumage becomes black, with a white triangular patch noted during flight under the patagium (Figs. 36–1, 36–2).

Condors possess a powerful broad-shaped beak, which can shear and tear tissue, and a serrated tongue,

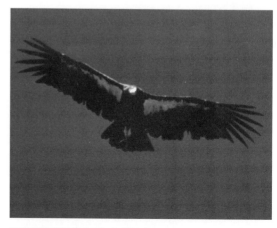

FIGURE 36–2. Adult California condor in flight reveals white triangular patches beneath the wings.

TABLE 36–1. Total Population of California Condors

Location	Male	Female	Total
San Diego Wild Animal Park	11	15	26
The Los Angeles Zoo	14	12	26
World Center for Birds of Prey	20	21	41
In the wild/California			
Lion Canyon	7	12	19
Ventana Wilderness Area	3	2	5
In the wild/Arizona	8	7	15
Totals*	**63**	**69**	**132**

*Totals as of March 1997.
Data from D. Jones, personal communication, 1997.

which rasps shreds of meat from a carcass. Condors do not have talons or grasping feet, but their nails are relatively sharp. They have good leg strength, which will permit them to drag or tear at a carcass while firmly positioning their feet.

Condors have a crop in the cervical esophagus where food passage is delayed. When full, the skin overlaying the crop appears distended and devoid of feathers. The stomach has a proventriculus or glandular compartment that produces hydrochloric acid, mucus, and pepsin, and there is a gizzard or muscular compartment where gastric proteolysis takes place.[45] When not searching for food, condors roost at traditional sites close to foraging grounds or nesting areas to allow digestion.

Males and females nearing or at maturity will form pair bonds thought to last for many years. A pair selects a nest site in sheltered cavities in cliffs or, more rarely, in a tree cavity. The same or similar alternate nest sites will be used again and again by a breeding pair.[43]

Courtship behavior in captivity, which begins in September/October with breeding in January/February, results in the female laying a single egg on the bare ground at a nest site. Each bird shares incubation duties, often for days at a time. After nearly 2 months of incubation, the chick hatches. Parents take turns brooding and regurgitating food into the mouth of their chick. As the chick matures, it learns how to stand on larger chunks of regurgitant, tearing and ingesting bits of food on its own.

A chick will fledge or take its first flight at about 5.5 months of age and in the wild will remain with the parents during the next year, curtailing successful courtship in most cases until the succeeding year. The oldest birds reintroduced in California in 1995 (hatched in 1994) will approach maturity in 2000.

The population numbers as of March 1998 are listed in Table 36–1.

CAPTIVE MANAGEMENT AND HUSBANDRY

Housing

Aviaries for maintaining California condors are patterned after structures built for Andean condors at the Patuxent Wildlife Research Center.[34] They are large outdoor free-flight wire mesh enclosures with catch pens, roosting perches, and nesting areas.[47] Keeper personnel are able to view birds and work with a minimum of contact or visual disturbance. Enclosures measure 12 × 24 m or larger and 6 to 7 m or more in height. Each enclosure has pools for drinking and bathing. There are elevated indoor roosts with adjacent nest sites. Enclosures and nest sites are monitored by remote television cameras.

Feeding

At the San Diego Wild Animal Park (SDWAP), juveniles and adults, fed generally in pairs, receive a diet of 1.5 pounds Nebraska Brand Feline Diet (Central Nebraska Packing Inc., North Platte, NE), two rainbow trout (*Oncorhynchus mykiss*), 1.5 pounds beef spleen, and one rabbit or two rats. Birds are fasted 2 days each week to allow time for food digestion and roosting behavior observed historically in the wild and to prevent obesity. Adult birds rearing chicks are not fasted.

Breeding Strategy

Before California condors were reintroduced in 1992, a conservative plan was approved to maximize the genetic resources of the 14 founder individuals. Pedigree of each member of the captive population, results of DNA fingerprinting, and release suitability of chicks are reviewed annually. From this information, recommendations are made for pairing, re-pairing, and selection of candidates for release and movement of birds between institutions.[9, 37, 38]

TRANSPORTATION

Birds are transported individually in standard fiberglass or plastic kennel-type carriers. They are lightweight and easily carried and offer seclusion. Front and side ventilation panels can be covered with a lightly woven fabric to provide a visual barrier yet allow good air flow. For extended trips, a sandy substrate or decomposed granite provides firm footing for a bird. Condors are capable of shredding and ingesting fabric, cardboard, or pebble substrate.

Food and water are not necessarily required for even long periods of travel. On occasion, birds have remained comfortable in carriers for up to 3 or 4 days without showing interest in food or water although offered after 12–24 hours. Vehicles used for travel should have heating and, in particular, good cooling and ventilation capabilities to prevent birds from overheating.

A bird in transit should periodically be evaluated visually, especially young birds that have had no transport experience. In 1988, a juvenile Andean condor intended for release in California was found dead in its carrier, presumably because of stress during transport from a breeding facility to a release site enclosure.

QUARANTINE PROCEDURE

At the SDWAP and The Los Angeles Zoo (LAZ), birds transferred from other breeding institutions are housed in a separate facility for 30 days before joining the captive collection. The birds are weighed in their transport container on arrival. There is an initial period of acclimatization, during which 3 to 4 days may pass before birds show interest in food. Birds that are reluctant to eat may be enticed to do so by the offering of organ or muscle meat. This has been especially true for juveniles or recent fledglings that have known only one institution. This has been the case with birds recaptured from the wild that have demonstrated a poor probability of survival or questionable behavior or health. The LAZ has observed birds returning from the wild to readily eat upon arrival.

In some cases, after physical examination, the quarantine period has been shortened when socialization with other birds has been critical in easing the acclimatization process. If food consumption of a new arrival is in question, the bird's weight is taken and compared with the arrival weight.

A few days after arrival and review of past medical records, quarantined birds are given a physical examination that includes diagnostic sample screening (see Annual Examination) and, in the case of a bird arriving from the wild, a whole body radiographic study. A bird returned to captivity from the wild because of a suspected health problem should have its blood lead level evaluated immediately upon arrival to rule out lead toxicity, previously discussed as a factor in the death of wild condors. On completion of quarantine, birds are reweighed and transferred to the collection facility.

CLINICAL TECHNIQUES

Physical Restraint

For elective procedures requiring physical restraint, a California condor should be fasted 1 day before to reduce the probability of regurgitation during handling. Physical manipulation should be restricted to a cool period of the day to prevent hyperthermia during restraint (Fig. 36–3).

Restraint of condors requires special skills and a minimum of two individuals. To facilitate handling, a bird is initially captured with a standard hand-held hoop net, allowing the bird to remain standing. While one person secures the wings folded against the body and grasps and flexes the legs against the body, the second individual first restrains the head from outside the net, then reaches under the net to guide the head out from under the net. In restraining the head, it is important to place the palm of one hand behind the bird's head while encircling the beak with the other hand, maintaining control of the head and neck. Whereas a bird's toes may scratch a handler, a beak can inflict a serious wound. Once apprehended, the bird can be placed in lateral recumbency on an examination table with the legs flexed against the body or extended toward the tail feathers.

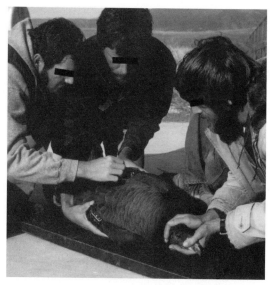

FIGURE 36–3. Field biologists restrain a wild-caught juvenile condor after application of patagial radiotransmitters.

A securely held bird will not struggle. Some birds are more comfortable if their eyes are lightly covered with a small towel in a manner that enables the handler to monitor the oral cavity for signs of airway obstruction from regurgitant or evidence of respiratory distress. Birds destined for release should have their eyes covered to prevent visual contact with humans, and they should not hear human voices during restraint.

Restrained condors initially display hurried respirations and a rapid heart rate, but they relax after 15 to 20 seconds. A particularly stressed bird's heartbeat can be heard 2 to 3 feet away as an audible click. Should this persist, the procedure should be terminated and the bird released. Birds with previous restraint experience adjust quickly. Young birds, 2.5 to 5 months of age, are prone to stress. One such chick died of stress during restraint in 1980 at a nest site while being examined by a single individual (Fig. 36–4).

Time of restraint should be held to a minimum of 10 to 12 minutes, which is adequate for a general examination and collection of routine diagnostic samples. Wild-caught and captive birds, however, have been held for up to 1 hour without harmful effects. There are no documented cases of exertional myopathy in California condors.

ANNUAL EXAMINATION

At the SDWAP and LAZ, birds from the captive breeding collection undergo annual examination in the late summer or early fall before annual courtship behavior. Birds are physically restrained for 10 to 12 minutes (Fig. 36–5).

First, a bird's microchip implant number (Trovan Transponder; Infopet Identification Systems, Inc., 517 W. Travelers Trail, Burnsville, MN) is validated. An aerobic cloacal culture (Culturette; Becton Dickinson &

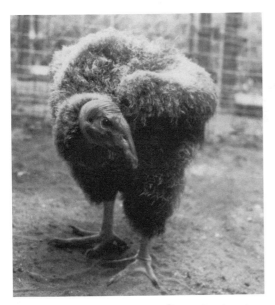

FIGURE 36–4. A condor chick at 2 1/2 months of age is susceptible to stress during manual restraint.

Co., Cockeysville, MD) is taken, followed by recording the cloacal temperature (Tele-Thermometer; Yellow Springs Instrument Co., Yellow Springs, OH), which ranges from 101° to 104°F in a calm bird and up to 106°–107°F in birds exercised before apprehension. Misting with a water sprayer will help cool a bird. The abdominal air sacs, lungs, and heart are auscultated. During restraint, the normal heart rate ranges between 120 and 180 beats per minute, and the respiratory rate

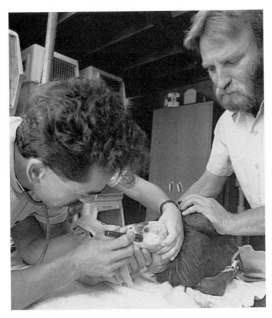

FIGURE 36–5. Manual restraint of a California condor during annual examination.

ranges from 15 to 30 breaths per minute. Keel musculature and the abdomen are palpated. Routine abdominal palpation at LAZ revealed an intracoelomic egg in one case and an encapsulated egg remnant abscess in the other.

Before the bird is manipulated further, a blood sample is obtained from the medial metatarsal vein as it courses superficially along the medial shaft of the tarsometatarsus. The skin is initially scrubbed with antiseptic soap (Nolvasan, Fort Dodge Labs, Fort Dodge, IA), and venipuncture is achieved with the use of a 21 g × 0.75 × 12 inch tubing infusion butterfly (Abbott Laboratories, North Chicago, IL).

For annual examination purposes, 10 ml of blood is taken for the tests listed in Table 36–2. Additional blood is taken for ongoing research on vitamin E levels, endocrinology studies, and serum archiving, and at the LAZ for bile acids, cholinesterase, and serology studies for aspergillosis, influenza, and mycoplasma. In healthy birds weighing 17 to 23 pounds, up to 20 to 25 ml of blood has been taken routinely without causing harmful effects. The LAZ has collected 30–36 ml from healthy adult birds without any harmful effects.

The examination continues with a general visual inspection of the head, including the external eye, adnexa and globe, external ear canal, nares, beak, and oral tissues. The general plumage and skin are examined for evidence of ectoparasites. The limbs are inspected and palpated. Patagial wing tags for identification, if present, are inspected at their point of attachment to evaluate any evidence of local irritation.

After examination, the bird is placed in standing position in a preweighed transport container to obtain a total body weight. A bird may be detained in the container to obtain a fecal specimen for parasite ova evaluation and stool culture.

At the SDWAP, if a bird is being examined in preparation for transfer to a reintroduction site, a total body radiographic study is desirable for survey information at this time. In this event, the examination and radiographic procedure are more effectively completed under general anesthesia.

Anesthesia

Indications for general anesthesia include radiographic examination, wound care, assistance in accurate place-

TABLE 36–2. Sample Sizes and Collection Tubes Required for Annual Examination and Blood Tests

Test	Sample Required	Minimum Amount
CBC	Heparin blood/navy EDTA Whole blood smears	0.5 ml
Biochemistry profiles	Red top tube—Serum	0.5 ml
Lead	Navy top tube—EDTA	1.25 ml
Zinc	Navy top tube—EDTA	1.25 ml

CBC, complete blood count; Chem, X; EDTA, ethylene diaminetetraacetic acid.

ment of patagial identification tags or radiotransmitter devices, coaptation procedures, and surgery.

Adults and juveniles should be fasted for 24 hours whenever possible to reduce crop volume and prevent regurgitation and aspiration. In the case of prefledglings or chicks, the crop volume may be palpated and the contents aspirated if regurgitation is deemed a risk.

Inhalation anesthesia is preferable to parenteral anesthesia. Ketamine hydrochloride (Ketaset), 15 mg/kg intramuscularly (IM), has been used successfully by the author on wild-caught and released adult Andean condors in Peru for abdominal laparoscopy procedures. Anesthesia induced by xylazine (Rompun; 1 mg/kg body weight IM) and ketamine (10 mg/kg IM) has been described in turkey vultures (*Cathartes aura*) to evaluate the effects of tolazoline (Priscoline) to stimulate arousal and return to mobility.[1]

Isoflurane is the anesthetic of choice because of its wide margin of safety. Once the various parameters apparent to the individual case are assessed to determine the risk, the condor is restrained in upright position, and induction is accomplished with a face mask. Intubation is achieved in most cases with a 5- to 6-mm tube in adults and juveniles; a Cole tube (Rush, Germany) has been successful in chicks (Fig. 36–6).

Anesthesia is monitored through the standard techniques of observing rate and depth of respiration, response of the cornea and palpebrae to stimulus, toe pinch and withdrawal, and cloacal sphincter tone. Heart rate and oxygen saturation are monitored with pulse oximetry (Nellcor N-3000; Nelcor, Inc., Pleasanton, CA) (Fig. 36–7). Accuracy of oxygen saturation measurements in condors has not been determined.

In procedures lasting up to 1 hour, it is appropriate to give fluids intravenously by slow drip throughout anesthesia. The medial metatarsal vein is catheterized

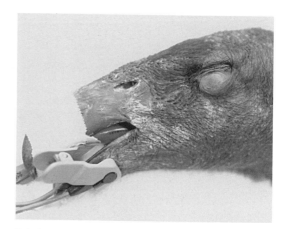

FIGURE 36–7. Pulse oxymetry sensor clip placement on the lower beak of a juvenile California condor under general anesthesia.

for fluid administration. Normal body temperature should be maintained and can be monitored by cloacal probe.

In field procedure situations, when general anesthesia is required, a portable isoflurane vaporizer (Ohmeda Isotec 3; Ohmeda Station Road, Steeton, West Yorkshire, England) can be used with an E cylinder oxygen tank, flow meter, and a Norman elbow or other nonrebreathing system. Portable pulse oximetry (Nellcor N-20; Hayward, CA) can be used to monitor anesthesia under field conditions.

RADIOGRAPHIC IMAGING

Indications for radiographic procedures on condors include evaluation for heavy metal ingestion, prerelease screening, and traumatic injury to limbs; as a diagnostic aid in abdominal disease of adults and chicks; and in near hatch eggs to evaluate embryo position. General anesthesia facilitates radiographic studies and reduces stress to condors.

In cases of suspected toxicity from ingestion of lead, a whole body radiograph is indicated. Appearance of a small irregular radiopaque object in the gastrointestinal tract, usually the gizzard, supports a tentative diagnosis of lead ingestion. A case involving the death of a free-ranging Griffon vulture (*Gyps fulvus*) in Spain caused by lead ingestion from an eroded lead shot or bullet fragment was documented.[31] A metallic object in the gastrointestinal tract must be differentiated from lead imbedded in body tissue from shooting.

Whole-body radiographs of condors before release serve to screen birds for the incidental appearance of small pebbles in the gizzard, which are probably swallowed while feeding and may assist in the digestive process. A survey film helps to familiarize the clinician with the radiographic anatomy of a species infrequently studied. In one case involving a captured, previously released condor, an enlarged heart was a suspected radiographic finding; however, this discovery was most likely normal for the species.

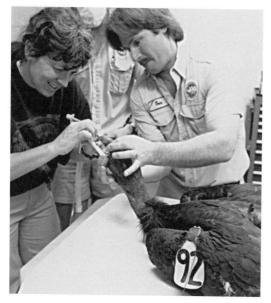

FIGURE 36–6. Placement of endotracheal tube after face mask induction with isoflurane gas anesthesia.

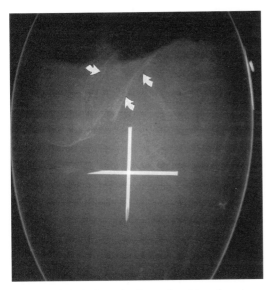

FIGURE 36–8. Radiograph of normal position of condor embryo at day 55 of incubation. *Arrows* denote head/beak position upside down beneath air cell.

At The LAZ, there have been two cases of a palpable abdominal mass in two female condors causing infertility and in time most probably death. In each incidence, radiographic imaging that included a barium swallow contrast study to define the masses proved beneficial before successful surgical removal of an intracoelomic egg in one case and an encapsulated egg remnant abscess in the other (R. Izaza, personal communication, 1997).

Radiographic imaging has been used to more critically evaluate chick position in near-hatch California condor eggs at the SDWAP and The LAZ.[7] This procedure was undertaken to determine embryo position when conventional candling techniques failed to determine if an abnormality or malposition near hatch was suspected. In cases in which a fatal malposition is identified with the likelihood of a failure to hatch, intervention by artificially pipping an egg near the chick's head to assist hatching may prevent the chick's demise if discovered early.

From 1990 to 1993, seven incubating California condor eggs, 7 cm in thickness, were exposed to a vertical x-ray beam (56 kVp and 100 mA) for 1/30 second at the distance of 101.6 cm. At least two films were made; the second image with the egg rotated 90 degrees from the first. Films made "end on" of an egg or in vertical axes did not assist in clarifying embryo position. Cronex 10T (E.I. Dupont DeNemours & Co. Inc., Wilmington, DE) and Kodak (MIN-R M MRM-1) Diagnostics Film (Eastman Kodak, Rochester, NY) were used in this study. Three of the eggs that were radiographed resulted in live hatches. In these eggs, embryo position appeared normal on radiographic images. Studies of the remaining four eggs in which the embryos did not survive revealed two with malpositioned embryos. The remaining two embryos were in apparently normal radiographic position; however, one

came from an egg with a previously cracked shell that consequently was incubated in a vertical rather than a horizontal position; the other came from an egg with the air cell at the small rather than large end of the egg (Figs. 36–8, 36–9).

There have been four cases of yolk sac infection with coelomitis in hatched California condor chicks and in a fifth case that died near hatch, at the SDWAP and LAZ. Radiographs of two of these chicks revealed the presence of gas within a space-occupying abdominal mass. An infected yolk sac and coelomitis was confirmed in two of these cases at surgery. Yolk sac infections have been an infrequent finding; however, radiographic imaging is indicated in suspected cases to support a diagnosis (Fig. 36–10).

SURGERY

In 1976, a severely weakened California condor was brought to the LAZ with gunshot wounds to one wing. The bird died of postoperative complications after surgical amputation of the limb (G. Kuehn, personal communication, 1997).

Because limb trauma was thought to be a likely possibility during the 1980s when cannon netting procedures were initiated to trap wild condors, a study was undertaken to critically describe the limb anatomy of this species. This anatomic and surgical study used the

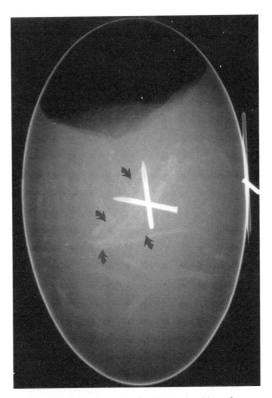

FIGURE 36–9. Radiograph of a fatal malposition of a condor embryo at day 54 of incubation. *Arrows* denote head/beak position distant to the air cell.

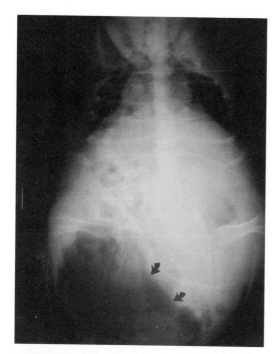

FIGURE 36–10. Radiograph of a 3-day-old condor chick with a yolk sac infection. *Arrows* denote gas within a space-occupying abdominal mass.

turkey vulture and other avian species as models and resulted in an atlas on the anatomy and surgical approaches to the thoracic and pelvic limbs that could be applied to the California condor as well as other species.[36]

As noted earlier, there have been four cases of yolk sac infection in condor chicks. In two of these cases, abdominal surgery to amputate and remove the infected yolk sac was attempted as previously described in other avian species.[18] In these two cases, one at the SDWAP and the other at The LAZ, coelomitis was a complication, making dissection and removal of the yolk sac difficult. One chick died intraoperatively, and the second was euthanized 2 days after surgery. In one case at The LAZ with an egg at 53 days of incubation, a chick required manual assistance to hatch as a result of a malposition. In this case, veterinarians successfully amputated an unretracted yolk sac at its stalk (C. Stringfield, personal communication, 1998). As previously mentioned, the two abdominal surgeries performed at The LAZ to remove abdominal masses resulted in successful reproduction by both adult females the next year.

Captive and released California condors are outfitted with patagial identification tags. Released condors have a combination patagial tag/radiotransmitter attached to each wing. Application of these devices is not considered a surgical procedure, but if incorrectly applied, they may lead to complicating infection. In the field, United States Fish and Wildlife Service personnel apply tag/transmitters by using a leather hole-punch tool that has been placed in a solution of Nolvasan for at least

10 minutes and wiped with 70% isopropyl alcohol. The patagial site for application is cleaned with a povidone-iodine scrub (Betadine; Purdue Frederick Co., Norwalk, CT) and wiped with 70% isopropyl alcohol before hole punch and tag/transmitter application. General anesthesia is desirable in reducing stress to birds and to facilitate correct tag placement.

Captive and released condors have Trovan microchip identification implants placed at the base of the neck. This has become an administrative procedure necessary to identify young birds before they are large enough to outfit with patagial tags or transmitters.

REPRODUCTION

Historically, in the wild, California condors lay eggs from late January through April. The same observation is made of captive pairs.

Before condors were bred in captivity, eggs removed as early as 1983 from wild breeding pairs were incubated and hatched through artificial techniques.[25] From 1983 to 1990, The LAZ and Zoological Society of San Diego incubated 37 eggs artificially. Thirty-two were fertile and 28 hatched (fertility, 86.5%; hatchability, 87.5%).[26] In 1988, the first egg laid in captivity successfully hatched at the SDWAP.

The results of captive California condor egg production from 1988 through 1997 are listed in Table 36–3.

The California condor egg is asymmetric. The air cell appears normally at 1 to 2 days of incubation at the large end of the egg. As a comparison, ostrich eggs are generally symmetric; therefore, the air cell may appear at either end of the egg.[28] Current general incubation parameters at the SDWAP include a dry bulb temperature of 97.5° to 98°F and a relative humidity range up to 52% produced by a Petersime Model #1 forced air incubator. (Some of these parameters change after the egg pips). An egg weight loss goal of 14% is desirable. At near hatch, the normal position of the California condor is not unlike that of other avian embryos. That is, the head is tucked upside down under the right wing (Fig. 36–11).

The incubation period for California condor eggs incubated in captivity is 55 to 58 days. The chick's head enters the air cell at 52 to 55 days, after which it takes 24 to 60 hours to pip. The pip-to-hatch interval is 72 hours. At the SDWAP, a chick is assisted from its

TABLE 36–3. Captive California Condor Egg Production: 1988 through 1997

Location	Laid	Infertile	Fertile	Hatched
San Diego Wild Animal Park	84	16	68	57
The Los Angeles Zoo	86	6	80	67
World Center for Birds of Prey	21	18*	3	2
Totals	**191**	**40**	**151**	**126**

*High infertility is most likely associated with the young breeding pairs at this facility.

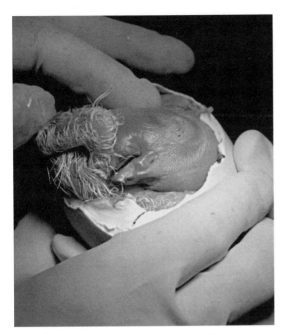

FIGURE 36–11. Condor chick being assisted from its egg. Note the head position beneath the right wing.

shell 72 hours after pip to reduce stress on the chick if it is judged to be not making sufficient progress toward hatch. In some cases, the drying eggshell membrane of pipped chicks appears to constrict or strangulate the chick if left too long in its shell. For this reason, pipped eggs are transferred from forced air to still-air incubators. Continued modification of incubation parameters has resulted in fewer chicks requiring assistance at hatch (Fig. 36–12). The LAZ has reduced the prevalence for manual assistance at hatch by placing the eggs at pip in high-humidity forced-air incubators (S. Kasielke, personal communication, 1998).

Condor reproductive conduct once studied in the wild is now observed in captivity at the SDWAP and LAZ.[12-14] Keeper personnel at the SDWAP have noted on at least three occasions females that have acted as if about to lay an egg and then did not. Facility personnel refer to this as *phantom egg behavior.*

MEDICAL CONDITIONS OF CHICKS AT HATCH

Previously mentioned was a condition known as fatal or lethal malposition, in which some cases may be diagnosed by radiographic imaging. This condition may be the result of a variety of problems, including inbreeding or incorrect or insufficient egg turning during incubation.[27, 48] In one case of a suspected fatal malposition diagnosed with radiographic imaging at the SDWAP, the egg was artificially pipped with a rotary power tool (Craftsman; Sears Roebuck & Co., Chicago, IL) to open a 1-cm² window over the chick's head. Through a 2.7-mm rigid endoscope (Richard Wolf Medical Instruments

Corp., Rosemont, IL), the chick's head was visualized in the air cell; however, it had already died.

After hatch of an artificially incubated egg, whether or not the chick was assisted at hatch, aerobic culture swabs are taken from the eggshell membrane, cloaca, and umbilicus. Results of these cultures have almost always yielded "no growth." Positive growth may become meaningful should the chick fail to thrive at 2 to 3 days after hatch. The umbilicus or umbilical seal is painted with a povidone iodine solution. Chicks given assistance at hatch sometimes require ligation of the umbilical vessels. In these chicks, the umbilicus may be open and appear in need of a purse-string suture to close. The periumbilical skin is quite edematous and will easily tear when attempting to close with suture against an abdomen distended because of a full yolk sac. It is best in these cases to apply a small sterile gauze soaked in povidone iodine solution against the open umbilicus that the chick can rest upon. An open umbilicus of 3 to 5 mm will usually close within a few hours.

Chicks may hatch with their eyes open or closed. They may or may not be vocal. Most often, new hatches are fatigued and need to rest. They cannot thermoregulate, so after brief inspection they should be placed immediately into an incubator set at 95°F. The respiratory rate for a newly hatched chick is approximately 20 breaths per minute, and if a chick shows labored respiration, the incubator may be too warm. Chicks are initially housed individually in incubators for the first 30 days. At The LAZ the incubator temperature is reduced 1°F daily, allowing chicks to be transferred to an open box at room temperature (75°F) by 3 weeks of age (S. Kasielke, personal communication, 1998).

Occasionally, an assisted hatch chick will have a very edematous head that can be partially elevated with

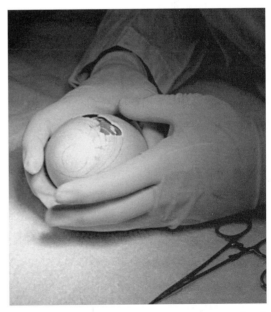

FIGURE 36–12. Condor egg in which the chick has pipped but is unable to hatch by itself.

a folded towel. The edema becomes mobilized in the first 24 hours (Fig. 36–13).

A chick's weight should be recorded in the first hour after hatch, and any debris left on the chick from hatching should be rinsed free with warm sterile saline. At the SDWAP, chicks are initially monitored 24 hours a day for any problems. Post-hatch weights range from 160 to 190 g. Chicks are offered food 24 hours after hatch or earlier in some cases. Initial feedings consist of 1 to 2 minced pinkie mice with one gram (a pinch) of calcium carbonate powder per feeding given every hour from 6:00 AM until 9:00 PM. Before each feeding, the crop is palpated. A chick with a crop that is not emptying is offered an oral pediatric electrolyte maintenance solution (Abbott Laboratories, Ross Products Division, Columbus, OH). Overfeeding may result in slow crop emptying or regurgitation, in which case a chick can be fasted for several feedings. If dehydration occurs, skin over the head, neck, and feet becomes more wrinkled. Chicks can be rehydrated orally with an electrolyte maintenance solution or, if necessary, by clysis with 2.5% dextrose and lactated Ringer's solution, 3 to 4 ml every 3 to 4 hours.

Chicks should show interest in food, but at times they appear listless or sleepy. At 5 to 7 days of age, chicks consume 7 to 10 minced pinkie mice per feeding. Whole pinkies and sliced fuzzy mice torsos are fed at 7 to 9 days of age, at which time most chicks are eating on their own and the calcium carbonate supplement is discontinued.

In the four cases of omphalophlebitis or yolk sac infection, chicks were reluctant to feed, listless, and prone to regurgitate as early as 24 hours after hatch. An increase in abdominal tension was a prominent finding in at least two cases. The source of the infection was uncertain in view of the strict sanitation routines used[55] (Fig. 36–14).

Daily weight gains are approximately 10% of body

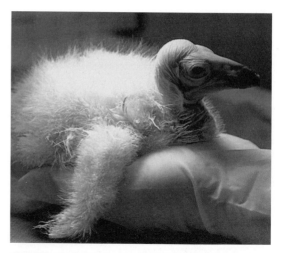

FIGURE 36–14. Three-day-old chick with yolk sac infection. Note the wrinkled skin over the head and neck caused by dehydration.

weight. As chicks grow, the amounts fed are increased until 30 days of age, when the chicks are essentially placed on an adult diet fed in small pieces and portions.

After the first 1 to 2 weeks of age, condor chicks adapt readily to a routine. Chicks identified as candidates for the reintroduction program are managed under a strict husbandry protocol designed to eliminate human visual and auditory stimulation. There have been relatively few medical problems with chicks, although a few are worthy of discussion.

Spraddle Legs

This condition manifests in the first few days. The legs appear to abduct and require simple taping or use of soft gauze dressing to help adduct the limbs to the correct posture. Limb position returns to normal in a few days.

Swollen Toes

Edema of the toes during the first 2 weeks has been noted, perhaps resulting from restricted movement in an incubator. This condition can lead to skin cracks and subsequent infection. Stimulating chicks to exercise in their confined surroundings should prevent the problem (Fig. 36–15).

Bacterial Enteritis

At the SDWAP, there have been two episodes of diarrhea in condor chicks resulting in illness manifested by a slow feeding response, dehydration, poor weight gain or loss, and lethargy. In the first episode involving three chicks at 1 week of age, *Salmonella* species, group C2, was isolated from cloacal cultures from two of the chicks. All three chicks were placed on antibiotic therapy—either gentamicin sulfate, 3.5 mg/kg IM once

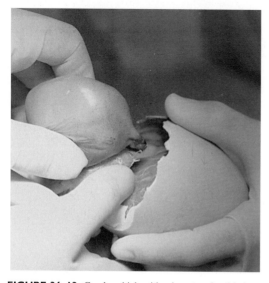

FIGURE 36–13. Condor chick with edematous head being assisted at hatch.

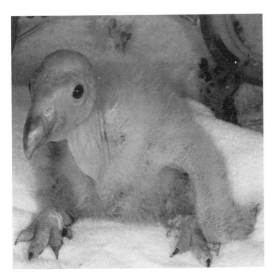

FIGURE 36–15. One-week-old condor chick with edematous feet.

daily for 3 days, or ampicillin sodium oral suspension (Omnipen), 35 mg/kg by mouth TID for 7 days. When required, fluid replacement was provided by clysis. All three birds responded, and follow-up cloacal cultures were negative for enteric pathogens (Fig. 36–16).

In a second episode, *Campylobacter jejuni* was isolated from two chicks with diarrhea. Only one of the two birds displayed illness and required antibiotic treatment. In the untreated bird, weekly cloacal cultures remained positive and then became negative.

Of interest, *Salmonella* species was cultured from

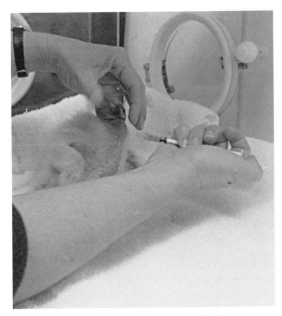

FIGURE 36–16. Week-old condor chick with diarrhea (caused by *Salmonella* species) receiving oral antibiotic medication.

day-old domestic chicks and commercially prepared meat rations fed to juvenile and adult condors at the SDWAP. In the *Salmonella*-positive condor chicks, day-old domestic chick yolk sacs had been fed after hatch.

A review of medical records indicates that on several occasions, *Salmonella* species and *C. jejuni* have been isolated from cloacal cultures of healthy chicks. This has also been a finding on several adult condors on annual examination. Currently at the SDWAP, asymptomatic chicks are not treated and adult birds have not demonstrated illness associated with either of these organisms. Rules of sanitation and personal hygiene are closely followed by facility personnel.

Trauma

One condor chick at the SDWAP was euthanized because of injuries sustained from a brooding adult bird. Another chick was cannibalized by the parent birds for unknown reasons.

Summary

There have been relatively few medical problems in condor chicks. When illness has occurred, it has been readily identified in hand-reared birds. As the captive population of condors grows, emphasis is seen shifting to produce chicks from parent-incubated eggs and chicks subsequently parent reared. This may result in chicks with greater survival skills and most likely better adapted for reintroduction. It will become more challenging to monitor the health of chicks under these circumstances.

SEX DETERMINATION

There are no external distinguishing features to differentiate male from female California condors. From 1982 until 1994, sex of condors was determined through the use of a modified leukocyte and chromosome preparation technique at the Center for the Reproduction of Endangered Species (CRES) at the Zoological Society of San Diego (A. Kumamoto, personal communication, 1997).[3] From 1994 until the present, DNA probe sex determination has been performed at the same facility through DNA-probe methodology. This can be completed by using DNA extracted from blood left in eggshell membranes after hatching or from a few drops of blood drawn from chicks[30] (L. Chemnick, personal communication, 1997). Blood samples from chicks are readily obtained from the right jugular vein.

PATHOLOGY

For nearly 20 years, the pathology department of the Zoological Society of San Diego has provided a necropsy service for specimens submitted from the SDWAP, LAZ, and Condor Recovery Team members, who worked initially with the wild condor population and are now working with reintroduced condors in

California and Arizona. This service includes sending tissue specimens to various appropriate agencies and investigators. The rapid dissemination of information to program participants has been vital to husbandry, management, and veterinary personnel.

Necropsy findings (B. Rideout, personal communication, 1998) from 1980 to 1998 are found in Table 36–4.

Brief Summary of Necropsy Findings

Of the 39 accessions, 15 condors were submitted from the wild population. Of the 15, 10 were reintroduced birds. Of the 10 reintroduced, 7 were lost to trauma. Of the remaining 5 submitted birds, which were hatched and living in the wild, 4 died from toxicity or poisoning—3 of which were caused by lead ingestion.

Of the 24 accessions submitted from captivity, 17 were eggs or eggs at or near hatch. The balance were chicks. Of the 17 eggs, 8 were malpositions. Of the remaining 7 chicks, 4 died from yolk sac infections and associated coelomitis. There have been no fatalities from the juvenile or adult captive populations.

Two reintroduced birds in California disappeared in 1996. Their remains were not located. One of the birds vanished during a forest fire. In Arizona, one reintroduced bird has disappeared.

ENVIRONMENTAL CONTAMINANTS AFFECTING CONDOR HEALTH

As noted at the beginning of this chapter, it is difficult to reliably measure the impact of historical environmental poisons such as strychnine and compound 1080 on the wild condor population. Eggshell thinning of California condor eggs caused by DDE, a breakdown metabolite of the pesticide DDT, occurred in the 1950s and 1960s.[19, 21, 50–52] The full impact of DDT on condors will remain unknown; however, because DDT has been banned for domestic use since 1972, it should no longer be a factor in condor survivability.

More recently, in 1983, one wild juvenile bird died from cyanide poisoning most likely intended for a coyote. This was a single documented loss, as was that of a captive bred and released condor that died in 1992 from ethylene glycol toxicosis.[33] The source of the ethylene glycol remains uncertain.

In 1996, organophosphate toxicity was suspected, although unconfirmed, in two of four juvenile condors confined together at a release site in preparation for reintroduction to the wild. These birds had ataxia, regurgitation, and depression. They were taken to The LAZ for further examination, where they demonstrated crop stasis and bradycardia. Blood lead levels were within normal limits. Because these birds each responded dramatically to a single dose of atropine (7.5 mg) given intramuscularly, organophosphate toxicity remained the presumptive diagnosis. The source of this toxicosis was thought to be contaminated food. Other suspected causes for this illness included botulism and ingested algae from the local water supply. Studies of cholinesterase levels in affected and normal condors did not prove helpful in elucidating this condition (C. Stringfield, personal communication, 1998).

Ingested lead was mentioned earlier as a cause of death in at least three wild condors in the 1980s. It is of interest that in the 1960s, both a wild-caught Andean condor taken from South America to the Patuxent Wildlife Research Center and a long-lived Andean condor at the San Diego Zoo died from ingesting lead from contaminated food.[10] This should not be a problem for captive or recently released California condors being provisioned on reliable food sources. When released birds forage into areas heavily hunted, however, exposure to lead is almost certain.

In 1997, up to 10 reintroduced condors were observed feeding on a hunter-shot carcass. Three days later, 8 of the birds were tested for blood lead levels. One the basis of elevated lead levels and radiographic evidence of ingested lead, 3 birds were taken to The LAZ. None demonstrated clinical illness. After chelation therapy, all 3 were released to the wild (C. Stringfield, personal communication, 1998).

The outcome of lead ingestion by condors may not be clear in every case. History of lead ingestion, radiographic evidence, elevated blood lead levels, and clinical depression together will help determine whether chelation therapy is appropriate. A blood lead concentration higher than 30 mg/dl should be a matter of concern. Because of high fatalities associated with lead toxicosis, if a condor is suspected of lead ingestion, diagnostic confirmation and treatment should begin as soon as possible.

With reintroduced birds that are monitored with radiotelemetry, it will become easier for biologists to locate dead birds and subsequently learn the cause of death.

BACTERIAL PATHOGENS

Reference has already been made to bacterial enteritis of condor chicks in captivity caused by *Salmonella* species and *C. jejuni*. Stool or cloacal cultures in healthy birds may reveal either of these bacteria.

Anecdotal references regard vultures as being relatively disease resistant, perhaps because of their historical place as scavengers in the food chain. A review of the medical records at the SDWAP did not demonstrate any bacterial disease unique to condors. A variety of bacteria have been isolated from fecal or cloacal cultures on annual examinations or during the course of handling for a variety of reasons. They are *Pseudomonas cepacia* and *aeruginosa*, *Plesiomonas shigelloides*, *Escherichia coli*, *Edwardsiella tarda*, *Enterobacter* species, *Proteus mirabilis*, *Enterococcus* species, *Staphylococcus* species, *Klebsiella* species (*pneumoniae* and *oxytoca*), and *Streptococcus fecalis*.

Respiratory disease in California condors has not appeared clinically; therefore, choanal flora has not been studied.

TABLE 36–4. Necropsy Findings from 1980 through 1997

Year	Necropsy No.	Necropsy Finding	Comments
1980	RP 1129	Shock, cardiac failure	Wild, chick; died during handling at nest site
1983	RP 2656	Cyanide poisoning	Wild, juvenile; likely encounter with coyote poison
1984	RP 2747	Lead poisoning—copper-coated lead fragment in gizzard	Wild, juvenile; likely lead ingestion from carcass
1984	20509	Malposition with congenital defects	Captive, near-hatch chick
1984	20535	Yolk sac infection, coelomitis	Captive, 3-day-old chick
1985	RP 3213	Lead poisoning	Wild, juvenile; cause of death based on tissue lead levels
1986	22398	Lead poisoning	Wild, adult; died during treatment, clinical diagnosis based on blood lead levels and radiographic findings
1990	RP 4223	Visceral and articular gout	Captive, chick; died at hatch
1991	RP 4407	Malposition	Captive, chick; died at hatch
1991	RP 4418	Malposition	Captive, chick; died before hatch
1991	RP 4477	Shock, cause undetermined	Captive, chick; sudden death
1992	RP 4670	Malposition	Captive, chick; died before hatch
1992	RP 4671	Bacterial infection, developmental abnormalities	Captive, chick; died before hatch
1992	RP 4886	Ethylene glycol toxicity	Reintroduced, juvenile; hatched in captivity
1993	RP 4994	Omphalophlebitis associated with *Streptococcus faecalis*	Captive, chick; died near hatch
1993	RP 5053	Malposition and congenital deformities	Captive, chick; died near hatch
1993	RP 5057	Electrocution	Reintroduced, juvenile; hatched in captivity, hit high power line
1993	RP 5078	Trauma	Reintroduced, juvenile; hatched in captivity, likely hit power line or vehicle
1993	RP 5145	Trauma	Reintroduced, juvenile; hatched in captivity, likely hit power line or pole
1994	RP 5228	Yolk sac infection, coelomitis, associated with *Streptococcus faecalis*	Captive, 2-day-old chick
1994	RP 5230	Cause of death unknown	Captive; early embryonic death
1994	RP 5232	Congenital deformities, malposition	Captive, chick; died at hatch
1994	RP 5233	Cause of death unknown	Captive, chick; died near hatch
1994	RP 5253	Trauma, source unknown	Reintroduced, juvenile; hatched in captivity
1994	RP 5280	Neoplasia, round cell tumor, with respiratory aspergillosis as a late secondary event	Reintroduced, juvenile; hatched in captivity
1995	35400	Cause of death uncertain	Captive, 10-day-old chick; reared by parents and was cannibalized
1995	35605	Euthanasia	Captive, chick; parent reared and parent traumatized; permanent eye damage, subsequently hand reared until injury fully appreciated
1995	36718	Euthanasia associated with yolk sac infection, coelomitis, sepsis	Captive, chick; surgical removal of infected yolk sac
1996	RP 5853	Malposition	Captive, chick; died near hatch
1996	RP 5854	Malposition, albumen aspiration	Captive, chick; died near hatch
1996	RP 5860	Congenital abnormalities	Captive, chick; died near hatch
1996	RP 5867	Yolk sac infection, coelomitis, associated with *Streptococcus faecalis*	Captive, 11-day-old chick; died during operation to remove infected yolk sac
1997	RP 6227	Trauma	Reintroduced, juvenile; hatched in captivity, possibly attacked by a golden eagle
1997	RP 6254	Emaciation	Reintroduced, juvenile; hatched in captivity, recaptured because of weakened condition
1997	RP 6364	Congenital abnormalities, euthanasia	Captive, chick; euthanized in ovo at pip after 54 days of incubation
1997	RP 6376	Advanced postmortem autolysis	Captive, chick; died in ovo after 53 days of parent incubation
1997	RP 6443	Trauma	Reintroduced, adult; hit power lines
1997	RP 6467	Cause of death unknown	Captive, chick; died in ovo after 52 days of incubation
1997	RP 6608	Trauma	Reintroduced, adult; trauma from hitting power lines is suspected

Data from B. Rideout, personal communication, 1998.

FUNGAL DISEASE

Aspergillosis in California condors has been documented in one case at necropsy (RP 5280) as a late secondary event in a reintroduced juvenile that died from a round cell tumor. At the SDWAP, serologic assays (CF and AGID) during the years have yielded negative results.

PARASITOLOGY

During the 1980s, when five California condors from the wild population were submitted for necropsy, no examples of internal parasitism appear. During the same period, only one of the four chicks removed from nest sites for the captive breeding program had feather lice. It is possible that other chicks could have had lice that were overlooked during brief examination.

In the captive population at the SDWAP, feather lice are a common finding during annual examinations. The source of these ectoparasites may have originated from wild-caught birds or from wild turkey vultures that roost on the top of the condor breeding facility. Because birds are examined only once a year, it may be impossible to eliminate this infestation.

At The LAZ, nematode ova have been demonstrated on fecal flotation examination. These birds receive ivermectin (Equalan) at the dose of 2 mg by mouth.

CLINICAL EVALUATION OF A SICK CONDOR

In captivity, a condor for unknown reasons may demonstrate anorexia for 2 to 3 days. Harsh weather can precipitate anorexia. A bird thought to be anorectic should eat vigorously after a fast day.

Trauma to feet from flying up against the wire mesh enclosure may produce cuts or abrasions to feet, resulting in discomfort, lameness, and anorexia. Unseen split nails or beak tip injuries also result in anorexia that may last several days. Deep open wounds to the feet require topical care, dressing, and treatment with oral or parenteral antibiotic therapy to prevent serious infection.

A bird that appears ataxic or depressed and anorectic for several days should be examined. The same guidelines for an annual examination should be followed. Caution should be exercised during examination of birds 2½ to 5 months of age. The heart rate in these birds can exceed 240 beats per minute, and the respiratory rate can exceed 40 breaths per minute, resulting in critical stress.

There are no published hematologic and serum biochemical values for the California condor. However, there are comparable reference values for birds in published exotic animal formularies.[5, 17] California condors demonstrate a unique stress leukogram, whereby white blood cell counts commonly range between 25 and 30 × 10³, thus masking leukocytosis associated with infection. Condors have one diagnostic advantage as a result of their size: as an aid to rule out sepsis, adequate blood can be drawn for blood culture (Pedi-Bact; Aerobic Culture Bottle, Organon Teknika Corp., Durham, NC).

In one such case, an anorectic and depressed adult male condor was seen with a history of its enclosure being recently repaired with new galvanized wire mesh. Zinc toxicosis was suspected. Radiographs were negative for metallic foreign body. A blood culture was positive for *Streptococcus uberis* (viridans group) with susceptibility to ampicillin. While waiting for results of plasma zinc levels, the bird was treated initially with ampicillin sodium, 25 mg/kg IM twice daily, then orally, 55 mg/kg twice daily, by medicating a food item for 4 days. When a plasma zinc value of 1632 μg/L was reported (expected value, 550 to 1400 μg/L) (Nichols Institute Reference Laboratories, personal communication, 1994), the bird was treated for suspected zinc toxicosis with edetate calcium disodium (Calcium Disodium Versenate) at a rate of 45 mg/kg IM twice daily for 2 days. The bird's appetite continued to improve, and therapy was discontinued. After this case, a survey of other condors revealed plasma zinc levels within and just above the expected value range. It is uncertain that this bird had zinc toxicosis. After treatment for sepsis, however, a second blood culture was found to be negative.

Supportive care to sick, anorexic adult or juvenile condors must involve intravenous fluid therapy. In such cases, an indwelling intravenous catheter in the medial metatarsal vein is well tolerated.

MEDICAL TREATMENT FOR RELEASED CONDORS

The third revision of the Recovery Plan for the California Condors[20] published in 1996, along with the Species Survival Plans, details the species status, including all known condors from 1966 to present, their genetic analyses, pedigree, and the current recovery strategy.[23, 24] It is remarkable that in the decade since the last wild condor was brought into the captive breeding program, this species has so successfully reproduced that it has been reintroduced in California and Arizona. It will become equally if not more challenging to provide medical care to birds released to the wild.

Currently, a staff veterinarian at The LAZ coordinates veterinary assistance to biologists monitoring reintroduced birds in California and Arizona. This person provides information to local veterinarians who may be called upon to examine a reintroduced bird. After consultation, a decision is made as to whether a bird is to be transported to The LAZ or DSDWAP for further examination, treatment, and release or held for long-term care (C. Stringfield, personal communication, 1998). A decision to capture a bird for medical examination based on behavior will be difficult because further confinement for diagnosis and treatment of a medical problem may compromise its survivability after release. As the geographic range of released condors broadens, more veterinarians will be required to become knowledgeable of the medical problems of this unique species.

Acknowledgments

The author would like to thank Donald J. Sterner, Lead Keeper at the San Diego Wild Animal Park, for his assistance in the preparation of this manuscript; Drs. Cynthia Stringfield, Romero Isaza, Gary Kuehn, and Charles Sedgwick at The Los Angeles Zoo for sharing their clinical experience; Susie Kasielke, Curator at The Los Angeles Zoo; Dr. Bruce Rideout, Department of Pathology at the Zoological Society of San Diego; and Sandy Walton, Administrative Assistant at the San Diego Wild Animal Park, for manuscript preparation.

REFERENCES

1. Allen JL, Oosterhuis JE: Effect of tolazoline on xylazine-ketamine–induced anesthesia in turkey vultures. J Am Vet Med Assoc 189:1011–1012, 1986.
2. American Ornithologists' Union: 41st supplement to the AOU checklist of North American birds (7th ed.). AUK 114:542–552, 1997.
3. Biederman BM, Lin CC: A leukocyte culture and chromosome preparation technique for avian species. In Vitro 18(4):415–418, 1982.
4. Carpenter JW: Medical and husbandry aspects of captive Andean condors: a model for the California condor. Proceedings of the American Association of Zoo Veterinarians, New Orleans, pp 13–19, 1982.
5. Carpenter JW, Mashima TY, Rupiper DJ: Exotic Animal Formulary. Manhatten, KS, Greystone Publications, 1996.
6. Ensley PK: Veterinary aspects of the California condor (*Gymnogyps californianus*) recovery program. Proceedings of the Student Chapter of the American Veterinary Medical Association, Symposium, University of California at Davis, pp 421–424, 1988.
7. Ensley PK, Rideout BA, Sterner DJ: Radiographic imaging to evaluate chick position in California condor eggs. Proceedings of the American Association of Zoo Veterinarians, Pittsburgh, pp 132–133, 1994.
8. Erickson RC, Carpenter JW: Captive condor propagation and recommended release procedures. In Wilbur SR, Jackson JA (eds): Vulture Biology and Management. Berkeley, University of California Press, pp 385–399, 1983.
9. Geyer CJ, Ryder OA, Chemnick LG, Thompson EA: Analysis of relatedness in the California condors, from DNA fingerprints. Mol Biol Evol 10:571–589, 1993.
10. Griner LA: Pathology of Zoo Animals. Zoological Society of San Diego, pp 172–176, 1983.
11. Harrison EN, Kiff LF: Apparent replacement clutch laid by wild California condor. Condor 82:351–352, 1980.
12. Hartt EW, Harvey NC, Leete AJ, Preston K: Effects of age at pairing on reproduction of captive California condors (*Gymnogyps californianus*). Zoo Biol 13:3–11, 1994.
13. Harvey NC, Hartt EW, Leete AJ, Preston K: Changes in incubation sharing in one pair of captive California condors (*Gymnogyps californianus*). Zoo Biol 13:157–165, 1994.
14. Harvey N, Preston KL, Leete AJ: Reproductive behavior in captive California condors (*Gymnogyps californianus*). Zoo Biol 15:115–125, 1996.
15. Janssen DL, Oosterhuis JE, Allen JL, et al: Lead poisoning in free-ranging California condors. J Am Vet Med Assoc 189:1115–1117, 1986.
16. Johnson WW: A flap over how to save the condor. Smithsonian 14(9):72–81, 1983.
17. Johnson-Delaney CA: Exotic Companion Medicine Handbook. Lake Worth, FL, Wingers Publishing, 1996.
18. Kenny D, Cambre RC: Indications and technique for the surgical removal of avian yolk sac. J Zoo Wildl Med 23(1):55–61, 1992.
19. Kiff LF: DDE and the California condor (*Gymnogyps californianus*): the end of the story? In Meyburg BU, Chancellor RD (eds): Raptors in the Modern World. Berlin, World Working Group on Birds of Prey, pp 477–480, 1989.
20. Kiff LF, Mesta RI, Wallace MP: Recovery Plan for the California Condor. U.S. Fish and Wildlife Service, Portland, OR, 1996.
21. Kiff LF, Peakall DB, Morrison ML, Wilbur SR: Eggshell thickness and DDE residue levels in vulture eggs. In Wilbur SR, Jackson JA (eds): Vulture Biology and Management. Berkeley, University of California Press, pp 440–458, 1983.
22. Koford CB: The California Condor. Natl Audubon Soc Res Rep 4:1–154, 1953.
23. Kuehler C: California Condor (*Gymnogyps californianus*) Studbook. Escondido, CA, San Diego Wild Animal Park, 1989.
24. Kuehler C: California Condor (*Gymnogyps californianus*) Studbook. Boise, ID, The Peregrine Fund, 1995.
25. Kuehler C, Whitman P: Artificial incubation of California condor eggs removed from the wild. Zoo Biol 7:123, 1988.
26. Kuehler CM, Sterner DJ, Jones DS, Usnik RL, et al: Report on captive hatches of California condors (*Gymnogyps californianus*): 1983–1990. Zoo Biol 10:65–68, 1991.
27. Landauer E: The hatchability of chicken eggs as influenced by environment and heredity. Storrs, CT, Storrs Agricultural Experimental Station, University of Connecticut, 1967.
28. Ley DH, Morris RF, Smallwood JE, Loomis MR: Mortality of chicks and decreased fertility and hatchability of eggs from a captive breeding pair of ostriches. J Am Vet Med Assoc 189:1124–1126, 1986.
29. Lieberman A, Rodriquez JV, Paez JM, Wiley J: The reintroduction of the Andean condor in Colombia, South America: 1989–1991. ORYX 27(2):83–90, 1993.
30. Longmire JL, Maltbie M, Pavelka RW, et al: Gender identification in birds using microsatellite DNA fingerprint analysis. Auk 110(2):378–381, 1993.
31. Mateo R, Molina R, Grifols J, Guitart R: Lead poisoning in a griffon vulture (*Gyps fulvus*). Vet Rec 140(2):47–48, 1997.
32. Miller AH, McMillan I, McMillan E: The current status and welfare of the California condor. Natl Audubon Soc Res Rep 6:1–61, 1965.
33. Murnane RD, Meerdink G, Rideout BA, Anderson MP: Ethylene glycol toxicosis in a captive-bred released California condor (*Gymnogyps californianus*). J Zoo Wild Med 26(2):306–310, 1995.
34. Olsen GH, Carpenter JW: Andean condor medicine, reproduction, and husbandry. Proceedings of the American Association of Veterinarians, Reno, NV, pp 147–152, 1995.
35. Oosterhuis J: Veterinary involvement in the California condor recovery program. Proceedings of the American Association of Zoo Veterinarians, Chicago, p 93, 1986.
36. Orosz SE, Ensley PK, Haynes CJ: Avian Surgical Anatomy: Thoracic and Pelvic Limbs. Philadelphia, WB Saunders, 1992.
37. Ryder O, Kuehler C, Ralls K: In Kuehler C (ed): California Condor (*Gymnogyps californianus*) Studbook. Zoological Society of San Diego, P.O. Box 551, San Diego, CA, 1993.
38. Ryder OA: California condor parentage inference employing hypervariable DNA sequence analysis. Report prepared for the California Condor Recovery Team, the California Department of Fish and Game, and the Greater Los Angeles Zoo Association, 1989.
39. Shima AL, Gonzales B: Veterinary involvement in the California and Andean condor recovery and release projects. Proceedings of the American Association of Zoo Veterinarians, Calgary, Alberta, Canada, pp 90–97, 1991.
40. Sibley CG, Mallette RD, Borneman JC, Dalen RS: California Condor Surveys, 1968. Calif Fish Game 55:298–306, 1969.
41. Snyder NFR, Hamber JA: Replacement-clutching and annual nesting of the California condors. Condor 87:374–378, 1985.
42. Snyder NFR, Johnson EV: Photographic censusing of the 1982–1983 California condor population. Condor 87:1–13, 1985.
43. Snyder NFR, Ramey RR, Sibley FC: Nest-site biology of the California condor. Condor 88:228–241, 1986.
44. Snyder NFR, Snyder H: Biology and conservation of the California condor. In Powers DM (ed): Current Ornithology, vol 6. Santa Barbara, CA, Santa Barbara Museum of Natural History, pp 175–267, 1989.
45. Tabaka CS, Ullrey DE, Sikarski JG, et al: Diet, cast composition and energy and nutrient intake of red-tailed hawks (*Buteo jamaicensis*), great horned owls (*Bubo virginianus*), and turkey vultures (*Cathartes aura*). J Zoo Wildl Med 27(2):187–196, 1996.
46. Terres JK: The Audubon Society Encyclopedia of North American Birds. New York, Alfred A Knopf, p 958, 1980.
47. Toone WD, Risser AC: Captive management of the California condor (*Gymnogyps californianus*). International Zoo Yearbook 27:50, 1988.
48. Toone CK: Causes of embryonic malformation and mortality. Pro-

ceedings of the American Association of Zoo Veterinarians, Tampa, FL, pp 167–170, 1983.

49. Wallace MP, Temple SA: Releasing captive-reared Andean condors to the wild. J Wildl Mgmt 351:541–550, 1987.
50. Wiemeyer SN, Jurek RM, Moore JR: Environmental contaminants in surrogates, foods and feathers of California condors (*Gymnogyps californianus*). Environ Monitor Assess 6:91–111, 1986.
51. Wiemeyer SN, Kryntsky AJ, Wilbur SR: Environmental contaminants in tissues, food and feces of California condors. *In* Wilbur SR, Jackson JA (eds): Vulture Biology and Management. Berkeley, University of California Press, pp 427–439, 1983.
52. Wiemeyer SN, Scott JM, Anderson MP, et al: Environmental contaminants in California condors. J Wildl Mgmt 52:238–247, 1988.
53. Wilbur SR: The California condor, 1966–76: a look at its past and future. U.S. Fish and Wildlife Service, North America Fauna, No. 72, 1978.
54. Wilbur SR: Estimating the size and trend of the California condor population, 1965–1978. Calif Fish Game 66:40–48, 1980.
55. Witman P: Techniques and problems in a brooder facility. Proceedings of the American Association of Zoo Veterinarians, Tampa, FL, pp 183–189, 1983.

SUGGESTED READINGS

Mundy PJ: The Comparative Biology of Southern African Vultures. Johannesburg, South Africa, the Vulture Study Group, 1982.
Mundy P, Butchart D, Ledger J, Piper S: The Vultures of Africa. Johannesburg, South Africa, Acorn Books, 1992.
Redig PT, Cooper JE, Remple DJ, Hunter BH (eds): Raptor Biomedicine. Minneapolis, University of Minnesota Press, 1993.
Wilbur SR, Jackson JA: Vulture Biology and Management. Berkeley, University of California Press, 1983.

CHAPTER 37

Water Quality for a Waterfowl Collection

RICHARD C. CAMBRE

Adequate water quality is essential for healthy captive waterfowl. Esthetics, breeding potential, maintenance requirements, and cost are some of the controllable factors that affect site selection and design criteria of waterfowl exhibits. All water amenities, whether natural or artificial, require periodic to frequent maintenance to prevent deleterious changes such as algal overgrowth, sedimentation, and eutrophication. A body of water cannot be built, stocked with birds, and left to fend for itself. Costly, unpleasant, and sometimes devastating consequences have resulted when water quality has been ignored. Diseases that can decimate a waterfowl collection, such as avian botulism, may occur when water quality is compromised.

TYPES OF WATER AMENITIES

Zoos, aviaries, and public and private waterfowl collections have used every conceivable type of water amenity in their exhibits, from opportunistically situated natural bodies of water to constructed lakes, ponds, pools, and streams. Each type offers its own advantages and disadvantages. Private breeders and hobbyists often completely surround their waterfowl enclosures with mesh or other material to discourage predation from ground or sky and to allow their birds to remain

flighted. Birds in zoos or aviaries, on public property such as municipal parks, and in certain private collections such as on corporate property or estates are generally deflighted and exhibited out in the open. This attracts wild waterfowl and other bird species to the area, which leads to increased usage of the lake or pond, affects water quality, and invites the introduction of diseases from the wild.

Natural Lakes and Ponds

Some properties holding waterfowl are graced with natural lakes and ponds. When mature, these constitute diverse biologic communities that are home to rich aquatic flora and fauna and that attract migratory and resident bird life. If deep enough and continually replenished with fresh water, these bodies can remain a viable asset to the property indefinitely with only routine maintenance. In contrast, problems may ensue with bodies of water that are shallow, that do not receive a constant infusion of new water, or that have not been adequately maintained through the years.

Artificial Lakes and Ponds with Natural Bottoms

Lakes and ponds built by people mandate even greater care and maintenance. Rarely do these enjoy continual natural replenishment, and in some instances they receive their water (of questionable quality) from a local storm drainage system or from precipitation and runoff from the surroundings. Often these bodies are not deep enough to begin with, which leaves them open to rapid sedimentation. Poor water circulation is another major problem, robbing the pond or lake of oxygen and compromising water clarity and quality. These bodies often lack the diverse biota of natural waters.

Natural Bottom Ponds with Membrane Liner

A relatively new innovation in pond design, membrane-lined ponds offer the benefits of reduced construction time and cost, ease of drainage for cleaning, reduction or elimination of seepage, and improved water clarity.

Concrete Ponds and Pools

While offering relative ease of draining and cleaning and the opportunity for continuous water flow, concrete ponds and pools often suffer from high construction cost and unnatural appearance unless sided with expensive artificial rockwork or heavily planted (Fig. 37–1). These frequently are drain-and-fill pools, which can lead to labor-intensive routine maintenance, costly water bills, and waste of water, a sometimes scarce and always precious resource.

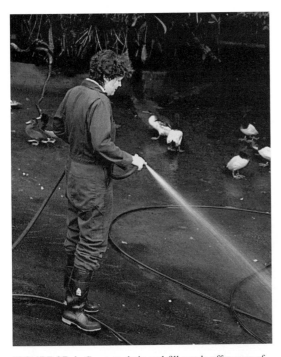

FIGURE 37–1. Concrete drain-and-fill ponds offer ease of cleaning but have the disadvantages of water wastage and unnatural appearance. Heavy plantings and dark-colored concrete help to naturalize the pond's look.

Interconnecting Streams

Waterfowl ponds in many zoo exhibits and private collections are linked sequentially through a series of streams that have concrete, artificial rock, gravel, or natural bottoms and sides. Although efficient in saving water and allowing for filtration and recirculation, interconnecting streams also permit the rapid spread of disease or harmful substances from one pond to the next.

FACTORS IN WATER QUALITY

Water amenities within exhibits are dynamic entities. The interplay of many physical, chemical, and biologic processes determines the water quality. Uncontrollable variables such as climate and weather affect the quantity and quality of water in all exhibits exposed to the elements. The source of exhibit water is another sometimes uncontrollable factor. Among natural sources are rivers, streams, groundwater springs, surface runoff, and precipitation. Artificial sources include municipal water supplies and drainage ditches. Water from these different sources varies markedly in its chemical composition. Once collected into a body, water becomes subject to physical and biologic phenomena that further alter its nature. A detailed review of the principles of water quality is beyond the scope of this chapter, but certain major factors that directly affect water quality within waterfowl exhibits merit discussion.

Clarity and Color

The full spectrum of water clarity can be seen in captive waterfowl exhibits, from totally clear to turbid, sometimes so much so that resident fish are invisible unless they come to the surface. Turbidity and color are functions of suspended particulate matter ranging in size from colloidal to coarse, which decreases the ability of water to transmit light. Clay and soil particles, dissolved organic matter, and plankton are some of the particulates that contribute to water turbidity and color. During phytoplankton blooms in particular, water may be tinted any of a variety of colors.[2]

Depth

Water depth in waterfowl exhibits ranges widely, depending on the nature of the enclosure and the types of birds kept. Maintaining depth is sometimes a difficult problem. Loss of water to seepage, leakage, and evaporation and loss of original pond or lake depth to sedimentation are major contributors to this problem. Seepage varies among ponds and is often the factor that determines replacement inflow to maintain water levels. It accounted for 87% of water lost from aquaculture ponds on a fish culture research station at Gualaca, Panama.[2] Lakes and ponds with heavy clay soil bottoms seep less. The introduction of membrane liners to natural-bottom pools offers one potential solution to this problem. However, leakage of concrete zoo ponds and pools remains an all-too-familiar occurrence. Adding replacement water from municipal water supplies or other sources is often necessary and can prove costly if done frequently. Maintaining adequate depth is essential for preventing harmful concentrations of numerous substances, such as ions, minerals, nutrients, phytoplankton, and toxic metabolites.

Temperature

Air temperature directly affects water temperature. Ambient temperature is dictated by solar radiation and varies widely by latitude. As light passes through water, its solar energy is absorbed as heat, primarily in surface layers. Water in turbid ponds has a higher temperature than water in clear ponds because the total heat absorbed by dissolved organic substances and suspended particulates is greater.[2] Higher temperatures directly affect biologic productivity of water systems, oxygen consumption, and growth of plants and animals and create favorable conditions for the emergence and perpetuation of some diseases, such as botulism.

Circulation

An often problem-filled area in waterfowl pond quality is water circulation. In stagnant bodies of water, motion is minimal, allowing thermal and chemical stratification and poor oxygenation of subsurface waters. Even in lakes and ponds with continuous water inflow and outflow, dead zones can develop if circulation does not occur. The aquaculture industry has pioneered many innovative water circulation devices, ranging from mechanical aerators that both oxygenate and circulate to subsurface baffle levees that force water to move around them in traveling between inflow pump and outflow pipe.[2]

Oxygenation

Oxygen is critical to the health of a body of water. Physical, chemical, and biologic processes interact to affect the concentration of dissolved oxygen. Diffusion from air to water accounts for part of the total concentration and is greater in natural waters, in which turbulence increases the surface area at the air-water interface, helping to distribute oxygen into deeper layers. In quiescent waters, typical of shallow exhibit lakes and ponds, this distribution to deeper layers does not occur, limiting diffused oxygen to a thin film at the surface in actual contact with air. The amount of oxygen that a body of water might receive in runoff, groundwater, or precipitation varies and depends on the inherent chemistry of the water as well as on climate and weather conditions.

In pond water, therefore, biologic processes surpass physical ones in importance in regulating dissolved oxygen concentrations.[2] A dynamic flux exists between organisms that produce oxygen through photosynthesis (phytoplankton) and those that consume it through respiration (plants and animals). The rate of photosynthesis and the amount of oxygen production in water in turn depend on several controlling factors, such as light, temperature, clarity, nutrient concentration, and plant species and density. Ponds show a daily cycle of oxygen concentration, highest during the daylight hours, when photosynthesis is at its peak, and lower at night, when respiration predominates. When phytoplankton density is too high, organic production and respiration rates increase, and the increased water turbidity restricts light and photosynthetic oxygen production to the shallower depths. In such conditions, factors that reduce photosynthesis even for short periods may cause severe depletion of dissolved oxygen. Another major source of oxygen consumption in ponds is the aerobic decomposition of organic matter by bacteria.

Nutrient Load

Nutrients enter a body of water from external sources and from internal generation. In the case of waterfowl lakes or ponds, the congregation of birds in large numbers can be a major source of external nutrient loading (Fig. 37–2). In some settings, this can be significant enough to affect water quality negatively, even to the point of hastening the sedimentation and eutrophication

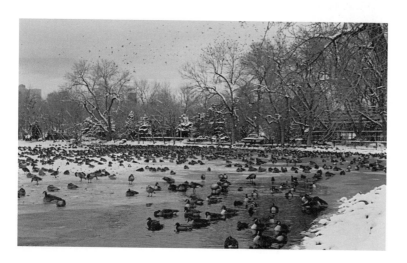

FIGURE 37–2. Congregation of migratory and resident wild waterfowl by the hundreds on a zoo lake. Feces add significantly to the lake's nutrient load.

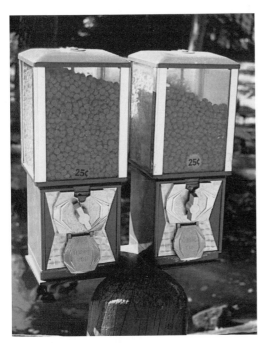

FIGURE 37–3. Selling dog kibble as duck food added to the nutrient load of the lake and encouraged congregation of wild birds.

of the lake or pond.[8, 10] In a study of a small (15-hectare) waterfowl lake in southwestern Michigan, an estimated 6500 Canada geese and 4200 ducks annually contributed, through feces, 69% of all carbon (4462 kg), 27% of all nitrogen (280 kg), and 70% of all phosphorus (88 kg) that entered the lake from external sources, resulting in poor water quality. The research team calculated that in a study plot on the frozen lake in winter, the average Canada goose defecated 28 times per day and considered this a grossly conservative figure, inasmuch as wild-caught geese defecated up to 92 times per day at the same food-scarce time of year. Their conclusion was that nutrient loading by the birds was probably far greater than their calculations permitted.[10] Other natural external sources of nutrients include watershed runoff, precipitation, leaves, and other parts of trees and plants.

Feeding of captive birds on the water can further encourage congregation of wild ones and add to nutrient loading through contribution of uneaten food and additional feces. The practice of selling "bird food," which is often dog kibble (Fig. 37–3), or of encouraging visitors to bring food to feed the birds can significantly compound the problem and should be discouraged.

Internally generated nutrient loading results from microbial degradation of organic matter in sediment and, in the natural setting, constitutes the main source of nutrients in the water, particularly ammonium nitrite, nitrate, and phosphate radicals. Primary producers, both plant and animal, consume the major part of these products. If these nutrients are not consumed, they accumulate. The result is sedimentation, poor water quality, and, ultimately, eutrophication.[6]

Biota

PLANTS

The plant life of a lake or pond can be a significant factor in its water quality. Species range from phytoplankton (algae, diatoms, and dinoflagellates) to macrophytes (macrophytic algae; submersed, floating, and emergent vascular plants). Discussion of the dynamics and interactions of these plant communities with each other and with resident animal life is beyond the scope of this chapter. Problems ensue when any of these plants overpopulates or dies as a result of an imbalance in water quality.

ANIMALS

The animal life of a mature lake or pond is classified into two main divisions: benthic organisms, which live in bottom mud, and nektonic organisms, which live in the water column and range from protozoa to crustaceans and fish. Their fate is intricately linked to the water's quality. Aquatic animals concentrate substances, including toxins, and move them up the food chain. In some instances, the death of these organisms is directly linked to morbidity and mortality in waterfowl that share the lake or pond (see later section on avian botulism).

WATER QUALITY MAINTENANCE

Regardless of the type of water amenity in a waterfowl exhibit, routine maintenance is essential. Facilities use a number of techniques to maintain high-quality water in their exhibits. The frequency and intensity of effort required vary by location and climate.

Cleaning

Drain-and-fill pools have long been the standard in zoo waterfowl exhibits, where the daily press of visitors mandates a high standard of cleanliness. This technique can be applied to concrete ponds as well as to membrane-lined ones. A major benefit is that bottom debris can be removed and cleaning and disinfecting agents applied. Household bleach (5.25% sodium hypochlorite) is commonly used. In view of today's resource conservation ethic and the high cost and scarcity of water in some areas of the world, the luxury of discarding large volumes of water on a regular schedule is rapidly becoming impractical. Skimming of leaves from the surface of natural and artificial lakes and ponds, and clearing away of plant and other organic debris from the water's edge, may reduce nutrient loading and delay the sedimentation process.

Water Exchange

Less drastic than complete drain-and-fill are systems that exchange water on a periodic or as-needed basis.

Water exchange helps prevent phytoplankton blooms through flushing excess nutrients and phytoplankton themselves, removing toxic metabolic wastes, and diluting excess salinity. Drawing the water level down and then immediately replacing the desired volume is considered the most beneficial method of water exchange.[2] Continually pumping in new water and discharging old through an overflow inevitably loses some new water and does nothing to alleviate dead zones within the pond if circulation is poor. The volume of water and the frequency of exchange necessary to achieve the desired water quality in the pond vary by location and may need to be determined through trial and error.

Filtration

Filtration offers the benefit of being able to recycle and conserve water. Initial investment of funds for equipment and supplies returns long-term savings. Filtration systems in water amenities range from simple to elaborate, depending on the nature and construction of the body of water and the economic realities of the facility. All three of the major types of water filtration systems—mechanical, chemical, and biologic—have been applied to waterfowl ponds.[14] Natural systems such as reed filter beds can be found in some of the larger waterfowl sanctuaries.

Aeration

Aeration is an effective method for supplying supplemental oxygen to water. At least two types of aerators are applicable to waterfowl exhibits: mechanical and gravity. A wide array of mechanical aerators has been developed for use in wastewater treatment and in intensive aquaculture systems, in which critically low oxygen levels can be reached at night. Fixed-position sprayers, which pump and spray pond water at high velocity into the air, are sometimes seen in waterfowl exhibits but are usually not of a size or type powerful enough to add significant oxygen, especially in larger ponds

and lakes. Mechanical devices that both aerate and circulate water by creating turbulence are more efficient at adding oxygen. Examples include propeller-aspirator-pump aerators and paddlewheel aerators.[2, 3] Subsurface aerators, commonly called *bubblers,* pump compressed air to a diffuser on the lake or pond bottom. The rising air bubbles efficiently oxygenate water and provide some degree of turbulence (Fig. 37–4). Gravity aerators work by allowing water to fall through a system of stacked screens, lattices, perforated trays, or similar devices before entering the pond.

Sediment Removal

Designs of new waterfowl lakes or ponds should include provisions for periodic removal of sediment from their bottoms. The frequency of sediment removal from any body of water, new or existing, is determined through regular monitoring of water depth and quality and assessment of the health of its residents. It is far more prudent and less costly to remove manageable amounts of sediment throughout the life of a body of water than to have it fill in to a fraction of its former depth and face the prospect of an expensive, labor-intensive, protracted major dredging operation (Fig. 37–5).

Phytoplankton Control

A variety of chemical, biologic, and mechanical measures have been used in an attempt to control blooms of phytoplankton and other vegetation in ponds. Although effective in lowering the density of phytoplankton, algicides such as copper sulfate are potentially toxic to fish when used at high concentrations and to other aquatic life at recommended concentrations. Their duration of effect is often limited, necessitating repeated applications, and the resulting decomposition of dead algae may deplete dissolved oxygen in the water. In ponds where the nutrient load is high, algal blooms are likely to recur over and over despite repeated applica-

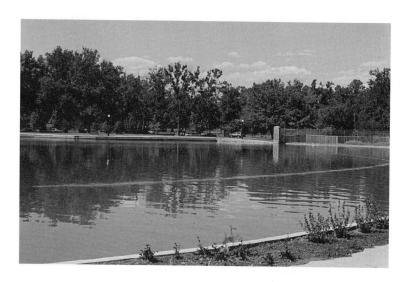

FIGURE 37–4. A bubbler aerator disperses tiny air bubbles from the lake bottom that percolate to the surface in line, improving both water circulation and oxygenation.

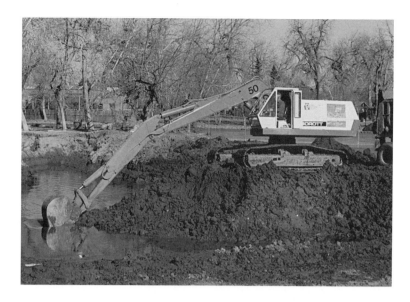

FIGURE 37–5. Dredging of a sedimented lake requires heavy machinery and is a time-consuming and costly process. Periodic sediment removal on a regular schedule precludes a major effort later.

tion of algicide. The use of aluminum sulfate (alum) and calcium sulfate (gypsum) to precipitate phosphorus, thereby limiting plankton growth, has been studied in aquaculture systems and in water treatment plants. The addition of filter-feeding fish such as carp and tilapia has been suggested as a possible means of biologic algae control but has resulted in some cases in even higher plankton density and a greater demand on dissolved oxygen. Water hyacinths have also been studied as possible biologic control agents for phytoplankton, on the basis of their competition for phosphorus and their water-shading effects. Finally, exchange of half of a pond's water with rapid refill has proved an effective mechanical means of reducing phytoplankton blooms.[2]

WATER-RELATED DISEASES

Avian Botulism

Although predominantly a disease of wild waterfowl in wetland areas, avian botulism has ravaged zoo, aviary, public, and private waterfowl collections on numerous occasions. It is intimately linked to water quality. Like outbreaks among wild waterfowl, outbreaks in captive collections are probably grossly underreported. What follows is not intended to be an in-depth review of all aspects of this disease (see the second edition of *Zoo and Wildlife Medicine,* page 349, for a thorough review). This discussion focuses on practical lessons learned by the author in dealing with botulism in a municipal zoo waterfowl collection during 10 consecutive summers.

ETIOLOGY

The circumstances under which avian botulism has emerged in captive collections are as varied as the facilities in question. It is puzzling how this disease could suddenly appear, as if out of nowhere, in the middle of a crowded city, miles from any wetlands

known to have experienced avian botulism for more than 30 years. The answer is found in the biologic processes of the bacterium that produces the paralyzing neurotoxin. *Clostridium botulinum* type C is an obligately anaerobic, spore-forming, gram-positive motile bacillus that is ubiquitous in soil and in lake, pond, and estuary bottoms throughout the world.[5, 9, 15] In the unlikely event that the bacterium is not present in the soil of a particular body of water, it is easy to imagine its being introduced in the excreta of migratory birds (not necessarily waterfowl) or in insects that can carry the bacterium in their intestines with impunity. If the new environment proves unfavorable to the organism, it can simply encyst into a spore and remain indefinitely in the lake or pond sediment, without causing harm, until favorable conditions occur.

When macroenvironmental and microenvironmental conditions are favorable, the organism germinates, multiplies, and produces its lethal toxin. Macroenvironmental factors that allow botulism to occur within a body of water include shallow depth, warm temperature, poor circulation, anaerobic conditions, salinity, nutrient-rich sediment, and a sudden change in water level. The microenvironment consists of invertebrate or vertebrate carcasses sharing many of the same factors and dead of any number of causes, often unrelated to botulism. Artificial lakes and ponds that have not received periodic maintenance such as sediment removal, often the case in municipal parks, are at risk for outbreaks. However, these same favorable environmental conditions can also occur in concrete-bottom pools and streams, especially after a botulism outbreak has begun in the area.

TRANSMISSION

For the toxin to be distributed to susceptible birds, a delivery system is needed. The primary means is through fly larvae (maggots) that feed on decaying carcasses of birds that have died of botulism or on those of any dead vertebrate in which *C. botulinum* type

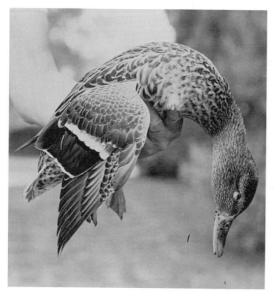

FIGURE 37–6. A mallard duck in late-stage botulism poisoning. Leg, wing, neck, and head muscles exhibit total flaccid paralysis. The lower eyelid is swollen.

C toxin is being produced. Maggots can concentrate the botulinum toxin to the extent that a bird that eats even one or two of them receives a potentially lethal dose. Less understood possible routes of exposure involve birds' ingesting the toxin directly from the water, especially in the vicinity of a carcass, or feeding on dead invertebrates in the bottom sediment. Whether toxico-infection (spontaneous toxin production by *C. botulinum* within the intestine of a live bird) occurs in waterfowl as in poultry is not clear.[5] Also unclear is how the toxin can spread around a zoo or aviary to nonwaterfowl species such as cranes housed in open-air pens or to pheasants in screened pens where the presence of maggot-laden carcasses is impossible. Living flies that have fed on toxin-laden carcasses are probably the source in these instances.[15]

When a body of water and its environs become heavily contaminated with bacteria, spores, and toxin, the disease is likely to recur with regularity unless appropriate, and sometimes drastic, control measures are taken.

TREATMENT AND PROPHYLAXIS

The highly potent neurotoxin of *C. botulinum* type C paralyzes the bird's legs, wings, and neck and head (Fig. 37–6). Severely affected birds soon drown. A high percentage of birds caught before reaching this stage can be saved with gavage, first with water or electrolyte solutions, followed by a gruel made of waterfowl pellets, until they are able to feed themselves. A non-commercial *C. botulinum* type C antitoxin produced by the US Fish and Wildlife Service has been credited with contributing to high rates of recovery in some waterfowl species,[9] but it did not help alter the fatal course of intoxication in cranes and pheasants when used by the author.

Since 1992, the author has used a *C. botulinum* type C bacterin-toxoid labeled for mink (Botumink, United Vaccines, Inc., Madison, WI) in hundreds of zoo birds of four orders (Anseriformes, Galliformes, Gruiformes, Pelicaniformes). One milliliter was administered to birds of all sizes subcutaneously on the dorsum between the wings, twice the first year (1 month apart), with yearly boosters thereafter. Injections were given in late spring and early summer. This proved highly and rapidly successful in protecting waterfowl, even in an active botulism outbreak in which wild birds were dying and maggot-infested carcasses were present in the same pond.[4]

CONTROL

Prompt carcass removal is a proven control measure in field outbreaks of avian botulism and is equally applica-

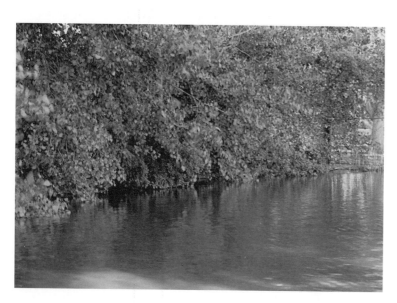

FIGURE 37–7. Low-lying branches along a zoo lake's shore provided cover for sick and dying birds during a botulism outbreak. Vegetation should be kept cut well above the water's surface to eliminate hiding places.

ble to the captive setting. Low-lying trees, bushes, and shrubs should be cut to eliminate hiding places at water's edge, where sick birds or maggot-ridden carcasses might escape notice and perpetuate an outbreak (Fig. 37–7). Long-term control measures must include a major effort to return the lake's or pond's waters to high quality, including dredging and deepening and installation of an aeration system, all aimed at rendering the environment unfavorable to botulism toxin production.

Other Toxicoses

Lead and zinc intoxication results from contamination of waterfowl lakes and ponds by objects that contain these elements. Certain waterfowl species, such as smew, seem especially prone to consumption of shiny metal objects. Removal of the objects, through any combination of surgery, endoscopic retrieval, or gavage, coupled with chelation therapy, is the preferred method of treatment. Algal blooms in shallow waters have resulted in occasional die-offs due to toxin liberation.[12]

Infectious Diseases

Two major infectious diseases of waterfowl with a water connection are fowl cholera (pasteurellosis) and duck plague (duck virus enteritis [DVE]). These diseases are discussed in detail in Chapter 38. Only their relation to water is discussed here.

In both the bacterial disease (pasteurellosis) and the viral one (DVE), environmental persistence is thought to be prolonged. Body fluids discharged from the mouths and other orifices of birds dying of either disease, and from their decaying carcasses, contaminate the environment. *Pasteurella multocida* was able to survive for 3 weeks in pond water, 4 weeks in soil, and 3 months in decaying carcasses.[7] Its survival was increased in water with high concentrations of calcium and magnesium.[13] The DVE virus was recovered from water held for 60 days at 4°C after a major outbreak in South Dakota.[1]

Measures suggested for reducing environmental con-

tamination from both diseases include prompt, head-first removal of dead birds (to minimize fluid discharge), double bagging of carcasses in plastic, and incineration. Ponds were scrubbed with chlorine bleach after an outbreak of DVE at the National Zoological Park in 1975 and refilled with water chlorinated to 3 ppm with calcium hypochlorite.[11]

REFERENCES

1. Brand CJ: Duck plague. *In* Friend M (ed): Field Guide to Wildlife Diseases. Washington, DC, US Fish and Wildlife Service, pp 117–127, 1987.
2. Boyd CE: Water Quality in Ponds for Aquaculture. Alabama Agricultural Experiment Station, Auburn University, 1990.
3. Boyd CE, Ahmad T: Evaluation of Aerators for Channel Catfish Farming. Bulletin 584, Alabama Agricultural Experimentation Station, Auburn University, 1987.
4. Cambre RC, Kenny D: Vaccination of zoo birds against botulism with mink botulism vaccine. Proceedings of the American Association of Zoo Veterinarians, St. Louis, p 383, 1993.
5. Eklund MW, Dowell VR (eds): Avian Botulism. Springfield, IL, Charles C Thomas, 1987.
6. Escaravage V: Daily cycles of dissolved oxygen and nutrient content in a shallow fishpond: the impact of water renewal. Hydrobiologia 207:131–136, 1990.
7. Friend M: Avian cholera: a major new cause of waterfowl mortality (Fish and Wildlife Leaflet 13.2.5). *In* Waterfowl Management Handbook. Washington, DC, US Fish and Wildlife Service, 1989.
8. Gere G, Andrikovics S: Effects of waterfowl on water quality. Hydrobiologia 243/244:445–448, 1992.
9. Locke LN, Friend M: Avian botulism: geographic expansion of a historic disease (Fish and Wildlife Leaflet 13.2.4). *In* Waterfowl Management Handbook. Washington, DC, US Fish and Wildlife Service, 1989.
10. Manny BA, Johnson WC, Wetzel RG: Nutrient additions by waterfowl to lakes and reservoirs: predicting their effects on productivity and water quality. Hydrobiologia 279/280:121–132, 1994.
11. Montali RJ, Bush M, Greenwell GA: An epornitic of duck viral enteritis in a zoological park. J Am Vet Med Assoc 169:954–958, 1976.
12. Olsen JH: Anseriformes. *In* Ritchie BW, Harrison GJ, Harrison LR (eds): Avian Medicine: Principles and Application. Lake Worth, FL, Wingers Publishing, pp 1237–1275, 1994.
13. Price JI, Yandell BS, Porter WP: Chemical ions affect survival of avian cholera organisms in pond water. J Wildl Manage 56:274–278, 1992.
14. Stoskopf MK: Veterinary issues in aquatic exhibit design. Proceedings of the American Association of Zoo Veterinarians, Pittsburgh, pp 173–178, 1994.
15. Wobeser GA: Diseases of Wild Waterfowl. New York, Plenum Press, 1981.

CHAPTER 38

Caring for Oiled Birds

ERICA A. MILLER
SALLIE C. WELTE

HISTORY AND BACKGROUND

Oil and its additives and contaminants, through simple physical contact, inhalation, ingestion, and transcutaneous absorption, have been demonstrated to have deleterious effects on birds.[8] The effects associated with oil include, but are not limited to, contamination of feathers and damage to vital organ systems, including the lungs and air sacs, kidneys, liver, heart, blood, and gastrointestinal tract.[11, 15, 18]

This chapter summarizes the effects of oil on birds and provides a general overview of the basic treatment protocols, the rehabilitation and husbandry techniques, and the criteria for prerelease evaluation currently used by Tri-State Bird Rescue & Research, Inc. These techniques are based on Tri-State's 20 years of experience in caring for oiled birds, as well as extensive literature research and colleague consultation.

Rehabilitation efforts focus primarily on the adverse physiologic effects of oil on individual birds. The primary objective is to care for injured animals and, once they have recovered, release them to their natural environment. Wildlife rehabilitation addresses two purposes in an oil spill response:

1. Philosophically or morally, it provides a humane response to wild animals harmed through human-related activities.
2. Biologically, it attempts to treat and return animals harmed by human activities to breeding populations in the wild. Rehabilitation efforts are important particularly when endangered or threatened species are contaminated.

LEGALITIES OF HANDLING OILED BIRDS

Under Federal Regulation 50 CFR 21 (revised March 1984), federal permits are required from the U.S. Fish and Wildlife Service to capture, transport, or possess migratory birds (Migratory Bird Treaty Act, 16 U.S.C. 703–711). Most native species are classified under the "protected" designation; introduced species, including the Rock dove (pigeon), European starling, and English sparrow, are exempt. Federal permits are obtained from the permit section of the U.S. Fish and Wildlife Service headquarters in each region.

State permits may also be required and may be obtained from the state Department of Natural Resources or an equivalent agency.

Other legal responsibilities during a spill response include compliance with Occupational Safety and Health Administration (OSHA) guidelines, including right-to-know issues (potential hazards of the spilled product), basic first aid and/or emergency notification instruction in case of exposure to the product, the use of proper protective equipment as advised for the spilled product, and the prevention and treatment of potential hazards involved in working with wildlife. All persons working with wildlife should also be instructed in proper procedures for handling the animals, both to prevent injury and to prevent the spread of zoonotic disease.

Specific health and safety concerns and regulations may be obtained through OSHA offices and have been addressed elsewhere.[28]

NATURAL RESOURCES DAMAGE ASSESSMENT

Natural resources damage assessment (NRDA) is the process of evaluating damages to natural resources as a result of an oil spill and estimating eventual recovery costs. State and federal wildlife agents, as the designated legal trustees for wildlife, are responsible for performing NRDA; however, the veterinarian and/or wildlife rehabilitator providing care for oiled wildlife may be asked to assist with several of the NRDA responsibilities. These responsibilities vary from region to region and between individual spills. The local trustees should be contacted in order to determine which data should be collected.

Chain of Evidence. In some spill responses, the trustees may require that every animal retrieved, live or dead, be assigned a custody number. Each animal or carcass must be accounted for from the time of admission until it is released or turned over to the trustees. In other instances, chain of evidence records may be required only for carcasses.

Feather Sampling. Frequently, the trustees require that feather samples and swabs of legs be collected from each bird. These samples are usually collected during the initial examination, wrapped in aluminum foil (shiny side in), labeled, and frozen. Feather and leg samples may later be analyzed and used as a means of verifying oil contamination from a specific source.

Necropsy Specimens. Any bird that does not recover should be subjected to necropsy after permission for necropsy is obtained from the trustees. Necropsy findings may be a necessary part of NRDA inquiries and may provide documentable information related to the spill. Necropsies during oil spills may also provide a means of measuring disease frequency or prevalence in a population or in a geographic region and may help quantify the physiologic effects of specific types of oil and of any prescribed treatments.

WILDLIFE REHABILITATION NEEDS IN MAJOR SPILLS

This chapter concentrates on the rehabilitation of the individual oiled bird, although references are made to handling large numbers of birds. Oil spills that contaminate a large number of birds present a greater challenge. In view of the intense human labor, the immediacy of the effort, and the need for special equipment, significant use of resources and an experienced team are needed to manage the response. A spill involving 100 or more birds taxes the resources of even the professionals who like to think they are always prepared for oil spills.

For example, a facility receiving 50 Canada geese a day needs an area 800 feet square for initial housing of the oiled birds, a second large enclosed area for washing the birds, a third area for housing the cleaned birds, and yet another area for performing physical examinations, administering medical treatments, and maintaining records. Additional needs include a way to produce over 6000 gallons of 103°F water at 60 psi and provisions for legal disposal of 1000 gallons of oiled waste water.

THE EFFECTS OF OIL ON BIRDS

The effects of oil on birds can be generally characterized as environmental, external, and internal.

Environmental Effects

Environmental effects are perhaps the broadest category and include immediate contamination of the food source biomass, reduction in the breeding animals and plants that provide future food sources, contamination of nesting habitat, and reduction in reproductive success through contamination and reduced hatchability of eggs.[1, 12]

In a number of spills, the environmental effects of the oil may be minimal (acute and temporary), whereas the physiologic effects on the individual animals and/or local populations may be severe (either acute or chronic and often long-lasting). For example, a barren rocky coastline that is contaminated by oil early in a spill may exhibit damages that are largely temporary, in that certain types of oil may flush off the rocks after only one or two tidal cycles. However, if that coastline is the nesting site of colonial birds such as common murres (*Uria aalge*; pelagic birds that do not breed until they are 4 years old and lay only one egg a year), oil contamination may have long-lasting effects on regional populations.

External Effects

The external effects of oil are the most noticeable and most immediately debilitating. Birds that are most often affected by oil spills include those that remain on the water, such as ducks, loons, and grebes; those that feed in the water, such as gulls, terns, and herons; and birds of prey, including bald eagles and ospreys. Oil can contaminate the entire bird or only parts of the bird, depending on the amount of oil in the water and the bird's natural behavior (swimming, wading, diving) in the water.

The interlocking structure of the barbicels of intact feathers provides the primary waterproofing and insulating properties of plumage (Fig. 38–1A). Oil, by dis-

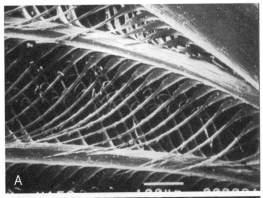

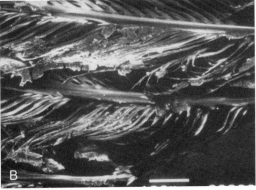

FIGURE 38–1. *A,* Scanning electromicrograph of clean feather structure. (Courtesy of H. Bryndza.) *B,* Scanning electromicrograph of oiled feather. (Courtesy of H. Bryndza.)

rupting this interlocking structure, destroys these properties (see Fig. 38–1*B*). The oiled bird may not be able to thermoregulate, may be unable to fly, or may be unable to remain afloat in the water. Experimental studies have demonstrated that eider ducks *(Somateria mollissima)* with only external oil contamination increased their metabolic rates by 400% when maintained on water.[10] Depending on the degree of impact, an oiled bird may also have difficulty obtaining food or escaping predators. The decreased foraging ability of the animal, combined with the presence of oil in the environment, usually results in a loss of attainable food and water sources.

Hypothermia is the most immediately life-threatening effect of oil contamination for most seabirds. The disrupted feathers allow cold water to penetrate the plumage and contact the skin, quickly lowering the body temperature and forcing the bird to beach itself and seek cover. Depressed body temperatures may directly affect other body functions, adding to the physiologic and biochemical stresses on the bird.

Other external effects of oil contamination include chemical burns and irritation to the skin and inflammation and ulceration of the conjunctivae, nictitans, and corneal surfaces of the eyes.

Internal Effects

Direct, toxic effects of oil on the lungs, gastrointestinal tract, pancreas, and liver have all been documented[12, 13, 18]; however, more recent studies suggest that there are no gross or microscopic lesions that can be directly attributed to oil intoxication in birds.[11] Stress, hypothermia, and dehydration are nonetheless often present, regardless of the cause, in oiled birds, and must be quickly diagnosed and treated as part of the care regimen.

Stress and/or ingestion of oil during preening may result in ulceration and hemorrhaging within the mucosa of the gastrointestinal tract.[9] This damage may prevent the absorption of sodium and water and may be clinically evident by the presence of diarrhea and/or blood in the feces. Injury to the mucosa may thus contribute to dehydration, anemia, and depressed total plasma protein levels.

Several types of pneumonia may occur in birds affected by oil. Pulmonary hemorrhage and edema appear to be the direct results of exposure to volatile components of certain oils.[1, 11, 18] Aspiration pneumonia is not uncommon and can occur when birds, while attempting to clean their feathers through preening, aspirate droplets of oil. Aspiration pneumonia may also occur during treatment, when birds regurgitate and aspirate liquid diets.

Kidney damage, a common finding in oiled birds, is believed to occur both as a direct effect of the toxins in the oil and secondary to severe dehydration.[18, 21] Contamination of food and water and the inability to seek other sources of water greatly reduce a bird's fluid intake. Dehydration may result in compromised kidney function and potential renal damage, with the ultimate sequelae of visceral gout, acidosis, clinical shock, and death.

Evidence of other internal effects of oil ingestion include an increase in mixed-function oxidase (MFO) activity in the liver, possible alterations of the osmoregulatory function of nasal salt glands, alterations of estrogen cycles and prolactin levels (and the resulting reduction of fertilization rates), suppressed growth rates, and possible suppression of the function of the adrenal glands and other endocrine organs.[9, 12]

Oil ingestion has also been shown to have toxic effects on the hematopoietic system. Birds often become severely anemic 4 to 6 days after ingestion of crude oils; this anemia is consistent with primary oxidant chemical damage to the hemoglobin of red blood cells and has not been observed in birds contaminated with diesel or home heating oils.[12] The initial packed cell volume (PCV) may not reflect an anemic condition because of the false elevation created by dehydration. As the bird is rehydrated and the spleen removes damaged red blood cells, the PCV may drop as much as 10% to 12% in 3 days[24] (Tri-State Bird Rescue & Research, Inc., unpublished records).

Secondary stress or the oil itself may have a suppressive effect on immune function by decreasing the proportion of lymphocytes among circulating white blood cells of birds that have ingested oil.[12] Suppression of the immune system renders the birds more susceptible to secondary bacterial and fungal infections.

Aspergillosis is a common secondary complication, particularly in pelagic species, which have little resistance to this fungal infection. *Aspergillus fumigatus* colonization may already be established in the oiled birds when they are presented for washing, or it may develop within rehabilitation centers if animals are bedded in moist straw or organic material or are left in damp areas. *A. fumigatus* growth is frequently found on the lungs or air sacs, but it can disseminate quickly throughout the body, occluding the trachea, surrounding the heart, penetrating the cornea, or infiltrating the liver, kidneys, or central nervous system.

Other secondary (captive-related) health problems that develop during rehabilitation of oiled birds include pododermatitis, hock (intratarsal joint) swelling, and keel sores from improper perching or cage substrate; feather damage from improper material on cage walls; and dermal, respiratory, and gastrointestinal infections from overcrowding or inadequate ventilation, including candidiasis, avian pox, colibacillosis, erysipelas, and chlamydiosis.[11, 24]

TREATMENT OF OILED BIRDS

Rapid retrieval, stabilization, and cleaning of oil-soaked birds are vital to successful treatment. Stabilization efforts may be initiated in the field, but complete medical care is often not provided until the birds arrive at the clinic. If transportation to the washing facility takes more than 1 hour, captured animals should be examined and stabilized at a field station (staging facility); if animals are captured less than an hour's distance from the washing facility, they may be stabilized upon arrival, in a designated medical area of that facility.

Stabilization

Initial examination begins with the identification of each bird through the use of a temporary numbered plastic leg band and a corresponding individual record. Baseline data collected from each animal include weight, body temperature, and minimal blood values (packed cell volume, total plasma proteins (TP), and blood glucose levels). (Normal ranges: temperature, 102° to 106°F; PCV, 35% to 55%; TP, 3.5 to 5.5 g/dL; glucose level, 150 to 250.[4])

Depending on the initial findings, stabilization efforts are directed toward any of the four primary conditions of concern: dehydration, hypothermia, traumatic injury, and disease.

Dehydration. Unless clinical signs indicate otherwise, all oiled birds are considered to be a minimum of 10% dehydrated by the time they are captured, transported, and presented for treatment. Any bird that is able to maintain head carriage is given an oral electrolyte solution (e.g., Pedialyte or lactated Ringer's solution and 2.5% dextrose), which also serves to flush any ingested oil from the intestinal lumen. Fluid quantities are calculated in order to provide the 10% rehydrating fluids over a 72-hour period, as well as the 5% (of body weight) maintenance fluids needed on a daily basis for washing.[27] Ongoing fluid losses resulting from diarrhea, regurgitation, and stress must also be considered.

A single dose of the enteric coating agent bismuth subsalicylate (Pepto-Bismol) is administered via crop tube immediately after the first bolus of oral fluids. The enteric coating agent, at a dosage of 2 to 5 ml/kg, is given to reduce the mucosal inflammation and to decrease further absorption of toxic components of the oil.[26] International Bird Rescue & Research Center, an oiled bird rehabilitation center based in Berkeley, California, recommends the use of an activated charcoal slurry (Toxiban; Vet-A-Mix, Shenandoah, IA) delivered via gavage at a dose of 52 mg/kg.[24] (Note: weak birds that cannot maintain head carriage or may not be able to swallow should *not* be given oral fluids.)

For a severely dehydrated bird, aggressive fluid therapy is instituted as soon as possible after retrieval. Parenteral fluid administration must be done as aseptically as possible so as to not introduce any contaminants, including bacteria and petroleum products, into the bird. The principles of fluid therapy have been addressed elsewhere[20, 27] and usually involve bolus injections into the medial tarsal or cutaneous ulnar vein at a rate of 15 to 35 ml/kg, three times a day.[26] Intravenous or intraosseous catheters may be placed in the medial tarsal vein and the distal ulna or in the proximal tibiotarsus, respectively, in order to provide fluids over the course of several days. The authors have chosen to use indwelling catheters only as a "last resort" approach to rehydration, because isolation of the animal is usually required in order to prevent catheter removal by conspecifics; also, washing should be delayed until catheters are removed and the placement site has healed.

Hypothermia. An early return to normal core body temperature (102° to 106°F) may be crucial to the animal's survival; all attempts to stabilize the body temperature should be made before oral fluid administration or washing. Although a bird may be rapidly warmed or cooled by many methods, gradual changes in the body temperature are much less stressful. Slow warming is best achieved through the use of heat lamps placed so that the bird can move away from the direct beam to avoid overheating. Hot water bottles and heating pads placed under a portion of the cage/holding box are also very effective for warming smaller birds; hot water bottles can also assist in core warming when placed under the wings (i.e., along the body). Wrapping the bottles in towels prevents thermal burns to any exposed skin. Birds that are moderately to severely hypothermic (<95°F) have compromised circulation and thus require administration of intravenous fluids to restore blood volume. Warm fluids (98° to 100°F) are usually administered in a slow bolus of 2% to 3% of body weight. Supplementing the fluids with dextrose provides an energy source for the increased metabolic needs. Hyperthermic birds (>108°F) can be gradually cooled by lowering the ambient temperature (air conditioners or indirect fans) or by placing cold water bags in the cage or holding box—but they must not be placed directly against the body.

Traumatic Injury. A precursory examination reveals any major traumatic injuries. It may be difficult, if not impossible, to adequately clean and successfully treat large wounds and compound fractures that are contaminated by oil. In cases such as this, or when large numbers of birds are involved and resources are limited, the feasibility of treating the individual animal must be assessed, and some animals may have to be humanely euthanized. Federal wildlife trustees must be consulted before a member of any threatened or endangered species is euthanized.

Injuries that are determined to be treatable should be addressed as soon as possible. Common traumatic injuries include bite wounds from predators, shoulder luxations from improper capture and handling techniques, and wing injuries from improper capture or transportation methods. Injured birds may have to be isolated or given extra supportive care, which may delay their washing. A less common injury that may be seen on presentation or several days afterward is capture myopathy.[32]

Disease. Initial examination should also include checking for evidence of any potentially epidemic or zoonotic disease. In spills involving large numbers of birds, a herd-health approach may need to be used, and diseased birds may have to be isolated or euthanized.

If this initial stabilization is performed at a field site, the animals may then be carefully boxed and transported in a properly ventilated vehicle to the washing facility, where they should again be examined and administered any necessary treatments. If the stabilization is performed at the washing facility, the treated animals should be placed in a warm, quiet, well-ventilated area away from people and noise.

Medical Treatment

Once the bird is stable, the physical examination is continued. Mucosal membranes are cleaned by removing oil from the mouth and the nares with cotton swabs and by flushing the eyes with warm sterile saline or other ophthalmic irrigation solution; irrigating the eyes also allows for evaluation of function of the nictitating membrane. The skin on the ventral patagia is examined to evaluate the extent of contact irritation from the petroleum product. The vent is checked for oil and matted feathers, which could contribute to cloacal impaction. The overall body condition is assessed, and any minor injuries or feather damage is noted and treated accordingly.

Because some components of petroleum products can be absorbed through the skin with possible toxic results to the kidneys and liver, all attempts should be made to stabilize and wash the animals within 8 to 24 hours of capture. If washing cannot be accomplished within 8 hours of capture, the birds should continue to receive oral fluids and other medical care necessary to reach and/or maintain a stable state until washing can occur.

Blood values (PCV and TP) are monitored every 3 to 4 days. If PCVs are below 25% or decrease more than 10% between sampling, iron dextran can be given at doses of 10 mg/kg every 5 to 7 days.[30] In cases of severe anemia (PCV < 20%), whole blood and plasma transfusions have been tried with varying degrees of success.[30] Hyperproteinemias have been observed in some oiled birds and may reflect a combination of dehydration, stress, and inflammatory response.[29] No specific treatment other than general supportive care has been suggested in the literature.

Seabirds and other birds considered to be at a high risk to aspergillosis are immediately given prophylactic doses of flucytosine, itraconazole, and/or amphotericin B.[7] Other complications often observed in oiled birds include transitory enteritis, acid-base imbalance, respiratory compromise, and problems secondary to captive conditions, including pododermatitis and keel lesions. Appropriate treatment is provided as indicated by clinical manifestation.

Removing the Oil from the Feathers

Because a bird's abilities to fly and to remain waterproof are dependent on the interlocking structure of feather barbs, barbules, and barbicels, oil must be removed from the feathers without damaging or leaving a residue on these structures.

Approximately 100 gallons of water, 103° to 105°F (40° to 45°C), is needed over a 30-minute period to wash one duck. Although the detergent is more effective in hot water (>102°F), water warmer than 105°F may overheat and stress the bird or result in thermal burns to the skin already sensitized by contact with the petroleum product. Water that is cooler than 102°F should also be avoided because it may cause hypothermia.

A cleaning agent must be nonirritating to both animals and humans and yet able to lift the oil, maintain it in suspension, and rinse quickly and completely from the feathers. In a series of reproducible, quantifiable tests of cleaning agent efficacy, Dawn dishwashing detergent (Procter & Gamble, Cincinnati, Ohio, 45202) has produced the best results.[3] (Note: it is available in Canada and in Central and South America under the name Joy and in England and South Africa under the name Fairy Liquid; in the authors' experience, green Dawn has not been as effective as the blue, clear, or yellow formulations).

Each bird is cleaned by a team of two to four people in a warm, quiet area, free from drafts. Large tubs, holding 10 to 20 gallons of a solution of 1% to 5% Dawn and water at 103° to 105°F, are used (Table 38–1).

Although modifications are made for each species, the basic techniques (as described here for waterfowl) remain the same. The entire bird, except for the head and a portion of the neck, is submersed in the tub. To prevent it from ducking into the soapy water, the bird's head is gently restrained by gently grasping the bases of the jaw or, temporarily, by holding the bill. Many waterbirds have soft bills, so this hold should be used with caution.

It is not advisable to tape a bird's bill closed during cleaning or any other portion of the care process. Many seabirds do not have external nares and can suffocate if their bills are taped; other species may have difficulty breathing with taped bills because of inflammation or oil-plugged nares. Birds respond to stress by open-mouth breathing and occasionally by regurgitating; taping a bird's bill can result in additional stress, suffocation, and/or aspiration.

The bird's body is held with feet supported; a weighted log may be placed in the bottom of the tub for long-legged waders (e.g., herons, egrets) to grasp. The wings are held securely against the body and are individually extended only for cleaning.

Soapy water is agitated through the feathers by hand, systematically addressing every portion of the bird's body and concentrating on belly, underwings, vent, and legs. Washcloths may be used to stroke the feathers in

TABLE 38–1. Detergent Concentrations (Cups/Gallon and Ounces/Gallon)

% Solution	Cups/1 Gal	Oz/1 Gal	Cups/5 Gal	Oz/5 Gal	Cups/10 Gal	Oz/10 Gal	Cups/15 Gal	Oz/15 Gal
1%	0.2	1.3	0.8	6.4	1.6	12.8	2.4	19.2
2%	0.3	2.6	1.6	12.8	3.2	25.6	4.8	38.4
3%	0.5	3.8	2.4	19.2	4.8	38.4	7.2	57.6
4%	0.6	5.1	3.2	25.6	6.4	51.2	9.6	76.8
5%	0.8	6.4	4	32	8	64	12	96

the direction of feather growth and to force contact of the detergent solution with all areas of the feathers.

The head is gently cleaned with rayon/polyester squares (Nugauze; Johnson & Johnson Products, Inc., New Brunswick, NJ), a soft toothbrush or dental swab, and, depending on the species and type of oil, a periodontal irrigator. The eyes are flushed frequently with a sterile saline solution to remove soap and oil. The entire head and beak must be thoroughly cleaned; otherwise, the body will become recontaminated when the bird preens.

Successive tubs containing an equivalent or lower detergent concentration are used as the water becomes saturated with oil. The bird is lifted quickly and gently out of the soiled water and placed in the next tub, where the entire cleaning process is repeated. As many as eight or ten tub washes may be required for large, heavily oiled birds. Cleaning must be thorough, but efforts should be made to clean animals as quickly as possible. When the detergent water is no longer discolored by the washing process, the bird is determined to be free of oil and is taken to a rinsing station.

Rinsing Cleaning Agents from the Feathers

Once all oil is removed from all parts of the feathers, the bird is completely rinsed with warm, clean water. Rinsing is carried out by a spray of clean water at 103° to 105°F and 40 to 60 psi, beginning with the head and face (40 psi) and progressing systematically down the neck, back, wings, breast, abdomen, and tail (all at 60 psi) in order to push the detergent in one direction off of the bird. Rinsing continues until beads of water roll freely from the feathers, and the down feathers fluff up and actually appear dry.

The failure to rinse a bird adequately is probably the most common cause of unsuccessful rehabilitation efforts. Because even minute quantities of oil or detergent (by its hydrophilic nature) can impede waterproofing, all cleaning station materials are clearly marked. Clean buckets and hoses are kept separate from buckets and hoses used to transfer soapy water or waste water.

A newly rinsed bird is blotted with clean, dry towels and placed in a clean holding pen to complete the drying process. The bird should not be returned to its original, contaminated housing. Solid-sided, netting-topped pens of various sizes from 8 × 8 × 4 feet on up may be used. Soft-sided baby playpens can be used as drying pens for individual birds or pairs of birds. Net-bottomed pens, especially when used in conjunction with forced air dryers, allow for air circulation from below and provide more thorough drying for seabirds that are naturally sternally recumbent. The pen walls are lined with sheets or tightly woven towels and are curtained to minimize external stimuli, particularly human intrusion. Ventilation is provided to individual pens and/or rooms as needed. Free access to and egress from heat lamps allow a bird to find a comfortable ambient temperature. Drying birds are closely monitored for signs of heat stress. Cleaned birds, if warm and not stressed, usually begin to preen immediately and dry in a short time.

Restoration of Waterproofing

In general, within 24 hours of being cleaned, the birds are given access to freshwater pools. Ramps or platforms must be present in all pools to permit access into and egress out of water so the birds can actively swim and preen at will. Because contaminants can lower the surface tension of the water enough to penetrate the feathers, a bird can become wet from oil and other debris released into the water through droppings.[23] Pools must be kept clean; constant overflow and/or filtration are recommended.

Waterbirds usually enter the water readily, exiting to preen when they begin to get wet. As a bird continues its efforts to swim and then preen, it realigns its feathers to restore the original feather structure, which ensures waterproofing. Some species of waterfowl require uropygial gland secretions to waterproof their feathers; in many species, however, the feather structure does not require the application of preen-gland wax.[14] This natural oil seems to assist in maintaining the feather alignment, much as hair spray might hold a hairstyle. The oil also prevents the feathers from becoming dry and brittle, thus keeping them strong, flexible, and waterproof.[21]

On birds that are waterproof, water beads on their feathers. Waterbirds are also able to remain buoyant in the water without getting wet or chilled (both covert and down feathers should be dry).

Excessive preening is a sign that a bird is not yet waterproof and needs to be examined for evidence of persistent oiling, feather damage, or other reason for loss of feather integrity (Table 38–2).[21]

WATER HARDNESS AS A DETERMINING FACTOR IN WATERPROOFING

One vital consideration for diving birds is the hardness of the rinse and swimming water. The mineral salts (calcium and magnesium in hard water, sodium chloride in saline water) are deposited on the microscopic feather structure and prevent proper realignment of the feathers (Fig. 38–2). These deposits of mineral salts or the gummy detergent residues (the result of these cations' combining with detergent) prevent the bird from restoring waterproofing, despite heavy preening and/or swimming. A bird rinsed in hard water looks well-rinsed; when placed in a swimming pool, it appears waterproof for 6 to 12 hours but gradually becomes wet. The bird needs rewashing to remove the unseen mineral salts, followed by a thorough rinse and subsequent pool swims in water between 2 to 3 grains of hardness (30 to 50 mg/L).[3] The birds should be kept in softened water for 24 hours before being moved to hard water or salt water; this applies even to birds that naturally swim in salt water.[5] Once the feather structure is restored, an impenetrable barrier is formed, and harder water and salt water do not seem to cause any problems.

Pelagic species (all seabirds) must be rinsed in water

TABLE 38–2. Causes of Wet Feather in Waterfowl

Cause	Clinical Signs	Treatment

Lack of preening
  Sickness
  Debilitation
  Behavioral causes
	Feather vanes become disrupted and are not rearranged by preening	Diagnosis and treatment of underlying problem: preening can sometimes be stimulated by gently spraying with water

Soiling of feathers
  Fecal material
  Mud
  Dirty or dusty bedding
  Plant oils or spores
	Feather structure is clogged with dirt	Correction of environment; allow access to clean, shallow water for bathing and preening (often called "weathering"). Birds that have become waterlogged may drown in water a few centimeters deep.

Chemical contaminants
  Oil
  Surfactants
	Oil clogs the feather structure and causes them to clump together; surfactants reduce surface tension and break down the air-water interface in the feather structure	Light contamination may be treated as for soiling; heavy contamination requires washing; sea ducts, sawbills and seabirds rarely respond to weathering and are best washed

Physical damage to feathers	Interlocking barbs and barbules broken; lattice structure lost	If severe and widespread, waterproofing will not return until after the next molt, when new feathers emerge
Infestation with shaft lice (*Holomenopon* species)	Intense irritation causes excessive preening and feather damage	Diagnose by examining a freshly plucked feather with a hand lens; treat with acaricides

From Robinson I: Feathers and skin. *In* Beynon PH (ed): Manual of Raptors, Pigeons and Waterfowl. Ames, Iowa State University Press, p 308, 1996.

of 2 to 3 grains of hardness. The degree of waterproofing must then be evaluated by observing the birds swimming in sizable pools with a minimum depth of three times the bird's body length. As these species dive, their feather structure is subjected to the pressure of the surrounding water, and so waterproofing cannot be evaluated by spraying alone, as it can with raptors or songbirds.[23]

Conversely, "waterbirds" that spend very little time actually in the water (e.g., cormorants [*Phalacrocorax auritus*] and anhingas [*Anhinga anhinga*]) appear to retain more water within their feathers and lack water repellency even when the feathers are clean and intact. These species require access to water for diving and preening, but they may appear wet afterward. This lack of water repellency has been attributed to a structural difference in the feather composition, and experience with these species is required to distinguish this normal wetting from excessive wetting caused by oil or other contaminants.[16]

HUSBANDRY CONSIDERATIONS FOR OILED BIRDS

A potentially high number of different species of birds could be contaminated after an oil spill. Housing and dietary needs may vary greatly from one species to another; local wildlife rehabilitators can often provide information about the precise needs of individual families or species of birds. Several rehabilitation and natural history references may also be helpful.[2, 25, 31]

Stress Reduction. The most important factor in the rehabilitation procedure is the reduction of stress and all sources of stressful stimuli. Stress reduction is accomplished mainly through two objectives: (1) minimizing any unusual inputs to the birds' senses (e.g., sights, sounds, smells) and (2) maximizing any simulation of the birds' natural environment, including appropriate diet, housing, social groupings, and ventilation.

Nutrition. Because of the stress, dehydration, potential gastrointestinal damage, and other illness or injury potentially present in oiled birds, special considerations must be made when diets are prescribed. The diets should contain appropriate levels of macronutrients (fat, protein, and carbohydrates) as well as micronutrients (vitamins and minerals) for each species. Both complex dietary components and damage to the gastrointestinal tract decrease nutrient absorption, whereas both simple dietary components and an intact gastrointestinal tract enhance absorption.[6] On the basis of these concerns, all birds are fed, through gavage, balanced isotonic liquid

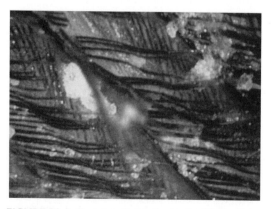

FIGURE 38–2. Scanning electromicrograph of feather from Canada goose residing on a saline retention pond. (Courtesy of H. Bryndza.)

diets (enterals) high in calories until the gastrointestinal function appears intact and the birds are determined to be sufficiently self-feeding. Assessment of adequate self-feeding is made through daily observations of behavior and droppings and monitoring of body weight changes.

Initial oral fluids should consist of clear electrolyte solutions. Nutrients should gradually be added to successive oral tubing solutions, and tube feeding repeated every 4 to 6 hours until the bird is allowed free access to food and water (after washing). Caloric needs can be calculated from the predicted basal metabolic rates (BMR) and resting energy expenditure (REE) based on natural diets (differs for carnivores and herbivores).[6] Enterics, such as Osmolite or Ensure (Ross Laboratories, Columbus, OH) can be given beginning 24 hours after admission, and no amount greater than 5% of the animal's body weight should be given at one feeding. Foods should be warmed to near body temperature and should include high levels of vitamin A and K, because the requirements for both may be elevated after ingestion of oil.[22] Specifics on tube feeding and oral diets are addressed in section 3 of *Oiled Bird Rehabilitation*.[26] After washing and evaluation, the birds may gradually be introduced to solid foods. The addition of cultured yogurt or lactobacillus products (Benebac; PetAg Corporation, Elgin, IL) may enhance digestion and nutrient absorption.

Once a bird has been stabilized and cleaned, it is allowed free access to a variety of appropriate foods.

All diets must be prepared fresh and must be nutritionally balanced and provide the necessary calories for the recovering birds. Piscivorous birds should be offered a variety of fresh, appropriate-sized, whole fish, similar to those on which they would naturally feed (e.g., freshwater fish for freshwater birds, saltwater fish for seabirds). Because many fish contain endogenous thiaminases, vitamin B_1 supplementation should be provided at 25 to 30 mg/kg of fish.[19] Fish with high natural oil content (such as sardines, tuna, and mackerel) should be avoided, because the resulting oily feces of the birds may recontaminate feathers and water sources.

Food placement, quantity, and quality, as well as time of feeding (especially for nocturnal birds) and access to food, are all important factors in getting wild birds to eat in captivity; for example, a large number of feeding stations should be provided to minimize competition, and the use of live fish may be necessary to entice a piscivorous bird to eventually accept dead fish. The birds are monitored to see which ones are self-feeding. The droppings are checked for the presence of blood or oil; birds in which blood is present or in which oil persists for more than 24 hours are treated with antibiotics and Pepto-Bismol, and fed enteric diets that are easily absorbed (e.g., Osmolite, Ensure) through gavage.

Fluid Support. All oiled birds experience some degree of dehydration (as a result of stress, lack of clean water to drink, diarrhea, and other fluid loss). Rehydration fluids are necessary to maintain blood pressure, assist digestion, and flush the gastrointestinal tract, liver, and kidneys. All birds receive intravenous and/or oral rehy-

drating fluids at approximately 4-hour intervals before being washed and possibly after washing, depending on the degree of dehydration and the birds' ability to drink unassisted. Birds are allowed access to only small bowls of water before washing, to prevent chilling and contamination of the water. After being washed, all birds are allowed free access to drinking water and, when dried, free access into and egress from pools.

Housing. Housing needs vary greatly with each species and should meet with the *Minimum Standards for Wildlife Rehabilitation*.[17] Soft-sided baby playpens provide adequate initial housing for most waterfowl, shorebirds, and seabirds. Large numbers of birds can be group-housed in constructed pens or entire rooms, if available. Pelagic birds that cannot stand or spend very little time standing (e.g., loons, gannets, shearwaters, petrels) must be housed on padded surfaces or net-bottomed cages to prevent keel lesions; netting provides the additional benefit of keeping feces and urates away from feathers, thus preventing additional feather damage. The proper size and style of perches must be provided for cormorants, ospreys, pelicans, eagles, and other perching birds. After being washed and dried, the birds can be housed in outdoor cages for acclimatization. These cages must contain the proper ground substrate: sand, gravel, Astro-Turf, or similar substrate for shorebirds and waterfowl; rocks for certain seabirds; and perches as needed.

All waste material and papers or linens used to line cages must be properly disposed as biohazardous waste before washing. After the birds have been washed, cage refuse may be disposed of according to the particular city ordinance for animal waste. Containers used to transport oiled birds should be disposed of as hazardous petroleum waste, as should all contaminated towels or sheets.

Pools. As discussed earlier, all cleaned birds must be allowed access to and egress from pools of the proper hardness and salinity to prevent problems with the interlocking structure of the feathers. The pools must also be deep enough for an animal to submerse itself, if that is part of the animal's normal behavior; for example, wading birds and many species of waterfowl need only submerse their legs and ventral abdomen, whereas diving birds must be able to fully immerse themselves to experience the increased water pressure on the feathers as they dive. Birds should also be misted with water at least three times daily to stimulate preening and evaluate waterproofing, especially if access to pools is limited. Misting can be done with either a spray bottle or a fine mist attachment for a garden hose.

Salt Water. Birds that live on the ocean or its coastline have a well-developed supraorbital or nasal salt gland that enables them to consume salt water in place of fresh water in their diets. The desalted water can then be used to fulfill the animal's dietary needs for fresh water. Seabirds placed on a fresh water diet in captivity may experience difficulties in converting salt water when returned to an ocean environment. Truly pelagic birds kept on fresh water diets for more than a few days should have salt reintroduced in their diets before being released back to the ocean. Specifics on this procedure are described in section 6 of *Oiled Bird Rehabilitation*.[26]

Social Grouping. Colonial species such as murres, pelicans, and many geese must be housed in contact or at least in sight of other conspecifics. Group housing should allow approximately 3 square feet (1 m²) of floor space per bird, in order to avoid overcrowding. Solitary species such as ospreys must be housed individually. Natural predators or competitors must not be housed in the vicinity of one another.

Temperature. Most oiled birds lose their ability to regulate their core body temperatures. Oiled birds must be housed in an environment that allows them to maintain their normal body temperature. In cold weather, heat lamps, hot water bottles, heating pads, and insulating layers of newspaper and blankets on the floor can be used to warm a hypothermic animal. In hot weather, hyperthermic birds can be slowly cooled with the use of fans, shaded pens, and, in the case of heat stress or heat stroke, gradual submersion into cool (not cold) water.

Ventilation. To reduce the odors and toxicants of petroleum, the potential of zoonotic disease, and the potential spread of disease among the oiled birds, all rooms, buildings, and cages should be well ventilated but draft free. Portable room air filter units are recommended, especially for pelagic birds and raptors, which are more susceptible to respiratory infections. Ideally, 15 air exchanges per hour should occur in order to minimize concentrations of hydrocarbons and fungal spores.[24]

Prerelease Examination. All prerelease medical examinations should be performed by an experienced wildlife veterinarian. This examination includes weighing the animal, evaluating body condition and waterproofing, examining for the presence of any infectious disease, determining that all injuries have resolved and blood values fall within the normal range, and observing that the animal can function normally to survive in the wild. Birds with any signs of disease or debilitation should not be released into wild populations. A U.S. Fish and Wildlife Service band may be placed on birds before release, and releases must be made in an uncontaminated environment with a food source adequate for the number and species of animals. The release should take place early enough for the animal to adjust before nightfall, and the release team should remain in the area long enough to observe that the birds are behaving normally.

Acknowledgments

The authors thank Lynne Frink and Joshua Dein for their pioneering work in the area of oiled bird rehabilitation. These individuals, and many others, have dedicated their skill, knowledge, and years of their lives in order to provide humane and increasingly successful care to wildlife affected by oil spills. Their moral and technical support are greatly appreciated in the production of this chapter.

REFERENCES

1. Albers PH: Oil spills and the environment: a review of chemical fate and biological effects of petroleum. *In* White J, Frink L (eds): The Effects of Oil on Wildlife: Research, Rehabilitation and General Concerns. Hanover, PA, Sheridan Press, International Wildlife Rehabilitation Council, pp 1–12, 1991.
2. Barnard WR, Clumpner, C, Albro R, et al: Wildlife Rescue Volunteer & Shoreline Oil Spill Training Manual. Olympia, WA, Department of Community, Trade and Economic Development-Fire Protection Services, 1994.
3. Bryndza HE: Surfactant efficacy in removal of petrochemicals from feathers. *In* White J, Frink, L (eds): The Effects of Oil on Wildlife: Research, Rehabilitation and General Concerns. Hanover, PA, Sheridan Press, International Wildlife Rehabilitation Council, pp 78–94, 1991.
4. Campbell TW: Avian Hematology and Cytology. Ames, Iowa State University Press, pp 7, 9, 1988.
5. Clumpner C: Water hardness and waterproofing of oiled birds: lessons from the Nestucca, Exxon Valdez and the American trader spills. *In* White J, Frink, L (eds): The Effects of Oil on Wildlife: Research, Rehabilitation and General Concerns. Hanover, PA, Sheridan Press, International Wildlife Rehabilitation Council, pp 101–102, 1991.
6. Donoghue S: Nutrition support of oil contaminated wildlife: clinical applications and research potentials. *In* White J, Frink L (eds): The Effects of Oil on Wildlife: Research, Rehabilitation and General Concerns. Hanover, PA, Sheridan Press, International Wildlife Rehabilitation Council, pp 103–112, 1991.
7. Flammer K: Antimicrobial therapy. *In* Ritchie B, Harrison G, Harrison L (eds): Avian Medicine: Principles and Application. Lake Worth, FL, Wingers Publishing, pp 451–454, 1994.
8. Frink L, Miller EA: Principles of oiled bird rehabilitation. *In* Frink L, Ball-Weir K, Smith C (eds): Wildlife and Oil Spills: Response, Research, and Contingency Planning. Newark, DE, Tri-State Bird Rescue & Research, pp 61–68, 1995.
9. Greth A, Rester C, Gerlach H, et al: Pathological effects of oil in seabirds during the arabian gulf oil spill. *In* Frink L, Ball-Weir K, Smith C (eds): Wildlife and Oil Spills: Response, Research, and Contingency Planning. Newark, DE, Tri-State Bird Rescue & Research, pp 134–141, 1995.
10. Jenssen BM, Ekker M: Effects of plumage contamination with crude oil dispersant mixtures on thermoregulation in common eiders and mallards. Arch Environ Contam Toxicol 20:389–403, 1991.
11. Jessup DA, Leighton FA: Oil pollution and petroleum toxicity to wildlife. *In* Fairbrother A, Locke LN, Hoff, GL (eds): Noninfectious Diseases of Wildlife, 2nd ed. Ames, Iowa State University Press, pp 141–156, 1996.
12. Leighton FA: The toxicity of petroleum oils to birds: an overview. *In* White J, Frink L (eds): The Effects of Oil on Wildlife: Research, Rehabilitation and General Concerns. Hanover, PA, Sheridan Press, International Wildlife Rehabilitation Council, pp 43–57, 1991.
13. Levin P, Skolnik S: The embryotoxicity and teratogenicity of oil on aquatic birds. Unpublished paper, 1990.
14. Lucas AM, Stettenheim PR: Avian Anatomy. Integument. Agricultural Handbook 362. Washington, DC, U.S. Department of Agriculture, 1972.
15. Lusimbo WS, Leighton, FA: Effects of Prudhoe Bay crude oil on hatching success and associated changes in pipping muscles in embryos of domestic chickens (*Gallus gallus*). J Wildl Dis 32(2):209–215, 1996.
16. Mahaffy L: The question of avian water-repellency: why are some birds more difficult to rehabilitate? *In* White J, Frink L (eds): The Effects of Oil on Wildlife: Research, Rehabilitation and General Concerns. Hanover, PA, Sheridan Press, International Wildlife Rehabilitation Council, pp 95–100, 1991.
17. Miller EA, White J (eds): NWRA/IWRC Minimum Standards for Wildlife Rehabilitation. St. Cloud, MN, National Wildlife Rehabilitators Association, 1994.
18. Pierce V: Pathology of wildlife following a #2 fuel oil spill. *In* White J, Frink L (eds): The Effects of Oil on Wildlife: Research, Rehabilitation and General Concerns. Hanover, PA, Sheridan Press, International Wildlife Rehabilitation Council, pp 78–94, 1991.
19. Pokras M: Clinical management and biomedicine of seabirds. *In* Rosskopf WJ, Woerpel R (eds): Diseases of Cage and Aviary Birds, 3rd ed. Baltimore, MD, Williams & Wilkins, pp 981–1001, 1996.
20. Redig PT: Medical Management of Birds of Prey, 3rd ed. Minn-

eapolis, MN, The Raptor Center at the University of Minnesota, 1993.

21. Robinson I: Feathers and skin. *In* Beynon PH (ed): Manual of Raptors, Pigeons and Waterfowl. Ames, Iowa State University Press, pp 305–311, 1996.

22. Sarafin JA: Nutrition and disease relationships that may serve as models for feeding oiled birds. *In* Rosie D, Barnes SN (eds): The Effects of Oil on Birds: A Multi-discipline Symposium. Newark, DE, Tri-State Bird Rescue & Research, pp 139–142, 1983.

23. Thorne KM: Is your bird waterproof? Int Wildl Rehab Council J (9)2:7–10, 1986.

24. Tseng, FS: Care of oiled seabirds: a veterinary perspective. Proceedings of the 1993 International Oil Spill Conference, American Petroleum Institute, Washington, DC, pp 421–424, 1993.

25. Walraven E: Rescue and Rehabilitation of Oiled Birds. New South Wales, Australia, Zoological Parks Board of New South Wales, 1992.

26. Welte SC: Oiled Bird Rehabilitation: A Guide for Establishing and Operating a Treatment Facility for Oiled Birds. Newark, DE, Tri-State Bird Rescue & Research, pp 3.5, 3.14, 16, 1990.

27. Welte SC: Principles of Fluid Therapy. Natl Wildl Rehab Assoc Q 13(3):13–16, 1996.

28. Welte SC, Bryndza H, Embick JR: Notes on health and safety concerns when handling oil contaminated wildlife. *In* White J, Frink L (eds): The Effects of Oil on Wildlife: Research, Rehabilitation and General Concerns. Hanover, PA, Sheridan Press, International Wildlife Rehabilitation Council, pp 73–77, 1991.

29. White J: Protocol for the rehabilitation of oil-affected waterbirds. Proceedings of the 1990 Annual Conference of the American Association of Zoo Veterinarians, South Padre Island, TX, pp 153–174, 1990.

30. White J: Current treatments for anemia in oil-contaminated birds. *In* White J, Frink L (eds): The Effects of Oil on Wildlife: Research, Rehabilitation and General Concerns. Hanover, PA, Sheridan Press, International Wildlife Rehabilitation Council, pp 67–72, 1991.

31. Williams AS: Rehabilitating Oiled Seabirds: A Field Manual. Washington, DC, American Petroleum Institute, 1983.

32. Williams ES, Thorne ET: Exertional myopathy (capture myopathy). *In* Fairbrother A, Locke LN, Hoff, GL (eds): Noninfectious Diseases of Wildlife, 2nd ed. Ames, Iowa State University Press, pp 181–193, 1996.

CHAPTER 39

Avian Analgesia

VICTORIA L. CLYDE
JOANNE PAUL-MURPHY

Limited information regarding avian pain perception and analgesia is available. The studies that have been performed suggest that pain perception in birds is mediated by neural pathways and neurotransmitters that are similar to those in mammals.[11] Clinical experience also indicates that pain perception in birds differs little from that in mammals and that many analgesics used in mammalian medicine may be used in birds. Unfortunately, specific dosages and effects of these drugs in avian species are not well described.

An inherent difficulty in the discussion of avian analgesia is the effect of species differences. Chickens and pigeons have been used most commonly in comparative pain research, whereas psittacines have been the focus of clinical work since the 1980s. Some studies have indicated differences in response to an analgesic agent between different breeds of chickens and between species of a given order of birds.[5] It is apparent that no single drug or dose works adequately or safely in every bird. Nonetheless, veterinarians are ethically bound to recognize and reduce pain in their patients whenever possible. This chapter is intended to be a guide to assist veterinarians in this quest and to stimulate further discussion and research in this area.

PAIN PERCEPTION AND MODULATION

Peripheral Nervous System

Sensitivity to pain is proportional to the number of pain receptors (nociceptors) present in a given tissue. Nociceptors are afferent nerve fibers that respond to noxious stimuli such as pressure, crushing, stretching, heat, burn, inflammation, or irritating chemicals. Two types of afferent pain fibers are generally described. Myelinated, modality-specific A-δ fibers typically respond to acute or sharp pain whereas slower conducting, polymodal, unmyelinated C fibers respond to mechanical, thermal, or chemical insults. Both fiber types can be activated by the same noxious stimulus, and differences in their nerve conduction times result in a double sensation of an initial sharp, prickling pain, which is carried by the A-δ fibers, followed by a dull, nonlocalizing, aching or burning sensation, carried on the C fibers.

Nociceptors are strongly activated by irritating chemicals that cause tissue injury. These chemicals are called *algogens*, and examples include organic acids, vasoactive amines (histamine), proteolytic enzymes, and products of the inflammatory cascade (prostaglandins and leukotrienes).[26, 27] Prostaglandins, especially prostaglandin E_2, can accentuate pain by sensitizing nociceptors. Sensitization is the result of a decreased threshold of activation of the pain fiber, secondary to activation of adenylate cyclase and altered calcium fluxes.

Central Nervous System

Activated nociceptors make synaptic connections with one of three types of postsynaptic cells in the dorsal horn of the spinal cord: *projection neurons* transmit the stimulus to higher brain centers; *excitatory* and *inhibitory neurons* (often called *internunciary neurons*) relay or control passage of the nociceptive stimulus to other cells within the spinal cord. The convergence of many nociceptive fibers on fewer projection cells causes an increase in the receptive field of each transmitting projection cell. This increase in receptive field size may be responsible for the poor localizability of pain. Convergence of both somatic and visceral fibers onto the same projection cell may also be a cause for referred pain, in which visceral pain is felt more cutaneously.[26]

Multiple centers in the brain, including areas in the brain stem, thalamus, and sensory cortical regions, are involved in pain perception and in the response to pain. Connections in the brain stem represent a phylogenetically older system that regulates the response of the autonomic nervous system to pain through the release of catecholamines, which activate the cardiovascular, gastrointestinal, and exocrine systems. The resultant effect includes elevation in heart rate, respiratory rate, and blood pressure to support a fight or flight response. The thalamus and associated regions play an important role in the discrimination of pain (localization, nature, and intensity). Both the midbrain and the cortex are involved in behavioral responses to pain. These pathways are given here as generalities; the exact localization of pathways in birds remains to be mapped.

Pain Modulation

The perception of pain may be modulated at many points along the pathway. Nociceptors differ from other sensory neurons in that sensitization, not habituation, is a common response to continued stimulus. Continuation of a stimulus facilitates the conversion of high-threshold nociceptors to low-threshold nociceptors, thus allowing the pain receptor to be activated by a milder stimulus.

Sensitization occurs by the release from an activated nociceptor of chemicals such as substance P that enhance nociception. Continued activation of a receptor induces an expansion of its nociceptive field. Eventual hypersensitization of spinal neurons allows continued pain perception even with lessened nociceptor stimulation. This sensitization of the entire pain perception system highlights the importance of analgesic timing. Early provision of adequate analgesia lessens the degree to which pain conduction is facilitated. Whenever possible, preemptive analgesia should be used to prevent activation of nociceptors before a pain stimulus. Al-

though this is not possible in most cases of trauma, it underscores the importance of a preoperative analgesic plan. Presurgical anti-inflammatory medication or nerve blocks markedly reduce postoperative pain and thereby lessen the need for additional analgesics.[3]

Endogenous analgesia is partially achieved by the descending antinociceptive system. This system is a dense set of neurons found in the brain and dorsal horn of the spinal cord, which release endogenous opiates (endorphins and enkephalins) in response to activation of the nociceptive system. Endogenous opiates stimulate the release of neurotransmitters (serotonin and norepinephrine), which then inhibit nociceptive conduction both presynaptically and postsynaptically. Analgesic modalities such as acupuncture, transcutaneous electrical nerve stimulation, and counterirritation work by activation of the descending antinociceptive system.

Exogenous analgesia occurs through the blocking of the nociceptive stimulus along the pain perception pathway. Several sites are available for interruption of the pain stimulus. Anti-inflammatory medications stop the release of chemical mediators that cause tissue damage, preventing the sensitization of the nociceptors. Local anesthetics block peripheral nerve conduction and prevent the activation of nociceptors. Opiates and alpha$_2$-adrenergic agonists decrease the sensitivity of both peripheral and central nociceptors by changing the threshold for receptor activation.

RECOGNITION OF PAIN IN BIRDS

Pain is a subjective experience which in humans is assessed from verbal statements of pain. In animals, the assessment of pain is usually based on observed behaviors. Active behaviors stimulated by acute pain, such as writhing or vocalizations, are easily interpreted. However, these behaviors may be stimulated only by severe or acute pain. Assessment of pain based solely on these readily observed behaviors consistently underestimates many instances of pain. The age or species of an animal modulates its ability or likelihood to demonstrate certain behaviors; for example, prey species exhibit signs of pain or disability less readily than predatory species. Likewise, the expression of pain in a social species is affected by the probable response of the other members within a social group (i.e., support and assistance, or ostracism). Therefore, careful observation of subtle behaviors, behavioral changes, and the absence of normal behaviors is necessary for assessing pain in animals.

Birds react to pain in many ways. Pain often evokes avoidance behavior in which the bird attempts to remove itself from the stimulus. If effective retreat is not possible, the bird may become anxious, display restless behaviors, vocalize, struggle, or become aggressive. A painful area may be guarded, resulting in a decreased interest or active avoidance of social interactions. The bird may exhibit abnormal, stiff, or crouched postures. A site of irritation may be overgroomed, resulting in feather loss, feather picking, or self-mutilation.

Birds may respond to a strong pain stimulus with

tonic immobility. This dramatic lack of reaction should not be interpreted as a lack of pain: it represents just the opposite. Low-grade or chronic pain in birds may produce withdrawal behaviors such as decreased appetite, irritability, lethargy, dyspnea, constipation, weight loss, or poor grooming. The bird may appear preoccupied, becoming less interested in external stimuli as it focuses on an internal source of pain or discomfort.

Accurate assessment of behavioral changes indicative of pain requires the veterinarian to be familiar with the normal behavior of both the individual bird and its species, as well as being aware that the observed changes in behavior may be the result of pain. In many situations, it is helpful to ask the following questions:

1. Would the lesion be painful in a human?
2. Does the lesion induce tissue damage?
3. Is the bird displaying aversive responses such as changes in temperament or posture or a decrease in normal behaviors?

If the answer to any of these questions is yes, the veterinarian should assume that the bird is in pain, and an analgesic plan should be instituted.[15]

ANALGESIC AGENTS

Analgesics are substances that decrease or eliminate the perception of pain without loss of consciousness. Analgesics work by a variety of methods, including modulation of the inflammatory process, blockade of nociceptor activation, and elevation of the activation threshold of a nociceptor. The quality of analgesia induced by different mechanisms may vary, and combination analgesia obtained by concurrent use of different classes of analgesic agents may produce a superior result.[18]

Each category of analgesics is summarized as follows, and specific references to birds are provided where available. The dosages listed herein are a compilation of doses reported in the literature and from personal communications from zoo and avian veterinarians. Many are extrapolations of mammalian dosages that appear to be clinically effective in limited case numbers. The dosages listed are given not as specific recommendations for use, but to disseminate information and to stimulate further studies in the area of avian analgesia.

Opioids

Opioids are a diverse group of natural and synthetic drugs with morphine-like action that combine reversibly with specific receptors in the central nervous system. Although considered the most effective class of centrally acting analgesics for sharp or acute pain, marked species differences in required dosages and clinical effects have been noted. These differences may be attributable to variations in the subclasses of opioid receptors present in the forebrains of different species. Multiple receptor subclasses have been described, and drugs that activate the mu and kappa subclasses produce analgesia. Mixed agonist-antagonist opioids, characterized by ago-

nist activity at kappa receptors and minimal or antagonist activity at mu receptors, are often used in veterinary medicine for pain relief. Mixed agonist-antagonist opioids have a lower abuse potential and as such are usually nonscheduled drugs.

Birds possess opioid receptors and are able to recognize and respond to a variety of opioids. However, early studies of opioids in pigeons and chickens yielded conflicting data on the sensitivity of birds to this class of drugs. The sensitivity to opioids is affected by both age and strain of chicken studied. Autoradiographic studies show a marked predominance of kappa receptors in the forebrain of pigeons, in comparison to the mammalian species studied.[21] Some evidence suggests that birds may not possess distinct mu and kappa receptors. In experimental studies, pigeons were unable to discriminate between mu and kappa agonists.[13] The administration of either a kappa or a mu agonist to isoflurane-anesthetized chickens produced similar reductions in the isoflurane concentration necessary to block response to a noxious stimulus.[4]

If other species of birds have an increased percentage of kappa receptors in the forebrain similar to those in pigeons, mu agonists should be less effective than mixed agonist-antagonists with kappa activity.[19] Buprenorphine, a partial agonist that binds avidly to mu receptors, produced minimal analgesic effect when given to African gray parrots, even at extremely high dosages of 2 mg/kg intramuscularly (IM) (J. Paul-Murphy, unpublished data). Better efficacy may be expected from mixed agonist-antagonists with kappa activity, such as butorphanol, pentazocine, and nalbuphine. Only butorphanol has been investigated in birds to date. The analgesic effect of butorphanol was assessed by measuring its isoflurane-sparing effect.[6] After administration of butorphanol, 1 mg/kg IM, the effective dose (ED$_{50}$) of isoflurane was decreased in cockatoos and African gray parrots (25% and 11%, respectively) but did not change significantly in blue-fronted Amazon parrots.[5, 6] In studies on awake African gray parrots, half the birds showed a higher threshold to noxious stimuli after receiving butorphanol, 1.0 mg/kg IM, evidence of an analgesic effect in birds (J. Paul-Murphy, unpublished data). Current recommendation for an empirical dosage range in psittacines has been reported as 1 to 4 mg/kg.[15, 29] Butorphanol has a short duration of action, and frequent redosing at 2- to 4-hour intervals is needed to maintain analgesia.

Adverse effects of opioids include respiratory and cardiovascular depression, increased intracranial pressure, behavioral effects, and development of tolerance. Few of these effects have been well studied in birds. Clinical trials in budgerigars given butorphanol, 3 mg/kg IM, produced mild motor deficits in half the birds, with no significant changes in heart rate or respiratory rate.[2] Other studies have measured heart rate and respiratory rate changes in anesthetized birds after opioid administration. Isoflurane-anesthetized cockatoos receiving IM butorphanol showed reductions in heart rate and tidal volume with a concomitant increase in respiratory rate.[6] However, heart rate and mean arterial pressures did not change in isoflurane-anesthetized chickens after the administration of either morphine or a kappa agonist.[4] Similarly, no changes in heart rate or respiratory rate were observed in turkeys anesthetized with halothane in a nitrous oxide–oxygen mixture after butorphanol administration.[24] Tolerance to opioid analgesia after several days of treatment has been noted in mammals, but no such information is available for birds.

Alpha₂-Adrenergic Agonists

Alpha₂-adrenergic agonists induce sedation, analgesia, anxiolysis, and muscle relaxation in mammals, although these effects vary considerably between species.[20] Limited data suggest that these drugs have similar effects in birds. Xylazine, 1 to 4 mg/kg IM, provides sedation for ketamine anesthesia and has been used in doses up to 10 mg/kg for sedation in small psittacines.[23, 28] Detomidine, 0.3 mg/kg IM, produced marked sedation in chickens, but data on duration, cardiopulmonary effects, or complications were not given.[22] Medetomidine, 0.1 mg/kg IM, produced drowsiness without immobilization in ostrich chicks. Again, no information concerning duration or cardiopulmonary effects was given, other than a statement that an unquantified drop in heart rate was seen in all birds.[31] Medetomidine, 0.05 to 0.10 mg/kg intravenously (IV) or 0.075 to 0.15 mg/kg IM, has been used in a small number of birds as an adjunct to ketamine anesthesia.[14] Unfortunately, analgesia was not assessed directly in these studies, but this class of drugs should be able to provide analgesia and warrants further investigation.

Possible complications of alpha₂-adrenergic agonists include a short duration of analgesia, hypotension, bradycardia, and hypothermia. Hypoxemia and hypercapnia were observed in Pekin ducks given xylazine.[19] Reversal agents for alpha₂-adrenergic agonists appear to be effective in birds. Yohimbine, 0.1 mg/kg IV, and tolazoline, 15 mg/kg IV, have been used for reversal of ketamine/xylazine anesthesia in raptors.[1, 7] Preliminary trials suggest that IM atipamezole is effective in birds when given at a dose five times that of medetomidine (weight:weight).[14]

Anti-Inflammatory Drugs

Anti-inflammatory drugs are indicated for the relief of pain induced by inflammation. Although not adequate as single agents for sharp or acute pain, anti-inflammatory drugs are synergistic with other classes of analgesic agents and may be used effectively in combined analgesic regimens.[16] Preoperative use of anti-inflammatory drugs lessens the need for postoperative opioids.[18] Two classes of anti-inflammatory agents, corticosteroids and nonsteroidal anti-inflammatory drugs (NSAIDs), are recognized.

CORTICOSTEROIDS

Corticosteroids suppress connective tissue response to chemical, thermal, traumatic, anaphylactic, or inflammatory injury. Inflammation is reduced as a result of suppression of fibroblastic and leukocytic activity, by

stabilization of lysosomal membranes in leukocytes and damaged tissue with a resultant decrease in release of proteolytic enzymes, and by suppression of edema formation.[27] Dexamethasone (1 to 2 mg/kg IM), betamethasone (0.1 mg/kg IM), and methylprednisolone acetate (0.5 to 1.0 mg/kg IM) have been used in a variety of species.[9, 25] Possible immunosuppression and other complications of corticosteroids make NSAIDs preferable in many situations.

NONSTEROIDAL ANTI-INFLAMMATORY DRUGS

NSAIDs act by inhibiting cyclooxygenase and the subsequent production of prostaglandins. Several categories of NSAIDs exist, few of which have been investigated in birds:

1. Carboxylic acid group contains derivatives of
   a. Salicylic acid (aspirin)
   b. Acetic acid (indomethacin, tolmetin)
   c. Propionic acid (naproxen, ibuprofen, ketoprofen)
   d. Fenamic acid (meclofenamic acid, flunixin meglumine)
2. Enolic acid group contains derivatives of
   a. Pyrazoline (phenylbutazone, dipyrone)
   b. Oxicam (piroxicam)

NSAIDs of different categories may have different effects. For example, salicylate derivatives often provide good analgesia for peripheral joint pain but are inadequate for deep or visceral pain.[27] This may underlie the observation that acetylsalicylic acid, 5.0 mg/kg PO TID, does not appear to be as effective as other NSAIDs in birds.[25] Clinically derived dosages include flunixin meglumine, 1.0 to 10.0 mg/kg IM SID, and meclofenamic acid, 2.2 mg/kg PO SID (S.E. Orosz, personal communication).[15, 25]

A potential complication of NSAIDs is gastrointestinal ulceration, which occurs through direct mucosal irritation and by inhibition of prostaglandin synthesis, thereby reducing mucosal integrity. Gastrointestinal side effects are not frequently recognized after use of these agents in birds. Administration of high-dose flunixin meglumine (10 mg/kg IM) to budgerigars resulted in initial regurgitation and tenesmus.[2] The birds resumed eating immediately after regurgitation, and continued straining was not apparent. An African crowned crane passed droppings containing fresh blood after a month-long course of daily injections with flunixin meglumine (J. Stover, personal communication). Droppings cleared upon cessation of treatment, and no further adverse gastrointestinal side effects were noted.

Renal ischemia with resultant damage may be the most serious complication with the use of NSAIDs in birds. In an experimental trial with northern bobwhite quails, daily administration of flunixin meglumine for 7 days at treatment levels ranging from 0.1 to 32 mg/kg IM produced renal disease in all birds.[17] The distribution and severity of the lesions increased with increasing dose. No hematologic or clinical chemistry changes were noted. Whooping cranes, Siberian cranes, and red-crowned cranes treated with flunixin meglumine have died as a result of acute necrotizing glomerulitis, gout tophi in the renal tubules, and visceral gout (F.J. Dein and J. Langenberg, personal communication). Currently, clinical use of flunixin meglumine in cranes is contraindicated, and caution should be used in treating other species with this drug. Use of the lowest possible therapeutic dose for the shortest duration along with supplemental hydration is advisable. Additional studies are needed to assess species differences and to investigate the effects of other NSAIDs on the avian renal system.

Local Anesthetics

Local anesthetics block ion channels, stopping the transmission of pain impulses. This blockade interferes with nociceptor sensitization and prevents central changes that are secondary to activation of pain pathways. Use of a local nerve block before tissue trauma significantly reduces postoperative pain, and blockade before nerve transection in amputation decreases the prevalence of so-called phantom pain in humans.[3] Lidocaine may be used for local anesthesia in birds, as long as the dose does not exceed 4 mg/kg.[19] Administration of this dose to small birds requires dilution of the commercially available solutions. Overdosage may result in seizures and possible cardiac arrest.

Little information was found on the use of longer acting local anesthetics, such as bupivacaine, in birds. Topical administration of bupivacaine and dimethyl sulfoxide (50:50) to the cut portion of chicken beaks immediately after trimming eliminated the reduction in food intake typically observed.[12] Similar improvements were seen with application of a mixture containing phenylbutazone, isopropylaminophenazone, and dimethyl sulfoxide.[12]

IV, epidural, and intrathecal routes of administration of local anesthetics, often in combination with opioids or alpha$_2$-adrenergic agonists, have provided superior analgesia in mammals.[16] These routes have not been investigated in avian patients.

Adjunctive Medications

Although sedatives and tranquilizing agents do not provide analgesia, the induced behavioral changes and reduction in limbic activity can decrease pain perception and allow for improved efficacy of concurrent analgesics. Diazepam, 0.5 to 2.0 mg/kg IV or IM, and midazolam, 1.0 to 2.0 mg/kg IM, have been used in birds.[19, 28, 30] In addition, both drugs provide skeletal muscle relaxation, which affords pain reduction in appropriate cases. Muscle relaxation may also be obtained with methocarbamol, 50 mg/kg IV BID.[8] The hypnotic metomidate has been used as a premedicant in birds at 5 to 15 mg/kg IM.[10]

TREATMENT OF PAIN IN BIRDS

When evidence of pain is noted in an avian patient, or when tissue trauma has occurred, an analgesic plan should be designed and instituted. The analgesic plan should incorporate multiple methods of pain reduction,

and simple, nonchemical methods of analgesia should not be overlooked. The source of pain should be identified and treated. The removal of fear and anxiety reduces muscle tension and central nervous system activation. Anxiolytics, tranquilizers, and muscle relaxants should be used judiciously along with environmental modifications. A dry, warm, quiet, comfortable, and nonstressful environment is essential.

Mechanical forms of analgesia provided by good nursing care are important. The first mechanical consideration should be rest for the traumatized area. The affected area should be bandaged or splinted if necessary to provide protection and support. Perches should provide easy and comfortable footing without the need for excessive gripping. Food and water should be readily available to the bird without the need for excessive movement. Other mechanical methods of analgesia (alternating heat and cold, massage, physical therapy, controlled exercise, and transcutaneous electrical nerve stimulation) should be considered, although they may not be applicable to all patients.

The chemical forms of analgesia selected should be appropriate for the type of pain. Acute, sharp pain is best treated by opioids or alpha$_2$-adrenergic agonists. Kappa agonists, such as butorphanol, appear beneficial in birds, although the short duration of action necessitates multiple redosing. Inflammatory or chronic pain is usually treated by NSAIDs. In chronic situations, a gradual increase in dosage is recommended until pain control is achieved. Although flunixin meglumine has been used safely in many birds, investigations revealing kidney damage even at low dosages raise concerns about extended use and species sensitivity. Information regarding other NSAIDs is needed. Corticosteroids can provide pain relief and temporary euphoria, which may stimulate appetite.

Basic principles of analgesia should be reviewed when an analgesic plan is formulated. The earliest possible disruption of the pain pathway is beneficial in order to reduce sensitization of pain pathways. Preemptive analgesia before the onset of pain stimulation should be implemented when possible. Nerve blockade with infiltration of a local anesthetic is recommended before nerve transection. Combinations of drugs that interrupt the pain pathway at different steps may improve the level of analgesia afforded to the patient.

The field of avian analgesia is in its infancy. Numerous additional studies are needed to clarify species differences, optimal drugs, and optimal dosages and to elucidate possible complications of analgesic medications in birds.

REFERENCES

1. Allen JL, Oosterhuis JE: Effect of tolazoline on xylazine/ketamine-induced anesthesia in turkey vultures. J Am Vet Assoc 189:1011–1016, 1986.
2. Bauck L: Analgesics in avian medicine. Proceedings of the 1990 Annual Conference of the Association of Avian Veterinarians, Phoenix, AZ, pp 239–244, 1990.
3. Coderre TJ, Katz J, Vaccarino AL, et al: Contribution of central neuroplasticity to pathological pain: review of clinical and experimental evidence. Pain 52:259–285, 1993.
4. Concannon KT, Dodam JR, Hellyer PW: Influence of a mu and

kappa opioid agonist on isoflurane minimal anesthetic concentration in chickens. Am J Vet Res 56:806–812, 1996

5. Curro TG: Evaluation of the isoflurane-sparing effects of butorphanol and flunixin in psittaciformes. Main Conference Proceedings, Association of Avian Veterinarians, Reno, NV, pp 17–19, 1994.

6. Curro TG, Brunson D, Paul-Murphy J: Determination of the ED50 of isoflurane and evaluation of the analgesic properties of butorphanol in cockatoo (*Cacatua* spp.). Vet Surg 23:429–433, 1994.

7. Degernes LA, Kreeger TJ, Mandsager R, et al: Ketamine-xylazine anesthesia in red-tailed hawks with antagonism by yohimbine. J Wildl Dis 24:332–336, 1988.

8. Done LB, Ialeggio DM, Cranfield M: Therapeutic use of methocarbamol in a demoiselle crane (*Anthropoides virgo*) with severe ataxia and lateroflexion of the neck. Proceedings of the Annual Conference of the American Association of Zoo Veterinarians, St Louis, MO, pp 137–138, 1993.

9. Duncan IJH, Beatty ER, Hocking PM, et al: Assessment of pain associated with degenerative hip disorders in adult male turkeys. Res Vet Sci 50:200–203, 1991.

10. Galvin C: Avian Drugs and Dosages. Suisan, CA, Internl Wildl Rehab Council, 1976.

11. Gentle M: Behavioural and physiological responses to pain in the chicken. Acta XX Cong Internatl Ornith 3:1915–1919, 1990.

12. Glatz PC, Murphy BL, Preston AP: Analgesic therapy of beak-trimmed chickens. Aust Vet J 69:18, 1992.

13. Herling S, Coale EH Jr, Valentino RJ, et al: Narcotic discrimination in pigeons. J Pharm Exp Ther 214:139–146, 1980.

14. Jalanka HH: New alpha-2 adrenoceptor agonists and antagonists. *In* Fowler ME (ed): Zoo and Wild Animal Medicine: Current Therapy 3. Philadelphia, WB Saunders, pp 479–480, 1993.

15. Jenkins JR: Postoperative care of the avian patient. Seminars in Avian and Exotic Pet Medicine 2:97–102, 1993.

16. Kehlet H, Dahl JB: The value of "multimodal" or "balanced analgesia" in postoperative pain treatment. Anesth Analg 77:1048–1056, 1993.

17. Klein PN, Charmatz, Langenberg J: The effect of flunixin meglumine (banamine) on the renal function in northern bobwhite (*Colinus virginianus*): an avian model. Proceedings of the Annual Conference of the American Association of Zoo Veterinarians, Pittsburgh, PA, pp 128–131, 1994.

18. Livingston A: Physiological basis for pain perception in animals. Fifth International Congress of Veterinary Anesthesia, pp 1–6, 1994.

19. Ludders JW, Matthews N: Birds. *In* Thurmon JC, Tranquilli WJ, Benson GJ (eds): Lumb & Jones' Veterinary Anesthesia, 3rd ed. Baltimore, Williams & Wilkins, pp 645–669, 1996.

20. MacDonald E, Virtanen R, Salonen J: Chemistry and pharmacokinetics of the alpha-adrenoreceptor agonists. *In* Short CE, Van Posnak A (eds): Animal Pain. New York, Churchill Livingstone, pp 181–200, 1992.

21. Mansour A, Khachaturian H, Lewis ME, et al: Anatomy of CNS opioid receptors. Trends Neurosci 11:308–314, 1988.

22. Mohammad FK, Al-Badrany MS, Al-Hasan AM: Detomidine-ketamine anaesthesia in chickens. Vet Rec 133:192, 1993.

23. Muir WM III, Hubbell JAE: Handbook of Veterinary Anesthesia. St. Louis, CV Mosby, pp 234–244, 1989.

24. Reim DA, Middleton CC: Use of butorphanol as an anesthetic adjunct in turkeys. Lab Anim Sci 45:696–698, 1995.

25. Ritchie BW, Harrison GJ: Formulary. *In* Ritchie BW, Harrison GJ, Harrison LR (eds): Avian Medicine: Principles and Application. Lake Worth, FL, Wingers Publications, pp 457–481, 1994.

26. Sackman JE: Pain: Part I. The physiology of pain. Compend Sm Anim 13:71–79, 1991.

27. Sackman JE: Pain: Part II. Control of pain in animals. Compend Sm Anim 13:181–191, 1991.

28. Sinn LC: Anesthesiology. *In* Ritchie BW, Harrison GJ, Harrison LR (eds): Avian Medicine: Principles and Application. Lake Worth, FL, Wingers Publications, pp 1066–1080, 1994.

29. Tully TN: Formulary. *In* Altman RB, Clubb SL, Dorrenstein GM, et al (eds): Avian Medicine and Surgery. Philadelphia, WB Saunders, pp 671–688, 1997.

30. Valverde A, Honeyman VL, Dyson DH, et al: Determination of a sedative dose and influence of midazolam on cardiopulmonary function in Canada geese. J Am Vet Assoc 51:1071–1074, 1990.

31. Van Heerden J, Keffen RH: A preliminary investigation into the immobilising potential of a tiletamine/zolazepam mixture, metomidate, a metomidate and azaperone combination and medetomidine in ostriches (*Struthio camelus*). J S Afr Vet Assoc 62:114–117, 1991.

PART IV

MAMMALS

CHAPTER 40

Contraception

CHERYL S. ASA

Controlling reproduction in captive animals may be important for limiting numbers or for genetic management to prevent inbreeding or to balance founder representation. Permanent sterilization or gonadectomy may be the safest and most effective way to accomplish these goals. However, if reversible contraception is necessary, the choices are more difficult, because no method is completely effective and all carry some degree of risk. This risk, however, should be weighed against the risks associated with pregnancy and parturition, not against those of the nonpregnant state. This chapter focuses on the results of research and analysis of surveys (Contraception Advisory Group [CAG] Database),[2] as well as on considerations for deciding among the various methods. Where available, information regarding implementation, monitoring, and reversal is also included. Historical information for captive and free-ranging wildlife have been published previously.[1]

PERMANENT METHODS

Gonadectomy

Male castration is simple except in species with undescended or partially descended testes.[42] However, effects on secondary sex characteristics caused by the decline in testosterone may involve complete loss (e.g.,

lion manes) or disruption of the seasonal cycle (e.g., deer antlers that stay in velvet). After castration, especially in sexually experienced males, libido may decline slowly if at all. Likewise, declining testosterone may result in reduced aggression, but learned behavior patterns may persist.

Ovariectomy or ovariohysterectomy of females may be preferable in species in which male sterilization may lead to repeated infertile cycles that can be associated with uterine and/or mammary disease. This is especially true for induced ovulators, in which repeated pseudopregnancies would result.

Sterilization

Vasectomy is an option for males in which maintenance of secondary sex characteristics and masculine behavior is desirable. Although potentially reversible, the technique is specific to human vasa, requiring highly skilled microsurgery, and carries an enormously variable success rate. Thus for captive wildlife, vasectomy should be considered permanent. As an alternative to surgery, permanent obstruction of sperm passage also can be accomplished by injection of a sclerosing agent into the cauda epididymis[33, 35] or vas deferens.[18] Although chemical sterilization also can be achieved with very low doses of cadmium chloride,[42] possible deleterious effects include lesions of the sensory ganglia.[20]

Female tubal ligation also should be considered permanent. Indeed, if permanent birth control is desired, the added health benefits of gonadectomy render gonadectomy preferable to sterilization except perhaps for very long-lived species, in which potential decrease in bone density pursuant to the loss of estrogen may become problematic. Unfortunately, no nonhuman data regarding this possibility currently exist.

REVERSIBLE CONTRACEPTION

Synthetic Steroid Hormones

The female-directed contraceptives most commonly used by zoos are steroid-hormone based, particularly the Silastic implants containing melengestrol acetate (MGA) according to Dr. E. Plotka and the American Zoological Association (AZA) Contraception Advisory Group. Other synthetic progestins include levonorgestrel implants (Norplant; Wyeth-Ayerst), medroxyprogesterone acetate injections (Depo-Provera; Upjohn Co.), and oral megestrol acetate (Ovaban; Shering Corp.). MGA also can be incorporated into feed for oral administration.

Progestins may act at any of several points in the reproductive process, including thickening cervical mucus, which impedes passage of sperm; interrupting sperm and ovum transport in the uterus and oviducts; interfering with aspects of implantation; and blocking the luteinizing hormone (LH) surge necessary for ovulation.[13, 15] Because progestins are not particularly effective in hindering follicle development, physical and behavioral signs of estrus or even ovulation may occur in individual animals with adequate contraception.[12, 26, 41] Thus signs of estrus cannot be used to judge the efficacy of a progestin-based contraceptive.

Birth control pills contain a combination of synthetic estrogen and progestin, with formulations that vary by manufacturer. (Provera is also available as the "mini-pill" but is not as widely used.) In general, estrogens are much more effective than progestins at blocking ovulation, but they also seem to be associated with more side effects. It is thought that the addition of progestin, especially in a regimen that includes a withdrawal period every fourth week, sufficiently counters the deleterious effects of estrogen. Because of the very high levels of endogenous gonadal hormones in the nonhuman primate family Cebidae, a combination estrogen/progestin Silastic implant was tested. Biopsies were used to monitor possible deleterious uterine effects that may occur because regular hormone withdrawal is not possible with an implant.

The synthetic androgen mibolerone (Cheque; Upjohn Co.), approved for use in domestic female dogs, may be effective in other taxa, but possible resultant increases in aggression remain a concern.

Gonadotropin-Releasing Hormone (GnRH) Analogs

Also sometimes called luteinizing hormone–releasing hormone (LHRH), GnRH stimulates the cascade of pituitary and gonadal hormonal events that results ultimately in ovulation or spermatogenesis. Analogs of GnRH can effect contraception either by blocking the action of GnRH (antagonists) or by first overstimulating and then suppressing the system through negative feedback (agonists). Because GnRH initiates reproduction in both males and females, this approach is theoretically effective in both. The functional result is equivalent to reversible gonadectomy. Most GnRH analog contraceptive development has concentrated on agonists such as leuprolide (Lupron; TAP), available only in injectable form. Although it failed to adequately suppress spermatogenesis in humans, Lupron has been used in males of various species with some success. Other GnRH agonists, incorporated in implants, are currently being tested but are not yet commercially available in the United States.

Vaccines

Although the early contraceptive promise[8] of antibodies to sperm, chorionic gonadotropin, follicle-stimulating hormone (FSH), and LH has not been realized, porcine zona pellucida (PZP) vaccines continue to be tested and used with some success.[25] A vaccine against bovine GnRH was commercially available in Australia until 1996 (Vaxstrate; Webster), and other such vaccines are currently under development.

Antispermatogenics

Several classes of drugs have been shown to reversibly block spermatogenesis. Bisdiamine has undergone the most extensive testing and has been shown to be safe and effective in rhesus monkeys, humans, several rodent species, dogs, and gray wolves.[9, 16] However, it is not commercially available except in very expensive laboratory grade (Fertilysin; Aldrich). Although successful in rodents,[46] pilot tests of several indenopyridine analogs in domestic cats were associated with mild but unacceptable side effects, including lethargy and occasional bloody diarrhea.[17] Busulfan also can suppress spermatogenesis,[44] but concomitant bone marrow suppression makes it unacceptable for contraception.[45]

Mechanical Devices

Occlusion of the vas deferens, such as through vas plugs, can successfully block the transport of sperm but should currently be considered nonreversible. Although little information regarding the use of intrauterine devices (IUDs) in nonhuman species exists, their safety in humans, if properly inserted, suggests that they may be appropriate for great apes.[14]

DELIVERY SYSTEMS

Delivery methods for currently available contraceptives include implants, injections, and pills. Obvious advantages to implants include a relatively long period of delivery per handling episode. Steroids are most amenable to this route of administration because they diffuse easily from Silastic rods. Peptide analogs have proved more difficult in this regard, although newer forms appear more reliable.

Problems with implants include loss and migration. Loss can be minimized by gas sterilization of Silastic implants followed by thorough degassing, sterile insertion, and, for social species, separation of the individual from the group until incision is healed. The smaller entry site left by a trocar (e.g., Norplant insertion) reduces chances of loss by grooming. Formation of sterile abscesses that contribute to implant loss may be common in perissodactyls and necessitates further study.

For solid implants, confirming presence and monitoring position, especially if migration is suspected, can be facilitated by addition of radiopaque material or an identity transponder microchip. Solid implants can also be sutured to the muscle to impede migration. However, these modifications are not recommended for implants fashioned from Silastic tubing (e.g., Norplant), because hormone release rate may be altered.

Slow-release preparations for injection can be formulated to release either peptide or steroid hormones. A single injection may be effective for 1 month (e.g., Lupron Depot) to 3 months (e.g., Depo-Provera). Vaccines also are administered by injection. Although remote delivery through dart is possible for injectables, certainty of complete injection can be problematic.

A disadvantage of oral preparations is that they typically must be administered daily, but they can usually be incorporated into food. Confirmation of ingestion is critical and can be difficult, especially in great apes.

EFFICACY

Latency to Effect

Progestins probably reach contraceptive levels in the blood within 1 hour (Norplant) to 3 days (MGA) of implant insertion and probably even sooner with injectable and oral forms. However, if follicles are present when treatment is initiated, the progestin may not be able to block ovulation for that cycle. Thus individuals should be considered fertile for at least 2 weeks after initiation of treatment.

Although castration and vasectomy immediately eliminate the source of sperm and antispermatogenics may interrupt spermatogenesis within hours, viable sperm may remain in the vas deferens for many weeks. Latency to clearance of sperm from the tract or until sperm death varies by species.[33, 34] As a conservative measure, males should not be considered sterile for at least 6 weeks after treatment. Ejaculation may hasten elimination of sperm from the vas, by electroejaculation, masturbation, or mating with a contraceptive-protected female. Flushing at the time of vasectomy immediately clears sperm from the tract.[19]

Animals treated with PZP or other vaccines should not be considered contraceptively protected until after the last booster is administered. The typical regimen is three injections about a month apart.

Efficacy Problems

Excepting delivery problems, such as implant loss, incomplete injection, or refusal to consume, progestins appear to be effective in all mammalian genera given an adequate dose, except in equids. Unfortunately, dose-response studies have not been conducted in nondomestic species other than the black lemur.[37] Assessment of efficacy is confounded by the likelihood of follicle growth and the possibility of ovulation in animals administered progestin. Furthermore, progestin-only contraception is especially difficult to accomplish in New World primates, apparently because of their high endogenous steroid levels, which leave the pituitary and hypothalamus less sensitive to steroid feedback. For example, the average human Depo-Provera dose is about 2 mg/kg body weight, whereas that needed for callitrichids may be as high as 20 mg/kg body weight (CAG Database).

Duration of Efficacy and Reversal

Experience with MGA implants indicates they are effective for at least 2 years (CAG Database), whereas Norplant implant systems are effective in humans for 5 years. After implant removal, reversal may be immediate, although there are undoubtedly individual differences in latency to first ovulation. Females are potentially fertile within a week after cessation of birth control pill administration, although time to first ovulation varies.

Depo-Provera injections are effective for at least 2 to 3 months; the variability is perhaps a result partly of dosage—that is, higher dosages may maintain blood levels above the efficacy threshold for a longer period. However, extremely variable reversal times have been reported, ranging from 2 months to almost 2 years.[41, 50]

Reports in the CAG Database indicate that the efficacy of PZP may last less than a year and possibly as short as 6 months, which is still adequate for species with a breeding season of less than 6 months. However, there is growing evidence that seasonal breeders may continue to cycle longer than previously believed, probably because, historically, females placed with males conceived within a few cycles. Cycling may not have been evident in those not with males, which led to an underestimation of the actual period of fertility. This explanation is more consistent with the data than is the possibility of a shift in the breeding season after withdrawal from contraception.

The length of the species-specific spermatogenic cycle determines latency to reversal for antispermatogenic compounds. Although data are unavailable for most species, 34 to 74 days are reported for the domestic and laboratory species studied.[48]

DELETERIOUS EFFECTS

The effects of progestins on uterine and mammary tissue of felids and canids have been described.[7, 29] In addition, an association with diabetes mellitus has been reported, at least in canids,[43] as well as a tendency for weight gain in all taxa. The results from canids and felids may apply to carnivores in general. Deleterious effects in primates appear limited,[30, 37] but the severity and implications for these species require further study. The few data available for ungulates have revealed no problems at this time, but as yet unexplained are occasional reports of either hair loss[22] or exaggerated hair growth over MGA implants (CAG Database).

Deleterious effects associated with PZP may be caused by the adjuvant or by the antibody itself. The adjuvant most effective at provoking an immune response (Freund's complete adjuvant) also causes subsequent positive tests for tuberculosis and is associated with other local or systemic reactions, especially in felids.[28] Some evidence also suggests that long-term PZP contraception may not be reversible, at least in some species.[27]

CONTRACEPTION DURING PREGNANCY OR LACTATION

Early association in humans of combination (estrogen/progestin) birth control pills with teratogenesis and virilization of female fetuses has not been corroborated, possibly because later doses were much lower. However, data from primates and ungulates showed that MGA implants are occasionally associated with abortion or stillbirth.[8, 37, 39] Although MGA can block parturition and prolong gestation in white-tailed deer,[36] MGA-implanted primates and domestic cows have given birth normally.[8, 37, 51] This discrepancy may be a result of dosage or species differences.

One of two Przewalski mares aborted when given PZP during early pregnancy, and one of three PZP-treated banteng cows gave birth prematurely.[25] These results argue against treating pregnant females with PZP until more data are available for other taxa.

Bisdiamine is teratogenic to developing embryos,[47] and so separation of males from potentially pregnant females is important during administration. No deleterious effects of bisdiamine in males has been found.[9]

Although estrogens (in combination pills) can suppress lactation, progestins have been found to have no effect or to actually increase milk production.[11] PZP appears to have no effect on lactation.

PREPUBERTAL CONTRACEPTION

Because virtually all contraceptive research has focused on humans or models for humans, and because prepubertal humans are not candidates for contraception, there are no available data on long-term reproductive and health effects for individuals in this age class. Because of potential deleterious effects on future fertility, contraception of prepubertal animals should be avoided when possible.

SOCIAL CONSIDERATIONS

As mentioned, the effects of castration on behavior may be extremely variable, depending on age and experience. Ovariectomy should eliminate sexual behavior, except for species that show independence from gonadal hormones, such as primates and horses.[5, 10] Sexual behavior in some primates may be truly hormone-independent,[21] but in horses, adrenal sex steroids can support estrous behavior.[6] In other species, ovariectomy is associated with masculinized behavior in some females, probably as a result of adrenal androgens.

Although progestins might be expected to have potentially profound social effects,[3, 4] systematic studies have as yet revealed no differences.[22, 40] The persistence of sexual interactions and external signs of estrus, such as perineal swelling or reddening, varies in progestin-treated females,[22, 37, 38, 40] probably in relation to the degree of follicle suppression. The placebo or pill-free week of birth control pill administration also is associated with signs of cycling.

ABORTION

During the first trimester, suction alone or suction plus curettage can be guided with ultrasonography after cervical dilation.[24] Such procedures are generally applicable for nonhuman primates as well.[8] Prostaglandin $F_{2\alpha}$ can be used to induce abortion in early pregnancy in hoofstock and other species in which the corpus luteum is sensitive to prostaglandin's luteolytic effect. Although prostaglandin has been used, prolactin inhibitors, such as cabergoline, are effective in the dog and cat, with fewer side effects, when given during the second half of gestation.[23, 31, 32, 49]

REFERENCES

1. Asa CS: Contraceptive development and its application to captive and free-ranging wildlife. Proceedings of the Annual Meeting of the American Association of Zoological Parks & Aquaria, Toronto, Canada, pp 71–75, 1992.
2. Asa CS: Structure and function of the AAZPA Contraception Committee. Proceedings of the Annual Meeting of the American Association of Zoo Veterinarians, St. Louis, pp 281–283, 1993.
3. Asa CS: The effects of contraceptives on behavior. In Seal US, Plotka ED, Cohn PN (eds): Contraception in Wildlife, Book 1. Lewiston, NY, Edwin Mellen Press, pp 157–170, 1996.
4. Asa CS: Physiological and social aspects of reproduction of the wolf and their implications for contraception. In Carbyn L, Fritts SH, Seip DR (eds): Ecology and Conservation of Wolves in a Changing World. Edmonton, Alberta, Canadian Circumpolar Institute, pp 283–286, 1996.
5. Asa CS, Goldfoot DA, Garcia MC, et al: Sexual behavior in ovariectomized and seasonally anovulatory mares. Horm Behav 14:46–54, 1980.
6. Asa CS, Goldfoot DA, Garcia MC, et al: Dexamethasone suppression of sexual behavior in the ovariectomized mare. Horm Behav 14:55–64, 1980.
7. Asa CS, Porton I: Concerns and prospects for contraception in carnivores. Proceedings of the Annual Meeting of the American Association of Zoo Veterinarians, Calgary, Alberta, Canada, pp 298–303, 1991.
8. Asa CS, Porton I, Plotka ED, et al: Contraception. In Kleiman DG, Allen ME, Thompson KV, Lumpkin S (eds): Wild Mammals in Captivity, Vol. 1: Principles and Techniques of Captive Management, Section A: Captive Propagation. Chicago, University of Chicago Press, pp 451–467, 1996.

9. Asa CS, Zaneveld LJD, Munson L, et al: Efficacy, safety and reversibility of a bisdiamine as a male-directed oral contraceptive in gray wolves (*Canis lupus*). J Zoo Wildl Med 27:501–506, 1996.

10. Baum MJ, Everitt BJ, Herbert J, et al: Hormonal basis of proceptivity and receptivity in female primates. Arch Sex Behav 6:173–192, 1977.

11. Benagiano G, Fraser I: The Depo-Provera debate. Contraception 24:493–528, 1981.

12. Brache V, Alvarez-Sanchez F, Faundes A, et al: Ovarian endocrine function through five years of continuous treatment with Norplant subdermal contraceptive implants. Contraception 41:169–177, 1990.

13. Brache V, Faundes A, Johansson E, et al: Anovulation, inadequate luteal phase and poor sperm penetration in cervical mucus during prolonged use of Norplant implants. Contraception 31:261–273, 1985.

14. Chi I: What we have learned from recent IUD studies: a researcher's perspective. Contraception 48:81–108, 1993.

15. Diczfalusy E: Mode of action of contraceptive drugs. Am J Obstet Gynecol 100:136–163, 1968.

16. Drobeck HP, Coulston F: Inhibition and recovery of spermatogenesis in rats, monkeys, and dogs medicated with bis(dichloroacetyl)-diamines. Exp Molec Pathol 1:251–274, 1962.

17. Fail PA, Asa CS, Kunze D: Testing indenopyridines as a male-directed oral contraceptive in felids. Final report to AZA Conservation Endowment Fund, 1997.

18. Freeman C, Coffey DS: Sterility in male animals induced by injection of chemical agents into the vas deferens. Fertil Steril 24:884–890, 1973.

19. Frenette MD, Dooley MP, Pineda MH: Effect of flushing the vasa deferentia at the time of vasectomy on the rate of clearance of spermatozoa from the ejaculates of dogs and cats. Am J Vet Res 47:463–470, 1986.

20. Gabbiani G: Action of cadmium chloride on sensory ganglia. Experientia 22:261–262, 1966.

21. Goldfoot DA, Wiegand SJ, Scheffler G: Continued copulation in ovariectomized adrenal-suppressed stumptail macaques (*Macaca arctoides*). Horm Behav 11:89–99, 1978.

22. Hayes KT, Feistner ATC, Halliwell EC: The effect of contraceptive implants on the behavior of female Rodrigues fruit bats, *Pteropus rodricensis*. Zoo Biol 15:21–36, 1996.

23. Jöchle W, Jöchle M: Reproduction in a feral cat colony and its control with a prolactin inhibitor, cabergoline. J Reprod Fertil Suppl 47:419–424, 1993.

24. Kaunitz AM, Grimes DA: First-trimester abortion technology. *In* Corson SL, Derman RJ, Tyrer LB (eds): Fertility Control. Boston, Little, Brown, pp 63–76, 1985.

25. Kirkpatrick JF, Zimmermann W, Kolter L, et al: Immunocontraception of captive exotic species: I. Przewalski's horses (*Equus przewalskii*) and banteng (*Bos javanicus*). Zoo Biol 14:403–416, 1995.

26. Kirton KT, Cornette JC: Return of ovulatory cyclicity following an intramuscular injection of medroxyprogesterone acetate (Provera). Contraception 10:39–45, 1974.

27. Mahi-Brown CA, Yanagimachi R, Nelson ML, et al: Ovarian histopathology of bitches immunized with porcine zonae pellucidae. Am J Reprod Immunol Microbiol 18:94, 1988.

28. Munson L, Harrenstein LM, Haslem CA, et al: Update on diseases associated with contraceptive use in zoo animals. Proceedings of the Joint Conference of the American Association of Zoo Veterinarians/Wildlife Disease Association/American Association of Wildlife Veterinarians, East Lansing, MI, pp 398–400, 1995.

29. Munson L, Mason RJ: Pathological findings in the uteri of progestogen-implanted exotic felids. Proceedings of the Annual Conference of the American Association of Zoo Veterinarians, Calgary, Alberta, Canada, pp 311–312, 1991.

30. Murnane RD, Zdziarski JM, Walsh TF, et al: Melengestrol acetate–induced exuberant endometrial decidualization in Goeldi's marmo-

sets (*Callimico goeldii*) and squirrel monkeys (*Saimiri sciureus*). J Zoo Wildl Med 27:315–324, 1996.

31. Onclin K, Silva LDM, Donnay I, et al: Luteotrophic action of prolactin in dogs and the effects of a dopamine agonist, cabergoline. J Reprod Fertil Suppl 47:403–409, 1993.

32. Onclin K, Silva LDM, Verstegen JP: Termination of unwanted pregnancy in dogs with the dopamine agonist cabergoline in combination with a synthetic analog of PGF$_{2\alpha}$, either cloprostenol or alphaprostol. Theriogenology 43:813–822, 1995.

33. Pineda MH, Dooley MP: Surgical and chemical vasectomy in the cat. Am J Vet Res 45:291–300, 1984.

34. Pineda MH, Reimers TJ, Faulkner LC: Disappearance of spermatozoa from the ejaculates of vasectomized dogs. J Am Vet Med Assoc 168:502–503, 1976.

35. Pineda MH, Reimers TJ, Faulkner LC, et al: Azoospermia in dogs induced by injection of sclerosing agents into the caudae of the epididymides. Am J Vet Res 38:831–838, 1977.

36. Plotka ED, Seal US: Fertility control in deer. J Wildl Dis 25:643–646, 1989.

37. Porton I: Results for primates from the AZA contraception database: Species, methods, efficacy and reversals. Proceedings of the Joint Conference of the American Association of Zoo Veterinarians/Wildlife Disease Association/American Association of Wildlife Veterinarians, East Lansing, MI, pp 381–394, 1995.

38. Porton I, Asa CS, Baker A: Survey results on the use of birth control methods in primates and carnivores in North American zoos. Proceedings of the Annual Meeting of the American Association of Zoological Parks & Aquaria, Indianapolis, pp 489–497, 1990.

39. Porton I, Hornbeck B: A North American contraceptive database for ungulates. Internatl Zoo Yrbk 32:155–159, 1993.

40. Portugal MM, Asa CS: Effects of chronic melengestrol acetate contraceptive treatment on perineal tumescence, body weight, and sociosexual behavior of Hamadryas baboons (*Papio hamadryas*). Zoo Biol 14:251–259, 1995.

41. Schwallie PC, Assenzo JR: The effect of depo-medroxyprogesterone acetate on pituitary and ovarian function, and the return of fertility following its discontinuation: a review. Contraception 10:181–197, 1974.

42. Setchell BP: The Mammalian Testis. Ithaca, NY, Cornell University Press, 1978.

43. Sloan JM, Path MRC, Oliver IM: Progestin-induced diabetes in the dog. Diabetes 24:337–344, 1975.

44. Stellflug JN, Leathers CW, Green JS: Antifertility effect of busulfan and DL-6-(N-2-pipecolinomethyl)-5-hydroxy-indane maleate (PMHI) in coyotes (*Canis lupus*). Theriogenology 22:533–543, 1984.

45. Sternberg SS, Phillips FS, Scholler J: Pharmacological and pathological effects of alkylating agents. Ann N Y Acad Sci 68:811–825, 1958.

46. Suter KE: Effects of an indenopyridine derivative, compound 20-438, on spermatogonial stem cells of the rat. Arch Toxicol Suppl 7:171–173, 1984.

47. Taleporos P, Salgo MP, Oster G: Teratogenic action of a bis(dichloroacetyl)diamine in rats: patterns of malformations produced in high incidence at time-limited periods of development. Teratology 18:5–16, 1978.

48. Van Tienhoven A: Reproductive Physiology of Vertebrates, 2nd ed. Ithaca, NY, Cornell University Press, 1983.

49. Verstegen JP, Onclin K, Silva I, et al: Abortion induction in the cat using prostaglandin F$_{2\alpha}$ and a new anti-prolactinic agent, cabergoline. J Reprod Fertil Suppl 47:411–417, 1993.

50. Zänartu J: Long-term contraceptive effect of injectable progestogens: inhibition and reestablishment of fertility. Internatl J Fertil 13:415–426, 1968.

51. Zimbelman RG, Lauderdale JW, Sokoloski JH, et al: Safety and pharmacologic evaluations of melengestrol acetate in cattle and other animals: a review. J Am Vet Med Assoc 157:1528–1536, 1970.

MONOTREMES AND MARSUPIALS

CHAPTER 41

Diseases of Koalas

ROSEMARY J. BOOTH
WENDY H. BLANSHARD

GENERAL PHYSIOLOGY

The koala, *Phascolarctos cinereus,* is an arboreal folivorous marsupial. Koalas derive food, water, and shelter almost exclusively from selected Eucalyptus trees, which discourage folivory with fibrous leaves containing toxic phenolics and oils. These "antinutrients" provide little energy, can interfere with digestion, require energy for detoxification, and dilute the nutritional components of the diet.[21] Koalas have adapted to overcome these plant protective mechanisms with specialized dentition, efficient hepatic detoxification mechanisms, and prolonged particle retention time in the proximal colon and elongated cecum, where bacterial fermentation and tannin-protein complex degradation occur.[20] Energy conservation is achieved with a low basal metabolic rate[23] and an activity cycle that includes resting or sleeping for up to 19 hours per day.[36] Although the koala is biologically successful, the foundation of its success is precarious because of its limited energy budget.[22] Factors such as habitat degradation with wild populations and inappropriate husbandry with captive animals alter activity patterns, which can compromise the koalas' energy budget and predispose it to disease.

A high incidence of neoplasia and opportunistic infections suggests that koalas may be immunodeficient.[68] Koalas may be constitutionally immunodeficient in comparison with eutherians. In vitro and in vivo tests on small numbers of animals revealed delayed humoral immune responses to a range of antigens.[7, 29, 64, 65] However, another in vivo study on three animals demonstrated apparently normal humoral responses apart from prolonged immunoglobulin M (IgM) production.[28] Cell-mediated immune responses to bacille Calmette-Guérin (BCG) are comparable with those seen in eutherians.[28, 65] Clearly, a larger sample of animals and antigens is required in order to characterize normal koala immune responses and to determine the relevance of standard immune function tests in this species. Koalas may acquire immunodeficiency through retroviral infection[68] or exposure to pollutants.[37] Lack of coevolution with pathogens may also contribute to disease susceptibility.

Table 41–1 shows selected physiologic data for normal koalas.

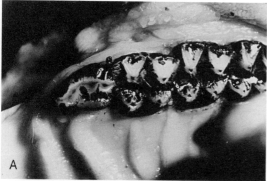

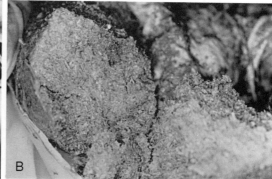

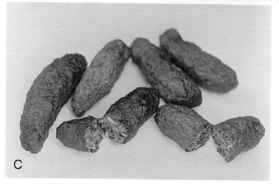

FIGURE 41–1. *A,* The upper teeth of a 4-year-old koala with minimal wear of the premolar blade and molar cusps. *B,* The stomach contents of a koala of the same age with leaf masticated into fine particles. *C,* The fecal pellets of a koala with effective mastication.

Severe tooth wear in old age is the principal factor limiting longevity of otherwise healthy koalas. The age at which tooth wear becomes incompatible with effective mastication varies from approximately 10 to 19 years. Figure 41–1 shows the effect of tooth wear on gastric particle size and on undigested fiber content in fecal pellets. Body condition should be assessed by palpation of the contour and bulk of the scapular muscles.[24, 67] Normal koalas tend to have inelastic skin, and so hydration status is best assessed by the ease of skin sliding over the scapulae.[4] Normal koalas sometimes pass red pigment in urine and mauve or grey fecal pellets. Calcium carbonate–like crystals and unidentified small rectangular crystals were seen in 12 of 20 urine samples from normal koalas.[12] Urine dipstick analyses yield false-positive readings for protein and ketones in koala urine.[12] Reference ranges for hematology and serum biochemistry are presented in Tables 41–2 and 41–3.

TABLE 41–1. Selected Physiologic Data for Normal Koalas

Parameter	Range	Reference
Body temperature	35.5°–36.5°C	23
Resting pulse rate	65–90/minute	4
Resting respiratory rate	10–15/minute	24
Urine specific gravity	1.062–1.135	13
Thermoneutral zone	15°–25°C	23
Basal metabolic rate	151 kJ/kg$^{0.75}$/day	23

PRINCIPLES OF SUPPORTIVE CARE

Injured or diseased koalas often suffer from anorexia, which leads to negative water and energy balance. It is critical to focus supportive care on establishing positive water and energy balance, in addition to providing any specific therapy required.

Positive Water Balance

1. Feed younger leaves.
2. Feed fresh leaves and maintain stems in water.
3. Spray leaves with water throughout the day.
4. Offer water or glucose/electrolytes via syringe.
5. Administer fluids subcutaneously (SQ) or intravenously (IV) if required. Indwelling catheters may be placed in the cephalic or caudal tibial veins. Use an injection port, and attach a burette two to three times daily when the koala can be supervised, or else it can become entangled in drip tubing. Use small animal principles for rate and volume.
6. Monitor hydration status, packed cell volume (PCV), total protein (TP), and electrolytes.

Positive Energy Balance

1. Feed younger leaves of most palatable species. Observe individual preferences.
2. Position leaves within easy reach, and reposition during the day as required.

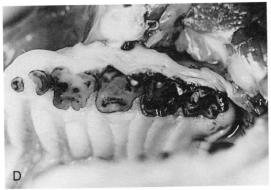

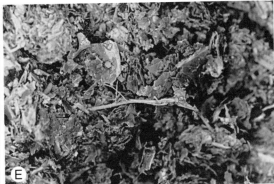

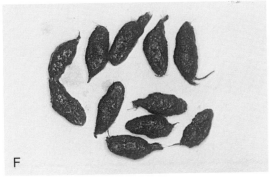

FIGURE 41–1 *Continued D,* The teeth of a 13-year-old koala with the premolar worn to two roots and obliteration of molar cusps. *E,* The stomach contents of the same koala with poorly masticated coarse leaf fragments. *F,* The fecal pellets of the same koala with unmasticated fibrous strands.

TABLE 41–2. Hematologic Values* Based on Blood Samples from Over 200 Apparently Normal Wild and Captive Koalas in Eastern Australia

Parameter	Units	Mature Koalas		Juveniles (<2 yrs)	
		Males	Females	Males	Females
PCV	%	41.5 (1.0)	37.4 (1.0)	379.0 (1.0)	35.9 (0.8)
Hb	g/dl	13.0 (0.4)	11.3 (0.2)	11.1 (0.3)	10.9 (0.2)
RBC	$\times\ 10^{12}$/L	3.85 (0.1)	3.39 (0.1)	3.46 (0.1)	3.31 (0.1)
MCV	fl	110.0 (5.2)	111.7 (3.9)	112.9 (6.3)	108.0 (4.9)
MCH	pg	34.4 (1.9)	35.1 (1.0)	33.4 (1.6)	33.1 (1.3)
MCHC	g/dl	31.3 (0.5)	30.6 (0.6)	29.3 (0.4)	30.5 (0.4)
Reticulocytes	%	1.6 (0.4)	1.5 (0.2)	2.6 (0.4)	3.5 (1.1)
nRBC	% WBC	14.0 (12.7)	17.4 (6.6)	3.9 (1.2)	4.4 (1.3)
Howell-Jolly bodies	% WBC	7.7 (2.8)	7.7 (6.1)	5.9 (4.8)	7.1 (4.0)
Total WCC	$\times\ 10^9$/L	8.5 (0.5)	8.0 (0.5)	7.8 (0.6)	7.0 (0.5)
Differential (abs)					
Neutrophils	$\times\ 10^9$/L	3.6 (0.3)	3.5 (0.6)	2.4 (0.4)	2.8 (0.5)
Lymphocytes	$\times\ 10^9$/L	4.3 (0.5)	4.0 (0.4)	5.0 (0.5)	4.0 (0.4)
Monocytes	$\times\ 10^9$/L	0.3 (0.07)	0.3 (0.04)	0.2 (0.01)	0.2 (0.05)
Eosinophils	$\times\ 10^9$/L	0.2 (0.02)	0.3 (0.02)	0.1 (0.01)	0.1 (0.02)
Basophils	$\times\ 10^9$/L	0.03	0.02	0.03	0.03
Differential (ref)					
Neutrophils	%	44.6 (4.2)	39.6 (3.5)	31.2 (3.8)	39.6 (4.7)
Lymphocytes	%	49.5 (3.9)	52.9 (3.3)	63.9 (4.6)	55.5 (4.8)
Monocytes	%	3.5 (0.6)	3.8 (1.3)	3.3 (0.7)	3.3 (0.9)
Eosinophils	%	2.2 (0.6)	3.8 (0.9)	1.2	1.2 (0.3)
Basophils	%	0.1 (0.0)	0.2	0.4	0.5

PCV, packed cell volume; Hb, hemoglobin; RBC, red blood cell count; MCV, mean cell volume; MCH, mean cell hemoglobin; MCHC, mean cell hemoglobin concentration; nRBC, nucleated red blood cell; WBC, white blood cells; WCC, white blood cell count.
*Values presented are means, with standard errors in parentheses.
Data from Dickens RK: The koala in health and disease. *In* Fauna, Proceedings No. 36, Post Graduate Committee in Veterinary Science. Sydney, New South Wales, Australia, University of Sydney, pp 105–117, 1978.

TABLE 41–3. Reference Ranges for Biochemical Values in Koalas

Parameter	Units	Reference Ranges	
		Dickens† (1978)	VPS‡ (1994)
Glucose	mmol/L	2.2–4.4	3.2–6.0
Urea	mmol/L	1.1–10.7	2.3–6.0*
Creatinine	mmol/L	0.09–0.13	0.05–0.12
Total protein	g/L	60–75	60–80
Albumin	g/L	29–38	30–40
Globulin	g/L		30–40
Albumin/globulin ratio			0.8–1.4
Total bilirubin	μmol/L	1.7–12	0–3
Alkaline phosphatase	U/L	30–200	50–200
Aspartate aminotransferase	U/L	10–50	25–120
Alanine aminotransferase	U/L	30	15–65
Lactate dehydrogenase	U/L	150–250	
Gamma-glutamyl transferase	U/L		1–8
Creatine phosphokinase	U/L		100–300
Cholesterol	mmol/L	2.1–2.8	1–3
Calcium	mmol/L	2.5–2.6	2.5–3
Inorganic phosphate	mmol/L	1.13–1.62	1.2–2.5
Sodium	mmol/L	133–140	136–146
Potassium	mmol/L	5.0–5.8*	4–5.5
Chloride	mmol/L	96–103	95–110
Bicarbonate	mmol/L		18–24
Anion gap	mmol/L		18–27

*Indicates a range that, in the opinion of the authors, more closely represents values expected from healthy captive koalas.
†Modified from Dickens, 1978.
‡Veterinary Pathology Services Pty Ltd, Brisbane, Australia, personal communication, 1994.

3. Provide supplementary feed if required.
4. Administer fluids containing glucose and/or amino acids if required.
5. Establish a routine, and minimize unfamiliar stimuli.
6. Maintain the koala in a thermoneutral environment.
7. Monitor body condition, body weight, food intake, and fecal output.
8. Identify and treat specific illness or injury.

Supplementary Feeding

Low-lactose milk powders—such as Portagen (Mead Johnson),[66] Prosobee (Mead Johnson),[66] and Di-Vetelact (Sharpe)—are the most commonly used energy supplements. Powders are mixed to a thick paste with water and slowly administered orally via a catheter-tipped syringe. Supplementation is usually well accepted, but some animals may strongly resist and may expend more energy than they gain. If they cannot be gradually accustomed to this method, it is better to rely on parenteral nutrition rather than fluids. Adult koalas eating no foliage can be maintained if they receive 60 ml of paste daily in three divided doses. Finely blended eucalyptus leaf can be added to the paste mixture to provide some fiber and to ensure that the specialized bacteria in the proximal colon and cecum are not totally deprived of their normal substrate. Koalas that are still eating but with reduced intake may require 20 to 40 ml daily.

Smaller quantities administered to adult animals do not usually have a demonstrable effect on body weight.

Principles of Specific Therapy

Although the koala has a low metabolic rate, its ability to metabolize drugs in the liver may be underestimated by metabolic scaling of dose rates. Koalas have a significantly faster rate of bromosulphthalein (BSP) clearance than do macropods and sheep.[48] Although no pharmacokinetic trials have been published for koalas, a range of therapeutic agents have been successfully used at dose rates extrapolated from domestic species and humans.

SIGNIFICANT INFECTIOUS DISEASES

Chlamydiosis

Etiology. Initially the causative agent was classified as *Chlamydia psittaci*, but it has been reclassified as two agents, *Chlamydia pecorum* and *Chlamydia pneumoniae*, according to sequence homology of surface antigen genes.[30] Both species cause ocular and urogenital disease. *C. pecorum* appears to be more prevalent and more virulent than *C. pneumoniae*, and combined infections suggest that cross-immunity does not occur (P. Timms, personal communication, 1996).

Epizootiology. Sexual transmission has been proposed as the most likely route of infection,[7, 45] on the basis of the extremely low incidence of infection in sexually immature koalas.[31] Transmission by close contact, fomites, arthropod vectors, at parturition, or during pap feeding have not been ruled out. In a transmission trial involving inoculation of four animals with 10^3 to 10^5 elementary bodies, the incubation period to development of conjunctivitis was 7 to 19 days, and for urogenital disease, 8 to 119 days.[7] Three of the four koalas in this trial developed conjunctivitis after urogenital inoculation with the organism. The fourth koala received direct ocular inoculation and developed conjunctivitis in 7 days.

In vitro, koala *C. pneumoniae* can remain infective for cell culture after 3 days' exposure on eucalyptus leaves.[52] Sheep blowflies *(Lucilia cuprina)* were found to be capable of carrying infectious particles for up to 1 hour and transmitting them to uninfected solutions of transport medium.[61] The seroprevalence and clinical prevalence vary markedly between wild populations, as does the effect of the disease on fertility and mortality.[63] Despite ample opportunity for transfer, there is no evidence that chlamydiosis in koalas is a zoonosis.[4]

Clinical Signs. There are three main clinical syndromes.

1. Keratoconjunctivitis: the initial signs are epiphora and erythema followed by chemosis (Fig. 41–2*A*). Granular hyperplasia of the conjunctiva and the nictitating membrane and mucopurulent discharge may occlude the entire palpebral fissure. Keratitis is common in chronic cases.[44]

2. Urinary tract disease: infection of the bladder mucosa causes dysuria and incontinence, which stains the fur of the cloacal region and rump orange-brown ("dirty tail"; see Fig. 41–2*B*). At necropsy, the bladder mucosa may be thickened with scattered petechial hemorrhages, or it may be deeply ulcerated. In addition to cystitis, there may be urethritis, cloacitis, and ascending bacterial pyelonephritis.[43, 44]

3. Reproductive tract disease: unilateral or bilateral cystic ovarian diverticulitis may cause infertility in the presence of normal ovaries. Salpingitis, hydrosalpinx, metritis, pyometron, vaginitis, and pyovagina have also been recorded in females, often with secondary bacterial involvement.[43, 44]

Diagnosis

1. Clinical pathology: there are no consistent hematologic or biochemical abnormalities, although anemia and hypoproteinemia may occur.[16, 44] Urine may contain erythrocytes, leukocytes, cellular debris, bacteria, and/or yeasts.[16, 44]

2. Advanced cysts can be detected by palpation of the region anterolateral to the free end of the epipubic bones in anesthetized koalas.

3. Radiography with negative contrast (pneumoperitoneum[6]) or ultrasonography may detect female reproductive tract anomalies.

4. Cell culture demonstrates the presence of viable organism and has high sensitivity and specificity.[59] Strict attention must be paid to specimen collection, transport, and storage. Aluminium-shafted plain cotton swabs are nontoxic to the organism. Specific chlamydial transport medium is essential. Swabbing must be vigorous enough to obtain multiple host epithelial cells. It is advisable to swab both conjunctiva, the urogenital sinus in females, and the penile urethra in males. The first swab may contain mostly superficial secretions; to maximize organism yield, two swabs can be taken from the same site and both included in one vial of transport medium.[59]

5. Conjunctival or urogenital swabs can be used to detect chlamydial DNA by polymerase chain reaction (PCR) amplification.[30]

6. Antibody enzyme-linked immunosorbent assay (ELISA) with rabbit anti–koala immunoglobulin G (IgG) conjugated to horseradish peroxidase is now available and is at least 16 times more sensitive than the

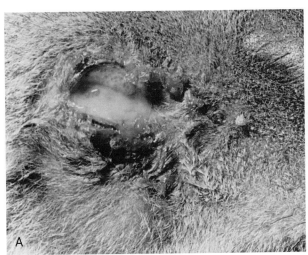
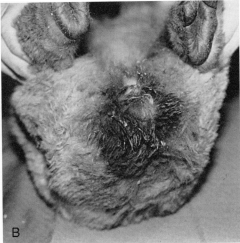

FIGURE 41–2. *A,* Chronic chlamydial conjunctivitis with purulent ocular discharge and chemosis. *B,* The stained rump fur of a koala with chlamydial cystitis ("dirty tail").

complement-fixation test (CFT; sheep antigen), which is not a reliable indicator of individual animal infection.[28]

7. Antigen ELISA: of six antigen-detection ELISA kits evaluated in a field study for use in koalas, Clearview (Unipath Ltd.) was the most sensitive (91%), followed by IDEIA Chlamydia Test (Boots-Celltech Diagnostics Ltd.; 88%) and Surecell (Eastman Kodak Company; 73%).[59]

8. Antigen detection through direct immunofluorescence: two test kits were evaluated as useful in detecting chlamydia in koalas: Chlamydia-Cel Vet IF Test (Cellabs Diagnostics)[14] and IMAGEN Chlamydia Test Kit (Boots-Celltech Diagnostics).[31] These kits were generally less sensitive than the ELISA kits.[59]

9. For histopathology, Giemsa or Macchiavello stains are used. Detection rates can be improved with immunologic stains.[15]

Treatment. Success of treatment is dependent on early diagnosis and initiation of therapy. Chronic cases are refractory to treatment and recurrence of clinical signs after treatment is common. Oxytetracycline and erythromycin, useful drugs for treating chlamydiosis in other species, are not recommended for use in koalas because they have been repeatedly associated with severe weight loss (up to 30%) and mortality, which has been presumed to result from their effects on gut microflora.[9]

A number of antimicrobials have been used to treat conjunctivitis and/or cystitis in koalas. Those treated with fluoroquinolones and tetracyclines have been supplementarily fed during therapy to minimize weight loss associated with anorexia. Dose rates used include enrofloxacin syrup 5 mg/kg SID PO for 5 to 60 days (E. O'Connor, personal communication, 1996); ciprofloxacin 10 mg/kg BID PO for a minimum of 10 to 14 days; chloramphenicol 30 mg/kg BID SQ for a minimum of 10 to 14 days[4]; oxytetracycline 5 mg/kg intramuscularly (IM) every 7 days (R. Osawa, personal communication, 1992); doxycycline 5 mg/kg IM every 7 days for 6 weeks (P. Wilson, personal communication, 1994).

Topical tetracycline eye preparations have also been used with success to treat conjunctivitis before it has reached the proliferative stage. Surgical excision of proliferative conjunctival tissue may be a useful adjunct to topical and/or systemic chemotherapy in chronic cases.

Control. Fly screening of koala quarantine facilities is recommended. Disinfectants effective at destroying chlamydiae infecting koalas include Parvocide (Arthur Webster; glutaraldehyde, 150 g/L plus dimethyl benzyl ammonium chloride 100 g/L) at 1% *dilution*, and Halasept (Intervet; chloramine 100%) at 0.3% *concentration*.[61]

Rhinitis/Pneumonia Complex

Etiology. Potential primary or secondary microbial pathogens isolated from the respiratory tract of captive koalas include *Bordetella bronchiseptica*, *Pseudomonas aeruginosa*, other *Pseudomonas* species, alpha-hemolytic *Streptococcus* species, *Corynebacterium* species, *Enterobacter agglomerans*, *Proteus* species, diphthe-

roids, *Pasteurella* species, *Micrococcus* species, *Staphylococcus aureus*, *Escherichia coli*, *Acinetobacter lwoffi*, *Cryptococcus neoformans*, *Aspergillus* species, and unidentified yeasts.[4, 5, 17, 42, 53, 67]

B. bronchiseptica, *P. aeruginosa*, *Streptobacillus moniliformis*, *Staphylococcus epidermidis*, *C. neoformans*, and *Nocardia asteroides* have been isolated at necropsy from wild koalas with pneumonia or other respiratory tract disease.[2, 4, 41, 53, 62]

Epizootiology. Respiratory disease may affect individual animals or groups. Captive colonies of koalas may experience outbreaks of respiratory disease,[17, 41, 49, 67] and cases are known to have occurred simultaneously at different sanctuaries.[5] The etiology of many outbreaks of respiratory disease remains unclear. In an outbreak in a captive colony, 23 of 26 koalas in one enclosure and three koalas in other enclosures showed clinical signs, but no consistent bacterial pathogen could be isolated from nasal or pharyngeal swabs. Affected koalas showed no clinical signs of ocular or urogenital disease, and all CFTs yielded negative results for chlamydia after the outbreak. A primary pathogen may have remained undetected and may have been a virus.[4]

Clinical Signs. Frequent or paroxysmal sneezing or coughing, unilateral or bilateral mucopurulent nasal discharge, pharyngeal inflammation, and regional lymph node enlargement (submandibular, facial) may be apparent. Stridor may indicate nasopharyngeal swelling or bronchitis. Peracute bronchopneumonia may lead to sudden death. Radiography may be required for assessing lung involvement, because it is difficult to effectively auscultate or percuss the chest.

Treatment. Because of the great variation in microbial isolates from clinical cases, culture and sensitivity testing is essential for selecting an appropriate antimicrobial agent. If the severity of the disease necessitates treatment before the results of culture and sensitivity tests are available, broad-spectrum antibiotics such as amoxicillin/clavulanic acid, trimethoprim/sulfamethoxazole, or chloramphenicol should be used. With systemic antibiotic treatment for rhinitis or bronchitis, responses may be slow, and relapses are not uncommon. Nebulization has been more effective than systemic antibiotic therapy in resolving clinical signs of rhinitis or bronchitis. Gentamicin sulfate at 2 mg/kg can be added to 2 to 3 ml saline and nebulized through a child-size face mask SID or BID for an average of 5 days (Fig. 41–3). Depending on culture and sensitivity test results, ampicillin, 10 mg/kg, may be nebulized alone or alternated with gentamicin; the latter is inactivated by penicillins in vitro.[35] In cases of pneumonia, concurrent nebulization and systemic antibiotic therapy are advised. In addition, pseudoephedrine hydrochloride, 1 mg/kg every 8 to 12 hours PO, or bromhexine hydrochloride, 2 mg/kg every 12 hours (5 days) PO followed by 1 mg/kg every 12 hours, may relieve clinical signs.

Control. All koalas in one large captive colony were vaccinated with an inactivated, cell-free extract of *B. bronchiseptica*, Canvac-BB (CSL). Each koala received a primary course of two SQ doses given 4 weeks apart and then annual boosters. In the 5 years preceding

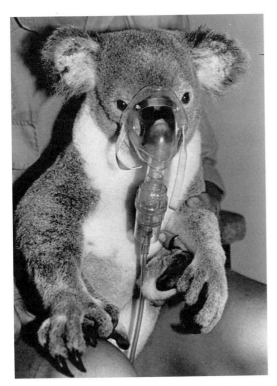

FIGURE 41–3. Treatment of rhinitis by nebulization.

administration of the first vaccinations, mortality from pneumonia in which *B. bronchiseptica* was confirmed by culture (n = 4) or suspected from the presence of gram-negative coccobacilli in histologic sections of affected lung (n = 1) accounted for 9.1%, 0%, 13.3%, 0% and 28.6% of annual deaths, respectively. This compared to none in each of the following 5 years in which annual revaccination was carried out. Although mortality from respiratory disease was reduced by vaccination against *B. bronchiseptica*, the incidence of clinical respiratory disease was not obviously changed.

Septicemia

Etiology. A range of gram-negative pathogens has been isolated in pure culture from antemortem or postmortem blood samples, including *Salmonella typhimurium, Salmonella sachsenwald, Morganella morganii,* and *E. coli.* Mixed cultures of *P. aeruginosa* or *Aeromonas hydrophila* with *E. coli* have also been obtained.[4] *Salmonella bovis-morbificans* has been incriminated as a cause of sudden deaths in a captive colony.[24]

Epizootiology. Septicemia occurs in both wild and captive koalas. It may be primary, or it may be secondary to another illness. There is no age or sex predilection. In captive animals, the most likely route of infection is ingestion of leaves inadvertently contaminated with bacteria. Cut browse should be prevented from touching the ground wherever possible. Septicemia caused by *E. coli* in emergent pouch young is occasionally observed in association with recent pap feeding. Secondary septi-

cemia has occurred in koalas with peracute pneumonia caused by *B. bronchiseptica*, and with oropharyngeal ulceration, enteritis, and leukemia.

Clinical Signs. Septicemia is a peracute illness with neurologic signs or sudden death. Lethargy, ataxia, nystagmus, flaccidity, localized tremor, convulsions, and vocalizations may occur. Body temperature may be increased, normal, or decreased. Profound leukopenia with leukocyte levels as low as 0.1×10^9/L is sometimes apparent.

Treatment. Treatment should be initiated before diagnosis is confirmed. No cases of successful treatment are known. Survival time has been extended up to 10 days with the following protocol:

1. Collect blood aseptically for culture and sensitivity, hematology and biochemistry.
2. Place an IV catheter and infuse an isotonic electrolyte solution at a rate to sustain moderate diuresis.
3. Administer prednisolone sodium succinate, 10 mg/kg IV. Repeat dose (5 to 10 mg/kg) after a few hours.
4. Administer canine anti-lipopolysaccharide antiserum to gram-negative bacterial endotoxin, 1.0 to 2.5 ml/kg slowly IV (Nerotect, Simvex), if available, before any antibiotic is administered. Repeat dose (1.0 ml/kg) after 24 hours.
5. Administer ticarcillin sodium, 45 to 50 mg/kg IV. Repeat dose every 4 to 6 hours pending results of culture and sensitivity testing. Alternatively, administer staggered doses of gentamicin sulfate, 2 to 4 mg/kg IV, and ampicillin, 5 to 10 mg/kg IV. Repeat gentamicin IM or SQ every 8 hours, and ampicillin IV every 6 hours, pending results of culture and sensitivity testing.
6. Administer flunixin meglumine, 1.0 mg/kg IV. Repeat dose after 24 and 48 hours.
7. Administer diazepam, 0.25 to 1.0 mg/kg IV or IM, to manage tremor and convulsions, and to reduce distress.
8. Consider using mannitol, 1 to 2 g/kg as a slow infusion IV, if neurologic signs continue to worsen.
9. Monitor body temperature frequently, and modify the environment appropriately.

Cryptococcosis

Etiology. *C. neoformans* var. *gattii* and var. *neoformans* are two biotypes of saprophytic, spherical, yeast-like fungi that form characteristic mucopolysaccharide capsules.[1]

Epizootiology. Infection often occurs opportunistically and is not contagious. *C. neoformans* var. *gattii* is associated with Eucalyptus trees and their flowers, particularly although not exclusively *E. camaldulensis, E. tereticornis, E. rudis,* and *E. gomphocephala*.[27] *C. neoformans* var. *neoformans* is commonly found in soil contaminated with bird excreta, particularly from pigeons.[1]

Infection of humans and animals occurs after inhalation of spores from the environment or, less commonly, by direct inoculation of the skin.[1] Aerosol formation after desiccation of contaminated substrate enhances the risk of inhalation. The incubation period is unknown. Ingested spores may be excreted unchanged in the feces.[26]

Of 8 isolates from clinically affected koalas that were biotyped, 5 were var. *gattii* and 3 were var. *neoformans*. In a captive colony with a high incidence of the disease, 9 of 28 nasal or interdigital swabs from apparently healthy koalas were found to contain cryptococci; all were var. *gattii*. There is no difference in the clinical presentation or course of the disease with each biotype; however, biotyping may help determine the source of infection. The incidence of mortality caused by cryptococcosis in koalas varies and is unusually high in one captive colony, representing 10% of 31 mortalities between 1991 and 1996.

Clinical Signs. Respiratory and neurologic signs are the most common manifestations of cryptococcosis in koalas. Nasal discharge, tachypnea, dyspnea, coughing, and sneezing may be observed. Of cryptococcal lesions at necropsy in 29 free-ranging and captive koalas, 55% were in the lungs, 34% in the nasal cavity, 24% in the central nervous system, 10% in the viscera, 10% in the skin, and 3% in the musculoskeletal system.[38] Eight of the 29 koalas (28%) had disseminated infections.[38]

Diagnosis

1. Smears of aspirates can be stained with new methylene blue, Gram stain, India ink, or fluorescent antibody to detect the presence of the encapsulated fungus.

2. Culture of clinical samples collected directly onto Sabouraud's glucose agar or bird seed agar increases detection rates. Biotyping usually requires specialized mycology facilities.

3. The latex cryptococcal antigen agglutination test (LCAT) is used to detect capsular polysaccharide antigen in serum or cerebrospinal fluid and is highly sensitive and specific. This test is potentially useful for screening captive populations. Titers of 1:2 or higher are considered positive. In a study of 58 infected animals of mixed species, including two koalas, serum LCAT titers positively correlated with disease severity and were highest in animals with disseminated skin and lymph node involvement.[39] The decline in LCAT titer lags behind clinical improvement but provides a useful quantitative indication of clinical progress.[39] In other species with cryptococcal meningitis, an LCAT titer on cerebrospinal fluid is almost always positive when it may not be in serum (Veterinary Pathology Services Pty Ltd, personal communication, 1994).

4. Histopathology sections can be stained with periodic acid–Schiff stain or with fluorescent antibody.

5. Diagnostic imaging: radiology, computed tomographic scan, and nuclear magnetic resonance imaging may be useful to localize pulmonary and soft tissue lesions.

Treatment. Successful treatment depends on early diagnosis and failure is common. The azole antifungal agents ketoconazole, itraconazole, and fluconazole have been used to treat cryptococcosis in koalas with mixed success. Although ketoconazole is relatively inexpensive, itraconazole and fluconazole are preferred for use in koalas. Itraconazole has the highest therapeutic index[33] and has successfully resolved cryptococcal lesions in koalas with no apparent side effects after 90 days of therapy. Fluconazole disseminates into the cerebrospinal fluid to a greater extent than the other azoles[33] and is the drug of choice for central nervous system lesions.

Dose rates used in koalas are as follows: ketoconazole, 10 mg/kg SID PO; itraconazole, 20 to 40 mg/kg SID or BID PO; and fluconazole, at up to 100 mg/koala twice daily PO (R. Malik, personal communication, 1995). Capsule contents or crushed tablets can be mixed into a paste of low-lactose milk powder for administration. Treatment should continue until the LCAT titer is negative.

Control. Disinfect the environment with 5% sodium hypochlorite solution.[1] Pigeon control may be indicated if *C. neoformans* var. *neoformans* has been identified. Monitoring captive populations with a combination of LCAT and culture, to allow early treatment of clinical cases, may be indicated in endemic areas. Environmental cultures to identify problem areas and tree species may also be indicated.

Dermatomycosis

Dermatomycosis is the most common skin infection in captive koalas but is rarely severe. Dermatophytes such as *Microsporum* species and *Trichophyton mentagrophytes* have been isolated from skin lesions, but often soil saprophytes such as *Acremonium* species and ubiquitous fungi such as *Penicillium* species appear to act as opportunistic pathogens. Damp environmental conditions predispose to infection. Lesions have occurred secondary to sarcoptic mange and chlamydial conjunctivitis. Nonpruritic, sharply demarcated alopecia with or without peripheral erythema and crusting commonly occur on the digits and nose. Treatment with topical povidone-iodine, chloramine, miconazole, or enilconazole is effective.

NONINFECTIOUS DISEASES

Tubulointerstitial Nephrosis

Renal disease unrelated to chlamydiosis is not uncommon. A number of zoos have reported a high incidence of chronic renal failure.[58] A specific etiology has not been determined, but many cases were characterized by tubulointerstitial nephrosis and fibrosis with degrees of renal oxalosis. In 16 cases with similar histopathologic processes, oxalate crystals were identified in 9 and were prominent in 5. The histologic sections from the most severe case were forwarded to the U.S. Armed Forces Institute of Pathology for review, where it was considered that the crystals were less prominent than would be expected with primary oxalosis.[60] Oxalate crystals may occur as a nonspecific response to renal necrosis in all species.[60] In koalas they may occur as a secondary response to renal disease or may reflect a physiologic or dietary predilection. There are a number of potential dietary sources for oxalate in koalas. These include naturally occurring calcium oxalate in eucalyptus leaves, particularly young growing tip, or contamination of leaf with oxalate-producing fungi *Aspergillus flavus, Aspergillus niger,* or *Penicillium* species.[34]

Although the cause of this apparent syndrome is unclear, it is possible that clinical dehydration leads to a reduction in the glomerular filtration rate, which may allow a myriad of dietary toxins to exert a local effect on the kidney. Any tendency to form crystals would be exacerbated by the koala's naturally concentrated urine. Dehydration may be precipitated by inappropriate maintenance of browse, which can lose water rapidly during storage. The institution for captive animals with the highest incidence of this disease had the least rigorous leaf storage system, whereas the condition has never been observed in a large captive colony for which leaf is cut fresh daily.

Diagnosis

1. Clinical signs: anorexia, lethargy, dehydration, polydipsia, polyuria or oliguria.
2. Clinical pathology: azotemia (urea up to 84 mmol/L), hypercalcemia, hyperphosphatemia, hemoconcentration.
3. Urinalysis: low specific gravity and crystalluria (including calcium oxalate, calcium carbonate, sulfur, and/or uric acid).
4. Histopathology: bilateral tubular dilation, interstitial nephrosis or nephritis, and fibrosis. Calcium oxalate crystals that are birefringent and stain with Pizzolato's peroxide silver stain may be present.[11]

Treatment. Aggressive IV fluid therapy and prophylactic antibiotic therapy are indicated. The prognosis is guarded if azotemia is severe for prolonged periods.

Control. Koalas should be fed fresh leaves, and there must be ready access to drinking water in their enclosure. Browse branches should be cut cleanly on an angle to facilitate water uptake after cutting; to avoid contamination, leaf should be transported in covered air-conditioned vehicles that are used for no other purpose. Browse should be stored with stems in fresh water soon after cutting. If stored for more than 24 hours, cold storage or overhead sprinklers should be used. Heat stress of animals should be avoided in hot weather with a combination of shade, ventilation, and overhead sprinklers.

Neoplasia

Neoplasia accounted for 7.5% of 253 captive and free-living koala mortalities in New South Wales over a 9-year period, or 12% of wild mortalities excluding trauma cases.[10] The reason for this high incidence is not clear. A C-type retrovirus that may be immunosuppressive or oncogenic has been isolated from affected and normal koalas.[19, 51, 68] The most commonly reported neoplasms are lymphoid neoplasia, craniofacial tumors of mixed cartilage and bone, and serosal proliferations.

LYMPHOID NEOPLASIA

Clinical signs may be highly variable and may include anorexia, lethargy, variable body condition, localized or generalized lymphadenopathy, swelling of the face and neck, swelling of the hind legs with abdominal enlargement, spontaneous hemorrhage, and acute shifting lameness.

Diagnosis

1. Hematology: leukocytosis, anemia, thrombocytopenia, and leukemia, are common.[16] "Atypical" lymphocytes may precede frank leukemia. Leukemic cells vary in morphology from relatively well differentiated to blasts.
2. Biochemistry: inconsistent findings may include hypoalbuminemia with or without hypoproteinemia, elevated urea, lactate dehydrogenase, gamma-glutamyltransferase, and aspartate aminotransferase.[16]
3. Cytology: neoplastic cells in smears made from fine needle aspirates of peripheral lymph nodes or solitary masses, from fluid obtained by abdominal paracentesis, or from bone marrow biopsy specimen.
4. Necropsy: affected lymph nodes may be enlarged; nodules or masses may be present in many organs; areas of necrosis may be obvious in affected bone (especially the femoral and/or humeral head); histologically extensive lymphoid infiltration may be present in tissues and organs that appear grossly normal.
5. Histochemistry and immunophenotyping may be useful to determine neoplastic cell lineage.

CRANIOFACIAL TUMORS OF MIXED CARTILAGE AND BONE

Koalas may have nasal or naso-ocular discharges, epistaxis, facial distortions, or palatine swelling. Tumors typically involve the bones of the nasal cavity and paranasal sinuses and have been described as benign and expansive.[18] Histologically, the masses consist of irregular compartments of hypertrophying chondrocytes embedded connective tissue, with variable degrees of calcification and ossification. Radiographically, they appear as dense masses with speckled appearance and distinct, rounded outlines.[18] Tumors that have been surgically removed have recurred.

SEROSAL PROLIFERATIONS

A range of tumors variously described as mesothelioma, fibrosarcoma, myxofibrosarcoma, and nodular granulomatous peritonitis have been grouped as serosal proliferations.[13] Affected koalas may have abdominal distension, anorexia, lethargy, and weight loss. At necropsy, serosal surfaces of affected body cavities bear white thickened areas that may extend 10 mm into underlying organs, in addition to large numbers of smooth, glistening white or red nodules, 1 to 10 mm in diameter, firmly attached to the serosa. The peritoneal cavity has been the primary site in all but one case. The pelvic cavity, pleural cavity, or pericardial sac may also be affected. Excess turbid, viscous, red-tinged peritoneal fluid is present when the abdominal cavity is affected. Histologically, most nodules are fibrous with low cellularity; some others are highly vascular or contain areas of hemorrhage.[13]

PARASITES

The parasites found in koalas and their clinical significance are summarized in Table 41–4.

THE POUCH AND YOUNG

Normal Development of Young

Pouch young first emerge for brief periods at age 6 to 7 months, when body weight is about 300 to 450 g.[4]

Around this time they consume a special unformed maternal feces known as "pap."[47] Greenish-brown semisolid paste or liquid feces are excreted in response to juveniles persistently nuzzling their mother's cloaca. Pap is consumed intermittently for 1 to 5 weeks, and juveniles usually first eat eucalyptus leaf within a few days or weeks of initial pap feeding. It is assumed that pap inoculates the juvenile's proximal colon and cecum with specialized bacteria necessary for digestion and detoxification of the adult diet. High counts of *viable* tannin-protein complex degrading enterobacteria were cultured from the pap of 10 females, but could be

TABLE 41–4. The Ectoparasites and Endoparasites Recorded for the Koala

Parasites	Species	Comments
Ectoparasites		
Fleas	*Ctenocephalides felis*	Occasionally fleas have been found on debilitated or orphaned wild koalas which have been cared for in private dwellings.[4]
Ticks	*Ixodes holocyclus* *I. cornuatus* *I. hirsti* *I. tasmani* *Haemophysalis bancrofti* *H. longicornis*	Ticks can be present in moderate numbers without causing harm. Heavy burdens may cause anemia.[54] Tick paralysis may occur in naive koalas translocated from paralysis tick–free areas to endemic areas. *I. holocyclus, I. cornuatus,* and *I. hirsti* may be capable of causing paralysis.[50,57]
Mites	*Austrochirus perkinsi*	A small fur-dwelling mite, possibly host specific. No records of associated pathology exist.[3]
	Sarcoptes scabiei	Two published reports; the first involved transmission in a wildlife shelter from an infected wombat.[3] The second describes an outbreak of disease associated with debility and mortality in a captive colony.[8] Has also been confirmed in wild koalas with mange lesions, particularly on the front paws. Not a common pathogen of koalas.
	Demodex species	Incidental finding on skin scraping in one animal.[4]
	Notoedres cati	Single report of these mites causing raised scabby lesions on the ventrum of captive koalas.[3]
Flies	Blowflies	Cutaneous myiasis of areas soiled by exudate, urine, or diarrhea (e.g., the pouch, conjunctival sac, external ear canal, perineum, or open wounds) has been observed.[4]
Endoparasites		
Cestodes	*Bertiella obesa*	The only common endoparasite of koalas, found in the small intestine.[55] A host-specific anoplocephalid tapeworm that has been associated with debility when present in large numbers. Arthropods may act as intermediate hosts; free-living soil mites (Orabatidae) have ingested eggs in vitro (T. Warren, personal communication, 1994). Treat with praziquantel 5 mg/kg PO.
Nematodes	*Marsupostrongylus longilarvatus*	Single report of a mild interstitial pneumonia associated with numerous 3- to 4-mm nematodes. There were no gross lesions; histologic study revealed nematodes in the airways.[40,56]
	Durikainema species	An incidental finding in koalas identified in histologic sections of lung.[56] Tightly spiraled worms up to 2 mm long have been located in the pulmonary arteries (D. Spratt, personal communication, 1994).
	Breinlia (Breinlia) cf. *mundayi*	Two filaroid nematodes were located free in the peritoneal cavity of a wild Victorian koala (D. Spratt, personal communication, 1992).
	Johnstonema species	The same koala also had a filaroid nematode in the chamber of its left ventricle, similar in appearance to worms found in the heart of a spotted cuscus (D. Spratt, personal communication, 1992).
Protozoans	Coccidia	Incidental finding on fecal floatation in one captive koala. A single elliptical oocyte measured 42.5×20 μm and was unsporulated.
	Cryptosporidium species	Four mortalities reported from duodenitis, enteritis, and colitis in two adults and two young from one captive facility (P. Whiteley and J. Phelan, personal communication, 1996). Transient *Cryptosporidium* infection has also been observed at another zoo.[68]
	Toxoplasma gondii	Three mortalities recorded in captive koalas; signs included acute tachypnea, tachycardia, pyrexia, and lymphocytosis or sudden death, caused by disseminated *T. gondii* infection.[25,32]

isolated only in much lower numbers from the normal feces of 6 of these females, which suggests that pap is an efficient inoculum.[47] Juveniles 8 to 8.5 months old weigh at least 700 g and are physically too large to return to the pouch. Back young are usually weaned by the time they are 12 months old and weigh at least 2.2 to 2.5 kg.[4]

Morbidity and Mortality of Pouch Young

Misadventure. Healthy pouch young that fall from their mothers for any reason may die of exposure, especially as their time of first emergence tends to be in winter or early spring. Even if the mother descends to the ground in response to the young's distress vocalizations, the young may not be well coordinated enough to regain the safety of her pouch. Pouch young may be killed accidentally by trauma during mating attempts if adult males are housed with mothers.

Pouch Infection. Discharge from the pouch opening, offensive odor, death of the pouch young, or pouch young with wet soiled fur are indications for microbiologic culture. Normally, it is not possible to culture viable microorganisms from the koala's pouch lining,[46] and so growth of organisms from a swab is an indication for careful extraction of the young and physical examination of both the pouch and the young. Pathogens cultured from the pouch include *P. aeruginosa,*[67] *Klebsiella* species, *Proteus* species, *Serratia marcescens, Enterococcus faecalis, Streptococcus bovis, E. coli, A. lwoffi, Candida albicans,* and unidentified yeasts. Small young that die in the pouch for any reason may be in an advanced state of decay when noticed. Whenever a pouch young dies, the pouch should be examined, disinfected, and then rechecked within a few days, as inflammation of the lining may progress to pyoderma. Ceftazidime, 15 mg/kg BID SQ, and ketoconazole, 10 mg/kg SID PO, have resolved pouch pyodermas caused by *P. aeruginosa* and *C. albicans,* respectively.

Mastitis. Mortality of pouch young has been associated with mixed cultures of *S. marcescens* with beta-hemolytic *Streptococcus* species, and of *E. coli* with *Klebsiella pneumoniae,* isolated from milk.

Enteritis. Soiling of fur around the pouch opening or visible on the young koala's head may signal that a problem exists. On extraction, the joey may be damp and soiled by its own diarrhea. Yeasts and/or bacteria can be cultured from both the joey's feces and the pouch lining. An association with the onset of pap feeding in some cases may indicate that the causal organisms were ingested in pap. After being washed, dried, and returned to the pouch, young may be treated in situ with oral antimicrobial agents, as indicated by culture and sensitivity results, by maneuvering the joey's head around to the pouch opening to allow drug administration.

Candidiasis. Oral thrush with shallow erosions or white curd-like accumulations on the tongue and palate is common in hand-raised young. Gastritis caused by *C. albicans* has been observed in mother-reared young that failed to thrive and in hand-raised young concurrently with severe oral thrush. *Candida* species have been cultured from pouch young with diarrhea. Nystatin, 5000 U/kg TID PO, is used as treatment.

Hand-Raising of Young

If hand-raising is required, koalas should be given a low-lactose milk formula. One person should assume the role of primary caregiver. It is important to establish an environment that emphasizes familiarity and security and avoids any sudden changes in routines. Orphan koalas acquired as unfurred or lightly furred pouch young, before the age at which they would normally consume pap, should be given fresh feces collected from a number of healthy adult koalas (males or females). Fresh cecal contents from healthy koalas that have died suddenly from trauma (e.g., as road kill; from dog attack) also may be a valuable potential source of "substitute pap" for hand-raised young. The organisms in freshly collected pap remain viable for at least 8 hours if stored anaerobically at 4°C; freezing is not suitable (R. Osawa, personal communication, 1992). Pap or adult feces should be made into a slurry and fed, or added to the milk formula, on several occasions over a 1- to 4-week period, commencing at the time the first molars begin to erupt.

Acknowledgments

The authors are grateful to Richard Malik, Elizabeth (Liz) O'Connor, Ro Osawa, Jim Phelan, Dave Spratt, Peter Timms, Ted Warren, Pam Whiteley, Peter Wilson, and Veterinary Pathology Services Pty Ltd (Brisbane, Queensland) whose unpublished information enhances these notes. The authors also thank Jeff McKee for editorial assistance.

REFERENCES

1. Ajello L, Padhye AA: Systemic mycoses. *In* Beran GW (ed): Handbook of Zoonoses, 2nd ed., Section A: Bacterial, Rickettsial, Chlamydial and Mycotic. Boca Raton, FL, CRC Press, pp 491–492, 1994.
2. Backhouse TC, Bolliger A: Morbidity and mortality in the koala (*Phascolarctos cinereus*). Aust J Zool 9(1):24–37, 1961.
3. Barker IK: *Sarcoptes scabiei* infestation of a koala (*Phascolarctos cinereus*), with probable human involvement [Letter]. Aust Vet J 50(11):528, 1974.
4. Blanshard WH: Medicine and husbandry of koalas. *In* Wildlife, Proceedings No. 233, Post Graduate Committee in Veterinary Science, University of Sydney, Sydney, New South Wales, Australia, pp 547–626, 1994.
5. Booth RJ, Blanshard WH: Rhinitis in koalas. Presented at the Annual Meeting of the Wildlife Disease Association (Australasian Section), Lake Eucumbene, New South Wales, Australia, 1989.
6. Brown AS, Carrick FN, Gordon G, Reynolds K: The diagnosis and epidemiology of an infertility disease in the female koala *Phascolarctos cinereus* (Marsupialia). Vet Radiol 25:242–248, 1984.
7. Brown AS, Grice RG: Experimental transmission of *Chlamydia psittaci* in the koala. *In* Oriel JD, Ridgway GL, Schachter J, et al (eds): Chlamydial Infections. Proceedings of the 6th International Symposium on Human Chlamydial Infections, Sanderstead, Surrey. Cambridge, UK, Cambridge University Press, pp 349–352, 1986.
8. Brown AS, Seawright AA, Wilkinson GT: The use of amitraz in

the control of an outbreak of sarcoptic mange in a colony of koalas. Aust Vet J 58(1):8–10, 1982.

9. Brown S, Woolcock J: Epidemiology and control of chlamydial disease in koalas. *In* Australian Wildlife, Proceedings No. 104, Post Graduate Committee in Veterinary Science, University of Sydney, Sydney, New South Wales, Australia, pp 495–502, 1988.

10. Canfield PJ: Diseases affecting captive and free-living koalas and their implications for management. *In* Lunney D, Urquhart CA, Reed P (eds): Koala Summit: Managing Koalas in New South Wales. Proceedings of the Koala Summit, Sydney. Hurstville, New South Wales, Australia, New South Wales National Parks and Wildlife Service, pp 36–38, 1990.

11. Canfield PJ, Dickens RK: Oxalate poisoning in a koala (*Phascolarctos cinereus*). Aust Vet J 59(4):121–122, 1982.

12. Canfield PJ, Gee DR, Wigney DI: Urinalysis in captive koalas. Aust Vet J 66(11):376–377, 1989.

13. Canfield PJ, Hartley WJ, Gill PA, et al: Serosal proliferations in koalas. Aust Vet J 67(9):342–343, 1990.

14. Canfield PJ, Love DN, Mearns G, Farram E: Evaluation of an immunofluorescence test on direct smears of conjunctival and urogenital swabs taken from koalas for the detection of *Chlamydia psittaci*. Aust Vet J 68(5):165–167, 1991.

15. Canfield PJ, Love DN, Mearns G, Farram E: Chlamydial infection in a colony of captive koalas. Aust Vet J 68(5):167–169, 1991.

16. Canfield PJ, O'Neill ME, Smith EF: Haematological and biochemical investigations of diseased koalas *(Phascolarctos cinereus)*. Aust Vet J 66(9):269–272, 1989.

17. Canfield PJ, Oxenford CJ, Lomas GR, Dickens RK: A disease outbreak involving pneumonia in captive koalas. Aust Vet J 63(9):312–313, 1986.

18. Canfield PJ, Perry R, Brown AS, McKenzie RA: Cranio-facial tumours of mixed cartilage and bone in koalas (*Phascolarctos cinereus*). Aust Vet J 64(1):20–22, 1987.

19. Canfield PJ, Sabine JM, Love DN: Virus particles associated with leukaemia in a koala. Aust Vet J 65(10): 327–328, 1988.

20. Cork SJ, Sanson GD: Digestion and nutrition in the koala: a review. *In* Lee AK, Handasyde KA, Sanson GD (eds): Biology of the Koala. Chipping Norton, New South Wales, Australia, Surrey Beatty and Sons, pp 129–144, 1990.

21. Cork SJ, Foley WJ: Digestive and metabolic strategies of arboreal mammalian folivores in relation to chemical defenses in temperate and tropical forests. *In* Palo RT, Robbins CT (eds): Plant Chemical Defenses Against Mammalian Herbivory. Boca Raton, FL, CRC Press, pp 133–166, 1991.

22. Degabriele R: The physiology of the koala. Sci Am 243(1):94–99, July 1980.

23. Degabriele R, Dawson TJ: Metabolism and heat balance in an arboreal marsupial, the koala (*Phascolarctos cinereus*). J Comp Physiol 134:293–301, 1979.

24. Dickens RK: The koala in health and disease. *In* Fauna, Proceedings No. 36, Post Graduate Committee in Veterinary Science, University of Sydney, Sydney, pp 105–117, 1978.

25. Dubey JP, Hedstrom O, Machado CR, Osborn KG: Disseminated toxoplasmosis in a captive koala (*Phascolarctos cinereus*). J Zoo Wild Anim Med 22(3):348–350, 1991.

26. Ellis DH, Pfeiffer TJ: Ecology, life cycle, and infectious propagule of *Cryptococcus neoformans*. Lancet 336:923–925, 1990.

27. Ellis DH, Pfeiffer TJ: The distribution of *Cryptococcus neoformans* var. *gattii* among the species of *Eucalyptus*. Australasian Mycol Newsl 15(3):47–51, 1996.

28. Emmins JJ: The Victorian koala: genetic heterogeneity, immune responsiveness and epizootiology of chlamydiosis. Ph.D. Thesis, Department of Pathology and Immunology, Monash University, Clayton, Victoria, Australia, 1996.

29. Girjes AA, Ellis WAH, Carrick FN, Lavin MF: Some aspects of the immune response of koalas (*Phascolarctos cinereus*) and in vitro neutralization of *Chlamydia psittaci* (koala strains). FEMS Immunol Med Microbiol 6:21–30, 1993.

30. Glassick T, Giffard P, Timms P: Outer membrane protein 2 gene sequences indicate that *Chlamydia pecorum* and *Chlamydia pneumoniae* cause infections in koalas. Syst Appl Microbiol 19:457–464, 1997.

31. Handasyde KA, Martin RW, Lee AK: Field investigations into chlamydial disease and infertility in koalas in Victoria. Australian Wildlife, Proceedings No. 104, Post Graduate Committee in Veterinary Science, University of Sydney, Sydney, pp 505–515, 1988.

32. Hartley WJ, Dubey JP, Spielman DS: Fatal toxoplasmosis in koalas (*Phascolarctos cinereus*). J Parasitol 76(2):271–272, 1990.

33. Heit MC, Riviere JE: Antifungal and antiviral drugs. *In* Adams HR (ed): Veterinary Pharmacology and Therapeutics, 7th ed. Ames, Iowa State University Press, pp 861–868, 1995.

34. James LF, Johnnson AE: Oxalate accumulators. *In* Howard JL (ed): Current Veterinary Therapy: Food Animal Practice II. Philadelphia, WB Saunders, pp 396–398, 1986.

35. Laurence DR, Bennett PN: Clinical Pharmacology, 5th ed. Edinburgh, UK, Churchill Livingstone, p 237, 1980.

36. Lee AK, Martin RW: The Koala, A Natural History. Kensington, New South Wales, Australia, New South Wales University Press, pp 61–62, 1988.

37. Lees N, Eccleston J, McKee J: Lead levels in koalas: can feeding browse from roadside eucalyptus compromise the health of koalas (*Phascolarctos cinereus*)? Proceedings of the Australian Koala Foundation Annual Conference, Greenmount, Queensland, Australia, pp 174–184, 1995.

38. Ley C: Cryptococcosis in the koala (*Phascolarctos cinereus*). Faculty of Veterinary Science Final Year Essay, University of Sydney, New South Wales, Australia, 1993.

39. Malik R, McPetrie R, Wigney DI, et al: A latex cryptococcal antigen agglutination test for diagnosis and monitoring of therapy for cryptococcosis. Aust Vet J 74(5):358–364, 1996.

40. McColl KA, Spratt DM: Parasitic pneumonia in a koala (*Phascolarctos cinereus*) from Victoria, Australia. J Wildl Dis 18(4):511–512, 1982.

41. McKenzie RA: Observations on diseases of free-living and captive koalas (*Phascolarctos cinereus*). Aust Vet J 57(5):243–246, 1981.

42. McKenzie RA, Wood AD, Blackall PJ: Pneumonia associated with *Bordetella bronchiseptica* in captive koalas. Aust Vet J 55(9):427–430, 1979.

43. Obendorf DL: Pathology of the female reproductive tract in the koala, *Phascolarctos cinereus* (Goldfuss), from Victoria, Australia. J Wildl Dis 17(4):587–592, 1981.

44. Obendorf DL: Causes of mortality and morbidity of wild koalas, *Phascolarctos cinereus* (Goldfuss), in Victoria, Australia. J Wildl Dis 19(2):123–131, 1983.

45. Obendorf DL: The pathogenesis of urogenital tract disease in the koala. Australian Wildlife, Proceedings No. 104, Post Graduate Committee in Veterinary Science, University of Sydney, Sydney, pp 649–655, 1988.

46. Osawa R, Blanshard WH, O'Callaghan PG: Microflora of the pouch of the koala (*Phascolarctos cinereus*). J Wildl Dis 28(2):276–280, 1992.

47. Osawa R, Blanshard WH, O'Callaghan PG: Microbiological studies of the intestinal microflora of the koala, *Phascolarctos cinereus:* II. Pap, a special maternal faeces consumed by juvenile koalas. Aust J Zool 41:611–620, 1993.

48. Pass MA, Brown AS: Liver function in normal koalas and macropods. Aust Vet J 67(4):151–152, 1990.

49. Rahman A: The sensitivity of various bacteria to chemotherapeutic agents. Br Vet J 113(4):175–188, 1957.

50. Roberts FHS: Australian Ticks. Melbourne, Commonwealth Scientific and Industrial Research Organisation, p 162, 1970.

51. Robinson W, O'Brien T, Hanger J, McKee J: Lymphoma/leukaemia in koalas: the presence of viral particles in cultured lymphocytes. Proceedings of the Australian Koala Foundation Conference on the Status of the Koala in 1996, Greenmount, Queensland, Australia, pp 97–99, 1997.

52. Rush CM, Timms P: In vitro survival characteristics of koala chlamydiae. Wildl Res 23:213–219, 1996.

53. Russell EG, Straube EF: Streptobacillary pleuritis in a koala (*Phascolarctos cinereus*). J Wildl Dis 15(3):391–394, 1979.

54. Spencer A, Canfield P: Haematological effects of heavy tick infestation in koalas (*Phascolarctos cinereus*). Proceedings of the Annual Meeting of the Wildlife Disease Association (Australasian Section), North Stradbroke Island, Queensland, Australia, pp 41–42, 1993.

55. Spratt DM: Note on the cestode (*Bertiella obesa*) in the koala. *In* Bergin TJ (ed): The Koala. Proceedings of the Taronga Symposium on Koala Biology, Management and Medicine. Sydney, New South Wales, Australia, Zoological Parks Board of New South Wales, p 200, 1978.

56. Spratt DM: Further studies of lung parasites (Nematoda) from Australian marsupials. Aust J Zool 32(2):283–310, 1984.

57. Stone BF: Ticks and wildlife: interactions, particularly of the Australian paralysis tick *Ixodes holocyclus*, with koalas, bandicoots and fruit bats. Proceedings of the Annual Meeting of the Wildlife Disease Association (Australasian Section), Warrumbungles National Park, New South Wales, Australia, p 17, 1992.

58. Theile G: Chronic renal failure in koalas at Perth Zoo. Proceedings of the Australasian Society of Zookeeping Conference, Auckland, New Zealand, pp 78–81, 1990.
59. Timms P, Wood M: Monitoring chlamydial disease in koalas: which tests are easy and reliable? *In* Gordon G (ed): Koalas—Research for Management. Proceedings of the Brisbane Koala Symposium. Brisbane, Queensland, Australia, World Koala Research, Inc., pp 56–61, 1996.
60. U.S. Armed Forces Institute of Pathology: Accession 2330591, Wednesday slide conference #23, March 18, 1992. Washington D.C., U.S. Armed Forces Institute of Pathology, Department of Veterinary Pathology, 1992.
61. Wati S: Transmission and control of *Chlamydia psittaci* in koalas. Bachelor of Applied Sciences, Honors Thesis, School of Life Science, Queensland University of Technology, Brisbane, Queensland, Australia, 1991.
62. Wigney DI, Gee DR, Canfield PJ: Pyogranulomatous pneumonias due to *Nocardia asteroides* and *Staphylococcus epidermidis* in two koalas, *Phascolarctos cinereus.* J Wildl Dis 25(4):592–596, 1989.
63. Whittington R: Chlamydiosis of koalas. *In* Williams B, Barker IK,

Thorne T (eds): Infectious Diseases of Wild Mammals. Ames, Iowa State University Press, in press.
64. Wilkinson R: Characterisation of immune responses of the koala. Ph.D. Thesis, Department of Microbiology and Immunology, University of Adelaide, South Australia, Australia, 1996.
65. Wilkinson R, Kotlarski I, Barton M: Further characterisation of the immune response of the koala. Vet Immunol Immunopathol 40:325–339, 1994.
66. Wood A: The use of supplements in breeding captive koalas. Proceedings of the 3rd Koala Management Conference, Currumbin, Queensland. Brisbane, Queensland, Australia, Australian Koala Foundation, 1987.
67. Wood A: The diseases of the captive koala. *In* Bergin TJ (ed): The Koala. Proceedings of the Taronga Symposium on Koala Biology, Management and Medicine. Sydney, New South Wales, Australia, Zoological Parks Board of New South Wales, pp 158–165, 1978.
68. Worley M, Rideout B, Shima A, Janssen D: Opportunistic infections, cancer and hematological disorders associated with retrovirus infection in the koala. Proceedings of the Annual Meeting of the American Association of Zoo Veterinarians, St. Louis, pp 181–182, 1993.

Sedation and Anesthesia in Marsupials

AMY L. SHIMA

Marsupials represent a diverse and fascinating group of mammals found in Australasia and the Americas. With the exception of the North American opossum (*Didelphis virginiana*), representatives of this order commonly found in zoological collections are primarily from Australia and New Guinea. Many species of marsupials can be safely handled with manual restraint for brief examination and simple procedures (e.g., obtaining venous blood samples). Techniques for physical restraint of marsupial species have been adequately covered elsewhere.[2, 5, 6, 9–11] Chemical restraint is necessary for more extensive procedures and for safe handling of some larger species. A number of anesthetic and tranquilizing agents have been employed to immobilize marsupials in both captive and free-ranging settings. Variable tolerances to general anesthetics in different species of marsupials have been previously reported,[11, 21] and a wide range of doses and protocols have been used in the immobilization and anesthesia of marsupials. Current protocols for use of calming agents and immobilizing or anesthetic agents in Australasian marsupials are discussed here.

GENERAL CONSIDERATIONS

In general, anesthetic procedures in marsupials can be approached in the same manner as for eutherian mam-

mals. Whenever possible, preanesthesia fasting for 12 to 24 hours should be practiced for foregut-fermentative, ruminant-type marsupials (kangaroos, wallabies, rat kangaroos) and hindgut-fermentative species such as wombats and koalas. Koalas may, if necessary, be safely anesthetized after 6 hours of fasting. Before anesthesia is induced, however, the abdomen should be palpated to ascertain the degree of stomach "fill." If the stomach still feels full, delaying the anesthetic procedure may be advisable. Preanesthesia fasting for dasyurids and nonruminant herbivores (possums, cuscuses) should follow guidelines for similarly sized eutherian mammals.

Because a number of effective anesthetic protocols could be used in marsupials, the method of choice should be based on considerations such as extent of the planned procedure, desired length and depth of anesthesia, options for managing the animal during recovery from anesthesia, ability to safely handle the animal for intravenous (IV) injections or induction through an inhalation agent, and the age, temperament, and condition of the animal.

ANESTHETIC MONITORING

Assessment of the anesthetized marsupial is the same as monitoring of eutherian mammal anesthesia. Moni-

TABLE 42–1. Injectable Immobilization Agents Used in Marsupials

Drug or Drug Combination	Species	Dose (mg/kg)	Route	Comments
Ketamine Xylazine	Macropods	10–25 5	IM	
Ketamine Medetomidine	Not specified	2–3 0.05–0.1	IM	Reverse medetomidine with atipamezole, 0.05–0.4 mg/kg IV
Ketamine Xylazine	Koalas, other marsupials	5 5	IM	Reverse with yohimbine, 0.2 mg/kg IV, or atipamezole, 0.05–0.4 mg/kg IV
Diazepam Ketamine	Bandicoots	0.5–1.0	IM	
	Potoroos	30	IM	~ 1 hr duration
Tiletamine-zolazepam	Kangaroos, wallabies	3–10	IM	Induction 2–15 minutes; duration 30–45 minutes
Tiletamine-zolazepam	Tree kangaroos	1.5–5.0	IM	Induction 2–15 minutes; duration 30–45 minutes; use high end of dose range if animal is very agitated or aggressive, low end of dose range for induction
Tiletamine-zolazepam	Possums	10–20	IM	Higher doses (20 mg/kg) needed in free-ranging animals under field conditions
Tiletamine-zolazepam	Dasyurids	10	IM	
Tiletamine-zolazepam	Wombats	2–8	IM	Recovery 1–5 hours; use high end of dose range if animal is very agitated or aggressive
Tiletamine-zolazepam	Koalas	5–10 2.5	IM IV	Induction ~3 minutes; surgical anesthesia ~6 minutes; duration 20–30 minutes; recovery 1–2 hours
Tiletamine-zolazepam Xylazine	Not specified	5 0.5	IM	Useful for induction then maintenance on gas anesthesia; reversal with yohimbine, 0.2 mg/kg IV, or atipamezole, 0.05–0.4 mg/kg IV
Tiletamine-zolazepam Xylazine	Not specified	3–4 1–2	IM	For short anesthetic procedures; reversal with yohimbine, 0.2 mg/kg IV, or atipamezole, 0.05–0.4 mg/kg IV

toring of respiratory and cardiac rates, degree of muscle tone, mucous membrane color, and pain, righting, and corneal reflexes is done in the usual manner. Pulse oximetry can be a useful tool in monitoring anesthesia in marsupials. The oximeter may be attached to the pinna, digit, tongue, cheek, pouch wall, or scrotum. Since many marsupials have a slightly lower mean body temperature than eutherian mammals, special attention should be paid to monitoring body temperature during anesthesia and appropriate means taken to avoid hypothermia.

INJECTABLE AGENTS

A variety of injectable anesthetic agents have been used with success in marsupials under both free-ranging and captive conditions. The advantages of injectable agents are that they can be administered by remote injection, they generally have a wide margin of safety, and, in some cases, their effects can be reversed with specific antagonists. The dose can be adjusted according to whether the desired result is simple sedation and immobilization or surgical anesthesia. Injectable agents can be used in conjunction with inhalation anesthetics for prolonged procedures. IV anesthetics can be administered to animals that can safely be manually restrained. Under suitable manual restraint, IV anesthetics can be

administered into the cephalic or saphenous vein in koalas and into either the lateral coccygeal vein or the medial saphenous vein in macropods.

The tranquilizing, immobilizing, and anesthetic protocols considered to be most effective and in contemporary use are listed in Table 42–1.

NEUROLEPTICS AND TRANQUILIZERS (CALMING AGENTS)

A variety of neuroleptic agents and tranquilizers have been used in a number of species of marsupials. These agents have proved useful in the management of nervous, flighty animals, for temporary confinement of free-ranging wild animals, during translocation or transfer between enclosures, and for the temporary confinement of animals for medical treatment[3, 13, 14, 16, 18] (Table 42–2).

DISSOCIATIVE AGENTS

Dissociative agents have been widely used in marsupials (see Table 42–1). They are potent anesthetic agents with a high therapeutic index. There is wide variation in reported dose ranges according to whether the desired

TABLE 42–2. Calming Agents Used Intramuscularly in Marsupials

Drug	Dose (mg/kg)	Duration	Comments
Diazepam	0.5–2.0	~6 hours	May be used orally at 2 mg/kg
Azaperone	1–2	Variable: 90 minutes to 24 hours	Induction time 15–20 minutes
Perphenazine enanthate	0.5–5.0	~7 days	Not available in US
Zuclopenthixol decanoate	10	Up to 10 days	Not available in US
Pipothiazine palmitate	10	Up to 10 days	Not available in US
Haloperidol lactate	0.1–0.3	~12 hours	
Haloperidol decanoate	1.0–4.5	7–30 days	Onset of action in 24–48 hours

result is simple sedation and immobilization or surgical anesthesia. These agents can be used in conjunction with inhalation anesthetics for prolonged procedures.

Historically, ketamine hydrochloride at doses ranging from 15 to 50 mg/kg given intramuscularly (IM) has been used in marsupials.[1, 15–17] Reddacliff[16] reported species variation, with phalangers requiring 30 to 50 mg/kg ketamine and dasyurids, macropods, wombats, and koalas requiring 25 mg/kg IM for light anesthesia. Problems with muscular rigidity and poor visceral analgesia associated with ketamine anesthesia prompted exploration of combination drug protocols with alpha$_2$-adrenergic agonists such as xylazine and medetomidine. Combinations of ketamine and xylazine or ketamine and medetomidine have been reported as achieving sedation in a number of species of macropods and other marsupials.[2, 3, 7, 10, 14] Reversal of the alpha$_2$-adrenergic agonist component of this combination can be achieved with either yohimbine, 0.2 mg/kg IV, or atipamezole, 0.05 to 0.4 mg/kg IV.

Tiletamine-zolazepam is considered by some to be the injectable agent of choice for immobilization of marsupials. It produces rapid (2–12 minutes), smooth induction, a duration of approximately 30 minutes, and recovery in 1.5 to 4 hours.[18, 19] The combination has been used in a variety of species in both field and captive conditions.[4, 8, 12, 18–20] Although induction with tiletamine-zolazepam is rapid in marsupials, waiting a minimum of 15 minutes before handling the animal generally decreases the incidence of undesirable reactions and gives better overall results. Supplemental doses of ketamine at 10 to 25 mg/kg IM or 5 to 10 mg/kg IV (to effect) may be given if the procedure is prolonged. Additional doses of tiletamine-zolazepam should not be given, because this may result in a prolonged or difficult recovery. After anesthesia induction with tiletamine-zolazepam, animals may be maintained on inhalation agents such as isoflurane.

Undesirable effects seen with dissociative agents include excessive salivation, muscle rigidity, prolonged recovery time, response to noxious stimuli, hyperexcitability, and "paddling" during recovery. Undesirable reactions and prolonged recovery are seen more frequently with higher doses of tiletamine-zolazepam. Response to noxious stimuli, hyperexcitability, and muscular activity while immobilized may occur if handling is attempted before induction is complete. Salivation can be controlled by glycopyrrolate (0.01 to 0.02 mg/kg IM, IV, or subcutaneously [SQ]), or atropine (0.02 to 0.04 mg/kg IM, IV, or SQ). Muscle relaxation is variable and is time and dose dependent.

OTHER INJECTABLE AGENTS

The use of a combination of butorphanol (0.3 to 0.5 mg/kg), detomidine (0.05 to 0.08 mg/kg), and midazolam (0.3 to 0.4 mg/kg) is under investigation (R. Wack, personal communication, 1997). It shows promise as a combination that provides smooth induction and reversible injectable anesthesia. The addition of glycopyrrolate or atropine to counteract bradycardia and respiratory depression may be necessary. This combination can be reversed with the administration of yohimbine (0.3 to 0.4 mg/kg IV) and naltrexone (0.5 to 0.6 mg/kg IV).

Alfaxalone-Alfadolone Acetate

Alfaxalone-alfadolone acetate (Saffan) is a steroid combination that has been used for many years in Great Britain, Australia, and Canada. It produces good immobilization for approximately 20 minutes and can be supplemented IV as needed. It has been used in koalas and other marsupials at doses of 0.1 to 0.2 ml/kg IV or 0.25 to 0.5 ml/kg IM.[2, 3]

Propofol

IV propofol (Diprivan 1%) given as a 0.25 to 0.3-mg/kg IV bolus then titrated to effect has been used in koalas.[2] It is not an irritant if injected perivascularly but is impractical for IM use because of its rapid metabolization. Induction and recovery are rapid and smooth. Propofol has been used for induction of anesthesia before maintenance with an inhalation agent or for short procedures in which good relaxation and fast recovery are desirable.

INHALATION ANESTHETICS

Volatile anesthetic agents such as isoflurane and halothane have been widely used with good results in marsupials. The low blood solubility, which allows for rapid induction and recovery, low potential to produce organ toxicity, and relative lack of toxicity to humans make isoflurane the preferred inhalation agent for use in marsupials. Inhalation agents are frequently used after induction with an injectable agent. Inhalation agents are safe and effective and allow good control over the depth and duration of anesthesia. Animals can be manually restrained and anesthesia induced with isoflurane administered through a standard, appropriately sized, tight-fitting cone-style mask. Care must be taken that the animal is adequately restrained to prevent injury to itself or to personnel during the induction phase. In general, mask induction with isoflurane at 3% to 5% followed by maintenance at 1% to 3% in oxygen provides adequate anesthesia for most marsupials.

INTUBATION

The relatively narrow dental arcarde and limited access possible with most marsupial mouths can make endotracheal intubation challenging. The location of the larynx in many marsupials requires that a relatively long endotracheal tube be used. With practice, one can safely intubate macropods, koalas, and other marsupials by using a long (4- to 6-inch), narrow-bladed laryngoscope or a long, curved transilluminator to visualize the epiglottis.

With the animal in a relatively deep plane of anesthesia, two pieces of roll gauze or soft cord are used to pull the mouth open. The tongue is grasped and pulled out of the way with a piece of gauze. In species such as the koala, the soft palate obscures the epiglottis from direct view. Positioning the animal in dorsal recumbency may help, but intubation can be achieved with the animal in any position. The tip of the endotracheal tube can be used to push the palate out of the way to visualize the epiglottis. Once the epiglottis is visualized, the endotracheal tube can be passed through it during inspiration in the usual manner. Because of the narrowness of the marsupial mouth, introducing the endotracheal tube often obscures the view of the epiglottis. In this case, once the laryngeal opening is visualized, a long (22-inch) polypropylene catheter (5F or 8F) can be passed into it. The laryngoscope can then be removed and the endotracheal tube passed over the catheter into the epiglottis. The catheter is removed and the endotracheal tube secured and, if appropriate, the cuff inflated. Care must be taken to ensure that the endotracheal tube fits over the polypropylene catheter; in some cases, the flared tip of the catheter may need to be trimmed. Threading the endotracheal tube onto the catheter before placement is sometimes helpful. If a long, narrow-bladed laryngoscope is not available, intubation can be achieved through the use of a curved transilluminator to visualize the larynx. The mouth is pulled open with two pieces of roll gauze or soft cord, the tongue is pulled out of the way, and the soft palate is pushed out of the way with the tip of the endotracheal tube, the tip of the transilluminator, or the end of the polypropylene catheter. Once the epiglottis is visualized, the

endotracheal tube or the polypropylene catheter can be passed into it.

Retrograde intubation has been described,[3] but, in the experience of this author, intubation can be achieved without having to resort to such an invasive procedure.

REFERENCES

1. Beck CC: Vetalar® (ketamine hydrochloride): A unique cataleptoid anesthetic agent for multispecies usage. J Zoo Anim Med 7:11–37, 1976.
2. Blanshard W: Medicine and husbandry of koalas. Proceedings of the Post-Graduate Committee in Veterinary Science, University of Sydney, No. 233, pp 547–623, 1994.
3. Blyde D: Advances in anaesthesia and sedation of native fauna. Proceedings of the Post-Graduate Committee in Veterinary Science, University of Sydney, No. 233, pp 243–245, 1994.
4. Boever WJ, Stuppy D, Kane K: Clinical experience with tilazol (CI744) as a new agent for chemical restraint and anesthesia in the red kangaroo (*Macropus rufus*). JZAM 8:14–17, 1977.
5. Booth R: Medicine and husbandry: monotremes, wombats and bandicoots. Proceedings of the Post-Graduate Committee in Veterinary Science, University of Sydney, No. 233, pp 395–420, 1994.
6. Booth R: Medicine and husbandry: dasyurids, possums and bats. Proceedings of the Post-Graduate Committee in Veterinary Science, University of Sydney, No. 233, pp 423–441, 1994.
7. Booth R: Macropod restraint. Proceedings of the Post-Graduate Committee in Veterinary Science, University of Sydney, No. 233, pp 443–447, 1994.
8. DeWildt DE, Obrien SJ, Graves JAM, et al: Anesthesia and reproductive characteristics of free-ranging male koalas (*Phascolarctos cinereus*). Proceedings of the American Association of Zoo Veterinarians, Toronto, pp 109–111, 1988.
9. Finnie EP: Monotremes and marsupials: Restraint. *In* Fowler ME (ed): Zoo and Wild Animal Medicine, 2nd ed. Philadelphia, WB Saunders, pp 570–572, 1986.
10. Finnie EP: Restraint and anesthesia in monotremes and marsupials. Proceedings of the Post-Graduate Committee in Veterinary Science, University of Sydney, No. 36, pp 49–52, 1976.
11. Fowler ME: Restraint and Handling of Wild and Domestic Animals. Ames, IA, Iowa State University Press, pp 183–188, 1978.
12. Holz P: Immobilization of marsupials with tiletamine and zolazepam. J Zoo Wildl Med 23:426–428, 1992.
13. Holz P, Barnett JEF: Long-acting tranquilizers: Their use as a management tool in the confinement of free-ranging red-necked wallabies (*Macropus rufogriseus*). J Zoo Wildl Med 27:54–60, 1966.
14. Keep JM: Marsupials: Anaesthesia. Proceedings of the Post-Graduate Committee in Veterinary Science, University of Sydney, No. 36, pp 123–134, 1976.
15. Ludders JW, Ojerio AD: Brief observations on handling and chemical restraint of the rat kangaroo (*Potorus tridactylus*). J Zoo Anim Med 11:106–108, 1980.
16. Reddacliff G: Therapeutic index—marsupials. Proceedings of the Post-Graduate Committee in Veterinary Science, University of Sydney, No. 39, Vol 2, pp 1037–1042, 1978.
17. Robinson PT: A review of thirty-three Queensland koala (*Phascolarctos cinereus adustus*) immobilization procedures. J Zoo Anim Med 12:4:121–123, 1981.
18. Shima A, McCracken H, Booth R, et al: Use of tiletamine-zolazepam in the immobilization of marsupials. Proceedings of the Annual Meeting of the American Association of Zoo Veterinarians, St. Louis, pp 171–174, 1993.
19. Smeller J, Bush M, Custer R: The immobilization of marsupials. J Zoo Anim Med 8:16–19, 1977.
20. Viggers KL, Lindenmayer DB: The use of tiletamine hydrochloride and zolazepam hydrochloride for sedation of the mountain brushtail possum *Trichosurus caninus* Ogilby (Phalangeridae: Marsupialia). Austral Vet J 72:215–216, 1995.
21. Watson CRR, Way JS: The unusual tolerance of marsupials to barbiturate anaesthetics. Int Zoo Yearb 12:208–211, 1972.

CHAPTER 43

Medical Management of Tree Kangaroos

MITCHELL BUSH

RICHARD J. MONTALI

Tree kangaroos (*Dendrolagus* species) are a unique and attractive group of marsupials because of their arboreal adaptation, colorful hair coat, interesting behavior, and the fact that they are cute. There is some disagreement on the taxonomy of tree kangaroos. The general consensus is there are eight species from New Guinea, including Matschie's (*D. matschiei*), Goodfellow's (*D. goodfellowi*), grizzled (*D. inustus*), Doria's (*D. dorianus*), Scott's (*D. scottae*), lowland (*D. spadix*), Vogelkop (*D. ursinus*), and black and white (*D. mbaise*). Bennett's (*D. bennettianus*) and Lumholtz's (*D. lumholtzi*) are species of Queensland, Australia. Their habitat is the rainforest; therefore, all species are considered vulnerable or threatened because of the classic reasons of habitat destruction and being hunted as a protein source. Tree kangaroos are totally dependent on mature forests containing trees large enough to support their weight.

The Matschie's, Goodfellow's, Doria's, and grizzled are the species currently maintained in approximately 40 collections worldwide. This chapter focuses on the medical management of the relatively docile Matschie's tree kangaroo; this management can be extrapolated to the other species. At present, Matschie's is the most commonly exhibited tree kangaroo species, and it is being fairly well maintained by captive breeding programs.

The anatomy and physiology of marsupials were reviewed by Finnie[6] and are applicable to tree kangaroos. Their metabolic rate and body temperature are lower than those of eutherian mammals, and the epipubic bone is present in both sexes. The retina of marsupials is a transition between those of monotremes and those of placental mammals, with few large vessels on the fundus and a group of fine vessels associated with the optic disc. The biology and management of this species have been compiled in a tree kangaroo workbook[7] and in edited proceedings of an American Association of Zoological Parks and Aquariums regional conference.[13]

Although captive tree kangaroos are usually considered crepuscular, they may be nocturnal in the wild, which is unique for animals with relatively small eyes. They are mainly arboreal but may come to the ground to eat and breed. The tail is used for a counterbalance or as a prop in the trees rather than for locomotion. Other adaptations for their arboreal lifestyle include stout muscular hindlegs and forelegs of comparable size, and they are the only macropods that can move their hind legs independently. Their strong claws and large granular footpads make them adept climbers. The Queensland species are generally more agile; the New Guinea species are heavier and stouter. Adult weights range from 6.5 to 11 kg for males and 7.5 to 9 kg for females. The females have a well-developed pouch with four mammae. A sternal gland, which is larger in males, is present. Their vocalizations include clicking, chuffing, and whistling.

HUSBANDRY

The enclosure should provide vertical height with trees and horizontal branches or runways 15 to 30 cm in diameter, with a roughened bark or scored surface for traction. Resting platforms and horizontal branches with forks should be located at intervals on the horizontal runways for resting and feeding platforms. The substrate should be soft because the animals leap down from considerable heights to escape. The animals need to be protected from direct sunlight, especially in warm climates, and provided with heat or indoor enclosures in cold climates. Their comfort range appears to be 18° to 24°C, with at least 50% humidity.

Although tree kangaroos are usually mild mannered and "laid back," they manifest stress by nasal discharge, licking of the forelegs, or both. Gastric ulcers seen at necropsy may also be manifestations of stress. Loud noises, changes in their routine, and illness are common stressors. It is important for keepers and veterinarians to understand that tree kangaroos may exhibit individualist behavior; a behavior typical of one individual animal can indicate in other individuals that they are not feeling well.

Free-living tree kangaroos are thought to be solitary and nongregarious, so in captivity they are usually housed alone except for breeding. It is recommended that they not be housed with avian species because of the danger of avian tuberculosis; tree kangaroos have also been reported to capture and eat certain birds. Any plants and trees in the exhibit require protection from the tree kangaroos.

Individual identification, which is critical to medical and management programs, is accomplished by tattoos, subcutaneous transponders on the midline between the scapulae, and individual markings on the face or tail. Ear tags are not ideal because the animals' ears are small and thick.

REPRODUCTION

Tree kangaroos appear to be polyestrous (cycle length, 51 to 79 days), with young born year round. Females become sexually mature at about 2 years; successful births have occurred in animals as old as 15 years. Courtship and breeding in captivity have been noted on the ground. The average gestation is 44 days, which is the longest of any marsupial. There are no reports of postpartum copulation or embryonic diapause.

An extremely high death rate of pouch young occurs by expulsion from the pouch if the mother is not isolated. The male should be removed 40 days after copulation to avoid interference with parturition. At the National Zoological Park, a 73% mortality rate in animals under 2 years of age reflected primarily the deaths of joeys. The expulsion may occur because of the presence of cage mates or because of a nervous mother. Pouch inspection at 50 days is recommended to allow isolation of the mother with a joey. If a joey is not present, the male is returned for breeding. This management procedure has markedly decreased joey mortalities.

In the Matschie's tree kangaroo, the joey's head emerges from the pouch at 22 weeks of age, with total emergence at about 28 weeks of age. The joey feeds alone at 28 weeks of age and is independent of the pouch at 41 weeks of age, but it will continue to nurse until 14 months of age. Platforms in the enclosure reduce injuries and deaths of joeys from falls.

NUTRITION

Tree kangaroos are browsing herbivores with a large sacculated stomach for foregut fermentation; good-quality browse is a major part of their diet. The type of browse depends on geographic location. They eat the leaves and strip the bark from browse, which should be placed in elevated feeding stations. Their diet should also include a variety of fruits and vegetables. The daily hand-feeding of treats by the keepers allows close daily observations, and treats can be a vehicle for oral medication. Tea leaves are added to the diet weekly as a source of tannic acid to maintain condition and coat color. Feeding a high-fiber apple biscuit (Marion Zoological, Inc., Marion, KS), developed for leaf-eating primates, has markedly decreased the incidence of dental problems that have plagued some collections.

A multivitamin supplement is used in many collections. Reports of a myopathy associated with vitamin E

and selenium deficiencies[8, 10] has led to dietary supplementation with vitamin E.

Tree kangaroo feces should be firm pellets. The urine color may be reddish brown and is affected by the choice of browse. Tree kangaroos regurgitate food and re-chew as part of their normal feeding. There is also some indication of coprophagy, primarily between mother and joey.

PHYSICAL RESTRAINT

Physical restraint should be used for some short, non-painful procedures. The animal is captured with a net or by grabbing the tail base to stop the animal and allow further manipulation or to direct it into a transfer crate. The animal must not be lifted by the tail. When entering the enclosure, the animals may leap to the ground to escape. Further restraint for nail trimming or pouch checking requires at least three keepers working together: one holds the tail while supporting the spine; the second person, using gloves, grasps and stabilizes the front legs, which can scratch; and the third person performs the procedure. A tree kangaroo bite is mainly a pinch, but it can be painful. Nail trimming, shifting to a crate, injection of medication or anesthetic, and pouch checking for young are the most common procedures performed with physical restraint.

ANESTHESIA

Anesthesia for tree kangaroos is usually induced with a dissociative anesthetic in combination with a tranquilizer or sedative. The tree kangaroo tail is grasped and elevated, and the injection is given in the rear leg. The two choices are a ketamine/xylazine combination or tiletamine/zolazepam (Telazol). The dose ranges reported are 5 to 25 mg/kg of ketamine with 1 to 5 mg/kg of xylazine.[7] The dose range for Telazol is 2 to 8 mg/kg.[4] Telazol produces a dose-dependent level of anesthesia. Surgical anesthesia usually requires the higher dosages, but the recovery can be prolonged (up to 3 hours). If a low dosage is used, the animals can usually be handled for minor procedures, and the anesthesia can be deepened with inhalational anesthesia (isoflurane or halothane) by face mask if necessary.

For a prolonged procedure, the animal is intubated. Tracheal intubation of tree kangaroos is difficult because of their limited mouth opening and relatively small trachea (a 3.5- to 4.0-mm tube should be used for an adult). Topical anesthetic applied to the vocal cords facilitates intubation. Respiratory secretions that may be present can be controlled by atropine, postural drainage, or suction.

Anesthesia can be induced with inhalation anesthetic (isoflurane or halothane) in a chamber or by face mask. This may be additionally stressful for the animal, but recovery is more rapid than with dissociative anesthetics.

Anesthesia monitoring is assisted by pulse oximetry; the sensors are placed on the external skin of the pouch in females and on the vessels at the base of the scrotum in males or just above the hock in the skin area anterior to the achilles tendon. Indirect blood pressure can be measured on the forelimb.

During recovery from dissociative anesthetics, the animals are monitored to prevent self-injury from chewing. Before release to their enclosure, the animals should be fully recovered to prevent injury from falls.

CLINICAL PATHOLOGY

Blood collection sites in tree kangaroos include the jugular, cephalic, lateral tail, and recurrent tarsal veins. It may be difficult to perform venipuncture with the jugular vein because the animals have such short necks. The peripheral veins will more easily bleed if the leg is warmed with water.

Table 43–1 reports the standard clinical laboratory values for tree kangaroos from the National Zoological Park. In most cases of illness, these values are maintained within a narrow reference range, making their

diagnostic and prognostic use somewhat limited. It is not uncommon to observe nucleated red blood cells in the peripheral blood smear in normal animals.

BACTERIAL INFECTIONS

Tree kangaroos are probably susceptible to most of the same bacterial infections noted in eutherian mammals, but the incidence of mycobacterial infections is very high.[5, 9, 12] More than 90% are caused by *Mycobacterium avium* complex (MAC); other environmental mycobacteria account for the remaining cases. For this discussion, both types are considered mycobacteriosis (MCB). The observed increased susceptibility may be attributed to a lowered cellular immune response seen in these species compared with eutherian mammals and other marsupials.[5] Mycobacteriosis has been reported in three species (Matschie's, Goodfellow's, and grizzled). Mycobacteriosis is 2.5 times more common in male Matschie's, which indicates a sex predilection.

TABLE 43–I. Hematology and Serum Chemistry Values of Matschie's Tree Kangaroos at the National Zoological Park

Parameters	Adult Males		Adult Females	
	Average (Range)	Number	Average (Range)	Number
Erythrocytes, RBC ($\times 10^6/\mu$l)	5.96 (4.69–8.3)	44	5.71 (4.11–7.62)	36
Hemoglobin (g/dl)	16.58 (13.5–20)	42	16.63 (12.2–22.3)	30
Hematocrit (%)	45.5 (36–55)	44	45.3 (33–61)	36
Mean corpuscular volume (μ^3)	75.8 (66–85)	44	78.6 (73–84)	36
Mean corpuscular hemoglobin (/g)	27.7 (24–31)	42	28.9 (27–32)	30
Mean corpuscular hemoglobin concentration (%)	36.4 (34–40)	42	36.8 (34–39)	30
Leukocytes, WBC ($\times 10^3/\mu$l)	4.6 (1.9–10.6)	44	4.4 (2.1–8.2)	36
Nucleated RBC (/100 WBC)	2.65 (1–17)	23		
Segmented neutrophils ($\times 10^3/\mu$l)	2.5 (0.8–8.5)	43	2.5 (0.8–5.8)	36
Segmented neutrophils (%)	51.5 (26–83)	43	54.8 (26–78)	38
Band neutrophils ($\times 10^3/\mu$l)	0	43	0	36
Lymphocytes ($\times 10^2/\mu$l)	1.7 (0.6–6.0)	43	1.5 (0.5–3.0)	36
Lymphocytes (%)	37 (12–60)	43	36.6 (12–62)	38
Monocytes (/μl)	203 (0–672)	43	160 (0–492)	36
Monocytes (%)	4.4 (0–12)	43	3.9 (0–8)	38
Eosinophils (/μl)	271 (0–1008)	43	193 (0–690)	36
Eosinophils (%)	6.3 (0–18)	43	4.5 (0–15)	38
Basophils (/μl)	30 (0–122)	43	12 (0–76)	36
Basophils (%)	0.6 (0–2)	43	0.3 (0–2)	38
Total protein (g/dl)	7 (6.1–8.3)	42	7.1 (6.1–7.8)	38
Fibrinogen (mg/dl)	118 (0–400)	44	108 (0–300)	36
Albumin (g/dl)	4.3 (3.4–5.8)	40	4.4 (3.5–5.6)	36
Blood urea nitrogen (BUN) (mg/dl)	25.6 (16–33)	40	25.2 (17–36)	37
Creatinine (mg/dl)	1.1 (0.7–1.7)	41	1.3 (0.8–1.7)	37
Glucose (mg/dl)	74 (50–114)	41	83 (55–132)	37
SGOT/AST (IU)	63 (26–349)	41	59 (16–135)	37
SGPT/ALT (IU)	6 (0–26)	41	4 (0–11)	37
Alkaline phosphatase (IU)	824 (282–2310)	41	769 (321–2950)	37
CPK (IU)	60 (19–167)	16	70 (32–257)	20
Calcium (mg/dl)	9.1 (8.1–10.4)	41	9.2 (6.7–11.0)	37
Phosphorus (mg/dl)	4.6 (2.2–10.4)	41	5.1 (1.8–10.8)	37
Sodium (mEq/l)	141 (136–146)	41	140 (135–146)	37
Potassium (mEq/l)	3.9 (2.8–4.9)	41	4.3 (3.3–6.0)	37
Total bilirubin (mg/dl)	0.13 (0–0.8)	39	0.08 (0–0.3)	35

RBC, red blood cell; WBC, white blood cell; SGOT/AST, serum glutamate oxaloacetate transaminase/aspartate aminotransferase; SGPT/ALT, serum glutamate pyruvate transaminase/alanine aminotransferase; CPK, creatine phosphokinase.

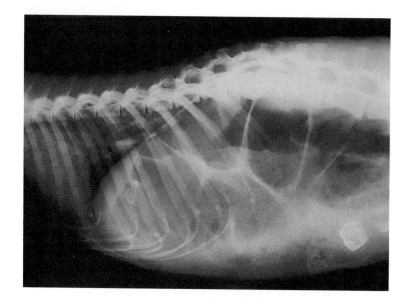

FIGURE 43–1. Radiograph of an aged adult female Matschie's tree kangaroo, demonstrating pneumonia caused by mycobacteriosis, as seen by the increased density in the diaphragmatic lobes. Also visible are a small trichobezoar, several gallstones, and spondylosis of the lumbar vertebra.

A disease survey reported an 8% incidence of MCB in animals older than 2 years of age. A review of the Matschie's tree kangaroo deaths at the National Zoological Park (Washington, D.C., and Front Royal, Virginia) found that of 28 deaths between 1975 and 1995, 25% of animals older than 2 years had MCB infections. Mycobacteriosis is the major infectious disease and cause of death of these species. The disease is further complicated by the tree kangaroo's apparently impaired immune reactivity, which probably affects the infection rate, course of the disease, and response to therapy. Some evidence suggests that a possible deficiency of cell-mediated immunity occurs in some marsupials with tuberculosis.[11] It appears that the lowered immune response for MAC does not predispose to other bacterial or fungal infections, inasmuch as the reported rate of these infections is not elevated.

Even with this high incidence, MCB is probably underreported because diagnosis is difficult, both before and after death. The tuberculin skin tests with avian mycobacterial antigens are inconclusive and are currently not recommended because they may alter immunologic evaluations. Causative organisms have been cultured from tracheal washes of several clinically normal animals that have remained normal for more than 3.5 years, which further confuses diagnostic tests and screening.

It is prudent to consider any ill tree kangaroo as possibly having MCB until proven otherwise, because the presenting signs may include weight loss, dyspnea, lameness, abscesses, neurologic problems, or blindness. Radiography aids in detecting pneumonia (Figs. 43–1, 43–2) and osteomyelitis (Fig. 43–3) caused by MCB. Radiographic signs of osteomyelitis can occur within 2 weeks of the initial lameness; therefore, repeat radiographs are indicated. In tree kangaroos, the hemogram often appears unresponsive even in advanced disease; the white blood cell and fibrinogen levels remain within expected normal limits. A diagnosis of MCB is made after the identification of the acid-fast organism by culturing or DNA probe from the suspected lesion.

Treatment of MCB is difficult, prolonged, and currently only moderately successful because the organisms are resistant to many antitubercular drugs; therefore, combinations of several drugs are required.[5] Treatment regimens include amikacin, 3 mg/kg BID; rifabutin, 20 mg/kg SID orally; ethambutol, 20 mg/kg SID orally; and azithromycin, 20 mg/kg SID orally. Amikacin is discontinued after 10 to 12 weeks. The oral medications have been continued for more than 3 years with no adverse effects, but mycobacterial organisms are still cultured from tracheal washes. The further suppression of the cellular immune responses occurs during the clinical course of the disease. Several appar-

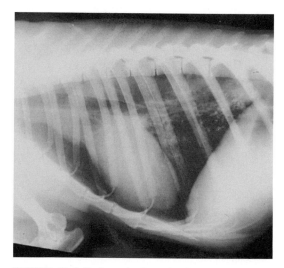

FIGURE 43–2. Radiograph of an adult female Matschie's tree kangaroo with extensive pneumonia in the apical and diaphragmatic lobes, caused by mycobacteriosis.

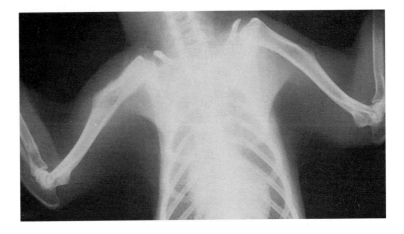

FIGURE 43–3. Radiograph of an adult female Matschie's tree kangaroo with osteomyelitis of the left humerus, caused by mycobacteriosis. In a radiograph taken 2 weeks before this radiograph, the humerus appeared normal.

ent "cures" have occurred in animals that had an isolated bone lesion that was completely curetted in addition to systemic multidrug therapy.[3]

Currently, tree kangaroos with MCB are not considered especially infectious to other tree kangaroos because the serotypes and DNA types of the MAC from diseased animals are usually diverse, indicating an environmental source (J. N. Maslow, personal communication, 1996). However, an infected individual excreting high concentrations of mycobacterial organisms from an osteomyelitis fistula or coughing animals in close contact might transmit the disease to another tree kangaroo.

The MAC organisms are common environmental organisms cultured from many sources (water, soil); therefore, tree kangaroos have continuous exposure to them. Prevention is being directed toward immunostimulation or vaccination of young animals.

VIRAL INFECTIONS

There are no documented reports of viral infections causing deaths in tree kangaroos.

PARASITIC PROBLEMS

Tree kangaroos can become infested with the same spectrum of intestinal parasites as other marsupials and eutherian mammals.[2] Parasites reported include protozoa, roundworms, and tapeworms, which respond to standard therapy with common anthelmintics. Parasitic problems are rarely encountered in established collections.

There are isolated reports of tree kangaroos' becoming infested with ticks, which were removed manually.

GASTROINTESTINAL PROBLEMS

In a 1989 survey, the major problems reported in tree kangaroos were related to the digestive system, with 35% involving the mouth and 18% associated with gastric trichobezoars.

Dental problems are not uncommon and range from receding gums to abscesses of the teeth and surrounding tissue. Treatment includes systemic antibiotics and surgical intervention to remove severely affected teeth and provide drainage. Exposure to the teeth is difficult because the mouth does not open wide, so the clinician's sense of smell is important in detecting infected teeth. Teeth with exposed roots can be salvaged if the tooth remains solid and the root is cleaned of tarter by dental treatments every month.

Trichobezoars are not an uncommon finding in the stomach of older tree kangaroos and may indicate impaired mastication and excessive grooming[15] (Fig. 43–4; see also Fig. 43–1). Trichobezoars are diagnosed by radiography or abdominal palpation. Their presence usually causes no clinical signs, and they need not be removed. In a radiographic survey of 29 Matschie's tree kangaroos at the National Zoological Park, 25% had at least one trichobezoar. If clinical signs of weight loss and decreased appetite develop, the trichobezoar can be removed via a gastrotomy.

The digestive system of tree kangaroos is surprisingly hardy. The authors have given broad-spectrum antibiotics to treat MCB for prolonged periods with minimal digestive upset. When digestive upset occurs (bloating and/or diarrhea), it is usually secondary to other medical problems and usually contributes to a poor prognosis.

Bacterial enteritis is not uncommon; *Salmonella* and *Yersinia* organisms have been identified as enteric pathogens causing death in tree kangaroos.

High iron storage has been seen in the livers of several aged animals, which poses the question of acquired hemochromatosis. It is speculated that some tree kangaroos may store iron very efficiently, as do other rainforest species, so systemic iron supplements should be used with caution or not at all. Gallstones are incidental findings on radiographs in aged animals.

RESPIRATORY PROBLEMS

The major respiratory problem is mycobacterial infections, but other pathogenic bacteria have caused fatal

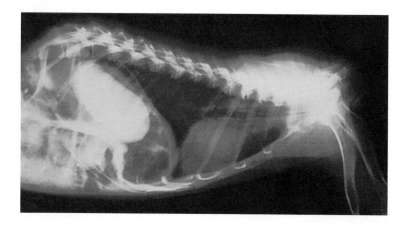

FIGURE 43–4. Radiograph of an aged female Matschie's tree kangaroo with a large gastric trichobezoar. This animal had no clinical signs.

pneumonia. There are several reports of fatal pulmonary toxoplasmosis, which is also seen in other marsupials. When respiratory problems are combined, they account for the second highest cause of medical problems in tree kangaroos.

CARDIOVASCULAR PROBLEMS

An increased incidence of myocardial problems is seen in tree kangaroos. Cardiomyopathy has resulted in several acute deaths of animals within 3 days of an anesthetic episode, and there are several other reports of acute heart failure. Diagnosis of an enlarged heart can be a problem because the chest cavity is relatively small in these species. Other heart problems observed are microinfarcts and arterioscleroses.[14]

MUSCULOSKELETAL PROBLEMS

Tree kangaroos develop the same maladies with age that other mammals do, including arthritis of the spine and pelvis. Infectious problems such as osteomyelitis are usually associated with MCB. Nutritional myopathy caused by the lack of selenium or vitamin E is still reported in several collections.

PREVENTIVE MEDICAL PROCEDURES

Newly arrived animals should be quarantined for at least 30 days before entry into an established collection. During this period, at least two fecal samples are examined and found negative for parasites. A complete physical examination is performed with the animal under general anesthesia, with particular attention to the teeth. Radiographs of the chest and long bones are obtained to screen for MCB. If suspect lung lesions are observed, a tracheal wash is performed and cultured for mycobacteria and examined cytologically with stains for acid-fast bacteria. Nails should be examined and trimmed if necessary each time the animal is under anesthesia.

Long nails get caught during climbing and break off or lead to a fracture of the toe. If the nails are cut too short, they bleed. Some collections vaccinate with tetanus toxoid and clostridium bacterins.

A complete necropsy with cultures for mycobacteria and other suspected pathogens is an important component of the preventive medical program for tree kangaroos.

MISCELLANEOUS PROBLEMS

Tree kangaroos are long-lived marsupials, with a life expectancy of 10 to 12 years. The life span of male tree kangaroos is shorter than that of females; this phenomenon is also reported in dasyurid marsupials (*Antechinus stuartii*).[1] Neoplasms occur but at a lower incidence than in other marsupials.

The tail can become dry and scaly and may reflect dietary or humidity problems. The dryness responds to application of petroleum jelly or A & D ointment. Many animals have a hairless area just below the base of the tail, which is a normal wear spot associated with their sitting posture. The blood supply to the tail seems to be marginal, and tail wounds appear to heal slowly. If an injury leads to amputation, it is not uncommon for delayed healing at the surgery site, which in turn may necessitate further surgery.

REFERENCES

1. Barker IK, Beveridge I, Bradley AJ, et al: Observations on spontaneous stress-related mortality among males of the dasyurid marsupial *Antechinus stuartii* Macleay. Aust J Zool 26:435–447, 1978.
2. Beveridge I: Marsupial parasitic diseases. *In* Fowler ME (ed): Zoo and Wildlife Medicine: Current Therapy 3. Philadelphia, WB Saunders, pp 288–291, 1993.
3. Burns DL, Wallace RS, Teare JA: Successful treatment of mycobacterial osteomyelitis in a Matschie's tree kangaroo (*Dendrolagus matschiei*). J Zoo Wildl Med 25:274–280, 1994.
4. Bush M, Graves J, O'Brien SJ, et al: Dissociative anesthesia in free-ranging male koalas and selected marsupials in captivity. Aust Vet J 67:449–451, 1990.
5. Bush M, Montali RJ, Murray S, et al: The diagnosis, treatment and prevention of tuberculosis in captive Matschie's tree kangaroos (*Dendrolagus matschiei*). Proceedings of the American Association of Zoo Veterinarians, East Lansing, MI, pp 312–314, 1995.
6. Finnie EP: Monotremes and marsupials (Monotremata and Marsu-

pialia). *In* Fowler ME (ed): Zoo and Wild Animal Medicine, 2nd ed. Philadelphia, WB Saunders, pp 555–562, 1986.

7. Vasey N, Frank ES (eds): Tree Kangaroo Husbandry Resource Manual. San Diego, in press.

8. Goss LJ: Muscle dystrophy in tree kangaroos associated with feeding of cod liver oil and its response to alpha-tocopherol. Zoologica 25:523–524, 1940.

9. Kennedy S, Montali RJ, James AE Jr, et al: Bone lesions in three tree kangaroos. J Am Vet Med Assoc 173:1094–1098, 1978.

10. MacKenzie W, Fletcher K: Mega-vitamin E responsive myopathy in Goodfellow's tree kangaroos associated with confinement. *In* Montali RJ, Migaki G (eds): Pathology of Zoo Animals. Washington, DC, Smithsonian Institution Press, pp 34–39, 1980.

11. Moriarty KM: A possible deficiency of cell-mediated immunity in the opossum in relation to tuberculosis. N Z Vet J 21:167–169, 1973.

12. Ott-Joslin J: Mycobacterial infections in tree kangaroos. *In* Proceedings of the American Association of Zoo Veterinarians, South Padre Island, TX, pp 35–42, 1990.

13. Roberts M, Hutchins M (eds): Bulletin No. 1: The Biology and Management of Tree Kangaroos. Wheeling, WV, AAZPA Marsupial and Montreme Advisory Group, 1980.

14. Schoon HA, Rosenbrunch M, Ruempler G: Systemic arterial calcinosis in a grey tree kangaroo *Dendrolagus inustus*, resembling Monckeberg type arteriosclerosis in man. J Comp Pathol 95:319–324, 1985.

15. Zdziarski JM, Bush M: Clinical Challenge Case 3. J Zoo Wildlife Med 22:507–509, 1991.

CHIROPTERA

CHAPTER 44

Medical Management of Megachiropterans

DARRYL J. HEARD

The mammalian order Chiroptera is subdivided into Microchiroptera and Megachiroptera. Although this classification implies "little" and "big" bats, there are some relatively large microchiropterans (for example, the false vampire bat, *Vampyrum spectrum*, 145 to 190 g) and small megachiropterans (for example, the dog-faced fruit bat, *Cynopteris brachyotis*, 30 g). The Megachiroptera includes a single family of fruit- and nectar-feeding bats, the Pteropodidae, with 42 genera and 166 species.[13] This family is confined to the subtropical and tropical regions of the Old World, east to Australia and the Caroline and Cook islands.[19] The term *flying fox* is generally applied to the large bats of the genera *Pteropus* and *Acerodon;* many of the other species are called *fruit bats*.

In 1994, there were 12 megachiropteran species in North American zoological institutions (Table 44–1). There are seven flying fox species listed in Appendix 1 of the Convention on International Trade in Endangered Species (CITES): Truk (*Pteropus insularis*); Marianas (*P. mariannus*); Ponape (*P. molossinus*); Mortlock (*P. phaeocephalus*); large Palau (*P. pilosus*); Samoan (*P. samoensis*); and insular (*P. tonganus*).[8] All other megachiropterans belonging to the genera *Pteropus* and *Acerodon* are listed in Appendix 2 of the CITES publi-

cation.[8] In the United States, all *Pteropus* spp. are classified as injurious wildlife; a permit is required from the U.S. Fish and Wildlife Service for their possession. This permit requires that they be housed and transported in double-wired enclosures. Additionally, a permit is required from the Centers for Disease Control and Prevention (CDC) for importation and movement of bats within the United States.

CLINICAL MANAGEMENT

Housing

It is unfortunate that many zoological institutions have historically housed megachiropterans in dark, humid, cool cave exhibits without consideration for their true environmental and behavioral requirements. Although many megachiropterans seek concealed roosting sites, others roost in trees (for example, *Pteropus, Acerodon,* and *Eidolon*).[13] Some of these roost aggregations may number in the thousands. Although some seasonally disperse, many species use the same roosting sites year-round.[13] Although mostly nocturnal, some megachiropterans may be active during the day even in bright

TABLE 44–1. Megachiropteran Species at North American Zoological Institutions in 1994

Common Name (Species)	Distribution*
Dog-faced fruit bat *(Cynopteris brachyotis)*	Sri Lanka, Andaman and Nicobar Islands, southern Burma, Thailand, southern China, Indochina, Malay Peninsula, Sumatra and nearby islands, Java, Kangean Islands, Borneo and many associated islands, Bali, Sulawesi, Philippines
Straw-colored fruit bat *(Eidolon helvum)*	Southwestern Arabian Peninsula, most of the forest and savannah zones of Africa south of the Sahara, and Madagascar; most widely distributed of African fruit bats
Wahlberg's epauleted bat *(Epomophorus wahlbergi)*	Cameroon and Somalia south to South Africa
Indian flying fox *(Pteropus giganteus)*	Pakistan, India, Nepal, Sikkim, Bhutan, Burma, Sri Lanka, Maldive Islands (Indian Ocean)
Island flying fox *(Pteropus hypomelanus)*	Sulawesi and on small islands from the Bay of Bengal and the Malay Peninsula to New Guinea and the Solomons
Grey-headed flying fox *(Pteropus poliocephalus)*	Southeastern Queensland, New South Wales, Victoria
Golden-mantled flying fox *(Pteropus pumilus)*	Palmas, Balut, Tablas, and Mindoro islands (Philippines)
Rodrigues island flying fox *(Pteropus rodricensis)*	Rodrigues island (Indian Ocean)
Malayan flying fox *(Pteropus vampyrus)*	Southern Thailand and Indochina, Tenasserim, Malaysia, Indonesia, Philippines
Pemba Island flying fox *(Pteropus voeltzkowi)*	Pemba Island off northeast coast of Tanzania
Egyptian fruit bat *(Rousettus aegyptiacus)*	Turkey and Cyprus to Pakistan, Arabian Peninsula, Egypt, most of Africa south of the Sahara
Ruwenzori long-haired fruit bat *(Rousettus lanosus)*	Sudan, northeastern Zaire, Kenya, Uganda, Rwanda

*Data from reference 19.

sunlight. As flying mammals, bats require adequate space for roosting and exercise; prolonged confinement to small cages will render them flightless. Treatment requires graded periods of flight in increasingly larger cages. It is also necessary to provide a route from the cage floor back to the roost sites. Circular rather than square cages promote flight. Megachiropterans are sensitive to cold and hot environmental temperatures; their thermoneutral zone is approximately 20° to 30°C. As the temperature rises, they spread and flap their wings, and at high temperatures, they urinate on and lick themselves to encourage evaporative cooling. Prolonged restraint in a hot environment, exacerbated by high humidity and confinement of the wings to the body, results in hyperthermia and death.

Physical Restraint

Megachiropterans will rapidly deliver a powerful defensive bite when restrained. Their thumbs and associated claws will scratch an unprotected handler and are used to pull a finger in close for a bite. The digital claws are also very sharp. Long-sleeved leather gloves are indicated for restraint of large species. An appropriately sized towel or drape is also recommended to confine the wings. Restraint time should be minimized to prevent hyperthermia and stress. Prolonged restraint produces marked elevations in cortisol and glucose.[29]

Anesthesia

In island flying foxes (400 to 600 g), ketamine alone (30 to 37.5 mg/kg intramuscularly [IM]) produced short-term chemical restraint, but poor muscle relaxation and struggling during recovery.[5] A xylazine (2 mg/kg IM) and ketamine (10 mg/kg IM) combination produced short-term immobilization (30 minutes) with good muscle relaxation and quiet recovery.[5]

Inhalation anesthesia is recommended for short-term and long-term restraint. Isoflurane (5% by mask decreased to 2.5% when relaxed) provides rapid (1 to 2 minutes) induction and recovery as well as easily adjusted anesthetic depth. Megachiropterans larger than 350 g are intubated with a 2-mm or larger internal diameter endotracheal tube. Good anesthetic relaxation and dorsal recumbency facilitate intubation. For visualization of the glottis, gauze is placed around the upper and lower jaws to open the mouth, and the tongue is displaced forward (Fig. 44–1). A laryngoscope with a small straight pediatric blade is used for illumination. Topical anesthetic applied to the glottal opening decreases reflex coughing. Glycopyrrolate (0.01 mg/kg IM) administered before induction will reduce the sometimes profuse pharyngeal secretions. Heart rate and rhythm and peripheral blood flow are monitored with a Doppler flow probe secured over the tibial artery behind the knee or the pedal artery on the palmar surface of the feet. Temperature is monitored with a probe placed in the rectum or esophagus; the latter is preferred because it more accurately reflects core body temperature. To prevent hypothermia, the wings are folded to the body, and the animal is placed on a circulating water blanket and, when possible, wrapped in a blanket or bubble-wrap. Electric and chemical heating pads should be avoided because they have caused severe burns. For recovery, bats are wrapped in a drape and left in a quiet cage to prevent struggling and wing-flapping; the animals are usually sufficiently recovered when they crawl out of the wrap.

Hematology

Venipuncture is facilitated by anesthesia. In megachiropterans 150 g or larger, blood volumes are collected

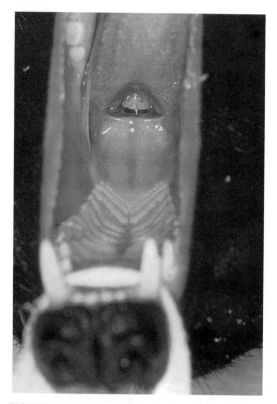

FIGURE 44–1. The oral cavity of a dorsally recumbent, anesthetized island flying fox (*Pteropus hypomelanus*) before intubation. Gauze has been placed around the upper and lower jaws to open the mouth, and the tongue has been pulled forward and upward. The epiglottis is visible at the base of the tongue.

from the median artery or vein on the lateral aspect of the humerus (Fig. 44–2). Small blood samples are collected into microhematocrit tubes from the cephalic vein, which extends along the leading edge of the patagium (Fig. 44–3), and from pedal veins. I prefer heparinized blood samples for biochemical analysis; this allows the blood to be centrifuged immediately after collection and the plasma to be removed from the blood cells and frozen until analysis. If the plasma remains in contact with the red cells, for even a few hours, there will be marked spurious elevations in potassium and decreases in sodium, chloride, and glucose concentrations.

Surgery and Postoperative Care

Megachiropterans aggressively lick and chew sutures, bandages, and external fixators. Where possible, sutures are buried. Lightweight Elizabethan collars will prevent access to surgical wounds and external fixators (Fig. 44–4). These collars need to be of large diameter to prevent access to many parts of the body. Consequently, care must be taken to ensure the animal is able to feed and drink. Use of an Elizabethan collar in a golden-mantled flying fox (*P. pumilus*) was associated with

paraphimosis caused by strangulation of the penile blood supply by entrapped hairs at the base of the penis. This was assumed to be caused by the animal's inability to adequately groom itself. The wing membranes make bandaging difficult, and their incorporation into a bandage will cause ischemic necrosis of those membranes.

Common injuries include wing-tip trauma, bite wounds, and thumb injuries from identification bands. Wing-tip trauma is a captive disease caused by inadvertent contact with the cage wire and exacerbated by small enclosures and lack of suitable perches. Square cages result in more wire contact, particularly with large bats, because it is difficult to turn in flight. Suitable perches include a variety of wooden branches and thick ropes. Although most wing-tip injuries resolve without treatment, healing may be prolonged and granulation tissue response pronounced; exposed bone is amputated. Bite wounds are treated as in other mammals; antibiotics are indicated for large wounds and delayed healing. Thumb bands will frequently produce strangulation and should be routinely checked.

The use of excessive force when extracting subadult animals from wire will result in distal femur epiphyseal fractures (Fig. 44–5). The digits have a locking mechanism associated with a tendon that causes pedal flexion. The epiphyseal fractures are repaired with a cross-pinning technique. Wing amputation, although rendering an animal flightless, does not preclude its inclusion back in the colony. Wing membrane burns occurred in

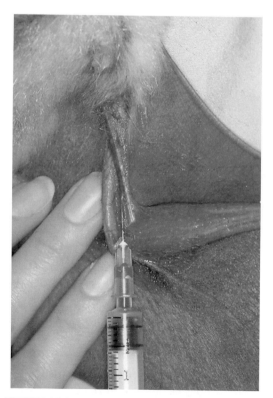

FIGURE 44–2. Venipuncture in a golden-mantled flying fox (*Pteropus pumilus*). The needle has been introduced into the median vein as it passes over the left humerus.

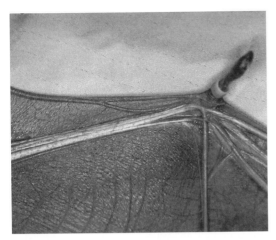

FIGURE 44–3. The left wing of a golden-mantled flying fox (*Pteropus pumilus*). The cephalic vein is visualized along the leading edge of the wing membrane. This vessel is used in small bats for blood collection into microhematocrit tubes after perforation with a small needle.

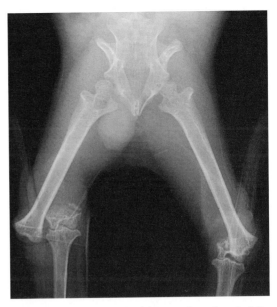

FIGURE 44–5. Radiograph of the upper legs of a subadult island flying fox (*Pteropus hypomelanus*). Note the bilateral epiphyseal fractures caused by excessive pulling force used during removal of the bat from a wire enclosure.

one anesthetized animal in which a chemical heat pack was placed directly against the skin. This injury initially produced large blisters and weeping wounds, and then dry areas in the wing membranes that sloughed, leaving fistulas. These subsequently scarred and closed over. Small to medium lacerations in the wing membranes will usually heal spontaneously and, surprisingly, completely close over. Excessive scarring will decrease membrane elasticity and cause wing contracture. Lacerations involving the wing edges will not heal without suturing because forces will keep the wound distracted.

Pharmacology

There is no pharmacokinetic information available for any drugs used in bats; dosages are extrapolated from those used for other small mammals. Megachiropterans readily ingest fruit-flavored drug preparations. Intramuscular injections into the forearms are avoided to prevent muscle damage. Bats do not have a wide sternum, as birds do, and pectoral injections can result in inadvertent thoracic injection.

Preventive Medicine

All bats should be examined at least once a year. There are no currently recommended vaccinations; this may change with the identification of potentially zoonotic paramyxoviruses and lyssaviruses in Australian flying foxes (see next section). Parasite control is directed at detection and treatment and appropriate and frequent sanitation of housing. For transport, the CDC requires that bats be free of rabies and *Histoplasma capsulatum*. Bats from captive collections should be quarantined a minimum of 90 days. During quarantine, a minimum of three fecal floatations should be performed to detect nematode ova. Additionally, pooled rectal fecal samples are cultured for *H. capsulatum*.

DISEASES

Bacterial

Bite wounds are usually infected (streptococci, staphylococci, and occasional anaerobes), and osteomyelitis

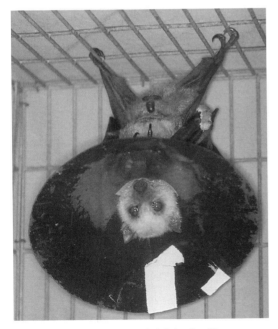

FIGURE 44–4. A golden-mantled flying fox (*Pteropus pumilus*) with an Elizabethan collar to prevent self-trauma to an external fixator placed on a fractured thumb (digit 1). The collar is constructed of used radiograph film and is relatively large.

may result from deep wounds. Septic arthritis and disseminated abscesses caused by bacteremia occur in juvenile and immunocompromised bats. Fatal septic arthritis and meningoencephalitis associated with *Listeria monocytogenes* have been observed in a juvenile Rodrigues island (*Pteropus rodricensis*) and an island flying fox (*P. hypomelanus*). A possible source of *L. monocytogenes* was rotting fruit and vegetable remnants in the enclosure.

Parasitic

Ectoparasites are common in wild bats and include many tick, mite, and fly species.[3, 28] They are usually reported as incidental findings rather than pathogens,[28] and most infestations in captivity are self-limiting. However, it is important that all ectoparasites be removed; they may transmit hemoparasites and zoonotic viruses.

Several megachiropteran hemoparasites have been identified. *Hepatocystis* species was observed in golden-mantled flying foxes (*P. pumilus*) imported from the Philippines. The parasites were not associated with disease and disappeared from the blood during a 12-month period. *Hepatocystis levinei*, identified in the grey-headed flying fox (*P. poliocephalus*), is transmitted by *Culicoides nubeculosus*.[14] A study of trypanosomiasis in 247 East African bats found 21% infected, but none were megachiropterans.[30] However, *Trypanosoma megachiropterorum* has been described from *P. tonganus* from Tonga.[17] This was the first report of a bat *Megatrypanum* outside America and Africa, and the first of a Pacific bat trypanosome.[17]

The nematode *Toxocara pteropodis* is found in southeast Asian and Australian flying foxes. Adult parasites live in the upper gastrointestinal tract of suckling pups.[20] Eggs passed in the feces of the pups are ingested by adult flying foxes during grooming and feeding.[20] Fertile eggs are ovoid to spheroid, 80 to 110 μm in diameter, and the outer layer is pitted.[21] The ova are bulkier than those of related ascaridoids because of a thicker external coat that, although not providing mechanical strength, is thought to protect against dessication.[21] The eggs hatch, and the larvae pass through the portal system to the liver where they encyst. In adult male bats, the larvae do not develop any further. In adult female bats, the larvae are activated at the end of parturition; during lactation they migrate to the mammary gland, where they pass in the milk to the suckling pup to complete the cycle. The adult worms are shed from the pup when it ceases to suckle and begins to eat solid food. There are usually only a few adult worms per pup (5 or fewer), and they rarely cause morbidity or mortality. However, a captive island flying fox pup died of an intestinal volvulus associated with more than 20 worms.[7] Furthermore, two *P. poliocephalus* pups died from worms obstructing the upper airway and gallbladder, respectively.[22] Despite these examples, it is questionable whether it is necessary to treat *T. pteropodis* in captivity. *T. pteropodis* was once thought to be a possible cause of human hepatitis, but this has subsequently been disproved. Several filarid species

have been identified in the peritoneum of the Malayan (*P. vampyrus*) (*Litomosa maki* and *L. miniopteri*)[27] and island *P. hypomelarus* (*Makifilaria inderi*)[12] flying foxes from Malaysia. Ivermectin (400 μg/kg IM) and fenbendazole (50 to 100 mg/kg orally) have been used for the treatment of nematode infections.

Viral

Until recently there was very little information on megachiropteran viruses. However, recent events in Australia and Africa have precipitated an increased interest because of their suspected role in harboring several zoonotic viruses.

LYSSAVIRUSES (RABIES)

Bat lyssaviruses have been reviewed by Constantine.[1] Within the family Rhabdoviridae the genus *Lyssavirus* contains five serotypes: classic rabies virus (serotype 1), Lagos bat virus (serotype 2), Mokola virus (serotype 3), Duvenhage virus (serotype 4), and European bat virus (serotype 5).[3] All can cause rabies or rabies-like diseases in infected animals.[4] In 1996 in Australia, a 5-month-old female black flying fox (*Pteropus alecto*) was found, unable to fly, under a tree.[4] Histologic examination of brain tissue revealed a severe nonsuppurative encephalitis. A second case, in 1995, was identified after retrospective examination of archived paraffin-embedded tissues.[4] The affected animal, a juvenile female of the same species, was reported to be more aggressive than usual and was euthanized. Although the encephalitis was very mild, many eosinophilic cytoplasmic inclusion bodies were present in various parts of the brain. An indirect immunoperoxidase test for rabies performed on paraffin-embedded tissues with an antirabies monoclonal antibody showed positive reactions over wide areas of the brains of both bats. Similar reactions were observed in neuronal cytoplasms in gastrointestinal nerve plexuses. Electron microscopy examination of ultrathin sections of hippocampus from the 1996 bat showed aggregates of viral nucleocapsids within the cytoplasm of cell bodies. Virus was isolated from a weanling mouse injected with tissue homogenate. Sequence comparisons were done by using the nucleocapsid proteins of known lyssaviruses and the virus now designated pteropid lyssavirus. Phylogenetic analysis of both the nucleotide and amino acid sequences showed that the virus is closely related to the European bat virus as well as to the classic street rabies strains. The virus has subsequently been identified by immunohistochemical techniques in five bats in three different virus isolations.[4] Some of these bats were from another species, the little red (*P. scapulatus*) and from locations as far apart as 1700 km along the Australian East Coast. After the discovery of the virus in flying foxes, the virus was isolated from a Queensland woman in whom the virus produced neurologic disease, coma, and death. The woman was a rehabilitation worker who was scratched by a sick fruit bat. Studies at the CDC indicate that human, veterinary, and subunit vaccines protect against lyssavirus, and sera of rabies-vaccinated persons neutralizes the virus, as does hyperimmune reference sera.

BAT PARAMYXOVIRUS (EQUINE MORBILLIVIRUS)

Two outbreaks of a previously unknown disease occurred in humans and horses in 1994 in Queensland, Australia.[31] The outbreaks occurred within 1 month of each other at two locations approximately 1000 km apart. In one incident, 14 of 21 infected horses died or were euthanized because of severe acute respiratory disease. One of two humans with less well-defined clinical signs also died. In the second incident, one person and two horses died. A paramyxovirus isolated from four of the horses and one human was designated equine morbillivirus. Serologic sampling (neutralizing antibody) demonstrated antibody in all four Australian flying fox species—spectacled (*P. conspicillatus*), black (*P. alecto*), little red (*P. scapulatus*), and grey-headed (*P. poliocephalus*)—with a prevalence rate of about 9%. A virus indistinguishable from equine morbillivirus and defined as bat paramyxovirus was subsequently isolated. This virus has not been associated with disease in flying foxes or in persons who have had extensive exposure to bats. Research is ongoing into the biology of this virus and its mode of transmission.

FILOVIRUSES (EBOLA)

Filoviruses are best known for their propensity to cause fatal hemorrhagic disease of humans with person-to-person spread.[25] This lethality suggests primates are incidental victims of infection and not true reservoir hosts. To determine the possible source, a wide range of vertebrates, invertebrates, and even plants were injected with Ebola Zaire isolated from a human patient.[25] This study was based on the principle that animals able to survive with circulating virus for prolonged periods without becoming ill were suspected reservoirs. The virus replicated in microchiropteran and megachiropteran bats. Virus antigen was detected in the lung tissue of one bat and on day 21 from the feces of a megachiropteran (*Epomorphus wahlbergi*).

KASOKERO (YOGUE)

A virus related to the unclassified virus Yogue was implicated as the cause of a mild to severe illness in four laboratory workers in Uganda.[11] The virus was originally isolated by mouse inoculation from the blood of Egyptian fruit bats (*Rousettus aegyptiacus*) collected from Kasokero cave in Uganda.[11] Serologic studies concluded that the isolates from bats and laboratory workers were strains of the same virus.

NUTRITIONAL

Nutrition is a major problem area in the captive management of bats because of bat diversity, the limited knowledge of nutrient requirements, the small size of most bats, and adaptation for flight. Bat nutrition is reviewed in Chapter 45.

Hypovitaminosis E

Hypovitaminosis E has been associated with dilated cardiomyopathy in flying foxes (see cardiovascular section).[6] The animals had been in captivity for about 2 to 3 years before the development of clinical signs. Significant findings included unmeasurable plasma vitamin E levels in affected bats and low to unmeasurable levels in many bats without dilated cardiomyopathy $(0.10 \pm 0.18 \mu g/ml)$. Tissue levels of alpha tocopherol were much lower in the affected than the unaffected bats. Additionally, gamma tocopherol levels were undetectable in affected bats. The diet was calculated to contain 56 IU/kg (dry basis) of vitamin E. Increasing dietary levels to 240 or more mg/kg appeared to resolve the problem. An important natural source of vitamin E is green leaves. Although large flying foxes have traditionally been thought to feed exclusively on fruits or flowers, it has recently been shown that some species chew leaves and ingest the fiber-free juices.[15] These leaves may be an important source of essential nutrients lacking in a purely frugivorous diet. Captive flying foxes have been observed crawling to the ground to consume or chew grasses.

Fluorosis

Fluorosis-induced multicentric hyperostosis has been reported in three species of flying fox (*P. giganteus, P. poliocephalus,* and *R. aegyptiacus*) from the same facility.[2] All affected bats were more than 2 years old, and the pectoral limb bones were most frequently involved. The initial lesions were discrete, eccentric, asymmetric bone proliferations that frequently coalesced into large raised firm areas. Articular bone surfaces were not involved, and tendons and ligaments diverted around the nodules. Skin overlying the nodules was swollen, taut, warm, smooth, hairless, and predisposed to abrasions. Necropsy bone specimens had markedly raised fluoride levels (2200 to 4700 ppm) compared with similar samples from another collection (290 to 320 ppm). Diet analysis revealed shrimp meal (1400 $\pm$ 200 ppm) and dicalcium phosphate (1900 $\pm$ 300 ppm) to be the main fluoride sources.

Metabolic Bone Disease

Metabolic bone disease was observed in twin Malayan flying fox pups and their mother. Significant clinicopathologic and radiographic findings included decreased cortical bone density, multiple appendicular fractures, and moderate hypocalcemia. This disease problem was attributed to the increased calcium requirement for suckling two pups, a rare occurrence, and marginal dietary content. All animals responded to oral calcium supplementation.

Obesity

Marked obesity has been observed in several island and Rodrigues island flying foxes. This appears to be the result of the reluctance of some animals to exercise and of dominance over the feed bowls in a large group enclosure.

SYSTEMS MEDICINE

Cardiovascular

Cardiovascular anatomy and physiology are reviewed by Kallen.[10] Bat hearts are large relative to body weight (for example, 0.94% for the straw-colored fruit bat [*Eidolon helvum*]). In large megachiropterans, the cardiac apex is moderately inclined to the left and rotated slightly around its anteroposterior axis (Fig. 44–6). In smaller bats, the heart is more inclined and rotated. A bicuspid valve is present where the caudal vena cava enters the large, thin-walled right atrium. Resting heart rates are related to environmental temperature and size; they plateau across the thermoneutral range and increase at low and high temperatures. The electrocardiogram is typically mammalian. All bats have paired, large cranial venae cavae and a single caudal vena cava of moderate to reduced size above the diaphragm. Below the diaphragm the caudal vena cava is huge, very thin walled, and in megachiropterans paired. In pteropids, the internal and external jugular veins are of similar size. Many arteriovenous anastomoses are present in the wing membranes and terminal digits. Lymph nodes are inconspicuous, particularly in the mesentery, and the spleens are relatively large and elongate.

Dilated cardiomyopathy of unknown origin was reported in an Indian flying fox (*P. giganteus*).[18] Dilated cardiomyopathy has also been diagnosed in six island and one Rodrigues island flying fox associated with concurrent hypovitaminosis E.[6] Clinical signs were consistent with decreased myocardial function and development of congestive heart failure: lethargy, reluctance to fly, exercise intolerance, hypothermia, tachyarrhythmias, and, in the later stages, anorexia/cachexia, hepatomegaly (see Fig. 44–6), and cranial edema (Fig. 44–7). Several bats were found dead without previous clinical signs. Diagnosis was based on clinical signs, enlarged cardiac silhouette on thoracic radiographs (see Fig. 44–6), and ultrasonographic evidence of cardiac dilatation, impaired contractility, and hepatomegaly. Cardiac ultrasonography was difficult because of the close apposition of the ribs. Treatment, when attempted, was directed at decreasing cardiac afterload (diltiazem) and circulatory volume (furosemide) and improving contractility (digoxin). Although myocardial damage was irreversible, large doses of injectable vitamin E were administered to prevent further damage.

Respiratory

Although the left lung is undivided, there is an observable shallow, poorly defined notch in some species; the right lung is subdivided into cranial, middle, caudal, and accessory lobes.[16] The maximal aerobic capacities of flying bats and birds of the same size are essentially the same.[16] Even the minimal metabolic requirement of a bat or a bird in level flight is at least 1.5 times greater than the maximal aerobic capacity of a nonflying mammal of the same size.[16] Consequently, megachiropterans at rest are not likely to manifest overt clinical signs until respiratory dysfunction is well advanced. Although respiratory disease is uncommon, I have observed unilateral lung abscesses in several Wahlberg's epaulated fruit bats (*Epomorphus wahlbergi*). Sneezing associated with a clear nasal discharge is relatively common in flying foxes.

Gastrointestinal

Megachiropteran teeth are structurally unique among mammals.[9] The incisors are small; canines are always present; and the cheek teeth are elongated and generally flat.[9] The dental formula varies from (I 2/2, C1/1, PM 3/3, M 2/3) × 2 = 34 in *Pteropus* and *Rousettus* to (I 1/0, C 1/1, PM 3/3, M 1/2) × 2 = 24 in *Nyctimene* and *Paranyctimene*.[19]

The gastrointestinal anatomy of black and grey-headed flying foxes was investigated by dissection and by light and electron microscopy[26]; there was little variation between the two species. The stomach has an elongated terminal part and expanded cardiac and fundic regions that display a relatively thick gastric mucosa and abundant parietal cells.[9, 26] A cecum and appendix are absent. The large intestine is short and features prominent longitudinal folds; the mucosa undergoes a gradual transition, with number and size of villi decreasing in the distal part of the intestine. Although a distinct rectum cannot be distinguished, the colonic mucosa is restricted to a short segment. These anatomic features are postulated to allow fruit bats to process large quantities of food rapidly.[26] This is an obvious advantage to a flying mammal by reducing bulk carried in the digestive tract, enabling it to reduce the energy expenditure associated with foraging flights.

Megachiropterans ingest food, chew it, swallow the fluids and soft material, and disgorge the pulp. Gastrointestinal transit times are very rapid. In black and grey-headed flying foxes, minimum food transit time varied from 12 to 34 minutes for cultivated fruits, but this was extended to 44 minutes by the addition of barium.[26] The fecal composition reflects the diet and may vary from semi-formed to a voluminous liquid. The rectal bacterial flora of four flying fox species was observed to be predominantly gram positive and aerobic (D. J. Heard, unpublished data, 1997). Gastrointestinal disease is uncommon. The teeth of flying foxes, especially wild caught, frequently have areas of discoloration associated with enamel defects; this may reflect dietary calcium deficiency.

Integumentary

Integumentary anatomy and physiology are reviewed by Quay.[23] Bat skin is characterized by the large flight membrane or patagium. This area is subdivided into

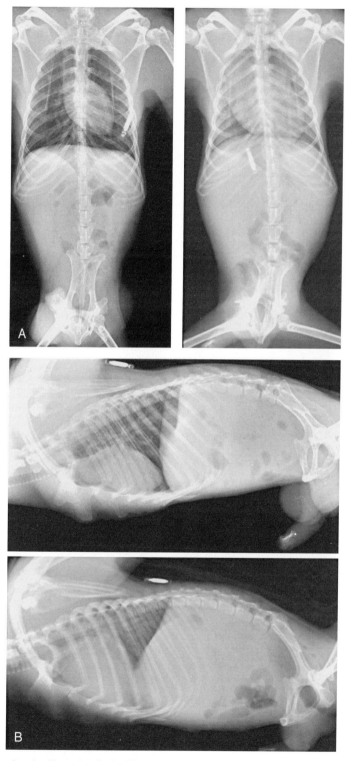

FIGURE 44–6. *A*, Ventrodorsal radiographs of a healthy *(left)* and a male island flying fox *(Pteropus hypomelanus)* with dilated cardiomyopathy *(right)* caused by hypovitaminosis E. *B*, Lateral radiographs of a healthy *(top)* and a male island flying fox *(Pteropus hypomelanus)* with dilated cardiomyopathy *(bottom)* caused by hypovitaminosis E. Note the marked cardiomegaly and abdominal distention resulting from ascites and hepatomegaly.

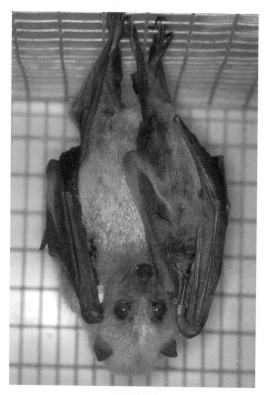

FIGURE 44–7. A golden-mantled flying fox (*Pteropus pumilus*) with cranial edema resulting from hypoproteinemia caused by glomerulonephropathy. Cranial edema has also been observed in bats with congestive heart failure. Note also the single large pup suckling from an axillary mammary gland.

five parts: the propatagium (prebrachium or antebrachial membrane) on the leading edge of the wing; plagiopatagium between the body and digit 5; dactylopatagium between the digits; uropatagium between the legs; and the epiblema, small keel, and skin fold or flap extending from the calcar. The epidermis is thin, but similar to that of other mammals.[23] Elastic fibers form special bands and bundles in the flight membranes, partly in association with slender striated muscle bands that may insert on them. Bat skin contains abundant and diverse nerves and nerve endings. Sebaceous glands in bats are coextensive with hair follicles. Although sudoriferous (sweat) glands are widespread in the skin, sweating is not of significance in thermoregulation. Bats have distinctive and pronounced odors originating from either food materials (for example, the juice of rotten fruit), urine, feces, or skin secretions. Most bats molt once a year, with waves of hair loss and replacement.

The most common integumentary problem is trauma from bite wounds or collision. Alopecia is occasionally observed in juvenile and small megachiropterans. Many of these alopecias spontaneously resolve or appear nonspecifically responsive to increases in dietary micronutrients. Malassezia-like yeasts have been observed in otherwise normal skin biopsies.

Musculoskeletal

The structure and organization of the musculoskeletal system reflects adaptation for flight. These adaptations include reductions in the size and thickness of skeletal elements, the promotion of a sturdy yet lightweight support system, and tremendous elongation of the forelimb elements.[9] The humerus, radius, and all the digits but the thumb are extremely long and slender and serve as a supporting framework for the wing membranes. The hindlegs are rotated 180 degrees at the coxofemoral joint such that the knee appears to bend in the opposite direction (see Fig. 44–6). In most bats, the thoracic vertebrae fit tightly together and form a fairly rigid unit. The rib cages are large and are usually broader than deep. The sternebrae of the body of the sternum are fused into a single structure that in some species is keeled. The manubrium is greatly enlarged and is shaped like a T; the lateral arms connect with the clavicula and first costal cartilages. The scapula acromion is large and strongly built and serves in part to anchor the distal end of the clavicula. The coracoid process is greatly enlarged. The megachiropteran humerus is relatively unspecialized, and the radius is approximately twice as long as the humerus. The ulna is greatly reduced and consists of proximal fusiform and distal thread-like sections. The metacarpals are the longest segments of the digits. The femur is roughly the same length as the tibia. Bat feet are unspecialized and retain the primitive mammalian phalangeal formula (2, 3, 3, 3, 3). The greatest foot specialization is the calcar, a slender bone that articulates proximally with the posterolateral surface of the calcaneus and projects into the adjacent border of the uropatagium. This bone is aerodynamically important by bracing the posterior part of the uropatagium and keeping it taut. Skeletal abnormalities encountered in megachiropterans have included fractures, osteomyelitis, septic arthritis, and fluorosis; these are discussed elsewhere in this chapter. Hypovitaminosis E was associated in several island flying foxes with skeletal muscle myositis and fibrosis.[6]

Renal

The kidneys are essentially the same as other mammals; they are short, tending to a more or less convex shape with a slight concavity at the hilar depression where the ureter and blood supply enter. The kidneys are located lower in the peritoneal cavity in relation to the overall body length than is the case with other mammals of similar size.[9] Some megachiropteran species drink sea water, probably for the minerals and trace elements. I have observed two cases of glomerulonephritis, both of which were associated with polyuria. One animal developed cranial edema secondary to hypoproteinemia caused by urinary protein loss (see Fig. 44–7). The edema spontaneously resolved after treatment with furosemide and glucocorticoids. A funnel is used to catch urine for urinalysis when the bats are first restrained. Occasionally, urine can be collected by cystocentesis.

Reproductive

Reproduction and development are reviewed by Hill and Smith[9] and by Kunz and Pierson.[13] Some megachiropterans appear to have continuous breeding patterns, but the majority are seasonal breeders.[13] This seasonality may be altered in captivity because of photoperiod differences and continuous access to abundant nutrition. Little is known regarding ovulation in megachiropterans; most are thought to spontaneously ovulate.[9] However, the Indian flying fox and *Rousettus leschenaulti* have been shown to be induced ovulators.[9] Mating is usually from behind and associated with much vocalization. Delayed implantation occurs in the African megachiropteran *E. helvum*, with blastocyst implantation coinciding with peak rainfall and maximum fruit availability.[13] Gestation (3 to 6 months) and lactation are relatively long; megachiropterans nurse until they are adult size. Megachiropterans generally have one very large (12% to 15% of maternal body weight) offspring a year. Pregnancy is assessed by abdominal palpation in the anesthetized bat. A small cyst is initially palpated, which enlarges to a large ball. In the later stages of pregnancy, the pup assumes a transverse abdominal position (Fig. 44–8). In some pteropids, parturition is preceded by enlargement and a white discharge from the perivulvar glands and licking of the genital area. Most megachiropterans are born in the head-first position, and the legs are well-developed to facilitate gripping to the mother. They are born well haired and alert, with their eyes open and pointy milk teeth. There are single bilateral axillary nipples and mammary glands. The pups grip the nipples tightly; a blunt probe gently placed in the commissure of the mouth is required to release the pup, if necessary (see Fig. 44–7). The pups are carried for the first few weeks to months by the mother. Mothers will respond to distress calls and retrieve uninjured fallen pups from the cage floor. Male megachiropterans possess penile bacula.

Reproductive disease is uncommon, and fecundity and neonatal survivability are remarkably high with appropriate housing and diet. Dystocia, resolved by either manipulation or cesarean section, has been observed several times in one female Rodrigues island flying fox. Bacterial placentitis has twice been associated with abortion in island flying foxes. Foreign pups will be killed if they are incorrectly placed on the wrong mother. In some megachiropterans, it may be necessary to separate males from females to prevent reproductive aggression, which may result in pup death. Castration and vasectomy have been used for contraception; the testicles readily retract into the abdomen.

Special Senses

Vision and chemoception are the predominant senses. Echolocation only occurs in the genus *Rousettus*.[13] They use these calls only for orientation, and like other megachiropterans, they rely on vision and olfaction for locating food. The anatomy of the megachiropteran eye was reviewed by Suthers.[24] The eyes are large and have unique choroidal papillae with contours that are matched by the retina. Highly specialized pathways lead from the retina to the midbrain. The retina does not possess its own circulation; the central artery is absent and nourishment presumably occurs by diffusion from choroidal capillaries. As would be expected for nocturnal mammals the retina consists almost entirely of rod cells. Color vision and a tapetum lucidum that causes the eyes to shine bright red in a spotlight are present in many megachiropterans. The ethmoturbinal plates are well developed, resulting in elongation of the nasal cavity, which gives them a dog- or fox-like face.

When exposed to light, the pupils are pinpoint. To allow retinal examination it is necessary to dilate the pupils with two applications of 1 drop each of 1% tropicamide (Mydriacyl) and a combination of 10% phenylephrine and 0.3% scopolamine (Murocol) given 45 minutes apart. This regimen will provide dilatation for less than 24 hours, and the bats are maintained in darkness until the pupils return to normal size. The most common ophthalmic problem is traumatic ulceration, which is managed with application of a topical antibiotic ointment. Keratoconjunctivitis sicca of unknown origin has been observed in an island flying fox.

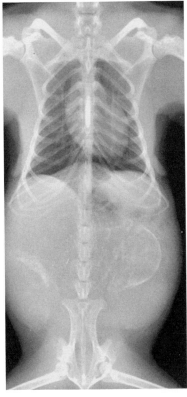

FIGURE 44–8. Radiograph of late-term pregnant island flying fox (*Pteropus hypomelanus*) showing the typical transverse position of a very large fetus.

Acknowledgments

Published as LuBee Foundation Publication Series No. 42.

REFERENCES

1. Constantine DG: Bat medicine, management, and conservation. *In* Fowler M (ed): Zoo and Wild Animal Medicine: Current Therapy 3. Philadelphia, WB Saunders, pp 310–321, 1993.
2. Duncan M, Crawshaw GJ, Mehren KG, et al: Multicentric hyperostosis consistent with fluorosis in captive fruit bats (*Pteropus giganteus*, *P. poliocephalus* and *Rousettus aegyptiacus*). J Zoo Wildl Med 27(3):325–338, 1996.
3. Fain A: The Acari parasitic on bats, biology, pathogenic importance, specificity, parallel evolution of parasites and hosts. Ann Speleologie 31:3–25, 1976.
4. Fraser GC, Hooper PT, Lunt RA, et al: Encephalitis caused by a Lyssavirus in fruit bats in Australia. Emerging Infect Dis 2(4):327–331, 1996 (http://www.cdc.gov/ncidod/EID/eid.htm).
5. Heard DJ, Beale C, Owens J: Ketamine and ketamine: xylazine ED_{50} for short-term immobilization of the island flying fox (*Pteropus hypomelanus*). J Zoo Wildl Med 27(1):44–48, 1996.
6. Heard DJ, Buergelt CD, Snyder PS, et al: Dilated cardiomyopathy associated with hypovitaminosis E in a captive collection of flying foxes (*Pteropus* spp.). J Zoo Wildl Med 27(2):149–157, 1996.
7. Heard DJ, Garner M, Greiner E: Toxocariasis and intestinal volvulus in an island flying fox (*Pteropus hypomelanus*). J Zoo Wildl Med 26(4):550–552, 1995.
8. Hemley G (ed): International Wildlife Trade: A CITES Sourcebook. Washington, DC, Island Press, 1994.
9. Hill JE, Smith JD: Bats: A Natural History. Austin, University of Texas Press, 1992.
10. Kallen FC: The cardiovascular system of bats: structure and function. *In* Wimsatt WA (ed): Biology of Bats. New York, Academic Press, pp 289–483, 1977.
11. Kalunda M, Mukwaya A, Lule M, et al: Kasokero virus: a new human pathogen from bats (*Rousettus aegyptiacus*) in Uganda. Am J Trop Med Hyg 35(2):387–392, 1986.
12. Krishnasamy M, Singh M, Iyamperumal R: *Makifilaria inderi* gen. et sp. nov. (Filarioidea: Onchocercidae) from the island flying fox, *Pteropus hypomelanus* (Temminck) in Malaysia. Southeast Asian J Trop Med Public Health 12(2):185–188, 1981.
13. Kunz TH, Pierson ED: Bats of the world: an introduction. *In* Nowak M (ed): Walker's Bats of the World. Baltimore, Johns Hopkins University Press, pp 1–46, 1994.
14. Landau I, Humphrey-Smith I, Chabaud AG, et al: Description and experimental transmission of the haemoproteid *Hepatocystis levinei* n. sp., a parasite of Australian Chiroptera. Ann Parasitol Hum Comp 60(4):373–382, 1985.
15. Lowry FB: Green-leaf fractionation by fruit bats: is this feeding behaviour a unique nutritional strategy for herbivores? Aust Wildl Res 16:203–206, 1989.
16. Maina JN, Thomas SP, Hyde DM: A morphometric study of the lungs of different sized bats: correlations between structure and function of chiropteran lung. Phil Trans R Soc Lond B 333:31–50, 1991.
17. Marinkelle CJ: *Trypanosoma* (*Megatrypanum*) *megachiropterorum* sp. n. from the flying fox, *Pteropus tonganus* (Quoy & Gaimard). J Protozool 26(3):352–353, 1979.
18. Miller RE, Gaber CE, Williams GA, et al: Cardiomyopathy in a fruit bat. Proceedings of the American Association of Zoo Veterinarians, Chicago, pp 133–134, 1986.
19. Nowak M (ed): Walker's Bats of the World. Baltimore, Johns Hopkins University Press, 1994.
20. Prociv P: Larval migration in oral and parenteral *Toxocara pteropodis* infections and a comparison with *T. canis* dispersal in the flying fox, *Pteropus poliocephalus*. Int J Parasitol 19(8):891–896, 1989.
21. Prociv P: Observations on the morphology of *Toxocara pteropodis* eggs. J Helminthol 64(4):271–277, 1990.
22. Prociv P: Aberrant migration by *Toxocara pteropodis* in flying foxes—two case reports. J Wildl Dis 26(4):532–534, 1990.
23. Quay WB: Integument and derivatives. *In* Wimsatt WA (ed): Biology of Bats. New York, Academic Press, pp 1–56, 1970.
24. Suthers RA: Vision, olfaction and taste. *In* Wimsatt WA (ed): Biology of Bats. New York, Academic Press, pp 265–309, 1970.
25. Swanepoel R, Leman PA, Burt FJ, et al: Experimental inoculation of plants and animals with Ebola virus. Emerging Infect Dis 2(4), 1996 (http://www.cdc.gov/ncidod/EID/eid.htm).
26. Tedman RA, Hall LS: The morphology of the gastrointestinal tract and food transit time in the fruit bats *Pteropus alecto* and *P. poliocephalus* (Megachiroptera). Aust J Zool 33(5):625–640, 1985.
27. Tibayrenc M, Bain O, Ramachandran CP: Two new species of *Litomosa* (Filarioidea) from bats. Bulletin du Museum National d' Histoire Naturelle, Paris, 4th series 1(sect A):183–189, 1979.
28. Whitaker JO: Collecting and preserving ectoparasites for ecological study. *In* Kunz TH (ed): Ecological and Behavioral Methods for the Study of Bats. Washington, DC, Smithsonian Institution Press, pp 459–474, 1988.
29. Widmaier EP, Kunz TH: Basal, diurnal, and stress-induced levels of glucose and glucocorticoids in captive bats. J Exp Zool 265:533–540, 1993.
30. Woo PTK, Hawkins JD: Trypanosomes and experimental trypanosomiasis in East African bats. Acta Tropica 32(1):57–64, 1975.
31. Young PL, Halpin K, Selleck PW, et al: Serologic evidence for the presence in *Pteropus* bats of a paramyxovirus related to equine morbillivirus. Emerging Infect Dis 2(3):239–240, 1996 (http://www.cdc.gov/ncidod/EID/eid.htm).

CHAPTER **45**

Advances in Fruit Bat Nutrition

JANET L. (REITER) DEMPSEY

The order Chiroptera comprises more than 900 species that account for one fourth of the world's living mammals. The order is divided into two suborders: Megachiroptera, consisting of one family (Pteropodidae), and Microchiroptera, consisting of 16 highly diverse families. Megachiroptera are limited to the Old World tropics and subtropics, and Microchiroptera are found throughout the world. The extreme ecologic, behavioral, and physiologic diversity of the numerous species has made bats increasingly popular subjects for research and as exhibit animals in zoological parks. This diversity, and the lack of knowledge on environmental and physiologic requirements, limits the species that can be successfully maintained in captivity. Bats may be categorized by food habits as insectivores, frugivores, nectarivores, carnivores, piscivores, or sanguinivores. Their specialization in feeding strategy and dietary habits is particularly limiting for maintenance of bats in captivity, because actual nutrient requirements remain unknown.

Pteropodidae (of the Megachiroptera) and Phyllostomidae (of the Microchiroptera) are composed primarily of frugivorous and nectarivorous species that have been maintained in captivity with the greatest success, primarily because of their preference for soft, sweet fruits. Captive fruit bat diets have traditionally been based on feeding habits in the wild. Studies on wild bats have attempted to collect and analyze food items and determine food intake through identification of fecal or stomach contents. These data, although important, do not quantify the nutrient requirements of fruit bats. The purpose of this chapter is to present recent research on nutrient requirements and interactions and to provide practical considerations for formulating diets for captive fruit bats. The nutrition and husbandry of other chiropteran species have been discussed previously.[2, 33]

CHARACTERISTICS OF FEEDING AND DIGESTION

Fruit bats are highly efficient at extracting the liquid portion of their chosen foods. They pulverize bites of fruit with specialized dentition, squeezing out and swallowing the juices. The remaining fibrous portion is virtually devoid of moisture and is spit out in tightly compressed pellets (ejecta). Therefore, to meet nutrient needs, fruit bats have daily food intakes that range as high as 2.5 times body mass.[4, 9, 12, 16, 25, 30] Rapid transit times (ranging from 15 to 100 minutes) allowed such large volumes of food to be processed through the digestive tract.[16, 29]

The gastrointestinal tract of fruit bats is highly modified in comparison with other bat species. The stomach is large and complex; the small intestine is long and convoluted; the cecum is absent; and the large intestine is short, nearly indistinguishable from the small intestine.[10, 28, 29] These large compartments do not serve as fermentation vats, because fruit bats do not have appreciable levels of intestinal microflora.[11] Instead, this specialization allows greater surface area for increased absorption of nutrients from the large volumes of liquid consumed.

NUTRIENT CONTENT OF FOODS

Fruit, when consumed alone, is considered a poor quality diet because of the low concentrations of many nutrients. However, a distinction should be made between cultivated and native fruits. Cultivated fruits tend to be higher in moisture and carbohydrate content and lower in energy, protein/nitrogen, fiber, and ash than native fruits (Table 45–1). In addition, cultivated fruits have lower concentrations of many essential minerals (Table 45–2). Cultivated fruits may also be lower in vitamin content than native fruits, although published values for native fruits are nearly nonexistent in the literature.

Fruit bats in the wild appear to meet their nutrient needs by consuming large quantities of mixed native fruits. In captivity, we must rely on readily available, cultivated fruits for use in bat diets. Therefore, it is necessary to supply many of the essential nutrients through use of nutritionally complete feeds. To do this we must know what nutrients are essential to fruit bats and in what amounts they should be supplied.

TABLE 45–1. Comparison of the Macronutrient Composition of Cultivated and Native Fruits

Fruit Type	Moisture (%)	Expressed on a Dry Matter Basis						
		Gross Energy (kcal/g)	Protein (%)	Nitrogen (%)	Fat (%)	Fiber (%)	Carbo-hydrates (%)	Ash (%)
Cultivated*†								
Apple	84.50	3.61	1.03	0.16	2.00	3.55	95.46	1.55‖
Banana	74.30	3.58	4.08	0.63	2.06	2.06	91.03	3.11‖
Cantaloupe	91.00	3.44	8.88	1.38	2.69	3.33	85.55	5.68‖
Orange	86.80	3.52	7.58	1.21	0.54	3.26	88.25	3.47‖
Native								
Fig (*Ficus ovalis*)‡	78.50	4.08	2.10	0.60	0.80	35.4	43.40	5.20
Fig (*Ficus sycomorous*)§	83.70	3.60	3.50	0.56	2.10	5.20	84.70	4.50
Piper fruit (*Piper amalago*)‡	73.00	3.95	6.00	1.90	1.40	10.90	86.70	23.0
Carob (*Ceratonoia siliqua*)§	20.50	3.90	6.50	1.04	0.95	7.60	82.40	2.60

*Data from reference 23.
†Fruit without skin or peel, includes seeds.
‡Data from reference 9.
§Data from reference 12.
‖Data from reference 32.

TABLE 45–2. Comparison of the Mineral Content of Cultivated and Native Fruits

Fruit Type	Moisture (%)	Expressed on a Dry Matter Basis			
		Ca (%)	P (%)	Fe (ppm)	Se (ppm)
Cultivated*†					
Apple	84.50	0.03	0.05	4.52	0.03
Banana	74.30	0.02	0.08	11.94	0.04
Cantaloupe	91.00	0.10	0.16	23.66	0.03
Orange	86.80	0.30	0.15	9.20	0.10
Natural‡					
Fig (*Ficus pertusa*)					
Ripe fruit	77.20	2.89	0.11	238.13	0.04
Fig (*Ficus trigonata*)					
Unripe fruit	83.70	0.74	0.23	49.93	0.10

*Data from reference 23.
†Fruit without skin or peel, includes seeds.
‡Data from reference 6.

NUTRIENT REQUIREMENTS

Despite differences in diet and feeding strategy among species, all mammals have similar qualitative nutrient needs for tissue metabolism. This, presumably, includes fruit bats. Approximately 50 nutrients have been identified as dietary essentials (must be obtained through diet or gastrointestinal microbes) because they cannot be synthesized in appropriate quantities to meet animal needs.[31]

Water

Water is the easiest and least expensive essential nutrient provided in captivity. Availability of fresh water is critical because of the variety of functions it performs in the body. The need for water is affected by a number of variables, including ambient air temperature, solar and thermal radiation, metabolic rates, feed intake, and dietary water content.[26] Fruit bats have been maintained in laboratory settings on mixed fruit diets without free access to water, and they presumably can obtain what they need from their high-moisture diets. However, many species have been observed to actively consume water in captivity and in the wild. Therefore, because of limited food choices and in some cases fluctuating environmental conditions, it is advisable to provide free access to fresh water in captivity.

Protein

Proteins are major constituents of the animal body and are vital to all tissues. Amino acids are the functional building blocks that make up protein. Animals with relatively simple stomachs and little or no capacity for fermentation require a dietary source of ten essential amino acids.[26, 31] Individual amino acid requirements for most species are not known, nor is the amino acid composition of many foods. Instead, researchers use estimates of crude protein to evaluate foods and estimate animal requirements. Because the amino acids

that make up protein contain nitrogen, and proteins are typically 16% nitrogen, crude protein content is determined by analyzing the nitrogen content and multiplying the result by 6.25. However, this is a crude estimate because not all nitrogen is contained as amino acids in protein, and the exact ratio between nitrogen and protein may not always be known.[26]

Fruit as the sole diet constituent has been considered a poor quality diet by many researchers. This opinion persists because of the low protein content of fruit when compared to other plant and animal food sources. It has been argued that both pteropodid and phyllostomid fruit bats must supplement their fruit diets with relatively higher protein items such as insects,[16] pollen,[14] or leaves[13, 15, 34] to meet protein needs. However, other researchers maintain that fruit bats can meet their protein requirements on exclusively fruit diets.[9, 27, 30]

Recent research supports the hypothesis that fruit bats are able to meet their protein needs consuming fruit alone. These studies have been conducted using diets that approximate the low protein content of fruits (both cultivated and native) or using native fruits alone. The author conducted a study measuring dry matter intake and body mass in a group of captive adult male *Artibeus jamaicensis* (phyllostomids).[25] A total protein requirement of 0.28 g/day/bat for maintenance was determined. The bats in this study adjusted their dry matter intake, irrespective of dietary energy content, to meet protein needs and maintain constant body mass. The experimental diets used were isocaloric, varying in protein and dry matter content.[25] This protein intake is supported by earlier estimates of 0.30 g protein/day/bat[16] as well as by data yet to be published (M. Delorme, personal communication, 1996) for the same species.

Delorme and Thomas determined nitrogen and energy requirements of another phyllostomid, *Carollia perspicillata*.[4] The total protein requirement for maintenance of nonreproductive, adult bats was 0.14 g/day/bat, which is lower than previously reported for this species.[9] The diets fed varied in protein, energy, and dry matter. The bats in this study adjusted their metabolic rates to maintain body mass because body mass changes were not correlated with energy intake. It was concluded that nonreproductive fruit bats of this species meet their protein requirements on low-protein diets because of metabolic fecal nitrogen losses, which are the lowest yet reported for any eutherian species.

Korine and colleagues conducted a study in which they fed nonreproductive, adult pteropids (*Rousettus aegyptiacus*) five different diets consisting of a single native fruit.[12] This study was designed to determine protein and energy balance on each diet. The bats maintained positive nitrogen balance on all but one of the single-fruit diets. The average total protein intake for maintenance was 0.16 g/day/bat for the four diets where positive nitrogen balance was achieved. This protein intake is lower than previously reported for other pteropids maintained on mixed diets.[4, 14, 27] It is interesting to note that these bats also exhibited low nitrogen excretion, which suggests an adaptation to low-protein diets.

Energy

Energy, in the form of calories (1000 cal = 1 kcal), is required to drive all active body functions, including basal metabolism, activity, thermoregulation, growth, reproduction, and lactation. Energy is not a discrete nutrient but is derived from the metabolism of other required nutrients. Because of their high concentration in plants, carbohydrates are quantitatively the most important sources of energy in captive diets. The second-most important source of energy is derived from dietary fats. In addition, excess protein in the diet may be broken down to provide energy in the absence of carbohydrates. The average amount of energy supplied by each of these nutrient classes is termed the *physiologic fuel value*. These values are 4.0 kcal/g for carbohydrates, 9.0 kcal/g for fats, and 4.0 kcal/g for proteins.

Fruit bats presumably have no difficulty meeting energy needs because they consume large amounts of high-carbohydrate fruits, both in captivity and in the wild. There is controversy among researchers as to whether fruit bats must over-ingest energy as a consequence of meeting protein requirements. This is due to the relatively high energy:protein ratio of most fruits, both cultivated and native. Stellar and Thomas determined that the feed intake of pteropids necessary to meet protein needs provided excess energy.[27, 30] In contrast, Herbst determined that *C. perspicillata*, a phyllostomid, did not have to ingest excess energy to meet protein needs.[9]

Estimates of maintenance energy requirements have been made by a number of researchers. The author[25] estimated a maintenance energy requirement of 17.17 kcal/day/bat for *A. jamaicensis,* which is higher than the previous estimate of 14.3 kcal/day/bat by Morrison[16] but lower than the estimate by Delorme (unpublished data, 1996). Estimates of maintenance energy requirements for *C. perspicillata* are 16.1 kcal/day/bat.[4] Korine and colleagues determined a metabolic energy requirement of 40.1 kcal/day for *R. aegyptiacus*.[12] Care must be taken when interpreting these data; much of the information is based on estimates of energy expenditure

for various activities of fruit bats, and a low-protein diet may artificially elevate apparent energy needs.

Apart from serving as a source of dietary energy, fats also provide essential fatty acids. Fatty acids function as structural components of cell membranes and precursors to the synthesis of metabolites that regulate tissue functions throughout the body (i.e., prostaglandins). The most important fatty acids are linoleic and arachidonic acid. Quantitative requirements for essential fatty acids have been demonstrated in a number of species, although actual levels remain largely unknown. Fruit bats are likely to have fatty acid requirements similar to other mammals. The recommendation for most mammals is to include essential fatty acids in the diet at 1% to 2% of the total caloric intake; however, this varies with the age and physiologic state of the animal.[26, 31]

Vitamins and Minerals

Specific vitamin and mineral requirements have not been determined for fruit bats. Information is available that may be used to formulate captive diets. The National Research Council (NRC) has established vitamin and mineral requirements for a variety of domestic and laboratory animals. The range of these requirements is relatively small (Table 45–3). Until specific requirements are determined, captive bat diets may be presumed safe and effective if formulated to provide vitamin and mineral levels within the range for other nonruminant mammalian species. Bats lack the ability to synthesize vitamin C and require a dietary source.[1]

Qualitative information on vitamin and mineral requirements of fruit bats is available from observations of deficiencies or toxicities in captivity. Careful consideration of methodology must occur when interpreting such results. A recent report described dilated cardiomyopathy in pteropid fruit bats as a result of hypovitaminosis E.[7] Although the diagnosis was based on low plasma and tissue vitamin E levels, the diet had a vitamin E content considered adequate for other nonruminant mammalian species (56 mg/kg dry diet). Because diet intake and digestibility were not measured, actual vitamin E intake was not determined. Therefore, the inference that fruit bats may require higher levels of vitamin E than other mammalian species requires further research.

Hemochromatosis (iron storage disease) has recently been reported in three species of pteropid fruit bats (*Rousettus aegyptiacus, Pteropus giganteus,* and *P. poliocephalus*) as a result of dietary overload.[3] The analyzed iron content of the diet fed was 400 mg/kg dry diet, approaching what would be considered toxic levels for some domestic species.[17] The main source of iron was dicalcium phosphate, used as a mineral supplement. In addition, excessive vitamin C supplementation (estimated intake per bat of 7500 mg/kg dry diet) may have compounded the problem by enhancing iron uptake.

Investigation into the cause of nodular bone lesions in the same three species of pteropid fruit bats identified fluoride toxicity as the probable cause.[5] The diet contained shrimp meal, which is naturally high in fluoride; dicalcium phosphate, which may contain fluoride as an

TABLE 45–3. Vitamin and Mineral Requirements of Domestic and Laboratory Species (Dry Matter Basis)

Species	Vitamins			Minerals							
	A (IU/g)	D (IU/g)	E (mg/kg)	Ca (%)	P (%)	K (%)	Mg (%)	Fe (ppm)	Zn (ppm)	Se (ppm)
Cat	4.0	0.5	30.0	0.8	0.6	0.4	0.04	80.0	15.0	0.1
Dog	5.0	0.5	50.0	0.6	0.4	0.4	0.04	32.0	36.0	0.1
Lab mouse	0.5	0.15	20.0	0.4	0.4	0.2	0.05	25.0	30.0	—
Lab rat	4.0	1.0	30.0	0.5	0.4	0.4	0.04	35.0	12.0	0.1
Nonhuman primate	10.0–15.0	2.0	50.0	0.5	0.4	0.8	0.15	180.0	10.0	—
Pig	1.3	0.15	11.0	0.5	0.4	0.2	0.04	40.0	50.0	0.1
Range	1.3–15.0	0.15–2.0	11.0–50.0	0.4–0.8	0.4–0.6	0.2–0.8	0.04–0.15	25.0–180.0	10.0–50.0	0.1

Data from references 17 to 22.

impurity; and fruit and other supplements. Although the concentration of fluoride in the total diet was not reported, the estimated amounts of fluoride consumed by the bats were well above maximum tolerable levels reported for other species.[17] Although quantitative fluoride requirements have not been established for most species, excessive levels have been shown to cause bone and tooth lesions, anorexia, lameness, necrosis of gastrointestinal mucosa, and cardiac failure.[17]

CAPTIVE DIETS FOR FRUGIVOROUS AND NECTARIVOROUS BATS

When formulating diets for captive fruit bats, we must determine what foods are available and appropriate for meeting probable nutrient needs. The same diets may be used for captive frugivorous and nectarivorous bats. Nutritionally complete nectar formulas may be included in diets for species that consume large amounts of nectar in the wild. Cultivated fruits are readily accepted, but these items are low in many nutrients, particularly protein, fat, vitamins, and minerals. An alternate source of these nutrients must be provided to formulate diets that have nutrient levels within the range for other nonruminant mammalian species. The preferred method for supplying essential nutrients lacking in cultivated fruits is to provide nutritionally complete feeds, such as low-fiber, dry primate diets or dry diets formulated for frugivorous birds. These feeds should be rationally formulated and meet the current requirements of the species for which they have been developed. The use of individual nutrient supplements, such as vitamin and mineral compounds, is not recommended. Oversupplementation and undersupplementation are common, as are the resulting toxicity and deficiency problems.

The nutritionally complete feed used should be as finely ground as possible to promote adequate consumption. Mixing fruit nectar, such as peach or apricot, with the ground feed will soften or dissolve the diet and encourage consumption—fruit bats tend to be attracted to fruit nectar. Fruit may also be added to this mixture, but it is advisable to chop the fruit into very small pieces or mix ingredients in a blender so bats cannot preferentially consume fruit only. Behavioral enrichments in the form of hanging whole fruits may be used to encourage natural foraging behavior.

Nutritionally complete nectar formulas may be offered in addition to fruit and other nutritionally complete feeds. A number of homemade nectar formulas used successfully in captivity have been described in the literature.[24] However, these formulations contain a variety of supplements and can be dangerous if misused. Nutritionally complete nectar powders formulated for hummingbirds are currently available (with varying protein content) and may be appropriate for nectarivorous bats. The total diet offered should still be formulated to provide nutrient levels that meet probable requirements.

SUMMARY

Although specific nutrient requirements for frugivorous and nectarivorous bats remain nearly unknown, information exists that provides practical guidelines for formulating captive diets. This information must be reviewed critically, applied sensibly, and compared with what is known for other mammalian species until more specific research is conducted. Opportunities for research in bat nutrition abound and, in view of the diversity of species, may provide important information for comparison with other species with similar dietary habits and feeding strategies.

REFERENCES

1. Ayaz KM, Birney EC, Jennes R: Inability of bats to synthesize L-ascorbic acid. Nature 260:626–628, 1976.
2. Constantine DG: Insectivorous bats. *In* Fowler ME (ed): Zoo and Wild Animal Medicine, 2nd ed. Philadelphia, WB Saunders, pp 650–655, 1986.
3. Crawshaw G, Oyarzun S, Valdes E, et al: Hemochromatosis (iron storage disease) in fruit bats. Proceedings of the Annual Meeting of the Nutrition Advisory Group of American Zoo and Aquarium Association, Toronto, Ontario, Canada, pp 136–147, 1995.
4. Delorme M, Thomas DW: Nitrogen and energy requirements of the short-tailed fruit bat (*Carollia perspicillata*): fruit bats are not nitrogen constrained. J Comp Physiol [B] 166:427–434, 1996.
5. Duncan M, Crawshaw GJ, Mehren KG, et al: Multicentric hyperostosis consistent with fluorosis in captive fruit bats (*Pteropus giganteus, P. poliocephalus* and *Rousettus aegyptiacus*). J Zoo Wildl Med 27(3):325–338, 1996.
6. Edwards MS: Comparative adaptations to folivory in primates. Ph.D. dissertation, Michigan State University, 1995.
7. Heard DJ, Buergelt CD, Snyder PS, et al: Dilated cardiomyopathy associated with hypovitaminosis E in a captive collection of flying foxes (*Pteropus* spp.). J Zoo Wildl Med 27(2):149–157, 1996.
8. Herbst LH: Nutritional analyses of the wet season diet of *Carollia perspicillata* (Chiroptera: Phyllostomidae) in Parque Nacional Santa Rosa, Costa Rica. M.S. thesis, University of Miami, 1983.
9. Herbst LH: The role of nitrogen from fruit pulp in the nutrition of the frugivorous bat *Carollia perspicillata*. Biotropica 18(1):39–44, 1986.
10. Hill JE, Smith JD: Food habits and feeding. *In* Bats: A Natural History. Austin, University of Texas Press, pp 60–72, 1984.
11. Klite PD: Intestinal bacterial flora and transit time of three neotropical bat species. J Bacteriol 90(2):375–379, 1965.
12. Korine C, Arad Z, Arieli A: Nitrogen and energy balance of the fruit bat *Rousettus aegyptiacus* on natural fruit diets. Physiol Zool 69(3):618–634, 1996.
13. Kunz TH, Diaz CA: Folivory in fruit-eating bats, with new evidence from *Artibeus jamaicensis* (Chiroptera: Phyllostomidae). Biotropica 27:106–120, 1995.
14. Law BS: The maintenance nitrogen requirements of the Queensland blossom bat (*Syconycteris australis*) on a sugar/pollen diet: is nitrogen a limiting resource? Physiol Zool 65(3):634–648, 1992.
15. Lowry JB: Green-leaf fractionation by fruit bats: is this feeding behaviour a unique nutritional strategy for herbivores? Aust Wildl Res 16:203–206, 1989.
16. Morrison DW: Efficiency of food utilization by fruit bats. Oecologia 45:270–273, 1980.
17. National Research Council: Mineral tolerance of domestic animals [Publication No. 3022]. Washington, DC, National Academy of Sciences, 1980.
18. National Research Council: Nutrient requirements of laboratory animals [Publication No. 2767]. Washington, DC, National Academy of Sciences, 1978.
19. National Research Council: Nutrient requirements of nonhuman primates [Publication No. 2786]. Washington, DC, National Academy of Sciences, 1978.
20. National Research Council: Nutrient requirements of dogs [Publication No. 3496]. Washington, DC, National Academy of Sciences, 1985.
21. National Research Council: Nutrient requirements of cats [Publica-

tion No. 3682]. Washington, DC, National Academy of Sciences, 1986.

22. National Research Council: Nutrient requirements of swine [Publication No. 3779]. Washington, DC, National Academy of Sciences, 1988.

23. Pennington JAT, Church HN (eds): Bowes & Church's Food Values of Portions Commonly Used, 14th ed. Philadelphia, JB Lippincott, pp 74–80, 209, 220, 1985.

24. Rasweiler JJ: American leaf-nosed bats. *In* Fowler ME (ed): Zoo and Wild Animal Medicine, 2nd ed. Philadelphia, WB Saunders, pp 638–644, 1986.

25. Reiter JL: The intake of captive adult, male fruit bats (*Artibeus jamaicensis*) fed diets of differing protein content. M.S. thesis, University of Illinois at Chicago, 1993.

26. Robbins CT: Wildlife Feeding and Nutrition, 2nd ed. New York, Academic Press, 1993.

27. Stellar DC: The dietary energy and nitrogen requirements of the grey-headed flying fox *Pteropus poliocephalus* (Megachiroptera). Aust J Zool 34:339–349, 1986.

28. Stevens CE, Hume ID: The mammalian gastrointestinal tract. *In* Comparative Physiology of the Vertebrate Digestive System, 2nd ed. New York, Cambridge University Press, pp 55–58, 1995.

29. Tedman RA, Hall LS: The morphology of the gastrointestinal tract and food transit time in the fruit bats *Pteropus alecto* and *P. poliocephalus* (Megachiroptera). Aust J Zool 33:625–640, 1985.

30. Thomas DW: Fruit intake and energy budgets of frugivorous bats. Physiol Zool 57(4):457–467, 1984.

31. Ullrey DE, Allen ME: Principles of zoo animal nutrition. *In* Fowler ME (ed): Zoo and Wild Animal Medicine, 2nd ed. Philadelphia, WB Saunders, pp 516–532, 1986.

32. United States Department of Agriculture: Composition of Foods. Agricultural Handbook No. 8, 1975.

33. Wimsatt WA: Vampire bats. *In* Fowler ME (ed): Zoo and Wild Animal Medicine, 2nd ed. Philadelphia, WB Saunders, pp 644–649, 1986.

34. Zortea M, Mendez SL: Folivory in the big fruit-eating bat, *Artibeus lituratus* (Chiroptera, Phyllostomidae) in eastern Brazil. J Trop Ecol 9:117–120, 1993.

CHAPTER 46

Rodent and Small Lagomorph Reproduction

DENNIS A. MERITT, JR.

Rodents occupy almost every niche on every land mass, are found on most islands, and can be characterized as one of the most successful mammalian life forms ever known. They have dispersed over the earth's surface, some forms far from their native haunts, as stowaways on ships, in containers on airlines, and as passengers attached to oceanic flotsam. There are more than three dozen families and several hundred genera of rodents. Rodents occupy most available ecologic niches: they are gliding, terrestrial, subterranean, aquatic, and arboreal; they are diurnal, nocturnal, or crepuscular in their activity cycle; and although preferring seeds, fruit, bark, and other plant material, they have diverse food requirements. Traditional zoo rodents include several species of arboreal or gliding squirrels, woodchucks, prairie dogs, kangaroo rats, beavers, springhaas, various mice and rats, gerbils, naked mole rats, jerboas, porcupines, cavies and guinea pigs, capybaras, pacaranas, pacas, agoutis and acouchis, and chinchillas.

Lagomorphs—hares, pikas, and rabbits—are also found in a worldwide range of habitats. Pikas are colonial, but most hares and rabbits are not. Pikas seek shelter and security in crevices or in burrows. Rabbits construct burrows or prepare nests, and hares take shelter or seek protection in grasses and other areas of dense vegetation. Pikas are diurnal, whereas most hares and rabbits are active late in the day or are nocturnal. All lagomorphs are terrestrial and feed on grass, plants, and vegetation.

Because of specialized requirements, lagomorphs, especially wild forms, are uncommon in zoo exhibits. However most zoos use domestic rabbits as demonstration animals that can be handled in interpretive programs. At least one lagomorph, the volcano rabbit of Mexico, is seriously endangered.

A wealth of useful lagomorph and rodent reproductive information, including gestation periods, the usual number of young produced per litter, and details of maternal care and behavior can be found elsewhere,[1, 20, 29, 33] as is detailed and specific information about North American lagomorph and rodent reproduction.[5, 10] Monogamy in mammals with reference to a number of rodent forms has been detailed by Kleiman.[8]

361

ECOLOGY, BEHAVIOR, AND REPRODUCTION

Lagomorph

Pikas (*Ochotona* species) are vocal, colonial, ground-dwelling lagomorphs that are active year-round. They clip, harvest, and prepare grasses and other plant material during the late summer and early fall for use as food during times of shortage, usually winter. Pikas become sexually mature in their first year. Mating occurs in the spring and summer, and litters are born about 30 days later. The young are born naked and helpless in a secluded, protected nest of soft grasses. The multiple offspring are weaned within 2 weeks and attain adult size and weight within 3 months. More than one litter may be born each year.

Hares (*Lepus* species) and rabbits are flighty, secretive lagomorphs that are usually found alone or as a small group consisting of mother and young. They are active year round and do not prepare or store food temporarily or for the annual period of food shortage. A signaling or warning behavior of note is their ability to drum or thump their feet. Hares also grind their teeth as a warning signal.

Rabbits are born nest bound, naked, and blind, whereas young hares are fully haired, sighted, and capable of independent activity. In both cases, the offspring are multiple. Multiple litters within a year are not infrequent, especially in years of favorable weather conditions and food availability. Rabbits are born in a nest prepared by the mother and lined with hair plucked from her abdomen. Hares do not prepare nests; they simply give birth in a secluded spot. Sexual maturity is reached within the first year for rabbits and before the end of the second year in hares.

Increased male activity, territorial disputes, and active pursuit of females signal lagomorph reproductive behavior. Males frequently dribble urine and attempt to caress the female during courtship. Gestation periods vary with the genera but range from just under 30 days for rabbits to less than 50 days for hares.

Rodents

Woodchucks (*Marmota monax*) are large, solitary, diurnal, ground-dwelling, burrowing rodents found throughout North America. In preparation for winter, large amounts of fat are stored in late summer and fall. In the more northern parts of their range, Woodchucks hibernate.

Woodchucks seek sexually receptive mates in early spring when the weather warms. The gestation period is slightly more than 30 days but less than 45. Multiple offspring are produced in an underground, vegetation-lined nest. They have teeth and hair but are sightless at birth. Within 4 to 6 weeks, they young begin exploration outside of the burrow. Adult mass and sexual maturity are reached in most animals in the second year.

Prairie dogs (*Cynomys* species) are North American, diurnal, gregarious, colonial, terrestrial, burrowing rodents that live in complex underground communities called towns. They are vocal, vigilant mammals that carefully maintain the burrow system, with particular attention to the entrance on a small hilltop or crest. Trevino-Villarreal[25] has detailed the annual life cycle of the Mexican prairie dog, *Cynomys mexicanus*.

Prairie dogs mate in late winter, producing multiple offspring about 30 days later. At birth the young are haired and capable of coordinated movement but are sightless. Weaning occurs within the first 2 months, and offspring are sexually mature by the end of the second year after birth. Females may remain within their social unit, but males are usually forced out.

So named because of their hopping method of locomotion, kangaroo rats (*Dipodomys* species) are nocturnal, burrowing rodents of arid and desert regions of North America. They collect seeds in cheek pouches and store this food in or near their home burrow. Their ability to conserve water is remarkable.

Kangaroo rats have a gestation period of about a month, have multiple offspring, and may produce more than one litter a year under favorable conditions. Sexual maturity is reached within the first year.

North American beavers (*Castor canadensis*) are large (~30 kg), aquatic rodents found in forested temperate regions. They are easily recognized by the broad, flat, scaled tail they use to slap the water surface in an alarm response. Beavers are best known for their ability to build dams and to store food underwater. They may be found as pairs, family units, or extended family groups called colonies.

Beavers become sexually mature in their second year and usually mate in mid-winter. Under ideal conditions, a single litter of multiple offspring is produced annually.

Springhaas (*Pedetes capensis*) are nocturnal, terrestrial, burrowing rodents found in arid regions of Africa that locomote by hopping. The forelegs are smallish, and the rear legs are strong and elongated. Springhaas appear kangaroo-like in sitting or moving profile. Butynski[2] has reported on the nocturnal ecology of this rodent in Botswana.

The gestation period of springhaas is from 75 to 80 days.[28] They produce young singly. At birth, the offspring is capable of coordinated movement, may or may not be sighted, is fully haired, and has teeth. Rosenthal and Meritt[22] have provided details of springhaas bred and reared in captivity. Reproductive patterns in harvested animals from the Orange Free State have been reported by van der Merwe and colleagues.[27] The reproductive ecology of this species in a free-ranging state in the Kalahari Desert has been comprehensively detailed by Butynski.[3]

The North American porcupine (*Erethizon dorsatum*) is a terrestrial and arboreal, diurnal and nocturnal mammal of forested areas of a significant portion of the North American continent. Preferred habitat is mixed coniferous and deciduous forests. Porcupines are usually found singly but may come together during extreme weather in tree hollows, which may be used year after year. The most notable feature of this rotund mammal is its system of quills, which are used as protection and defense against predators.

North American porcupines mate in the early winter,

producing a single young after a gestation period of about 7 months. The offspring is born with soft quills, which harden within a few days. At birth, the animal is sighted, can hear, is capable of coordinated motion, including climbing, and can eat solid food within several days. Sexual maturity is reached before the third year.

African crested porcupines (*Hystrix* species) have the longest quills of any extant porcupine. Found throughout sub-Saharan Africa, these burrowing, ground-dwelling rodents are patchy in their distribution. They are intermittently active by day or night, depending on available food resources. They may be found singly, in small groups, or in extended family groups.[26] They are capable of rapid movements, which can be surprising for an animal of this form and size.

African crested porcupines produce multiple offspring, usually two to four, after a gestation period of less than 4 months. The young are precocious—able to stand, walk, and run from birth. The quills are flexible at birth but soon become firm and useful in defense. More than one litter per year may be produced under ideal conditions. Gosling[7] has provided reproductive details about the related Indian form, *Hystrix hodgsoni*, held in captivity in England.

Cavies (*Kerodon rupestris*) are members of the neotropical family Caviidae, which includes the well-known guinea pig (*Cavia* species). The common name, rock cavy, refers to where the animals are usually found, seeking escape and shelter from predators among rocky outcroppings and in rock piles. In some respects their form is more rabbit-like than are the other rodent family members.

Rock cavies produce litters of one to three offspring after a gestation period of about 75 days.[11] Offspring are precocial and reach adult size and weight at approximately 7 months of age.[11, 12] Details of this species' reproductive biology and development in a captive environment can be found in the work of Roberts and associates.[21]

Patagonian cavies (*Dolichotis patagonum*) are terrestrial, burrowing, diurnally active rodents of the semiarid areas of northwestern Argentina. Cavies practice enurination, the spraying of urine on conspecific animals, either as a defensive act or, more likely, to assist in the recognition of familiar animals. Captive behavior and management have been reported on by MacNamara.[13]

Male Patagonian cavies are relentless in their pursuit of prospective mates and may enurinate the female while standing in a crouched position. More than one young may be produced at a time—usually two but as many as four. The young look identical to the adults in every way except size and are capable of eating solid food within a few days of birth. Kleiman and coworkers[9] have reported that Patagonian cavies experience a postpartum estrus.

Capybaras (*Hydrochaerus hydrochaeris*), the largest rodent (adults weigh 100–140 Ib), are aquatic and Neotropical. They are found in shallow bodies of water, frequently in association with birds and reptiles. Males are easily identifiable by a conspicuous hairless nose flap, which becomes most exaggerated during the breeding season. Capybaras are sexually dimorphic in size as well: females are larger and heavier than males. They are most often found in extended multifamily groups numbering up to several dozen animals of various ages. Schaller and Crawshaw[23] have published detailed population and behavioral information about animals from the Pantanal in Brazil.

Capybara males compete for females and copulate in the water. After a gestation period of slightly less than 6 months,[31] multiple offspring are produced, usually 2 to 4 in young mothers and 4 to 12 in more mature females. Sexual maturity is reached in the second year of life. Chapman[4] and Zara[32] provided detailed information on reproduction in captivity.

Pacaranas (*Dinomys branicki*), the only extant members of the family Dinomyidae, are found on the eastern slopes of the Andes Mountains in western South America. Little is known about the species' ecology and behavior in nature. Although pacaranas are uncommon in captivity, captive studies have provided some details about behavior and breeding.[6] They are short-legged, robust rodents that are nocturnally active. They are also contact animals in that captive creatures lie next to one another, touching or close together.

Pacaranas produce single or multiple young after a gestation period of about 8.5 months. The young look identical to adults in every way except size and, in addition, can hear, see, walk, climb awkwardly, and chew solids within hours of birth. By 1 week of age, infants are capable of self-cleaning and grooming and begin to eat solid food.[18]

Pacas (*Cuniculus paca*) are found throughout Central and South America, although the distribution is patchy and dependent on suitable habitat. This nocturnal, terrestrial rodent is usually solitary, but mothers and young may be seen together. Pacas are frequently sought as food by indigenous peoples.[19] They are sexually dimorphic, males being larger and heavier than females. Captive management and care under natural conditions have been reported on by Matamoros and Pashov.[15]

Like agoutis and Patagonian cavies, male pacas spray females during courtship. Pacas produce a single offspring or, rarely, twins after a gestation period of 114 to 118 days.[9, 14, 15] Solid food is consumed within the first 5 to 7 days after birth, and suckling continues for at least 5 weeks. Two litters can be produced per year under favorable conditions. The mean interbirth interval for captive animals is 178 days. Sexual maturity for both males and females occurs at just under 2 years of age in pacas bred and raised in captivity.[19]

Agoutis (*Dasyprocta* species) are Neotropical, forest-dwelling, terrestrial, diurnally active rodents.[24] They may be found as individuals, as pairs, as mothers with offspring, or in small matriarchal groups. Agoutis clean, eat, and store a variety of tropical fruits, seeds, and nuts. The act of burying a single cleaned nut or seed is described as scatterhoarding. These individually buried food items are retrieved during times of food shortage, much as North American squirrels retrieve acorns.[16]

Agoutis produce single or multiple offspring after a gestation period of less than 127 days, which is the shortest recorded interbirth interval. The one to three young are precocial and in captivity have been born in every month of the year.[17] Females experience a postpartum estrus.[30] Additional reproductive characteristics of these and other hystricomorph rodents can be found in the work of Weir.[31]

REFERENCES

1. Asdell SA: Patterns of Mammalian Reproduction, 2nd ed. Ithaca, NY, Cornell University Press, 1964.
2. Butynski TM: Nocturnal ecology of the springhare, *Pedetes capensis,* in Botswana. M.S. Thesis, East Lansing, Michigan State University, pp 1–54, 1975.
3. Butynski TM: Reproductive ecology of the springhaas, *Pedetes capensis,* in Botswana. J Zool Lond 189:221–232, 1979.
4. Chapman CA: Reproductive biology of captive capybaras. J. Mammal 72:206–208, 1991.
5. Chapman JA, Feldhamer GA: Wild Mammals of North America. Baltimore, Johns Hopkins University Press, 1990.
6. Collins LR, Eisenberg JF: Notes on the behavior and breeding of pacaranas. Int Zoo Yearb 12:108–114, 1972.
7. Gosling LM: Reproduction of the Himalayan porcupine (*Hystrix hodgsoni*) in captivity. J Zool Soc Lond 192:546–549, 1980.
8. Kleiman DG: Monogamy in mammals. Q Rev Biol 52:39–69, 1977.
9. Kleiman DG, Eisenberg JF, Maliniak E: Reproductive parameters and productivity of caviomorph rodents. *In* Eisenberg JF (ed): Vertebrate Ecology in the Northern Neotropics. Washington, DC, Smithsonian Institution Press, pp 173–183, 1979.
10. Kurta A: Mammals of the Great Lakes Region, Rev ed. Ann Arbor, University of Michigan Press, 1995.
11. Lacher TE: Rates of growth in *Kerodon rupestris* and an assessment of its potential as a domesticated food source. Papeis Avulsos de Zoologia, Sao Paulo, 33:67–76, 1979.
12. Lacher TE: The comparative social behavior of *Kerodon rupestris* and *Galea spixii* and the evolution of behavior in the Caviidae. Bull Carnegie Mus Nat Hist 17:1–71, 1981.
13. MacNamara M: Notes on the behavior and captive maintenance of mara, *Dolichotis patagonum,* at the Bronx Zoo. Zoologisher Garten N F, Jena 50:422–426, 1980.
14. Matamoros Y: Investigaciones preliminares sobre la reproduction, comportamiento, alimentacion y manejo del tepezcuente (*Cuniculus paca*) en cautiverio. *In* Salinas PJ (ed): Zoologia Neotropical Actas del VIII Congreso Latinoamericano de Zoologia. pp 961–992, 1982.
15. Matamoros Y, Pashov B: Ciclo estral del tepezcuinte (*Cuniculus paca*) en cautiverio. Brenesia 22:249–260, 1984.
16. Meritt DA: The natural history and captive management of the Central American agouti, *Dasyprocta punctata* and agouti, *Dasyprocta agouti.* Annual Conference Proceedings of American Association of Zoological Parks and Aquariums, Wheeling, WV, pp 177–190, 1978.
17. Meritt DA: Preliminary observations on reproduction in the Central American agouti, *Dasyprocta punctata.* Zoo Biol 2:127–131, 1983.
18. Meritt DA: The pacarana, *Dinomys branickii. In* Ryder OA, Byrd ML (eds): One Medicine. New York, Springer-Verlag, pp 154–161, 1984.
19. Meritt DA: The husbandry and management of the paca at Lincoln Park Zoo, Chicago. Int Zoo Yearb 28:264–267, 1989.
20. Nowak RM: Walker's Mammals of the World. Baltimore, Johns Hopkins Press, 1991.
21. Roberts M, Maliniak E, Deal M: The reproductive biology of the rock cavy, *Kerodon rupestris,* in captivity: A study of reproductive adaptation in a trophic specialist. Mammalia 48:253–266, 1984.
22. Rosenthal MA, Meritt DA: Handrearing springhaas. Int Zoo Yearb 13:135–137, 1972.
23. Schaller GB, Crawshaw PG: Social organization in a capybara population. Sonderdrucke aus Saugetierkundliche Mitteilungen, BLV Verlagsgesellschaft, Munchen 40, 29 Jhg. Heft 1, Seite 3–16, 1981.
24. Smythe N: The natural history of the Central American agouti, *Dasyprocta punctata. In* Smithsonian Contributions to Zoology 257, Washington, DC, Smithsonian Institution, 1978.
25. Trevino-Villarreal J: The annual cycle of the Mexican prairie dog (*Cynomys mexicanus*). Occasional Papers Museum of Natural History. Manhattan KS, University of Kansas, 139:1–27, 1990.
26. van Aarde RJ: Reproduction in the Cape porcupine, *Hystrix africaeaustralis:* An ecological perspective. Suid-Afrikaanse Tydskrif vir Wetenskap 83:605–607, 1978.
27. van der Merwe M, Skinner JD, Millar RP: Annual reproductive pattern in the springhaas, *Pedetes capensis.* J. Reprod. Fertil 58:259–266, 1980.
28. Velte FF: Hand-rearing springhaas, *Pedetes capensis,* at the Rochester Zoo. Int Zoo Yearb 18:206–208, 1978.
29. Walker EP: Mammals of the World, vol 2. Baltimore, Johns Hopkins University Press, 1968.
30. Weir BJ: Some observations on reproduction in the female agouti, *Dasyprocta aguti.* J. Reprod Fertil 24:203–211, 1971.
31. Weir BJ: Reproductive characteristics of hystricomorph rodents. *In* Rowlands IW, Weir BJ (eds): The Biology of Hystricomorph Rodents. Symp Zool Soc Lond, 34:265–301, 1974.
32. Zara JL: Breeding and husbandry of the capybara, *Hydrochaeris hydrochaeris.* Int Zoo Yearb 13:137–139, 1973.
33. Zuckerman S: The breeding seasons of mammals in captivity. Proc Zool Soc Lond 122:827–947, 1952.

PRIMATES

CHAPTER 47

Diseases of Prosimians

RANDALL E. JUNGE

The term *prosimian* is used to refer to the group of more evolutionarily primitive primates. The order Primata is divided into two suborders: Prosimii, containing lemurs, lorises, and tarsiers; and Anthropoidea, containing New and Old World monkeys, apes, and humans. The Asian and African prosimian families include Tarsiidae (tarsiers), Loridae (pottos and lorises), and Galagonidae (galagos). The Malagasy prosimians include five extant families: Cheirogaleidae (mouse lemurs and dwarf lemurs), Lemuridae (lemurs), Megaladapidae (sportive lemurs), Indiridae (sifakas and indris), and Daubentoniidae (aye-ayes).[20] Both Asian and African prosimians have been displayed in zoos, and the galago has been used as a research primate as well. Of the Malagasy prosimians, a number of species of lemurs are commonly displayed, including *Lemur catta* (ring-tailed lemur), *Eulemur* species (black lemur and brown lemur), and *Varecia* (ruffed lemurs). Nocturnal species, such as mouse lemurs and dwarf lemurs, are also displayed, but less commonly than the diurnal lemurs. Recently, aye-ayes have been established in small numbers in captivity. Some species, such as bamboo lemurs and some sifaka species, continue to present medical and husbandry (often diet) problems that have prevented sustained captive propagation attempts. There has been increasing interest in establishment of Malagasy prosimians in captivity because of the unstable condition of their natural populations. Many of these species are subject to rapidly decreasing habitat as human populations expand and turn forest into agricultural lands.

The discussion of diseases in this chapter will be focused mainly on Malagasy prosimians because of their predominance in zoological collections and the preponderance of medical information. Although prosimians are certainly susceptible to a wide variety of disease syndromes, discussion will be limited to conditions with unique significance to prosimians. Information on medical conditions of galagos can be found in laboratory primate sources.[9]

Clinical diseases and pathology have been reviewed for lemurs in captivity[1, 4, 8, 10] and in the wild.[11]

DISEASES OF THE GASTROINTESTINAL SYSTEM

Loose or abnormal stool was the most common cause for medical intervention in two surveys of diseases of lemurs.[4, 10] A variety of enteric pathogens have been associated with enteritis and colitis in lemurs. Bacteria isolated from lemurs with evidence of gastrointestinal disease include *Yersinia enterocolitica,* producing ulcerative colitis[3]; *Campylobacter fetus jejuni, Salmonella typhimurium,* and enteropathogenic *Escherichia coli* as the cause of enteritis[4]; and *Klebsiella pneumoniae* as the agent of necrotizing enterocolitis.[1] As with any species, the results of fecal culture must be evaluated in light of the clinical presentation of the animal, and medical intervention must be determined accordingly. With cases of bacterial enteritis that are associated with profuse or persistent diarrhea, dehydration, electrolyte imbalances, and secondary bacterial infections must be considered.

Trichobezoars may occur in captive lemurs, especially ruffed lemurs (*Varecia*). Surgical intervention may be required to alleviate gastric obstruction in severe cases. Regular administration (weekly or biweekly) of laxatives or lubricants (such as oral cat laxatives) will prevent the occurrence. Trichobezoars have not been reported from wild lemurs, and it is likely that components in the natural diet prevent accumulation of hair in the stomach.

Hemochromatosis (hepatic iron storage disease) has historically been considered a common problem in lemurs in captivity, most commonly in *Eulemur* species. Hemochromatosis is the development of pathologic changes in the liver as a result of excess iron storage. The condition is suspected to be the result of the combination of excess dietary iron, excess ascorbic acid, and lack of tannins in the diet. The natural diet of lemurs contains tannin-containing leaves that bind iron, reducing the amount available for absorption. The presence of ascorbic acid in the diet in captivity enhances the reduction of Fe^{3+} to Fe^{2+}, a more readily absorbable form. Recognition of this problem and its mechanism has resulted in lowering the iron content of primate chows and eliminating the feeding of citrus fruits with chow, which has greatly reduced the incidence of hemochromatosis in the past 10 years. A common sequela to iron storage disease was the initiation of neoplastic transformation of the damaged cells, which resulted in a high incidence of hepatic neoplasia. With the decrease in hemochromatosis, a concomitant decrease in hepatic neoplasia appears to have occurred.

Gastrointestinal parasitism is a common cause of diarrhea in captive lemurs. Protozoal parasites are most commonly associated with clinical diarrhea. Commonly identified organisms include *Entamoeba, Trichomonas, Giardia,* and *Balantidium*. Protozoal infestation is identified by direct fecal examination; infestation responds to treatment with metronidazole (25 mg/kg BID for 7 days) or paromomycin (12.5 mg/kg BID for 5 days). Potentiated sulfas and tetracyclines have also been used.

Common nematode parasites include organisms in the genera *Strongylus, Strongyloides, Gongylonema,* and *Physaloptera* as well as ascarids. Gastrointestinal nematodes are readily identified by fecal flotation and respond to a variety of anthelmintics (ivermectin, 0.2 mg/kg orally or subcutaneously once; mebendazole, 10 to 20 mg/kg orally for 3 days; thiabendazole, 50 mg/kg, and pyrantel, 5 to 10 mg/kg orally for 3 days; any of these treatments may be repeated in 10 to 14 days for persistent infestations). *Physaloptera* may present a challenge for diagnosis and treatment. The eggs of this gastric nematode are shed intermittently and may be difficult to find in fecal flotations. In addition, it appears to be resistant to standard anthelmintic regimes. Treatment with ivermectin, 0.2 mg/kg orally once daily for 7 days, or levamisole, 2.5 mg/kg orally once daily for 14 days, has been successful.

No viral enteric diseases have been documented in lemurs.

DISEASES OF THE RESPIRATORY SYSTEM

Bacterial pneumonia in lemurs is not common under good management conditions; however, in stressful conditions, or when animals are acclimating to a new environment, it can occur. Cases have been reported in newly captive animals that have been exposed to environmental changes. These animals were also likely to be stressed and may have been in a poor nutritional state as well. Clinical signs can include fever, inappetence, and labored breathing. Incidences of *Klebsiella pneumoniae* pneumonia are often peracute and fulminant, resulting in rapid fatalities.

The incidence of tuberculosis in prosimians is extremely low. There have been three reports involving seven lemurs (one ring-tailed lemur,[18] three mongoose lemurs,[13] and three unidentified lemurs[6]). Only one of these involved a lemur living in a North American zoo (ring-tailed); the others were recent imports (mongoose) or in captivity in Madagascar. Lesions were described as typical tuberculosis granulomas in lungs, liver, spleen, kidney, and lymph nodes, with acid-fast bacilli.[6, 13, 18] Culture results were only listed as "typical human-type tubercle bacilli."[13] Only three of these animals were tuberculin tested. One was positive, one equivocal, and one negative. The most advanced case had radiographic changes typical of pneumonia.[13]

Pleural effusions have been reported several times in ring-tailed lemurs. Effusions have been related to systemic fungal disease,[5] but they have also been spontaneous. Effusions have been isolated to one hemithorax. Spontaneous cases have been managed conservatively with repeated thoracocentesis and have resolved. Cytologic examination and culture of aspirates have identified the fluid as a sterile transudate.

No viral respiratory diseases have been documented in lemurs.

DISEASES OF THE MUSCULOSKELETAL SYSTEM

Two significant skeletal diseases have been reported in lemurs. A familial bone disease involving periarticular new bone formation coincident with progressive renal failure has been described in 12 black lemurs (2 males, 10 females) in two family lines.[12] This disease, described as periarticular hyperostosis, has occurred in animals ranging from 3 to 27 years of age. The earliest clinical signs are nonpainful enlargement of knee and ankle joints. Radiographs reveal the enlargement to be periosteal new bone proliferation at the metaphyseal regions of the involved bones (Fig. 47–1). Results of complete blood cell counts are normal, and serum bio-

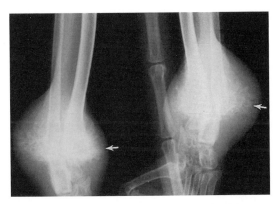

FIGURE 47–1. Periarticular hyperostosis in a black lemur. Radiograph of ankles show periosteal bone proliferation at the distal tibial and fibular diaphyses (*arrows*) and soft tissue swelling.

chemical profiles reveal a twofold to threefold increase in serum alkaline phosphatase activity. As the disease progresses, bone proliferation continues at the affected site, and the wrist joints, proximal femora, digits, and elbow joints may become involved. Levels of alkaline phosphatase remain elevated, and evidence of renal compromise (elevated blood urea nitrogen and creatinine) occur. Proliferation of bone and degeneration of kidneys continue throughout the course of illness. Cases typically progress to death, caused by end-stage renal disease, or euthanasia in 6 to 12 months. Histologic examination of bone indicates that the proliferation is periosteal new bone. Histologic examination of renal tissue indicates chronic interstitial nephritis or glomerulonephritis, with no indication of cause.

The etiology of periarticular hyperostosis in lemurs is not known. This syndrome bears similarities to hypertrophic osteopathy, but differs in distribution of lesions, association with renal disease, and familial component. The association of renal and skeletal disease suggests secondary hyperparathyroidism; however, the histopathology of the lesions and examination of hormone profiles indicate that this is not the underlying cause.

A second syndrome was described in ruffed lemurs (*Varecia variegata*), and is characterized by irregular periosteal bone proliferation along the diaphyses of long bones (primarily tibia, fibula, radius, and ulna). This syndrome has been theorized to be a nonspecific inflammatory response.[19]

Age-related degenerative arthritis is not common in this group. When it does occur, a variety of analgesic drugs have been used with apparent success. Traumatic skeletal injury also occurs infrequently, and seems to respond well to standard techniques of fracture repair, including external stabilization by casting. Internal fixation with pins works well.

DISEASES OF THE INTEGUMENTARY SYSTEM

The most common cause for medical intervention for the integumentary system—and for all systems com-

bined—is traumatic injuries to the skin (lacerations and abrasions). Although lacerations are usually superficial fight wounds, they may be caused by enclosure features (e.g., cage wire or metal edges) as well. Occasionally, they are deep and involve other tissues. Most heal well with little intervention; however, suturing and prophylactic antibiotics may be appropriate. Bite wounds inflicted by lemurs do not appear to be prone to abscessation.

Cutaneous mycosis occurs rarely. In species that scent mark frequently (such as black lemurs), areas of alopecia may occur at scent gland areas (wrists, anogenital, forehead) as a result of excessive rubbing.

DISEASES OF THE UROGENITAL SYSTEM

Age-related renal degeneration is a common cause of mortality in aged lemurs. Glomerulonephritis, glomerulosclerosis, and chronic interstitial nephritis are diagnosed at postmortem examination of aged individuals. Urethral obstructions also have occurred but are not common. However, urethral obstructions caused by coagulum plugs may occur after electroejaculation. In these cases, coagulum material produced by electroejaculation becomes lodged in the urethra at the ischial arc and requires surgical intervention for removal.

DISEASES OF THE NERVOUS SYSTEM

Seizures may occur in relation to several generalized or system illnesses. Epilepsy (recurrent seizures of unknown etiology) may occur rarely, and in cases where the incidence of seizures is high, anticonvulsant therapy with phenobarbital is effective (2 mg of phenobarbital orally once daily resulted in significant reduction of seizures in a 3.2-kg male).

Encephalitis may be caused by bacteria or virus. A case of nonsuppurative meningoencephalitis in a ruffed lemur was caused by a herpesvirus. The clinical signs associated with the disease included intermittent rear limb lameness, progressing to seizures, coma, and death.[14] Bacterial meningitis and encephalitis has been associated with *K. pneumoniae* in a ruffed lemur and a black lemur.

A cerebrovascular accident (stroke) was diagnosed in a male black lemur. The animal was suspected to have experienced a seizure, but when he regained consciousness, he continued to have no function of the left forelimb or rear limb. Improvement in use occurred gradually over several months, to the point that the forelimb had good function and the rear limb had moderate use.

DISEASES OF THE CARDIOVASCULAR SYSTEM

Dissection and rupture of aortic aneurysms have been one of the most common causes of mortality among captive lemurs in Madagascar.[2, 6] Aneurysms occurred as the result of migration of the parasite *Spirocerca lupi*. This parasite has a dung beetle–dog cycle, but can apparently complete the cycle in lemurs as well. After ingestion, the larvae migrate through the wall of the thoracic aorta and may lead to rupture of the aorta.

This disease scenario does not occur in North America, probably because of the lack of access to infected beetles and because of hygiene practices that would remove contaminated feces. However, dissecting aneurysms and cardiac tamponade have occurred, and they were suspected to result from hypertension based on signs of cardiac hypertrophy.[1]

SYSTEMIC DISEASES AND MISCELLANEOUS CONDITIONS

Lemurs are quite sensitive to serious disease associated with *Toxoplasma gondii* infection. Toxoplasmosis is most common in ring-tailed lemurs, probably because they are a more terrestrial species. Deaths are often peracute; in some instances, death may follow a 1- to 2-day course of nonspecific signs such as depression and inappetence. Clinical pathology may reflect the multisystemic nature of the infection, with elevated liver and renal function indices. Diagnosis is conclusively made by histologic examination of tissues in animals that die. Tachyzoites may be seen in many tissues and may initiate inflammatory reactions or necrosis. In animals that survive, determination of toxoplasmosis titers in paired serum samples confirms the diagnosis. No treatment is effective. The disease is transmitted via ingestion of oocysts from infected cat feces; therefore, effective sanitation should prevent occurrence.

Malaria parasites have been identified in blood samples of *Eulemur* species in Madagascar. Several species of *Plasmodium* have been described, including *P. girardi* and *P. foleyi* in *Eulemur fulvus rufus*; *P. uilenbergi* in *Eulemur fulvus fulvus*; and *P. pereyarnhami*, *P. bucki*, and *P. coulangesi* in *Eulemur macaco*. These organisms are not pathogenic in the lemur hosts and do not infect humans.[15]

Arbovirus infections of lemurs have been investigated in an effort to determine if lemurs serve as a natural reservoir for human diseases. Lemurophilic mosquito species (*Mansonia uniformis, Aedes aegypti,* and *Culex watti*) are also anthropophilic, establishing a potential transmission route. Serologic surveys of lemurs have found titers to West Nile Fever virus and other alphaviruses and flaviviruses in a small percentage of free-ranging lemurs in some areas of Madagascar.[16] In no cases was virus isolated from lemurs, and in experimental inoculations with West Nile fever virus and yellow fever virus, transient viremia existed without clinical signs of illness. Antibody titers remained detectable, but virus could not be isolated after the initial viremia.[17] This suggests that these viruses are not sig-

nificant health concerns for lemurs, and captive lemurs do not pose a risk for exposure except for newly imported animals.

Cases of toxicosis are unusual in lemurs. This may be because of discretion in foraging habits. Three ruffed lemurs were apparently poisoned by hairy nightshade (*Solanum sarrachoides*) when introduced into a new exhibit.[7] In another incident, aflatoxin poisoning was suspected for three acute deaths in brown lemurs fed peanut meal as part of the ration.

REFERENCES

1. Benirschke K, Miller C, Ippen R, et al: The pathology of prosimians, especially lemurs. Adv Vet Sci Comp Med 30:167–208, 1985.
2. Blancou J, Albignac R: Note sur l'infestation des lemuriens malagaches par *Spirocerca lupi* (Rudolphi, 1809). Rev Elev Med Vet Pays Trop 29:127–130, 1976.
3. Bresnahan JF, Whitworth UG, Hayes Y, et al: *Yersinia enterocolitica* infection in breeding colonies of ruffed lemurs. J Am Vet Med Assoc 185:1354–1356, 1984.
4. Brockman DK, Willis MK, Karesh WB: Management and husbandry of ruffed lemurs, *Varecia variegata*, at the San Diego Zoo: III. Medical considerations and population management. Zoo Biol 7:253–262, 1988.
5. Burton M, Morton RJ, Ramsay E, et al: Coccidioidomycosis in a ring-tailed lemur. J Am Vet Med Assoc 189:1209–1211, 1986.
6. Coulanges P, Zeller H, Clerc Y, et al: Bacteries, virus, parasites pathologie et pathologie experimentale des lemuriens malagaches: Interet pour l'homme. Arch Inst Pasteur Madagascar 47:201–219, 1978.
7. Drew ML, Fowler ME: Poisoning of black and white ruffed lemurs (*Varecia variegata*) by hairy nightshade (*Solanum sarrachoides*). J Zoo Wildl Med 22:494–496, 1991.
8. Griner LA: Pathology of Zoo Animals. San Diego, Zoological Society of San Diego, 1983.
9. Haines DE: The Lesser Bushbaby (*Galago*) as an Animal Model: Selected Topics. Boca Raton, FL, CRC Press, 1982.
10. Junge RE: Medical management of the black lemur (*Eulemur macaco macaco*) in captivity [unpublished manual written for the Black Lemur SSP Committee]. St. Louis: St. Louis Zoo, 1997.
11. Junge RE, Garell D: Veterinary evaluation of ruffed lemurs (*Varecia variegata*) in Madagascar. Primate Conservation 16:44–46, 1995.
12. Junge RE, Merhen KG, Meehan TP, et al: Periarticular hyperostosis and renal disease in six black lemurs of two family groups. J Am Vet Med Assoc 205:1024–1029, 1994.
13. Knezevic AL, McNulty WP: Tuberculosis in *Lemur mongoz*. Folia Primatol (Basel) 6:153–159, 1967.
14. Kornegay RW, Baldwin TJ, Pirie G: Herpesvirus encephalitis in a ruffed lemur (*Varecia variegatus*). J Zoo Wildl Med 24:196–203, 1991.
15. Landau L, Lepers JP, Rabetafika R, et al: Plasmodies des lemuriens malagaches. Ann Parasitol Hum Comp 64:171–184, 1989.
16. Rodhain F, Clerc Y, Albignac R, et al: Arboviruses and lemurs in Madagascar: a preliminary note. Trans R Soc Trop Med Hyg 76:227–231, 1982.
17. Rodhain F, Petter JJ, Albignac R, et al: Arboviruses and lemurs in Madagascar: experimental infection of *Lemur fulvus* with Yellow Fever and West Nile Viruses. Am J Trop Med Hyg 34:816–822, 1985.
18. Schmidt RE: Tuberculosis in a ringtailed lemur (*Lemur catta*). J Zoo Anim Med 6:11–12, 1975.
19. Weber MA, Lamberski N, Heriot K: An idiopathic proliferative disease of bone in two subspecies of ruffed lemur (*Varecia variegata variegata* and *Varecia variegata rubra*). Proceedings of the Joint Conference of the American Association of Zoo Veterinarians, Wildlife Disease Association, and American Association of Wildlife Veterinarians, East Lansing, MI, p 268, 1995.
20. Wilson DE, Reeder DM (eds): Mammal Species of the World, 2nd ed. Washington, DC, Smithsonian Institution Press, 1993.

CHAPTER 48

Diseases of the Callitrichidae

RICHARD J. MONTALI

MITCHELL BUSH

Marmosets, tamarins, and Goeldi's monkeys (*Callimico goeldii*) are small neotropical primates indigenous to Central and South America. The taxonomy of a number of these species and subspecies appear to be under continual revision, but according to current International Species Information System (ISIS) usage, the three groups are classified as Callitrichidae. Earlier classification of marmosets and tamarins as Callithricidae is no longer the acceptable form; Goeldi's monkeys have also been categorized as Callimiconidae. Genera in these families include *Callithrix*, the marmosets (pygmy marmosets have been classified also as *Cebuella*); *Saguinus* and *Leontopithecus*, the tamarins; and *Callimico*, the Goeldi's monkeys.

Marmosets are smaller than tamarins and have specialized lower incisors for gathering tree sap (exudates)[44] (Fig. 48–1). Tamarins are a diverse group and contain the most species, including the endangered cotton-top tamarin, *Saguinus oedipus*, and four species of lion tamarins, *Leontopithecus* species, which are endemic to the Atlantic coastal rain forests of Brazil and also endangered. These include the golden lion tamarin, *L. rosalia*, from Rio De Janeiro, the golden-headed lion tamarin, *L. chrysomelas*, from southern Bahia, the black

lion tamarin, *L. chrysopygus*, from São Paulo, and the rare black-headed (or black-faced) lion tamarin, *L. caissara*, most recently described as a new species near São Paulo and on the island of Superagui. The highest profile species of lion tamarin in zoological collections is the golden lion tamarin, which has been propagated under captive conditions, ex situ, and reintroduced successfully into natural habitat during the last decade.[27] Goeldi's monkeys are the most primitive of the three groups.[13, 19, 39]

Callitrichids usually live in family groups, lending themselves to interesting exhibitry in zoo collections. Although adaptable, marmosets, tamarins, and Goeldi's monkeys are delicate and require careful management for successful display and propagation. Callitrichids are subject to a number of infectious and noninfectious diseases that need to be controlled or prevented. A recent comprehensive review by Potkay summarizes the world literature on diseases of Callitrichidae,[43] and includes descriptions of infectious, parasitic, nutritional/metabolic disease, tumors, and diseases of special organ systems. Several additional disease surveys of various species of callitrichids have also been published.[12, 15, 28, 49, 54]

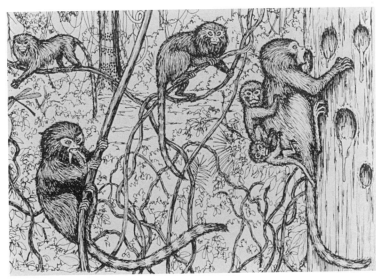

FIGURE 48–1. Graphic depiction of callitrichid food gathering habits: tamarins catching and eating insects (*left*), and a marmoset gouging for tree exudates (*right*). (From Fleagle JG: Primate Adaptation and Evolution. New York, Academic Press, 1988, p 146.)

This chapter will discuss and illustrate some important diseases of marmosets, tamarins, and Goeldi's monkeys that occur commonly in zoological collections. Sources include pathology surveys of diseases affecting callitrichids derived from a 20-year pathology database at the National Zoological Park (NZP), Species Survival Plan (SSP) and studbook records for the golden lion tamarin,[2] and the available literature. Conditions improved by medical intervention or management changes will be emphasized.

INFECTIOUS DISEASES

Viral

Herpesvirus tamarinus (herpesvirus T or *Herpesvirus platyrrhinae*) and *Herpesvirus simplex* (HSV-1 and HSV-2), both alphaherpesviruses, can cause acute, disseminated disease characterized by oral and cutaneous ulceration, lethargy, and death in several days. Squirrel monkeys, *Saimiri sciureus,* are the reservoir host for herpes-T, which usually remain asymptomatic while carrying the virus. *Herpesvirus simplex* has clearly been implicated in fatalities in callitrichid species associated with owners or keepers with open herpetic lip or mouth ulcers.[7, 25] Latent gammaherpesviruses, including *Herpesvirus saimiri* in squirrel monkeys, *Herpesvirus ateles* in spider monkeys, *Ateles* species, and the human herpes Epstein-Barr virus (EBV or human herpesvirus 4), can experimentally induce lymphoproliferative conditions in callitrichids and potentially cause lymphomatous conditions in these species. Such fatal neoplastic conditions have occurred in a colony of common marmosets, *Callithrix jacchus,* in which EBV was implicated.[46] Preventing callitrichid herpesvirus infections can be achieved by avoiding any form of direct or indirect contact or mixed exhibits with cebids and callitrichids. In addition, humans symptomatic for HSV infections or EBV should not be allowed to have any contact with callitrichids.

Lymphocytic choriomeningitis virus (LCMV), the etiologic agent of callitrichid hepatitis (CH), is characterized by an acute onset with lethargy, anorexia, elevated liver enzymes, and variably jaundice and grand mal seizures. The case-fatality rate is high, with a direct association with feeding mice that are latently infected with LCMV. Historically, supplementing callitrichids with neonatal mice (pinkies) (Fig. 48–2) led to sporadic outbreaks of this disease throughout U.S. zoos in the 1980s and early 1990s, with a high incidence in golden lion tamarins. In addition, cases of CH can also occur from the callitrichids catching wild mice in their exhibits and eating and sharing them (Fig. 48–3). The clinical signs and characteristic findings of a viral type of hepatitis with acidophilic bodies and immunohistochemical evidence of LCMV antigens are diagnostic for this disease.[35]

No cases or evidence of previous exposure to LCMV have been reported from research colonies of callitrichids nor have they been identified in a comprehensive serosurvey of wild golden lion tamarins in their natural habitat in Brazil.[51] Seroconversion to LCMV, a zoonotic

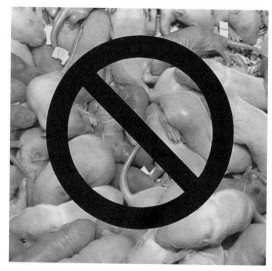

FIGURE 48–2. Neonatal mice (pinkies) should *never* be fed to callitrichids because they can carry lymphocytic choriomeningitis virus, the cause of callitrichid hepatitis.

disease, has occurred in several callitrichid caretakers but without evidence of clinical disease. Control of CH can be achieved by avoiding the feeding of mice to callitrichids and by vigilant rodent extermination; however, eradication of the disease requires zero-level contact of the callitrichids with wild mice.[36]

Hepadenoviruses and other hepatotropic viral diseases of callitrichids are covered in *Zoo and Wild Ani-*

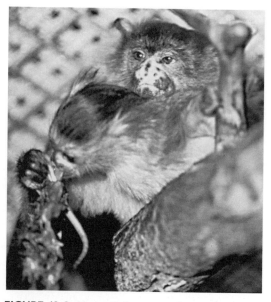

FIGURE 48–3. Black-tailed marmoset shown with a decapitated wild mouse it caught in its exhibit with cagemate waiting behind to share. This behavior can lead to callitrichid hepatitis, toxoplasmosis, yersiniosis, and other infectious diseases. Stringent rodent control is necessary wherever callitrichids are kept. (Courtesy of Lee Miller.)

mal Medicine: Current Therapy 3.[47] Other fatal viral diseases sporadically reported in callitrichids include measles[29, 30] and encephalomyocarditis virus.[56] Types of clinically relevant viral diseases documented in laboratory and research callitrichid colonies include an inclusion body hepatitis seen in *S. fuscicollis*,[55] parainfluenza type 1 (Sendai), and a paramyxovirus distinct from measles.[20]

Bacterial Diseases

Streptococcus zooepidemicus septicemia outbreaks in callitrichids can occur from exposure to contaminated uncooked horse meat fed to carnivorous species kept in mixed exhibits or from cross-contamination during food preparation. This occurred in golden lion tamarins, red-bellied tamarins, *S. labiatus,* and Goeldi's monkeys.[52] Animals developed cervical suppurative lymphadenitis, splenitis, and enteritis that usually terminated in fatal sepsis; one animal treated with fluids and antibiotics survived. Raw meat products used in mixed exhibits with susceptible species should be cooked or not fed; sanitary precautions should be taken to prevent cross-contamination by food pans or other fomites during food preparation.

Yersinia pseudotuberculosis and *Y. enterocolitica* harbored by rodents and birds can cause sporadic or high mortalities in callitrichids. Animals are often found dead and show severe suppurative enteric and hepatic lesions containing massive colonies of organisms, which is nearly diagnostic. The virulence of the *Yersinia* varies and has been found to be related to certain plasmids in callitrichids.[4] Rodent and avian pest management is important in the control of yersiniosis. Some zoos, particularly in Europe, have resorted to autologous vaccines, with some anecdotally reported success.

Pasteurella species cause disease in callitrichids, including pneumonia, hepatitis, tooth infections, and septicemia. Chronic tooth root abscesses mainly of the canine teeth have occurred in black-tailed marmoset, *C. argentata melanura,* and golden lion tamarins, with signs as vague as lethargy and anorexia to obvious facial fistulas from infected tooth roots. Outbreaks of fatal septicemia caused by *Pasteurella multocida* have occurred in Goeldi's monkeys in association with oral gongylonemiasis.[11]

Other important bacterial diseases of callitrichids include *Bordetella bronchiseptica* pneumonia in common marmosets; *Klebsiella* species infections[43] and sporadic or singular cases of leptospirosis[48]; listeria meningitis (NZP golden-headed lion tamarin); and peritonitis associated with *Aeromonas hydrophilia.*[6] Mycobacterial diseases are uncommon; a case of *Mycobacterium avium* complex was reported in a common marmoset *(C. jacchus),*[17] and an outbreak of an undetermined type of tuberculosis was recorded in golden lion tamarins.[9]

Infectious Versus Noninfectious Causes of Diarrhea, Colitis, and Wasting Disease

Diarrhea is relatively common in callitrichid species. It is sometimes related to diets with too high a ratio of fruit or vegetables, selective feeding by individuals, and colony social or physiologic stress factors. A complete history of the callitrichid patient followed by a physical examination and laboratory evaluation should be initiated. Fecal cytology for white blood cells, Gram staining and morphology of the microflora, examination for parasites and occult blood, and culturing for bacterial pathogens should be performed before antibiotic treatment.

Colitis and so-called wasting marmoset syndrome (WMS) may have been more common in laboratory colonies where animals were usually not housed in family units. Results of a survey addressing this syndrome, however, indicated that WMS continues to be a significant cause of morbidity in callitrichid collections. The etiology is likely multifactorial, with dietary factors being important considerations.[22] WMS and colitis are mentioned in other sections of this chapter on infections, parasitisms, and neoplastic conditions.

The most common causes of infectious forms of diarrhea in zoo callitrichids include *Salmonella enteritidis,* other salmonellae, and yersiniosis; shigellosis appears to be more of a problem in laboratory colonies of callitrichids. *Campylobacter jejuni* is commonly isolated from well animals and animals with diarrhea, but clinical interpretation of this organism can be difficult. It has been isolated from golden lion tamarins at NZP without clinical disease, but it has been associated with inflammatory bowel disease in other callitrichid colonies.[43] Enterohemorrhagic colitis occurred in common marmosets associated with enteroadherent *Escherichia coli* (Dr. James Thompson, Wisconsin Regional Primate Center, unpublished observations). Some viral agents, including coronaviruses[50] and adenovirus in pygmy marmosets[40] of questionable pathogenicity, have been observed in callitrichids with enteric diseases.

Management and Treatment of Suspected Infectious Diarrheas

Therapy for diarrhea should not be delayed pending an etiologic diagnosis because callitrichids are fragile, with limited reserves (like birds), and require immediate support. Initially, warmth and a quiet environment should be provided, and food intake should be restricted to remove any item that may have initiated or could aggravate the diarrhea. Adequate water intake is essential; drinking should not be discouraged by adding medication to the water source.

Unless the condition appears life-threatening, handling and medication should be withheld for 8 to 12 hours with the animal under close observation, after which intestinal protectorants such as kaolin or barium sulfate can be administered. The use of anticholinergics may be contraindicated unless spasmodic pain accompanies the diarrhea.

Depending on the circumstances, fluid and electrolyte replacement may be initiated subcutaneously or via stomach tube, especially in protracted cases, to restore potassium. If unresponsive, the patient may need to be rehydrated by the intravenous or interosseous route. The initial choice and route of the antibiotic depends on whether septicemia is also a factor, and it might change depending on the culture and sensitivity results. Antibiotic should be continued for 3 to 5 days beyond abatement of symptoms. During prolonged use of antibiotics, feces should be monitored by cytologic examination for yeast overgrowth. Yogurt or lactobacillus can be given during and for several days after the antibiotic treatment to aid in restoring normal intestinal flora.

Parasitism

PROTOZOA

Toxoplasma gondii occurs sporadically in marmosets and tamarins. Acute enteric and pulmonary forms of toxoplasmosis have occurred in clusters of golden lion tamarins[16, 24, 34] at North American and European Zoos. Clinical signs can resemble an acute toxicosis, with affected animals showing respiratory distress from pulmonary edema or found dead with typical pathologic findings of acute toxoplasmosis. Sources of the disease are usually through contamination of food or living quarters by cat feces or from callitrichids catching and eating mice containing toxoplasma cysts (see Fig. 48–3). Best prevention is by rodent and feral cat control.

Trypanosoma cruzi, the cause of Chagas' disease of humans, can be carried by natural callitrichid hosts, although any public health risks reside where triatomid bugs exist in tropical areas.[43] Neotropical primates are commonly found to be infected (subclinically), but monitoring of these natural trypanosomal infections has been inadequate. Golden lion tamarins positive for *T. cruzi* have been identified from preserves in Brazil that have provided stock for SSP programs; however, no reported clinical signs or disease implication for other animals or humans have been documented (J. Dietz, University of Maryland, personal communication, December, 1997).

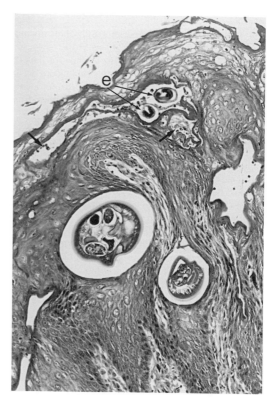

FIGURE 48–5. Photomicrograph of cross sections of *Gongylonema* nematodes and embryonated eggs *(e)* from the tongue of a Goeldi's monkey. Hematoxylin and eosin stain; original magnification, ×150. (From Duncan M, Tell L, Gardiner CH, et al: Lingual gongylonemiasis and pasteurellosis in Goeldi's monkeys, *Callimico goeldii.* J Zoo Wildl Med 26[1]:102–108, 1995.)

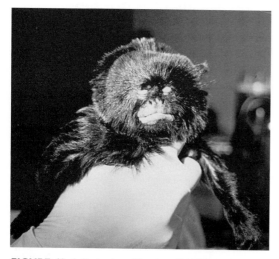

FIGURE 48–4. Perioral swelling in a Goeldi's monkey caused by severe *Gongylonema* (tongue worm) infection. (From Duncan M, Tell L, Gardiner CH, et al: Lingual gongylonemiasis and pasteurellosis in Goeldi's monkeys, *Callimico goeldii.* J Zoo Wildl Med 26[1]:102–108, 1995.)

NEMATODES

Three spirurid nematodes carried by cockroaches and copraphageous beetles represent an important group of helminths pathogenic for callitrichid species. *Pterygodermatites nycticebi* (formerly *Rictularia* species) emerged as a significant intestinal spirurid in captive callitrichids, primarily in golden lion tamarins,[32] but it has been found also in other tamarin species. *Trichospirura leptostoma* is a commonly found spirurid in the pancreatic duct of callitrichids; it is usually considered incidental, but it has been implicated in WMS.[41] *Gongylonema pulchrum,* previously considered to be an innocuous spirurid of the oral cavity with a wide host range, recently emerged as a clinically important parasite of the tongue and other oral tissues in Goeldi's monkey and pygmy marmosets; it is also associated with chronic ptyalism[11] (Figs. 48–4, 48–5).

These three forms of pathogenic spirurids in callitrichids are diagnosed by finding typical thick-shelled embryonated eggs (Fig. 48–6) by fecal flotation, although distinguishing the different nematodes by the eggs is difficult. Gentle scraping of tongue and oral mucosa for similarly appearing eggs, however, provides evidence of oral spirurid infection. Periodic (monthly,

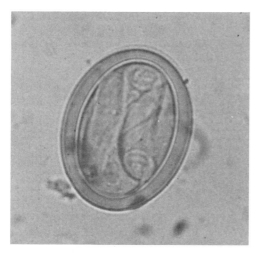

FIGURE 48–6. Characteristic appearance of a spirurid egg from a fecal flotation; note thick shell with embryonated center. Unstained; original magnification, × 500. (From Jones TC, Mohr U, Hunt RD [eds]: Nonhuman Primates II, Monographs on Pathology of Laboratory Animals. International Life Sciences Institute. Berlin, Springer-Verlag, pp 69-70, 1993.)

quarterly, or biannually depending on the degree of infection) treatment with mebendazole (Telmin) orally at 15 mg/kg for 3 consecutive days appears to be efficacious for the enteric and perhaps the pancreatic spirurids, but at the time of this writing this product was being removed from the market. Fenbendazole, 40 to 60 mg/kg orally for 5 consecutive days, or ivermectin, 200 to 250 μg/kg subcutaneously, appears to be similarly effective. The oral spirurids appear to be much more resistant; they respond best to periodic treatment with mebendazole, up to 70 mg/kg consecutively for 3 days, but not very well to ivermectin. Levamisole has been used successfully in treating saki monkeys, *Pithecia pithecia,* for clinical oral spiruridiasis with 4 to 5 mg/kg orally for 6 days, after which worms and eggs were no longer detectable.[26] Heavy parasitism with any of these spirurids can be associated with heavy cockroach infestation, so vigilant roach control is essential.

Cerebrospinal nematodiasis (larva migrans) in callitrichids is associated with aberrant migration of larvae of *Baylisascaris* species, the natural hosts of which are raccoons, skunks, and badgers. Larvae cannot be distinguished between the three, but *B. procyonis* from raccoons is considered the most common source. Affected animals show a variety of central nervous system deficits, including ataxia, head tilt, blindness, and circling, weeks to months after direct ingestion or from food contaminated with feces of the definitive host that contained *Baylisascaris* eggs. Antemortem diagnosis is difficult and postmortem proof is required; immunologic diagnostic methods are still experimental. This condition appears to be on the increase in zoo callitrichids, probably because of the continuing urbanization of raccoons and their latrine habits of exposing scats in trees and on the ground. The incidence in lion tamarins in North American zoos appears to be increasing. Pre-

vention includes control of raccoons and other wildlife and judicious planning of facilities so that fecal contamination of exhibits does not occur.[14, 21]

ACANTHOCEPHALA

The thorny-headed worm, *Prosthenorchis elegans*, also borne by cockroaches, has remained a cause of fatal peritonitis from gastric penetration by the parasite in some zoo callitrichid collections.[28] To prevent this parasite from causing death, aggressive treatment is required, with mebendazole up to 100 mg/kg of body weight for alternate weeks together with a special surgical technique to remove adult and juvenile worms embedded in the intestinal tracts of affected callitrichids.[57] Rigid control of roaches is also an essential step in controlling this parasite.

NONINFECTIOUS DISEASES

Congenital/Familial

A low percentage of congenital anomalies, including facial and cephalic malformations, cleft palate, and hydrocephalus, were recognized predominantly in neonatal golden lion tamarins from SSP mortality records.[2]

A relatively high frequency of retrosternal diaphragmatic defects leading to herniation occurred in the early ex situ propagation stages of golden lion tamarins, possibly associated with the use of over-represented founders occultly affected by the condition.[36] Subsequently, diaphragmatic defects were reported anecdotally in a golden-headed lion tamarin and were also observed in a black lion tamarin originating from the wild (Dr. F. Simon, personal communication, 1988). A true genetic mode could never be established for these diaphragmatic abnormalities, and the incidence of overt defects decreased markedly after breeding management changes.

However, a familial basis for such defects is still very likely, and an inverted radiographic contrast peritonealogram was developed to score variations in diaphragm contour that were inapparent by conventional methods. Golden lion tamarins evaluated for reintroduction potential are screened, and those with a score above 3 (range, 0 to 5), which is indicative of an abnormal contour or protrusions at the retrosternal attachments of the diaphragm (Fig. 48–7), are withdrawn from the program.[5]

Hyperbilirubinemia resembling the Dubin-Johnson syndrome, a nonlethal disturbance in the metabolism of bilirubin in humans, occurs in female golden lion tamarins.[53] The animals have persistent hyperbilirubinemia (1 to 8 mg/dl, mostly conjugated) and may appear slightly jaundiced and retain bromsulphalein, but otherwise remain healthy with no evidence of liver enzyme elevation or illness. Animals necropsied (for unrelated conditions) show dark brown to black, reticulated livers containing a melanin-like pigment low in iron content. Although it is benign, tamarins identified with this condition should be removed as breeders and from reintroduction programs.

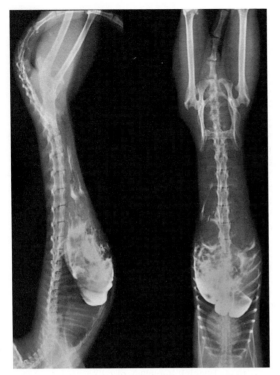

FIGURE 48–7. Inverted contrast peritonealogram in a golden lion tamarin shows moderate protrusion (grade 4) of the diaphragm at the retrosternal attachments indicating a propensity for herniation. (From Bush M, Beck BB, Dietz J, et al: Radiographic evaluation of diaphragmatic defects in golden lion tamarins, *Leontopithecus rosalia rosalia:* implications for reintroduction. J Zoo Wildl Med 27[3]:346–357, 1996.)

Emergency Conditions

Gastric bloat occasionally occurs usually for unknown reasons in callitrichids and requires immediate relief via gastric lavage and supportive treatment. Hypoglycemic episodes are characterized by finding animals at the bottom of their cage and weak. This also may be life-threatening and can usually be reversed with 20% dextrose by stomach tube or, in milder cases, by feeding fruit.[7]

Organ-Specific Entities

GASTROINTESTINAL

Gastrointestinal diseases, including gastric ulcers, ulcerative and lymphoplasmacytic colitis, intussusception, and rectal prolapse, were observed in different NZP callitrichid species. Peritonitis of unknown etiology was observed in NZP pygmy marmosets.

An unusually high prevalence of cystine choleliths and septate gallbladder occurs in lion tamarin species and marmosets. Biliary obstruction is an uncommon sequela. Calculi are slight radiopaque and are usually found incidentally at necropsy as light to dark gray and measuring 1 to 5 mm in diameter. The pathogenesis of these cystine-rich stones is unknown, and a familial trend has not been established for this condition. Stone formation may be related to bile flow stasis associated with interference from the incomplete mural septae in the gallbladder.[42]

URINARY

Callitrichids have a relatively high incidence of glomerulonephropathies. Glomerulonephritis has been attributed in some species older than 6 months of age to immunoglobulin M deposition in glomeruli via immune-mediated mechanisms.[3] Renal disease in pygmy marmosets resembles forms of hypertensive nephropathy associated with vascular lesions. Cardiomegaly and ascites are indicative of congestive heart failure.[8] A progressive nephropathy in Goeldi's monkeys may have a different pathogenesis from these renal conditions and requires further study.

REPRODUCTIVE

Subcutaneous contraceptive implants of melengestrol remaining in female Goeldi's monkeys for 2 to 7 years led to extensive decidualization of the endometrial stroma. This caused extensive thickening of the uterine wall, mimicking neoplastic growth that resulted in clinical disease. This form of steroidal contraception is discouraged.[37]

Dystocias with fetal and maternal mortalities have occurred in golden-headed lion tamarins, possibly related to pelvic diameter and fetal size incompatibilities.

Nutritional and Metabolic

Metabolic bone disease and other micronutrient deficiencies have been reported in callitrichids and still remain important considerations under captive conditions. Much higher circulating levels of vitamin D metabolites occur in wild and captive callitrichids (greater than 50 ng/ml 25-hydroxyvitamin D_3) than in humans and other primates, suggesting higher requirements in callitrichids for this vitamin. Therefore, furnishing adequate ultraviolet light (UV-B) for indoor exhibits balanced with exposure to sunlight and providing cholecalciferol, the bioavailable form of vitamin D, are necessary for good bone health in all callitrichid species. Callitrichids also require good sources of vitamin C and E.[1, 31, 45]

Toxic and Miscellaneous

Toxic exposures in callitrichids are sporadic and uncommon. Organophosphate poisoning has been reported in marmosets. One significant event occurred at the NZP with inadvertent exposure to brodifacoum, a third-generation anticoagulant rodenticide. Four golden lion tamarins ingested this substance and died of a coagulopathy.

Iron accumulation in callitrichid livers is common with baseline levels reported as high as 6182 mg/g (dry weight) in common marmosets.[32] It is most likely related to factors associated with dietary iron, a high iron-absorption threshold, and low or lack of natural protective or regulating factors. As with many other species in captive settings, iron metabolism is not well understood in callitrichids. Iron feeding trials in laboratory marmosets for up to a year resulted in mortalities in a high-dose group and hepatic iron levels below baseline in the low-dose group.[31a] Therefore, hepatic iron accumulation may be detrimental in callitrichids over the long term; fruit and vitamin C and its derivatives enhance gut absorption of iron, and these should be fed judiciously to these species.

Tumors

A number of sporadic tumors are reported in callitrichids, but the most highly characterized tumor is colonic adenocarcinoma of cotton-top tamarins. This lesion has been associated with ulcerative colitis and represents a model for colitis and cancer in humans; etiologic agents, including viruses, have not been identified.[23] Callitrichids seem also to have a higher predilection for endocrine tumors, particularly benign pheochromocytomas and benign thyroid and pituitary neoplasms, than do Old World primates.[10] Tumors observed with two or more occurrences in golden lion tamarins included biliary adenocarcinomas. Lymphosarcoma was observed in a golden lion tamarin and a common marmoset, and an unusual melanotic ependymoma occurred in a Goeldi's monkey neonate.[38]

Hepatic myelolipomas have been observed in Goeldi's monkeys from NZP and from several other sources[18] (Dr. L. Phillips, unpublished observations, University of California at Davis) and in adrenals of other callitrichid species.[43] The pathogenesis of these quasi-neoplasms is unknown.

CONCLUSION

Callitrichids are subject to many infectious and noninfectious conditions that can limit success rates for good exhibitry and breeding programs. One unifying theme in the infectious category is the association of the number of viral, bacterial, and parasitic diseases with roaches, mice (see Fig. 48–3), and other vermin that the callitrichids seek out in their exhibits and regularly eat. Therefore, zoo veterinary staff members must be very familiar with these issues and must participate in their control. Pest control programs should be established at all zoos.

Many of the noninfectious conditions seen may also be products of ex situ conditions that can be rectified by management decisions relating to species selection, breeding choices, and sensitivity to the special needs of these delicate callitrichids. Veterinary advisors from the SSP and Taxon Advisory Groups (TAGs) for the Callitrichidae are a good source of biomedical knowledge and can be readily consulted for more detailed information about any of these species. Special quarantine procedures before reintroduction have been developed for lion tamarins[34] and are available through the International Golden Lion Tamarin Studbook Keeper.[2]

REFERENCES

1. Allen ME, Montali RJ: Nutrition and disease in zoo animals. Verh ber Zootiere 37:215–231, 1995.
2. Ballou JD: International Studbook Keeper, Golden Lion Tamarin, *Leontopithecus rosalia rosalia.* Washington, DC, National Zoological Park, 1983–1995.
3. Brack M: IgM-mesangial nephropathy in callitrichids. Vet Pathol 25:270–276, 1988.
4. Brack M, Hosefelder F: In vitro characteristics of *Yersinia pseudotuberculosis* of nonhuman origin. Zbl Bakt 277:280–287, 1992.
5. Bush M, Beck BB, Dietz J, et al: Radiographic evaluation of diaphragmatic defects in golden lion tamarins, *Leontopithecus rosalia rosalia:* implications for reintroduction. J Zoo Wildl Med 27(3):346–357, 1996.
6. Chalifoux LV, Hajema EM, Lee-Parritz DL: *Aeromonas hydrophila* peritonitis in a cotton-top tamarin, *Saguinus oedipus,* and retrospective study of infections in seven primate species. Lab Anim Sci 43(4):355–358, 1993.
7. Cicmanec JL: Medical problems encountered in a callitrichid colony. *In* Kleiman DG (ed): The Biology and Conservation of the Callitrichidae. Washington, DC, Smithsonian Institution Press, pp 331–336, 1977.
8. Cooley AJ: Hypertension in Pygmy marmosets (abstract). Annual Proceedings of the American College of Veterinary Pathology, Baltimore, p 51, 1989.
9. Crandall LS: Management of Wild Mammals in Captivity. Chicago, University of Chicago Press, pp 101–106, 1964.
10. Dias JLC, Montali RJ, Strandberg JD, et al: Endocrine neoplasia in New World primates. J Med Primatol 25:34–41, 1996.
11. Duncan M, Tell L, Gardiner CH, et al: Lingual gongylonemiasis and pasteurellosis in Goeldi's monkeys, *Callimico goeldii.* J Zoo Wildl Med 26(1):102–108, 1995.
12. Eulenberger VK, Krische G, Adler J, et al: Keeping, reproduction, and diseases of common marmosets *(Callithrix jacchus)* in Leipzig Zoo. Verh ber Erkr Zootiere 29:225–238, 1987.
13. Fleagle JG: Primate Adaptation and Evolution. New York, Academic Press, pp 114–157, 1988.
14. Garlick DS, Marcus LC, Pokras M, et al: *Baylisascaris* larva migrans in a spider monkey, *Ateles* sp. J Med Primatol 25:133–136, 1996.
15. Gozalo A, Montoya E: Mortality causes of the moustached tamarin, *Saguinus mystax,* in captivity. J Med Primatol 21:35–38, 1991.
16. Griner LA: Pathology of Zoo Animals. San Diego, Zoological Society of San Diego, p 334, 1983.
17. Hatt JM, Guscetti F: A case of mycobacteriosis in a common marmoset, *Callithrix jacchus.* Annual Proceedings of the American Association of Zoo Veterinarians, Pittsburgh, pp 241–243, 1994.
18. Hauser BR, Baumgartner R: Colonic adenocarcinoma and hepatic myelopipomas in a Goeldi's monkey, *Callimico goeldii.* Folia Primatol 57:52–56, 1991.
19. Hershkovitz P: Living New World Monkeys *(Platyrrhini),* with an Introduction to Primates, vol 1. Chicago, University of Chicago Press, pp 397–450, 1977.
20. Hunt RD, Blake DJ: Gastroenteritis due to paramyxovirus. *In* Jones TC, Mohr U, Hunt RD (eds): Nonhuman Primates II, Monographs on Pathology of Laboratory Animals. International Life Sciences Institute. Berlin, Springer-Verlag, pp 32–37, 1993.
21. Huntress SL, Spraker T: *Baylisascaris* infection in the marmoset. Annual Proceedings of the American Association of Zoo Veterinarians, Scottsdale, AZ, p 78, 1985.
22. Ialeggio M, Baker AJ: Results of a preliminary survey into wasting marmoset syndrome in callitrichid collections. Proceedings of the First Annual Conference of the Nutrition Advisory Group of the American Zoo and Aquarium Association, Ontario, Canada, pp 148–158, 1995.
23. Johnson LD, Ausman LM, Sehgal PK, et al: A prospective study of the epidemiology of colitis and colon cancer in cotton-top tamarins, *Saguinus oedipus.* Gastroenterology 110:102–115, 1996.
24. Juan-Salles C, Prats N, Marco AJ, et al: Fatal acute toxoplasmosis in three golden lion tamarins, *Leontopithecus rosalia.* J Zoo Wildl Med 29(1), 1998.
25. Juan-Salles C, Ramos-Vara JA, Prats N, et al: Spontaneous herpes simplex virus infection in common marmosets, *Callithrix jacchus.* J Vet Diagn Invest 9:341–345, 1997.
26. Klaver PSJ, Hobbelink ME, Erken AHM, et al: *Gongylonema pulchrum* infection and therapy in a pale-head sake, *Pithecia pithecia:* a case report. Verh Erkrg Zootiere 36:409–413, 1994.

27. Kleiman DG, Beck BB, Baker AJ, et al: The conservation program for the golden lion tamarin. Endang Sp Update 8(1):82–85, 1990.
28. Letcher J: Survey of *Saguinus* mortality in a zoo colony. J Med Primatol 21:24–29, 1992.
29. Lorenz D, Albercht P: Susceptibility of tamarins, *Saguinus*, to measles virus. Lab Anim Sci 30:661–665, 1980.
30. Lowenstine LJ: Measles virus infection, non-human primates. *In* Jones TC, Mohr U, Hunt RD (eds): Nonhuman Primates I, Monographs on Pathology of Laboratory Animals. International Life Sciences Institute. Berlin, Springer-Verlag, pp 108–118, 1993.
31. Meehan TP, Crissey SD, Langman CB, et al: Vitamin D related disease in infant primates. Annual Proceedings of the American Association of Zoo Veterinarians, Puerta Vallarta, Mexico, pp 91–93, 1996.
31a. Miller GF, Barnard DE, Woodward RA, et al: Hepatic hemosiderosis in common marmosets, *Callithrix jacchus*: effect of diet on incidence and severity. Lab Anim Sci 47(2):138–142, 1997.
32. Montali RJ: *Pterygodermatites nycticebi*, tamarins. *In* Jones TC, Mohr U, Hunt RD (eds): Nonhuman Primates II, Monographs on Pathology of Laboratory Animals. International Life Sciences Institute. Berlin, Springer-Verlag, pp 69–70, 1993.
33. Montali RJ: Congenital retrosternal diaphragmatic defects, golden lion tamarins. *In* Jones TC, Mohr U, Hunt RD (eds): Nonhuman Primates II, Monographs on Pathology of Laboratory Animals. International Life Sciences Institute. Berlin, Springer-Verlag, pp 132–133, 1993.
34. Montali RJ, Bush M, Hess J, et al: Ex situ diseases and their control for reintroduction of the endangered lion tamarin species, *Leontopithecus* spp. Verh Erkrg Zootiere 37:93–98, 1995.
35. Montali RJ, Connolly BM, Armstrong DL, et al: Pathology and immunochemistry of callitrichid hepatitis, an emerging disease of captive new world primates caused by lymphocytic choriomeningitis virus. Am J Pathol 148:1441–1449, 1995.
36. Montali RJ, Scanga CA, Pernikoff D, et al: A common-source outbreak of callitrichid hepatitis in captive tamarins and marmosets. J Infect Dis 167:946–950, 1993.
37. Murnane RD, Zdziarski JM, Walsh TF, et al: Melengestrol acetate–induced exuberant endometrial decidualization in Goeldi's marmosets, *Callimico goeldii*, and squirrel monkeys, *Saimiri sciureus*. J Zoo Wildl Med 27(3):315–324, 1996.
38. Nichols DK, Dias JLC: Melanotic ependymoma in a Goeldi's marmoset, *Callimico goeldii*. J Med Primatol 24:49–51, 1995.
39. Nowak RM: Order, Primates. *In* Walker's Mammals of the World, 5th ed, vol 1. Baltimore, Johns Hopkins University Press, pp 435–444, 1991.
40. Paul-Murphy J, Cooley AJ, Krugner-Higby: Epidemic of enteritis and colitis in a pygmy marmoset, *Cebuella pygmae*, colony. Annual Proceedings of the American Association of Zoo Veterinarians, Puerta Vallarta, Mexico, pp 214–217, 1996.
40a. Pessier A, Stringfield C, Tragle J, et al: Cerebrospinal nematodiasis due to *Baylisascaris* sp. in golden lion tamarins *(Leontophithecus chrysomelas)*: Implications for management. Annual Proceedings of the American Association of Zoo Veterinarians, Houston, TX, pp 245–247, 1997.

41. Pfister R, Heider B, Illgen B, et al: *Trichospirura leptostoma*: a possible cause of wasting disease in the marmoset. Z Versuchstierkd 33:157–161, 1990.
42. Pissinatti AJ, Batista da Cruz M, Dias do Nascimento R, et al: Spontaneous gallstones in marmosets and tamarins (*Callitrichidae*, primates). Folia Primatol 59:44–50, 1992.
43. Potkay S: Diseases of the Callitrichidae: a review. J Med Primatol 21:189–236, 1992.
44. Power ML, Oftedal OT: Differences among captive callitrichids in the digestive responses to dietary gum. Am J Primatol 40:131–144, 1996.
45. Power ML, Oftedal OT, Savage A, et al: Assessing vitamin D status of callitrichids: baseline data from wild cotton-top tamarins, *Saguinus oedipus*, in Columbia. Zoo Biol 16:39–46, 1997.
46. Ramer JC, O'Rourke C, Thomson JA: Fatal lymphoproliferative lymphosarcoma in a captive population of common marmosets, *Callithrix jacchus*. Annual Proceedings of the American Association of Zoo Veterinarians, Puerta Vallarta, Mexico, pp 206–207, 1996.
47. Ramsay E, Montali RJ: Viral hepatitis in new world primates. *In* Fowler ME (ed): Zoo and Wild Animal Medicine: Current Therapy 3. Philadelphia, WB Saunders, pp 355–358, 1993.
48. Reid HAC, Herron SJ, Hines ME, et al: Leptospirosis in a white-lipped tamarin, *Saguinus labiatus*. Lab Anim Sci 43(3):258–259, 1993.
49. Rothe H, Darms K, Koenig A: Sex ratio and mortality in a laboratory colony of the common marmoset, *Callithrix jacchus*. Lab Anim 26:88–99, 1992.
50. Russell RG, Brian DA, Lenhard A, et al: Coronavirus-like particles and *Campylobacter* in marmosets with diarrhea and colitis. Dig Dis Sci 30(12):72S–77S, 1985.
51. Scanga CA, Holmes KV, Montali RJ: Serological evidence of infection with lymphocytic choriomeningitis virus, the agent of callitrichid hepatitis, in primates in zoos, primate research centers, and a natural reserve. J Zoo Wildl Med 24(4):469–474, 1993.
52. Schiller CA, Wolff MJ, Munson L, et al: *Streptococcus zooepidemicus* infections of possible horsemeat source in red-bellied tamarins and Goeldi's monkeys. J Zoo Wildl Med 20(3):322–327, 1989.
53. Schulman FY, Montali RJ, Bush M, et al: Dubin-Johnson–like syndrome in golden lion tamarins, *Leontopithecus rosalia rosalia*. Vet Pathol 30:491–498, 1993.
54. Scullion FT, Brown PJ, Potts E: A survey of the pathology in a breeding group of cotton top tamarins, *Saguinus o. oedipus*. Verh Erkr Zootiere 29:239–245, 1987.
55. Stiglmair-Herb MT, Scheid R, Haenichen T: Spontaneous inclusion body hepatitis in young tamarins: I. Morphological study. Lab Anim 26:80–87, 1992.
56. Wells SK, Gutter AE, Soike KF, et al: Present status of encephalomyocarditis virus at the Audubon Zoo. Annual Proceedings of the American Association of Zoo Veterinarians, Chicago, p 24, 1986.
57. Wolf P, Pond J, Meehan T: Surgical removal of *Prosthenorchis elegans* from six species of *Callitrichidae*. Annual Proceedings of the American Association of Zoo Veterinarians, South Padre Island, TX, pp 95–97, 1990.

CHAPTER 49

Emerging Viral Diseases of Nonhuman Primates

JOSEPH T. BIELITZKI

The concept of emerging diseases is well known to zoo veterinarians, who should always be aware of any new and previously unreported diseases and syndromes. Zoos house a variety of animal species, including those from many geographic areas, often held in close proximity. Many naturalistic zoo exhibits allow for contact between zoo and feral animals. People, including the zoo staff, and to a lesser extent the zoo visitor, are also brought into contact with the zoo animals. These situations provide opportunities for exposure to new infectious agents and subsequent disease emergence.

Examples of interspecies transfers of disease within zoological parks include eland fatally infected with malignant catarrhal fever when exposed to wildebeest carriers of the virus, the introduction of tuberculosis into captive hoofstock populations from feral deer, and the spread of simian hemorrhagic fever from patas monkeys and baboons to susceptible Asian nonhuman primates.

Emerging infectious diseases can be caused by either a new agent that results from genetic change or by previously described pathogens that are increasing in a population or are introduced into a new species. From an evolutionary point of view, when an interaction of a pathogen with a susceptible host is recent, the disease consequences are more likely to be more serious. However, care must be taken in evaluating changing prevalence of a disease; new laboratory methodologies make diagnosis possible or more accurate and create an apparent increase in prevalence. On the other hand, a lack of appropriate diagnostic techniques may curtail a diagnosis of actively emerging agents. Additionally, the small size of many captive populations hampers the identification of new diseases and syndromes. Because of the potential for human-animal interaction in the zoo, anthropozoonoses and zooanthropozoonoses should always be considered.

For human pathogens, several factors are considered critical to emergence. These include changing human behavior and demographics, changing land use and economic development, increased international travel and commerce, microbial adaptation and change, and a breakdown of public health programs.[23] These factors may also be applicable to captive animal populations.

Perhaps most important to the potential for disease emergence in zoological parks are environmental factors. These can include interspecies exhibits, changes in local flora and fauna (including vectors) caused by changing land use practices, or changes in wildlife migratory patterns that can also affect carrier or vector populations. Likewise, changes in the human population may affect the diversity and load of the local pathogens.

These environmental factors should be closely monitored, and management practices that minimize the transfer of microbial organisms should be used. In addition to the factors noted above, care should be taken to avoid substandard handling of food supplies and the use of modified live virus (MLV) vaccines. Vaccines attenuated for one species may be fatal for others; for example, many cases of rabies in nonhuman primates have been caused by MLV rabies vaccines produced for use in canids. The use of human MLV vaccines may present an additional threat if the virus is shed into an animal population.

As population and genetic management dictates more animal moves between zoos, the need for disease monitoring and control becomes more important. Appropriate quarantine and disease testing can minimize disease transmission, but obviously, evaluation must be carried out for the appropriate infectious agents. Given the small numbers of animals of a species in most zoo populations, it is critical that zoo clinicians identify new diseases or syndromes in their collections; in order to identify larger epidemiologic patterns, this information must also be quickly transmitted to others.

The number of nonhuman primate viruses that are reported in the literature continues to grow. A previous review of emerging viral disease of nonhuman primates described hepatitis A, simian retrovirus type D, and the primate filoviruses.[25] These agents continue to affect primates, but will be discussed here only as an update.

ARENAVIRUS

During the early 1980s, callitrichid hepatitis (CH) was identified as a cause of hepatitis in marmosets and tamarins.[28, 38] It was later reported in other species of the Callitrichidae and Callimiconidae families, and it came to prominence in the late 1980s when the affected population was the highly endangered golden lion tamarin (*Leontopithecus rosalia*).[39]

Research identified the etiologic agent to be the lymphocytic choriomeningitis virus (LCMV).[46] This arenavirus is a lipid-enveloped RNA virus carried inapparently by the common mouse (*Mus musculus*) and the house mouse (*Mus domesticus*). Experimentally infected animals showed a rapid onset of symptoms, including anorexia, depression, and lethargy within 7 days. Mild lymphocytosis and serum chemistry profiles indicative of hepatocellular damage were reported. Clinical deterioration was rapid and required euthanasia.[30] In naturally occurring infections within the zoo, seropositive animals were identified as long as 1.5 years after the last clinical case.[44]

Histologically, multiple organs are affected, but severe liver damage is characteristic. Necrosis has also been reported in the spleen, abdominal lymph nodes, adrenal cortex, and intestinal tract.[29] Encephalitis and gliosis was more pronounced in the pygmy marmoset (*Callithrix pygmaea*) than in the golden lion tamarin.[31]

The introduction of LCMV into callitrichid populations appears to be associated with the feeding of infected neonatal mice.[42] Most sources of rodents for research maintain breeding stock that are specific pathogen free (SPF) for LCMV; other sources provide randomly bred rodents that harbor LCMV. The inapparent nature of the infection in rodents makes clinical detection difficult. Feral populations of mice also carry LCMV.[31] Rodent reservoirs may pass the virus inapparently to their offspring and shed the virus in urine and oral secretions, providing additional routes of transmission within the zoo.

Serologic surveys of New and Old World primates species housed within zoos showed 4.5% of all nonhuman primates to be seropositive for LCMV. Of those serologically positive for LCMV, 97% had originated or were housed in facilities that had experienced a CH outbreak.[42] The members of Callithricidae seem to be most sensitive for the development of severe clinical signs and mortality. Clinical disease has not been reported in other nonhuman primate species.

The antiviral agent ribavirin has been used to treat animals showing clinical signs of LCMV infection. A dose of 150 mg/kg intramuscularly was administered, but all treated cases were late in their clinical course and a clinical response was not noted.[31]

LCMV is recognized as a zoonotic disease associated with exposure to infected hamsters and gerbils. In humans, the early and most frequent signs are similar to that of influenza and may progress to the neurologic symptoms of aseptic meningitis. Transmission of LCMV from infected marmosets and tamarins to human caretakers is possible. Two cases of LCMV seroconversion in zoo staff have been reported, but were not related to clinical disease.[30] Appropriate biosafety measures should be employed when working with colonies that are affected.

Callitrichid hepatitis is prototypical for the concepts of emergence. Lymphocytic choriomeningitis virus is an RNA virus with high mutation rates and significant strain variation. It is an Old World virus, from a point of origin perspective, and causes severe clinical disease in New World nonhuman primates. Mice are inapparent carriers, and neonatal mice are frequently a preferred food item for captive marmosets and tamarins. Infected mice can come from infected rodent supplies or feral populations in the zoo.

The number of laboratories working with arenaviruses with nonhuman primates is limited. The infection first occurred in a small number of animals, and although promptly reported, it took a significant duration of time to identify the urgency of the problem. It was finally diagnosed through serologic evidence; electronmicroscopy findings that were highly suggestive of LCMV; and isolation of virus from feeder mice and infected primates. Strain variation and antigenic variability always makes final diagnosis difficult. The emergence of this disease also illustrates the potential consequences of infection for species involved in reintroduction programs (see Chapter 48).

OTHER VIRAL HEPATITIS INFECTIONS

Infections caused by hepatitis A virus (HAV), a picornavirus, are well documented.[22, 25] Spontaneous infections have been reported in the common chimpanzee (*Pan troglodytes*), long-tail macaques (*Macaca fascicularis*), stump-tail macaques (*M. arctoides*), rhesus macaques (*M. mulatta*), the African green monkey (*Cercopithecus aethiops*), and the New World owl monkey (*Aotus trivirgatus*).[1] Genotypes isolated from nonhuman primates are restricted to types IV, V, and VI.[43] Human and primate strains of HAV exist and cross-infection is possible, but the development of clinical disease in the primate is variable. With the exception of chimpanzees and marmosets, nonhuman primates are less susceptible to human genotypes.[8] Antibody to HAV has been detected in members of the genera *Papio*, *Saguinus*, *Callithrix*, and *Saimiri*.[1] Virus is shed in feces, making the chance of transmission to human caretakers and other primate species a distinct possibility.[8, 35] Hepatitis B virus (HBV) is an orthohepadnavirus in the family Hepadnaviridae. The virus is common in humans, with infection rates as high as 25% in some populations; humans serve as the primary reservoir for nonhuman primate infections. Nonhuman primates may be chronically infected. The chimpanzee (*P. troglodytes*), the orangutan (*Pongo* species), the white-handed gibbon (*Hylobates lar*), and the long-tailed macaque (*M. fascicularis*) have developed infections.[14, 20] Although most individuals infected with HBV develop antibody and good immunity with a rapid removal of antigen, individuals remaining antigenemic become chronic carriers and may pose significant zoonotic risk to animal caretakers and veterinary staff.

Although the frequency of HBV infections in zoological collections is low, the identification of a unique HBV in a chronically antigenemic white-handed gibbon (*H. lar*) and a genotypically distinct variation of the gibbon virus in a common chimpanzee (*P. troglodytes*)[34] raises the potential for strain adaptation to nonhuman primates and the need for surveillance.

Hepatitis C infections have also been reported in nonhuman primates. Chronic infections in the chimpanzee may result in chronic active hepatitis, cirrhosis, or hepatocellular carcinoma (HCC).[33] Carrier states with persistent antigenemia are associated with chronic infection. RNA polymerase chain reaction has been used experimentally for screening suspect cases in the chimpanzee. Several vaccine trials currently being conducted in nonhuman primates have not provided total protection.[9] To prevent accidental transmission to other nonhuman primates and staff, carrier animals must be identified.

Nonhuman primates have been experimentally infected by the recently described hepatotropic viruses. Hepatitis E is an enterically transmitted hepatitis virus. Although active infections have been seen only in humans, feral macaques have been antibody positive when tested. The broad distribution of the virus and the fecal shed places this virus in the position for emergence.[51] Hepatitis F is another enteric virus that has been transmitted to macaques. The virus is shed in stool, and the enteric route makes this virus a potential pathogen for nonhuman primates. Hepatitis G is a blood-borne pathogen that causes acute hepatitis in humans after transfusion. Early transmission studies in nonhuman primates have shown that nonhuman primates are susceptible. The GB agent, a flavi-like virus, was successfully transmitted to tamarins. The GB agent causes acute hepatitis. The number of agents causing hepatitis will continue to increase.[5, 12] The susceptibility of nonhuman primates to infection causes concern and points to the need for appropriate and accurate evaluation of liver disease in nonhuman primates.

PARAMYXOVIRUS

Paramyxoviridae contains three distinct genera, the morbilliviruses, the pneumoviruses, and the paramyxoviruses. These are single-stranded RNA viruses, making the potential for genetic variation associated with transcriptional errors more likely. Viruses from each of the genera have been reported in nonhuman primates, and emergence is probable if infected hosts come into proximity to either captive or feral populations of nonhuman primates.

Measles is caused by a morbillivirus and has been reported in New World and Old World primate species, including the great apes.[27] Species susceptibility to the virus is variable. Callitrichids[26] and members of the genus *Colobus*[43] appear more susceptible and show higher mortality. Infection in feral animals or recently transported animals is often associated with human contact. Serologic surveys have shown many newly imported animals carry titers to measles virus. Symptoms may be mild and resemble influenza, and rashes may not always be present.[55] Morbidity is high; mortality is variable. The highest acute mortality was associated with pneumonia, and additional deaths were associated with diarrhea and dehydration. Measles-associated encephalitis has not been documented in nonhuman primates. Measles vaccine has been used successfully in colonies where exposure has occurred[40] and in feral groups.[17] As an alternative to human measles vaccine, a MLV canine distemper/measles vaccination has been used in nonhuman primates. On subsequent challenge of macaques, two strains of measles virus failed to produce illness (M. Ratterree, personal communication, Tulane Regional Primate Research Center, Covington, LA, 1997). The apparently mild clinical signs associated with some reports of measles infection raises the potential for further emergence and the possibility for subclinical infections.

Several other paramyxoviruses have also been associated with clinical disease. Canine distemper virus (CDV), also a morbillivirus, caused fatal encephalitis in a Japanese macaque (*M. fuscata*). Antibodies to CDV were detectable in other members of the group but antibodies to measles virus were not detectable.[57]

Simian virus 5 (SV5) is related to human parainfluenza virus, mumps virus, and the canine parainfluenza virus. The virus does not cause clinical disease in nonhuman primates but has been isolated from monkey kidney cells. Sequencing data suggest that this virus should survive equally well in human, simian, and canine hosts. This situation is conducive for emergence of the agent as a pathogen in any or all hosts.[3] Infected primates may serve as inapparent carriers, with the potential to transmit the agent to susceptible canine populations within the zoo.

The Murayama virus has been isolated from long-tailed macaques (*M. fascicularis*) with respiratory disease. The virus failed to demonstrate any antigenic relationship to mammalian viruses of the paramyxovirus group; however, Murayama virus is related to avian paramyxovirus type 2 and has the ability to emerge in nonhuman primates.[21] The virus's relationship to the avian paramyxoviruses raises questions concerning the initial mode of transmission to nonhuman primates and whether avian species may act as an inapparent host for the virus.

FILOVIRUS/EBOLA RESTON

Ebola Reston was first described as an epizootic in newly imported long-tailed macaques (*M. fascicularis*) from the Philippines. Mortality and morbidity was high and complicated by a secondary infection with simian hemorrhagic fever. The epizootic attracted immediate attention because human outbreaks caused by the Sudan and Zaire strains of Ebola virus were associated with hemorrhagic illness and high mortalities. Ebola Reston is distinct from the Sudan and Zaire strains of the virus and has not caused clinical disease in humans. However, serologic evidence suggests that subclinical infections may occur in both humans and the nonhuman primate.[4]

Ebola Reston is not a persistent or latent virus in affected nonhuman primate populations. High titers to Ebola Reston develop 14 to 21 days after infection in survivors. Viral clearance coincides with the development of filovirus-specific antibody.[13] The reservoir of Ebola Reston remains unidentified; antibodies have been detected in Chinese rhesus macaques (*M. mulatta*),[4] suggesting that filoviruses may have a wider geographic distribution.

EBOLA COTE-D'IVOIRE

In 1995, wild chimpanzees living in the Tai National Park in the western part of the Côte-d'Ivoire developed clinical signs of hemorrhagic disease. Of 40 animals within the group, 12 died during a 3-week period; all had similar clinical signs.[32]

The group had been under observational study for an extended period of time, and a postmortem examination of one of the affected animals was conducted. Uncoagulated blood was found surrounding a number of internal organs, indicating the possibility of hemorrhagic fever. Eight days after the postmortem examination, one of the human participants in the necropsy developed acute diarrhea, high fever, and a pruritic rash, but recovered without sequelae.[24]

Serologic screens for known hemorrhagic agents were negative. Co-cultivation failed to demonstrate cytoplasmic effects by day 12 of incubation. Hematoxylin and eosin staining of the culture revealed cytoplasmic inclusion bodies characteristic of the filoviruses.[24] Histologic evaluation of tissues from the affected chimpanzees was consistent with changes seen with Ebola infection in human cases and experimentally infected rhesus monkeys. Ebola Côte-d'Ivoire represents the first identified Ebola virus with documented zoonotic potential. As with the other reported strains of Ebola, no reservoir has been identified. Because of the high fatality rate in infected chimpanzees, it should be considered a recent emergent disease. The geographic restrictions of the agent are undetermined.[45]

HERPESVIRUSES

The herpesviruses as a group are both persistent and latent, characteristics that provide potential for emergence into other species. Encephalitis associated with an unidentified herpesvirus was reported in the ruffed lemur (*Varecia variegata*).[19] Although no definitive etiology was identified, the alphaherpesviruses have a strong neurotropism and should be considered in the differential diagnosis of neurologic disease. A herpesvirus-associated malignant lymphoma was reported in a slow loris (*Nycticebus coucang*), based on an uncharacterized herpesvirus in mononuclear cells seen on electron microscopy. The oncogenic herpesviruses cause malignant transformation of a number of cells; the epidemiology of the case suggested the exposure to an infected human was a possible route of transmission.[47]

Herpes B virus has long been a concern for those handling macaque species. Macaques are often inapparent carriers and can shed virus with or without clinical signs of infection. Herpes B virus also poses a threat to other nonhuman primate species; an outbreak occurred in a group of DeBrazzas monkeys (*Cercopithecus neglectus*). The affected animals had classic herpes vesicles on the nares, oral cavity, and conjunctiva and signs of respiratory involvement; the mortality was greater than that anticipated for macaques. Several animals remained antibody positive for an extended period after primary infection.[50] Such occurrences should serve as a continuous warning concerning the potential for common viral infections to be transmitted to atypical species.

PAPILLOMAVIRUS

Papillomaviruses are in the family Papovaviridae. Members of the family are nonenveloped double-stranded DNA viruses. Many are capable of tumor induction under appropriate conditions.[7] Papillomas associated with a viral etiology have been reported in the rhesus macaque (*M. mulatta*)[36] and the Colobus monkey (*Colobus guereza*).[48] The rhesus papillomavirus type 1 (RhPV-1) has been associated with a squamous cell carcinoma and was transmitted sexually.[36] Additionally, a colony of long-tailed macaques have recently been reported with papillomatous growths in the vaginal vault that prevented intromission and successful copulation. A viral etiology is suspected but not confirmed.[16]

Recent isolations of a papillomavirus from bonobos (*P. paniscus*) located in two separate facilities[49, 52] has indicated that further attention should be given to this group. In each case, oral focal epithelial hyperplasia was the presenting sign. The affected bonobos had a common point of origin and have been removed from the breeding pool to prevent sexual transmission of the infection. The isolated virus is similar to human papillomavirus 13 and the chimpanzee papillomavirus.[52, 53]

On the basis of the number of reported cases, the papillomaviruses do not constitute a significant problem, but it is likely that improved diagnostics will lead to increased identification. The venereal route of transmission and the cell-transforming ability of the virus with oncogenic capability[49] further increases the potential for emergence.

MIXED VIRAL INFECTIONS

Among the clinical syndromes affecting nonhuman primates, a number are related to infections by two different viruses. These multiple infections are drawing greater attention and may present as emergent disease syndromes.

Most notable are viral infections that cause immune suppression or viral transformation that predispose nonhuman primates to secondary challenge by a variety of etiologic agents. These infections should not be confused with those associated with incompetent viruses that need an additional viral agent to be pathogenic, such as hepatitis D, the delta agent. Although the list of emerging mixed infections is growing, several seem to clearly represent the pattern.

Malignant T cell lymphomas have been reported in the colony of hamadryas baboons (*Papio hamadryas*) at the Institute of Medical Primatology, formerly located in Sukhumi, Abkhazia, Georgia. Infection may be linked to studies done in the 1960s, where human blood from leukemic patients was transfused to several animals. These transfused animals remained within the colony, and a second unexposed group failed to develop a similar prevalence of lymphoma. All affected animals are seropositive for simian T cell lymphotrophic virus (STLV), and 90% are positive for herpesvirus papio. An Epstein-Barr–like agent has been reported.[18, 56] Simian T lymphotrophic virus appears to have a worldwide distribution and may be endemic in some nonhuman primate populations. The virus is related to human T cell lymphotrophic virus (HTLV) and may cross species lines.[10, 54] The isolation of a novel STLV from a bonobo (*P. paniscus*) that closely resembles an African strain of HTLV indicates that emergence is continuing for the agent.[11, 15]

Simian immunodeficiency virus (SIV) and simian retrovirus type D (SRV-D) can also predispose nonhuman primate species to secondary viral infections. Long-tailed macaques (*M. fascicularis*) with active SRV infections and coinfected with simian parvovirus (SPV) developed fatal anemia.[6] Simian parvovirus is one of two members of the genus *Erythrovirus* within the family Parvovirinae; the other member of this genus is the human parvovirus 19. Parvovirus 19 and SPV show a high degree of homology, and each has a trophism for bone marrow precursor cells.[37] Rhesus macaques (*M. mulatta*) infected with SIV also developed fatal enteric disease associated with adenovirus infection.[2] Adenoviruses may cause enteric disease, but the clinical course is rarely fatal in the uncompromised individual.

Infectious processes involving more than one pathogen will continue to cause significant morbidity in animal collections such as the zoological garden. The isolation of a single etiologic agent may mislead the clinician in developing preventive measures. Viral etiologies that are persistent and latent pose a greater potential for emergence. Likewise, when evaluating a previously undescribed syndrome, agents that may be endemic within a population should not be discounted. The close and intimate relationship among human caretaker, visitor, and the zoo animal underlines the potential for disease transmission and risk of emergence.

REFERENCES

1. Balayan MS: Natural hosts of hepatitis A virus. Vaccine 10(Suppl 1):S27–S31, 1992.
2. Baskin GB, Soike KF: Adenovirus enteritis in SIV-infected rhesus monkeys [Letter]. J Infect Dis 160(5):905–907, 1989.
3. Baty DU, Southern JA, Randall RE: Sequence comparison between the haemagglutinin-neuraminidase genes of simian, canine and human isolates of simian virus 5. J Gen Virol 72(12):3103–3107, 1991.
4. Becker S, Feldman H, Will C, Slenczka W: Evidence for occurrence of filovirus antibodies in humans and imported monkeys: do subclinical filovirus infections occur worldwide? Med Microbiol Immunol (Berl) 181(1):43–55, 1992.
5. Bowden DS, Moaven LD, Locarnini SA: New hepatitis viruses: are there enough letters in the alphabet? Med J Aust 164(2):87–89, 1996.
6. Brown KE, O'Sullivan MG, Young NS: Simian parvovirus. Semin Virol 6(5):339–346, 1995.
7. Butel JS: Papovaviruses: neurological disease and therapy. *In* McKendall RR, Stroop WG, et al (eds): Handbook of Neurovirology, vol 27. New York, Marcel Dekker, pp 339–354, 1994.
8. Cederna JB, Stapleton JT: Hepatitis A virus. *In* Murray PR, Barron EJ, Pfaller MA, et al (eds): Manual of Clinical Microbiology, 6th ed. Washington, DC, American Society of Microbiology, pp 1025–1032, 1995.
9. Choo Q-L, Kuo G, Ralston R, et al: Vaccination against hepatitis C virus infection: miles to go before we sleep. Hepatology 20:758–765, 1994.
10. Crandall KA: Multiple interspecies transmissions of human and simian T-cell leukemia/lymphoma virus type I sequences. Mol Biol Evol 13(1):115–131, 1996.
11. Dekaban GA, Digilio L, Franchini G: The natural history and evolution of human and simian T cell leukemia/lymphotropic viruses. Curr Opin Genet Dev 5(6):807–813, 1995.
12. Fackelmann K: The hepatitis G enigma: researchers corner new viruses associated with hepatitis. Sci News 149(15):238–239, 1996.
13. Fisher-Hoch SP, Perez-Oronoz GI, Jackson EL, et al: Filovirus clearance in non-human primates. Lancet 340(8817):451–453, 1992.
14. Gallagher M, Fields HA, de la Torre N, et al: Characterization of HBV2 by experimental infection of primates. *In* Hollinger FB, Lemon SM, Margolis H (eds): Viral Hepatitis and Liver Disease. Baltimore, Williams & Wilkins, pp 227–229, 1991.
15. Giri A, Markham P, Digilio L, et al: Isolation of a novel simian T-cell lymphotropic virus from *Pan paniscus* that is distantly related to the human T-cell leukemia/lymphotropic virus types I and II. J Virol 68(12):8392–8395, 1994.
16. Grabber JE: Papillomas in Long Tailed Macaques. Madison, WI, Association of Primate Veterinarians, 1996.
17. Hastings BE, Kenny D, Lowenstine LJ, Foster JW: Mountain gorillas and measles: ontogeny of a wildlife vaccination program. Annual Proceedings of the American Association of Zoo Veterinarians, Calgary, Alberta, Canada, pp 198–205, 1991.
18. Indzhiya LV, Yakovleva LA, Overbaugh J, et al: Baboon T cell lymphomas expressing the B cell-associated surface proteins CD40 and Bgp 95. J Clin Immunol 12(3):225–236, 1992.
19. Kornegay RW, Baldwin TJ, Pirie G: Herpesvirus encephalitis in a ruffed lemur (*Varecia variegatus*). J Zoo Wildl Med 24(2):196–203, 1993.
20. Kornegay RW, Giddens WE Jr, Van Hoosier GL Jr, Morton WR: Subacute nonsuppurative hepatitis associated with hepatitis B virus infection in two cynomolgus monkeys. Lab Anim Sci 35(4):400–404, 1985.
21. Kusagawa S, Komada H, Mao X-j, et al: Antigenic and molecular properties of Murayama virus isolated from cynomolgus monkeys: the virus is closely related to avian paramyxovirus type 2. Virology 194(2):828–832, 1993.
22. Lapin BA, Shevtsova ZV: Sensitivity of the Old World monkeys to hepatitis A virus (spontaneous and experimental infection). Exp Pathol 36(1):63–64, 1989.
23. Lederberg J, Shope RE, Oaks SC (eds): Emerging Infections: Microbial Threats to Health in the United States. Washington, DC, Institute of Medicine, National Academy Press, 1992.
24. Le Guenno B, Formentry P, Wyers M, et al: Isolation and partial characterization of new strain of Ebola virus. Lancet 345(8960):1271–1274, 1995.
25. Lerche NW: Emerging viral diseases of nonhuman primates in the wild. *In* Fowler ME (ed): Zoo and Wild Animal Medicine: Current Therapy 3. Philadelphia, WB Saunders, pp 340–344, 1993.
26. Levy BM, Mirkovic RR: An epizootic of measles in a marmoset colony. Lab Anim Sci 21:33–39, 1971.
27. Lowenstine LJ: Measles virus infection, nonhuman primates. *In* Jones TC, Mohr U, Hunt RD (eds): Nonhuman Primates I. Berlin, Springer-Verlag, pp 108–118, 1993.
28. Lucke VM, Bennett AM: An outbreak of hepatitis in marmosets in a zoological collection. Lab Anim 16:73–77, 1982.
29. Montali RJ, Connolly BM, Armstrong DL, et al: Pathology and immunohistochemistry of callitrichid hepatitis, an emerging disease of captive New World primates caused by lymphocytic choriomeningitis virus. Am J Pathol 147(5):1441–1449, 1995.
30. Montali RJ, Ramsay EC, Stephenson CB, et al: A new transmissible viral hepatitis of marmosets and tamarins. J Infect Dis 160(5):759–765, 1989.
31. Montali RJ, Scanga CA, Pernikoff D, et al: A common-source outbreak of callitrichid hepatitis in captive tamarins and marmosets. J Infect Dis 167(4):946–950, 1993.
32. Morrell V: Chimpanzee outbreak heats up search for Ebola origin. Science 268(5213):974–975, 1995.
33. Muchmore E, Popper H, Peterson DA, et al: Non-A non-B hepatitis-related hepatocellular carcinoma in a chimpanzee. J Med Primatol 17(5):235–246, 1988.
34. Norder H, Ebert JW, Fields HA, et al: Complete sequencing of a gibbon hepatitis B virus genome reveals a unique genotype distantly related to the chimpanzee hepatitis B virus. Virology 218(1):214–223, 1996.
35. Ochs A, Rietschel W, Schiller W-G: Hepatitis A: risk by contact with primates. Kleintierpraxis 40(1):5–8, 1995.

36. Ostrow RS, McGlennen RC, Shaver MK, et al: A rhesus monkey model for sexual transmission of a papillomavirus isolated from a squamous cell carcinoma. Proc Natl Acad Sci USA 87(20):8170–8174, 1990.
37. Pattison JR: A new parvovirus: similarities between monkeys and humans. J Clin Invest 93(4):1354, 1994.
38. Phillips LG: Suspected viral hepatitis in golden lion tamarins—case report. Proceedings of the American Association of Zoo Veterinarians, Seattle, WA, pp 34–35, 1981.
39. Ramsay E, Montali RJ: Viral hepatitis in New World primates. *In* Fowler ME (eds): Zoo and Wild Animal Medicine: Current Therapy 3. Philadelphia, WB Saunders, pp 355–358, 1993.
40. Roberts JA, Lerche NW, Anderson JH, et al: Epizootic measles at the California Primate Research Center [Abstract]. Lab Anim Sci 38(4):492, 1988.
41. Robertson BH, Jansen RW, Khanna B, et al: Genetic relatedness of hepatitis A virus strains recovered from different geographical regions. J Gen Virol 73(6):1365–1377, 1992.
42. Scanga CA, Holmes KV, Montali RJ: Serologic evidence of infection with lymphocytic choriomeningitis virus, the agent of callitrichid hepatitis, in primates in zoos, primate research centers, and a natural reserve. J Zoo Wildl Med 24(4):469–474, 1993.
43. Scott GBD, Keymer IF: The pathology of measles in Abyssinian colobus monkeys (*Colobus guerza*): a description of an outbreak. J Pathol 117:229–233, 1975.
44. Scott RAW, Holmes KV, Scanga CA, Montali RJ: An update on the epizootiology of callitrichid hepatitis. Proceedings of the American Association of Zoo Veterinarians, South Padre Island, TX, pp 261–262, 1990.
45. Simpson DIH: The filovirus enigma. Lancet 345(8960):1252–1253, 1995.
46. Stephenson CB, Jong YP, Blount SR: cDNA sequence analysis confirms that the etiologic agent of callitrichid hepatitis is lymphocytic choriomeningitis virus. J Virol 69:1349–1352, 1995.
47. Stetter MD, Worley MB, Ruiz B: Herpesvirus-associated malignant lymphoma in a slow loris (*Nycticebus coucang*). J Zoo Wildl Med 26(1):155–160, 1995.
48. Sundberg JP, Reichmann ME: Animal models of human disease: venereal papilloma and squamous cell carcinoma. Comp Pathol Bull 22(2):2–3, 1990.
49. Sundberg JP, Shima AL, Adkison DL: Oral papillomavirus infection in a pygmy chimpanzee (*Pan paniscus*). J Vet Diagn Invest 4(1):70–74, 1992.
50. Thompson SA, Hilliard JK, Lipper SL, Giddens WE Jr: Fatal herpesvirus infection in DeBrazzas monkeys [Abstract]. Contemp Top Lab Anim Sci 31(4):6, 1992.
51. Ticehurst J: Hepatitis E virus. *In* Murray PR, Barron EJ, Pfaller MA, et al (eds): Manual of Clinical Microbiology, 6th ed. Washington, DC, American Society of Microbiology, pp 1056–1067, 1995.
52. van Ranst M, Fuse A, Fiten P, et al: Human papillomavirus type 13 and pygmy chimpanzee papillomavirus type 1: comparison of genome organizations. Virology 190:587–596, 1992.
53. van Ranst M, Tachezy R, Opendakker G, Burk RD: Co-evolution of primate papillomaviruses and their hosts [Abstract]. Am J Primatol 30(4):353, 1993.
54. Voevodin A, Miura T, Samilchuk E, Schaetzl H: Phylogenetic characterization of simian T lymphotropic virus type I (STLV-I) from the Ethiopian sacred baboon (*Papio hamadryas*). AIDS Res Hum Retroviruses 12(3):255–258, 1996.
55. Welshman MD: Measles in the cynomolgus monkey (*Macaca fascicularis*). Vet Rec 124(8):184–186, 1989.
56. Yakoleva LA, Lennert K, Chikobava MG, et al: Morphological characteristics of malignant T-cell lymphomas in baboons. Virchows Arch 422(2):109–120, 1993.
57. Yoshikawa Y, Ochikubo F, Matsubara Y, et al: Natural infection with canine distemper virus in a Japanese monkey (*Macaca fuscata*). Vet Microbiol 20(3):193–205, 1989.

CHAPTER **50**

Great Ape Neonatology

BRENT SWENSON

NORMAL NEONATES

Much of the specialized expertise and technology available for human neonates is unavailable or must be creatively applied to infant great apes. Moreover, economic constraints often require that decisions are made and care is provided by generalists. Therefore, those responsible for management decisions should be able to distinguish normal from abnormal infants and to recognize suboptimal maternal care. In this way, informed judgments about the need for human intervention can be made.

The neonatal period is usually considered to encompass the first 4 weeks of life. The full-term infant ape is born with a moderately well-developed haircoat and a covering of vernix, a lanolin-like substance that pro-

tects the fetal skin in utero. A newborn great ape should be robust with a strong grip, an animated rooting reflex, and a hearty voice that becomes apparent when the infant is distressed. The Apgar scale used to score neonatal physical status in humans is not completely transferable to neonatal apes; however, it can provide a reasonable estimate of the infant's condition. The Apgar score is typically assessed at 1 and 5 minutes postpartum, and except for infants delivered by cesarean section, this is not feasible for most great ape births. In general, gestational age can be estimated with birth weight and haircoat development. Infants born more than 6 to 8 weeks preterm will have little or no hair and weigh less than 800 g. The amount of vernix tends to decrease with increasing fetal maturity. Birth weights average 1.73 ± .33 kg for chimpanzees (*Pan troglo-*

dytes). Orangutans (*Pongo pygmaeus*) and gorillas (*Gorilla gorilla*) tend to be smaller, at 1.60 ± .3 kg and 1.65 ± .43 kg, respectively. Although there is less experience with pigmy chimps (*P. paniscus*), normal birth weights fall within comparable ranges. Loss of up to 10% of birth weight during the first postpartum week with daily weight gain thereafter is normal. Rates of weight gain tend to be less for mother-reared than hand-reared infants. For chimpanzees, "normal" rates of weight gain, and possibly ages for dental eruption, vary by sex and among different colonies and environmental conditions.[4]

Apes born in captivity fall into two management categories: those born to competent mothers and those that are not. A competent mother cleans the infant and cradles it near a nipple to encourage suckling. She will actively move the infant to a nipple in response to its cries. An incompetent mother may abandon the infant or abuse it; however, there is a range of behaviors between the clearly normal and obviously incompetent.

There are, unfortunately, no clear standards for when to nursery-rear a newborn. Marginally competent mothers often carry their infants in abnormal positions. Normal infants can help the inexperienced dam learn proper mothering techniques. An attentive dam quickly perceives that the infant becomes calmer and less fussy in response to appropriate nurturing behaviors. Thus, the infant's behavior reinforces appropriate maternal care. Because of this feedback, aberrant maternal behavior in a previously competent female can indicate a health problem in the infant.

MOTHER-REARING

There are two options for managing the neonate: it may be left with the mother or removed to be hand-reared. A host of considerations enter into the decision to leave an infant with its mother or rear it by hand. These include (in no particular order of importance) previous maternal experience and competence, maternal social status (dominance and alliances with other group members), stability of the social group, availability of peers in a nursery setting, genetic value of the infant and need for future reproductive performance, sex, physical condition of the infant, and ease of observation. As a rule, mothers who were themselves mother-reared are more likely to be competent, although this seems to be less predictive for orangutans, and there are individuals of every great ape species that have successfully cared for infants even though they were hand-reared themselves. Also, mothers who are marginally competent sometimes rear their infants successfully in spite of bizarre behaviors (such as carrying the infant upside down). When the mother's competence is not obvious, the best criterion to apply is the apparent condition of the infant. The behavioral and social outcome is nearly always superior for infants reared by their mothers in normal social groups. Adult males, other females, and peers each provide social contributions that are vital to optimal infant development. However, the risk of injury or illness is also higher because they may subject the infant to kidnapping or aggression.

The mother and infant should be observed closely to evaluate the infant's status. Useful indicators include strength and muscle tone. Even the newborn should raise its head and grasp tightly with hands and feet. Neonatal eyes should be clear, and the lids should be squeezed tightly together when crying. Determining whether the infant is suckling and receiving adequate nourishment is difficult. Lactation is rarely optimal after parturition, but milk production increases over several days. Often, during the first few postpartum days, much of the nursing takes place at night. Passage of nonmeconium stools is presumptive evidence of suckling. An infant that fails to suckle or receives insufficient milk grows weaker and may become moribund as early as 2 to 3 days postpartum and sometimes as late as 10 to 14 days after birth. If no suckling is observed for several days, the condition of the infant should provide the ultimate basis for assessing whether it can remain with the dam. If necessary, nursing can often be confirmed by briefly anesthetizing the dam to check the adequacy of her milk flow and sample the infant's gastric contents. However, in general, it is preferable to avoid anesthetizing the dam during the first several postpartum days because of possible injury to the infant.

Breast milk contains relatively low levels of vitamin D. Rickets has occurred in mother-reared orangutan infants who had no access to natural sunlight. If the mother and infant do not have outdoor access, the infant should receive vitamin D supplementation.

HAND-REARING

Initial Management

The condition of hand-reared neonates is often compromised because of injury, illness, or exposure. The retrieved infant should undergo a triage process on the basis of physical examination. Adequacy of airway patency and ventilation should be confirmed. Sources of bleeding should be identified and controlled, and if necessary, vascular access obtained. The umbilical cord should be cleaned, disinfected, clamped, cut and tied, or clipped. These infants are often hypothermic and hypoglycemic. Intravenous, intraperitoneal, or nasogastric tube administration of 5% glucose may dramatically improve their condition. The infant should be bathed in warm water, thoroughly dried, and placed in a temperature-controlled isolator set at 90° to 95°F.

A more thorough examination should include an assessment of maturity and development, a general inspection for birth trauma, and icterus or petechial hemorrhage that could indicate sepsis. Although clinically apparent neonatal jaundice (bilirubin levels above 4 to 5 mg/100 ml) can be normal in humans, in apes it is much more likely the result of infection. In chimpanzees, jaundice may also be caused by neonatal hemolytic syndrome from maternal-fetal ABO blood type incompatibility. This can occur when the dam has type O blood and the infant is type A. Disease can occur with the first offspring, but it is usually mild and treatment is unnecessary.

The cranium should be palpated and assessed for

bulging fontanelles or fractures. The presence of congenital defects such as atresia of the nares or anus, hypospadia, craniofacial defects, and umbilical or inguinal hernia should be evaluated. The oral mucosa and perineal skin are good sites to assess the presence of cyanosis. The chest should be carefully ausculted for normal, bilateral, respiratory sounds, and heart sounds. Abdominal palpation should rule out organomegaly, masses, and distention. In the neonatal great ape, testicles are usually inguinal. Neurologic examination should evaluate alertness, muscle tone, bilaterality of function, suck and grasp reflexes, and cry-response.

Feeding

Bottle feeding can usually be initiated immediately. It is advisable to begin with water or 5% glucose and continue this for the first 24 hours. This ensures that the infant can coordinate nursing while minimizing the consequences of aspiration. The nipple's aperture should be large enough to facilitate easy flow, but small enough to limit the flow to a readily swallowed amount. Initially, quantities should be limited initially to 5 to 10 ml per feeding, then gradually increased until the infant is drinking ad libitum. For normal infants, feedings should be given every 1 to 2 hours for normal infants and every 1 to 2 hours for high-risk neonates. If the infant is unable to suckle effectively, gavage feedings may be necessary. These can be administered through a soft, 12-French, polyethylene, nasogastric feeding tube that is secured in place with tape. Feedings should be given initially in small amounts (2 to 3 ml) every 2 hours. Before feeding, the tube should be aspirated to estimate residual fluid from the previous feeding. If the residue is more than 1 to 2 ml, the feeding should be omitted and the cause of delayed gastric emptying investigated.

If feedings are uneventful during the first 24 hours, formula feedings may be initiated with commercially available human infant formulas. Formulas containing iron should be avoided during the neonatal period because of stimulation of bacterial growth. Formulas can be fed according to label directions. After the first several days, daily intake should provide approximately 100 to 120 kcal/kg.

Weights should be recorded daily. Proper nutrition results in daily incremental growth (usually after the first week of life). Recognition of an extended (more than 2 to 3 days) growth plateau or weight loss can signal inadequate nutrition or early illness. The amount of weight gain is less important than its steady progression.

Handling

Handling practices during the neonatal period are critical to later development. It is important to provide the infant with physical and sensory stimulation. Some experts advocate reproducing the natural environment as nearly as possible; for chimpanzees this would include mimicry of normal facial expressions and vocalizations and exposure to normal, conspecific adults.

Others advocate dressing the infants to provide continual stimulation of the skin. However, the benefits from such intervention are not clear. However, it is clear that exposure to sensory stimulation and physical contact with the caregiver are important for normal behavioral development. Where possible, infants should be carried in a sling during conduct of routine job duties by the caregiver. In addition, colorful objects can be suspended above the infant in its isolator. Minimally, the infant should be cradled and spoken to during feeding and cleaning. Diapers are usually used to facilitate sanitation. Diapers should be changed several times daily; like humans, great apes can develop skin irritation in response to prolonged skin contact with urine and feces. Drying agents such as talc or emollients such as zinc oxide-based ointments can be used as skin protectants, but they are not substitutes for attentive care.

Health Considerations

The first day, the first month, and the first year of life are three temporal milestones predictive of mortality in infant apes. Ninety percent of the mortality risk for great apes occurs in the first year and two thirds or more of the mortalities occur in the first month of life. Day 1 is the period of highest risk.

Parturient Complications

Although incompetent females will merely abandon infants, occasionally they actively injure the neonate. More commonly, neonatal trauma is inflicted by other members of the social group. Adolescent males are particularly dangerous in this regard—especially if they are of higher rank than the dam or if the dominant male is ineffectual. Primiparous females are not only less competent dams, but they also tend to have significantly longer labor than multiparous females. Both factors probably contribute in the higher mortality among infants of these females.

A pregnant female in a social group can pose management dilemmas. If she is experienced and the group has no history of infanticide, it is preferable to leave the group intact. If a group member is known to have injured infants, it should be removed from the group. Management of females that are marginally competent or of unknown history varies with the species. For chimpanzees, it is often safer to separate the pregnant female from the group near the time of parturition and then gradually reintroduce her after delivery. Gorillas and orangutans often fare better when other group members are present (for orangutans, this is likely limited to the sire and any juvenile offspring that are present).

Obstetric complications are not uncommon causes of neonatal deaths. Placenta previa or placental abruption can cause excessive maternal bleeding, placing both the dam and the neonate at risk. Hemorrhage at parturition resulting from placenta previa is an emergency that dictates immediate cesarean section. Ultrasound examination is helpful for diagnosis of placenta previa, and if possible, at least one prenatal examination should be performed. Identification of placenta previa warrants further examinations because the placental attachment sometimes moves away from the cervix as pregnancy progresses. If it remains situated over the internal cervical os, the infant should be delivered by cesarean section.

Depending on the extent and site of placental separation, placental abruption can produce obvious or occult bleeding. Because of the risks attendant to this condition and the difficulty of regular monitoring in apes, cesarean delivery should be considered as soon as the infant is viable.

In a prolonged gestation, the hypermature fetus can outgrow the capacity of the placenta to support it. Placental insufficiency and a large infant also increase the risk of neonatal mortality at birth. Dams with diabetes mellitus tend to deliver large infants, and dystocia increases the risk of mortality.

Any cause of parturient distress can stimulate the infant to defecate in utero. When combined with fetal hypoxia, the infant's premature attempts to breathe can result in aspiration of meconium and compromised ventilation after delivery. Treatment necessitates an oxygen-enriched environment.

Neonatal Sepsis

One of the most common causes of neonatal mortality is sepsis. This can result from contamination of the uterine interior, umbilical inoculation after birth, or exposure to invasive primary pathogens. Signs of sepsis include weakness, anorexia, vomiting, dehydration, pyrexia or hypothermia, petechial and ecchymotic hemorrhage, jaundice, hepatosplenomegaly, hypotension, and respiratory distress. Early neonatal sepsis is generally caused by enteric organisms or, more rarely, staphylococci or streptococci. Later infection is likely to be caused by either *Streptococcus pneumoniae* or *Haemophilus influenzae*. Both of these organisms cause pneumonia, meningitis, and septicemia. *Shigella* and *Campylobacter* species cause bacteremia, sepsis, and enteric disease. *Listeria* can cause neonatal sepsis in monkeys and has been reported to cause meningoencephalitis in an adult chimpanzee.[2]

Treatment of sepsis must be prompt, aggressive, and specific. Mortality from sepsis syndrome is high. Antimicrobial therapy should be based on results of blood cultures, but initial empiric therapy should not be delayed. A combination of a beta-lactam antibiotic and an aminoglycoside is recommended. Close attention should be paid to support of body temperature, respiration, and fluid and electrolyte balance. High-dose corticosteroids have long been promoted for treatment of sepsis and septic shock. However, several controlled human studies showed no clinical benefit, and one suggested increased severity of infection.[1, 7, 9]

Other Bacterial Infections

Bacteremia may lead not to sepsis but to local manifestations such as meningitis, pneumonia, or septic arthritis.

BACTERIAL MENINGITIS

Like sepsis, meningitis in the early postpartum period is most commonly caused by enteric bacteria and *S. pneumoniae* or *H. influenzae* later on. Clinical signs can be ambiguous, particularly in dam-raised infants, but early recognition and treatment are essential to a satisfactory outcome. Signs range from lethargy to grand mal seizures. More commonly, fine-muscle fasciculations signal meningeal irritation. Recognition of the infection is easier in hand-reared infants because rectal temperature is almost always elevated (102°F and often more than 104°F). Examination of cerebrospinal fluid (CSF) obtained by lumbar puncture is diagnostic. Initial treatment should be based on examination of Gram-stained CSF, followed by treatment based on antibiotic sensitivity results. Antibiotic levels in the CSF must be greater than the minimum bactericidal concentration for the etiologic agent. Most beta-lactam antibiotics achieve CSF concentrations that are 5% to 10% of serum concentrations in the presence of meningeal irritation.[8] Chloramphenicol is metabolized inconsistently in the neonate and should be avoided. Early treatment with dexamethasone can minimize postinfectious obstructive hydrocephalus. These infants require fluid and nutritional support and may need anticonvulsant therapy. Antipyretic agents such as acetaminophen may be needed if the rectal temperature exceeds 104°F.

PNEUMONIA

Most neonatal pneumonias are associated with formula aspiration. Prevention, as described, is better than treatment. Gradual introduction of formula, combined with patience by the caregiver, go a long way toward preventing aspiration pneumonia.

Neonatal pneumonia is usually caused by the same bacteria associated with sepsis. Although coughing occurs infrequently in neonates, pneumonia may be difficult to recognize in mother-reared neonates. Lethargy and weakness are most likely to be recognized. Increased respiratory effort can be seen, and in severe cases, the oral or perineal mucosa may be cyanotic. The large thymic shadow complicates the interpretation of radiography, and the small lungs offer less contrast than older animals. Blood culture is often more informative than sputum culture, which often yields multiple organisms, all of which might be contaminants. Sputum cultures serve an attempt to correlate cultured organisms with intracellular organisms seen in phagocytic cells. Treatment can begin with broad-spectrum antibiotics, but should then be based on antimicrobial-sensitive drugs. Supplemental oxygen may be necessary, and unless disease is extensive, the prognosis is good.

Viral respiratory disease is uncommon in neonates. When it does occur, it is toward the end of the neonatal period. Although great ape infants are susceptible to human respiratory agents, respiratory syncytial virus (RSV) is most likely to cause severe disease. Viral pneumonias must be managed supportively, and secondary bacterial infections should be treated appropriately.

One serious pulmonary infection seen in orangutans is hyperinfestation with *Strongyloides stercoralis*. This parasite exists in free-living and parasitic forms. Infectious larvae penetrate the skin, migrate through the lungs, then localize in the intestine. Ova produced in the intestine can hatch, and the larvae can become infectious before being expelled in the stool. This can result in a large volume of infectious larvae penetrating the bowel wall and migrating to the lungs, where they cause massive hemorrhage and tissue damage. Although more common in older infants, this can also occur in neonates. The disease is insidious. Although there are few recognizable early signs, the most common is marked lethargy or death with no premonitory illness. There is no successful treatment of pulmonary hyperinfestation syndrome in orangutans, but prevention by elimination of enteric infection of adults is feasible with intensive anthelmintic regimens that alternate imidazole drugs and ivermectin.

SEPTIC ARTHRITIS

Although uncommon, septic arthritis occurs when infectious agents localize in the joints of newborn apes. One joint or several can be affected. As with other disorders, arthritis is more readily noticed in hand-reared infants. Involved joints are hot, swollen, and extremely tender. Regional lymph nodes are usually enlarged. Unless it was preceded by trauma, infection rarely proceeds to osteomyelitis. *Staphylococcus aureus* or enteric organisms are most commonly isolated. Affected joints should be promptly drained by centesis or incision. Antibiotic treatment should be based on microscopic examination of Gram-stained exudate, culture, and sensitivity tests.

Diarrhea

Diarrhea, like fever, often occurs as a nonspecific response in neonatal apes. It can result from events ranging from benign dietary upsets or eruption of teeth, to life-threatening infections. It is important to be aware of the clinical context in which liquid stools occur. If there is no evidence of systemic illness, such as anorexia, fever, vomiting, or dehydration, diarrhea can be managed symptomatically. Concomitant systemic illness; persistence beyond 2 or 3 days; or the presence of blood, neutrophils, or mucus in the stools warrant more aggressive intervention.

Intolerances to lactose, milk protein, and fat have caused diarrhea in infant apes. Although they are not usually severe, they result in discomfort to the infant and slowed growth. They usually respond to a change to lactose-free or soy-based formulas.

Infectious agents that have been associated with diarrhea in great apes are numerous and include *Campylobacter, Shigella, Yersinia, Escherichia coli, Pseudomonas aeruginosa, Aeromonas hydrophila, Balantidium coli, Giardia lamblia, Strongyloides stercoralis, Entamoeba histolytica, Candida albicans,* and various viral agents.

Isolates of *E. coli* in particular should not be automatically assumed to constitute normal flora. Enterotoxigenic, enteroinvasive, enteropathogenic, enterohe-

morrhagic, and nontoxigenic colonizing strains are associated with diarrheal disease.[6] *Clostridium difficile* causes enterocolitis in humans but has not been reported in newborn apes. However, it should be considered when other causes have been ruled out. Similarly, other agents that have been associated with epidemic diarrhea in humans, such as rotavirus and *Cryptosporidium parvum,* should be assumed to be infectious for apes. Gorillas seem to be especially susceptible to invasive colitis caused by *B. coli* infection. This has typically occurred in animals older than neonates but should be considered in management of neonatal diarrhea as well.

Although dehydration and electrolyte imbalance can develop rapidly, commercial, oral rehydration solutions are highly effective for maintaining diarrheic neonates within physiologic ranges. Severe volume depletion warrants intravenous fluid support. Specific antiparasitic or antibacterial therapy should be instituted. When bacterial enteritis is suspected, therapy may be initiated with a combination of cotrimoxazole and erythromycin while culture and sensitivity tests are pending. An aminoglycoside may be appropriate as well if a pathogenic *E. coli* or *Yersinia* is suspected. Antibiotic-treated neonates and infants may be more prone than older animals to superinfection with *Candida albicans.* Treatment may require addition of nystatin, ketoconazole, or fluconazole.

MISCELLANEOUS OTHER DISORDERS

Herpesvirus Infection

Great apes are susceptible to disease caused by several herpesviruses. Generalized infection with *Herpesvirus hominis* type 1 was responsible for the death of a 13-day-old lowland gorilla in Switzerland,[3] and multiple cases of infection by *Herpesvirus hominis* type 2 have occurred in common chimpanzees and bonobos, including infants. In humans, the greatest risk for neonatal infection occurs if genital lesions from the dam's first infection are present at parturition. Transmission risk is substantially diminished if the lesions are recurrent. Transmission from human caregivers to hand-reared infants should also be considered, and appropriate hygienic measures should be used when handling neonates. If begun early in the infection, acyclovir is effective as the treatment for herpes simplex.

Chimpanzees and gorillas[5] are also susceptible to varicella (chickenpox). This seems generally to be a milder illness in apes than in humans, and it resolves in a few days without treatment.

Cytomegalovirus (CMV) can infect infant great apes, although exposure to this organism usually occurs later than the neonatal period. Cytomegalovirus has caused viral pneumonia in one infant chimpanzee in our colony and generalized lymphadenopathy in others. However, in immunocompetent animals, CMV disease is not likely to be life-threatening.

Congenital Defects

Congenital disorders such as Down's syndrome, hydrocephalus, and hypoplastic right heart syndrome have been observed, and there is no reason to expect that any defect recognized in humans could not occur in apes. However, birth defects are surprisingly rare in great apes.

REFERENCES

1. Bone RC, Fisher CJ, Clemmer TP, et al: A controlled clinical trial of high-dose methylprednisolone in the treatment of severe sepsis and septic shock. N Engl J Med 317:653, 1987.
2. Heldstab A, Ruedi D: Listeriosis in an adult female chimpanzee (*Pan troglodytes*). J Comp Pathol 92:609–612, 1982.
3. Heldstab A, Ruedi D, Sonnabend W, Deinhardt F: Spontaneous generalized *Herpesvirus hominis* infection of a lowland gorilla (*Gorilla gorilla gorilla*). J Med Primatol 10:129–135, 1981.
4. Marzke MW, Young DL, Hawkey DE, et al: Comparative analysis of weight gain, hand-wrist maturation, and dental emergence rates in chimpanzees aged 0–24 months from various captive environments. Am J Phys Anthropol 99:175–190, 1996.
5. Myers MG, Kramer LW, Stanberry LR: Varicella in a gorilla. J Med Primatol 23:317–322, 1987.
6. Schlager TA, Guerrant RL: Seven possible mechanisms for *Escherichia coli* diarrhea. Infect Dis Clin North Am 2:607–624, 1988.
7. Sprung CL, Caralis PV, Marcial EH, et al: The effects of high-dose corticosteroids in patients with septic shock: a prospective controlled study. N Engl J Med 311:1137, 1984.
8. Tauber MG, Sande MA: General principles of therapy of pyogenic meningitis. Infect Dis Clin North Am 4:661–667, 1990.
9. Veterans Administration Systemic Sepsis Cooperative Study Group: Effect of high-dose glucocorticoid therapy on mortality in patients with clinical signs of systemic sepsis. N Engl J Med 317:659, 1987.

CHAPTER 51

Veterinarian's Role in Monitoring the Behavioral Enrichment Standards of the Animal Welfare Act

RITA McMANAMON

REGULATORY REQUIREMENTS

All animal dealers, exhibitors, and research facilities that hold nonhuman primates and that are regulated and inspected by the United States Department of Agriculture (USDA) under the provisions of the Animal Welfare Act[26] must establish and follow "an appropriate plan for environmental enhancement adequate to promote the psychological well-being" of the nonhuman primates housed in that facility.[27] The licensed exhibitor or facility itself is held responsible for compliance with any regulation under the Act. However, the actual logistics and details of the plan are not delineated, and the regulations specifically hold the attending veterinarian responsible for implementing an enrichment plan. The reader is directed to the published regulations[27] for the precise wording. This chapter seeks to present the basic concepts of primate enrichment, to point out areas of concern, to anticipate issues that may involve challenges or precipitate conflict with other staff, to suggest potential approaches to these challenges, and to provide useful references to assist the veterinarian with formulating the plan.

Not only must a primate enrichment plan be developed and implemented, but the record must be made available to the USDA when requested. Specific concepts (social grouping, environmental enrichment, special considerations, and restraint devices) must be addressed. The plan must be adapted to each species involved, and it must be "in accordance with currently accepted professional standards as they are cited in appropriate" published literature.[27] The Special Considerations section lists several circumstances (such as research protocols that require restricted activity) or classifications of animals (for example, infants, great apes) where special attention to environmental enhancement is required.[28]

EXEMPTIONS TO THE REQUIREMENTS

The plan itself can provide special exceptions, such as for debilitated, vicious, or incompatible animals, or for situations involving contagious disease. In addition, the attending veterinarian may write individual exemptions to the plan if they are based on animal health, condition, or well-being. Such situations could include quarantine, controlled socialization/introduction procedures, or postsurgical hospitalization or treatment. Within research facilities, the Institutional Animal Care and Use Committee (IACUC)[2] can exempt individual nonhuman primates from all or parts of the plan, if the exemption was approved during the IACUC review process.

The structure of the regulations clearly discourages blanket exemptions for groups of animals or to the plan as a whole. Documentation should clearly indicate the reason(s) for the exemption and should separately address each conceptual area (social grouping, environmental enrichment, special considerations, or restraint devices) that falls under the exemption. These exemptions must be documented, reviewed, and signed on a regular basis. Unless the basis for the exemption is a permanent condition, in nonresearch situations this review must be performed by the attending veterinarian every 30 days. For research animals, the intervals may be set by the IACUC, but reviews must be performed at least annually.[27] Proper documentation must be maintained by the licensee (not the veterinarian) and must be available to USDA officials upon request. For research facilities, the records must also be made available to any pertinent funding federal agencies.[27]

MEDICAL ISSUES AND THE ENRICHMENT PLAN

Before the environmental enhancement plan is developed, the veterinarian should consider the available resources (discussed later in this chapter), assess their applicability to the facility, seek insight from animal managers and veterinarians of other institutions, anticipate financial and logistical challenges that may arise, and structure the plan so that it builds consensus and collaboration. Usually, the veterinarian discovers that intrinsic tension exists between the dual roles of "enrichment facilitator" and "protector of animal health." Although the veterinarian has a duty to minimize animal health risks, the regulatory authorities deliberately assigned both of these responsibilities to the veterinarian.

ADVANTAGES OF THE VETERINARIAN'S ROLE IN FACILITATING ENRICHMENT

The regulations provide little detail regarding plan development, nor any specific engineering or behavioral criteria that must be met. Section 3.81 (3)(c)(2) presents a particular challenge, because it requires special attention for "those that show signs of being in psychological distress through behavior or appearance."[28] No definition of "signs" is provided, nor whether providing "special attention" is considered adequate even if the "signs" persist.[28] Therefore, the regulations hold the facility's veterinarian responsible for the environmental enhancement plan, without providing clear criteria for decision making. Depending on the viewpoint(s) of the veterinarian and other facility staff, this lack of detail can be a blessing, a curse, or both.

This responsibility should be accepted with enthusi-asm. The veterinarian has an opportunity to suggest positive actions that might otherwise conflict with other provisions of the Animal Welfare Act. Thus, the regulations allow innovative husbandry opportunities in circumstances where the overall benefit-versus-risk assessment is judged acceptable by the veterinarian. For example, free-ranging opportunities have been provided to golden lion tamarins in zoos, even though their freedom increases the likelihood of injury or exposure to disease. This is acceptable because they are learning survival skills for reintroduction, and they have been judged to benefit from the enrichment opportunities experienced under supervision (J. Garbe, personal communication).

Additionally, a formal enrichment plan can ensure that husbandry tasks that may reduce health problems (such as the provision of browse or climbing opportunities) are considered vital parts of the daily routine. The types and variety of enrichment opportunities provided should be determined by species-specific needs, not by the charismatic nature of the animal or the time budget or motivation level of the keeper.

Zoo veterinarians are adept in adapting standard medical equipment to diverse species; this innovative thinking can easily be applied to developing safe toys or exercise apparatus for various primates. Working with a nutritionist (or Species Survival Plan [SSP] nutrition advisor), the veterinarian is also qualified to provide guidance on the types and amounts of food and bedding that will have minimal risk of gastrointestinal disruption if ingested.[1]

Potential Sources of Conflict

Some provisions of this section also set the stage for potential conflict between the veterinarian and other facility staff. Historically, most staff members have interacted with veterinarians in a traditional patient-client-doctor relationship. This experience can heavily influence the conscious and unconscious expectations of all parties when applied to the relatively new wellness paradigm in zoological medicine. Some veterinarians may also be uncomfortable with this new expectation. For consultant veterinarians, imposing directions on one's client instead of suggesting them can be especially challenging. Within the traditional relationship, the owner/client has an intrinsic motivation to limit the intrusion of the veterinarian into the human-animal bond, and the veterinarian is consulted primarily when something needs to be repaired. In some zoos, relationships can be strained when the veterinarian directs actions to be taken by other management personnel, particularly when there is no clear medical crisis to be solved. Indeed, to address this, some workers in this field have advanced the terminology of *behavioral husbandry* or *management* rather than *behavioral enrichment*.[4, 5]

While directing the plan, the veterinarian also runs the risk of alienating the behavioral scientist. Often, veterinarians are not sufficiently familiar with the methodology of behavioral studies and statistical analysis. On the other hand, some behaviorists are unaware of veterinarians' knowledge of behavioral patterns and how objective analysis underlies their diagnostic decisions.

In turn, thoughtful veterinarians acknowledge the limitations of their field, which emphasizes detection, prevention, and correction of dysfunction and frequently must combine the art and science of medicine. Veterinarians are more likely to report a single, dramatic incident of toxicity rather than the hundreds of innocuous exposures. And because anesthesia always carries some risk, most veterinarians prefer zero-risk scenarios and avoid even a single laparotomy for intestinal foreign bodies. Because the veterinarian is responsible for avoiding health risks, approving experiments with unquantifiable risk often creates an inherent conflict.

Acknowledgment of the potential for differences of opinion is often sufficient to avoid serious problems. In this regard, humility, collaboration, sharing of risk-assessment responsibilities, and communication are essential elements in implementing a successful enrichment plan.

RISK ASSESSMENT AND CONTROL

The veterinarian is frequently called on to evaluate enrichment strategies that have been successful in other zoos, but that may be particularly difficult in the situation at hand. For example, many sweet foods used as enrichments in northern climates will attract fire ants (*Solenopsis invicta*) in southern regions, creating a potentially painful experience for the animal. In another example, at Zoo Atlanta, we substitute bouillon cubes or whole fish for the frozen blood balls presented to carnivores at other zoos, believing that the latter is more likely to support the growth of *Salmonella* species and other intestinal pathogens. Ideally, keepers and curatorial staff should perform their own risk assessments, rather than adopt policies of other institutions without objective evaluation. The Shape of Enrichment[14] (Table 51–1) is an example of an extremely helpful newsletter

for sharing ideas. However, by design, its information is often published without broad-based expert review. Although this approach facilitates open discussion, it can also lead to inaccuracies if the conclusions are accepted without question.

In the author's practice, she has been frustrated when anticipating and measuring the potential for foreign body ingestion and balancing it against the benefit of many objects used in enrichment. These circumstances clearly illustrate the challenge of promoting enrichment while controlling risk. To date, the best solution appears to be a trial-and-error period of supervised experimentation and then evaluating results. Experimentation has proven that some previously rejected items were later deemed safe. Alternatively, close supervision has allowed keepers to remove items quickly when they were found to be unsafe. Careful selection of materials (stainless steel attachments rather than brass) reduce the likelihood of systemic consequences if ingestion occurs. The veterinarian should also check that cage furnishings are properly installed, because appendages can be easily caught in rope or hardware. Improper installation can also result in the failure of an apparatus and subsequent injury.

Another challenge lies in the assessment of potential disease transmission between human and nonhuman primates through the use of recycled materials. In a conservation-minded organization, recycling is desirable and these items are frequently in demand for enrichment of great apes. However, humans and great apes are frequently susceptible to the same viruses and bacteria.[30] So the circulation of used items from humans to nonhuman primates should be scrutinized, so that it does not negate quarantine and safety procedures. Some institutions refuse such donations altogether, or refuse them during influenza seasons, or make arrangements with companies to donate newly manufactured, excess stock. However, to the author's knowledge, proven disease transmission through the recycling of enrichment materials or foods to nonhuman primates has not been reported.

TABLE 51–1. Sources Mentioned in Text

National Animal Poison Control Center (NAPCC)
University of Illinois
2001 S. Lincoln Avenue
Urbana, IL 61801
1-800-548-2423

The Shape of Enrichment Newsletter
1650 Minden Drive
San Diego, CA 92111-7124
(619) 231-1515 x4272; (619) 279-4273

United States Department of Agriculture
National Agricultural Library
Animal Welfare Information Center
10301 Baltimore Boulevard
Beltsville, MD 20705
(301) 504-5755

TOXICITY

Because the toxic potential for many plants depends heavily on factors that are extrinsic to the plant itself,[11–13] all staff must recognize that plant toxicities are not always predictable. Compiling an approved safe browse list can be challenging. Subclinical toxicity can mimic simple indigestion, so incidents of toxicity may be underdiagnosed. In some zoos, highly toxic plant species have been fed regularly without incident (S. Winslow, personal communication), whereas in others, a small quantity may prove fatal (M.E. Fowler, personal communication). Animals that have recently been changed from impoverished to enriched environments, that have no previous exposure to certain browse materials, or that overindulge in some items are more likely to experience toxicity.[11–13] In such circumstances, extra caution is advised. Lists of approved browse species from other zoos warrant careful scrutiny by the veterinarian and horticultural experts. This is especially true when common names are used instead of taxonomic names or where regional variability in subspecies is likely. A fail-safe written procedure must be established to ensure that the plant is properly identified and that animal caretakers understand the correct procedure for obtaining and feeding approved browse items. This is especially critical with new personnel because they may assume that any plants being trimmed on zoo grounds are nontoxic. Additionally, the zoo veterinarians must keep abreast of newly reported toxicities.

Freshly cut browse can also serve as a mechanical vector for disease organisms (for example, *Mycobacterium avium, Toxoplasma* species) if contaminated by feces from free-living animals. To minimize this risk, the veterinarian should consult with medical experts and advise on proper disinfection procedures.

AVAILABLE RESOURCES

An effective plan should be based on a compilation of diverse resources available in this field. These include relevant institutional staff (veterinarians, behavioral scientists, curators, keepers, horticulturists, maintenance technicians, exhibit designers, volunteers, and students), experts outside the institution (SSP advisors, local universities and veterinary schools, other zoos, toxicologists, animal trainers, etc.), and published literature (including basic references on primate biology and ecology as well as those on laboratory animal science and applied behavioral biology).

Because the regulations require that the plan be species specific, broad-based primate references are extremely valuable.[19, 21, 23, 24] Currently, exponential growth is occurring within the published literature of applied behavioral science, relating to laboratory primates,[4–9, 21] and to those in zoos.[6, 15, 16, 18, 20–23, 25, 29] This necessitates frequent review in order to maintain a current database, which the regulations require. Fortunately, the USDA has established a national Animal Welfare Information Center[3] that publishes examples of enrichment plans, other relevant publications,[2, 9] and bibliographies.[3, 10] In addition, references such as Fowler[11, 12] and Oehme,[17] combined with regular, proactive consultation with the National Animal Poison Control Center (NAPCC) (see Table 51–1) can be extremely helpful in evaluating the potential toxicity of plants, paints, or other products used in exhibit enhancements/construction. The NAPCC maintains a unique databank, with expert veterinary toxicologists. In many instances, their knowledge, understanding of the limitations of applying standard therapeutic procedures to exotic animals, and willingness to extrapolate to a variety of species have been instrumental in avoiding and treating accidental poisonings.

DEVELOPING, DOCUMENTING, AND FOLLOWING THE ENRICHMENT PLAN

Publications by Bloomsmith and colleagues[4, 5] provide direction in setting up behavioral enrichment programs in a multiuser environment. Although a committee is vital to the planning process, holding a single person accountable for carrying ideas to implementation works best in many institutions. Even a well-thought out plan can quickly bog down if it does not realistically address work schedule needs, delegate tasks, mobilize volunteers to assist with labor,[20a] and provide for consistent record keeping and decision making. Ideas can and do become lost in the transition from brainstorming to implementation, and they can also be forgotten if responsible personnel change.

It is important that there is clear accountability of animal staff in carrying out the prescribed actions. Care must be taken that the most desirable and rewarding tasks do not fall to a few individuals and that appropriate credit is given to all involved; otherwise, the morale and effectiveness of the team will suffer.[20a] Currently, the Zoo Atlanta Behavioral Husbandry Committee is co-chaired by a veterinarian and a behavioral scientist. Permanent members include animal curators and representatives of the maintenance, horticultural, and exhibit design staff. Keeper members, balanced across animal areas and between supervisory and nonsupervisory positions, are rotated every 6 months. All personnel, however, are invited to attend indefinitely. Monthly meetings are held; minutes are distributed to all areas. The Committee serves primarily to facilitate communication and problem solving. Currently, coordination and record keeping duties are performed by a senior research associate; a volunteer crew assists the keeper staff with implementation. This basic structure can be modified and adapted to the specific needs of any institution.

EVALUATING THE EFFECTIVENESS OF THE ENRICHMENT PLAN

Other than stating that the plan should be responsive to the needs of the species,[27] the regulations do not delineate how the plan's effectiveness should be measured. Written plans can consist of specific tasks to be performed and how often; the success of accomplishing these tasks can be measured through records. This approach may be necessary in complex organizations or where voluntary compliance with directives is uncertain. Other institutions have written goal-oriented, philosophical plans that leave the details of enrichment tasks to the caretaker's imagination and the practicality of the season. The reasoning behind this approach is the concept that scheduled enrichment activities can become routine and do not reflect the variability of natural situations. At the time of this writing, USDA authorities appear to accept either approach, as long as reasonable documentation of activities is provided.

However, implementing tasks does not prove that the needs of an individual animal are satisfied nor increase behaviors that are appropriate to the species. A trained behavioral scientist should objectively examine the animal's behaviors, determine to what degree observed behaviors are appropriate to that species in nature, and evaluate the cost-effectiveness of the various activities. For example, large amounts of time and effort can be expended in preparing costly food items that are quickly consumed and contrary to desired nutritional goals or that provide amusement to the visiting public without facilitating species-typical behaviors. Cutting and scattering of food items can dramatically increase foraging behavior, but provisioning of whole foods might increase desirable food processing behaviors; the relative value of these conflicting strategies should be measured. Although human-animal interaction during training clearly falls within the definition of enrichment in these regulations, the types of behavior being promoted should again be evaluated for species-appropriateness.

SUMMARY

Ideally, evaluating the effectiveness of an enrichment plan involves setting clear behavioral goals for each species, designing innovative opportunities to elicit those behaviors, objectively measuring the results, and comparing them with the desired goals. Although not every activity needs to be subjected to such rigorous analysis, veterinarians should recognize and take advantage of well-designed precedents in the literature.[6, 8, 15, 16, 18, 20, 25, 29]

This review will also help ensure that time is primarily being expended to satisfy animal needs and that the enrichment plan does not become an unproductive staff activity. A broad-based, professional approach ensures that the best and most appropriate techniques are being consistently applied.

Acknowledgments

The author gratefully acknowledges the dedicated contributions of all members of the Zoo Atlanta Behavioral Husbandry Committee and Behavioral Husbandry Volunteers toward animal welfare.

REFERENCES

1. Allen ME, Oftedal OT: Nutrition and dietary evaluation in zoos. *In* Kleiman DG, et al (eds): Wild Mammals in Captivity. Chicago, University of Chicago Press, pp 109–116, 1996.
2. Allen T, Clingerman K: Animal Care and Use Committee. Beltsville MD, USDA National Agricultural Library, September 1992.
3. Swanson TC, Kreger MD, Berry BG, et al: Animal Welfare Information Center: Environmental Enrichment Information Resources for Nonhuman Primates. U.S. Dept of Agriculture, National Library of Medicine, U.S. Dept of Health and Human Services, Primate Information Center, University of Washington, 1987–1992.
4. Bloomsmith MA: Evolving a behavioral management program in a breeding/research setting. Annual Proceedings of the American Zoo and Aquarium Association, Wheeling, WV, pp 372–377, 1994.
5. Bloomsmith MA, Brent L, Schapiro SJ: Guidelines for developing and managing an environmental enrichment program for nonhuman primates. Lab Anim Sci 41:372–377, 1991.
6. Bloomstrand MA, Riddle K, Alford P, Maple TL: Objective evaluation of a behavioral enrichment device for captive chimpanzees (*Pan troglodytes*). Zoo Biol 1:243–250, 1982.
7. Box H (ed): Primate Responses to Environmental Change. New York, Chapman and Hall, 1991.
8. Chamove AL, Anderson JR, Morgan-Jones SC, Jones SP: Deep woodchip litter: hygiene, feeding, and behavioral enhancement in eight primate species. Int J Stud Anim Probl 3:308–319, 1982.
9. Clark BC: Applying Ecological Principles to Captive Primate Environments: Needs and Environmental Design for Colony Management. Toledo, OH, BC Clark, 1992.
10. Allen T: Ethical and Moral Issues Relating to Animals. Beltsville, MD, USDA National Agricultural Library, May 1993.
11. Fowler ME: Plant poisoning in captive nondomestic animals. J Zoo Anim Med 12:134, 1981.
12. Fowler ME: Plant poisoning in free-living wild animals: a review. J Wildl Dis 19:34, 1983.
13. Garland T, Bailey EM: Toxic ornamental and garden plants. *In* Bonagura JD (ed): Kirk's Current Veterinary Therapy XII. Philadelphia, WB Saunders, pp 217–222, 1995.
14. Hare VJ, Carlstead K, et al (eds): The Shape of Enrichment. San Diego, The Shape of Enrichment Newsletter, 1995.
15. Maple TL, Perkins LA: Enclosure furnishings and structural environmental enrichment. *In* Kleiman DG, Allen ME, Thompson KV, Lumpkin S (eds): Wild Mammals in Captivity. Chicago, University of Chicago Press, pp 212–222, 1996.
16. Mellen JD, Ellis S: Animal learning and husbandry training. *In* Kleiman DG, Allen ME, Thompson KV, Lumpkin S (eds): Wild Mammals in Captivity. Chicago, University of Chicago Press, pp 88–99, 1996.
17. Oehme FW: Information resources for toxicology. *In* Kirk RW (ed): Current Veterinary Therapy IX. Philadelphia, WB Saunders, pp 129–132, 1986.
18. Ogden JJ: A post-occupancy evaluation: naturalistic habitats for captive lowland gorillas. M.S. thesis, Georgia Institute of Technology, 1989.
19. Parker CE: Behavioral diversity in ten species of nonhuman primates. J Comp Physiol Psychol 87:930–937, 1969.
20. Perkins LA: Variables that influence the activity of captive orangutans. Zoo Biol 11:177–186, 1992.
20a. Porton I, Merz R, et al: Creating opportunities: some resourceful solutions to the challenges of management. Annual Proceedings of the American Zoo and Aquarium Association, Seattle, WA, pp 432–435, 1995.
21. Segal EF (ed): Housing, Care and Psychological Wellbeing of Captive and Laboratory Primates. Park Ridge, NJ, Noyes, 1989.
22. Seidensticker J, Doherty JG: Integrating animal behavior and exhibit design. *In* Kleiman DG, Allen ME, Thompson KV, Lumpkin S (eds): Wild Mammals in Captivity. Chicago, University of Chicago Press, pp 180–190, 1996.
23. Seidensticker J, Forthman DL: Second nature: environmental enrichment for captive animals. *In* Shepherdson D, Mellen J, Hutchins M (eds): Environmental Enrichment for Captive Animals. Washington, DC, Smithsonian institution Press, pp 15–29, 1997.
24. Smuts BB, et al (eds): Primate Societies. Chicago, University of Chicago Press, 1987.
25. Tripp JK: Increasing activity in captive orangutans: provision of manipulable and edible materials. Zoo Biol 4:225–234, 1985.
26. U.S. Department of Agriculture: Animal Welfare. 9 CFR, Chapter 1, Subpart D, Sections 3.75–3.92: 68–84, 1995.
27. U.S. Department of Agriculture: Animal Welfare, 9 CFR, Chapter 1, Subpart D, Section 3.81: 74–75, 1995.
28. U.S. Department of Agriculture: Animal Welfare, 9 CFR, Chapter 1, Subpart D, Section 3.81 (3)(c)(2): 75, 1995.
29. Wilson SF: Environmental influences on the activity of captive apes. Zoo Biol 1:201–209, 1982.
30. Kreger M, Swanson J, Jensen D: Zoonoses: Disease Transmission from Animal to Man. Beltsville, MD, USDA National Agricultural Library, May 1994.

CHAPTER 52

Tuberculin Responses in Orangutans

PAUL P. CALLE

Orangutans (*Pongo pygmaeus*) are susceptible to infection by pathogenic mycobacteria (*Mycobacterium tuberculosis, M. bovis,* and *M. avium*) and can develop disseminated disease.[18, 21, 24, 29] Orangutans in Indonesia that were previously pets have recently been documented with *M. tuberculosis* infection and *M. avium* infection has been documented in captive orangutans in Malaysia (W. Karesh and A. Kilbourn, personal communication, 1998). These orangutans developed clinical signs (cough, weight loss), pulmonary radiographic abnormalities (focal pulmonary consolidation without calcification), and responses to intradermal mammalian old tuberculin (MOT; Colorado Serum Co., Denver; distributed by Synbiotics Co., Kansas City, MO) similar to those developed by other nonhuman primates infected by pathogenic mycobacteria.

There are no reported cases of disease caused by nontuberculous mycobacteria in orangutans. However, similar to other nonhuman primates[7, 11, 26, 29, 34, 44] and humans,[45] they could probably develop illness after infection by nontuberculous mycobacteria. If disease developed, clinical signs would probably be similar to those caused by pathogenic mycobacteria and reflect the affected organ systems—respiratory or gastrointestinal signs with subsequent weight loss. Acquired leprosy has been reported in captive chimpanzees (*Pan troglodytes*).[17, 19]

Healthy captive orangutans, with no known exposure to pathogenic mycobacteria, frequently respond to tuberculin (MOT, avian old tuberculin [AOT; National Veterinary Service Laboratory, Ames, IA], and purified protein derivatives [PPD]) in the eyelid and other intradermal locations.[2, 21, 25, 32, 46] Tuberculin responses occur with similar frequency in Bornean, Sumatran, and subspecific hybrid orangutans, in females more commonly than in males, and in adults more frequently than in immature animals.[46] Intradermal palpebral tuberculin testing is most common, but other test sites include the arm, chest, or abdomen. Responses are most frequently observed in the eyelid and another intradermal location. Eyelid response, without a response in another location, is more common than a negative eyelid response with a positive response elsewhere.[46] This suggests that the eyelid may be more sensitive than other sites in the orangutan. Reliability of alternate sites should be investigated to determine optimal test location.

In contrast, macaques do not demonstrate a significant difference in tuberculin responses of palpebral, compared to abdominal, test sites, and a combination

of testing in both locations is more accurate than either one alone.[30] Limited evaluation of recently caught wild orangutans has also demonstrated responses to intradermal MOT, but at lower prevalence rates than occurs in the captive orangutan population in North America (W. Karesh and A. Kilbourn, personal communication, 1998). One published account documented tuberculin responses to MOT, but not a PPD designed for use in humans, in an orangutan with fulminating tuberculosis.[18] In another study, healthy orangutan tuberculin responders also did not respond to a similar PPD tuberculin (Aplisol; Parke-Davis, Morris Plains, NJ),[2] suggesting that this antigen does not aid in distinguishing specific from nonspecific tuberculin responses. It is a misconception that repeated tuberculin tests will induce responses; in fact, in other species repeated testing may promote anergy. Orangutans are not sensitized to tuberculin by tuberculin testing, and orangutans have responded to various tuberculins when first tested.[2]

A review of medical records for 80% (249 orangutans) of the North American orangutan Species Survival Plan (SSP) population for an 8-year period (1980–1988) failed to identify a single case of tuberculosis.[46] Necropsy records of 30 orangutans, 5 of which had a history of responding to various tuberculins and from which nontuberculous mycobacteria had been cultured several years before death, were also reviewed. None had gross or histologic evidence of tuberculosis,[46] but postmortem mycobacterial cultures were not performed in each case. Despite this apparent absence of tuberculosis in the SSP population, 62.5% (107) of the 171 orangutans tested responded to one or several tuberculins.[46] This prevalence of tuberculin responses in the population is similar to that reported at two different institutions whose healthy orangutan tuberculin responders were thoroughly evaluated.[2, 32]

Orangutans appear to be more susceptible than other nonhuman primates to the development of tuberculin responses without exposure to pathogenic mycobacteria, but the reasons for this are not known. Two possible explanations are sensitization to mycobacterial antigens by exposure to nontuberculous mycobacteria[2, 32, 46] or a greater sensitivity to tuberculin than other nonhuman primates possess.[46]

Nontuberculous and pathogenic mycobacteria share common antigenic determinants.[6, 13, 45] If the tuberculin responses observed in orangutans result from mycobacterial antigen cross-reaction, the responses are more properly described as nonspecific responses rather than false-positive reactions. Nonspecific tuberculin responses resulting from exposure to nontuberculous mycobacteria have been described in other nonhuman primates[23, 24, 34, 37, 41, 44] and humans.[5, 9, 13, 33, 36, 45] Nontuberculous mycobacteria (*M. avium, M. chelonai, M. flavescens, M. fortuitum, M. gordonae, M. kansasii, M. nonchromogenicum, M. parafortuitum, M. terrae*) have been isolated from samples obtained from healthy orangutans or their environments.[2, 25, 32, 46] It is possible that orangutans, compared with other nonhuman primates, are more sensitive to tuberculin skin test conversion when exposed to these environmental mycobacteria. Another possibility is that they naturally harbor mycobacteria as part of the endogenous bacterial flora of the respiratory tract (including the prominent laryngeal air sac) or gastrointestinal tract and have therefore been sensitized to mycobacterial antigens.[2] Alternatively, arboreal free-ranging orangutans may have limited natural exposure to saprophytic mycobacteria, and consequently are more likely to mount an immunologic response when exposed to these novel antigens. One or a combination of these possibilities may explain why tuberculin responses are so prevalent in orangutans.

Monkeys require 1000 to 10,000 times more tuberculin than humans to elicit a positive intradermal tuberculin test.[8, 28, 34, 42] The minimum recommended dose for tuberculin testing monkeys is 0.1 ml tuberculin containing at least 1500 tuberculin units (TU).[28] Mammalian old tuberculin, the formulation recommended for nonhuman primates, contains approximately 13,500 TU per 0.1 ml dose (C. Thoen, personal communication, 1997). In contrast, the recommendation for humans is 0.1 ml tuberculin containing 5 TU.[3, 5, 13] Because the response to a tuberculin skin test is dose related, increasing the dose when testing humans results in an increased frequency and size of nonspecific tuberculin responses.[13] Orangutans appear to have a greater sensitivity to tuberculin than do gorillas (*Gorilla gorilla*) or chimpanzees.[2, 25, 32] The antigenic concentrations of tuberculins used in nonhuman primates may be too great for orangutans, and they may respond because of a greater antigenic sensitivity.[46]

TUBERCULIN RESPONSE EVALUATION

There are no standardized, widely accepted protocols for evaluation of nonhuman primates that respond to tuberculin. Several approaches for investigation of nonhuman primate[26, 34, 35] and specifically orangutan[1, 2, 32, 46] tuberculin responders have been published. Recommendations for the control of tuberculosis in nonhuman primates housed in laboratory colonies are also available.[28]

Clinical evaluation of a tuberculin response in orangutans includes physical examination, blood tests, radiography, intradermal tuberculin testing, and mycobacterial cultures.[1, 2, 25, 32, 46] Orangutans that die should have a thorough necropsy, including histopathology, performed. If the individual or collection has a history of

tuberculin responses, mycobacterial cultures of lymph nodes and other organs are appropriate.

The following protocol reflects what is presently known about the evaluation of tuberculin responses in orangutans. It is intended as a guide to aid the zoo veterinarian in formulating an appropriate diagnostic approach for each individual situation. A major limitation in determining the optimal frequency, significance, sensitivity, and specificity of test procedures and interpretation of results is the absence of evaluations of these techniques in orangutans infected by pathogenic mycobacteria.[1] In addition, there have been a limited number of orangutans that have been evaluated with the same battery of tests. Compliance with recommendations for primate quarantine and preventive medical procedures[22, 38] and occupational health guidelines for personnel[39, 40] are encouraged.

EVALUATION PROTOCOL

History

A thorough evaluation of the tuberculosis histories of the individual specimen, contact animals, and the zoo's animal collection is necessary. Critical assessment should be made of the likelihood of exposure to pathogenic mycobacteria by contact with primates, the visiting public (and fomites such as food thrown into open exhibits), or zoo personnel. A review of the employee tuberculin testing program, individual test results, and consideration of additional staff tuberculin testing are important components of the assessment.

Examination

A complete physical examination of the orangutan should be performed with specific evaluations for respiratory disease, weight loss, lymphadenopathy, hepatomegaly, or splenomegaly.

Diagnostic Testing

Blood should be collected for complete blood count, serum biochemical profile, and serum banking (for serum enzyme-linked immunosorbent assay [ELISA][7, 31, 43] or other additional testing). Chest and abdominal radiographs are indicated. Vertical positioning (anteroposterior or posteroanterior views), as are standard for evaluation of humans,[5] improves the quality of thoracic radiographic detail, especially in adult and obese orangutans.[2, 20] It is advisable to take radiographs before tracheal wash or gastric lavage to avoid creation of artifactual radiographic lesions.

The optimal tuberculin, concentration, volume, test site, and test frequency for evaluation of orangutans has not been determined. Intradermal palpebral testing is typically used because it is easily read. Mammalian old tuberculin (0.1 ml undiluted) is most commonly used. It is the most sensitive but least specific tuberculin. When an orangutan responds to MOT, comparative testing should be performed to aid in determining the significance of the response. Tuberculins used include 0.1 ml each of undiluted MOT, AOT, purified protein derivative bovis (PPD-B), balanced purified protein derivative avian (BPPD-A), balanced purified protein derivative bovine (BPPD-B), medium control, and saline control. When an individual or collection has a history of responses to tuberculin, it is common to perform initial comparative intradermal palpebral testing with MOT and AOT. Avian tuberculin responses significantly greater than those to mammalian or bovine tuberculin are consistent with a nonspecific response. After a positive initial test, retest and comparative tuberculin testing should be performed immediately or within 2 weeks, in a different intradermal test site or repeated in the same site in 1 to 3 months. Palpebral testing is limited to one or two tuberculins; when more will be used all are given in the same nonpalpebral intradermal location (abdomen, chest, or arm are frequently used). The test is visually read at 24, 48, and 72 hours. For greater accuracy, palpation and measurement of test site diameter and skin thickness are conducted at 72 hours. Responses are characterized by erythema, swelling, induration, and infrequently by ulceration and serum exudation (Fig. 52–1). If it is suspected the response is a result of trauma, infection, or contamination, biopsy of tuberculin test sites will confirm a delayed-type hypersensitivity reaction.

Commonly collected samples for mycobacterial culture include tracheal wash, gastric lavage, feces, exudate from draining lesions, and lesion biopsy. Gastric lavage reflects both gastric flora and swallowed respiratory tract secretions. Tracheal wash cultures are indicated if the orangutan is ill or there is a suspicion that it has been exposed to pathogenic mycobacteria. In clinically ill orangutans, the affected organ system must be sampled (tracheal wash and gastric samples for respiratory disease, gastric and fecal samples for gastrointestinal disease, exudate from an abscess, lymph node biopsy, etc.). Apparently healthy orangutan tuberculin responders should at a minimum have fecal and gastric mycobacterial cultures and acid-fast stains done.

Mycobacterial cultures and acid-fast stains may be performed at local hospitals, regional mycobacterial laboratories, or the National Veterinary Service Laboratory.[1, 2] Because laboratory procedures and requirements vary, the laboratory of choice should be contacted in advance to determine cost as well as optimal sample collection, handling, and shipping procedures. All mycobacteria isolated should be speciated. Antibiotic sensitivity patterns for all pathogenic mycobacteria need to be determined if treatment will be attempted. This is especially important because of the development, spread, and high mortality rate of multiple drug resistant *M. tuberculosis* infection in the human population.[5, 12, 14]

Test results (isolation of *M. tuberculosis* from a tracheal wash sample of an ill orangutan with pulmonary radiographic abnormalities) may be diagnostic for pathogenic mycobacterial infection in an orangutan tuberculin responder; however, more common is the absence of confirmatory results. Although this suggests a nonspecific tuberculin response, it does not exclude infection by, or exposure to, pathogenic mycobacteria. Only after consideration of all historic information and

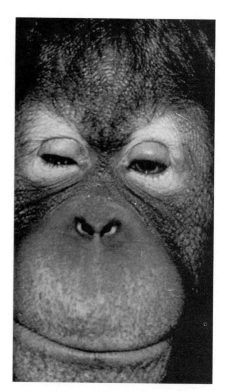

FIGURE 52–1. Tuberculin skin test responses in a 10-year-old female orangutan (*Pongo pygmaeus*) injected with balanced purified protein derivative of *Mycobacterium avium* (right eye) and balanced purified protein derivative of *Mycobacterium bovis* (left eye). The bilateral responses are characterized by moderate palpebral erythema and swelling (From Calle PP, Thoen CO, Roskop ML: Tuberculin skin test responses, mycobacteriologic examinations of gastric lavage, and serum enzyme-linked immunosorbent assays in orangutans [*Pongo pygmaeus*]. J Zoo Wildl Med 20[3]:307-314, 1989.)

diagnostic test results can the significance of a tuberculin response in an orangutan be determined. Additionally, determination that an orangutan has developed a nonspecific response does not preclude later infection by pathogenic mycobacteria. Protocols for future assessment of these orangutans are dependent on earlier evaluations and a comparison of current and previous test results.

MANAGEMENT OF RESPONDER ORANGUTANS

Although confirmed cases of tuberculosis are reportable, there are no national animal disease or public health regulations restricting the movement of orangutans that respond to a tuberculin test. Individual state animal disease or public health agency restrictions may occur, but they vary over time and on a state-by-state basis. If an orangutan tuberculin responder truly has tuberculosis, local public health regulations, potential zoonotic hazard, and risk to a new collection must be considered when animals are relocated. Specific state regulations of the shipping and receiving institutions should be verified before animal movement between institutions.

It is the professional and ethical obligation of individuals and institutions to inform potential recipients of the tuberculin responder status of an orangutan and to share pertinent historical and medical information. Specific procedures and tests to be included in the preshipment evaluation of an orangutan should be agreed upon before movement between institutions. Documentation of pathogenic mycobacteria in either a healthy or ill orangutan, or clinical illness resulting from infection by a nontuberculous mycobacteria, necessitates treatment or euthanasia as deemed appropriate. In these situations, isolation ability, physical facility, collection size, genetic value of the individual, clinical condition of the animal, organism isolation and identification, the isolate's antibiotic sensitivity pattern, and the ability to administer medications must all be taken into consideration. Prophylactic medication of healthy orangutans that respond to tuberculin, especially those with recent skin test conversions, may also be considered based on the likelihood of exposure to pathogenic mycobacteria.[32, 46]

FUTURE RESEARCH

Immunologic assays such as ELISA, lymphocyte transformation test (LT), and fused rocket immunodiffusion testing have been applied on a limited basis in orangutan tuberculin responders with mixed results.[2, 32, 46] Testing by ELISA and LT may be arranged by contacting Dr. Charles Thoen (Iowa State University; phone 515-294-7608; fax 515-294-8500). Fused rocket immunodiffusion testing is not presently available. These tests are probably sensitive and will rule out false-negative responses, but preliminary evaluations suggest that they are no more specific than the skin test.

Development and production of tuberculins from nontuberculous mycobacteria would likely improve the specificity of orangutan intradermal tuberculin testing. These antigens are not commercially available but have been periodically developed and used in nonhuman primates[25, 44] and humans.[45] The specificity and sensitivity of intradermal tuberculin testing are inversely related. Optimal tuberculin concentrations to minimize false-negative responses and maximize true positive responses have been determined by experience and evaluation of various tuberculins and concentrations in humans[4, 5, 13] and macaques.[28, 30, 34, 42] The significance of a tuberculin response in humans is determined by the size of the response, which is interpreted based on the individual's history and existence of predisposing risk factors.[5] The studies needed to similarly interpret the results in orangutans have not yet been conducted. Determination of the optimal tuberculin concentration for orangutans could be investigated with dilute MOT or PPD-B. Evaluation of the sensitivity and specificity of these preparations requires testing of healthy orangutan tuberculin responders. Their responses will then need to be compared with those of orangutans either known to be infected with pathogenic mycobacteria or those

experimentally sensitized to pathogenic mycobacterial antigens (such as by vaccination with bacillus Calmette-Guérin [BCG] or administration of Freund's complete adjuvant). A straightforward approach would be concurrent testing with serial dilutions of various tuberculins on an abdominal site to determine the optimal dilution to distinguish a nonspecific response from one diagnostic for pathogenic mycobacterial exposure. Simultaneous comparative testing of optimal tuberculin dilutions at eyelid and other intradermal locations would then be necessary to determine the most accurate site for intradermal tuberculin testing. It would also be of interest to perform comparative tuberculin testing on recently collected wild orangutans to determine if the captive environment contributes to the high tuberculin response rate observed.

Application of antigen 85 testing[15, 16] to orangutans may aid in the diagnosis of active mycobacterial infections. Antigen 85 complex proteins are major secretory proteins produced by actively proliferating mycobacteria (both pathogenic and nonpathogenic) that bind fibronectins. Sensitized T cells produce fibronectins that are associated with the initiation of delayed hypersensitivity reactions. Antigen 85 complex proteins are involved in the inactivation of T cell fibronectin and diminish antimycobacterial delayed hypersensitivity reactions. Antigen 85 results in a dose-dependent suppression of PPD tuberculin cutaneous delayed hypersensitivity responses in sensitized guinea pigs. An antigen 85 dot blot immunoassay has been developed that detected anergic, culture positive, *Mycobacterium tuberculosis* infections in humans[15, 16] and mycobacterial infections in zoological species.[27] This assay would likely be useful for the diagnosis of active mycobacterial infections in orangutans, but would be unlikely to differentiate a nonspecific tuberculin response from one resulting from previous exposure to pathogenic mycobacteria. Evaluation of this test in orangutans will require comparative testing of healthy orangutans that respond to tuberculin and those infected with, or exposed to, pathogenic mycobacteria.

Nucleic probe analysis and polymerase chain reaction testing for diagnosis of mycobacterial infections in humans and animals are also under development at a number of locations but are not widely available at this time.[10, 26, 31] These tests will probably aid in the diagnosis of active mycobacterial disease but not in differentiating nonspecific tuberculin responses from those resulting from pathogenic mycobacterial exposure.

Development of these techniques will increase our understanding and knowledge of tuberculin responses in orangutans. At this time, clinical interpretation of the results are difficult and determining the significance of an intradermal tuberculin response must take into consideration all factors surrounding the case and not depend solely on the presence of an intradermal tuberculin response. Despite the relatively high frequency of nonspecific tuberculin responses in orangutans, the possibility of infection by a pathogenic mycobacteria must always be considered. Final interpretation of the significance of a tuberculin response in an orangutan is up to the attending veterinarian after evaluation of all test results and consultation with veterinary and public health officials as appropriate.

REFERENCES

1. Calle PP: Tuberculin reactions in orangutans (*Pongo pygmaeus*). *In* American Association of Zoo Veterinarians Infectious Disease Reviews. Media, PA, American Association of Zoo Veterinarians, #3:1–7, 1992.
2. Calle PP, Thoen CO, Roskop ML: Tuberculin skin test responses, mycobacteriologic examinations of gastric lavage, and serum enzyme-linked immunosorbent assays in orangutans (*Pongo pygmaeus*). J Zoo Wildl Med 20(3):307–314, 1989.
3. Centers for Disease Control: Screening for tuberculosis and tuberculosis infection in high-risk populations. MMWR 39(RR-8):1–7, 1990.
4. Centers for Disease Control: The use of preventive therapy for tuberculous infection in the United States. MMWR 39(RR-8):9–12, 1990.
5. Centers for Disease Control: Core Curriculum on Tuberculosis, 3rd ed. Atlanta, U.S. Department of Health and Human Services, Public Health Service, 1994.
6. Chaparas SD, Brown TM, Hyman IS: Antigenic relationships of various mycobacterial species with *Mycobacterium tuberculosis*. Am Rev Respir Dis 117:1091–1097, 1978.
7. Corcoran KD, Thoen CO: Application of an enzyme immunoassay for detecting antibodies in sera of *Macaca fascicularis* naturally exposed to *Mycobacterium tuberculosis*. J Med Primatol 20:404–408, 1991.
8. Dannenberg AM: Pathogenesis of pulmonary tuberculosis in man and animals: protection of personnel against tuberculosis. *In* Montali RJ (ed): Mycobacterial Infections of Zoo Animals. Washington, DC, Smithsonian Institution Press, pp 65–75, 1978.
9. Des Prez R: Diseases due to mycobacteria: tuberculosis. *In* Wyngaarden JB, Smith LH (eds): Cecil Textbook of Medicine, vol 2. Philadelphia, WB Saunders, pp 1538–1554, 1982.
10. Dillehay DL, Huerkamp MJ: Tuberculosis in a tuberculin-negative rhesus monkey (*Macaca mulatta*) on chemoprophylaxis. J Zoo Wildl Med 21(4):480–484, 1990.
11. Fleischman RW, du Moulin GC, Esber HJ, et al: Nontuberculous mycobacterial infection attributable to *Mycobacterium intracellulare* serotype 10 in two rhesus monkeys. J Am Vet Med Assoc 181(11):1359–1362, 1982.
12. Frieden TR, Sterling T, Pablos-Mendez A, et al: The emergence of drug-resistant tuberculosis in New York city. N Engl J Med 328(8):521–526, 1993.
13. Glossroth J, Robins AG, Snider DE: Medical progress: tuberculosis in the 1980s. N Engl J Med 302(26):1441–1450, 1980.
14. Goble M, Iseman MD, Madsen LA, et al: Treatment of 171 patients with pulmonary tuberculosis resistant to isoniazid and rifampin. N Engl J Med 328(8):527–532, 1993.
15. Godfrey HP: T cell fibronectin and mycobacterial adversarial strategy. Int J Clin Lab Res 23:121–123, 1993.
16. Godfrey HP, Feng Z, Mandy S, et al: Modulation of expression of delayed hypersensitivity by mycobacterial antigen 85 fibronectin-binding proteins. Infec Immun 60(6):2522–2528, 1992.
17. Gormus BJ, Xu K, Alford PL, et al: A serologic study of naturally acquired leprosy in chimpanzees. Int J Leprosy 59(3):450–457, 1991.
18. Haberle AJ: Tuberculosis in an orangutan. J Zoo Anim Med 1(2):10–15, 1970.
19. Hubbard GB, Lee DR, Eichberg JW, et al: Spontaneous leprosy in a chimpanzee (*Pan troglodytes*). Vet Pathol 28:546–548, 1991.
20. Janssen DL: Diseases of great apes. *In* Fowler ME (ed): Zoo and Wild Animal Medicine: Current Therapy 3. Philadelphia, WB Saunders, pp 334–338, 1993.
21. Jones DM: Veterinary aspects of the maintenance of orangutans in captivity. *In* De Boer LEM (ed): The Orang Utan: Its Biology and Conservation. The Hague, The Netherlands, Dr W Junk Publishers, pp 171–199, 1982.
22. Junge RE: Preventive medicine recommendations. *In* American Association of Zoo Veterinarians Infectious Disease Reviews. Media, PA, American Association of Zoo Veterinarians #1:1–21, 1991.
23. Kaufmann AF, Anderson DC: Tuberculosis control in nonhuman primate colonies. *In* Montali RJ (ed): Mycobacterial Infections of Zoo Animals. Washington, DC, Smithsonian Institution Press, pp 227–234, 1978.
24. Kehoe M, Phin CS, Chu CL: Tuberculosis in an orang utan. Aust Vet J 61(4):128, 1984.
25. Kuhn USG, III, Selin MJ: Tuberculin testing in great apes. *In* Montali RJ (ed): Mycobacterial Infections of Zoo Animals. Washington, DC, Smithsonian Institution Press, pp 129–134, 1978.
26. Lamberski N: An update on tuberculosis testing in nonhuman primates. *In* American Association of Zoo Veterinarians Infectious Disease Reviews. Media, PA, American Association of Zoo Veterinarians, in press.
27. Mangold BJ, Raphael BL, Cook RA, et al: Detection of mycobacterial antigens in *Mycobacterium paratuberculosis* infected nondomestic ruminants. Proceedings of the Annual Meeting of the American Association of Zoo Veterinarians, East Lansing, MI, pp 132–134, 1995.
28. Manning PJ, Cadigan FC, Goldsmith EI, et al: Detection of tuberculosis. *In* Manning PJ, Cadigan FC, Goldsmith EI, et al (eds): Laboratory Animal Management: Nonhuman primates. Washington, DC, Institute of Laboratory Animal Resources, National Academy Press, vol 23, no. 2–3, pp 27–29, 1980.
29. McClure HM: Bacterial diseases of nonhuman primates. *In* Montali RJ, Migaki G (eds): The Comparative Pathology of Zoo Animals. Washington, DC, Smithsonian Institution Press, pp 197–218, 1980.
30. McLaughlin RM, Thoenig JR, Marrs GE: A comparison of several intradermal tuberculins in *Macaca mulatta* during an epizootic of tuberculosis. Lab Anim Sci 26(1):44–50, 1976.
31. Meunier LD, Rock FM, Morris TH, Rolf LL, et al: Enzyme-linked immunosorbent assay for detection of *Mycobacterium tuberculosis* in a colony of *Macaca fascicularis*. Lab Anim Sci 43(4):389–390, 1993.
32. Miller RE: Problems in interpretation of TB testing in an orangutan colony. Proceedings of the Annual Meeting of the American Association of Zoo Veterinarians, Louisville, KY, pp 89–91, 1984.
33. Ogunmekan DA: The sensitization of children by opportunistic mycobacteria in Lagos, Nigeria. J Hyg 80:321–325, 1978.
34. Ott JE: Tuberculin testing in primates. Proceedings of the Annual Meeting of the American Association of Zoo Veterinarians, Denver, CO, pp 75–83, 1979.
35. Ott-Joslin JE: Tuberculin testing recommendations for primates. American Association of Zoo Veterinarians Infectious Disease Committee, American Association of Zoo Veterinarians, 1983.
36. Palmer CE, Edwards LB: Tuberculin test in retrospect and prospect. Arch Environ Health 15:792–808, 1967.
37. Renquist DM, Potkay S: *Mycobacterium scrofulaceum* infection in *Erythrocebus patas* monkeys. Lab Anim Sci 29(1):97–101, 1979.
38. Roberts JA: Primates: quarantine. *In* Fowler ME (ed): Zoo and Wild Animal Medicine: Current Therapy 3. Philadelphia, WB Saunders, pp 326–331, 1993.
39. Shellabarger WC: Zoo personnel health program recommendations. *In* American Association of Zoo Veterinarians Infectious Disease Reviews. Media, PA, American Association of Zoo Veterinarians #7:1–21, 1994.
40. Silberman MS: Occupational health programs in wildlife facilities. *In* Fowler ME (ed): Zoo and Wild Animal Medicine: Current Therapy 3. Philadelphia, WB Saunders, pp 57–61, 1993.
41. Soave O, Jackson S, Ghumman JS: Atypical mycobacteria as the probable cause of positive tuberculin reactions in squirrel monkeys (*Saimiri sciureus*). Lab Anim Sci 31(3):295–296, 1981.
42. Stunkard JA, Szatalowicz FT, Sudduth HC: A review and evaluation of tuberculin testing procedures used for *Macaca* species. Am J Vet Res 32(11):1873–1878, 1971.
43. Thoen CO, Mills K, Hopkins MD: Enzyme-linked protein A: an enzyme-linked immunosorbent assay reagent for detecting antibodies in tuberculous exotic animals. Am J Vet Res 40(5):833–835, 1980.
44. Valerio DA, Dalgard DW, Voelker RW, et al: *Mycobacterium kansasii* infection in rhesus monkeys. *In* Montali RJ (ed): Mycobacterial Infections of Zoo Animals. Washington, DC, Smithsonian Institution Press, pp 145–150, 1978.
45. Wallace RJ, O'Brien R, Glassroth J, et al Diagnosis and treatment of disease caused by nontuberculous mycobacteria. Am Rev Respir Dis 142(4):940–953, 1990.
46. Wells S, Sargent EL, Andrews ME, et al: Tuberculosis and tuberculin testing in orangutans. *In* Wells S, Sargent EL, Andrews ME, Anderson DE (eds): Medical Management of the Orangutan. New Orleans, The Audubon Institute, Audubon Park and Zoological Garden, pp 53–63, 1990.

CHAPTER 53

Diabetes in Primates

CHRISTIAN WALZER

Diabetes mellitus can be differentiated clinically into insulin-dependent diabetes mellitus (IDDM) and non–insulin-dependent diabetes mellitus (NIDDM). Further categorization can be made along human pathologic and functional criteria, wherein type I diabetes mellitus occurs in humans with a genetic predisposition to an autoimmune disease (in most cases this is analogous to IDDM), and type II diabetes mellitus describes an inadequate functioning of insulin at the peripheral receptors, with ensuing modified beta-cell secretion. Although the causes of type II diabetes mellitus are often not clearly defined and understood, it is, in most cases, referred to as NIDDM.[15]

Diabetes mellitus has been described in numerous nonhuman primates. Most of these descriptions are derived from experimental data, in which diabetes was induced by beta-cell destruction either chemically with streptozotocin or surgically. Experimental diabetes mellitus has been described in rhesus macaques (*Macaca mulatta*),[17–19] baboons (*Papio anubis, Papio cyanocephalus,* and *Papio hamadryas*),[11, 36] Japanese macaques (*Macaca fuscata*),[43] and cynomolgus macaques (*Macaca fascicularis*).[12] Experimental infection with coxsackie B4 virus has induced diabetes in Patas monkeys (*Cercopithecus patas*).[44]

Nonexperimental spontaneous diabetes mellitus has also been observed in several nonhuman primates, among others, in rhesus monkeys,[10, 25] Celebes crested macaques (*Macaca nigra*),[3, 13, 14] cynomolgus macaques,[37] pig-tailed macaques (*Macaca nemestrina*),[30] chimpanzees (*Pan troglodytes*),[34] and in an orangutan (P. Klaver, personal communication, 1996).

Reports on diabetes in prosimians are rare.[24, 40] Howard and Yasuda[15] point out that very few cases are described in New World monkeys, great apes, and prosimians.

ETIOPATHOGENESIS

Type II diabetes mellitus, that which arises from a functional lesion, is the most common form of spontaneous diabetes mellitus in humans and nonhuman primates.[15] It has been described as a heterogeneous disorder with the occurrence of hypoinsulinemia and hyperinsulinemia, a variability of clinical symptoms, and impaired glucose tolerance that can cause hyperglycemia.[7, 39] The variable clinical presentation and the

often seemingly contradictory clinical pathologic parameters depend to a great degree on the stage at which the diabetes mellitus is initially evaluated.[39] Disease progression in most cases is gradual from onset to final overt ketoacidotic stage (Fig. 53–1). Diabetes mellitus progresses through various rather distinct stages. It is important to appreciate these various stages when examining a single animal and it is even more so when evaluating primate colonies.

The first disease stage is characterized by hormonal impairment and an increasing peripheral insulin resistance.[3] Age, obesity, species predilection, and a probable genetic component have all been associated with this onset.[2, 7, 20] This increased peripheral insulin resistance induces a compensatory hyperinsulinemia. With time, the pancreas is unable to maintain adequate insulin secretion and progression to the next disease stage, borderline diabetes, follows.[3] Onward progression to an overt diabetic stage with severe hypergylcemia, weight loss, ketosis, and acidosis correlates with the gradual decrease in beta cell secretion and the establishment of

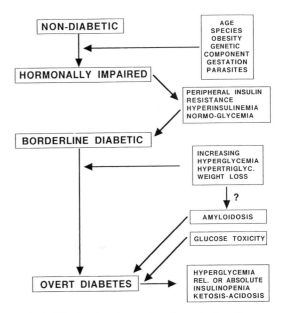

FIGURE 53–1. Etiopathogenetic pathways in Type II diabetes mellitus.

a relative or absolute insulinopenia. Progression from the hyperglycemic borderline diabetic to the overt stage may be enhanced by glucose toxicity and the secondary death of insulin-producing cells. Such models are presently discussed in humans, cats, and dogs.[29, 35]

Jen et al.[16] examined a group of aging, obese rhesus monkeys in which fasting plasma insulin levels correlated with body weight, reaching levels of 415 ± 84 μU/ml in the heaviest monkeys. Based on the sequential phases defined in the study, the monkeys deteriorated beyond this obese-hyperinsulinemic phase and exhibited decreased body mass, decreasing plasma insulin values, and increasing plasma glucose values.[13] Howard[14] identified a group of Celebes crested macaques that were obese and had hyperinsulinemia. In this group, values of 511 ± 42 μU/ml were recorded in the hyperinsulinemic monkeys. The monkeys appeared to have concurrent peripheral insulin resistance and an excessive insulin secretion. The author suggested that obesity is a necessary component in the development of diabetes in these monkeys.

Concurrent with the developing hyperglycemia, impairment of the insulin-dependent lipoprotein lipase often induces a hypertriglyceridemia at this stage.[39] Although the data available on type II diabetes mellitus in prosimians is limited, the disease progression seems to be similar. In the description of overt ketoacidotic type II diabetes in a ring-tailed lemur (*Lemur katta*),[40] hyperglycemia, hypertriglyceridemia, and subnormal to normal insulin values were recorded. The examination of other lemurs revealed an extremely obese ring-tailed lemur (5500 g) with marked hyperinsulinemia of 466 μU/ml. Two other moderately obese animals (3400 and 3500 g) were also hyperinsulinemic with values of 49.5 μU/ml and 93.4 μU/ml, respectively. As described previously, the hyperinsulinemic stage is an early hormonally impaired stage of type II diabetes, which is followed by the hypoinsulinemic late to end stage overt diabetes. The three obese lemurs are believed to fall into this hormonally impaired, borderline diabetic stage and, without intervention, will gradually progress to have overt diabetes mellitus.

The pathologic lesions associated with type I and type II diabetes mellitus at the onset differ considerably. As in humans, the main pancreatic lesion in nonhuman primates in type II diabetes mellitus is severe islet amyloidosis. One hypothesis is that polypeptide-derived amyloidosis precedes the progression from borderline diabetic to overt diabetes. This amyloid directly causes the destruction of the secretory beta cells.[15, 39] Type I diabetes presents with an inflammation of the islets of Langerhans that progresses to autoimmune-mediated destruction of the islets. Type I diabetes can further be characterized by the presence of autoantibodies toward the islet cells.[32]

GESTATIONAL DIABETES

A special form of type II diabetes is the spontaneous insulin-resistant gestational diabetes. This is defined as the development of hyperglycemia during pregnancy in individuals previously not diagnosed with diabetes

mellitus.[1] Apart from the various anecdotal reports from zoos concerning glucose intolerance and neonatal macrosomia, especially in squirrel monkeys (*Saimiri* species), detailed accounts of gestational diabetes have been reported in a cynomolgus monkey[22] and in a white-faced saki (*Pithecia pithecia*).[23] As in humans, the reported clinical problems in nonhuman primates associated with this transient form of type II diabetes are related to obstetric problems caused by macrosomia, often resulting in the death of the mother and infant. In the reported case in the saki, the postpartum recovery was spontaneous.[23] This resolution is consistent with most human cases, although many human cases result in subsequent adult type II diabetes.

PARASITE-INDUCED DIABETES MELLITUS

In some animals, pancreatic lesions are caused by parasites.[26, 42] At one institution, chronic pancreatitis and interstitial pancreatic fibrosis in titi monkeys (*Callicebus moloch*) have been related to infection with the spirurid *Trichospirura leptostoma*. If the diabetes mellitus described in another titi monkey of the same institution is due to chronic pancreatic disease secondary to *T. leptostoma* is still undetermined but deemed possible by the authors.[8] A further case, clinically indicative of exocrine pancreatic insufficiency and diabetes mellitus in a pied tamarin (*Saguinus b. bicolor*) caused by a parasitic chronic fibrosing pancreatitis, has been described. Although the actual parasite in the pancreas could not be identified, the authors suggest it could be *Pterygodermatites nycticebi*, which was isolated from the gastrointestinal tract of the same animal.[33] This parasite has been described in the pancreas in other cases.[27]

CLINICAL DIAGNOSIS

Clinical signs associated with diabetes mellitus in nonhuman primates are similar to those described in humans. These can include hyperglycemia, glucosuria, hyperlipidemia, polyuria, dysuria, polydipsia, polyphagia, weight loss, inappetence, and lethargy.[5, 15, 23, 40] However, the progression to clinically overt diabetes is gradual and can easily be overlooked.[15] This is especially true in larger colonies in naturalistic enclosures with enriched feeding protocols. A significant number of unsuspected cases have been diagnosed by routine blood sampling. Various tests are available to recognize potential diabetes at an early clinically inapparent stage. These tests are extremely valuable when screening larger groups of primates.

Serum Glucose

Serum glucose is the standard test for clinically overt diabetes. Most diabetic primates have persistent serum glucose values of more than 150 mg/dl, with severely diabetic primates having fasting serum glucose values of more than 300 mg/dl.[15] Other causes of hyperglycemia, such as hyperadrenocorticism, iatrogenic corticoids, glucagonoma, acromegaly, pheochromocytoma, chronic hepatic disease, and capture and manipulation stress, must be ruled out.[8, 15]

Urine Glucose

When the blood glucose concentration exceeds the renal threshold, glucosuria occurs. Glucosuria is easily detected by various dipstick methods. Severely diabetic primates can demonstrate a glucosuria in excess of 2000 mg/dl.[23] Proximal renal tubular dysfunction must be considered as a differential in persistent glucosuria.[21]

Ketonuria

Primate urine should be negative for ketones. Ketones are produced by lipolysis as occurs in end-stage diabetes mellitus. Ketonuria and concurrent hyperglycemia are diagnosed as diabetic ketoacidosis.[21] The acidosis can be further confirmed by an increased anion gap in serum electrolyte analysis.[39]

Glucose Tolerance Tests

Various test protocols have been described to measure glucose tolerance. One can differentiate between oral glucose tolerance tests (O-GTT) and intravenous glucose tolerance tests (IV-GTT). In GTT, after a glucose or dextrose administration (O-GTT: 2 to 4 g glucose/kg body weight; IV-GTT: 0.5 to 2.5 g glucose/kg body weight[15]; 750 mg dextrose/kg body weight[39]), the glucose elimination rate over a time frame is examined. Whereas in experimental settings primates have been trained to consume the necessary glucose loads,[15] in the normal clinical setting these procedures are invasive and require at least vigorous physical restraint or anesthesia. In all these tests, the influence of stress in physically restrained animals (catecholamine secretion suppresses insulin secretion[31]) and the potential drug influence in anesthetized animals must be considered.

Glycosylated Hemoglobin (HbA$_{1c}$)

Glycosylation of hemoglobin and plasma lipoproteins occurs when persistent high serum glucose condenses onto the various molecules.[8, 38] The advantage of measuring HbA$_{1c}$ rather than standard serum glucose is that the HbA$_{1c}$ value reflects the glucose levels over the past 4 to 12 weeks. Normal values have not been determined in many different nonhuman primate species, but values inflated by 10% or more can be considered elevated.[4, 8, 38] HbA$_{1c}$ measurement is also useful in determining the efficacy of therapy. The usefulness of various glycosylated lipoprotein concentration determinations in diabetes monitoring is currently being evaluated.[38]

Serum Fructosamine

Similar to HbA$_{1c}$, serum fructosamine has proven useful in the diagnosis and monitoring of diabetes mellitus in humans and nonhuman primates.[4, 38] In one study by Wagner and colleagues, diabetic cynomolgus monkeys had fructosamine values of 225 $\pm$ 30.7 μmol/L, whereas a control group had levels of 97.2 $\pm$ 12.3 μmol/L.[38]

Insulin Determination

Because the structure of insulin is identical in humans and monkeys,[28, 41] insulin determination is easily accomplished using the same radioimmunoassay as for humans. Fasting values ranging from 0 to 20 μU/ml in humans are considered normal, according to the Institute for Nuclear Medicine and Endocrinology in Salzburg. Howard and Yasuda[15] summarized various insulin control values for nonhuman primates in the 17- to 40-μU/ml range.

TREATMENT OF DIABETES MELLITUS

Evaluation of potential therapeutic strategies in treating diabetes mellitus depends on the stage at which the diagnosis is made. Asymptomatic primates may require only nutritional modifications. Overt ketoacidotic diabetes mellitus, on the other hand, requires intensive emergency management to correct the hydration status and the associated metabolic and electrolyte disorders.

Nutritional management should be geared not only to restrict caloric intake but also to limit the intake of simple sugars by providing a high-protein and high-fat diet.[23, 39] Caloric restriction and subsequent weight loss lead to a decrease in the peripheral insulin resistance with lower serum insulin levels and an increasing tolerance for carbohydrates.[39] Dietary management on its own is only sufficient for early stage diabetes or gestational diabetes.

As in human type II diabetes, the administration of oral hypoglycemic agents may be necessary. Some remnant endogenous secretion of insulin is necessary for these drugs to work. Reports on the use of these agents are sparse.[6, 8, 9] Tolbutamide in an initial dose of 250 mg daily and then 100 mg every second day has been used to treat a capuchin monkey (*Cebus apella*).[9] A second generation sulfonylurea, glipizide, has been used in the long-term therapy of a titi monkey at a rate of 1.25 mg/kg once a day. This dosage maintained the glucose levels at a stable 110 mg/dl. No side effects from the glipizide were noted at this rate.[8]

Because most cases of diabetes mellitus are diagnosed late in the disease progression, the most common therapeutic approach in nonhuman primates has been the subcutaneous or intramuscular administration of exogenous insulin. When using insulin, it is advisable to start with a lower dosage of 0.5 IU insulin per kilogram of body weight once a day and reevaluate based on blood glucose levels after a few days of stabilization.[15] When glucose control with a once daily approach is not possible, it is beneficial to split the total daily dose into two separate doses.[15, 38] Additionally, consideration must be given to the type of insulin used. Human insulin is given preference over the older porcine insulin products. Insulin is available in numerous forms and two concentrations (40 and 100 IU/ml). From the short-acting (regular or rapid), intermediate (longer acting), ultra lente (depot) to combination products consisting of short- and longer acting components. Treatment of diabetic cynomolgus monkeys with a combination of short-acting and longer acting insulin (70/30) at a dosage of 2.5 IU/kg divided into two daily doses has been described.[38] After the initial adjustments in the insulin dose have been made based on the serum glucose levels, it could be beneficial to monitor the long-term therapy using serum fructosamine or HbA_{1c}.[4] In the initial phases, close monitoring of the animals is essential because exogenous insulin-induced hypoglycemia is the most common fatal complication of treatment. If clinical signs of hypoglycemia (e.g., ataxia, lethargy, weakness tremor, or coma) are seen, intravenous glucose therapy must be initiated.[15]

REFERENCES

1. American Diabetes Association: Summary and recommendations of the second international Workshop-Conference on Gestational Diabetes Mellitus. Diabetes 34:123–126, 1985.
2. Bennett PH: Epidemiology of diabetes mellitus. *In* Rifkin H, Porte D (eds): Ellenberg and Rifkin's Diabetes Mellitus, Theory and Practice. Amsterdam, Elsevier Science Publishing, pp 357–377, 1990.
3. Berguido F, Kagey M, Howard CF: Insulin-like growth factor-1 levels decrease in the development of diabetes in *Macaca nigra*. Primates 36:423–429, 1995.
4. Cefalu WT, Wagner JD, Bell-Farrow AD: Role of glycated proteins in detecting and monitoring diabetes in cynomolgus monkeys. Lab Anim Sci 43:73–77, 1993.
5. Cesana G, Panza G, Ferraio M, et al: Can glycosylated hemoglobin be a job stress parameter? J Occup Med 27:357–360, 1985.
6. Davidson IWF, Lang CM, Blackwell WL: Impairment of carbohydrate metabolism in a squirrel monkey. Diabetes 16:395–401, 1967.
7. DeFonzo RA, Bonadonna RC, Ferrannini E: Pathogenesis of NIDDM: a balanced overview. Diabetes Care 15:318–368, 1992.
8. Gilardi KV, Valverde CR: Glucose control with glipizide therapy in a diabetic dusky titi monkey (*Callicebus moloch*). J Zoo Wildl Med 26:82–86, 1995.
9. Greenwood AG, Taylor DC: Control of diabetes in a capuchin monkey with tolbutamide. Vet Rec 101:407–408, 1977.
10. Hansen BC, Bodkin KL: Heterogeneity of insulin responses: phases leading to type 2 (non insulin dependent) diabetes mellitus in the rhesus monkey. Diabetologia 29:713–719, 1986.
11. Heffernan S, Phippard A, Sinclair A: A baboon (*Papio hamadryas*) model of insulin-dependent diabetes. J Med Primatol 24:29–34, 1995.
12. Honjo S, Kondo Y, Cho F: Oral glucose tolerance test in the cynomolgus monkey (*Macaca fascicularis*). Lab Anim Sci 26:771–776, 1976.
13. Howard CF Jr: *Macaca nigra* with fasting and secretory hyperinsulinemia. Am J Primatol 14:425, 1988.
14. Howard CF Jr: Obesity is an obligatory component for development of type II diabetes in predisposed monkeys: a testable hypothesis. Nutrition 5:51–52, 1989.
15. Howard CF Jr, Yasuda M: Diabetes mellitus in nonhuman primates: recent research advances and current husbandry practices. J Med Primatol 19:609–625, 1990.
16. Jen K-LC, Hansen BC, Metzger BL: Adiposity, anthropometric measures, and plasma insulin levels of rhesus monkeys. Int J Obes 9:213–224, 1985.
17. Jonasson O, Jones CW, Bauman A, et al: The pathophysiology of experimental insulin-deficient diabetes in the monkey. Ann Surg 201:27–39, 1985.
18. Jones CW, Cunha-Vaz JC, Zeimer RC, et al: Ocular fluorophotometry in the normal and diabetic monkey. Exp Eye Res 42:467–477, 1986.
19. Jones CW, West MS, Hong DT, et al: Peripheral glomerular base-

20. Kahn SE, Porte D: The pathophysiology of type II (noninsulin-dependent) diabetes mellitus: implication for treatment. *In* Rifkin H, Porte D (eds): Ellenberg and Rifkin's Diabetes Mellitus, Theory and Practice. Amsterdam, Elsevier Science Publishing, pp 436–456, 1990.
21. Lees GE, Willard MD, Green RA: Urinary disorders. *In* Willard MD, Tvendten H, Turnwald GH (eds): Small Animal Clinical Diagnosis by Laboratory Methods, 2nd ed. Philadelphia, WB Saunders, pp 126–127, 1994.
22. Litwak K, Wagner J, Carlson C, et al: Noninsulin dependent diabetes mellitus complicated by pregnancy in a cynomolgus monkey. Vet Pathol 32:581, 1995.
23. Lloyd ML, Susa JB, Pelto JA, et al: Gestational diabetes mellitus in a white faced saki (*Pithecia pithecia*). J Zoo Wildl Med 26:76–81, 1995.
24. Meier J: Diabetes mellitus in a ring-tailed lemur. San Diego Zoonooz 1:17, 1981.
25. Metzger BL, Hansen BC, Speegle LM, et al: Characterization of glucose intolerance in obese monkeys. J Obesity Weight Regul 4:153–167, 1981.
26. Montali RJ, Bush M, Hess J, et al: Ex-situ diseases and their control for reintroduction of the endangered lion tamarin species (*Leontopithecus* species). Verh ber Erkrg Zootiere 37:93–98, 1995.
27. Montali RJ, Gardiner CH, Evans RE, et al: *Pterygodermatites nycticebi* (Nematoda:Spirurida) in golden lion tamarin. Lab Anim Sci 33:194–197, 1983.
28. Naithani VK, Steffens GJ, Tager HS, et al: Isolation and amino-acid sequence determination of monkey insulin and proinsulin. Hoppe-Seyler's. Physiological Chemistry 365:571–575, 1984.
29. Nelson RW, Feldman EC: Noninsulin-dependent diabetes mellitus in the cat. Feline Pract 21:15–17, 1993.
30. Ohagi S, Nishi M, Bell I, et al: Sequences of islet amyloid polypeptide precursors of an Old World monkey, the pig tailed macaque (*Macaca nemestrina*) and the dog (*Canis familaris*). Diabetologia 34:555–558, 1991.
31. Porte D Jr, Robertson RP: Control of insulin secretion by catecholamines, stress, and the sympathetic nervous system. Fed Proc 32:1792–1796, 1973.
32. Riley WJ, Maclaren NK: Islet cell autoantibodies. *In* Samols E (ed): The Endocrine Pancreas. New York, Raven Press, pp 409–419, 1991.
33. Robert N, Carroll JB: Comparative pathological-clinical aspects of captive Callitrichids at the Jersey Wildlife Preservation Trust. *In* Pryce C, Scott L, Schnell C (eds): Marmosets and tamarins in biological and biomedical research. Salisbury, UK, DSSD Imagery, pp 102–109, 1997.
34. Rosenblum IV, Barbolt TA, Howard CF Jr: Diabetes mellitus in the chimpanzee (*Pan troglodytes*). J Med Primatol 10:93–101, 1981.
35. Sai P, Martignat L: Etio-pathogenesis of diabetes-mellitus in man and dog. Point Veterinaire 26:9–23, 1994.
36. Stout LC, Folse DS, Meier J, et al: Quantitative glomerular morphology of the normal and diabetic baboon kidney. Diabetologia 29:734–740, 1986.
37. Tanaka Y, Ohto H, Kohno M, et al: Spontaneous diabetes mellitus in cynomolgus monkeys (*Macaca fascicularis*). Exp Anim 35:11–19, 1986.
38. Wagner JD, Bagdade JD, Litwak KN, et al: Increased glycation of plasma lipoproteins in diabetic cynomolgus monkeys. Lab Anim Sci 46:31–35, 1996.
39. Wagner JD, Carlson CS, O'Brien TD, et al: Diabetes mellitus and islet amyloidosis in cynomolgus monkeys. Lab Anim Sci 46:36–41, 1996.
40. Walzer C, Kübber-Heiss A: Obesity in the development of diabetes mellitus in ring-tailed lemurs (*Lemur katta*); an obligatory component? Verh ber Erkrg Zootiere 37:143–148, 1995.
41. Wetekam W, Groneberg J, Leineweber M, et al: The nucleotide sequence of cDNA for preproinsulin from the primate *Macaca fascicularis*. Gene 19:179–183, 1982.
42. Wolff PL: Parasites of New World primates. *In* Fowler ME (ed). Zoo and Wild Animal Medicine: Current Therapy 3. Philadelphia, WB Saunders, pp 378–389, 1993.
43. Yasuda H, Harano Y, Kosugi K, et al: Development of early lesions of microangiopathy in chronically diabetic monkeys. Diabetes 33:415–420, 1984.
44. Yoon J-W, London WT, Curfman BL, et al: Coxsackie virus B4 produces transient diabetes in nonhuman primates. Diabetes 35:712–714, 1986.

CARNIVORES

CHAPTER 54

Emerging Viral Infections in Large Cats

SUZANNE KENNEDY-STOSKOPF

"Emerging diseases" has become an epidemiologic catch phrase. Implicit in the word "emerging" is a sense of newness. An emerging disease may be a newly recognized disease, a known disease that is affecting new hosts or expanding into new geographic ranges, or an "old" disease that is considered to be controlled but is re-emerging as a significant health problem. Many emerging diseases are caused by infectious agents. Multiple factors contribute to the emergence of an infectious disease. Travel-shrunk international borders, encroachment of susceptible hosts into endemic populations, increased drug resistance, and predisposing infections that cause immunodeficiency favor the infectious agent. Biotechnologic techniques that identify new infectious agents and better diagnostic assays for enhanced surveillance have contributed to a heightened awareness of the prevalence of infectious diseases.

For the clinician, the "newness" of an emerging infectious disease often causes confusion and frustration. Interpretation and significance of diagnostic tests can be perplexing. Assessing the risk of the infected individual to the population can be daunting. Lack of effective vaccines and therapeutics is depressing. For the veterinarian working with nondomestic species there is the added complexity of extrapolating what is known about a disease in the closest domestic counterpart and hoping it applies to a related species.

This chapter examines three "emerging" viral infections of large cats. Feline immunodeficiency virus (FIV), a retrovirus first isolated in the domestic cat in 1986 and subsequently found endemic in certain populations of free-ranging large cats, qualifies as a newly recognized infection of felids. Feline leukemia virus (FeLV), another retrovirus recognized in the domestic cat since the 1960s, apparently can infect nondomestic felids exposed to viremic cats encroaching their habitats. The epizootics of canine distemper virus (CDV) infections in large cats in both a captive and a free-range setting raises the issue of whether a canine pathogen is emerging as a feline pathogen. The chapter focuses on understanding the risks for infection, implications of infection, interpretation of diagnostic tests, and population management to prevent infection.

FELINE RETROVIRUSES

FeLV and FIV are retroviruses that cause persistent infections in the domestic cat. To assess the risk of feline retroviruses to large cats requires a fundamental understanding of the biology of these viruses. Familiarity with the retroviral proteins provides a basis for comprehending diagnostic tests and determining an appropriate plan of action for managing animals with positive results.

Retroviruses are RNA viruses with three major genes—*env*, *gag*, and *pol*—which code for the envelope proteins, the core proteins, and reverse transcriptase, respectively. The envelope proteins contain the antigenic determinants recognized by neutralizing antibodies. The *env* gene, however, is subject to a high degree of genetic mutation and recombination events during replication so that multiple genotypes exist in an infected host. Consequently, neutralizing antibodies may not recognize all the variants in circulation, thereby allowing the virus to persist. Core proteins are also immunogenic and elicit antibody production. Detection of the core proteins themselves in circulation and cell culture is evidence of virus replication. Reverse transcriptase can also be used as evidence of viral replication in cell culture. This polymerase transcribes RNA into DNA, which can either serve as a template for more infectious virus or remain latent within a target cell. This proviral DNA can be detected by a polymerase chain reaction (PCR) assay or via cocultivation with permissive target cells in culture. The proviral DNA is responsible for the so-called "Trojan horse" character of retroviruses, that is, the ability to hide free of detection from immune surveillance until conditions favor another assault.

Detection of both antibodies and viral antigens has been used to screen felids for exposure to retroviruses. Considering the replication strategies of retroviruses, the presence of virus-specific antibodies not only means exposure but also gives evidence of persistent infection. This is certainly true of FIV and probably should be considered true for FeLV. To further add to the clinician's dilemma, FIV- and FeLV-infected cats may remain asymptomatic for years and even have a normal life span. The concern, then, is for the magnitude of risk that these healthy, persistently infected animals pose to other cats.

Feline Leukemia Virus

FeLV belongs to the Retroviridae subfamily Oncovirinae, so named because of the association of these viruses with tumors. Not only does FeLV cause cytoproliferative diseases such as lymphoma and leukemia but it also causes cytosuppressive diseases. Currently, FeLV does not appear to be endemic in nondomestic felids in zoological and free-range settings. The lack of antigen-positive animals and absence of clustered clinical cases with FeLV-related diseases are evidence that the virus is not maintained in these populations. However, scattered reports exist to indicate that nondomestic felids are susceptible to FeLV infection.[13, 21, 30, 31] Free-ranging, zoo, and privately owned felids have been infected. In some animals, transient viremias developed and the animals remained free of disease; in others, clinical signs related to FeLV infection developed. In all cases, domestic and feral cats were suspected to be the FeLV source.

EPIZOOTIOLOGY

Virus is present in the saliva and nasal secretions of cats actively infected with FeLV. Close intimate contact, as occurs with grooming, and contamination of feeding and watering utensils are the most common routes of transmission in the domestic cat. Virus can also be found in urine and feces but this is a less important source of exposure because infectious virus does not survive long in such an environment. The virus is labile outside of the cat, so direct contact is necessary for efficient transmission to occur. Venereal transmission is possible in that virus or virus-infected cells have been detected in semen and vaginal fluids. Vertical transmission can occur, resulting in high neonatal mortality rates. More commonly, infected queens suffer from infertility because of fetal resorption during the first month of pregnancy. Blood is also infectious but probably does not play a significant role in natural transmission. Fleas are not implicated in transmission.[20, 42]

Several case reports suggest that nondomestic felids acquired FeLV infection from their domestic counterparts. A privately owned cougar (*Felis concolor*) that tested antigen positive and died of FeLV-associated diseases lived in a household with both domestic cats and other large felids.[31] One domestic cat and two Siberian tigers (*Panthera tigris*) were FeLV antibody positive and antigen negative, indicating virus exposure with no current virus shedding. FeLV was isolated from a testicular cell culture of a leopard cat (*Felis bengalensis*) that lived with domestic cats.[39] FeLV has also been isolated from a free-ranging European wildcat (*Felis silvestris*) in Scotland[30] and a free-ranging cougar in California.[21] The ability of the European wildcat and domestic cat to hybridize ensures that close intimate contact can occur to allow FeLV transmission. Consumption of FeLV infected domestic cats by larger, nondomestic felids would also be an effective way to transmit the virus. Urbanization encroaching the cougar's habitat and evidence of cats in cougar stomach contents make this a plausible scenario.[21]

The risk then of free-ranging, nondomestic felids becoming infected with FeLV from free-roaming, domestic cats depends on the prevalence of FeLV within the latter population and the likelihood that individuals within the two populations will encounter one another during a period of active viremia. Although sample sizes are small, the prevalence of FeLV in the European wildcat based on virus isolation was found to be similar to that of the domestic cat in Great Britain, around 5%.[30] Seroprevalence of FeLV antigen in free-ranging Florida panthers (n = 38)[40] and California mountain lions (n = 58)[36] is zero. Seroprevalence of FeLV antigen in asymptomatic, high-risk (outdoor, multicat households) cats in the United States is 6.8% (n = 15,374).[32] A serosurvey of lions (*Panthera leo*; n = 31), leopards (*Panthera pardus*; n = 18), and cheetahs (*Acinonyx jubatus*; n = 4) in Botswana detected no FeLV antigenemic animals.[34]

Documented cases of FeLV infection in felids maintained in zoos are rare. A transient FeLV antigenemia and a positive antibody response developed in a clouded leopard (*Panthera nebulosa*).[13] The feral cat population at this zoo was high and cited as a possible source of virus exposure. A 1993 survey of North American zoos to evaluate prevalence of feline retroviruses determined that FeLV infection was not a problem. Of the 87 institutions that responded, seven reported positive FeLV antigen tests in a total of 11 animals. Seven of these animals were negative when retested. Three were not retested and a male margay (*Felis wiedii*) that was older than 15 years died with no evidence of FeLV-related diseases. Of the seven transiently FeLV antigen-positive animals, only two pampas cats (*Felis colocolo*) were housed together. The significance of false-positive tests is discussed under Interpretation of Diagnostic Assays.

INTERPRETATION OF DIAGNOSTIC ASSAYS

Detection of FeLV antigen in peripheral circulation is the assay of choice for clinically managing infected felids. The presence of FeLV group-specific antigens, corresponding primarily to the major core *gag* gene-encoded protein p27, correlates with an active virus infection and thus potential virus transmission. The most commonly used diagnostic assay is the enzyme-linked immunosorbent assay (ELISA) for the detection of soluble p27 protein in serum, plasma, or whole blood. In an FeLV ELISA, mouse anti-p27 monoclonal antibodies non-covalently bound to a solid matrix trap FeLV antigen present in a test sample. A second enzyme-conjugated murine monoclonal antibody specific for a different epitope of p27 is then added so that a "sandwich" is formed. The addition of a chromogen substrate oxidizes the enzyme conjugate to form a visible color if p27 is present. The immunofluorescent antibody (IFA) assay uses acetone- or methanol-fixed blood smears and detects *gag* proteins within the cytoplasm of leukocytes and platelets.

Discordant ELISA and IFA results are the subject of much confusion.[4, 42] Numerous commercial ELISA kits exist for the detection of FeLV p27, and all claim high sensitivity and specificity. False-positive results can occur with improper washing between steps when using antibody-coated plastic microwells. This was a potential source of error when in-house ELISAs were first introduced. Concentration immunoassays that use a bioreactive filter to detect p27 antigen have helped to minimize this problem with in-house assays. Most zoos, however, use commercial laboratories to perform diagnostic assays for feline retroviruses. Of 60 zoos that screened for feline retroviruses, only nine tested in-house. False-positive ELISA reactions may also occur if the test animal has naturally occurring antibodies against mouse immunoglobulins. This was believed to be the cause of positive ELISA reactions in a Florida panther that had been vaccinated with a mouse brain–origin, killed rabies virus vaccine 2 weeks prior to testing.[28] Probably the most significant reason for false-positive reactions in nondomestic felids is low prevalence of FeLV in the population. When disease prevalence is low, even diagnostic tests with high sensitivity and specificity are poor predictors of infected animals. Consequently, nondomestic felids that test positive for FeLV antigen by ELISA should be retested. If the results remain positive, an IFA should be performed.

A positive IFA test indicates that the bone marrow is infected and active virus replication is occurring.[42]

False-negative IFA results can occur early in infection before bone marrow involvement and when antigen concentration is low or few infected cells are present. Rarely, virus is sequestered in sites other than bone marrow so leukocytes and platelets remain antigen negative. If discordant results (ELISA positive, IFA negative) are obtained, both tests should be repeated. Recommendations for repeat testing vary between 4 and 12 weeks. Enough time needs to elapse between tests to allow for virus to replicate in the bone marrow if the animal happened to be sampled early in the course of infection.

Furthermore, tests should be done to detect FeLV antibodies. There are several FeLV antibody assays. Serum neutralization measures the ability of antibody to inhibit virus replication in cell culture. This assay is highly specific and extremely sensitive but is cumbersome to perform. An ELISA that detects antibodies to the FeLV envelope glycoprotein gp70 is more commonly performed by diagnostic laboratories. An assay for feline oncornavirus-associated cell membrane antigen (FOCMA) is an indirect membrane immunofluorescence assay in which the test serum serves as the source of primary antibody, a fluorescein-labeled anticat antibody serves as secondary antibody, and an FeLV-infected, feline lymphoblastoid cell line (FL74), derived from a renal lymphoma, serves as the target cell. Although the nature of FOCMA remains controversial, antibodies against FOCMA (>1:8) appear to protect against tumor formation.[42]

Detection of antibodies to FeLV is additional evidence of virus exposure, which is helpful for interpreting conflicting or inconsistent FeLV antigen tests. Although an FeLV antigen-negative, antibody-positive cat is not infectious at that particular point in time, the possibility of latency and future recrudescence cannot be eliminated.

EXPRESSION OF CLINICAL DISEASE

Clinical disease does not develop in every cat that is infected with FeLV. The dogma of outcome of exposure to FeLV has been that approximately 30% of affected animals remain viremic and clinical disease develops, whereas neutralizing antibodies develop in 60% and these animals are not at risk for disease.[20] In approximately 30% of these 60%, a transient viremia develops. At issue is whether cats that are FeLV antigen-negative, antibody-positive have truly eliminated the virus or are latently infected and therefore potential virus shedders if the virus is reactivated. Virus can often be isolated from bone marrow and lymphoid tissues of these cats, and virus recrudescence can occur following experimental administration of adrenocorticosteroids and complement depletion.[20]

Multiple viral and host factors contribute to disease pathogenesis. Feline leukemia virus exists as many different genetic variants (genotypes) in nature. A cat is exposed to multiple genotypes within a virus inoculum, and, once infected, there is a high incidence of genetic mutation and recombination during virus replication. Three subgroups of FeLV exist and determine efficiency of virus transmission, establishment of viremia, and induction of particular diseases (proliferative versus immunosuppressive).[20] Subgroup A viruses are dominant in nature. They are replication competent and readily transmissible. Subgroups B and C arose from FeLV-A and appear to be more highly pathogenic, although less transmissible and less likely to establish a persistent viremia. In cats, FeLV-B and FeLV-C are only found in combination with subgroup A viruses. Cloned isolates of FeLV, representing a different virus subgroup, have induced either immunodeficiency syndrome, erythrocyte aplasia, myeloid leukemia, or thymic lymphoma. Little has been done to evaluate FeLV subgroups in nondomestic felids. Subgroup A viruses were isolated from the blood of a healthy, 12-month-old, free-ranging, male European wildcat[30] and from testicular fibroblast culture of a leopard cat.[39]

The host also plays a pivotal role in determining disease pathogenesis. Persistent viremia and subsequent disease are more likely to develop in young cats and immunocompromised cats. A captive cougar with FeLV-related disease was 14 months old,[31] and a symptomatic, FeLV-positive, free-ranging cougar was estimated to be 3 years of age based on dentition.[21] Although genetic makeup of the individual cat probably contributes to innate resistance to FeLV, gross differences in susceptibility of various breeds of domestic cats have not been identified.[20]

Multiple FeLV-related diseases exist.[20] The most common neoplastic disease caused by FeLV in the domestic cat is lymphoma. Three anatomic patterns of lymphoma are recognized: thymic (mediastinal), multicentric, and alimentary. Nonlymphoid leukemias and myeloproliferative disorders within the bone marrow also occur. Infection with FeLV can also lead to clinical immunodeficiency characterized by leukopenia, lymphopenia, variable degrees of anemia, progressive weight loss, and signs of opportunistic and secondary infections. Other FeLV-related diseases include enteropathy manifested by chronic diarrhea, infertility resulting from fetal resorption, and neurologic dysfunction, which can take many forms including lower motor neuron paralysis, behavioral and locomotor disorders, sensory and motor polyneuropathy (hyperesthesia, weakness, and proprioceptive defects), retinal degeneration, and anisocoria. Few case reports exist for FeLV-related diseases in nondomestic felids. In two published accounts in cougars, cytoproliferative (diffuse lymphoid hyperplasia)[21] and cytosuppressive (nonresponsive anemia, leukopenia, and thrombocytopenia)[31] disease patterns were reported.

PREVENTION

The domestic cat is the reservoir for FeLV. Large cats, particularly in zoological settings, do not appear to be at high risk for becoming infected with FeLV because intimate contact with their domestic counterparts is rare. Nondomestic felids maintained in private households and ranging in areas overlapped by domestic cats potentially are at higher risk for infection. Strategies then for preventing FeLV infection in captive animals is somewhat dependent on their environment.

First, monitoring is essential to determine the prevalence within a population. Because the prevalence of FeLV infection and disease appears to be low in nondomestic felids and the risk of false-positive ELISAs for FeLV antigen is potentially high, augmenting FeLV antigen testing with FeLV antibody testing seems prudent to document actual exposure to the virus. For a zoo population, this could be a single screening to ensure that no animal that was not antigenemic had previously been exposed to FeLV. New animals should be screened while in quarantine. The need for annual or periodic retesting for zoo felids is dependent on the perceived risk of FeLV infection and on development of clinical signs compatible with infection. Because antigenemia can be transient, antibody testing of free-ranging cats is a more sensitive indicator of actual exposure than antigen testing alone. The basis for antigen detection as the preferred diagnostic assay in the domestic cat is that FeLV-associated diseases usually develop in animals with persistent circulating antigen and that these animals are infectious for other cats. The issue of antigen-negative, antibody-positive cats being latently infected and subject to periodic reactivation with virus shedding is problematic. Insufficient data exist to establish whether this will be an issue for nondomestic felids.

Second, exposure of nondomestic felids to domestic cats should be minimized. Feral cat problems vary between institutions. Although control measures usually exist, concern remains that an FeLV antigen-positive cat might infect a captive, nondomestic felid. This raises the issue of FeLV vaccination. Multiple FeLV vaccines exist. Any one of them should be safe to administer to a nondomestic felid because they are either subunit or killed-virus preparations. Whether any one of the vaccines would actually protect the nondomestic felid is another issue and has been a source of lively controversy even with regard to domestic cats.[26] The first commercially available FeLV vaccine was shown to be immunogenic for cheetahs,[9] tigers, and servals (*Felis serval*)[14] but has since been shown to be ineffective in protecting domestic cats.[26] Even though seemingly efficacious vaccines exist, vaccinating zoo felids with minimal risk of exposure is probably not warranted. Furthermore, vaccinating would eliminate the use of antibody screening for FeLV exposure. Clinicians who see nondomestic felids in private households may wish to evaluate risk of infection versus benefit of vaccination on a case-by-case basis.

Feline Immunodeficiency Virus

Feline immunodeficiency virus belongs to the Retroviridae subfamily Lentivirinae. Lentiviruses cause so-called slow diseases because the time between infection and development of clinical signs can be months to years. Because these viruses persist, an unambiguous demonstration of virus-specific antibodies equates with infection. Diseases caused by lentiviruses include acquired immunodeficiency syndrome (AIDS), equine infectious anemia, visna-maedi, and caprine arthritis-encephalitis. The first FIV isolate was from the domestic cat in 1986.[37] Serologic surveys subsequently showed that certain populations of free-ranging and captive nondomestic felids had FIV antibodies.[5, 10, 33] Isolation and characterization of FIV from a lion,[11] mountain lion,[33] and Pallas cat (*Felis manul*)[6] demonstrated that the lentiviruses from these nondomestic species were sufficiently divergent from one another and domestic cat isolates to indicate that these viruses had been in their respective host populations for some time. Because the seroprevalence of FIV is so high in certain free-ranging populations of lions and mountain lions without overt clinical signs compatible with AIDS, the issue was raised whether the lentiviruses in these species were frankly pathogenic or were host-adapted and caused inapparent infections similar to simian immunodeficiency virus in *Cercopithecus* monkeys. There is no definitive answer but evidence is beginning to accumulate that suggests these lentiviruses may not be entirely benign.

EPIZOOTIOLOGY

In the domestic cat, transmission occurs primarily through bite wounds.[37] Saliva contains infectious virus as does blood. Grooming and contamination of feed and water bowls do not appear to be efficient modes of transmission in that seronegative cats are slow to seroconvert. Virus has also been isolated from semen[23] and milk[43] and has been transmitted by artificial insemination[22] and nursing,[43] respectively. At least one isolate can be transmitted in utero. The importance that these alternative sources of FIV play in natural transmission is not known. Similar FIV *pol* sequences were obtained from a female puma and her kitten in British Columbia and Wyoming, suggesting that vertical transmission can occur.[12] Like FeLV, FIV does not remain infectious for long outside its host and is readily inactivated with common disinfectants.

Seroprevalence varies greatly between species of nondomestic felids and between populations of a given species. Seroprevalence is highest for both free-ranging and captive lions. Infection appears to be endemic in certain East African (Serengeti National Park, Ngorongoro Crater, and Lake Manyara, Tanzania) and South African (Kruger National Park) populations with the number of antibody-positive animals ranging between 70% and 91%.[10, 33] Lions in Namibia (Etosha National Park) and in India (Gir forest) are seronegative. Physical barriers such as the Kalahari Desert between the neighboring countries of Namibia and South Africa and the geographic separation of continents probably restricts the virus to certain populations. However, one study reported that 8 of 31 lions tested in Botswana were FIV seropositive.[34] Because Botswana lies between South Africa and Namibia and contains the greatest proportion of the Kalahari ecosystem, concern exists about the possible spread of FIV westward into Namibia. In captive settings, 57% of African lions (30 of 53) in European zoos (n = 9)[29] have antibodies to FIV, whereas only 12% (5 of 43) in U.S. zoos[10] are seropositive. The seroprevalence in captive Asian lions was 73% (16 of 22),[27] but these lions were later determined to be African/Asian hybrids. The absence of FIV-seropositive, free-ranging and captive Asian lions in India strongly

suggests that the African lion was the source of virus introduction into this population.

Twelve different free-ranging populations of cougars (n = 205) in North America had seroprevalence rates ranging from 9% to 69%.[10] Only 4.5% of the captive population (5 of 111) had antibodies to FIV. The seroprevalence appears to be low in both free-ranging and captive cheetahs and leopards except in areas such as the Serengeti and Kruger where virus is endemic in the lion population.[10] The suggestion has been made that the solitary nature of cheetahs and leopards reduces the risk of transmission in natural settings compared to lions living in prides. Whether the virus in cheetahs and leopards is the same lentivirus that occurs in lions is under investigation. An FIV *pol* sequence from a South African leopard is sufficiently divergent from the lion sequences to suggest that leopards retain species-specific strains.[12] Additional species maintained in captive settings from which FIV antibodies have been detected include tigers, snow leopards (*Panthera uncia*), jaguars (*Panthera onca*), leopard cats, and flat-headed cats (*Felis planiceps*).[5, 10]

A frequent concern about FIV in captive, nondomestic felids regards the magnitude of risk of intraspecies and interspecies transmission. Transmission between species appears efficient, particularly in lions, for which more information is available. Within given populations, all animals are frequently seropositive and, when seropositive lions have been introduced into a population of known seronegative animals, seroconversion does occur, although it may take several years. Seroconversion also occurred in a female Pallas cat introduced to a seropositive male. The risk of a domestic cat transmitting FIV to a nondomestic felid is not known, and, prudently, no transmission studies have been conducted. An FIV *pol* sequence from a puma in a Peruvian zoo was more closely aligned with domestic cat sequences, suggesting that interspecies transmission may be possible under appropriate circumstances.[12] Domestic cats have been experimentally infected with isolates from nondomestic felids but no clinical disease has been reported.[33, 44]

INTERPRETATION OF DIAGNOSTIC ASSAYS

The presence of FIV antibodies correlates with persistent infection and the ability to transmit virus.[7, 37] For initial screening, commercial ELISA kits are available. Both microtiter plate and bioreactive filter tests exist. The source of antigen in these kits is either gradient-purified virus from cell culture or recombinant viral core proteins of FIV isolates from the domestic cat. Enough sequence homology usually exists between the major core proteins of domestic and nondomestic lentiviruses for cross-reactivity to occur. An exception has been found with ViraCHEK/FIV (Synbiotics) in which false-negative results occur, presumably because the antigen source is a highly specific viral peptide of domestic cat isolates. For this reason, it is important to know the exact assay being used by the diagnostic laboratory to which nondomestic felid samples are sent. Some commercial laboratories perform an IFA assay for FIV. This assay is somewhat more labor intensive because a source of FIV-infected cells is required. Test serum is added to infected cells present on a slide. Following an appropriate incubation, the slides are washed and then incubated with a fluorescein-conjugated anticat immunoglobulin G and evaluated for the presence of fluorescence.

A positive or equivocal ELISA or IFA result should be confirmed by an immunoblot (Western blot) assay. Not all commercial laboratories perform this assay because it is more cumbersome to conduct. Viral proteins separated by electrophoresis on a polyacrylamide gel are transferred to a nitrocellulose membrane, which is then incubated with a serum or plasma sample. Following appropriate incubation, the membrane is washed and incubated with an enzyme-linked anticat immunoglobulin G for several hours and the blot is developed with the addition of chromogen. Interpretation of positive results varies between laboratories. Some require the detection of antibodies against several *gag* core proteins as well as the envelope glycoprotein. This is not practical for nondomestic felid samples because the *env* proteins are the most variable, and a nondomestic felid would not be likely to have antibodies cross-reactive to these determinants. Concern has also been raised that domestic cat isolates may not be the best source of viral proteins for Western blots in nondomestic felids, particularly in cheetahs.[25] One study showed that puma lentiviral antigens appeared more sensitive than those from a domestic cat isolate for use in detecting seropositive lions, leopards, and cheetahs by Western blot.[34] For the sake of consistency in conducting and interpreting immunoblots, the felid taxonomic advisory group (TAG) of the American Zoological Association recommends that all samples for Western blot testing be sent to the Cornell Diagnostic Laboratory, Upper Tower Road, Ithaca, New York 14853. The recognition of two or more viral proteins is reported as a positive test. Detection of only one viral protein is reported as equivocal with a high probability that the sample is positive. FIV isolated from the Pallas cat is the source of viral antigen.

Primary virus isolation is difficult because usually peripheral blood leukocytes (PBL) from a seronegative animal of the same species must be added every 1 to 2 weeks to PBL cultures of the seropositive animal. Cultures need to be maintained for a minimum of 6 to 8 weeks and checked for the presence of reverse transcriptase activity or viral antigens in the culture supernatant. Only the Pallas cat virus replicated readily in domestic cat PBL and Crandell feline kidney cells.[6] The lion lentivirus originally isolated by cocultivation with PBL from seronegative lions[11] has been adapted to a feline lymphoid cell line[44] as has an isolate from a puma.[34] PCRs for proviral DNA can be performed by certain research laboratories but, again, results may vary depending on the primer sequences used.

EXPRESSION OF CLINICAL DISEASE

Considerable heterogeneity exists among FIV isolates from domestic cats, and the pathogenicity of these isolates is variable. A positive test for FIV antibodies

cannot predict when or if a cat will develop FIV-associated disease. Many experimentally infected domestic cats have remained asymptomatic for years despite changes in their immune system.[7] The suggestion has been made that these cats are sheltered from other infectious agents, but healthy FIV antibody-positive cats are also present in populations at large. As with FeLV, as more is learned about different FIV isolates and host responses, a better understanding of viral pathogenesis will emerge.

Clinical signs of FIV infection in the domestic cat are varied and often nonspecific.[37] Early in the course of infection, generalized lymphadenopathy, fever, depression, and neutropenia may occur. Following recovery of the initial stage of infection, cats enter the asymptomatic phase. During this time, major immunologic changes can be detected including depression of the $CD4^+$ and $CD8^+$ T-lymphocyte ratio, depressed mitogen and antigen-specific lymphoproliferative responses, and hypergammaglobulinemia. The duration of the asymptomatic phase is highly variable but, for most animals, is probably years. Following the asymptomatic period, approximately one third of the FIV-infected cats are seen with vague clinical signs including recurrent fever of undetermined origin, leukopenia, lymphadenopathy, anemia, unthriftiness, anorexia, intermittent weight loss, and nonspecific behavioral changes that could have any number of causes. Approximately another half of all FIV-infected cats are seen with chronic secondary infections, usually bacterial in origin. These cats often have chronic progressive infections of the mouth involving the gingiva, periodontal tissues, cheeks, oral fauces, or tongue. Chronic upper respiratory infections and chronic skin disorders are also seen. The health of these cats often declines over several months to years and a clinical picture consistent with human AIDS, characterized by wasting and opportunistic infections, can eventually develop. Numerous other disorders have been associated with FIV infection including ocular lesions, renal complications, higher incidence of cancer, and neurologic abnormalities. Both lymphoid and myeloid tumors have been reported. The neurologic abnormalities are primarily behavioral and include dementia, twitching movements of face and tongue, and psychotic behavior such as excessive aggression, sleep disorders, and compulsive roaming.

The clinical manifestations of FIV in domestic cats are vague, and the situation in nondomestic felids is not any more straightforward. Data are slowly accumulating in nondomestic felids that FIV-associated clinical signs can develop in antibody-positive animals. In zoo lions, lymphoma,[38] granulocytic leukemia,[27] and an inoperable tumor of unspecified origin[29] have been reported. In a survey of zoos that screened for the prevalence of FeLV and FIV, 6 of 18 FIV-positive lions (confirmed by Western blot assay) exhibited periodic behavior changes. Since that survey, an FIV-seropositive circus lion had to be retired from performing because of unpredictable behavior, and a seropositive zoo lion was euthanized because of progressive neurologic deterioration. The Pallas cat from which virus was originally isolated was euthanized because of severe wasting. Peripheral retinopathies associated with FIV infection have been observed in both captive and free-ranging seropositive lions. Approximately one fourth of the captive, FIV-seropositive lions surveyed had depressed CD4:CD8 ratios, and hypergammaglobulinemia has been seen.[24] The Pallas cat that was euthanized had very few CD4[+] lymphocytes in circulation, and the female that seroconverted following introduction had a depressed CD4:CD8 ratio. The data sets are limited and the prevalence of similar clinical signs and immunologic changes in FIV-seronegative populations is not fully known. However, until such knowledge is gained, preventing the spread of infection in captive populations is recommended. The impact on free-ranging populations in which FIV is endemic remains to be elucidated.

PREVENTION

The prevalence of FIV antibodies is low (<2%) in captive nondomestic felids other than lions, and, in U.S. zoos, that rate is only around 12% to 14%.[10, 24] Because a vaccine for FIV does not appear imminent, limiting the spread of infection by managing seropositive and seronegative animals as two separate populations is highly recommended. Theoretically, the virus could be eliminated from captive animals as seropositive animals leave the population. This recommendation is not without problems. Segregating an asymptomatic, seropositive animal is a frustrating proposition. Many of these animals live a normal life span without overt problems related to their infection. The only thing that appears certain is that this animal can transmit virus to a seronegative animal. Whether this animal in turn will remain free of FIV-associated illnesses cannot be predicted.

The delay between time of exposure and detection of virus-specific antibodies is also problematic. In the domestic cat, seroconversion occurs approximately 6 to 8 weeks after infection. In some nondomestic felids, seroconversion may take up to several years following virus exposure. An analogous situation occurs with visna-maedi in which sheep may be seronegative for several years yet are virus positive and fully infectious. This delay in the onset of detectable antibodies is a major impediment for eradication of the infection from a flock and means that repeated testing is required. Similar rigorous testing, particularly with seronegative, nondomestic felids with known exposure, is necessary if segregation is to succeed in the elimination of lentiviruses within captive populations. For populations at risk, annual testing by Western blot assay is recommended.

CANINE DISTEMPER VIRUS

CDV is a morbillivirus with a wide host range. The pathogenicity of CDV infection varies among species and may result in inapparent infection or cause high mortality rates. Carnivores, particularly in the families Canidae, Mustelidae, Procyonidae, and Ailuronidae, can experience high mortality rates. The epizootics of CDV in captive large felids in the United States and lions in the Serengeti-Mara ecosystem of East Africa have raised concern that canine distemper is an emerging disease of big cats. In 1992, clinical signs consistent with CDV infection developed in 35 of 74 nondomestic felids at the Wildlife Waystation in southern California.[3] Seventeen of the animals died. The 1994 epizootic of CDV in lions in the Serengeti was estimated to have reduced the population of approximately 3000 animals by 30%.[41] Previously, only a few isolated case reports existed of suspected or confirmed CDV infection in large felids.[8, 17, 18] To evaluate whether CDV is a significant, emerging health risk to large cats, certain questions must be addressed. What is the risk of transmission of CDV to large felids? Has the virus mutated to become more pathogenic to large felids? Are large felids particularly susceptible to CDV infection? What can be done to minimize the risk of CDV infection to large cats?

What Is the Risk of Transmission of CDV to Large Felids?

In carnivores, CDV is transmitted primarily through aerosolization of respiratory secretions during the acute phase of infection. All body excretions are infectious at this time, and virus is shed regardless of whether the animal is symptomatic. CDV is rapidly inactivated outside the host and is susceptible to all common disinfectants. Animals with naturally acquired immunity provide a level of "herd" protection in populations of unvaccinated dogs and wild carnivores. Periodic epizootics of CDV occur as the balance shifts between protected and unprotected animals.

Epizootics of CDV in neighboring carnivore populations preceded the two CDV epizootics in large cats in California and Africa.[3, 41] Raccoons and skunks were dying with CDV in the area around the Wildlife Waystation in southern California and were believed to be the source of virus infection for the felids. An increase in CDV seroprevalence in dogs living in villages around the Serengeti National Park preceded the lion epizootic. These dogs were unvaccinated, and the increased seroprevalence between 1991 and 1993 is consistent with a susceptible population acquiring immunity through infection. Although dog-to-lion transmission was considered unlikely, other carnivores such as the spotted hyena that ranges closer to human habitation could have disseminated the virus throughout the park. Transmission and amplification of virus could then readily occur at kill sites where carnivores congregated. The source of virus exposure is not as readily apparent in isolated cases of CDV in large felids, although, in one instance, a Bengal tiger cub was raised from birth in a household with multiple exposure to dogs[8] and another 4-month-old tiger had been in an animal shelter.[3]

A retrospective survey of more than 200 serum samples collected between 1985 and 1993 from different species of exotic felids at the National Zoological Park in Washington, D.C., demonstrated an absence of CDV antibodies except in two jaguars housed together.[3] A smaller survey of felids at the Los Angeles Zoo found CDV antibodies in a mountain lion and tiger but none in two jaguars, a snow leopard, or another mountain lion. Two different groups of performing tigers had CDV antibodies. Both groups had a previous history of enteric/respiratory diseases from which all animals recovered. A tiger that was born after the apparent CDV outbreak had no CDV antibodies.

Has the Virus Mutated to Become More Pathogenic to Large Felids?

With the recognition of phocine distemper virus (closely related to CDV) and morbilliviruses in dolphins and porpoises (closely related to ruminant morbilliviruses) as unique virus entities,[35] the possibility that canine distemper in large cats is caused by a morbillivirus adapted to felids is a legitimate concern. Based on cross-neutralization studies with CDV monoclonal antibodies in both the California and Serengeti epizootics[3, 41] and conservation of polymerase gene sequences between virus isolated from a Serengeti lion and a reference isolate of CDV,[19, 41] the felids in both epizootics were infected with CDV and not some new morbillivirus of cats. However, the multiple strains of CDV vary in virulence. Whether the biotypes isolated from the two large cat epizootics are particularly virulent is not known.

Natural infections with CDV have caused deaths in a surprising range of species other than terrestrial carnivores. The seal deaths in Lake Baikal in 1987 were due to CDV infection and not to the subsequently isolated phocine distemper virus from seals in the North Atlantic.[35] In 1989, javelinas (collared peccaries) in Arizona died of encephalitis from CDV infection.[1] Fatal encephalitis from CDV infection developed in a Japanese macaque (*Macaca fusata*).[46] This animal was housed in a facility adjacent to a small animal veterinary hospital. No restrictions existed between personnel entering the two facilities so that introduction of CDV-contaminated material or equipment from the hospital to the laboratory animal facility was considered the probable source of infection. The remaining 21 macaques in the colony were asymptomatic yet had antibodies to CDV and not to measles. Clearly, all animals were exposed but only one animal died. Individual host factors play a role in disease expression.

Are Large Felids Particularly Susceptible to CDV Infection?

Domestic cats experimentally infected with CDV remain asymptomatic and do not shed virus.[2] Natural exposure to CDV does occur in domestic cats in that CDV neutralizing antibodies can be detected in healthy animals. During the 1992 epizootic of CDV in California, the observation was made that 16 of 17 animals that died were Old World large cats—leopards, lions, and tigers. Only one jaguar, a New World cat, died. What may be more telling is that all these cats belong to the genus *Panthera*. Mountain lions, bobcats (*Felis rufus*), a serval cat, and a margay, all members of the genus *Felis* like the domestic cat, were present at the same facility and did not succumb. Only cats in the

genus *Panthera* have died from infection with CDV. Whether this represents increased susceptibility to the development of severe clinical disease in members of this genus or merely the overrepresentation of *Panthera* species in captive settings with increased risk of exposure to CDV remains to be determined.

As stated previously, infection with CDV can range from asymptomatic to profound clinical signs and death. In both epizootics, the most striking clinical signs were related to neurologic dysfunction, in particular, generalized seizure activity. Host factors can affect the outcome of infection. Puppies and old dogs are more likely to die with CDV infection because of age-related, compromised immune systems. Several individual case reports of fatal CDV infection exist in young tigers and lions as does one report involving two leopards, aged 14 and 19 years.[3, 8] During major epizootics, factors other than age can affect mortality rates. In both the California and East Africa epizootics, the seroprevalence of other infectious agents was evaluated to determine whether a concurrent infection may have favored a greater mortality rate. In both instances, the answer was "no." An unusual case presentation of suspected concurrent feline panleukopenia virus and CDV infection does exist for two snow leopards.[17]

Environmental factors that stress the host undoubtedly play a critical role on mortality rates but are seldom discussed because they are difficult to quantify. Population densities, availability of food and water, changes in food sources, extreme weather conditions, altered social dynamics, and exposure to toxicants are among the environmental variables that can impact an animal's response to an infectious agent. Sera collected from 77 lions in the Serengeti between 1984 and 1989 showed that 22 lions had antibodies to CDV, indicating that lions were exposed during this time without recognized CDV-related disease.[41] Whether the CDV strain in 1994 was more virulent or environmental factors such as population density contributed to the estimated 30% mortality rate is not easy to determine. Re-evaluation of the phocine distemper virus epizootic in the North Atlantic suggests that pre-existing, immunosuppressive, environmental contaminants contributed significantly to the high mortality rates.[15]

What Can Be Done to Minimize the Risk of CDV Infection to Large Cats?

The environment of large cats is a major factor in determining the risk of exposure to CDV. A lion housed in a moated zoo exhibit and denned inside every night is less likely to encounter CDV than a lion roaming in a national park surrounded by unvaccinated canines. Felids performing in circuses and nondomestic felids kept in private households are also at greater risk of exposure.

Canine distemper can be prevented by vaccination. Only modified live virus (MLV) vaccines are commercially available in the United States. The tragic consequences of MLV vaccine-induced distemper in some species of carnivores other than the domestic dog makes the use of MLV vaccines in felids a legitimate safety issue. Killed CDV vaccines provide only partial protection against infection and disease in dogs, prompting their withdrawal commercially. Their relative ineffectiveness has been attributed to an "incomplete" antibody response to the fusion (F) protein, which is responsible for the hemolytic activity of CDV.[16] The subunit CDV-ISCOM vaccine presents the F protein in a proper immunogenic form so that dogs and seals in experimental trials in Europe are protected against morbillivirus infection.[16, 45] This vaccine would be safe for felids, but it is not commercially available. Whether the commercially available MLV vaccines used in ferrets would be safe for felids is not known. Therefore, vaccinating zoo felids against CDV cannot be justified, particularly because the relative risk of exposure is low. In East Africa, vaccinating native dogs is being attempted to reduce the risk of CDV exposure in wild carnivores.

Finally, virus isolation is difficult in species other than canids. Diagnosis is usually based on demonstration of CDV in affected tissues immunocytochemically or by development of CDV antibodies. As CDV has undoubtedly caused clinical disease in nondomestic felids, it should be included as a differential diagnosis, particularly when enteric, respiratory, or neurologic signs of unknown origin develop in more than one felid in a setting. The nonspecific nature of these clinical signs also apply to FeLV and FIV. For all three viral infections, serologic assays are the fastest way to make a presumptive diagnosis and, given the inherent difficulties encountered for isolating these viruses, are often the only way. The importance of routine screening and maintaining a serum bank for retrospective evaluation of captive animals as well as conducting serosurveys in free-ranging populations cannot be overemphasized if the threat of emerging viral infections to populations of large cats is to be ascertained.

REFERENCES

1. Appel MJG, Reggiardo C, Summers BA, et al: Canine distemper virus infection and encephalitis in javelinas (collared peccaries). Arch Virol 199:147–152, 1991.
2. Appel MJG, Sheffy BE, Percy DH, et al: Canine distemper virus in domesticated cats and pigs. Am J Vet Res 35:803–806, 1974.
3. Appel MJG, Yates RA, Foley GL, et al: Canine distemper epizootic in lions, tigers, and leopards in North America. J Vet Diagn Invest 6:277–288, 1994.
4. August JR: Husbandry practices for cats infected with feline leukemia virus or feline immunodeficiency virus. J Am Vet Med Assoc 199:1474–1477, 1991.
5. Barr MC, Calle PP, Roelke ME, et al: Feline immunodeficiency virus infection in nondomestic felids. J Zoo Wildl Med 20:265–272, 1989.
6. Barr MC, Zou L, Holzschu DL, et al: Isolation of a highly cytopathic lentivirus from a nondomestic cat. J Virol 69:7371–7374, 1995.
7. Bendinelli M, Pistello M, Lombardi S, et al: Feline immunodeficiency virus: an interesting model for AIDS studies and an important cat pathogen. Clin Microbiol Rev 8:87–112, 1995.
8. Blythe LL, Schmitz JA, Roelke M, et al: Chronic encephalomyelitis caused by canine distemper virus in a Bengal tiger. J Am Vet Med Assoc 183:1159–1162, 1983.
9. Briggs MB, Ott RL: Feline leukemia virus infection in a captive cheetah and the clinical and antibody response of six captive cheetah to vaccination with a subunit feline leukemia virus vaccine. J Am Vet Med Assoc 189:1197–1199, 1986.
10. Brown EW, Miththapala S, O'Brien SJ, et al: Prevalence of exposure to feline immunodeficiency virus in exotic felid species. J Zoo Wildl Med 24:357–364, 1993.
11. Brown EW, Yuhki N, Packer C, et al: A lion lentivirus related to feline immunodeficiency virus: epidemiologic and phylogenetic aspects. J Virol 68:5953–5968, 1994.
12. Carpenter, MA, Brown EW, Culver, M, et al: Genetic and phylogenetic divergence of feline immunodeficiency virus in the puma. J Virol 70:6682–6693, 1996.
13. Citino SB: Transient FeLV viremia in a clouded leopard. J Zoo Anim Med 17:5–7, 1986.
14. Citino SB: Use of a subunit feline leukemia virus vaccine in exotic cats. J Am Vet Med Assoc 192:957–959, 1988.
15. De Swart RL, Ross PS, Vedder LJ, et al: Impairment of immune function in harbour seals (*Phoca vitulina*) feeding on fish from polluted waters. AMBIO 23:155–159, 1994.
16. De Vries P, Uytdehaag FGCM, Osterhaus ADME: Canine distemper virus (CDV) immune-stimulating complexes (iscoms), but not measles virus iscoms, protect dogs against CDV infection. J Gen Virol 69:2071–2083, 1988.
17. Fix AS, Riordan DP, Hill HT, et al: Feline panleukopenia virus and subsequent canine distemper virus infection in two snow leopards (*Panthera uncia*). J Zoo Wildl Med 20:273–281, 1989.
18. Gould DH, Fenner WR: Paramyxovirus-like nucleocapsids associated with encephalitis in a captive Siberian tiger. J Am Vet Med Assoc 183:1319–1322, 1983.
19. Harder TC, Kenter M, Appel MJG, et al: Phylogenetic evidence of canine distemper virus in Serengeti's lions. Vaccine 13:521–523, 1995.
20. Hoover EA, Mullins JI: Feline leukemia virus infection and diseases. J Am Vet Med Assoc 199:1287–1297, 1991.
21. Jessup DA, Pettan KC, Lowenstine LJ, et al: Feline leukemia virus infection and renal spirochetosis in a free-ranging cougar (*Felis concolor*). J Zoo Wildl Med 24:73–79, 1993.
22. Jordan HL, Howard J, Sellon RK, et al: Transmission of feline immunodeficiency virus in domestic cats via artificial insemination. J Virol 70:8224–8228, 1996.
23. Jordan HL, Howard J, Tompkins WA, et al: Detection of feline immunodeficiency virus in semen from seropositive domestic cats (*Felis catus*). J Virol 69:7328–7333, 1995.
24. Kennedy-Stoskopf S, Gebhard DH, English RV, et al: Clinical implications of feline immunodeficiency virus infection in African lions (*Panther leo*): preliminary findings. Proceedings of the Association of Reptilian and Amphibian Veterinarians and American Association of Zoo Veterinarians, Pittsburgh, PA, pp 345–346, 1994.
25. Killmar L, Grisham J (eds): Proceedings of the Cheetah SSP's Workshop on Feline Immunodeficiency Viruses (FIV), Cheetah Immunodeficiency Virus (CIV) and Feline Infectious Peritonitis (FIP), San Diego, CA, p. 22, 1995.
26. Legendre AM, Hawks DM, Sebring R, et al: Comparison of the efficacy of three commercial feline leukemia virus vaccines in a natural challenge exposure. J Am Vet Med Assoc 199:1456–1461, 1991.
27. Letcher JD, O'Conner TP Jr: Incidence of antibodies reacting to feline immunodeficiency virus in population of Asian lions. J Zoo Wildl Med 22:324–329, 1991.
28. Lopez N: Panther study provides new insight into FeLV tests. Feline Health Topics 3:5–6, 1988.
29. Lutz H, Isenbügel E, Lehmann R, et al: Retrovirus infections in non-domestic felids: serological studies and attempts to isolate a lentivirus. Vet Immunol Immunopathol 35:215–224, 1992.
30. McOrist S, Boid R, Jones TW, et al: Some viral and protozoal diseases in the European wildcat (*Felis silvestris*). J Wildl Dis 27:693–696, 1991.
31. Meric SM: Suspect feline leukemia virus infection and pancytopenia in a western cougar. J Am Vet Med Assoc 185:1390–1391, 1984.
32. O'Connor TP, Tonelli QJ, Scarlett JM: Report of the National FeLV/FIV Awareness Project. J Am Vet Med Assoc 199:1348–1352, 1991.
33. Olmsted RA, Langley R, Roelke ME, et al: Worldwide prevalence of lentivirus infection in wild feline species: epidemiologic and phylogenetic aspects. J Virol 66:6008–6018, 1992.
34. Osofsky SA, Hirsch KJ, Zuckerman EE, et al: Feline lentivirus and feline oncovirus status of free-ranging lions (*Panthera leo*), leopards (*Panthera pardus*), and cheetahs (*Acinonyx jubatus*) in Botswana: a regional perspective. J Zoo Wildl Med 27:453–467, 1996.

35. Osterhaus ADME, deSwart RL, Vos HW, et al: Morbillivirus infections of aquatic mammals: newly identified members of the genus. Vet Microbiol 44:219–227, 1995.
36. Paul-Murphy J, Work T, Hunter D, et al: Serologic survey and serum biochemical reference ranges of the free-ranging mountain lion (*Felis concolor*) in California. J Wildl Dis 30:205–215, 1994.
37. Pedersen NC, Barlough JE: Clinical overview of feline immunodeficiency virus. J Am Vet Med Assoc 199:1298–1304, 1991.
38. Poli A, Abramo F, Cavicchio P, *et al.*: Lentivirus infection in an African lion: a clinical, pathologic and virologic study. J Wildl Dis 31:70–74, 1995.
39. Rasheed S, Gardner MB: Isolation of feline leukemia virus from a leopard cat cell line and search for retrovirus in wild felidae. J Natl Cancer Inst 67:929–933, 1981.
40. Roelke ME, Forrester DJ, Jacobson ER, et al: Seroprevalence of infectious disease agents in free-ranging Florida panthers (*Felis concolor coryi*). J Wildl Dis 29:36–49, 1993.
41. Roelke-Parker ME, Munson L, Packer C, et al: A canine distemper virus epidemic in Serengeti lions (*Panthera leo*). Nature 379:441–445, 1996.
42. Rojko JL, Kociba GJ: Pathogenesis of infection by the feline leukemia virus. J Am Vet Med Assoc 199:1305–1310.
43. Sellon RK, Jordan HL, Kennedy-Stoskopf S, et al: Feline immunodeficiency virus can be experimentally transmitted via milk during acute maternal infection. J Virol 68:3380–3385, 1994.
44. VandeWoude S, O'Brien S, Langelier K, et al: Infectivity of lion and puma lentiviruses for domestic cats. Proceedings of the Third International Feline Retrovirus Research Symposium, Fort Collins, CO, p. 45, 1996.
45. Visser IKG, Vedder EJ, van de Bildt MWG, et al: Canine distemper virus ISCOMS induce protection in harbour seals (*Phoca vitulina*) against phocid distemper but still allow subsequent infection with phocid distemper virus-1. Vaccine 10:435-523, 1995.
46. Yoshikawa Y, Ochikubo F, Matsubara Y, et al: Natural infection with canine distemper virus in a Japanese monkey (*Macaca fuscata*). Vet Microbiol 10:193–205, 1989.

CHAPTER **55**

Giant Panda Management and Medicine in China

S. A. MAINKA

CAPTIVE PANDAS IN CHINA: HISTORY

Giant pandas have been held in captivity in China since 1953 when a panda was taken from Guanxian County to the Chengdu Zoological Gardens.[11] Two years later, the Beijing Zoological Gardens also added giant pandas to their collection. The first giant panda birth in captivity did not occur until 1963 at the Beijing Zoo when Li Li gave birth to a male, Ming Ming.[14] Since 1953, 32 Chinese city zoos, five nature reserve breeding centers, and two circuses have had giant pandas in their collections.[31]

In the late 1970s, both the Beijing and the Chengdu zoos began investigating artificial insemination (AI) techniques in the giant panda. The first successful birth by AI at Beijing Zoo was in 1978 and the first successful AI at Chengdu was in 1980. For the next 10 years, most Chinese institutions tried to perfect their AI techniques but the success of births from both natural mating and AI was low. Between 1980 and 1989, only 17 of 60 baby pandas born in Chinese zoos survived beyond 6 months of age,[31] the officially recognized demarcation of "infant survival."

By the late 1980s, emphasis was again shifting toward natural mating and the success of breeding increased exponentially. In 1992, 14 infants were born, 11 of which survived past 6 months. Survival rates of infants surpassed 50% for the first time in captive panda history. By alternating maternal and human care for each infant, the Chengdu Zoo became the first institution to successfully raise twin giant pandas. In 1993, the Beijing Zoo was the first institution to completely hand-raise an infant from birth. By 1993, there were 113 giant pandas in captivity in China in 25 institutions.[31]

MANAGEMENT

Housing

Most Chinese zoos holding pandas have only one or two animals, with each being housed separately. Even if a larger number of pandas is in the collection, adults are each held individually while weaned infants and juveniles up to the age of about 2 years may be housed together.

In all cases, both indoor and outdoor enclosures are provided, and outdoor enclosures have a pool and some climbing structure. Usually, only the younger pandas make use of the climbing structure. Many giant pandas prefer to sleep on a raised platform, and most institutions provide a wooden pallet or similar structure for this purpose.

Whenever possible, some access through mesh between adult males and females should be offered for several months before and during the breeding season.

The Beijing Zoo recommends keeping pandas in temperatures between 10° and 27°C and at a relative humidity of 55% to 65%.[28] Whereas pandas tolerate colder temperatures well, they appear uncomfortable in hotter, humid weather. Chinese zoos in warmer climates provide shade, bathing opportunities, and cool indoor pens for their pandas.

Enclosure maintenance is routine, including daily sweeping and weekly disinfection of floors.

Nutrition

Giant pandas show poor utilization of plant material and digest less than 20% of ingested bamboo dry matter.[5, 19, 27] Most Chinese zoos feed pandas both a concentrate, in the form of gruel or steamed bread, as well as bamboo. Although bamboo is offered on a free-choice basis several times a day, the concentrate is fed twice daily, morning and afternoon.[6] Some Chinese zoos do not have regular access to fresh bamboo and use substitutes such as carrots to provide the necessary fiber (Liu Weixin, personal communication).

An assessment of diets in five Chinese zoos, all having success breeding giant pandas, showed that, although the ingredients used in each institution's diet were different, the nutritional composition of the diets all approximated the established nutritional requirements for the domestic dog.[6]

In captive pandas fed diets with less than 60% bamboo (dry matter [DM] basis), accumulation of intestinal mucus develops, leading to constipation.[19] The panda may become anorexic and exhibit signs of abdominal discomfort in efforts to pass the mucous stool. At the Wolong Reserve, mucous stools may occur as often as twice a month in some pandas (Zhang Hemin, personal communication). To keep the incidence of mucous stool as low as possible, every effort must be made to provide steady supplies of bamboo.

MEDICINE

Immobilization

Only very young pandas can be manually restrained for physical examination or medical procedures. In most other cases, chemical restraint is required. Many different immobilization protocols have been used successfully on giant pandas in China. The most commonly used includes ketamine alone and ketamine and xylazine combinations, but this is primarily due to drug availability. A summary of reports on giant panda immobilization in China, including physiologic data, is listed in Table 55–1.

Use of diazepam and other drug combinations containing benzodiazepines in giant pandas has been re-

TABLE 55–1. Summary of Giant Panda Immobilization Reports from Chinese Institutions

Drug	Dose (mg/kg)	Comment	Reference
Ketamine	4–6	Induction time 5–8 minutes; body temperature 36.5 to 38.9°C	24
	2.4–4.4	Heart rate 86–106 beats/minute Respiratory rate 18–20 breaths/ minute	7
	4.5 ± 1.3	Induction time 16.4 ± 12 minutes Heart rate 90 ± 26 beats/minute Respiratory rate 31 ± 1 breaths/ minute Rectal temperature 38.1° ± 0.2°C	18
Ketamine/diazepam	6–8/0.2		24
	7.1 ± 2.1/0.2	Induction time 22.7 ± 8.7 minutes	18
Ketamine/fentanyl	5–6/0.02–0.04	Temperature 37° to 38.5°C	24
Ketamine/xylazine	3.9–8/0.39–0.7	Heart rate 32–89 beats/minute Respiratory rate 20–39 breaths/ minute Temperature 36.4 to 37.7	24
	4.8 ± 1.0/0.43	Induction time 8.8 ± 6.6 minutes Heart rate 82 ± 26 beats/minute Respiratory rate 29 ± 10 breaths/ minute Rectal temperature 37.8° ± 0.8°C used on animal with seizures	18
Sodium thiopental	6 mg/kg	Induction time 10.7 ± 5.5 minutes	29
Tiletamine/zolazepam	5.8 ± 1.3	Heart rate 134 ± 9 beats/minute Respiratory rate 42 ± 6 breaths/ minute Rectal temperature 38.0° ± 0.4°C	18

ported to cause excitement and result in using higher doses of immobilizing drugs.[18] Furthermore, after being given injections of diazepam as premedication for general anesthesia, several pandas have been noted to look for food and consume any available in the enclosure.

Clinical Pathology

Most giant panda clinical pathology reports from Chinese institutions are contained in case reports. The only summary report comes from the Wolong Nature Reserve (Table 55–2). Red blood cell counts and blood urea nitrogen values were linearly correlated with age. No difference was noted between adult male and female blood parameters except that male pandas had higher red blood cell values than females and females had higher triglyceride levels.[20] These differences were not dietary in origin but may have reflected seasonal changes.

Rouleaux formation and rapid erythrocyte sedimen-

tation rates are normal in giant pandas and are not useful indicators of inflammation.[10]

Diseases and Pathology

Giant pandas are subject to many of the infectious diseases of other carnivores including canine distemper, tuberculosis, and *Escherichia coli* septicemia.[25] Serum from several captive pandas showed serologic evidence of exposure to canine parvovirus, canine adenovirus, canine distemper virus, and canine coronavirus.[21] A few institutions in China have vaccinated their pandas for parvoviruses and other canid diseases using killed vaccines with no adverse effects. However, no research has been done in China to determine whether immunity develops in giant pandas as a result of these immunizations.

Since 1986, giant pandas have been diagnosed with a severe hemorrhagic enteritis. Many Chinese scientists believe this enteritis to be of viral origin, although only

TABLE 55–2. Hematological and Serum Biochemical Values for Captive Giant Pandas

	N	Mean ± SE	Minimum	Maximum
Hematology				
Red blood cells ($\times 10^6/\mu l$)	17	6.8 ± 0.2	5.2	8.0
Packed cell volume (%)	17	40.6 ± 1.3	32.0	49.0
Mean corpuscular volume (fl)	15	59.4 ± 2.6	43.9	83.2
White blood cells ($\times 10^3/\mu l$)	16	7.0 ± 0.7	4.0	14.5
Segmented neutrophils (%)	18	72 ± 2	61	84
Band cells (%)	18	1 ± 0.4	0	4
Lymphocytes (%)	18	18 ± 1	6	27
Monocytes (%)	18	7 ± 1	0	22
Eosinophils (%)	18	2 ± 1	0	14
Serum Chemistry				
Alanine aminotransferase (IU/L)	16	50 ± 5	25	82
Aspartate aminotransferase (IU/L)	16	62 ± 6	33	104
Creatine kinase (U/L)	16	221 ± 72	35	1105
Alkaline phosphatase (U/L)	16	125 ± 23	31	422
Gamma glutamyl transferase (U/L)	15	11.8 ± 1.8	5	28
Lactate dehydrogenase (U/L)	13	532 ± 93	7	1034
Glucose (mg/dl)	14	92.4 ± 6.1	69.0	156.2
Total protein (g/dl)	16	6.2 ± 0.2	5.0	7.5
Albumin (g/dl)	16	2.8 ± 0.1	2.1	3.3
Total bilirubin (mg/dl)	14	0.15 ± 0.02	0.05	0.31
Direct bilirubin (mg/dl)	13	0.08 ± 0.02	0.02	0.23
Creatinine (mg/dl)	16	1.6 ± 0.1	0.7	2.2
Blood urea nitrogen (mg/dl)	16	15 ± 2	6	33
Cholesterol (mg/dl)	13	191 ± 8	123	245
Triglycerides (mg/dl)	11	48 ± 7	24	95
Calcium (mmol/L)	15	2.5 ± 0.2	1.4	3.6
Phosphorus (mmol/L)	16	1.4 ± 0.1	1.0	3.0
Sodium (mmol/L)	16	128 ± 3	108	150
Potassium (mmol/L)	16	3.7 ± 0.3	2.0	6.0
Chloride (mmol/L)	16	94 ± 3	64	114
Magnesium (mmol/L)	16	1.1 ± 0.1	0.5	1.8
Serum Vitamins				
Retinol ($\mu g/ml$)	7	0.45 ± 0.07	0.11	0.63
Alpha-tocopherol ($\mu g/ml$)	7	8.5 ± 1.1	6.5	15.1

From Mainka SA, He T, Chen M, et al: Hematological and serum biochemical values for healthy captive giant pandas (*Ailuropoda melanoleuca*) at the Wolong Reserve, Sichuan, China. J Zool Wildl Med 26(3):377–381, 1995.

one case with coronavirus has been confirmed by virus isolation.[2] Research at the Chengdu Zoo reports that another of the etiologic agents involved in cases of hemorrhagic enteritis is *E. coli*.[16] A parvovirus is suspected to be the cause of many cases of hemorrhagic enteritis but has not yet been isolated from clinical cases.

The most common parasite of giant pandas in China is *Ascaridia schroederi* with wild pandas (77%) being more commonly affected than captive animals (12%).[25] Other parasites reported in pandas in China include *Ancylostoma caninum, Demodex ailuropodae, Chorioptes panda,* several *Ixodes* species, and several *Haemaphysalis* species.[13] Piperazine and ivermectin, administered at doses used for domestic canids, have been used to treat parasites in giant pandas.

Neoplasias, including hepatopancreatic, renal and uterine cancer, ovarian adenocarcinoma, and lymphosarcomas, have also been reported in giant pandas.[25]

In addition, giant pandas have been reported to have ringworm[1] and are prone to development of seizures of unknown origin.[25]

For both free-ranging and captive pandas, disease of the gastrointestinal system is most commonly involved (42% of cases) in deaths.[25] In particular, captive pandas are subject to intestinal disease, primarily enteritis and impaction.

REPRODUCTION

Mating Season

Giant pandas are seasonally monoestrous with mating season occurring in the spring. Males mature between 5.5 and 7.5 years of age and generally weigh 95 to 105 kg at that time.[8] The quality of semen and size of testicles in males vary with seasons, with optimal semen quality occurring during mating season.[9, 22] Panda semen has been cryogenically preserved and quality of semen on thawing is good.[26]

Female pandas become sexually mature between 5.5 and 6.5 years of age and may weigh as little as 40 to 55 kg.[8] Although estrous behavior may be seen as early as 2 years of age, pregnancy rarely occurs before 6 years of age. The youngest female to give birth was 5-year-old Guo Guo of the Chengdu Zoo.[31]

Female pandas are in estrus for only a few days each year. Behaviorally, estrous females are restless and have a decrease in appetite and an increase in vocalization. Physically, the primary visible change is enlargement and reddening of the vulva. Chinese scientists have been using vaginal cytology to help determine peak estrus and receptivity, with a cornified cell to noncornified cell ratio of greater than 3:1 being the indicator (Chen Meng, personal communication). In addition, urine hormones have been monitored to determine peak estrus,[3] but this technique requires equipment and technical expertise that is not universally available in Chinese zoos.

Captive giant panda breeding success is best at Chinese zoos where females can choose a mate from among several males. Compatibility of male and female

appears to be very important. For a few months before mating season, a female is allowed access to at least two males to allow her to demonstrate a preference of mate. Then, at peak estrus, the female is given access to her preferred male's pen and allowed a chance to investigate the scent marking left by the male. Finally male and female are introduced to each other. Mating is marked by many vocalizations, but at intromission there is a pronounced change in vocalization, from barking and bleating to chirping, by both male and female. Mating may last up to 20 minutes and is considered "unsuccessful" if it lasts less than 2 minutes

If artificial insemination is attempted, it must be carefully timed because there is some evidence that any immobilization may delay ovulation in giant pandas.[4]

Birth

Female pandas are provided with a nest, either tree or box, at least 1 month before expected delivery, which, for most females, occurs between August and October. The earliest recorded panda birth in China was on May 4 at the Fuzhou Zoological Gardens and the latest recorded birth was November 20, 1997, at the Wolong Reserve.

Gestation periods varied from 83 to 181 days.[8] The large discrepancy in gestation periods may be explained by the fact that giant pandas likely experience delayed implantation.[23]

There are no reliable physical indicators of impending birth other than marked restlessness and anorexia during the 24 to 48 hours before and some increase in licking the vulva. Some females display maternal behavior toward objects in their enclosure (e.g., apples, balls) for 10 to 20 days before delivery.[15] Delivery occurs without difficulty and, if there are twins, the second cub is usually delivered within 2 hours of the first. Of 81 litters produced in Chinese institutions between 1973 and 1992, 36 were twins; the remaining were single births.[31]

Females immediately begin care of their infants and may nurse up to 10 times per day for the first week. At birth, infant pandas are pink in color with a light white coat of lanugo. Black pigmentation does not begin until 7 to 10 days of age. Eyes and ears open after 1 month, and deciduous dentition is first seen after 2.5 to 3 months.[30]

For mother-reared infants, Beijing and Chengdu zoos also provide additional feedings of cow's milk to giant panda infants from 3 months onward. Mother-raised infants gain weight at an average of 71 g/day in the first 6 months.[30]

Most Chinese zoos holding pandas wean giant panda infants at about 6 months of age to allow the females to come into estrus and breed again in the following year. The most successful females produce offspring regularly, but they often have at least 1 year in 4 in which no young are produced.

Pseudopregnancy, including physical changes such as mammary swelling, vulva swelling, and milk production, has been reported in the giant panda in China.[4]

Hand-Rearing

The first successful hand-raising from birth (i.e., survival past 6 months of age) occurred in 1993 at the Beijing Zoo. Previously, the only successes were one infant that survived to 75 days at the Beijing Zoo in 1981 to 1982 and another that survived to 160 days at the Wolong Reserve in 1991 to 1992.[17]

Development of hand-raised infants is slower than that for mother-reared infants (daily weight gains average 50 g/day).[30] Initial incubator temperatures were maintained at 33° to 35°C. and humidity maintained at 65% to 75%.[15]

Giant panda milk samples have had very low lactose levels.[12] This has led to speculation that the giant panda is lactose intolerant and hand-rearing formulations should be lactose free. The Ueno Zoological Gardens in Tokyo has therefore developed a lactose-free panda milk formulation, which was successfully used, in combination with cow's milk powder, at the Wolong Reserve to hand-raise giant pandas.[15] During 5 months of hand-rearing, the formula averaged 13.4% dry matter, 6% crude protein, 5% crude fat, and 6% carbohydrate, with the formula being quite dilute (12% dry matter) for the first few weeks and then becoming progressively more concentrated.[15]

REFERENCES

1. Anon: Clinical observations of and experiments on ringworm in the giant panda. Chinese Zoo Yearbook 3:124–125, 1980.
2. Chen Y, Pan X: Etiological studies on acute enteritis in giant panda [Abstract]. Proceedings of the 3rd Asian Bear Conference, Harbin, China, p. 193, 1991.
3. Chen Y, Wang S, Li X, et al: Urinary estrogen concentrations at estrous in the giant panda. *In* Zhang A, He G (eds): Minutes of the International Symposium on the Protection of the Giant Panda (*Ailuropoda melanoleuca*), Chengdu, China, pp 243–246, 1994.
4. Chen Y: Pregnancy and pseudo-pregnancy in giant panda (*Ailuropoda melanoleuca*). Proceedings of the Conference of Chinese Zoos, vol 1, pp 8–13, 1990.
5. Dierenfeld ES, Hintz HF, Robertson JB, et al: Utilization of bamboo by the giant panda. J Nutr 112:636–641, 1982.
6. Dierenfeld, ES, Qiu X, Mainka SA, et al: Giant panda diets fed in five Chinese facilities: an assessment. Zoo Biol 14:211–222, 1995.
7. Fan Z, Ou Y, Chao Y: A discussion on anesthesia of the giant panda with the injection ketamine. *In* Proceedings of Therapeutics of the Giant Panda. China Forestry Publishing House, Beijing, China, pp 61–65, 1987. [In Chinese]
8. Feng W, Chang A: Reproductive physiology and artificial breeding of the giant panda. Sichuan, Sichuan University Publishing House, 1988. [In Chinese]
9. Feng W, Wang P, Wang C, et al: Semen character study in the giant panda (1) Observe the semen quality. Sichuan Univ J 28:93–101, 1991. [In Chinese]
10. Hawkey CM: Haematology. Trans Zool Soc London 33:99–101, 1976.
11. Hu J, Liu T, He G: Giant Pandas with Graceful Bearing. Sichuan, Sichuan Publishing House of Science and Technology, 1990.
12. Hudson GJ, Bailey PA, John PMV, et al: Composition of milk from *Ailuropoda melanoleuca*, the giant panda. Vet Rec 115:252, 1984.
13. Jeu M, Zhu C: Treatments and controls of parasitoses to the giant panda. Proceedings of Therapeutics of the Giant Panda, China Forestry Publishing House, Beijing, China, pp 1–9, 1987.
14. Kan O, Shu-hua T: In the Peking Zoo—the first baby giant panda. Animal Kingdom 57(2):44–46, 1964.
15. Kewen Z (ed): Hand-raising an infant giant panda: a study at the Wolong Nature Reserve. Sichuan, Sichuan Science Publishing House, 1993. [In Chinese with English abstracts]
16. Li G, Zhong S, Zhang A, et al: Studies on hemorrhagic enteritis of giant pandas [Abstract]. Proceedings of the 4th Giant Panda Conference, Chengdu, China, pp. 319–324, 1994.
17. Liu WX, Liu NL, Zhang HM, et al: Hand-rearing of new-born giant panda. Chinese Science Bull 39:514–519, 1994.
18. Mainka SA, He T: Immobilization of healthy male giant pandas (*Ailuropoda melanoleuca*) at the Wolong Nature Reserve. J Zoo Wildl Med 24(4):430–433, 1993.
19. Mainka SA, Zhao G, Li M: Utilization of a bamboo, sugar cane, and gruel diet by two juvenile giant pandas (*Ailuropoda melanoleuca*). J Zoo Anim Med 20:39–44, 1989.
20. Mainka SA, He T, Chen M, et al: Hematological and serum biochemical values for healthy captive giant pandas (*Ailuropoda melanoleuca*) at the Wolong Reserve, Sichuan, China. J Zoo Wildl Med 26(3):377–381, 1995.
21. Mainka SA, Qiu X, He T, et al: Serologic survey of giant pandas (*Ailuropoda melanoleuca*), and domestic dogs and cats in the Wolong Reserve, China. J Wild Dis 30(1):86–89, 1994.
22. Masui M, Hiramatsu H, Nose R, et al: Successful artificial insemination in the giant panda (*Ailuropoda melanoleuca*) at Ueno Zoo. Zoo Biol 8:17–26, 1989.
23. Monfort SL, Dahl KD, Czekala NM, et al: Monitoring ovarian function and pregnancy in the giant panda (*Ailuropoda melanoleuca*) by evaluating urinary bioactive FSH and steroid metabolites. J Reprod Fertil 85:203–212, 1989.
24. Qiu X: Anesthesia of the giant panda. J Sichuan Teachers College 11(2):114–117, 1990. [In Chinese]
25. Qiu X, Mainka SA. Review of mortality of the giant panda (*Ailuropoda melanoleuca*). J Zoo Wildl Med 24(4):425–429, 1993.
26. Seager SWJ, Dolensek EP, He G, et al: Giant panda (*Ailuropoda melanoleuca*) semen collection, evaluation and freezing in southwest China. *In* Asakura S, Nakagawa S (eds): Proceedings of the 2nd International Symposium of the Giant Panda. Tokyo, Tokyo Zoological Park Society, pp 123–126, 1990.
27. Wang XQ, Liu A, Chen R: The utilization of bamboo by the giant panda in captivity. *In* Smith AT, Hoffmann RS, Lidicker WZ, Schlitter DA (eds): Proceedings of the Symposium of Asian-Pacific Mammalogy [Abstract]. Beijing, China, Scientific Publishing House, 1988.
28. Wang W, Liao G: The keeping and management of the giant panda—Beijing Zoo. Proceedings of the 4th Giant Panda Conference, Chengdu, China, pp 84–89, 1994.
29. Yu B, Yu Z: Anaesthetic treatments of the giant panda. *In* Proceedings of Therapeutics of the Giant Panda. Beijing, China, China Forestry Publishing House, pp 51–53, 1987. [In Chinese]
30. Zhang G, Zhang H, Chen M, et al: Growth and development of infant giant pandas (*Ailuropoda melanoleuca*) at the Wolong Reserve, China. Zoo Biology 15:13–20, 1996.
31. Zhao Q, Fan Z, Gipps J, et al: The Giant Panda Studbook. Beijing Zoological Gardens, Beijing, China, 1993.

CHAPTER 56

Medical Management of a Cheetah Breeding Facility in South Africa

D. G. A. MELTZER

The conservation status of cheetahs (*Acinonyx jubatus*) in southern Africa as defined by the International Union for the Conservation of Nature and Natural Resources is "out of danger."[15] For many years, the "endangered" status of this animal has been an anomaly. The cheetah has been regarded as endangered by some and treated as vermin by others in many areas of the African continent as a result of its predation upon domestic livestock. Despite persecution by the farming communities, the free-ranging population of cheetahs still does well in Namibia, Botswana, Zimbabwe, and the bushveld areas of the Republic of South Africa. Survival of the cheetah depends on the conservation of its habitat and prey species. Successful captive breeding contributes to the conservation of the species by providing animals for in-depth research into the biology of the species and by making animals available for release into newly established conservation areas, zoological gardens, and safari parks.

The De Wildt Cheetah Centre, which was established by Ann van Dyk in collaboration with the National Zoological Gardens of South Africa in 1971, has led the way in breeding large numbers of cheetahs in captivity. A second large facility for the captive breeding of cheetahs, The Hoedspruit Research and Breeding Centre for Endangered Species, was established in 1989

in South Africa. Each of these centers manages a population of 60 to 80 cheetahs. In addition, there are two or three smaller breeding centers in southern Africa. The captive breeding potential of cheetahs is such that breeders in South Africa can produce far more animals than the market can accommodate.

Captive-bred cheetahs have been released into nature reserves.[12] Cheetahs from the Hoedspruit Centre were released onto a nearby military air base where they control the antelope population that tends to wander onto the landing strip.

The lack of genetic variation in cheetahs has given rise to concerns about their potential vulnerability to diseases and thus their survival.[9–11] However, it is apparent from the improved understanding of the status of the animal in nature, the success of efforts to breed cheetahs in captivity, and the potential for their release into nature reserves that cheetahs can indeed survive in a suitable habitat.

BIOLOGIC DATA

Data from the De Wildt Cheetah Centre for the period 1975 to 1984 are summarized in Table 56–1.

TABLE 56–1. Biologic Data from Captive Cheetahs Recorded at the De Wildt Cheetah Centre During the Period 1975 to 1984

	Mean	Range
Body mass—male (kg)	46	45–55
Body mass—females (kg)	39	35–45
Body temperature (°C)		38–39
Life span in captivity (years) (n = 98)	11.1	3,5–16
Age at first litter (years)	3.8	3–4
Gestation (days)	93.4	91–95
Mean litter size	3.5	1–8
Neonate mass (g)	412.6	350–500
Cub survival > 1 month (%) (10-year period)	57	0–96
Weaning—optimal minimum (months)	6.75	6–8
Cub production/female lifetime (n = 19)	10.4	1–25
Peak reproductive age (years)		6–8

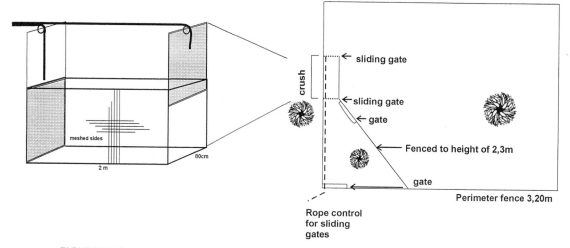

FIGURE 56–1. Design of the enclosure showing large and corner sections as well as detail of the crush.

HANDLING

Cheetahs can be handled differently when compared to any of the other felids. Even wild-caught animals can be approached within the confines of an enclosure immediately after capture. The animals hiss, growl, and attempt to slap with their forepaws, but they do not attack. Once habituated, the cheetahs can be herded and chased within their enclosure and moved down passageways of fenced paths to other areas if necessary.

Enclosure Design

The enclosures of the two southern African cheetah-breeding centers vary in size from 1500 square meters for animals kept singly to large enclosures of up to 5 hectares where groups of 8 to 10 male cheetahs may be kept. Enclosures are designed to permit capture and handling without the need for chemical restraint.

Entrance into each enclosure is gained by passing through a smaller corner enclosure. Resident animals have free access between the large and corner enclosures through a crush and soon become habituated to moving through the crushes in their enclosures as part of the daily routine. Sliding gates at each end of the crush are kept open but can be closed to trap the animal. The design of these corner camps and the attached crushes is shown in Figures 56–1 and 56–2.

Animals are fed in the corner enclosure and can be caught when handling or treatment is required. Wooden staffs of approximately 1.5 meters are used to restrain animals that have been confined in the crush. The staffs are placed through the meshed sides as a barrier to prevent movement when animals are vaccinated or injected. The placement of wooden staffs to restrain a cheetah in a crush is shown in Figure 56–3.

The animal may be pinned down within the crush, its hind leg pulled through the mesh, and an intravenous injection given. Figure 56–4 shows the administration of an intravenous injection to a cheetah in a crush.

Access roads used for feeding are used as routes through which cheetahs can be herded to other enclosures or to a central area where groups of animals undergo treatment. During the breeding cycle, males are released into the roadway between the female enclosures and left there for several weeks. Access into female enclosures can be controlled because animals must move through the smaller corner areas to enter the main enclosure.

ANESTHESIA
Intravenous Drug Administration

Alphaxolone and alphadolone acetate (Saffan, Janssen A. H. Halfway House, Republic of South Africa) can

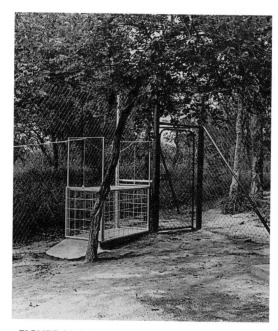

FIGURE 56–2. The crush and a section of the enclosure.

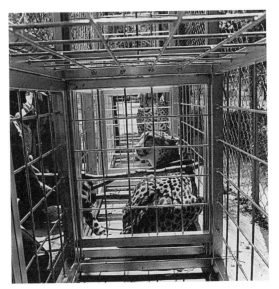

FIGURE 56–3. The restraint of a cheetah using wooden staffs in a crush.

be used in adult cheetahs as a hypnotic or anesthetic depending on the dose given (1 ml of Saffan contains 9 mg of alphaxolone and 3 mg of alphadolone acetate). With the animal restrained in a crush, the drug is administered intravenously. A bolus of 5 ml is sufficient to allow general handling, examination, and semen collection by electroejaculation. Anesthesia is induced by administering 6 to 8 ml as a bolus and then adding to effect. Transient apnea may follow when the higher dose is given. Induction is rapid and not accompanied by excitement. Muscular relaxation is excellent and the recovery is uneventful in adult animals. Cubs and juveniles may experience a period of excitement during recovery. Nevertheless, in South Africa, Saffan remains the drug of choice for use in cheetahs.

Darting or Intramuscular Injection

The cyclohexylamines—phencyclidine, ketamine, and tiletamine—all have a tendency to cause severe muscular hypertonicity, hyperthermia, and epileptiform convulsions at higher dosages. Phencyclidine has been reported to cause deaths in cheetahs as a result of these side effects[14] and it was only after the manufacture of ketamine and later tiletamine, derivatives of phencyclidine, that cheetahs could be immobilized with reasonable safety. The inclusion of a tranquilizer in the drug mixture is essential to reduce muscular hypertonicity.

A mixture of ketamine and xylazine is an effective combination for the immobilization of cheetahs. Medetomidine, which is a more potent alpha$_2$-agonist, has replaced xylazine in the drug mixture used. The greater potency of medetomidine makes it possible to immobilize cheetahs in combination with a reduced amount of ketamine. The recovery time is shortened by reversing the effects of the tranquilizer with an antidote after 45 to 60 minutes when the ketamine effects have worn off

to a degree. Atipamizole and yohimbine, which are alpha$_2$-antagonists, are the two most commonly used antidotes.

The drug combination of tiletamine and zolazepam is commonly used for the immobilization of carnivores. It is used in cheetahs at 2 to 3 mg/kg. Higher doses may cause apnea, which lasts for 15 to 60 minutes, and the response to stimulants such as doxapram is limited in these circumstances. It is advisable to have the full backup for anesthetic emergencies available at all times when using this drug in cheetahs.

Thiopentone sodium, a barbiturate, is a useful drug for use as an adjunct to immobilization with cyclohexylamine mixtures. It results in improved muscular relaxation and the control of epileptiform convulsions when given to effect in small doses of 1 to 2 ml of a 5% injectable solution.

Darting Accidents

Although infrequent, particularly when gas-powered projectors are used, darting accidents can have severe consequences. Femoral fractures have occurred in which the dart needle appears to have penetrated the shaft of the bone. Even though the damage caused by the needle is not great, spiral fractures of the femur have been seen in two animals. This suggests that, apart from the bone lesion, an associated severe muscular spasm sheers the bone in its length. It is advisable, therefore, to avoid darting close to the femur when aiming for the large muscle masses of the hind leg.

Tranquilization

Tranquilization is seldom necessary in cheetahs because they have a quiet disposition and lack aggression, but

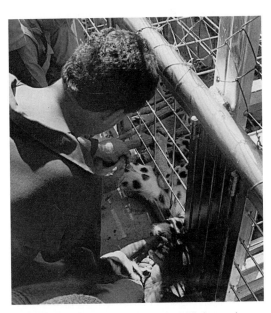

FIGURE 56–4. After restraint, the cheetah's leg can be pulled through the wire mesh and an intravenous injection given.

TABLE 56–2. Tranquilizers Used in Cheetahs

Drug	Dose/kg
Acetylpromazine	0.5–1 mg
Azaperone	0.5–1.5 mg
Medetomidine	50–100 µg
Xylazine	0.5–1 mg

it may be indicated when animals are new to an environment and are particularly anxious. The tranquilizers and dosages used are summarized in Table 56–2.

DISEASES

The lack of genetic variation and the suggested reduction in immunocompetence in cheetahs dictate that special attention be given to disease control measures and to the response of cheetahs to the treatment of disease.

Breeding groups of cheetahs should be kept as a closed population. The introduction of new animals into the facility should be undertaken with careful attention to disease prevention. All new acquisitions must be quarantined for at least 1 month. During this time, the new cheetahs must be examined thoroughly for the presence of infectious diseases and for internal and external parasites. Routine vaccinations, treatment with anthelmintics, and spraying with insecticides are part of the preparation of an animal for entry into the facility.

The management of food supplies and the control of leftover food is equally important. Rats, mice, and feral cats, which may enter the facility in search of food, are a continuous threat for the introduction of disease. Epidemics of rhinotracheitis brought in by cats are not uncommon, as are outbreaks of ringworm. Rats are a source of external parasites, and toxoplasmosis has been reported in captive cheetahs.[17]

A careful in-depth diagnostic workup should be undertaken in animals with signs of ill health. Hematologic and blood chemistry studies may be influenced by the sampling method and environmental factors, and it is advisable to collect this baseline data, which are unique to the facility, whenever possible. Published data may be used for comparison.[4, 5, 13]

Rational antibiotic therapy should be based on bacterial isolation and antibiotic sensitivities. Close monitoring of any animal in which antibiotic therapy is undertaken is essential to ensure that an optimal response is achieved.

Vaccination

In South Africa, all animals at the facility are vaccinated annually using a combined modified live vaccine for panleukopenia, infectious rhinotracheitis, and calicivirus (Felocell CVR, Pfizer Animal Health, Sandton, Republic of South Africa). Maternal antibodies have been shown to wane after 8 weeks in cheetah cubs.[16] These animals should be vaccinated at 8 weeks and 3 months of age, and then annually thereafter. In North America,

recommendations have been made that only killed vaccines be used at 6 to 8 weeks of age, at 10 to 12 weeks of age, and then annually thereafter. This is important because virulence and safety of vaccine strains may vary between manufacturers and on different continents.

Gastritis

The incidence of chronic gastritis may be high in some institutions (see Chapter 62).[7, 8] Animals suffering from gastritis lose weight, appear listless, and, often, the black spots in the skin lose color to become reddish brown. These animals tend to vomit. Immature animals are often stunted. The diagnosis is made by gastroscopic examination, a visual assessment of the condition of the gastric mucosa, and the examination of biopsy specimens taken from various areas of the stomach mucosa.

Control measures should include a gastroscopic survey of the entire cheetah population at the facility and follow-up gastroscopy of animals to assess their response to therapy.

Treatment with amoxicillin, metronidazole, and bismuth has been found to be effective. There are indications that treatment with the proton pump inhibitor, omeprazole, may result in a more rapid response, but information is limited and more investigation is needed.

Dermatomycosis

Ringworm infection within a large population of captive cheetahs, although uncommon, should be treated aggressively because infection is difficult to eradicate in large populations and signs of the infection are not easily seen in a group of animals. In some cases, animals may remain infected for several months. An epidemic in cheetahs caused by *Microsporum canis* was controlled using 0.2% enilconazole spray (Imaverol, Janssen Animal Health, Halfway House, Republic of South Africa) administered at intervals of 4 days. A 2% solution of captan (Kaptan powder, Kyron Laboratories, Benrose, Republic of South Africa) or a 0.5% solution of benzuldazic acid (Defungit, Novartis Animal Health, Isando, Republic of South Africa) has also given good results in this species. Scanning with an ultraviolet lamp is useful in identifying the presence of the active *M. canis* infections on cheetahs and other felids. The use of griseofulvin in this species may result in toxic side effects.[18]

Tuberculosis

Tuberculosis has been diagnosed in both captive and free-ranging cheetahs in southern Africa. An invasive proliferative granuloma in the lungs, from which *Mycobacterium bovis* was isolated, was seen in all of the animals. The signs in the captive animal were loss of appetite and condition with the development of dyspnea. Death followed rapidly and the diagnosis was only made postmortem.

All personnel working at the facility should be thoroughly screened to ensure that they are free from tuberculosis. Other sources of infection may be the meat fed to the animals, milk used in feeding cheetah cubs, and the visiting public.

Salmonellosis

Two epidemics of salmonellosis in captive cheetahs have resulted from infected meat being brought into the facility. In one epidemic, cheetah cubs were fed whole rabbit carcasses that had been minced. Two cubs died suddenly with a severe hemorrhagic diarrhea, and *Salmonella typhimurium* was isolated from their intestinal contents.

Infected meat from feedlot cattle carcasses was the source of infection in the second epidemic. Several cheetah cubs died of salmonellosis soon after birth. *S. typhimurium*, *Salmonella dublin*, *Salmonella muenchen*, and *Salmonella chile* were isolated from tissue collected at autopsy and in the feces of adult cheetahs. Of these, *S. typhimurium* was the most common. Antibiotic sensitivity testing showed these bacteria to be resistant to most of the commonly used antibiotics, but enrofloxacin (Baytril, Bayer Animal Health, Isando, Republic of South Africa) was identified as the antibiotic of choice. This problem was successfully controlled by ensuring adequate hygiene at the butchering of cattle that had died at the feedlot and by the treatment of pregnant cheetahs from which *Salmonella* species were found in fecal samples.

Cryptococcus neoformans

Two cases of *Cryptococcus neoformans* infection have been treated unsuccessfully in cheetahs. In a 4-year-old male, what appeared to be a subcutaneous abscess over the zygomatic arch did not respond to treatment with amoxicillin (Clamoxyl, Pfizer Animal Health, Sandton, Republic of South Africa). A biopsy sample was obtained and *C. neoformans* isolated. Treatment with nizoral (200 mg BID) was terminated when the animal stopped eating and became dehydrated, ataxia developed, and, finally, the animal was not able to walk. After supportive and fluid therapy, the animal appeared

to have recovered sufficiently and treatment with fluconazole was started. Once again, this treatment resulted in inappetence and dehydration, and the animal was euthanized when its chances of recovery were deemed to be poor. *C. neoformans* was found throughout the body. In the second case, otitis media and meningitis were treated in a two-year-old male, which was finally euthanized. Necropsy showed the cheetah to be suffering from meningeal and pulmonary cryptococcosis.

PARASITES

External Parasites

External parasites seen on captive cheetahs in South Africa are listed in Table 56–3. The two tick species that are found primarily on dogs, *Rhipicephalus sanguineus* and *Haemaphysalis leachi*, are common external parasites on cheetahs. Apart from the application of acaricides, it is important to control mice and rats that may thrive at a cheetah breeding facility because they act as hosts for these parasites.

Notoedres cati can be introduced into a facility on newly acquired animals that are not quarantined and examined carefully. It can also be introduced if rabbit carcasses are fed. Free-ranging cheetahs have died as a result of this infestation, but animals in captivity respond well to spraying with insecticide.

Hippobosca longipennis is found characteristically on cheetahs that emanate from Namibia. This parasite was imported into the De Wildt facility in 1974 and was finally eradicated several years later with the advent of synthetic pyrethroid insecticides, which were used in an intensive spraying campaign. *Hippobosca longipennis* was introduced into the United States during the 1970s.[1, 3]

Demodex was found in a skin scraping from a 1-year-old cheetah male with conjunctivitis and blepharitis. The animal was immobilized twice at an interval of 3 days and a 0.025% aqueous solution of amitraz (Triatix, Hoechst Ag-Vet, Halfway House, Republic of South Africa) applied. Recovery was uneventful.

TABLE 56–3. External Parasites Found on Captive Cheetahs

	Parasite	Common Name	Other Hosts
Fleas	*Ctenocephalides* species	Fleas	Dogs, cats, and other carnivores
	Tungu penetrans	Sand flea	Warm-blooded animals (in coastal areas)
Flies	*Stomoxys calcitrans*	Stable fly	Animals and humans
	Hippobosca longipennis	Louse fly	Wild carnivores
Lice	Not identified		
Mange	*Demodex* species	Demodectic mange	
Mites	*Notoedres cati*		Cats and rabbits
Ticks	*Rhipicephalus sanguineus*	Kennel tick	Dogs and wild carnivores; larvae and nymphae on primary host and also on mice, rats, shrews and hedgehogs
	Haemaphysalis leachi	Yellow dog tick	Dogs and wild carnivores; larvae and nymphae on mice and rats
	Amblyomma species	Bont tick	Domestic livestock and wild herbivores
	Hyalomma species	Bont-legged tick	Domestic livestock and wild herbivores

TABLE 56–4. Acaricides and Insecticides Used in Cheetahs

Compound	Trade Name	Parasite	Application
Amitraz 12.5% m/v	Triatix cattle spray (Hoechst Ag-Vet, Halfway House, Republic of South Africa)	Lice, mange mites, ticks	Spray or apply 1:500 dilution
Diazinon 30% m/v	Dazzel (Agricura, Silverton)	Fleas, lice, mites, and ticks	Spray 1:1000 dilution
Flumethrin 1% m/v	Deadline (Bayer, Isando, Republic of South Africa)	Ticks	Pour on 1 ml/5 kg at 14-day intervals
Flumethrin 2% m/v	Bayticol (Bayer, Isando, Republic of South Africa)	Ticks, flies	Spray 1:2000 dilution
Ivermectin 1% m/v	Ivomec (Logos Ag-Vet, Halfway House, Republic of South Africa)	Helminths, lice, mange mites, some ticks	Inject 200 µg/kg subcutaneously
Quinthiophos 50% m/v	Bacdip (Bayer, Isando, Republic of South Africa)	Fleas, mange mites, ticks	Spray 1:1000 dilution

M/V, mass/volume.

Other parasites may cause problems sporadically and their presence is often related to the location of the facility and, in some cases, to poor management practices. A plague of sand fleas caused several deaths from exsanguination in cheetahs kept at a facility situated in a tropical climate on the coast of South Africa.

CONTROL MEASURES

Routine spraying with acaricides is undertaken while the animals are captured in crushes. During the summer, when ticks in particular are active, spraying is done each month. During the winter, this interval is extended to once every 3 months. Regular monitoring of the animals makes it possible to adjust the intervals and the particular insecticide used to the needs of the situation at any one time. The acaricides and insecticides used on captive cheetahs in South Africa are listed in Table 56–4.

Banks of crushes are erected in strategic places within the facility for use when cheetahs that are kept in large groups are captured and sprayed with acaricides. Figure 56–5 illustrates the construction of these crushes, which accommodate up to four animals at one time.

Internal Parasites

The internal parasites of cheetahs are summarized in Table 56–5. Routine fecal analyses are conducted and anthelmintic treatment is applied when necessary. Anthelmintics are summarized in Table 56–6.

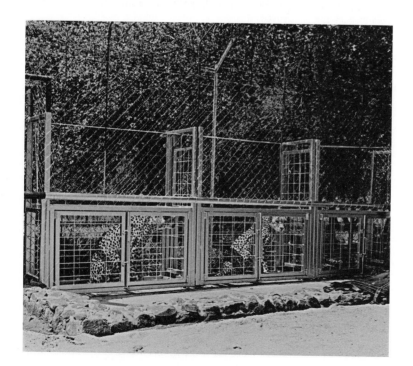

FIGURE 56–5. Cheetahs restrained in a row of crushes in preparation for spraying with acaricide.

TABLE 56–5. Helminth Parasites of Captive Cheetahs in South Africa

Nematodes

Ancylostoma species
Toxocara cati
Toxascaris leonina

Cestodes

Taenia species
Dipylidium caninum
Taenia species

NUTRITION

Basic Diet

Beef makes up the bulk of the diet fed to captive cheetahs but has the potential of being a vehicle for the introduction of disease. Meat that has been inspected by trained personnel at a recognized abattoir is preferred. It must be properly handled. Contamination of the carcass at slaughter has led to the introduction of salmonellosis into captive cheetah populations. The threat of tuberculosis or other diseases must not be overlooked. Meat obtained from feedlots may contain high levels of growth stimulants that can influence the animal's hormonal balance.

A supplement must be added to the beef. An analysis of the cheetah serum concentrations of vitamins and minerals and the levels of these in the basic diet should be undertaken. Specifications of the dietary requirements of domestic cats can be used as a guide to estimate the quantities of copper, thiamin, vitamins A and E, and essential fatty acids, commonly linoleic and linolenic acid, to be added in the supplement.[2] Fish oil as part of the formulation renders the supplement into an oily sticky paste that adheres to the meat. The ratio of calcium to phosphate in the diet must be adjusted to at least 1:1.

Adult cheetahs are fed approximately 2 kg of meat daily for 6 days and are fasted for 1 day each week. Daily feeding makes it possible to check each animal, its appetite, general condition, and state of health.

Feeding During Pregnancy and Lactation

Pregnant females should be fed an extra one third of the standard diet. During the cheetah's last month of pregnancy, the diet is changed gradually. The meat is cut into chunks and gradually changed until mince is fed. At the same time, commercial pelleted feed (Iams cat food, Spoor Products, Midrand, Republic of South Africa) is added in increasing quantities until up to 200 g is fed per day. This mixture is also fed during lactation, with an additional increase in quantity to provide for the extra needs of the female. This change in diet is made not only for the benefit of the pregnant female but also to make available a mixture that, when taken by the cubs as they grow older, is well mixed and balanced in terms of the supplement. If this is not done, osteodystrophy may develop as a result of the cubs taking meat without supplement from their mother's diet. Supplementation with copper (1 mg copper sulphate/day per cub) and thiamin (20 mg/day per cub) is essential in cubs aged 6 to 12 weeks.

Weaning takes place at 4 to 6 months and cubs are fed a mixture similar to that already discussed until they are fed the basic diet from the age of 8 to 10 months. Cubs of similar size can be kept together in groups of six to eight animals after weaning. Groups must be monitored carefully because, in some cases, animals are deprived of food as a dominance hierarchy develops and the animals compete for food.

BREEDING MANAGEMENT

A few fundamental principles govern the successful management of cheetahs to facilitate breeding in captivity.

1. Attend to the level and quality of the diet. Cheetahs are lean, active animals in nature, but, like other carnivores, they may become lazy and generally overweight in captivity.

2. Allow only intermittent contact between the sexes. When males and females are kept together for extended periods, they appear to become habituated to one another. The estrous cycle appears to be triggered

TABLE 56–6. Anthelmintics Used in Captive Cheetahs

Compound	Dose
Nematodes	
Ivermectin (Ivomec, Logos Ag-Vet, Halfway House, Republic of South Africa	200 μg/kg
Mebendazole (Telmin, Janssen Animal Health, Halfway House, Republic of South Africa)	50 mg/kg/day for 5 days—< 2-kg cubs 100 mg/kg/day for 5 days—> 2-kg
Pyrantel pamoate (Nemex-H, Pfizer Animal Health, Sandton, Republic of South Africa)	14.5–30 mg/kg
Cestodes	
Niclosamide (Lintex, Bayer, Isando, Republic of South Africa)	50 mg/kg
Praziquantel (Droncit, Bayer, Isando, Republic of South Africa)	5 mg/kg

by intermittent contact with cheetah males. Habituated cheetah males show little, if any, sexual interest in females.

3. Undertake the management of the breeding program during times when the cheetahs are less disturbed by human activity at the facility, for example, during periods when visitor numbers are low. Building programs and other activities must not be undertaken when breeding is under way.

Male Fertility

Constitutionally sound cheetah males should be used in the breeding program and they should be chosen based on their semen quality and their behavior when in contact with estrous females. Semen is collected by electroejaculation and evaluated using a standard protocol that includes examination of fresh semen after collection and an assessment of spermatozoal morphology.[6, 19–21]

Breeding behavior is assessed by observing the males when they roam freely in the access road between the female enclosures and come into contact with the females through the perimeter fence. Males that show aggression toward females should not be given direct access to females. Males that clearly show no interest in females at this time are not likely to mate if allowed into the females' enclosure.

Mating

Breeding activity is at a peak during the period from 1 hour before sunset until dark. Animals should be observed unobtrusively during this time and their activities managed with minimal human interference. It is preferable to release more than one male into the area because interaction between these animals and probably a sense of competition stimulate greater interest in the females. Males that are active and interested in the females appear to stimulate female sexual activity. At first, females move as far as possible away from any males in the road. Estrous females, however, then move to the perimeter of their enclosure adjacent to the road and attract males. Typical signs of estrus include rubbing against the fence, rolling, and lifting the tail to one side. Males are obviously interested and attempt to get to the female through the fence. They communicate with the female by making soft stuttering sounds through their nostrils and often an erection develops. A single male is allowed into the enclosure and mating occurs shortly thereafter. The pair of animals stay close together and often do not come for food during this time. After 1 to 2 days, their interest in one another wanes and the male can be let out of the enclosure into the road once again.

Observations at the De Wildt Centre have shown that cheetah females do not come into estrus when the males are first released into the area around their enclosures. The males are left in the area for 2 weeks or until it is seen that their interest has waned. They are then moved away for approximately 10 to 14 days

and brought back once again. Shortly after their arrival in the female area for the second time, cheetah females start coming into estrus. It is not uncommon to find more than one cheetah female in estrus at the same time.

The careful recording of the behavior observed during the interaction between males and females is essential because each animal's behavior and responses may differ. For example, records of observations of female behavior at De Wildt Centre have shown that some females do not show clear overt signs of estrus. Estrus may, however, be identified by a subtle change in behavior. A study of the breeding records is often the only way in which these animals can be identified and appropriate steps taken to enable successful mating when the next breeding session occurs. Pseudopregnancy is common in cheetahs after an infertile mating.

REFERENCES

1. Recent introduction of an ectoparasitic fly into North America (*Hippobosca longipennis*) on cheetahs. Foreign Animal Diseases Report October-November, 5:5–6, 1973.
2. Burger I (ed): Waltham Book of Companion Animal Nutrition. Oxford: Pergamon Press, 1993.
3. Bram RA: Alert for exotic pests (*Hippobosca longipennis*). J Am Vet Med Assoc 165:494, 496, 1974.
4. Caro TM, Holt ME, Fitzgibbon CD, et al: Health of adult free living cheetahs. J Zool (Lond) 212:573–584, 1987.
5. Hawkey CM, Hart MG: Haematological reference values for adult pumas, lions, tigers, leopards, jaguars and cheetahs. Res Vet Sci 41:268–269, 1986.
6. Howard JG, Bush M, Wildt DE, et al: Preliminary reproductive studies on cheetahs in South Africa. Proceedings of the Annual Meeting of the American Association of Zoo Veterinarians, Seattle, WA, pp 72–74, 1981.
7. Munson L: Diseases of captive cheetahs: results of the cheetah SSP pathology survey 1988–1992. Proceedings of the Annual Meeting of the American Association of Zoo Veterinarians, Oakland, CA, p 151, 1992.
8. Munson L: Diseases of captive cheetahs (*Acinonyx jubatus*): results of the cheetah research council pathology survey, 1989–1992. Zoo Biology 12:105–124, 1993.
9. O'Brien SJ, Roelke ME, Marker L, et al: Genetic basis for species vulnerability in the cheetah (mortality and feline infectious peritonitis). Science 227:1428–1434, 1985.
10. O'Brien SJ, Wildt DE, Goldman D, et al: The cheetah is depauperate in genetic variation. Science 221(4609):459–462, 1983.
11. O'Brien SJ, Wildt DE, Simonson JM, et al: On the extent of genetic variation of the African cheetah *Acinonyx jubatus*. Proceedings of the Annual Meeting of the American Association of Zoo Veterinarians, Seattle, WA, pp 74–77, 1981.
12. Pettifer HL: The experimental release of captive-bred cheetah (*Acinonyx jubatus*) into the natural environment. Proceedings of the Worldwide Furbearer Conference, Vancouver, BC, pp 1001–1026, 1981.
13. Pospisil J, Kase F, Vahala J: Basic haematological values in carnivores. 2. The Felidae. Comp Biochem Physiol [A] 87:387–391, 1987.
14. Seal US, Erickson AW: Immobilization of carnivora and other mammals with phencyclidine and promazine. Fed Proc 28(4):1410–1419, 1969.
15. Smithers RHN: The South African Red Data Book—Terrestrial Mammals. Project 125. Pretoria, South African Scientific Programmes, Foundation for Research Development, 1986.
16. Spencer JA, Burroughs R: Decline in maternal immunity and antibody response to vaccine in captive cheetah (*Acinonyx jubatus*) cubs. J Wildl Dis 28:102–104, 1992.
17. Van Rensburg IBJ, Silkstone MA: Concomitant feline infectious peritonitis and toxoplasmosis in a cheetah (*Acinonyx jubatus*). J S Afr Vet Assoc 4:205–207, 1984.
18. Wack RF, Kramer LW, Cupps W: Griseofulvin toxicity in four cheetahs (*Acinonyx jubatus*). J Zoo Wildl Med 23:442–446, 1992.

19. Wildt DE, Brown JL, Bush M, et al: Reproductive status of cheetahs (*Acinonyx jubatus*) in North American zoos: the benefits of
physiological surveys for strategic planning. Zoo Biology 12:45–
80, 1993.
20. Wildt DE, Bush M, Howard JG, et al: Unique seminal quality in

the South African cheetah and a comparative evaluation in the
domestic cat. Biol Reprod 29:1019–1025, 1983.
21. Wildt DE, O'Brien SJ, Howard JG, et al: Similarity in ejaculation-
endocrine characteristics in captive versus free ranging cheetahs of
two subspecies. Biol Reprod 35:351-360, 1986.

CHAPTER 57

Intrahepatic Cysts and Hepatic Neoplasms in Felids, Ursids, and Other Zoo and Wild Animals

K. CHRISTINA PETTAN-BREWER

LINDA J. LOWENSTINE

A variety of primary hepatic cystic and solid proliferative disorders of biliary, hepatocellular, and mesenchymal origin have been described in humans[15] and in
domestic[54] and captive wild animals of all vertebrate
orders.[41, 56, 64, 65] Some are incidental findings, whereas
others may be life-threatening. The etiology and pathogenesis of these lesions are not always certain. On the
basis of the human "model," it is thought that genetic,
infectious, dietary, iatrogenic, and environmental factors
may be involved. Because of the high incidence in
felids and ursids, these taxa receive special emphasis in
this discussion.

HEPATIC CYSTS AND CYSTADENOMAS (BILIARY CYSTADENOMA, BILE DUCT CYSTADENOMA, INTRAHEPATIC BILE DUCT CYSTADENOMA, CHOLANGIOMA)

Cystic lesions of the liver may be inflammatory, hyperplastic, or neoplastic. Of the inflammatory cysts, parasitic cysts caused by cestodes and trematodes are
common entities, particularly in wild-caught animals.
Hydatid disease caused by *Echinococcus* species is the
most common cause of parasitic cysts. Any mammalian
species can serve as an intermediate host, being infected
through ingestion of ova shed in the feces of carnivores.
These cysts may be unilocular (single) or multilocular

(compound) and may be solitary or multifocal. Diagnosis relies on identification of scolices and the characteristic histologic appearance of the cyst wall.[19] Other
cestodes (e.g., *Taenia* species) and biliary trematodes
(e.g., *Opisthorchis viverrini* and *Opisthorchis sinensis*)
can also cause hepatic cysts.[7, 32] Other hepatic inflammatory processes are rarely cystic, but there has been a
single report of *Mycobacterium avium* infection in wild
waterfowl that had multiple fluid-filled, thin-walled intrahepatic cysts.[57]

Noninfectious biliary cysts have been best described
in humans, in whom they occur in conjunction with
polycystic kidney disease inherited as either an autosomal recessive trait, which is lethal in infancy, or an
autosomal dominant trait, which is evident in adults.[20,
22, 36] Cysts may arise from either the intrahepatic or
extrahepatic bile ducts. The most accepted hypothesis
is that hepatic cysts generally arise as congenital abnormalities of the intrahepatic and extrahepatic biliary system as a result of malformation of embryonic bile ducts
that lack a connection to the main biliary system. These
bile ducts fail to involute during development and gradually undergo cystic dilatation with age. Additional predisposing factors for development of intrahepatic cysts
in humans include female gender, old age, cirrhosis,
multiple pregnancies, and contraceptive steroids.[22, 47, 62]

Solitary or multiple intrahepatic and extrahepatic
bile duct cysts have been described in animals.[61] One
of the authors (Lowenstine) has noted that multiple
biliary cysts, usually less than 2 mm in diameter, are
found in older squirrel monkeys (*Saimiri* species) and
occasionally in other nonhuman primates.

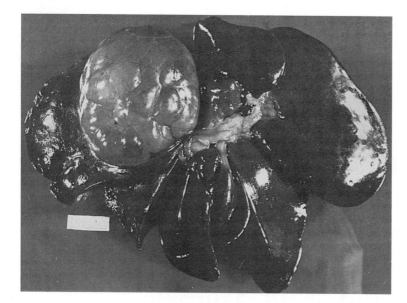

FIGURE 57–1. Liver of an elderly male dingo with a multiloculated biliary cyst.

Congenital biliary cysts in conjunction with renal and/or pancreatic cysts have been reported in a Nubian goat (*Capra hircus*)[35] and springbok (*Antidorcas marsupialis*)[31] and have been seen by one of the authors (Lowenstine) in a Barbary red deer fawn (*Cervus elaphus barbarus*). These cases resembled autosomal recessive polycystic kidney disease in human infants. A congenital extrahepatic biliary cyst was described in an 8-week-old Congo African gray parrot (*Psittacus erithacus erithacus*) with a history of abdominal enlargement since hatch.[49]

Polycystic liver disease has also been described as an incidental postmortem finding in adult white-tailed deer (*Odocoileus virginianus*),[53] red deer, and roe deer (*Capreolus capreolus*).[44] The authors have diagnosed hepatic cysts in an elderly male dingo (*Canis familiaris dingo*) (Fig. 57–1) and several felids from zoo collections.[52]

Hepatic cysts, especially if large and multifocal or multiloculated, must be distinguished from cystic hepatic neoplasms, especially biliary cystadenomas. Intrahepatic biliary cysts usually lack the extensive involvement of the parenchyma and the complexity of cystadenomas. Biliary cystadenomas are benign cystic neoplasms of the liver with an epithelial lining that produces mucinous fluid. They are believed to arise from the intrahepatic bile ducts and, less commonly, from the extrahepatic bile ducts.[54] The cystadenomas of bile ducts or ductules (cholangiomas) are composed of glandular structures and may be multilocular or papillary. They are single or multiple circumscribed tumors composed of irregularly sized tubules lined by cuboidal or flattened epithelium resembling that of the intrahepatic bile ducts.

Because of the variety and pleomorphism of developmental and congenital cysts, there is some controversy even in the literature on humans about whether true bile duct adenomas occur.[19] It is also unclear whether biliary cysts or cystadenomas are ever precancerous, although malignant transformation has occa-

sionally been documented.[10, 17] The etiology of true cystadenomas is not known, but they have been induced by carcinogenic chemicals in dogs,[3] pigs,[59] rats,[46] and rabbits.[68]

Cholangiomas associated with hemosiderosis and marked intrahepatic bile duct proliferation were reported in three lemurs (*Lemur catta, Lemur macaco,* and *Varecia varigata*).[8] Biliary cystadenomas have been identified in other primates as well, including guenons (blue monkey [*Cercopithecus mitis*] and mona monkey [*Cercopithecus mona*]) and a baboon (*Papio hamadryas papio*) and others.[38] The authors have diagnosed cystadenomas in an Asian cobra (*Naja naja*),[56] in an old privately owned llama (*llama glama*) (Fig. 57–2) and in wild felids from zoo collections.[52]

Hepatic cystic and proliferative lesions are fairly common findings in older ursids and felids including

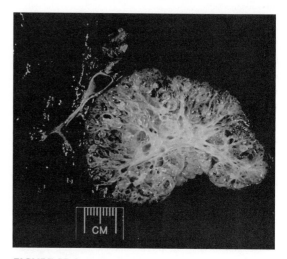

FIGURE 57–2. Biliary cystadenoma (cut surface) on the liver of an elderly llama.

domestic house cats (*Felis catus*),[55] and wild felids. In these species a spectrum of lesions from single to multiple cysts to a variety of true hepatic neoplasms are seen. Hepatic proliferative lesions in ursids and felids are discussed in detail below.

PRIMARY HEPATIC NEOPLASMS

The standard veterinary classification of primary neoplasms of the liver and biliary system is used.[32, 54]

Biliary Adenocarcinoma and Cystadenocarcinoma (Bile Duct Carcinoma, Intrahepatic Bile Duct Carcinoma, Cholangiocarcinoma)

In veterinary medicine, in contradistinction to the medical literature on humans, no distinction is made between adenocarcinomas arising from the bile ducts and those arising from the bile ductules.[12, 32, 54] Cystadenocarcinoma of the liver may either arise de novo or evolve from the malignant transformation from pre-existing cystadenomas, congenital liver cysts, and bile duct cysts,[17] and both cystadenomas and adenocarcinomas may arise in the same individual. It is not clear whether these observations apply to all species.

On gross examination, biliary adenocarcinoma is large and firm because of extensive connective tissue stroma. This feature aids in distinguishing the tumor from hepatocellular carcinoma, which tends to be soft and friable. It is usually lobulated, may extend above the surface of the liver, and may have a central depression. The tumor is frequently solid (adenocarcinoma) but may also be cystic (cystadenocarcinoma). Cystic spaces may contain mucin. The metastatic rate of biliary carcinoma is higher than that of hepatocellular carcinoma. Metastasis occurs primarily to the lung and regional lymph nodes, although widespread intrahepatic and extrahepatic metastasis are also common.

The etiology of spontaneous cystadenocarcinomas in humans and animals is unknown. An association between oral contraceptive use and biliary cystadenoma and cystadenocarcinoma with an increased level of estrogen receptor in the cystic epithelium has been observed in humans.[62] A possible association has been made in the United States between cholangiocarcinoma and host infection in humans and canids with helminths of the families Ancylostomidae and Trichuroidea.[28] Experimentally, cystadenocarcinoma (cholangiocarcinoma) has been induced in dogs given diethylnitrosamine,[29] a potent carcinogen that can be found in animal food. Similar experimental study was done in macaques with diethylnitrosamine and hepatitis B virus[26] and in rainbow trout with aflatoxin.[6] Usually, cholangiocarcinoma tends to occur spontaneously in older animals.[54] In dogs, 65% of the cases occur in animals older than 10 years.[51] In domestic cats, the occurrence of disease is also believed to be age-related.[2, 55] Cholangiocarcinoma (cystadenocarcinoma) has also been described in reptiles,[56] rodents and rabbits,[68] sheep and cattle,[54] margay

(*Felis wiedii*),[39] macaques,[38] capuchin monkey,[38] and California sea lions (*Zalophus californianus*).[30]

Hepatocellular Adenoma ("Hepatoma")

Hepatocellular adenomas are well-circumscribed, noninvasive, nonencapsulated, solitary lesions that compress the adjacent normal liver tissue. In animals, hepatomas may be single or multiple, in which case they are associated with chronic liver disease, resulting in fibrosis and nodular hyperplasia. On gross examination, these lesions are soft and light tan, sometimes with areas of red-brown hemorrhages or gray-white infarcts. Well-differentiated adenomas may be difficult to distinguish from normal liver tissue or nodular hyperplasia, except that portal structures are not present in hepatocellular adenomas.

Hepatocellular adenoma has been described in domestic and laboratory animals and exotic species, including mammals,[41, 64] birds,[65] reptiles,[56] and fish.[6] Nodular hyperplasia and hepatocellular adenomas are very common in small rodents, especially hamsters.[61]

The etiology of hepatocellular adenomas is often unknown; however, they have been associated with hepatocarcinogenic agents, including nitrosamines and aflatoxins.[58] It is reported to be the most frequent liver tumor in women worldwide who use contraceptive steroids.[47] A bacterium, *Helicobacter hepaticus*, has been associated with the spontaneous development of hepatocellular adenomas in laboratory rodents.[67]

Hepatocellular Carcinoma

The affected liver is characterized variably by discrete small lesions and large, diffuse, soft, friable, light tan to grayish masses that may be more than 10 cm in diameter.[15, 54] The larger lesions usually have an irregular shape with a multinodular surface and protrude above the surface of the liver. They are not umbilicated and may contain dark red areas of hemorrhage secondary to necrosis. On histologic examination, hepatocellular carcinoma is usually well-differentiated with malignant hepatocytes arranged in cords or trabeculae, separated by thin fibrous stroma, and abutting sinusoids. These neoplastic hepatocytes frequently produce bile, but as in adenomas, bile ductules are not present. Mitotic figures are often seen. These neoplasms may reach rather a large size before spreading by metastasis to hepatic lymph nodes and the lungs. Some hepatocellular carcinomas are so undifferentiated that the tumor cells no longer resemble hepatocytes and become difficult to identify. Sometimes, arrangement in a pseudoglandular pattern resembling ducts makes differentiation from bile duct adenocarcinoma difficult.

Hepatocellular carcinoma in humans is rare in the Western world and relatively frequent in sub-Saharan Africa and Asia, paralleling the incidence of viral hepatitis and diets high in "ground nuts." It is most frequent in males 70 to 80 years old, but in high-risk areas, age at presentation is 30 to 40 years.[20] Most human patients have long-standing alcoholic cirrhosis and/or hemochromatosis or a history of anabolic steroid use, chronic infection with hepatitis B virus (a hepadnavirus), or exposure to aflatoxins, often in diets high in peanuts.[20, 58, 69]

The etiology of spontaneous hepatocellular carcinoma in animals is not as well known. Hepadnaviruses similar to human hepatitis B virus have been associated with hepatocellular carcinomas in woodchucks[60] and ducks.[48] An association with *Schistosoma mansoni* was found in a chimpanzee.[1] Hepatocellular carcinomas experimentally induced by water or dietary exposure to diethylnitrosamine have been described in dogs,[29] and those induced by aflatoxin have been described in pigs,[59] primates,[69] rainbow trout,[6] and newborn and adult rats.[46] Aflatoxins and nitrosamines are common in the environment and may be potential causes for carcinomas in exposed zoo and wild animals. Both hepatomas and hepatocellular carcinomas have been reported in lemurs (*Lemur, Varecia,* and *Microcebus* species) and in zoo birds with hemosiderosis or hemochromatosis, but a causal relationship has not yet been proved.[3, 14, 38, 65] Other species with spontaneous hepatocellular carcinomas have included primates,[9, 38] dogs,[51] cats,[50] cows, fowl, and sheep.[54] These tumors are more frequent in older individuals in most species, but they have been reported in sheep and pigs less than 1 year old.[55, 59]

Hemangiosarcoma and Other Mesenchymal Tumors

The liver is a relatively uncommon primary site for hemangiosarcoma in comparison with other organs, but it is a relatively common site for metastasis of hemangiosarcoma from other organs, such as the spleen. Hepatic hemangiosarcomas are usually single, but intrahepatic metastasis may occur. Numerous blood-filled cystic spaces may be present in this tumor. Hemangiosarcoma must be distinguished from hemangioma, vascular hamartoma, and acquired telangiectasia or peliosis hepatis.[54]

In humans, endogenous and exogenous female sex hormones may have a role in development of hepatic vascular tumors. In addition, angiosarcoma (angioblastoma) of the liver in humans is associated with exposure to arsenic in chemical manufacturing facilities and pesticides, to vinyl chloride in plastic factories, and to Thorotrast (thorium dioxide), formerly used as contrast medium in radiography.[20]

In domestic cats, a study with 47 animals, 11% of nonepithelial intrahepatic neoplasms were metastatic hemangiosarcomas.[50] Hepatic vascular proliferations have been reported in marsupials[12] and in a palm civet (*Nandinia binotata*) which also had a hepatocellular carcinoma.[41] Domestic ferrets (*Mustela putorius furo*) seem especially predisposed to development of this neoplasm.[16]

Other sarcomas of the liver in domestic animals are very rare, and only a few have been reported as primary growths: leiomyosarcoma, fibrosarcoma, and osteosarcoma.[54, 55] In rodents, fibrosarcomas in the liver have been associated with parasitism by the *Cysticercus fasciolaris* larvae from the cestode *Taenia taeniaeformis*.[32]

Myelolipoma of the liver has been reported in domestic and captive wild felids[37] but not in other species of domestic animals.[32, 54] A report of myelolipomas in captive wild cats described seven cases, mostly in cheetahs, which suggests a species predilection.[37] Myelolipomas have also been seen occasionally in other zoo animals, such as in marsupials.[12] The authors and others have noted these tumors in Goeldi's marmoset (*Callimico goeldii*).

HEPATIC PROLIFERATIVE DISEASES IN URSIDS

Among captive wild mammals, ursids, particularly Asian bear species, seem overrepresented with regard to the occurrence of hepatic neoplasms. Biliary adenoma was described as an incidental finding in an old adult male Eurasian brown bear (*Ursus arctos*)[25] and a hepatoma presumed to be associated with aflatoxins has been described in a male Kodiak bear (*Ursus arctos middendorffi*).[64]

Biliary adenocarcinomas have been described in grizzly bears (*Ursus arctos horribilis*),[18, 43] polar bears (*Thalarctos maritimus*),[40] Malayan sun bear (*Helarctos malayanus*), and sloth bears (*Melursus ursinus*).[11, 18, 24, 34, 43] One Asiatic black bear (*Selenarctos thibetanus*) had both biliary and hepatocellular carcinomas.[21] Reports of two bears with primary hepatic neoplasms were found in the authors' files: a sloth bear with biliary adenocarcinoma (Fig. 57–3) and an American black bear with widely metastatic liver carcinoma.

Biliary adenocarcinomas in Asiatic bears commonly are of extrahepatic biliary origin and metastasize, often to the pancreas.[24, 42] Environmental and management factors, including dietary factors,[11] aflatoxins,[40] or hereditary factors, have been implicated, especially in sloth bears, which are largely insectivorous in the wild.[24] The incidence of hepatic neoplasms in aged wild bears has not yet been investigated, and comparisons between wild and captive populations may shed light on the pathogenesis of these tumors.

Interestingly, ursids produce a fairly unique bile acid, ursodeoxycholic acid (ursodiol),[27] which is being used increasingly in human medicine to treat gallstones, chronic biliary cirrhosis, cystic fibrosis, and other chole-

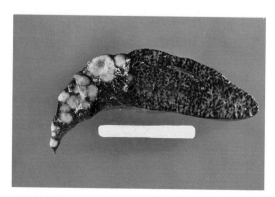

FIGURE 57–3. Liver (cut surface) of a sloth bear with intrahepatic metastatic biliary adenocarcinoma.

static liver diseases (over 700 references in University of California libraries' medical data base since 1989). It has also been found to be protective against colon cancer in experimental rodent models.[66] Whether these observations have relevance to the incidence of hepatic neoplasms in ursids remains to be seen.

HEPATIC PROLIFERATIVE DISEASES IN NONDOMESTIC FELIDS

Neoplasia is common in felids, both domestic and wild. Single or multiple nonparasitic intrahepatic cysts are considered to be an incidental postmortem finding in older domestic cats.[55] There is some confusion in the literature about the true nature of these lesions; other authors have called them *biliary cystadenomas* and suggested that they are an age-related proliferation of acquired biliary diverticula and are not precancerous.[2] A retrospective study of liver tumors in domestic cats revealed that biliary epithelial tumors are more common than those of hepatocytes and suggested that bile duct adenomas are precancerous.[50] Similar lesions have been seen in exotic felids presented to the Veterinary Medical Teaching Hospital pathology service at the University of California, Davis. To better understand the incidence, significance, and pathogenesis of liver cysts and tumors in nondomestic felids, the authors conducted a multi-institutional retrospective study.[52] Necropsy data from over 700 zoo-housed wild felids were reviewed. Of these animals, 4.5% had liver cysts or neoplasms, the majority of which (89%) were multifocal benign cysts or cyst adenomas. Malignancies identified included biliary cystadenocarcinomas and hepatocellular carcinomas. This study also identified other hepatic lesions, including several cases of veno-occlusive disease in species other than cheetahs or snow leopards and varying degrees of sinusoidal ectasia or telangiectasia; these lesions were examined as possible predisposing factors for hepatic cysts.

In addition to hepatic lesions, many other neoplasms or proliferative disorders were identified in cats in this study, several of which had more than one tumor type. These disorders included uterine and/or cervical leiomyomas; thyroid/parathyroid cystic hyperplasia, cystadenomas, and adenocarcinomas; pheochromocytomas; myelolipomas; ovarian papillary cystadenocarcinomas; pulmonary adenocarcinomas; pleural mesothelioma; lymphosarcoma with leukemia; mammary fibrosarcoma with metastases; pancreatic carcinoma; insulinoma; renal carcinoma; bladder leiomyoma; esophageal squamous cell carcinoma; Sertoli cell tumor; adrenal nodular hyperplasia; and myeloproliferative disease.

Hepatic cysts and cyst adenomas were usually incidental lesions diagnosed at postmortem examination in both domestic and wild cats, although in two cases in the authors' survey, ultrasonography or radiography had been used to make antemortem diagnoses. In contrast, animals with hepatocellular or biliary neoplasms had elevated liver enzymes or jaundice, and liver failure had prompted euthanasia.

On gross and histologic examination, the hepatic cysts and neoplasms resembled those reported in humans, dogs, and domestic cats. The cyst lining was confirmed to be of biliary origin by immunohistochemistry and electron microscopy studies. Immunohistochemistry was also used to confirm the histogenesis of the biliary cystadenocarcinomas and hepatocellular carcinomas.

The cysts were filled with clear to straw-colored, watery to mucinous fluid that occasionally contained mucopurulent exudate. In addition, blood-filled lesions, thought to be hematomas arising from telangiectatic foci, could be demonstrated by immunohistochemistry and electron microscopy to be the result of hemorrhage into biliary cysts.

The pathogenesis of cysts and neoplasms in nondomestic felids remains uncertain. These lesions appear predominantly in older animals (median age, 16 to 20 years), as has been observed in domestic cats. Among cats in this study with hepatic cysts and neoplasms, lions and leopards were significantly more affected than were other species. Although a heritable predisposition could not be proved, the institution from which the cats were reported or from which they originated was a significant association. This was not just a result of surveillance, as smaller collections without internal pathology departments were overrepresented. In contrast to humans, in which females treated with contraceptive steroids are at risk of developing hepatic cysts, there was no sex predisposition or association with contraceptive administration in wild felids in this study. This may be because the contraceptives used in zoo felids are progestogens, not estrogens.[4] Also in contrast to humans, hepatic cysts did not occur in the context of polycystic kidney disease. The data were insufficient for deciding whether cystadenomas were precancerous in wild felids or not.

There was no association in this study with parasites, hepatobiliary inflammation, fibrosis, cirrhosis, or veno-occlusive disease. Veno-occlusive disease was diagnosed in five leopards, two lions, one tiger, and one cheetah in this study. Veno-occlusive disease, best studied in cheetahs and snow leopards, occurs in U.S. zoos, ostensibly in association with the feeding of commercially prepared diets.[45] As mentioned, hepatobiliary tumors in bears are believed to be a result of environmental, especially dietary, factors; however, in this study, no association between type of diet and cystic lesions or hepatic neoplasms was found in the captive wild felids.

DIAGNOSIS OF HEPATIC CYSTS AND PROLIFERATIVE LESIONS

The diagnosis of hepatic cysts and neoplasms in humans is usually established by surgical exploration for a defined abdominal mass or by radiography, ultrasonography, computed tomography, magnetic resonance imaging, or percutaneous needle biopsy. Constitutional signs of illness, including jaundice, elevated levels of liver enzymes, or evidence of liver failure, are much more common in animals with malignancies but occur late in the course of disease. An increased awareness of the incidence of these tumors in zoo animals and routine physical examinations with abdominal palpation and ultrasonography or radiography may help identify more cases ante mortem.

TREATMENT AND PREVENTION

Several methods of therapy and prevention for hepatic proliferative lesions have been described and applied in human medicine, such as prevention of viral diseases that affect the liver (e.g., hepatitis B virus),[20, 58] withdrawal of contraceptives in women,[47] percutaneous drainage, surgery or albendazole therapy in parasitic cysts,[33] treatment with fluorodeoxyuridine and mitomycin,[5] enucleation, cyst aspiration or surgical excision of single lesions,[36] intraluminal brachytherapy,[23] and conservative or nonconservative surgical excision of neoplasms.[13]

The wisdom of applying several of these methods of treatment in zoo and wild animals is questionable, although some of them can be useful. Supportive therapy, in the form of administration of multiple vitamin B supplements, was shown to mildly improve the clinical status of a captive Asiatic black bear.[21] Surgical treatment of hepatic cysts and cystadenomas has been applied in domestic animals[63] and might be applied to zoo or wild animals in some cases.

CONCLUSIONS

Although hepatic cysts and neoplasms are well documented in captive wild animals, particularly ursids and felids, much more work needs to be done to confirm diagnosis and exact etiology and to dictate prophylactic or therapeutic possibilities. The lesions in felids are mostly benign, incidental, and not generally associated with mortality, although they may contribute to disability in elderly animals. In bears, however, the lesions are frequently malignant and lethal. As such, they may limit successful management, particularly of Asiatic bears, and are a concern of the Ursid Taxon Advisory Group. Areas for further investigation include identification of the occurrence of these lesions in free-ranging populations of bears, as well as investigations into the roles of diet, viruses, genetic factors such as altered tumor suppressor genes or expression of oncogenes, and association with ursodeoxycholic acid.

REFERENCES

1. Abe K, Kagei N, Teramura Y, et al: Hepatocellular carcinoma associated with chronic *Schistosoma mansoni* infection in a chimpanzee. J Med Primatol 22:234–239, 1993.
2. Adler R, Wilson DW: Biliary cystadenoma of cats. Vet Pathol 32(4):415–418, 1995.
3. Alison JB, Wase AW, Leathem JW, et al: Some effects of 2-acetylaminofluorene on the dog. Cancer Res 10:266–271, 1950.
4. Asa CH, Porton I: Concerns and prospects for contraception in carnivores. Proceedings of the annual meeting of the American Association of Zoo Veterinarians, Calgary, Alberta, Canada, pp 298–303, 1991.
5. Atiq OT, Kemeny N, Niedzwiecki D, et al: Treatment of unresectable primary liver cancer with intrahepatic fluorodeoxyuridine and mitomycin C through an implantable pump. Cancer 69:920–924, 1992.
6. Bailey GS, Williams DE, Hendricks JD: Fish models for environmental carcinogenesis: the rainbow trout. Envir Health Perspec 104(Suppl):15–21, 1995.
7. Barker IK, VanDreumel AA, Palmer N: The alimentary system. *In* Jubb K, Kennedy PC, Palmer N (eds): Pathology of Domestic Animals, 4th ed. New York, Academic Press, pp 258–316, 1995.
8. Benirschke K, Miller C, Ippen R, Heldstab A: The pathology of prosimians, especially lemurs. Adv Vet Sci Comp Med 30:167–208, 1985.
9. Borda JT, Ruiz JC, Sanchez-Negrette M: Spontaneous hepatocellular carcinoma in *Saimiri boliviensis*. Vet Pathol 33:724–726, 1996.
10. Callea F, Sergi C, Fabbretti G, et al: Precancerous lesions of the biliary tree. J Surg Oncol Suppl 3:131–133, 1993.
11. Canfield PJ, Bellamy T, Blyde D, et al: Pancreatic lesions and hepatobiliary neoplasia in captive bears. J Zoo Wildl Med 21:471–475, 1990.
12. Canfield PJ, Hartley WJ: A survey and review of hepatobiliary lesions in Australian macropods. J Comp Path 107:147–167, 1992.
13. Cherqui D: Treatment of benign tumors of the liver. Rev Prat 42:1616–1619, 1992.
14. Cork SC, Stockdale PHG: Carcinoma with concurrent hemosiderosis in an Australian bittern (*Botaurus poidiloptilus*). Avian Pathol 24:207–213, 1995.
15. Craig JR, Peters RL, Edmondson HA: Tumors of the liver and intrahepatic bile ducts. *In* Atlas of Tumor Pathology. Washington, DC, U.S. Armed Forces Institute of Pathology, pp 44–51, 1990.
16. Cross BM: Hepatic vascular neoplasms in a colony of ferrets. Vet Pathol 24(1):94–96, 1987.
17. Cruickshank AH, Sparshott SM: Malignancy in natural and experimental hepatic cysts—experiments with aflatoxin in rats and the malignant transformation of cysts in human livers. J Pathol 104:185–190, 1971.
18. Dorn CR: Biliary and hepatic carcinomas in bears at the San Diego Zoological Gardens. Nature 202:513–514, 1964.
19. Edmondson HA: Tumors of the Liver and Intrahepatic Bile Ducts. Washington, DC, U.S. Armed Forces Institute of Pathology, 1958.
20. Farber E, Phillips MJ, Kaufman N: Pathogenesis of Liver Diseases. Sydney, Australia, International Academy of Pathology, 1987.
21. Fitzgerald, SD: Clinical challenge. J Zoo Wildl Med 27(3):428–431, 1996.
22. Gabow PA, Johnson AM, Kaehny WD, et al: Risk factors for the development of hepatic cysts in autosomal dominant polycystic kidney disease. Hepatology 11:1033–1037, 1990.
23. Goldschmidt RP, Kotzen JA, Giraud RM: Intraductal hepatocellular carcinoma treated by intraluminal brachytherapy. Clin Oncol (R Coll Radiol) 5:118–119, 1993.
24. Gosselin SJ, Kramer LW: Extrahepatic biliary carcinoma in sloth bears. J Am Vet Med Assoc 185:1314–1316, 1984.
25. Griner LA: Pathology of Zoo Animals. San Diego, CA, Zoological Society of San Diego, 1983.
26. Gyorkey F: Experimental carcinoma of liver in macaque monkeys exposed to diethylnitrosamine and hepatitis B virus. J Natl Cancer Inst 59:1451–1467, 1977.
27. Hagey LR, Crombie DL, Espinosa E, et al: Ursodeoxycholic acid in Ursidae: bile acids of bears, pandas and related carnivores. J Lipid Res 34:1911–1917, 1993.
28. Hayes HM, Morin MM, Rubenstein DA: Canine biliary carcinoma: epidemiological comparison with man. J Comp Pathol 93:99–107, 1983.
29. Hirao K, Matsumara K, Imagawa A, et al: Primary neoplasms in dog liver induced by diethylnitrosamine. Cancer Res 34:1870–1882, 1974.
30. Howard EB, Britt JO, Simpson JG: Neoplasms in marine mammals. *In* Howard EB (ed): Pathobiology of Marine Mammal Diseases, vol 2. Boca Raton, FL, CRC Press, pp 95–162, 1983.
31. Iverson W, Fetterman G, Jacobson E, et al: Polycystic kidney and liver disease in springbok: I. Morphology of the lesions. Kidney Int 22:146–155, 1982.
32. Kelly WR: The liver and biliary system. *In* Jubb K, Kennedy PC, Palmer N (eds): Pathology of Domestic Animals, 4th ed. New York, Academic Press, pp 319–406, 1995.
33. Khuroo MS, Dar MY, Boda MI, et al: Percutaneous drainage versus albendazole therapy in hepatic hydatidosis: a prospective, randomized study. Gastroenterology 104:1452–1459, 1993.
34. Kingston RS, Wright FW: Bile duct carcinoma with widespread metastases in a sloth bear. J Zoo Anim Med 16:16–20, 1985.
35. Krotec K, Smith Meyer B, Freeman W, et al: Congenital cystic disease of the liver, pancreas, and kidney in a Nubian goat (*Capra hircus*). Vet Pathol 33:708–710, 1996.

36. Lerner ME, Roshkow JE, Smithline A, et al: Polycystic liver disease with obstructive jaundice: treatment with ultrasound-guided cyst aspiration. Gastrointest Radiol 17:46–48, 1992.

37. Lombard LS, Fortna HM, Garner FM, et al: Myelolipomas of the liver in captive wild felidae. Vet Pathol 5:127–134, 1968.

38. Lowenstine LJ: Neoplasms and proliferative disorders in nonhuman primates. *In* Benirschke K (ed): Primates—The Road to Self-Sustaining Populations. New York, Springer-Verlag, pp 781–814, 1986.

39. McClure HM, Chang J, Golarz MN: Cholangiocarcinoma in a margay (*Felis wiedii*). Vet Pathol 14:510–512, 1977.

40. Miller RE, Boever WJ, Thornburg LP, Curtis-Velasso M: Hepatic neoplasia in two polar bears. J Am Vet Med Assoc 187:1256–1258, 1985.

41. Montali RJ: An overview of tumors in zoo animals. *In* Montali RJ, Migaki G (eds): The Comparative Pathology of Zoo Animals. Washington, DC, Smithsonian Institution Press, pp 531–542, 1980.

42. Montali RJ, Hoopes PJ, Bush M: Extrahepatic biliary carcinomas in Asiatic bears. J Natl Cancer Inst 66:603–608, 1981.

43. Moulton JE: Bile duct carcinomas in two bears. Cornell Vet 51:285–293, 1961.

44. Munro R: Intrahepatic biliary cysts in deer. J Comp Pathol 105:105–107, 1991.

45. Munson L, Worley MB: Veno-occlusive disease in snow leopards (*Panthera uncia*) from zoological parks. Vet Pathol 28:37–45, 1991.

46. Naidu NR, Sehgal S, Bhaskar KV, et al: Cystic disease of the liver following prenatal and perinatal exposure to aflatoxin B1 in rats. J Gastroenterol Hepatol 6:359–362, 1991.

47. Olesen, LL, Vyberg M, Kruse V, et al: Hepatocellular adenoma after oral contraception. Ugeskr Laeger 154:2820–2823, 1992.

48. Omata M, Uchiumi K, Ito Y, et al: Duck hepatitis B virus and liver diseases. Gastroenterology 85:260–267, 1983.

49. Opengart KN, Brown TP, Osofsky SA, et al: Congenital extrahepatic biliary cyst in a Congo African grey parrot (*Psittacus erithacus erithacus*). Avian Dis 34:497–500, 1990.

50. Patnaik AK: A morphologic and immunocytochemical study of hepatic neoplasms in cats. Vet Pathol 29:405–415, 1992.

51. Patnaik AK, Lieberman PH, Hurvitz AI, et al: Canine hepatocellular carcinoma. Vet Pathol 18:427–438, 1981.

52. Pettan-Brewer KC, Lowenstine LJ, MacManamon R, et al: Biliary cysts and proliferative hepatic lesions in captive wild felids. Proceedings of the annual meeting of the American Association of Zoo Veterinarians, St. Louis, pp 214–219, 1993.

53. Picone JW, Williams JF, Wesley LR, et al: Polycystic liver disease in four white tailed deer. J Wildl Dis 17:395–400, 1981.

54. Popp, JA: Tumors of the liver, gall bladder, and pancreas. *In* Moulton JE (ed): Tumors in Domestic Animals. Berkeley, University of California Press, pp 436–457, 1995.

55. Post G, Patnaik AK: Nonhematopoietic hepatic neoplasms in cats: 21 cases (1983–1988). J Am Vet Med Assoc 201:1080–1082, 1992.

56. Ramsay EC, Munson L, Lowenstine LJ, Fowler ME: A retrospective study of neoplasia in a collection of captive snakes. J Zoo Wildl Med 27(1):28–34, 1996.

57. Roffe, TJ: 1989. Isolation of *Mycobacterium avium* from waterfowl with polycystic livers. Avian Dis 33:195–198.

58. Saracco G: Primary liver cancer is of multifactorial origin: importance of hepatitis B virus infection and dietary aflatoxin. J Gastroenterol Hepatol 10:604–608, 1995.

59. Shalkop WT, Armbrecht BH: Carcinogenic response of brood sows fed aflatoxin for 28 to 30 months. Am J Vet Res 35:623–627, 1974.

60. Snyder RL, Tyler G, Summers J: Chronic hepatitis and hepatocellular carcinoma associated with woodchuck hepatitis virus. Am J Pathol 107:422–425, 1992.

61. Somvanshi R, Iyer PKR, Biswas JC, et al: Polycystic liver disease in golden hamsters. J Comp Pathol 97:615–618, 1987.

62. Suyama Y, Horie Y, Suou T: Oral contraceptives and intrahepatic cysts and biliary cystadenomas having an increased level of estrogen receptor. Hepatogastroenterology 35:171–174, 1988.

63. Trout NJ, Berg RJ, McMillan MC, et al: Surgical treatment of hepatobiliary cystadenomas in cats. J Am Vet Med Assoc 206(4):505–507, 1995.

64. Wadsworth JR, Williamson WM: Neoplasms from captive wild species. J Am Vet Med Assoc 137:424–425, 1960.

65. Wadsworth PF, Majeed SK, Brancker WM, Jones DM: Some hepatic neoplasms in non-domesticated birds. Avian Pathol 7:551–555, 1978.

66. Wale RK, Frawley BP Jr, Hallmann S, et al: Mechanism of action of chemoprotective ursodeoxycholate in the azoxymethane model of rat colonic carcinogenesis. Cancer Res 55:5257–5264, 1995.

67. Ward JM, Fox JG, Anver MR, et al: Chronic active hepatitis and associated liver tumors in mice caused by a persistent bacterial infection with a novel *Helicobacter* sp. J Natl Cancer Inst 86:1222–1227, 1994.

68. Weisbroth SH. Neoplastic diseases. *In* Weisbroth SH, Flatt RE, Kraus AL (eds): The Biology of the Laboratory Rabbit. New York, Academic Press, pp 332–375, 1974.

69. Yan RQ, Su JJ, Huang DR, et al: Human hepatitis B virus and hepatocellular carcinoma: II. Experimental induction in tree shrews exposed to hepatitis B virus and aflatoxin B1. J Cancer Res Clin Oncol 122:289–295, 1996.

CHAPTER 58

Chemical Restraint and Immobilization of Wild Canids

TERRY J. KREEGER

Wild canids (family Canidae) are widely distributed throughout the world from deserts to the Arctic. Indeed, the gray wolf (*Canis lupus*) has the greatest natural range of any living terrestrial mammal other than humans. There are 16 genera containing 36 species.

Weights range from 1 kg (fennec fox. [*Fennecus zerda*]) to 80 kg (gray wolf).[43]

This chapter addresses chemical restraint and immobilization of canids, with discussion of physical means as appropriate. Canids are relatively easily immobilized and appear to respond physiologically in a similar manner to tranquilizers and anesthetics. Fortunately, adverse reactions are rare and are more of a result of the capture method than of the drugs used. Dozens of studies on canid immobilization have been reported in the literature, including reviews.[23, 24] The pharmacology of immobilizing drugs, equipment to administer drugs, methods of capturing, handling, and monitoring the patient, and medical concerns are considered here.

DRUGS USED FOR RESTRAINT AND IMMOBILIZATION

Neuromuscular Blocking Drugs

Neuromuscular blocking (NMB) drugs are some of the earliest drugs used for the chemical immobilization of canids.[12] There are two classes of NMB drugs—competitive and depolarizing. Competitive NMB drugs result in flaccid paralysis, whereas depolarizing NMB drugs cause an initial transient rapid firing of the muscles, which is quickly replaced by general paralysis. Overdosage of either class of drug results in diaphragmatic paralysis and death by asphyxia. The effects of competitive NMB drugs can be antagonized by anticholinesterase agents, but the effect of the antagonist may be dissipated before complete elimination or metabolism of the NMB drug, resulting in recycling and renewed paralysis. Also, overdosing resulting in death is possible with anticholinesterase drugs.

There are two major deficiencies of NMB drugs: (1) they have a low therapeutic index, and dosage errors of only 10% can result in either no effect or death; (2) they are virtually devoid of central nervous system effects. Thus, an animal paralyzed with NMB drugs is conscious, aware of its surroundings, fully sensory, and, as such, can feel pain and experience psychogenic stress but is physically unable to react. Although still used by some biologists and animal control personnel to capture feral dogs,[12] NMB drugs are not recommended for use on canids because superior modern drugs are available.

Opioids

Opioids have been used for animal immobilization since the 1960s and are the most potent drugs available for this purpose. Potential opioids for canid immobilization include fentanyl, etorphine, carfentanil, sufentanil, A3080, and butorphanol. Although these opioids have been used to immobilize a variety of wild canids,[1, 15, 17, 31, 34, 62] they are generally not recommended because of their adverse effects and the extraordinary safety and efficacy of cyclohexane combinations. The major drawback with the opioids is respiratory depression. For example, the author was unable to determine an effective immobilizing dose of carfentanil in wolves that did not also cause complete respiratory arrest for at least 1 minute. Sufentanil also caused prolonged apnea but not in all wolves at all doses. Although opioid "recycling" or "renarcotization" is seen more commonly with ungulates, it has been documented in wolves given sufen-

tanil,[31] and it is assumed that the same would apply to the more potent carfentanil.

A3080 is a synthetic opioid not yet on the market but undergoing the approval process. The potency of A3080 appears to be somewhat less than carfentanil but more than etorphine.[38] A3080 has been shown to be effective on ungulates; its usefulness for canid immobilization has not been determined. Butorphanol is a morphine analog that has mixed agonist-antagonist properties. Alone, butorphanol provides only "apathetic sedation," but when combined with xylazine, it is capable of immobilizing canids.[29]

Cyclohexanes

Also termed *cyclohexamines* or *dissociative anesthetics,* cyclohexanes (ketamine, tiletamine, phencyclidine) are the most widely used drugs for wildlife immobilization because of their efficacy and high therapeutic index, so their use is emphasized in this chapter. Phencyclidine is the most potent of these drugs but is no longer available in the United States because of abuse. Tiletamine is unavailable as a single product; it is combined in equal proportions with the diazepinone tranquilizer zolazepam (as Telazol, or Zoletil). The relative potencies of phencyclidine, tiletamine, and ketamine are approximately 5:2.5:1, respectively.[8]

If used alone, the cyclohexanes can cause rough inductions and recoveries, and convulsions are not uncommon. Thus, they are usually administered concurrently with tranquilizers. There is no complete antagonist for the cyclohexanes, although several drugs appear to overcome some of their effects.[32]

Tranquilizers

Tranquilizers are used primarily in wildlife immobilization as adjuncts to primary immobilizing agents (opioids, cyclohexanes) to hasten and smooth induction and recovery and to reduce the amount of the primary agent required to achieve immobilization. Phenothiazine tranquilizers (promazine, acepromazine), sometimes referred to as neuroleptics, are used frequently in combination with ketamine to anesthetize canids, although promazine is temporarily off the market in the United States.

Azaperone is a butyrophenone neuroleptic reported to counteract narcotic respiratory depression in wild animals.[40] Azaperone combined with fentanyl has been shown to be effective on some carnivores[63] and should be useful in canids. Benzodiazepine derivatives (midazolam, diazepam) are used primarily as anticonvulsant adjuncts to the cyclohexane anesthetics and are also excellent muscle relaxants. Benzodiazepines are useful in small canids,[36] but large canids, such as wolves, require large volumes when given intramuscularly (IM) to exert a beneficial effect.

Alpha-adrenergic agonists are potent tranquilizers that can be completely antagonized. They are usually used as adjuncts with cyclohexanes to hasten and smooth anesthetic induction, but they are capable of heavily sedating canids to the point of relatively safe handling.[25, 33] However, animals sedated solely with alpha-adrenergic agonists can generally be aroused with stimulation and are capable of directed attack. Caution should always be exercised in such situations, even though the animals appear harmless.

Antagonists

Some of the more notable pharmacologic developments relative to wild animal immobilization have been specific, long-lasting opioid and alpha$_2$-adrenergic antagonists. The ability to antagonize anesthesia and return the animal more quickly to physiologic normalcy offers many advantages, including (1) quicker restoration of any oxygen desaturation; (2) expedited correction of metabolic imbalances; (3) alleviation of problems associated with prolonged recumbency, such as nerve and muscle damage or hypothermia; (4) reduced probability of injury or death after recovery due to accident because there is no residual sedation or ataxia; (5) decreased probability of rejection or interspecific strife as a result of quicker return to parent or pack; and (6) decreased personnel and equipment time dedicated to monitoring the recovery process.

In general, opioid and alpha$_2$-adrenergic antagonists are safe, causing adverse effects only at higher doses. It should be remembered that antagonists act on the animal and not on the agonist. Thus, it does not necessarily follow that the more potent the agonist, the greater the amount of antagonist that needs to be administered. Increasing the dose of an antagonist usually does not decrease recovery times,[26] but higher doses could prolong antagonism by maintaining serum concentrations at higher levels. The preferred route for both opioid and alpha$_2$-adrenergic antagonists is intravenous (IV) administration, which provides the most rapid recovery. A slower (10 to 15 minutes) recovery occurs with IM injection.[60] A common practice is to give equal doses of the antagonist both IV and IM or subcutaneously (SQ).

Early opioid antagonists included nalorphine, levallorphan, pentazocine, nalbuphine, and diprenorphine. Some of these antagonists exhibit agonistic properties at higher doses, such as respiratory depression. Naloxone, nalmefene, and naltrexone are preferred antagonists because they exhibit only antagonistic properties at all opioid receptors.

Alpha-adrenergic antagonists are used to antagonize tranquilizers such as xylazine, detomidine, and medetomidine. Although both idazoxan and atipamezole are used for the antagonism of xylazine, only atipamezole should be used to antagonize the effects of medetomidine because yohimbine, tolazoline, and idazoxan may result in incomplete antagonism.

Benzodiazepine antagonists have been used on canids but, in and of themselves, do not appear to decrease immobilization times[39] or exert significant physiologic effects.[28]

Two drugs—4-aminopyridine and doxapram—appear to have some antagonist action against some anesthetics. They are not true antagonists in that they do not operate on the same receptors as do the agonists. None-theless, on administration of the drugs, a heightened level of arousal is often reported. Although they are incapable of effecting complete recovery in the anesthetized animal, they can help diminish some adverse effects of the anesthetic by increasing respiration or cardiovascular function. 4-aminopyridine has been used to antagonize a variety of chemical immobilizing agents; it can be used alone or as an adjunct to other antagonists, such as yohimbine.[19] Doxapram has been used to counteract xylazine sedation and to shorten barbiturate anesthesia in dogs. Its primary use is to stimulate respiration in cases of hypoventilation or apnea caused by injectable anesthetics, including ketamine (T. J. Kreeger, unpublished data, May, 1988) and carfentanil.[2]

Adjuvants

Adjuvants are substances added to drugs that affect the action of the main ingredient in a predictable way. They may be added to immobilizing drugs to decrease undesirable effects or to heighten desirable effects. Atropine and glycopyrrolate are often used to decrease salivation caused by cyclohexanes[34] or to increase heart rate depressed by alpha$_2$-adrenergic agonists.[25] Adjuvants should be used conservatively, however, because they are capable of producing undesirable effects if used incorrectly. For example, atropine increases heart rate and should be used judiciously when the animal has already been given other drugs that have cardioacceleratory properties, such as ketamine and yohimbine.[14]

EQUIPMENT AND TECHNIQUES FOR ADMINISTERING DRUGS

Oral Administration

Oral administration of drugs is usually not appropriate to capture wild canids. Effective doses are difficult to predict, and inductions are usually prolonged. There may be circumstances, however, in which an animal cannot be captured or darted. The author and colleagues have successfully immobilized a gray wolf by placing concentrated tiletamine-zolazepam (500 mg/2 ml) in bait. Phencyclidine has been used to sedate hyenas, but induction was lengthy (6 to 7 hours).[47]

Hand Injection

Wild canids are often physically restrained with a catch pole, forked stick, or large fishing net before drug administration. These techniques work for animals caught in foothold traps or, in captive situations, for those that have been maneuvered into a corner or kennel box. Once restrained, drugs can be safely and effectively administered either by hand or pole syringe. Small canids are probably best given injections by hand syringe to ensure accurate placement. For large or aggressive canids, a pole syringe (1 to 2 m) is the safest method. Large-bore needles (16 to 18 gauge) should be used to inject the drug rapidly into the large muscle masses of the hindquarters.

Blow Pipes

Blow pipes, whether powered by lung or compressed air/carbon dioxide, can effectively deliver immobilizing drugs to canids. Although used mostly on captive animals, blow pipes can be used to dart trapped canids. Darts used in blow pipes are generally limited to less than 3-ml volumes, which restricts their use to potent drugs or drugs that can be concentrated. Such darts also deliver their contents as a result of expanding compressed air or gas. This process normally takes 1 to 2 seconds to deliver all the drug during which canids are capable of removing the dart before the drug has been completely delivered. One company (Pneu-Dart) makes a blow pipe for its powder-charged, 0.50-caliber darts, which expel their contents in about 0.001 seconds, but volumes are limited to 1 to 2 ml. A major advantage of blow pipes is that dart impact energies are low, making them the dart delivery system of choice for small canids (<15 kg).

Dart Guns

Dart guns are probably the most versatile means of delivering drugs to wild animals. However, their use is limited to the larger-sized species (≥20 kg). Dart rifles can be used for captive or trapped canids or canids pursued by helicopter, whereas carbon dioxide–powered pistols can be useful for short-range capture situations (<20 m), such as for captive, trapped, or cornered (e.g., urban dogs) canids.

Darts of different manufacture vary greatly in weight for a given volume. The amount of energy delivered by the dart is a function of both mass and velocity, so fast darts, whether heavy or light, can be dangerous to canids.[24] Some darts have a tapered nosepiece as opposed to a flat or truncated nose, which may cause greater penetration on impact.

CAPTURING, HANDLING, AND MONITORING

Drugs can be administered to captive canids in a variety of ways. If unrestrained in a cage, darts can be delivered by blow pipe or dart gun. Smaller canids can be restrained in a large fishing net for subsequent hand injection.[30] Larger canids can be pinned with a forked stick or held with a catch pole and drugs administered through a short-handled pole syringe.[26]

Free-ranging canids are usually trapped before drug administration, although some species (e.g., African wild dogs) may be approached and darted from a vehicle.[44] In general, box, padded-jawed, or offset-jawed foothold traps are preferred.[37, 61] Some species rarely enter a box trap (e.g., red foxes), however, and others may not be effectively restrained by padded-jawed traps (e.g., gray wolves). Trapped canids fight the trap franti-

cally when approached by humans and may pull out of the trap or injure themselves during these efforts.

Gray wolves are probably one of the few canid species that can be safely pursued and darted from a helicopter because of their large size and their habitat of broken or open country.[6, 7, 27] African wild dogs can be captured by chasing a pack into a funnel-shaped boma of plastic sheeting with a helicopter. Once in the boma, the dogs can be chemically immobilized.[55]

In drug dose calculation, it is almost always better to estimate body weights on the heavier side so as not to underdose. If the animal received only a partial drug injection or is not satisfactorily immobilized within 10 to 15 minutes of the initial dose, half of the initial dose should be administered. If there are only minimal signs after this time, the entire initial dose is repeated. When using drug combinations (e.g., ketamine-xylazine), it is usually necessary to supplement with only the primary immobilizing agent (e.g., ketamine) and no additional tranquilizer.[49] Likewise, if the animal starts to awaken during the immobilization process and additional time is required, IM supplemental boosters of half the initial primary immobilizing agent can be administered repeatedly. When tiletamine-zolazepam combinations (e.g., Telazol) are used, recovery time can be shortened if boosters of ketamine instead of tiletamine-zolazepam are given.[34]

In very cold weather, drugs may freeze in the dart or syringe before they can be administered. Addition of a small amount of propylene glycol (0.5 to 1.0 ml) to the drug mixture can prevent or delay freezing.[27]

When the animal is down, it should be approached quietly. The inside of the animal's ear can be touched with a pole syringe or stick to evoke a twitch. If there is a twitch, the animal may not be completely immobilized, and more drugs may be required and caution used. If there is no ear twitch, the animal is probably safely immobilized. It should be positioned on its side, and a clear airway ensured. Vital signs must be quickly checked, with respiration and temperature being the most critical. A drug overdose can cause respiratory depression or arrest, and prolonged exertion in a trap can cause hyperthermia, particularly if respiration (and thus heat loss through panting) is decreased by chemical immobilization.

The animal should be moved out of direct sunlight or shaded with portable material. The eyes should be covered after the exposed cornea has been treated with an ophthalmic ointment or kept hydrated with sterile saline. Hobbling the legs or muzzling probably is not necessary unless the animal is only sedated or lightly anesthetized and additional control is required. Once the animal is stable and secure, it can be examined for wounds, ectoparasites, and general condition. If it was trapped, the roof of the mouth must be checked for jammed sticks. If a dart was used, it must be removed and the used wound treated appropriately.

Vital signs should be monitored continuously throughout the immobilization process. Rectal temperature can be monitored by mercury or digital thermometers. Portable vital signs monitors gauge not only temperature but also pulse, electrocardiogram, and blood pressure. Such units are expensive and probably not required for field immobilizations unless the animal is intrinsically or economically valuable. Respiratory efficiency is probably best monitored by a pulse oximeter. Intubation is generally not necessary, but it may be a wise precautionary step.

The immobilized animal should not be left unattended until it has recovered, unless it is in captivity or held in a manner that it can be kept away from other animals and hazards, such as in a crate. Ideally, someone should remain with the animal until it can walk in a relatively coordinated manner and can respond appropriately to humans, animals, and objects. Monitoring recovery is even more important when hazards such as water and precipices are in the immediate area.

For these reasons, in wild canids, the use of immobilizing drugs that can be antagonized are preferred. Antagonists are usually administered IV for a more rapid effect; IM administration is effective but less rapid. Preferred IV sites are the cephalic and jugular veins, although the femoral and saphenous veins can also be used. When alpha-adrenergic antagonists (e.g., yohimbine) are administered to canids immobilized with cyclohexane–alpha-adrenergic combinations (e.g., ketamine-xylazine), one should wait at least 30 minutes, and preferably 45 minutes, after the last injection of ketamine to administer the antagonist. Because there are no antagonists for cyclohexanes, failure to wait for most of the cyclohexane to be metabolized may result in the animal's becoming cataleptic, hyperthermic, and convulsant on recovery.[26, 32, 36]

MEDICAL CONCERNS

The primary medical concerns for immobilized canids are respiratory depression and hyperthermia. In the case of respiratory depression, supplemental oxygen from a portable tank can be delivered through an endotracheal tube. Alternatively, the animal can be placed in lateral recumbency and the chest firmly compressed 15 to 20 times per minute.[24] After artificial ventilation has returned normal color to the mucous membranes, ventilation is stopped for at least 1 minute to determine whether the animal will begin breathing on its own. If no respirations are noticed, the cycle is repeated. Doxapram can also be given to chemically stimulate respiration if the depression is thought to be due to drug overdose. If all else fails, the immobilizing drugs can be antagonized, which invariably results in increased respiration.

Hyperthermia is a constant concern with trapped or chased canids. Heavily furred animals can also build endogenous heat when under a warm sun, even in cold winter conditions. Hyperthermia should be suspected if the rectal temperature exceeds 40°C (104°F); treatment is mandatory if the temperature is 41.1°C (106°F) or higher. The best and most rapid method to cool canids is by whole-body immersion in water (e.g., pond, stream, stock tank). Alternatively, cooling can be achieved by spraying the entire animal with water (particularly the groin area and head), packing with ice or cold water bags, dousing with isopropyl alcohol, giving cold water enemas, or administering cold lactated Ringer's solution IV or intraperitoneally.[24]

Hypothermia is generally not a problem, unless the animal is kept immobilized for extended periods under cold conditions or has lost the insulating value of its fur (wet fur, hair loss). Hypothermic animals can be warmed by placing warm containers of water around them or by wrapping them in blankets or placing them under heat lamps or on heat pads or hand warmers. Recovery is slow because of impaired drug metabolism, so the animal may have to be confined to a crate to allow it to shiver and slowly arouse until it has reached normal body temperature.

Vomiting can occur in immobilized canids regardless of the drug or drugs used. Choking on large pieces of undigested food or aspiration of stomach contents presents a hazard. This usually is not a problem if the vomiting occurs during induction or recovery because the animal generally is capable of clearing the vomitus on its own. If the animal vomits when anesthetized, it should be placed sternally with its neck extended and head down. The animal's body is lifted, while its head is kept down, to help clear the vomitus. Captive animals should be fasted 24 hours before anesthetic administration.

Seizures are not uncommon in canids immobilized by ketamine or other cyclohexane drugs. Usually, one or two seizures of short duration are not cause for intervention. However, repeated seizures should be treated to prevent hyperthermia and other complications. Seizures can usually be controlled by administering 5 to 10 mg diazepam or midazolam IV or IM. Diazepam IV should be administered slowly (over 10 to 15 seconds) to prevent cardiac arrest due to propylene glycol solvent.

Other medical concerns, such as cardiac arrest, bloat, dehydration, and capture myopathy, are rare in canids. Wounds, on the other hand, are common because of the capture methods used (traps, darts). All wounds should be treated using standard veterinary techniques. Dart wounds should always be cleaned and treated (intramammary infusion devices work well) and antibiotics (preferably long-term penicillins) administered. Under cold climatic conditions, removal of hair to clean or visualize a wound should be minimized.

DRUG DOSES

All canids can be immobilized safely and effectively with ketamine combined with a tranquilizer. Tiletamine-zolazepam is also highly effective but can result in prolonged recoveries. Concentrated tiletamine-zolazepam (250 to 500 mg/ml) can be combined with xylazine to produce a potent anesthetic dose in a small volume.[27] With the exception of fentanyl, opioids are rarely necessary and often cause profound respiratory depression.

Ketamine and medetomidine promise to be a good combination, although specific doses for most of the canids have yet to be developed. The reason for this is that medetomidine greatly reduces the amount of ketamine required compared with other combinations, which results in smaller drug volumes and quicker and

TABLE 58–1. Dosages for Immobilization of Canids

Common Name (Genus)	Dosages	References
Wolves, coyotes, jackals *(Canis)*	4.0 mg/kg ketamine plus 0.08 mg/kg medetomidine; antagonize with 0.4 mg/kg atipamezole 10.0 mg/kg ketamine plus 2.0 mg/kg xylazine; antagonize with 0.15 mg/kg yohimbine 10.0 mg/kg tiletamine-zolazepam (Telazol) 10.0 mg/kg ketamine plus 0.1 mg/kg acepromazine	1–8, 10, 15–18, 23–25, 27, 29–32, 34, 35, 41, 42, 45, 48–52, 59, 62
Maned wolf *(Chrysocyon)*	6.6 mg/kg ketamine plus 1.25 mg/kg xylazine plus 0.05 mg/kg atropine 2.5 mg/kg ketamine plus 0.08 mg/kg medetomidine	21
Dhole *(Cuon)*	10.0 mg/kg tiletamine-zolazepam 20.0 mg/kg ketamine plus 0.1 mg/kg acepromazine	23, 24
Bush dog *(Speothos)*	10.0 mg/kg tiletamine-zolazepam 20.0 mg/kg ketamine plus 0.1 mg/kg acepromazine	23, 24
African hunting dog *(Lycaon)*	2.0 mg/kg ketamine plus 2.4 mg/kg xylazine plus 0.05 mg/kg atropine; antagonize with 0.2 mg/kg yohimbine 5.0 mg/kg ketamine plus 0.05 mg/kg medetomidine; antagonize with 0.25 mg/kg atipamezole 0.1 mg/kg fentanyl plus 1.0 mg/kg xylazine; antagonize with 0.04 mg/kg naloxone plus 0.15 mg/kg yohimbine	11, 13, 23, 24, 44, 46, 55–58
Raccoon dog *(Nyctereutes)*	5.0 mg/kg ketamine plus 0.1 mg/kg medetomidine; antagonize with 0.5 mg/kg atipamezole 6.6 mg/kg tiletamine-zolazepam	3, 23, 24
Small-eared dog *(Atelocynus)*	10.0 mg/kg tiletamine-zolazepam 20.0 mg/kg ketamine plus 0.1 mg/kg acepromazine	23, 24
Foxes *(Alopex, Vulpes, Otocyon, Cerdocyon, Fennecus, Urocyon, Dusicyon)*	10.0 mg/kg tiletamine-zolazepam 20.0 mg/kg ketamine plus 1.0 mg/kg xylazine; antagonize with 0.15 mg/kg yohimbine 20.0 mg/kg ketamine plus 0.1 mg/kg acepromazine	9, 20, 22–24, 36, 42, 49, 53, 54

more complete recoveries after medetomidine antagonism with atipamezole.[22]

Canids can also be heavily sedated (but not anesthetized) with either xylazine[33] or medetomidine.[25] These sedatives can be used to chemically restrain calm animals for short, nonpainful procedures (e.g., moving from pen to pen, vaccinations, blood sampling), with the advantage of rapid and complete antagonism with either yohimbine or atipamezole. With medetomidine, only atipamezole should be used for antagonism.[25]

With few exceptions, immobilization dosages for canids can be grouped by genus (Table 58–1). Readers unfamiliar with a species are encouraged to read the specific literature cited before attempting immobilizations.

Acknowledgments

Special thanks to Steve Osofsky, D.V.M., for reviewing sections of this chapter.

REFERENCES

1. Alford BT, Burkhart L, Johnson WP: Etorphine and diprenorphine as immobilizing and reversing agents in captive and free-ranging mammals. J Am Vet Med Assoc 154:701–705, 1974.
2. Allen JL, Janssen DL, Oosterhuis JE, et al: Immobilization of captive non-domestic hoofstock with carfentanil. Proceedings of the American Association of Zoo Veterinarians, Calgary, Alberta, Canada, pp 343–353, 1991.
3. Arnemo JM, Moe R, Smith RJ: Immobilization of captive raccoon dogs (*Nyctereutes procyonoides*) with medetomidine-ketamine and remobilization with atipamezole. J Zoo Wildl Med 24:102–108, 1993.
4. Baer CH, Severson RE, Linhart SB: Live capture of coyotes from a helicopter with ketamine hydrochloride. J Wildl Manage 42:452–454, 1978.
5. Bailey TN: Immobilization of bobcats, coyotes, and badgers with phencyclidine hydrochloride. J Wildl Manage 35:847–849, 1971.
6. Ballard WB, Ayres LA, Roney KE, et al: Immobilization of gray wolves with a combination of tiletamine hydrochloride and zolazepam hydrochloride. J Wildl Manage 55:71–74, 1991.
7. Ballard WB, Franzmann AW, Gardner CL: Comparison and assessment of drugs used to immobilize Alaskan gray wolves (*Canis lupus*) and wolverines (*Gulo gulo*) from a helicopter. J Wildl Dis 18:339–342, 1982.
8. Beck CC: Chemical restraint of exotic species. J Zoo Animal Med 3:3–66, 1972.
9. Brooks C, Morris, KD: Blood values and the use of ketamine HCl in the fox. Vet Med Small Animal Clin 74:1179–1180, 1979.
10. Cornely JE: Anesthesia of coyotes with ketamine hydrochloride and xylazine. J Wildl Manage 43:577–579, 1979.
11. De Vos V: Immobilization of free-ranging wild animals using a new drug. Vet Rec 103:64–68, 1978.
12. Dyson RF: Experience with succinylcholine chloride in zoo animals. Intl Zoo Yearb 5:205–206, 1965.
13. Ebedes H, Grobler M: The restraint of the Cape hunting dog *Lycaon pictus* with phencyclidine hydrochloride and ketamine hydrochloride. J So Afr Vet Assoc 50:113–114, 1979.
14. Faggella AM, Kreeger TJ, Seal US: Cardiovascular Effects of Xylazine HCl and Ketamine HCL Anesthesia in Dogs and Wolves. Midwest Anesthesia Conference, Urbana, University of Illinois, 1986.
15. Fuller TK, Keith LB: Immobilization of wolves in winter with etorphine. J Wildl Manage 45:271–273, 1981.
16. Fuller TK, Kuehn DW: Immobilization of wolves using ketamine in combination with xylazine or promazine. J Wildl Dis 19:69–72, 1983.
17. Green B: The use of etorphine hydrochloride (M99) in the capture and immobilization of wild dingoes, *Canis familiaris dingo*. Austral Wildl Res 3:123–128, 1976.

18. Hallett DL, Rhoades JD, Paddleford RR: Immobilization of coyotes with ketamine and propiomazine. J Am Vet Med Assoc 175:1007–1008, 1979.

19. Hatch RC, Clark JD, Booth NH et al: Comparison of five preanesthetic medicaments in pentobarbital-anesthetized dogs: antagonism by 4-aminopyridine, yohimbine, and naloxone. Am J Vet Res 44:2312–2319, 1983.

20. Indrebø A: Anestesi av blarev med Ketelar® og Rompun® [Anesthesia of blue foxes using ketamine and xylazine]. Nor Veterinæridsskr 101:767–770, 1989.

21. Jalanka HH: The use of medetomidine, medetomidine-ketamine combinations, and atipamezole at Helsinki Zoo—a review of 240 cases. Acta Vet Scand 85:193–197, 1989.

22. Jalanka HH: Medetomidine- and medetomidine-ketamine–induced immobilization in blue foxes (*Alopex lagopus*) and its reversal by atipamezole. Acta Vet Scand 31:63–71, 1990.

23. Kreeger TJ: A review of chemical immobilization of wild canids. Proceedings of the Joint Conference of the American Association of Zoo Veterinarians and American Association Wildlife Veterinarians, Oakland, CA, pp 271–283, 1992.

24. Kreeger TJ: Handbook of wildlife chemical immobilization. Laramie, WY, International Wildlife Veterinary Services, 1996.

25. Kreeger TJ, Callahan M, Beckel M: The use of medetomidine sedation with atipamezole antagonism in the management of captive gray wolves. J Zoo Wildl Med 27:507–512, 1996.

26. Kreeger TJ, Faggella AM, Seal US, et al: Cardiovascular and behavioral responses of gray wolves to ketamine-xylazine immobilization and antagonism by yohimbine. J Wildl Dis 23:463–470, 1987.

27. Kreeger TJ, Hunter DL, Johnson MR: Immobilization protocol for free-ranging gray wolves (*Canis lupus*) translocated to Yellowstone National Park and central Idaho. Proceedings of the Joint Conference of the American Association of Zoo Veterinarians and American Association of Wildlife Veterinarians, East Lansing, MI, pp 529–530, 1995.

28. Kreeger TJ, Levine AS, Seal US, et al: Diazepam-induced feeding in captive gray wolves (*Canis lupus*). Pharmacol Biochem Behav 39:559–561, 1991.

29. Kreeger TJ, Mandsager RE, Seal US, et al: Physiological response of gray wolves to butorphanol-xylazine immobilization and antagonism by naloxone and yohimbine. J Wildl Dis 25:89–94, 1989.

30. Kreeger TJ, Seal US: Immobilization of coyotes with xylazine hydrochloride-ketamine hydrochloride and antagonism by yohimbine hydrochloride. J Wildl Dis 22:604–606, 1986.

31. Kreeger TJ, Seal US: Immobilization of captive gray wolves (*Canis lupus*) with sufentanil citrate. J Wildl Dis 26:561–563, 1990.

32. Kreeger TJ, Seal US: Failure of yohimbine hydrochloride to antagonize ketamine hydrochloride immobilization in gray wolves. J Wildl Dis 22:600–603, 1986.

33. Kreeger TJ, Seal US, Callahan M, et al: Use of xylazine sedation with yohimbine antagonism in captive gray wolves. J Wildl Dis 24:688–690, 1988.

34. Kreeger TJ, Seal US, Callahan M, et al: Physiological and behavioral responses of gray wolves to immobilization with tiletamine and zolazepam (Telazol®). J Wildl Dis 26:162–194, 1990.

35. Kreeger TJ, Seal US, Faggella AM: Xylazine hydrochloride–ketamine hydrochloride immobilization of wolves and its antagonism by tolazoline hydrochloride. J Wildl Dis 22:397–402, 1986.

36. Kreeger TJ, Seal US, Tester JR: Chemical immobilization of red foxes (*Vulpes vulpes*). J Wildl Dis 26:95–98, 1990.

37. Kreeger TJ, White PJ, Seal US, et al: Pathological responses of red foxes to foothold traps. J Wildl Manage 54:147–160, 1990.

38. Lance WR: New Pharmaceutical Tools for the 1990's. Proceedings of the American Association of Zoo Veterinarians, Calgary, Alberta, pp 354–359, 1991.

39. Lemke KA, Tranquilli WJ, Thurmon JC, et al: Ability of flumazenil, butorphanol, and naloxone to reverse the anesthetic effects of oxymorphone-diazepam in dogs. J Am Vet Med Assoc 209:776–779, 1996.

40. Marsboom R: On the pharmacology of azaperone, a neuroleptic for the restraint of wild animals. Acta Zool Path Antver 48:155–161, 1969.

41. Mulde JB: Anesthesia in the coyote using a combination of ketamine and xylazine. J Wildl Dis 14:501–502, 1978.

42. Nielsen L, Haigh JC, Fowler ME (eds): Chemical Immobilization of North American Wildlife. Milwaukee, WI, Wisconsin Humane Society, 1982.

43. Nowak RM: Walker's Mammals of the World, 5th ed. Baltimore, Johns Hopkins University Press, 1991.

44. Osofsky SA, McNutt JW, Hirsch KJ: Immobilization and monitoring of free-ranging wild dogs (*Lycaon pictus*) using a ketamine/xylazine/atropine combination, yohimbine reversal and pulse oximetry. Proceedings of the Joint Conference of the American Association of Zoo Veterinarians and American Association of Wildlife Veterinarians, East Lansing, MI, pp 278–286, 1995.

45. Philo LM: Evaluation of xylazine for chemical restraint of captive Arctic wolves. J Am Vet Med Assoc 173:1163–1166, 1978.

46. Raath JP, Knox CM, Kernes D, et al: Anesthesia of free-ranging wild dogs (*Lycaon pictus*) with fentanyl and xylazine. Proceedings of the Joint Conference of the American Association of Zoo Veterinarians and American Association of Wildlife Veterinarians, East Lansing, MI, pp 287–289, 1995.

47. Rogers PS: The capture of large carnivores using orally administered drugs. In McKenzie AA (ed): The Capture and Care Manual. Pretoria, Wildlife Decision Support Services, pp 225–246, 1993.

48. Rowe-Rowe DT, Green B: Ketamine and acetylpromazine for black-backed jackal immobilization. So Afr J Wildl Res 10:153, 1980.

49. Seal US, Kreeger TJ: Chemical immobilization of furbearers. In Novak M, Baker JA, Obbard ME, et al (eds): Wild Furbearer Management and Conservation in North America. Toronto, Ontario Ministry of Natural Resources, pp 191–215, 1987.

50. Servin J, Huxley C, Vences M: The combined use of ketamine hydrochloride and xylazine hydrochloride for immobilization of the wild coyote *Canis latrans*. Acta Zool Mex 36:27–37, 1990.

51. Sillero-Zubiri C: Field immobilization of Ethiopian wolves (*Canis simensis*). J Wildl Dis 32:147–151, 1996.

52. Tobey RW, Ballard WB: Increased mortality in gray wolves captured with acepromazine and etorphine hydrochloride in combination. J Wildl Dis 21:188–190, 1985.

53. Travaini A, Delibes M: Immobilization of free-ranging red foxes (*Vulpes vulpes*) with tiletamine hydrochloride and zolazepam. J Wildl Dis 30:589–591, 1994.

54. Travaini A, Ferreras P, Delibes M, et al: Xylazine hydrochloride-ketamine hydrochloride immobilization of free-living red foxes (*Vulpes vulpes*) in Spain. J Wildl Dis 28:507–509, 1992.

55. Van Heerden J: Chemical capture of the wild dog, *Lycaon pictus*. In McKenzie AA (ed): The Capture and Care Manual. Pretoria, Wildlife Decision Support Services, pp 247–251, 1993.

56. Van Heerden J, Burroughs REJ, Dauth J, et al: Immobilization of wild dogs (*Lycaon pictus*) with a tiletamine hydrochloride/zolazepam hydrochloride combination and subsequent evaluation of selected blood chemistry parameters. J Wildl Dis 27:225–229, 1991.

57. Van Heerden J, de Vos V: Immobilization of the hunting dog *Lycaon pictus* with ketamine hydrochloride and a fentanyl/droperidol combination. So Afr J Wildl Res 11:112–113, 1981.

58. Van Heerden J, Swan GE, Dauth J, et al: Sedation and immobilization of wild dogs *Lycaon pictus* using medetomidine-ketamine hydrochloride combination. So Afr J Wildl Res 21:88–93, 1991.

59. Vilà C, Castroviejo J: Use of tiletamine and zolazepam to immobilize captive Iberian wolves (*Canis lupus*). J Wildl Dis 30:119–122, 1994.

60. Wallingford BD, Lancia RA, Soutiere EC: Antagonism of xylazine in white-tailed deer with intramuscular injection of yohimbine. J Wildl Dis 32:399–402, 1996.

61. White PJ, Kreeger TJ, Seal US, et al: Pathological responses of red foxes to box traps. J Wildl Manage 55:75–80, 1990.

62. Wiesner H, Rietschel W, Gatesman TJ: The use of the morphine-like analgesic carfentanil in captive wild mammals at Tierpark Hellebraun. J Zoo Animal Med 15:18–23, 1984.

63. Williams TD, Williams AL, Siniff DB: Fentanyl and azaperone produced neuroleptanalgesia in the sea otter (*Enhydra lutris*). J Wild Dis 17:337–342, 1981.

CHAPTER 59

Otter Anesthesia

LUCY H. SPELMAN

Respiratory depression (apnea, hypoxemia), hypothermia, and hyperthermia have been reported often in anesthetized otters.[1, 3, 4, 6–11, 15, 16, 18, 21–23, 28–31] However, detailed physiologic data is lacking for many of these studies, and the available data account for only the most common species (North American river otter, *Lutra canadensis;* Eurasian otter, *Lutra lutra;* small-clawed otter, *Aonyx cinerea;* and sea otter, *Enhydra lutris*). For the other otter species in the subfamily Lutrinae (Table 59–1), one report briefly mentioned ketamine-xylazine anesthesia in Amazonian otters.

GENERAL CONSIDERATIONS

Anatomy and Biology

Otters have a wide geographic range that includes both fresh water and marine habitats (see Table 59–1). Their dentition is typical of that of other carnivores, and otters can inflict serious bites, even in play. Adaptations for aquatic life include an elongate, streamlined body shape with short limbs, a stout tail, a relatively large thoracic cavity, and thick waterproof fur (Fig. 59–1). Otters lack subcutaneous fat stores and rely instead on their fur for thermoregulation.[25, 26] Their coat consists of two layers:

a short, dense underfur, which provides insulation by trapping air, and an outer layer of long, waterproof guard hairs. Regular grooming is essential. If the guard hairs are disrupted (shaved) or damaged (oiled) in such a way that the underfur becomes wet, hypothermia can develop rapidly and can predispose the otter to pneumonia. Dry otters on land are at risk for hyperthermia if subjected to prolonged physical exertion or dehydration.

Anesthetic Administration

Otters can be physically restrained with a net, a squeeze cage, or a restraint box. Restraint should be brief, and care should be taken to avoid oral cavity trauma (e.g., fractured canine teeth). Manual restraint of an otter is virtually impossible because of its great strength, stout neck, and loose skin. With experienced personnel, a deep narrow net can be used to restrain the otter for hand injection of anesthetic. A thick woven mat can be used for added protection.

Standard metal squeeze cages have been used for otters, but excessive struggling can lead to preanesthetic excitement or injury. Alternatively, a modified smooth-walled squeeze cage can be constructed of wood, polyvinylchloride (PVC) piping, or a small carrying crate

TABLE 59–1. The 13 Species of Otter in the Subfamily Lutrinae, Their Distribution, and Relative Size

Common Name	Scientific Name	Distribution	Size*
Cape clawless otter	*Aonyx capensis*	Africa	Large (up to 25 kg)
Asian small-clawed otter	*Aonyx cinerea*	Asia	Small
Congo clawless otter	*Aonyx congica*	Equatorial Africa	Small to medium
Sea otter	*Enhydra lutris*	North American Pacific coast, Soviet Union	Large (up to 45 kg)
North American river otter	*Lutra canadensis*	Canada, United States	Medium to large
Marine otter	*Lutra felina*	Pacific South America	Small to medium
Neotropical otter	*Lutra longicaudis*	Central and South America, Mexico	Medium
Eurasian otter	*Lutra lutra*	Europe, Asia, Northern Africa	Medium
Spotted-necked otter	*Lutra maculicollis*	Africa	Small to medium
Smooth-coated otter	*Lutra perspicillata*	Asia	Medium to large
Southern river otter	*Lutra provocax*	Argentina, Chile	Medium
Hairy-nosed otter	*Lutra sumatrana*	Southeast Asia	Medium
Giant otter	*Pteronura brasiliensis*	South America	Large (up to 32 kg)

*Small, 2 to 4 kg; medium, 5 to 9 kg; large, >10 kg.

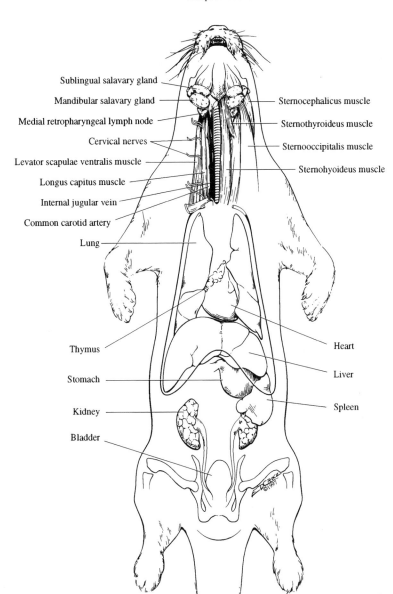

Sublingual salavary gland

Mandibular salavary gland

Medial retropharyngeal lymph node

Cervical nerves

Levator scapulae ventralis muscle

Longus capitus muscle

Internal jugular vein

Common carotid artery

Lung

Sternocephalicus muscle

Sternothyroideus muscle

Sternooccipitalis muscle

Sternohyoideus muscle

Thymus

Stomach

Kidney

Bladder

Heart

Liver

Spleen

FIGURE 59–1. General anatomy of the North American river otter (*Lutra canadensis*).

with a movable end piece.[13, 20] In order to habituate the otters, the squeeze cage may also be used as a den in an exhibit or as a transport box. Sea otters have been readily restrained with a V-shaped box for minor procedures, both with and without sedation.[27] For all species, anesthetics can also be delivered through pole syringe or nonmetal dart.

Deep intramuscular (IM) injection of anesthetic is essential, regardless of the method of administration. The otter's relatively loose skin increases the chance of inadvertent subcutaneous injection. Delayed onset of action and reduced potency can be expected with subcutaneous administration of most anesthetics. For smaller species, injection in the cranial thigh (quadriceps) is recommended to ensure IM delivery. The caudal thigh (semimembranosus-tendinosus) or paralumbar muscles may also be used in the larger otter species.

Anesthetic Monitoring

Relative oxyhemoglobin saturation should be recorded in anesthetized otters in addition to heart rate, respiratory rate, and rectal temperature whenever possible. Respiratory depression (apnea, bradypnea, tachypnea, hypoxemia) was the most common complication associated with injectable anesthesia during a multiyear study on North American river otters.[21–23] In eight anesthetic protocols evaluated in 256 river otters (ketamine, ketamine-diazepam, ketamine-midazolam, medetomidine-ketamine, ketamine-xylazine, tiletamine-zolazepam, fentanyl-azaperone, and fentanyl-azaperone-midazolam), apnea frequently developed within 5 minutes of induction. Respiratory pattern tended to improve with time and stimulation (tongue pull, nose pinch, minor surgery) but significant hypoxemia (relative oxyhemoglobin

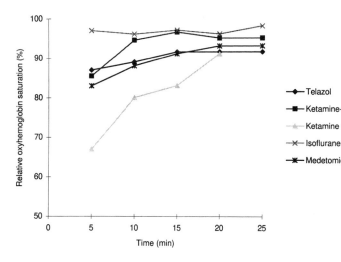

FIGURE 59–2. Median values (percentages) for relative oxyhemoglobin saturation for North American river otters (*Lutra canadensis*) anesthetized with isoflurane, ketamine, ketamine-midazolam, medetomidine-ketamine, and tiletamine-zolazepam (*n* = 16 per group).

saturation, <80%) persisted in otters given fentanyl combinations or ketamine-xylazine. Although less pronounced, hypoxemia (relative oxyhemoglobin saturation, <90%) was also present for the first 20 minutes of anesthesia in most otters given ketamine or tiletamine-zolazepam (Fig. 59–2). Respiratory depression was comparably mild in otters anesthetized with ketamine-midazolam or medetomidine-ketamine. Representative arterial blood gases also readily demonstrate different degrees of respiratory depression among anesthetic protocols in river otters (Table 59–2).

Finding a suitable probe site for pulse oximetry in an otter can be problematic. Most species have short ears, short and/or webbed digits, and relatively small tongues. Smaller species also tend to have high heart rates (especially if given a dissociative anesthetic), which contribute to signal artifact. Recommendations include a Nellcor D-25 probe (Nellcor, Inc.) folded over the tongue or digits and secured with a paperclip, or a Nellcor RS-10 reflectance probe modified as an esophageal or rectal probe (or any comparable probe). Indirect blood pressure can be readily measured with a small or neonatal cuff on the base of the tail. Placement of electrocardiograph (ECG) leads is routine.

Without established "normals" for physiologic parameters for a particular otter species, it may be difficult to determine "abnormal" parameters during anesthesia. Physiologic data from North American river otters that were masked down and maintained with isoflurane were used as the gold standard to generate baseline parameters for heart rate, respiratory rate, rectal temperature, relative oxyhemoglobin saturation, ECG data, and indirect blood pressure.[22] From these data, a series of anesthetic-related complications were defined for subsequent evaluation of other anesthetic protocols in this species (Table 59–3). Although generated for North American river otters, these reference values may be useful for related species such as the Eurasian otter and neotropical otter (*Lutra longicaudis*).

Anesthetic Recovery

During recovery from anesthesia, appropriate measures should be taken to maintain body temperature, with the use of either heating pads or cool packs as indicated. Access to a quiet, dark den box or a confined area facilitates smooth anesthetic recovery. Care should be taken to remove wire or sharp objects, to eliminate narrow crawl spaces, and to enable the otter to recover in a secure place.

TABLE 59–2. Representative Arterial Blood Gas Results from 6 River Otters Anesthetized with Different Protocols

Anesthetic Combination	PO$_2$ (mm Hg)	PCO$_2$ (mm Hg)	pH	HCO$_3^-$ (mEq/L)	SPO$_2$ (%)	SaO$_2$ (%)
Ketamine-midazolam	81.6	56.6	7.29	27.4	93	94.2
Tiletamine-zolazepam	69.3	51.9	7.32	27.2	93	91.8
Medetomidine-ketamine	68.8	54.2	7.29	26.4	93	90.9
Ketamine-diazepam	60.3	54.1	7.38	30.0	93	88.7
Fentanyl-midazolam	34.4	90.7	7.11	29.2	<50	44.6
Fentanyl-midazolam-azaperone	29.4	76.2	7.24	32.7	<50	42.0

PO$_2$, oxygen partial pressure; PCO$_2$, carbon dioxide partial pressure; HCO$_3^-$, bicarbonate radical; SPO$_2$, relative oxyhemoglobin saturation; SaO$_2$, oxygen saturation.

Samples were taken 20 minutes after initial anesthetic injection; supplemental oxygen was not provided.

TABLE 59–3. Anesthetic-Related Complications as Defined in North American River Otters (*Lutra canadensis*)

Physiologic Measure	Baseline (Range)	Increased	Decreased
Heart rate (beats/minute)	152 (130–178)	>180 (tachycardia)	<100 (bradycardia)
Respiratory rate (breaths/minute)	31 (10–60)	>40 (tachypnea)	<8 (bradypnea)
Relative oxyhemoglobin saturation (%)	97 (92–100)	NA	<80% (hypoxemia)
Mean arterial blood pressure (mm Hg)	63 (31–77)	<50 (hypotension)	>100 (hypertension)
Rectal temperature (°C)	38.4 (38.1–38.7)	>40.1 (hyperthermia)	<36.7 (hypothermia)

The baseline values for cardiopulmonary parameters were based on data from otters in which anesthesia was induced and maintained with isoflurane (mean and range at 10 minutes post induction) and on resting core temperature as determined by telemetry.

INJECTABLE ANESTHESIA

Ketamine

A wide dose range has been reported for ketamine when used alone for anesthesia in river otters and European otters (6 to 30 mg/kg).[8, 10, 13, 15, 16, 20, 22] Numerous complications have been reported in otters given ketamine, although this anesthetic is generally considered to have a high margin of safety in small carnivores. Apnea and hyperthermia were reported in early studies with river otters anesthetized with ketamine (6 to 14 mg/kg).[10] Poor myorelaxation, excitable state during recovery, tachycardia, and fatal hyperthermia were observed in European otters under ketamine anesthesia (7.8 to 16 mg/kg).[15, 16] Several authors reported successful surgical anesthesia with a higher dosage of ketamine (22 mg/kg), but no details of the anesthesia were provided.[13, 20] An exceptionally low dose of ketamine (0.9 to 1.2 mg/kg) was associated with death in three sea otters.[28] These otters were injured and debilitated at the time of anesthesia, which may have predisposed them to an adverse reaction. However, there are other accounts of severe anesthetic complications (hyperthermia, prolonged recovery, death) attributed to ketamine in sea otters (T. Williams, B. Joseph, personal communication, 1997).

In North American river otters given ketamine (10 mg/kg), anesthesia time was short (median, 17.4 minutes), and the quality of anesthesia was variable.[22] Most otters exhibited poor myorelaxation and motion. Hyperthermia (39.4° to 41.1°C) developed in one third of the otters. However, otters that were excited or struggled during restraint did not consistently develop higher body temperatures. In most otters, two or more of the following cardiopulmonary complications also developed: bradycardia (including second-degree atrioventricular block in one otter), tachycardia, apnea, bradypnea, tachypnea, and hypoxemia (see Table 59–3). Anesthetic recovery was relatively rapid and characterized by persistent ataxia. All otters were fully alert within 60 minutes from the start of anesthesia.

Ketamine-Diazepam and Ketamine-Midazolam

Ketamine-benzodiazepine combinations have the advantage of improved myorelaxation and longer anesthesia time. Ketamine (17 to 30 mg/kg) combined with diazepam (0.3 to 0.6 mg/kg) has been reported in North American river otters,[4] Eurasian otters,[11] and Asian small-clawed otters (dosage not given).[2, 12] Mild hyperthermia (40°C) and prolonged recovery (100 minutes) were noted in the Eurasian otter study. Lower dosages of ketamine (10 to 12 mg/kg) combined with diazepam (0.3 to 0.5 mg/kg) have been used by the author for anesthesia in river otters, Asian small-clawed otters, and Cape clawless otters (*Aonyx capensis*) with good results, although recovery was slow (L. Spelman, unpublished data).

Ketamine (6 to 16.7 mg/kg) combined with midazolam (0.1 to 0.5 mg/kg) was first reported for anesthesia in Asian small-clawed otters undergoing electrocardiography.[17] In river otters, ketamine (10 mg/kg) combined with midazolam (0.25 mg/kg) consistently produced short-term anesthesia (20 to 30 minutes) with excellent muscle relaxation, mild initial respiratory depression, and smooth recovery within 60 to 70 minutes from initial administration.[23] Hyperthermia developed in some otters, as in those anesthetized with ketamine alone. Tachycardia occurred in one third of the otters and was also reported in small-clawed otters. Both ketamine and midazolam can increase heart rate, and mild to moderate tachycardia can be expected with this combination.

Ketamine and midazolam have also been used successfully for short-term anesthesia in Cape clawless otters and small-clawed otters (L. Spelman, unpublished data). This combination is recommended by the author for use in all species of otter except the sea otter. Recommended dosages for medium-sized to large otters are similar to those used in river otters (ketamine, 10 mg/kg, and midazolam, 0.25 to 0.5 mg/kg). Smaller otters require higher dosages (ketamine, 15 mg/kg, and midazolam, 1.0 mg/kg). The only disadvantages of this combination are the cost of midazolam and the drug volume, which may exceed 4 ml for large otters. Because midazolam is metabolized very rapidly, flumazenil is not recommended as a partial antagonist for this combination. Not only would recovery time remain unchanged, but flumazenil could unmask the undesirable effects of ketamine (excitation, tonic-clonic seizures).

Tiletamine-Zolazepam

Tiletamine-zolazepam has been widely recommended for use in small carnivores, including mustelids. Potential advantages of this combination include small injection volume, rapid onset of action, and good muscle relaxation. However, both respiratory depression and prolonged recovery from anesthesia have been reported in otters. Sea otters anesthetized with 1.4 to 4 mg/kg of tiletamine-zolazepam became apneic and recovered very slowly.[18, 28] In river otters given tiletamine-zolazepam (4 mg/kg, combined), adequate muscle relaxation lasted for 20 to 30 minutes after injection, but complete recovery was prolonged (60 to 120 minutes), and most otters exhibited residual sedation.[21] Otters also exhibited respiratory depression similar in degree to that produced by ketamine. Apnea occurred with induction, followed by tachypnea, and relative oxyhemoglobin saturation remained below 90% for the first 15 minutes of anesthesia in most otters given tiletamine-zolazepam (see Fig. 59–2).[21] Tachycardia and hyperthermia developed, similar to those observed in river otters anesthetized with ketamine or ketamine-midazolam. Small-clawed otters require comparatively higher dosages of tiletamine-zolazepam (6 to 9 mg/kg)[14] (L. Spelman, unpublished data).

Because of prolonged recovery time, flumazenil was evaluated as a partial antagonist for river otters anesthetized with tiletamine-zolazepam.[21] In river otters given flumazenil 20 minutes after the start of anesthesia, mean recovery time was reduced from 89 to 65 minutes. No adverse effects of the dissociative anesthetic were observed, and no resedation occurred. However, because the relative half-lives of tiletamine and zolazepam vary among closely related species, the response to flumazenil is variable, and caution should be taken when this antagonist is used for the first time in any species. For prolonged recovery resulting from persistent heavy sedation, flumazenil should be administered no sooner than 60 minutes from the initial injection of tiletamine-zolazepam.

Another important consideration for otters anesthetized with any of the dissociative-benzodiazepine combinations is the tendency for respiratory depression to develop even if the anesthetic plane is light. Inadequate anesthetic depth may occur if the animal is underdosed or with subcutaneous administration. Supplemental ketamine (5 mg/kg) or isoflurane can be given to deepen anesthesia. Respiratory rates should be monitored carefully during this time. Supplemental doses of the benzodiazepines (or repeat dosing of tiletamine-zolazepam) are not recommended because they may significantly prolong recovery and further depress respiration.

Ketamine-Xylazine and Medetomidine-Ketamine

When combined with ketamine, alpha$_2$ agonists improve muscle relaxation and increase anesthetic depth in a manner similar to that of the benzodiazepines. The primary advantage of this combination is its potential reversibility. The disadvantages include respiratory depression, bradycardia, peripheral vasoconstriction, and variable changes in blood pressure (usually transient hypotension followed by normotension or hypertension). Thermoregulation may also be disrupted, thereby increasing the likelihood of hypothermia during long procedures. Without the use of an alpha$_2$ antagonist, recovery is prolonged.

There have been several reports of ketamine-xylazine anesthesia in otters,[1, 3, 6, 7, 31] and ketamine (10 mg/kg) combined with xylazine (1 to 2 mg/kg) has been generally recommended for mustelids.[19] Ketamine (17 mg/kg) combined with a low dose of xylazine (approximately 0.15 mg/kg) and acepromazine (approximately .07 mg/kg) produced short-term anesthesia in river otters but was associated with hypothermia and bradycardia, especially when supplemented with isoflurane.[6, 7] In the only account of anesthesia in Amazonian river otters (three neotropical otters, one giant river otter), xylazine (1.5 to 2 mg/kg) was used in combination with ketamine (8.5 to 10.6 mg/kg)[3]; mild hypothermia (37°C) developed in the neotropical otters, and prolonged recovery (6 hours) was noted in the giant river otter.

During a pilot study by the author designed to establish equipotent dosages of xylazine-ketamine and medetomidine-ketamine in river otters, severe respiratory depression developed with ketamine (10 mg/kg) and xylazine (1 to 2 mg/kg) (L. Spelman, unpublished data.) Light anesthesia was achieved with a lower dosage of ketamine (7.5 mg/kg) combined with xylazine (1.5 mg/kg), but muscle relaxation was variable, duration was short (15 to 20 minutes), and most otters remained hypoxemic. Similar problems (variable anesthetic depth, respiratory depression) also occurred with xylazine-ketamine in Asian small clawed otters at dosages (xylazine 3 to 5 mg/kg and ketamine 3 to 5 mg/kg) which work well in other small carnivores (L. Spelman, unpublished data). Yohimbine (0.125 mg/kg, intravenously [IV] or IM) rapidly reversed the respiratory depression, but residual ketamine effects were apparent in otters given higher ketamine dosages.

In contrast, medetomidine (25 µg/kg) combined with a low dose of ketamine (2.5 mg/kg) produced stable short-term anesthesia in river otters.[23] At this dosage, apnea occurred initially, but respiratory efforts improved with stimulation. Median relative oxyhemoglobin saturation throughout anesthesia was similar to that observed with ketamine-midazolam (see Fig. 59–2). Because of the low dosage of ketamine used in combination with medetomidine, anesthetic reversal with atipamezole (100 µg/kg) was rapid and complete within 15 minutes. Higher dosages of medetomidine (50, 75, and 100 µg/kg) combined with the same dose of ketamine extended anesthesia time beyond 25 minutes, but significant bradycardia, hypotension, and hypoxemia developed in most otters. Medetomidine and ketamine

with atipamezole reversal has also been used successfully by the author in Asian small-clawed otters (medetomidine, 50 μg/kg, and ketamine, 5 mg/kg) and in a
single giant otter (medetomidine, 30 μg/kg, and ketamine, 3 mg/kg). Similar dosages were reportedly effective in European otters during a reintroduction project
in Spain (medetomidine, 50 μg/kg, and ketamine, 5
mg/kg) (J. Fernandez Moran, personal communication,
1996). Higher dosages (medetomidine, 100–120 μg/kg,
and ketamine, 4 to 5 mg/kg) had been reported for
Asian small-clawed otters.[12]

Routine use of atropine with dissociative anesthetics
or dissociative–alpha₂ agonist combinations is not recommended unless airway secretions are excessive or
bradyarrhythmias develop. When given as a premedication, atropine does not necessarily prevent bradycardia
produced by xylazine or medetomidine. Hypertension
may develop with concurrent use of atropine and the
alpha₂ agonists. This effect can be potentiated by the
dissociative anesthetics, which also increase heart rate
and cardiac output.

Narcotics

Narcotic agonists have been used almost exclusively for
sedation and analgesia in sea otters.[5, 9, 18, 28–30] Initially,
a combination of meperidine (11 to 13 mg/kg) and
diazepam (0.22 to 0.55 mg/kg) with reversal by naloxone (0.01–0.05 mg/kg) was recommended for sea otters
undergoing minor procedures, including transmitter implantation.[9] More recently, protocols involving fentanyl
(0.1 mg/kg) with diazepam (0.5 mg/kg) and azaperone
(0.5 mg/kg) or acepromazine (0.05 mg/kg) were developed for long-term sedation during washing of oiled
otters after the Exxon Valdez oil spill.[18] Unfortunately,
conditions precluded physiologic monitoring, but sedation was adequate for up to 2.5 hours and was considered to pose less risk to the debilitated otters than was
general anesthesia. In a hospital setting, sea otters can
be sedated with diazepam with or without butorphanol
(0.5 mg/kg) or oxymorphone (0.3 mg/kg), and general
anesthesia can be induced by mask with isoflurane (T.
Williams, personal communication, 1996).

Dosages of fentanyl-azaperone or fentanyl-azaperone-midazolam comparable with those used in sea otters
were evaluated in river otters (L. Spelman, unpublished
data). Although river otters were sedated, severe muscle
rigidity was present and respiratory depression (apnea)
was pronounced (relative oxyhemoglobin saturation,
<50%). Arterial blood gases revealed severe hypox-
emia and respiratory acidosis (see Table 59–2). Reversal
with naloxone was instituted as soon as possible.
Clearly, the dosage combinations evaluated in river otters did not achieve the appropriate ratio of butyrophenone to narcotic in which respiratory depression is minimized. However, in view of the severe hypoxemia, it
was considered unsafe to continue the pilot study in
river otters.

INHALATION ANESTHESIA

Intubation in otters is straightforward, and isoflurane
(or halothane) delivered in oxygen can be used to supplement and maintain anesthesia. If a chamber is available, isoflurane can also be used as an induction agent.
Mask induction with the use of a net and manual restraint of the head is not generally recommended but
can be performed safely by experienced personnel. As
in most species, isoflurane can produce mild hypotension (secondary to vasodilation) and decrease heart rate
in otters. Significant respiratory depression is not expected with isoflurane and did not occur in river otters.[22]
Hypothermia may develop with longer procedures as a
result of the profound muscle relaxation that accompanies inhalation anesthesia.

Apnea has been described in river otters in which
anesthesia was induced with ketamine-xylazine-acepro-
mazine, supplemented with isoflurane via intubation,
and placed in dorsal recumbency.[7] In the author's experience, otters often become apneic both before intubation and after extubation, regardless of the injectable
agent used for induction. Typically, the anesthetic plane
is light, and decreased respiratory efforts appear to
result from increased muscle tension. Increasing anesthetic depth after intubation can be accomplished by
increasing the isoflurane concentration and/or brief administration of positive pressure ventilation. During recovery, extubation should be delayed as long as possible
and supplemental oxygen via face mask should be provided if a poor respiratory pattern is observed.

SPECIAL CONSIDERATIONS
FOR WILD OTTERS

Translocation Projects

Many of the earlier studies involving translocation and
telemetry in river otters,[4, 6, 7, 13, 31] sea otters,[29] and Eurasian otters[15, 16] were associated with relatively high
rates of mortality occurring from hours to days after
anesthesia. During the earlier studies, otters were typically anesthetized within hours of capture and released
immediately after transmitter implantation. Most anesthetic protocols included ketamine (15 to 22 mg/kg)
alone or in combination with diazepam, xylazine, or
acepromazine. Stress, injury, dehydration, and depleted
energy stores undoubtedly contributed to anesthetic-
related death. Otters found dead after relocation apparently died of inanition and, in some cases, pneumonia
or peritonitis.

On the basis of successful relocation projects in the
United States, several recommendations can be made
for relocated river otters that can also be applied to any
otter species. After capture, otters should be allowed to
adjust to their temporary captive environment for several days before anesthesia. Care should be taken during
transport and handling to avoid injury, especially to the
teeth. Appropriate holding cages should be constructed
of plastic-coated wire mesh or polyvinylchloride piping.
Fresh fish or other natural food items should be offered
on a daily basis. During anesthesia, physiologic parameters should be carefully monitored, especially respiratory rate and pattern. For longer procedures, measures
should be taken to avoid hypothermia. If surgery is
performed, a minor amount of fur should be shaved.

After anesthesia, otters should be confined at least 3 to 4 days to ensure that they are feeding well and exhibiting normal grooming behavior.

Oiled Otters

Sea otters should be sedated and lightly restrained for washing procedures, which may require several hours to complete. Because of the length of the procedure and the debilitated condition of oiled otters, general anesthesia is not recommended. Even isoflurane, generally regarded as the safest anesthetic, was associated with anesthetic-related death in four sea otters after the Exxon Valdez oil spill.[18] Although anesthetic recovery was uneventful, each of the otters died within 24 hours apparently because the volatile anesthetic solubilized the inhaled hydrocarbons.

For river otters undergoing simulated de-oiling procedures, light anesthesia was required for safe handling. Ketamine (10 mg/kg) and midazolam (0.25 mg/kg) or tiletamine-zolazepam (4 mg/kg, combined) were used with supplemental ketamine (5 mg/kg) if necessary. Regardless of warm or cool bath water temperature, body temperature dropped precipitously during the 90 minute washing procedure and decreased below 35°C in most otters.[24] Body temperature did not return to normal until drying of the fur was complete, which was aided by the use of a blowdryer.

CONCLUSIONS

Regardless of anesthetic protocol, respiratory depression can be expected in all anesthetized otters, particularly during induction with injectable anesthetics. An endotracheal tube should be available, and supplemental oxygen should be administered when possible. Regular monitoring of relative oxyhemoglobin saturation is strongly recommended.

For sea otters, minor procedures should be performed whenever possible with the use of a restraint box and a light narcotic or benzodiazepine sedation. Techniques for general anesthesia with injectable anesthetics in sea otters have not been well established, and there are numerous reports of fatal complications with dissociative anesthetics in these animals. Unless oiled, sea otters can be safely anesthetized by mask or chamber induction with isoflurane.

For all other otter species, dissociative-benzodiazepine combinations are recommended for short-term anesthesia. Ketamine combined with midazolam has several advantages over ketamine-diazepam or tiletamine-zolazepam. Ketamine (10 to 12 mg/kg) and midazolam (0.25 to 0.5 mg/kg) can be expected to produce rapid induction, 20 to 30 minutes of anesthesia, minimal respiratory depression, and smooth recovery. Smaller species may require higher dosages (ketamine, 15 mg/kg, and midazolam, 1 mg/kg). This combination is also useful as an induction agent before inhalation anesthesia. Ketamine (5 mg/kg) can be used as a supplement for ketamine-midazolam, ketamine-diazepam, or tiletamine-zolazepam.

Medetomidine (25 to 50 µg/kg) and ketamine (2.5 to 5 mg/kg) with atipamezole reversal may prove especially useful in the field when rapid remobilization is necessary. The appropriate dosage of medetomidine-ketamine must be established for each species because of the potent respiratory depressant effects of this combination. When administered at a dosage ratio of 5:1, atipamezole can be expected to produce full recovery within 15 minutes. Xylazine-ketamine is not recommended for field anesthesia in otters unless other combinations are unavailable. Xylazine (3 to 5 mg/kg) and ketamine (3 to 5 mg/kg) can be used for induction prior to isoflurane, but yohimbine should be administered after intubation to improve respiratory effort and minimize the risks of prolonged recovery and hypothermia.

REFERENCES

1. Arnemo JM: Chemical immobilization of European river otters (*Lutra lutra*). Norsk Vet 102(11):767–770, 1990.
2. Calle PP, Robinson PT: Glucosuria associated with renal calculi in Asian small-clawed otters. J Am Vet Med Assoc 187(11):1149–1153, 1985.
3. Colares EP, Best RC: Blood parameters of Amazon otters (*Lutra longicaudis, Pteronura brasiliensis*). Comp Biochem Physiol 99A(4):513–515, 1991.
4. Elmore RG, Hardin DK, Balke JME, et al: Analyzing the effects of diazepam in combination with ketamine. Vet Med 80:55–57, 1985.
5. Holmes AA: Immobilon in the otter. Vet Rec 95:574, 1974.
6. Hoover JP, Bahr RJ, Nieves MA, et al: Clinical evaluation and prerelease management of American river otters in the second year of a reintroduction study. J Am Vet Med Assoc 187:1154–1165, 1985.
7. Hoover JP, Jones EM: Physiologic and electrocardiographic responses of American river otters (*Lutra canadensis*) during chemical immobilization and inhalation anesthesia. J Wildl Dis 22:557–563, 1986.
8. Jenkins D, Gormon ML: Anesthesia of the European otter (*Lutra lutra*) using ketamine hydrochloride. J Zool 194:265–267, 1981.
9. Joseph BE, Cornell LH, Williams TD: Chemical sedation of sea otters, *Enhydra lutra*. J Zoo Anim Med 18:7–13, 1987.
10. Kane KK: Medical management of the otter. Proceedings of the Annual Meeting of American Association of Zoo Veterinarians, Denver, CO, pp 100–103, 1979.
11. Kuiken T: Anesthesia in the European otter (*Lutra lutra*). Vet Rec 123:59, 1988.
12. Lewis JCM: Reversible immobilization of Asian small-clawed otters with medetomidine and ketamine. Vet Rec 128:86–87, 1991.
13. Melquist WE, Hornocker MG: Ecology of river otters in west central Idaho. Wildl Monogr 47:10, 1983.
14. Petrini K: The medical management and diseases of mustelids. Proceedings of the Annual Meeting of American Association of Zoo Veterinarians, Oakland, CA, pp 116–131, 1992.
15. Reuther C: Immobilization of European otter with ketamine hydrochloride. Berl Munch Tieraztl Wochenschr 96:401–405, 1983.
16. Reuther C, Brandes B: Occurrence of hyperthermia during immobilization of European otter (*Lutra lutra*) with ketamine hydrochloride. Dtsch Tieraztl Wochenschr 91:66–68, 1984.
17. Samuels MS, Cook RA: Electrocardiography of the Asian small-clawed otter (*Aonyx cinerea*). Zoo Biol 10:277–280, 1991.
18. Sawyer DC, Williams TD: Chemical restraint and anesthesia of sea otters affected by the oil spill in Prince William Sound, Alaska. J Am Vet Med Assoc 208(11):1831–1834, 1996.
19. Seal US, Kreeger TJ: Chemical immobilization of furbearers. *In* Novak M, Baker JA, Obbard ME, Mallock B (eds): Wild Furbearer Management and Conservation in North America. Montreal, Ontario, Canada, Ministry of Natural Resources, Montreal, p 208, 1987.
20. Serfass TL, Peper RL, Whary MT, Brooks RP: River otter (*Lutra canadensis*) reintroduction in Pennsylvania: prerelease care and clinical evaluation. J Zoo Wild Anim Med 24(1):28–40, 1993.
21. Spelman LH, Sumner PW, Karesh WB, Stoskopf MK: Tiletamine-zolazepam anesthesia in North American river otters (*Lutra cana-*

densis) and partial antagonism with flumazenil. J Zoo Wildl Med 28(4):418–423, 1997.

22. Spelman LH, Sumner PW, Levine JF, Stoskopf MK: Field anesthesia in the North American river otter (*Lutra canadensis*). J Zoo Wildl Med 24(1):19–27, 1993.

23. Spelman LH, Sumner PW, Levine JF, Stoskopf MK: Medetomidine-ketamine anesthesia in the North American river otter (*Lutra canadensis*) and reversal by atipamezole. J Zoo Wildl Med 25(2):214–223, 1994.

24. Stoskopf MK, Spelman LH, Sumner PW: The impact of water temperature on core body temperature of North American river otters (*Lutra canadensis*) during simulated oil spill recovery washing protocols. J Zoo Wildl Med 28(4):407–412, 1997.

25. Tarasoff FJ: Anatomical adaptations in the river otter, sea otter, and harp seal. *In* Harrison RJ (ed): Functional Anatomy of Marine Mammals. New York, Academic Press, pp 111–141, 1974.

26. Turley PF, Macdonald S, Mason C (eds): Otters: An Action Plan for their Conservation (IUCN/SSC Otter Specialist Group). Broadview, IL, Kelvyn Press, pp 4–6, 1990.

27. Williams TD: A physical restraint device for sea otters. J Zoo Wildl Med 21(1):105, 1990.

28. Williams TD, Kocher FH: Comparison of anesthetic agents in the sea otter. J Am Vet Med Assoc 173(9):1127–1130, 1978.

29. Williams TD, Siniff DB: Surgical implantation of radiotelemetry devices in the sea otter. J Am Vet Med Assoc 183(11):1290–1291, 1983.

30. Williams TD, Williams AL, Siniff DB: Fentanyl and azaperone produced neuroleptanalgesia in the sea otter (*Enhydra lutris*). J Wildl Dis 17:337–342, 1981.

31. Woolf A, Curl JL, Anderson E: Inanition following implantation of a radiotelemetry device in a river otter. J Am Vet Med Assoc 185:1415–1416, 1984.

CHAPTER 60

Health Assessment, Medical Management, and Prerelease Conditioning of Translocated North American River Otters

GEORGE V. KOLLIAS

North American river otter (*Lutra canadensis*) populations are recovering from their markedly decreased numbers that resulted from the additive effects of wetland destruction, aquatic pollution, and unregulated trapping for the fur industry in the late 19th and early 20th centuries. Although a variety of conservation efforts throughout North America have been instrumental in improving population numbers, the International Union for the Conservation of Nature and Natural Resources (IUCN) Otter Specialist Group still considers population status determinations of high priority in states and provinces where trapping for fur is permitted. Two of the many conservation strategies implemented in a number of states are reintroduction and translocation. The first includes reintroduction of river otters from areas with dense populations to historic habitats with sparse or small populations and where introduction has previously been attempted. A second strategy includes translocation of river otters from densely populated areas to areas from which otters have been extirpated or are present in very small numbers. There are logistic, fiscal, and biologic advantages and disadvan-

tages to each strategy. Reintroduction may ultimately cost more money; it also presents the challenge of screening for and eliminating certain infectious diseases that may be of importance to other resident mustelids, and it may result in higher mortality rates following release. The monetary costs of translocation, even within a state, may also be relatively high (approximately $1000 per otter) depending on (1) the trapping methods, (2) the trapper (state wildlife biologists versus private trappers), (3) the method of transport (ground versus air transport), and (4) the health screening/treatment and preconditioning protocols that are implemented to maximize survival and, ultimately, reproductive success following release. Translocation of river otters within a state does have distinct biologic and logistic advantages over reintroduction. First, the probability of "foreign" diseases being introduced is low or minimal. Second, the stress of holding before transport is minimized as is the total transport time for individual otters.

This chapter describes health assessment/management, husbandry, and preconditioning methods used over a 3-year period in an ongoing collaborative river otter translocation project in the state of New York, which includes the New York State Department of Environmental Conservation (NYSDEC), the New York River Otter Project, Inc. (NYROP), and the College of Veterinary Medicine at Cornell University. This ongoing project has resulted in the successful release of 97 otters (92% of the individuals trapped) into five geographically separated sites in the western parts of the state. Although there have been similar projects undertaken in other states, only a few have addressed in detail health assessment, medical management, and infectious disease considerations for river otters.[1, 2, 4, 6, 10, 11]

TRIAGE, INITIAL ASSESSMENT, AND MEDICAL PLAN FOR TRANSLOCATED RIVER OTTERS

River otters are received at a Cornell University, Association for the Assessment and Accreditation of Laboratory Animal Care, International– (ALAC)-approved, specific pathogen-free (SPF) carnivore holding facility and strictly isolated from other wild and domestic animals. The building consists of an anteroom with platform scale, food storage and prep room, individual animal holding rooms, an examination/treatment/intensive care room, and a locker room for animal care personnel. Otters are received between September 1 and December 1. Upon arrival, they are weighed in their respective transport cages and visually examined. At the time of receipt, a complete history is obtained from the NYSDEC biologist transporting the otter whose report includes trapping location and technique, estimated time the otter remained in a particular trap, weather conditions, time and conditions of holding and transport, perceived condition of the otter, quantity of food and water accepted by the otter, if any, and any other relevant information that may be important to the health assessment and initial management of the individual otter. After visual examination, individual otters are either transferred from the transport cage to a portable small mammal restraint (squeeze) cage (Fig. 60–1) and administered (1) *Clostridium perfringens* types C and D antitoxin, ivermectin, trimethoprim-sulfamethoxazole, d-alpha tocopherol (vitamin E), selenium, and B-complex vitamins (to include minimally 10 mg/kg thiamin) (Table 60–1) or (2) a combination of ketamine hydrochloride and midazolam or ketamine hydrochloride and diazepam to chemically immobilize them. If there is evidence of soft tissue or skeletal trauma or if the otter appears depressed (usually a result of hypothermia, hypoglycemia, or generalized stress), it is given treatment for its specific problems. This initial prophylactic treatment protocol is based on clinical laboratory and necropsy findings on otters from year one of the NYROP and results of other similar projects.[6, 10]

HOUSING AND DAILY MAINTENANCE PROCEDURES

After their initial assessment, all otters are transferred and housed individually in double-tiered, stainless steel,

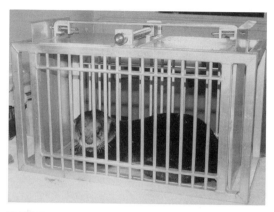

FIGURE 60–1. North American river otter being held in a portable small mammal restraint (squeeze) cage prior to chemical immobilization.

36-inch-square primate holding/restraint cages. They are offered food, water, and a measured amount (usually 500 ml) of an oral electrolyte/mineral/dextrose solution (Ora-Lyte; Butler, Inc.) in a separate crock. Each cage includes a 30- × 30-inch removable 1- × 1-inch mesh floor rack, 0.5-inch diameter/0.75-inch spaced door bars with a 10.5- × 12.0-inch guillotine door and solid top, sides, and back. A removable pan below the floor rack allows continued observation of feces (e.g., for volume and consistency) and urine production by each otter. Each cage is equipped with a 6.5-inch (D) × 26-inch (L) resting platform 10 inches above the floor rack. Water is provided in an 8-inch diameter, 4-inch deep ceramic crock, which is changed once or twice daily. Otters are provided daily with 1 to 2 clean terry cloth bath towels for them to rub and clean their fur, keeping it free from food particles, water, feces, or urine—factors critical to enable otters to maintain appropriate thermoregulation and buoyancy once released. Cages are located in rooms with environmental and timed lighting controls. Cages are arranged so that individual otters are in visual contact with other individuals within a room or run.

DAILY TREATMENT AND OBSERVATION

Antimicrobial therapy is continued orally for 7 to 10 days to treat apparent and nonapparent soft tissue trauma associated with capture and transport. (Gross evidence of soft tissue trauma to feet, toes, and occasionally teeth are evident only by physical examination.) In addition, because of a high prevalence of ivermectin-resistant *Crenosoma* species in New York State otters, fenbendazole is given for 3 consecutive days once the otters begin to accept food. Antibiotic tablets are placed inside a small (0.5 × 1.0 inch) piece of lake trout, and fenbendazole is injected into fish pieces and presented to otters on a blunt-pointed dowel through the cage bars. Acceptance of drug-laden fish pieces is 95% successful, particularly in otters in captiv-

TABLE 60–1. Drugs, Nutritional Supplements, and Biologics Used in the New York River Otter Project

	Dose	Route/Interval	Maximum
Antibiotics			
Enrofloxacin	2.5 mg/kg	IM, PO, BID	14 days
Metronidazole	25 mg/kg	PO, BID	7 days
Trimethoprim-sulfamethoxazole	20 mg/kg	PO, IM, or SQ (depending on formulation), BID	3 days (IM or SQ) 30 days (PO)
Parasiticides			
Fenbendazole	50 mg/kg	PO, SID	3 Days consecutively for *Crenosoma* species
Ivermectin	0.4 mg/kg	SQ (1 dose is usually efficacious)	2 Doses 10–14 days apart have infrequently been required to treat *Strongyloides* species and *Capillaria* species.
Vitamins/Minerals			
Thiamin	10 mg/kg	SQ, SID	3 Days consecutively (usually administered q 7 days)
Vitamin E (*d*-alpha-tocopherol)	40 IU/kg (300 IU minimum)	SQ, q 7 days	q 7 days × 4 weeks
Selenium	0.06 mg/kg	IM (once)	q 7 days × 3 weeks (generally given only once)
Biologics			
Clostridium perfringens Types C and D antitoxin (Equine origin)	3 ml	SQ (once)	q 7 days × 2 weeks
Oral Fluid Replacement (Electrolytes/Dextrose)			
*Ora-Lyte (Butler, Inc.)	500 ml (prepared per package insert)	PO, prn, BID	3–7 days (readily accepted)

IM, intramuscularly; PO, per os; SQ, subcutaneously.
*Contains NaCl, KCl, Ca gluconate, dextrose, Mg sulfate, Na citrate niacin, thiamin HCl, ascorbic acid, zinc sulfate, Fe sulfate.

ity for more than 24 to 48 hours. If attempts at treatment are unsuccessful, repeated coaxing and stimulation around the vibrissae and muzzle prompt the individual to accept the medicated fish. If an otter refuses medicated fish pieces, it is transferred to the small mammal restraint (squeeze) cage and injected with the antibiotic or it is slowly and carefully administered the fenbendazole by mouth with a dose syringe. Injections of B-complex vitamins (including thiamin) and vitamin E are given at 7- to 10-day intervals (minimally twice) or whenever an otter is chemically or physically restrained in the squeeze cage.

Complete medical records, in addition to daily food consumption records, are kept on all animals from admission until release. In addition, it is of particular importance to observe and record the character and volume of the otter's feces. Blood, mucus, or foamy light brown to gray coloring to the feces may be indicative of early or impending enteritis caused by intestinal nematodes (e.g., *Strongyloides* species or *Capillaria* species) or *Clostridium perfringens*.

FEEDING AND NUTRITION

A variety of feeding strategies have been reported successful for captive North American river otters.[9] Be-

cause the holding period is relatively short (12 to 50 days), providing diets most similar to natural prey avoids problems related to the disruption of normal intestinal microbial flora and the lack of recognition and rejection of new diets. Otters involved in the first year NYROP were offered a variety of freshwater fish species (e.g., perch, bullhead catfish, rainbow trout), but their diets were limited almost solely to lake trout the second and third year of the project. It is important to have fish analyzed for nutrient quantity and quality because their nutritional value may vary considerably if acquired locally or commercially (Table 60–2). The fish fed should be fresh or fresh frozen and not stored in the freezer for longer than 60 days. In addition, parenteral supplementation of individual otters or supplementation of the fish they are fed with thiamin, vitamin E, or other nutrients (as appropriate and based on the fish analysis or the species of fish being offered) is carried out weekly if administered to otters or daily if added to fish.

In general, minimally stressed otters accept fish immediately or within 24 hours of admission. Moderately to severely stressed or physically traumatized individuals may require "hand feeding" chunks of fish muscle offered on the end of a blunt dowel until they begin to eat food on their own volition, usually within 48 to 72

TABLE 60–2. Examples of Nutritional Content of Fish Fed to North American River Otters
(*Lutra canadensis*)

Analyte*	Lake Trout (Lake Erie)	Rainbow Smelt (Lake Erie)
DM	41.54%	21.00%
Ash	3.56%	1.78%
Fat	55.78%	14.94%
Protein	40.69%	71.83%
d-Alpha-tocopherol	245.58 µg/g	302.76 µg/g
τ-Tocopherol	16.05 µg/g	3.83 µg/g
Vitamin E activity (τ- + alpha-tocopherol)	368.30 IU/kg	333.42 IU/kg
Retinol	7.90 µg/g	3.55 µg/g
Vitamin A activity	26,333.33 IU/kg	11,833.30 IU/kg
Calories	664.78 kcal/100g	421.78 kcal/100g

Performed by E. S. Dierenfeld, Ph.D., Head, Department of Nutrition, Wildlife Conservation Society, Wildlife Health Center, Bronx, NY.
*All results on a dry matter basis except DM.

hours of admission. Otters that do not accept food on their own within 63 to 72 hours have serious medical problems that need to be addressed. In my practice, we offer 2 to 2.5 lb (0.9 to 1.4 kg) of fish daily in the afternoon. The amount consumed by 8 AM the following morning is recorded and the remaining fish or parts thereof are discarded. Smaller otters require fresh food twice daily.

CHEMICAL IMMOBILIZATION FOR HEALTH ASSESSMENT, MINOR SURGICAL PROCEDURES, AND DIAGNOSTIC PURPOSES

If not on the day of admission, all otters are chemically immobilized within 72 hours of admission or after they have accepted food for 2 consecutive days. Otters are transferred from their respective holding cages to the portable squeeze cage and placed on the examination room table. Once they are restrained in the squeeze cage, the otters are injected in any available muscle mass (usually the rectus femoris, quadriceps, triceps, or longissimus) with the ketamine (15 mg/kg)–midazolam (0.3 mg/kg) or ketamine (15 mg/kg)–diazepam (0.5 mg/kg) combination on the basis of their entrance weight. The squeeze cage is covered with a drape or towel to be light proof and environmental noise is kept to a minimum. A complete anesthesia record is kept during the procedure. Uniformly (based on more than 100 immobilizations), otters are completely immobilized in 10 to 12 minutes and remain immobilized for 30 to 45 minutes. If the procedure is extended beyond 35 to 45 minutes, an occasional individual will require additional 20 to 30 mg IV boluses of ketamine. The jugular, cephalic, and saphenous veins are easily accessible, but the thick pelage of some individuals must be wetted or clipped in order to visualize these veins. Because of the importance of the fur in thermoregulation, however, clipping should be kept to a minimum. Table 60–3 contains body weight ranges, heart and respiratory rates, and rectal temperatures of river otters chemically immo-

bilized with ketamine-midazolam or ketamine-diazepam combinations.

Otters requiring prolonged anesthesia are intubated and administered isoflurane-oxygen with intermittent positive pressure ventilation. Minimal monitoring with either technique includes heart, respiratory rate, and rectal temperature (see Chapter 59). Anesthetized otters are recovered in their holding cages that have been padded with towels and draped with a sheet to keep out light and reduce auditory stimuli. Complete recovery times range from 30 to 90 minutes. Occasionally during recovery, an otter goes through a hyperactive period, which soon subsides. If this becomes prolonged, there is a threat of hyperthermia and the animal may require additional sedation and other corrective measures.

HEALTH STATUS ASSESSMENT OF RECENTLY CAPTURED RIVER OTTERS

Protocol for assessing the health status of recently captured river otters includes a complete physical examination (including weighing) and detailing and addressing any observable problems including injuries to feet and teeth. Blood is routinely collected for packed cell volume (PCV), total solids (TS), and Knott's test (to screen for microfilaria) or complete blood count and biochemical profiling when needed to further assess the health status of the otter.[3, 6] In addition, blood is collected for vitamin and mineral analysis and for seroepidemiologic studies focusing on exposure to viral agents reported to be transmissible to North American river otters.[5, 7, 8, 12, 13] All otters are permanently identified with titanium microchips (AVID, Norco, CA) injected at a 45-degree angle into the fascia between the scapulae. In general, before physical examination, a fresh fecal sample is collected for examination for endoparasite ova or protozoal trophozoites, aerobic and anaerobic culture, and *C. perfringens* exotoxin assay. After this assessment and receipt of clinical laboratory results, a medical and surgical treatment plan is formulated and revised as dictated by the otter's progress.

While the otter is anesthetized, the drugs described

TABLE 60–3. **Physiologic Parameters Recorded in River Otters Immobilized With Ketamine/ Midazolam or Ketamine/Diazepam Combinations**

	Males (n = 34)		Females (n = 36)		Males and Females (n = 65)		
	Mean	Range	Mean	Range	Mean of Means	SD of Means	Range
Body weight (kg)	5.64	2.90–9.30	5.50	3.6–8.0			
Respiratory rate (breaths/ minute)					30.91	+ 8.53	12–56
Heart rate (beats/minute)					165.66	28.06	120–264
Rectal temperature (°F)					101.86	1.19	99.80–104.75

under Triage, Initial Assessment, and Medical Plan for Translocated River Otters are administered parenterally as appropriate.

Minor to moderate traumatic injuries (e.g., distal pharynx amputation, diffuse soft tissue debridement) are treated surgically or medically during this immobilization. Injured paws are treated and bandaged using nonadherent wound dressing pads, limited amounts of cast padding, and waterproof adhesive tape that extends onto the fur of the proximal part of the affected limb. If applied properly, this type of bandage remains on the leg for up to 5 days when it is manually removed. Most otters seem unconcerned about their bandage and do not attempt to remove it. Following the physical examination, otters are periodically weighed before their release to verify that they are experiencing continued weight gain. This can easily be performed without chemical restraint by using the transfer box depicted in Figure 60–2, which is also used to move otters when their cages require thorough cleaning.

MANAGEMENT OF MEDICAL PROBLEMS

Unless additional problems arise, the otters involved in the NYROP are held optimally for 10 to 15 days for assessment, treatment, and prerelease improvement of body condition. Using the nutritional and treatment plan described, the otters involved in this project have increased their admission body weight on average by 20% over the 10- to 15-day period.

Common medical problems observed during the assessment period include diarrhea (enteritis with or without blood) resulting from intestinal parasitism or overgrowth of *C. perfringens* and purulent nasal discharge (usually unilateral) associated with *Crenosoma* species (lungworm) infection or of undetermined etiology.

A third problem occurs in a small number of individuals (3% of the total) at 24 to 72 hours after admission. The affected individuals exhibit inactivity, including a marked reduction in normal grooming behavior, hypophagia and hypodipsia, profound hypothermia, and eventually coma. Once recognized, these individuals are so profoundly physically depressed that they can be handled and treated using only manual restraint. Response to aggressive therapy is dramatic. Therapy includes the administration of warmed 5% dextrose solution and half-strength saline in equal amounts or Isolyte solution IV, intraosseous (IO), or SQ, B-complex vitamins to include thiamin (10 mg/kg SQ), *d*-alpha-tocopherol (300 to 400 IU SQ), parenteral trimethoprim-sulfamethoxazole, and *C. perfringens* antitoxin (3 ml SQ, if it has not been recently given). Additional environmen-

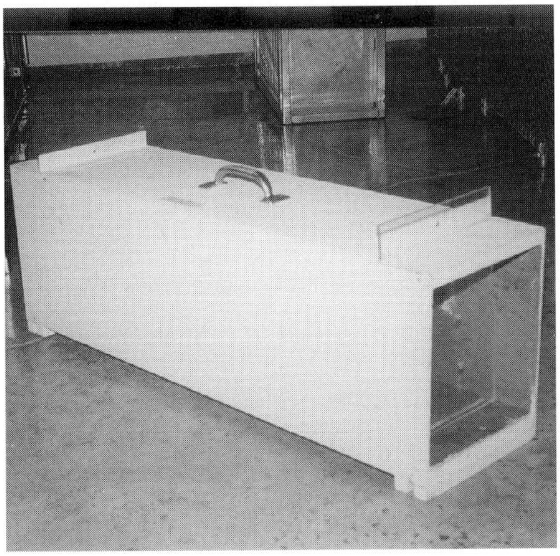

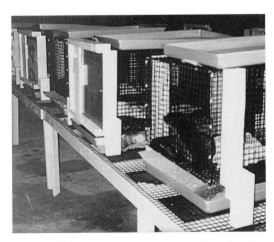

FIGURE 60–2. Wooden transfer box used to move otters from cage to cage and for purpose of obtaining periodic body weights (40 [L] × 9.5 [W] × 11 [H] inch; weight = 15 lbs).

FIGURE 60–3. Cages used to environmentally acclimatize otters in secondary holding facility prior to release (modified from the North Carolina River Otter Project, courtesy of Perry W. Sumner).

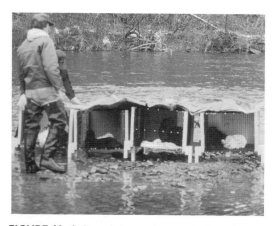

FIGURE 60–4. Otters in transport cages at release site. Note the tarp covering the cage tops, which is used to diminish visual stimulation.

tal heat is provided using an incubator or heat lamps with ceramic elements until the animals are recovered. Only one recurrence has been noted, and this animal again responded to treatment. The etiopathogenesis of this syndrome is unknown and it has not been reported in other similar projects involving river otters. Our hypothesis is that it may be a sequela to the stress of capture and transport, and may be precipitated by replication and subsequent exotoxin production by *C. perfringens* (which appears to be part of the normal intestinal flora of New York State otters).

Virtually all of the otters that have died in transport or shortly after admission (10 of 97, or 10.3%) have had evidence of heavy parasitism or severe exertional myopathy.

An occasional otter that refuses oral medications and is not drinking sufficient water may require parenteral injections of the appropriate drug or the administration of subcutaneous fluids. This usually can be performed by transferring the individual to the portable squeeze cage and administering the treatments with or without light sedation.

Two of the 97 otters released (approximately 2%) have required orthopedic surgery to correct problems associated with capture. Both had prolonged general anesthesia (4 to 6 hours), with extensive physiologic support and monitoring, and recovered rapidly without complications.

ENVIRONMENTAL ACCLIMATION AND CONTINUED SUPPORT BEFORE RELEASE

Following the average 10 to 15 days required for health assessment and medical care, otters (usually in groups of 6 to 12) are moved to a secondary facility in vinyl-coated wire and wood 19 (H) × 28 (W) × 39 (L) inch holding cages (Figure 60–3). These cages are taken to the release sites. This facility is totally enclosed and not heated but is equipped with bay doors that can be opened and closed, helping to simulate the environmental conditions under which the otters will be released. The vinyl coated wire holding cages have no resting platform but have a slightly larger floor space than the holding cages used in the medical facility. The otters are fed and offered water and dry towels in the same manner as described previously.

The environmental acclimation holding period before release varies between 3 and 7 days.

Before loading into covered, well-ventilated pickup truck cabs, the cages containing otters are reweighed to record an accurate release weight. All releases have been conducted in the morning between mid-October and mid-December. Transport time between the secondary holding facility and the release sites ranges 45 minutes to 3 hours, during which time otters remain calm, particularly if they are provided with visual barriers on the tops and/or sides of the transport cages (Figure 60–4).

Acknowledgments

The author would like to thank the New York River Otter Project, Inc., New York State Department of Environmental Conservation–Division of Wildlife, Drs. N. Abou-Madi, N. Gentz, B. Hartup, A. Hoogestyn, Mr. Kevin Kimber, my wife Heidi and my children George and Alexandra for their support, assistance, and interest in this project.

REFERENCES

1. Andrews RD, Reeved DA, Jackson LS: Reintroduction of river otters in Iowa. Proceedings Iowa Acad Sci 9391(abstr):93, 1986.
2. Beck TDI: River otter reintroduction procedures. Colo Div Wildl Res Rev 2:14–16, 1993.
3. Davis HG, Aulerich R, Bursian SJ, et al: Hematologic and blood chemistry values of the Northern River Otter (*Lutra canadensis*). Scientifur 16:267–271, 1992.
4. Erickson DW, Hamilton DA: Approaches to river otter restoration in Missouri. Trans North Am Wildl Nat Resource Conf 53:404–413, 1988.
5. Harwell G: Coccidioidomycosis in a river otter (*Lutra canadensis*). Proceedings of the Annual Meeting of the American Association of Zoo Veterinarians, Scottsdale, AZ, p 50, 1985.
6. Hoover JP, Bahr RJ, Nieves MA, et al: Clinical evaluation and pre-release management of American river otters in the second year of a reintroduction study. J Am Vet Med Assoc 187:1154–1161, 1985.
7. Hoover JP, Castro AE, Nieves MA: Serologic evaluation of vaccinated American river otters. J Am Vet Med Assoc 187:1162–1165, 1985.
8. Petrini K: The medical management and diseases of mustelids. Proceedings of the annual Meeting of the American Association of Zoo Veterinarians, Oakland, CA, pp 116–135, 1992.
9. Reed-Smith J: Diet. *In* Husbandry Notebook—North American River Otter (*Lutra canadensis*). Grand Rapids, MI, John Ball Zoological Garden, 1995.
10. Serfass TL, Peper RL, Whary MT, et al: River otter (*Lutra canadensis*) reintroduction in Pennsylvania: pre-release care and clinical evaluation. J Zoo Wildl Med 24:28–40, 1993.
11. Serfass TL, Brooks RP, Rymon LM: Evidence of long-term survival and reproduction by translocated river otters (*Lutra canadensis*) Can Field Nat 107:59–63, 1993.
12. Serfass TL, Whary MT, Peper RL, et al: Rabies in a river otter (*Lutra canadensis*) intended for reintroduction. J Zoo Wildl Med 26:311–314, 1995.
13. Wells GAH: Suspected Alentian disease in a wild otter. Vet Rec 125:232–235, 1989.

Assisted Reproductive Techniques in Nondomestic Carnivores

JoGAYLE HOWARD

Conventional methods of assisted reproduction include artificial insemination (AI; manual deposit of sperm into a female), in vitro fertilization (fertilization of an egg outside the body, producing an embryo), and embryo transfer (transfer of embryo produced by in vitro or in vivo fertilization into a surrogate host). These techniques have become routine procedures for human infertility and farm animal production. In fact, reproduction of some species (such as dairy cattle and turkeys) depends on techniques like AI. Advances in livestock and human reproductive biotechnology also have resulted in the development of additional methods, such as in vitro egg maturation (immature eggs are matured and fertilized outside the body) and intracytoplasmic sperm injection (sperm is manually injected into an egg and an embryo is produced). The potential of assisted reproduction is enhanced further by cryopreservation of sperm and embryos, which saves valuable genetic material for future generations. Strategies using these assisted reproductive techniques are being developed for the management and conservation of endangered carnivores.

BENEFITS OF ASSISTED REPRODUCTION

Assisted reproduction offers many advantages for species that are propagated under the auspices of an organized genetic management plan (such as a species survival plan; Table 61–1).[47, 50] Cooperating institutions breed animals on the basis of genetic value to maintain maximal genetic diversity in the population. For this, animals must be moved between zoos for breeding. It is less expensive to move sperm than living animals from one location to another. This strategy also provides an approach for improving reproductive efficiency in species that demonstrate poor breeding performance (e.g., the cheetah, [*Acinonyx jubatus*]) or male-female behavioral incompatibility (e.g., the clouded leopard, [*Neofelis nebulosa*]).

Cryopreservation techniques and the development of genome resource banks (repositories of sperm, eggs, and embryos) also would be beneficial in species conservation programs (see Table 61–1).[50] The combination of frozen germ plasm and in situ and ex situ populations can guarantee the greatest survival chance for an endangered species. For example, the combined use of assisted reproduction and germ plasm banks has enormous potential for infusing genetic material from wild populations into genetically stagnant captive populations. This would eliminate the need to capture wild animals for zoo breeding programs, leaving the animals instead to protect their native habitats. Furthermore, the transfer of sperm from captive to wild populations or between wild populations that are geographically separated could restore genetic vigor to wild populations that have become highly fragmented. The transfer of germ plasm into an in situ population would eliminate reintroduction or translocation of animals and would reduce the potential transmission of infectious diseases.

Although the concept of assisted reproduction is easily advocated for many of the 238 species in the order Carnivora, development of effective techniques has been difficult, primarily because of species-specific differences in reproductive processes. Knowledge of basic reproductive traits is critical for these techniques to be successful. In a few cases, reproductive biotech-

TABLE 61–1. Benefits of Assisted Reproductive Techniques and Genome Resource Banks for Population Management

Improve Reproductive Efficiency in Breeding Programs

Ensure reproduction in genetically valuable individuals
Enhance founder representation in small populations
Combat behavior incompatibility between individuals

Exchange of Genetic Material Between Populations

Between ex situ populations
  Avoid risk and expense of shipping animals for breeding
From in situ to ex situ populations
  Restore genetic vigor to captive populations
  Animals remain in the wild, protecting their habitat
From ex situ to in situ populations or between in situ
    populations
  Restore genetic vigor to fragmented wild populations
  Eliminate reintroduction or translocation of animals
  Avoid potential disease transmisson

TABLE 61–2. Impact of Sperm Morphology on Fertilization and Cleavage in Felids After In Vitro Fertilization

	Normal Sperm (%)	Fertilization (%)	Cleavage (%)	Reference
Tiger *(Panthera tigris)**	81.4	63.4	57.4	11
Cheetah *(Acinonyx jubatus)*	28.4	26.2	17.3	9
Puma *(Felis concolor)*	7.0	33.5	10.9	31

*Pregnancy (three cubs) produced following in vitro fertilization and embryo transfer.

niques have been adapted rapidly from one species to another, especially when a sound database was available from a related animal model. In general, however, the reliable use of assisted reproduction in carnivores has required that species receive individualized research attention.

IN VITRO FERTILIZATION AND EMBRYO TRANSFER

In vitro fertilization (IVF) has been used extensively in felids for understanding sperm-egg interaction and the relation of teratospermia (morphologically abnormal sperm) and sperm function.[19, 50] Most felid species produce high proportions of abnormal spermatozoa, a finding probably related to a loss of genetic variation.[19, 50] Using methods developed in the domestic cat model, it is possible to generate embryos by IVF in exotic felids. However, fertilization and cleavage rates are directly proportional to the number of normal sperm in the inseminate (Table 61–2).[18, 51] For example, the normospermic tiger produces greater than 80% normal sperm, and the rate of fertilization and embryo cleavage is high (>55%). In contrast, the teratospermic cheetah and puma produce less than 30% normal sperm and embryo cleavage is low (<18%).

Induction of Ovarian Activity

To generate oocytes for IVF, development of ovarian follicles can be induced with either equine chorionic gonadotropin (eCG) or follicle-stimulating hormone (FSH) followed by human chorionic gonadotropin (hCG).[9, 11, 12, 31, 36] Because of its long biologic half-life (~120 hours), a single injection of eCG elicits follicular activity in felids, whereas FSH must be administered in a series of daily injections because of its short circulatory persistence.[44] Although hCG is typically used to induce ovulation, it is injected in IVF procedures to stimulate final oocyte maturation within the follicle. An interval of more than 6 months between ovulation induction regimens is effective for preventing the production of neutralizing immunoglobulins to gonadotropins such as eCG and hCG.[43]

Laparoscopic Oocyte Recovery

A laparoscopic technique has been developed for IVF for transabdominal oocyte recovery (Fig. 61–1). The

procedure has been used effectively in numerous felid species, including the domestic cat,[18] leopard cat (*Felis bengalensis*),[17] tiger,[11, 12] puma (*Felis concolor*),[31] caracal (*Felis caracal*),[16] and cheetah.[9, 16] The ability to visualize ovaries and recover oocytes in carnivores, however, is species specific. For example, ovaries in felids are observed easily by laparoscopy for assessment of preovulatory follicles (flattened or slightly raised clear areas; Fig. 61–2) and aspiration of oocytes (see Fig. 61–1). In contrast, mustelid ovaries are embedded in adipose tissue and canid ovaries are enclosed within a bursa, prohibiting observation of ovarian activity or oocyte retrieval.

For laparoscopic oocyte recovery, anesthetized females are placed in a supine position and tilted head down at approximately 45 degrees. A pneumoperitoneum is created with carbon dioxide or room air instilled through a Veress needle. A 180-degree laparoscope (usually 5, 7.5, or 10 mm in diameter) is inserted through a midline skin incision cranial to the umbilicus and used to view the reproductive tract. Ovaries are evaluated for number and size (estimated using the 2-mm-diameter Veress needle) of ovarian follicles. The Veress needle also is used to position and secure the ovary for oocyte aspiration. A 22-gauge needle is attached to polyethylene tubing and rinsed with culture medium containing serum and heparin. A collection

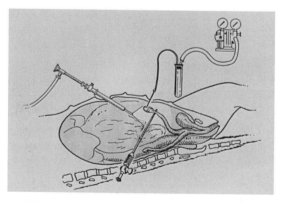

FIGURE 61–1. Laparoscopic oocyte recovery for in vitro fertilization. The laparoscope is used to identify the reproductive tract and ovarian follicular development. The ovary is elevated using a Veress probe, and a needle is punctured through the ventral abdominal wall and inserted into the follicle. Gentle negative pressure is applied with a vacuum pump as each follicle is aspirated and the oocyte recovered into a collection tube.

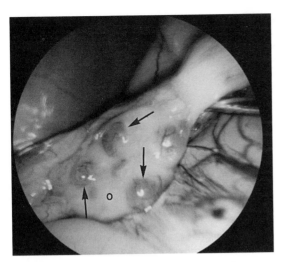

FIGURE 61–2. Clouded leopard ovary (O) containing follicles (*arrows*) after gonadotropin stimulation. (From Howard JG, Roth TL, Byers AR, et al: Sensitivity to exogenous gonadotropins for ovulation induction and laparoscopic artificial insemination in the cheetah and clouded leopard. Biol Reprod 56:1059–1068, 1997.)

tube is attached to the free end of the polyethylene tubing, and the aspiration system is driven by a vacuum pump. Distinct follicles are perforated with the needle while gentle negative pressure is applied with the vacuum pump. After follicles from one ovary are aspirated, the collection tube and aspiration needle are replaced and the procedure is repeated for the contralateral ovary. Collection tubes are emptied into separate culture dishes and examined by stereomicroscopy. In contrast to that of other mammals, the vitellus of carnivore oocytes typically is dark as a result of a high lipid content (Fig. 61–3A). After recovery, each oocyte–cumulus cell complex is evaluated and classified as mature (if cumulus oophorus cells are loose and expanded) or degenerate (if oocyte appears abnormal or lacks cumulus oophorus cells).

Oocytes are co-cultured with sperm for approximately 20 hours and assessed for fertilization and embryo cleavage about 30 hours after insemination (see Fig. 61–3B). Fertilization (i.e., the presence of pronuclei) in carnivores is more difficult to see than in other mammals because of the dark vitellus of the oocyte. Although oocytes can be stained to detect pronuclei, fertilization usually is determined by embryo cleavage to at least the two-cell stage of development. Although few attempts have been made to transfer IVF embryos in carnivores, offspring have been produced from Indian desert cat (*Felis silvestris ornata*)[36] and tiger (*Panthera tigris*)[11] embryos.

Gamete Rescue

It is possible to "rescue" oocytes from animals after death or ovariohysterectomy. Mature ovulated eggs have been collected from oviducts of foxes (*Alopex lagopus*) and fertilized in vitro.[14] Because the fertilizable life of an ovulated egg is usually less than 24 hours, however, time for gamete retrieval from oviducts is limited. For this reason, eggs typically are recovered from ovaries. Immature eggs obtained from ovaries of cheetahs, tigers, pumas, leopard cats, servals (*Felis serval*), bobcats (*Lynx rufus*), lions (*Panthera leo*), leopards (*Panthera pardus*), jaguars (*Panthera onca*), and snow leopards (*Panthera uncia*) have been matured in vitro.[28] Many of these oocytes were fertilized and developed in vitro. Recently, the biologic competence of domestic cat embryos produced after in vitro egg maturation and fertilization was demonstrated by the birth of live young after embryo transfer.[37]

ARTIFICIAL INSEMINATION

The relatively poor breeding history of many nondomestic carnivores in captivity resulted in the early application of AI technology. In the 1970s, AI success was achieved in timber wolves (*Canis lupus*) using frozenthawed semen previously collected by digital manipu-

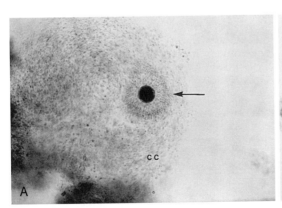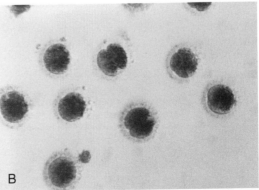

FIGURE 61–3. *A*, Mature tiger oocyte (*arrow*) with expanded cumulus cell (CC) mass collected by laparoscopic ovarian aspiration. *B*, Two- and four-cell stage, in vitro–fertilized tiger embryos after 30 hours of culture. (From Donoghue AM, Johnston LA, Seal US, et al: *In vitro* fertilization and embryo development *in vitro* and *in vivo* in the tiger (*Panthera tigris*). Biol Reprod 43:733–744, 1990.)

TABLE 61–3. Pregnancy Rates After Nonsurgical (Vaginal or Transcervical) Versus Laparoscopic (Intrauterine) Artificial Insemination

	Nonsurgical Vaginal/Transcervical Insemination	Laparoscopic Intrauterine Insemination	References
Domestic cat *(Felis catus)*	6/56 (10.6%)	9/18 (50.0%)	20, 35
Cheetah *(Acinonyx jubatus)*	0/23 (0%)	6/13 (46.2%)	23, 26, 51
European ferret *(Mustela putorius furo)*	0/10 (0%)	17/24 (70.8%)	46

lation.[40, 41] This semen collection technique is used routinely today in fox breeding programs.[1, 15] However, the need to handle nonsedated animals precludes use of this method for most nondomestic carnivores. AI techniques using sperm collected by electroejaculation have produced embryos obtained by flushing the uterine horns in a tiger[38] and a lion.[3] Various gonadotropins and their ability to stimulate ovarian activity and ovulation have been assessed for AI. Administration of eCG or FSH is effective for inducing folliculogenesis, whereas hCG or gonadotropin-releasing hormone (GnRH) induces ovulation.[32, 33, 38, 49] Initial AI success for propagating wild felids was achieved with a puma cub produced by in utero deposition of sperm at laparotomy in 1981[32, 33] and a Persian leopard cub *(Panthera pardus saxicolor)* that was born after nonsurgical, transcervical AI in 1982.[13] Nonsurgical inseminations also have been effective for producing pregnancies in the giant panda *(Ailuropoda melanoleuca)*.[34, 45]

Site of Insemination

Recent AI attempts in carnivores have demonstrated that success is highly influenced by the site of semen deposition (Table 61–3). Although pregnancies have been achieved in domestic cats after vaginal deposition of semen into anesthetized females, the incidence of pregnancy was only 10.6%.[35] Numerous AI attempts were conducted using nonsurgical (vaginal or transcervical) methods, but no pregnancies resulted after 23 inseminations in cheetahs, 11 AI attempts in tigers, and 7 attempts in clouded leopards.[22, 48, 51] It was determined later that the anesthesia event itself (necessary for most wild animals) compromises sperm transport in nonsurgically inseminated females.[48] To circumvent this problem, a laparoscopic intrauterine AI technique was devel-

oped for depositing sperm in the uterine horn near the site of fertilization (oviduct; Fig. 61–4).[20] This approach resulted in a higher pregnancy rate (~50%) in the domestic cat and cheetah (see Table 61–3).[20, 26]

AI trials in other carnivores, including the blue fox *(Alopex lagopus)* and silver fox *(Vulpes vulpes)*, have demonstrated that vaginal AI fails to result in pregnancies, whereas intrauterine sperm deposition results in pregnancy rates comparable to those obtained after natural breeding.[1, 15] In 1992, intrauterine AI using fresh semen was used to produce a litter of red wolves *(Canis rufus)* (W. Waddall, personal communication, September 1997). Vaginal deposition of sperm also was ineffective for producing pregnancies in the European ferret *(Mustela putorius furo;* see Table 61–3).[46] Use of the laparoscopic intrauterine AI technique to deposit fresh or frozen-thawed ferret semen in utero resulted in high pregnancy rates (70%), however.[25, 46] This AI method (using fresh or cryopreserved semen) also has been successful for producing pregnancies in Siberian polecats *(Mustela eversmanni)* and black-footed ferrets (Table 61–4).[24] Laparoscopic AI currently is being used in the Black-Footed Ferret Species Survival Plan program for overcoming behavioral incompatibility between selected pairs.

Laparoscopic Intrauterine Insemination

The laparoscopic insemination technique involves depositing sperm directly into the uterine horn by means of a catheter inserted through the abdominal wall in carnivores (see Fig. 61–4). Anesthetized females are subjected to laparoscopy, and ovaries are assessed for preovulatory follicles (flattened or slightly raised clear areas) (see Fig. 61–2) and postovulatory corpora lutea

TABLE 61–4. Ferrets Produced by Laparoscopic Intrauterine Artificial Insemination Using Fresh or Frozen-Thawed Semen

Species	Sperm Treatment	No. of Pregnancies	No. of Kits	Mean No. Kits/Litter (±SEM)	Reference
European ferret	Fresh	17/24 (70.8%)	85	5.2 ± 0.5	46
(Mustela putorius furo)	Thawed	7/10 (70.0%)	31	4.4 ± 1.0	21
Siberian polecat	Fresh	1/1 (100.0%)	6	6.0	24
(Mustela eversmanni)	Thawed	5/6 (83.3%)	26	5.2 ± 1.2	24
Black-footed ferret	Fresh	11/14 (78.6%)	32	2.9 ± 0.4	24
(Mustela nigripes)	Thawed	2/3 (66.7%)	3	1.5 ± 0.5	24

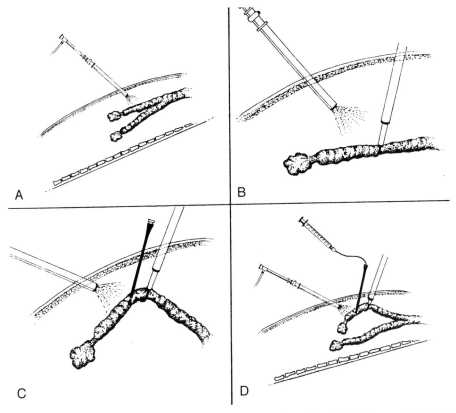

FIGURE 61–4. Laparoscopic intrauterine insemination. *A*, The laparoscope is used to identify the reproductive tract. *B*, Accessory forceps are used to grasp the uterine horn. *C*, The horn is elevated, and a catheter is punctured through the ventral abdominal wall and inserted into the uterine lumen. *D*, The stylet is withdrawn from the catheter, and tubing containing spermatozoa is guided through the catheter into the uterine lumen for sperm deposition. (From Howard JG, Barone MA, Donaghue AU, et al: The effect of pre-ovulatory anaesthesia on ovulation in laparoscopically inseminated domestic cats. J Reprod Fertil 96:175–186, 1992.)

(opaque, reddish yellowish structures raised above the ovarian surface) (Fig. 61–5).

To stabilize the uterine horn for cannulation and AI, an accessory grasping forceps is inserted lateral to the umbilicus and used to elevate each uterine horn to the ventral body wall. (In small species, such as ferrets, this step is not necessary.) The uterine horn is cannulated with a sterile 20-gauge indwelling catheter inserted percutaneously into the proximal aspect of the uterine lumen. The catheter stylet is removed and replaced with sterile polyethylene tubing containing the diluted spermatozoa. The tubing (attached to a 1-ml syringe) is inserted beyond the tip of the catheter and into the uterine lumen. The sperm suspension is expelled from the catheter and into the lumen using a minimal amount of air delivered from the syringe. The entire procedure is repeated on the contralateral uterine horn.

Transmission of Disease

The use of assisted reproductive techniques offers an approach for transferring genetic material without many of the health risks associated with transporting live animals. Reintroduction or translocation poses the risk of potential disease transmission among individuals or populations. With the increasing concern about the susceptibility of numerous species of carnivores to certain infectious viruses, including canine distemper virus, herpesvirus, feline immunodeficiency virus, and feline infectious peritonitis, assisted reproduction may become necessary for propagating valuable infected individuals. It is essential, however, that assisted breeding techniques themselves not serve as disease vectors. In domestic cats, feline immunodeficiency virus is present in cat semen and can be transmitted to females by laparoscopic intrauterine AI.[29, 30]

Numerous types of bacteria (gram-negative and gram-positive) have been detected in domestic cat and cheetah semen (Table 61–5).[25] Although these bacterial isolates constitute normal microflora with no detrimental impact on natural breeding, these organisms may compromise assisted reproduction. Initial AI attempts in felids and mustelids relied on vaginal deposition of raw (unwashed) semen. Laparoscopic intrauterine AI, developed to circumvent sperm transport problems, proved to be highly successful in mustelids using unwashed ejaculates mixed in egg yolk diluent.[21, 24, 46] Centrifugation of semen and removal of seminal plasma

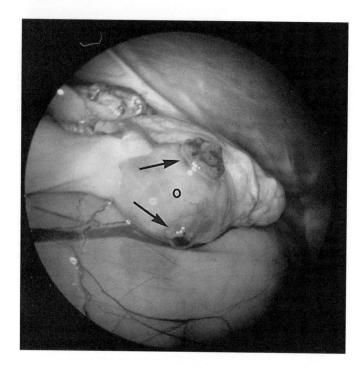

FIGURE 61–5. Cheetah ovary (O) containing fresh corpora lutea (*arrows*) after gonadotropin stimulation. (From Howard JG, Roth TL, Byers AR, et al: Sensitivity to exogenous gonadotropins for ovulation induction and laparoscopic artificial insemination in the cheetah and clouded leopard. Biol Reprod 56:1059–1068, 1997.)

appeared to be unnecessary to achieve high pregnancy rates in ferret species (see Table 61–4). In contrast, when a similar semen-processing method was used in domestic cats, pyometra developed in 4 of 10 (40%) females following laparoscopic intrauterine AI with un-washed semen, despite the fact that semen was diluted in culture media containing antibiotics (penicillin and streptomycin).[25] It was assumed that the seminal plasma of the cat sperm donors was contaminated because *Escherichia coli* (the most common type of bacteria in felid semen) was isolated from the uterus of each in-fected female. In a subsequent study, intrauterine AI

was performed on 53 domestic cat females using washed sperm after centrifugation and seminal plasma removal.[20] No uterine infections developed, and a 50% pregnancy rate was achieved. Laparoscopic intrauterine AI using washed sperm deposited in utero in 13 female cheetahs resulted in no bacterial infections and a 46% pregnancy rate.[26] Continued investigation of potential routes of disease transmission and of methods to elimi-nate the introduction of pathogens during assisted repro-duction is needed.

Time of Insemination

Inseminations traditionally are scheduled to occur be-fore ovulation. This timing is effective in mustelids, resulting in high rates of pregnancy when females are anesthetized and inseminated in utero before ovulation (see Table 61–4). For example, the European ferret is a reflex ovulator, in which ovulation occurs about 30 hours after an injection of hCG.[46] AI is highly success-ful in this species when preovulatory inseminations are conducted either at the time of hCG administration (75% pregnancy rate) or 24 hours later (67% pregnancy rate).[46] Similarly, pregnancies have been achieved in Siberian polecats and black-footed ferrets when AI was performed 0 to 24 hours after hCG administration.[24]

Interestingly, use of anesthesia and AI before ovula-tion compromises ovulation and pregnancy in felids. When domestic cats are anesthetized with a combina-tion of ketamine hydrochloride, acepromazine, and gas-eous halothane before ovulation, few females ovulate and the pregnancy rate is low (14%).[20] Conversely, if the interval from hCG administration to anesthesia is increased to 6 to 14 hours after ovulation has begun, all cats ovulate and 50% of these become pregnant

TABLE 61–5. Bacterial Isolates from the Semen of 40 Male Cheetahs

Number of males with bacteria in semen	26/40 (65%)
Number of males with no bacteria in semen	14/40 (35%)
Number of bacterial isolates*	
Gram-negative bacteria	
Escherichia coli (hemolytic)	7 (18%)
Escherichia coli (nonhemolytic)	3 (8%)
Enterobacter cloacae	1 (3%)
Aeromonas hydrophila	1 (3%)
Klebsiella oxytoca	4 (10%)
Pasteurella species	4 (10%)
Proteus species	6 (15%)
Pseudomonas aeruginosa	3 (8%)
Gram-positive bacteria	
Staphylococcus species (beta-hemolytic)	4 (10%)
Streptococcus species (beta-hemolytic)	1 (3%)
Streptococcus species, group D, *Enterococcus*	6 (15%)

*Number in parentheses indicates the percentage of males with the isolate.

TABLE 61–6. Pregnancy Rates After Preovulatory Versus Postovulatory Laparoscopic Intrauterine Artificial Insemination in Anesthetized Felids

	Time of Insemination		
	Preovulation	Postovulation	**References**
Domestic cat *(Felis catus)*	2/14 (14.3%)	9/18 (50.0%)	20
Cheetah *(Acinonyx jubatus)*	0/3 (0%)	6/13 (46.2%)	23, 26

and deliver live offspring (Table 61–6).[20] Compromised ovulation also has been observed in tigers anesthetized near the time of ovulation.[8] In preovulatory tigers treated with eCG and hCG followed by anesthesia and laparoscopy 39 to 42 hours later, three of the four animals (75%) never ovulated based on laparoscopic re-evaluation 4 weeks later.[8] A similar phenomenon has been detected in cheetahs, and pregnancies have occured only in females that underwent AI after ovulation (see Table 61–6).[23, 26] Based on these findings, it is apparent that the optimal time for AI in felids is after ovulation has commenced. However, the time of ovulation in felids differs among species (Table 61–7).

Hormonal Stimulation

Assisted reproduction success is linked to gonadotropin stimulation of ovarian activity. There appears to be rather remarkable differences in ovarian response among felids to gonadotropin dosages, and certain species demonstrate an extreme level of sensitivity to gonadotropins (see Table 61–7). Some eCG and hCG dosages result in an excessive number of ovulated follicles, whereas others impair ovulation. Both problems appear to be related to inadequate luteal development, which can fail to sustain a pregnancy.[2, 22, 23, 26] The optimal dosage of eCG required to elicit an ovarian

response mimicking normalcy is independent of body weight. For example, although 5 to 10 times larger in body weight, the cheetah and clouded leopard require about the same eCG dosage (100–200 IU) as the leopard cat (100 IU) to elicit comparable follicular growth.[22, 23, 26, 47] By contrast, the ocelot *(Felis pardalis)*, which is about half the size of the clouded leopard, requires 500 IU of eCG (five times the clouded leopard dosage) to mimic similar ovarian follicular activity.[22, 26, 42] These findings continue to emphasize the fundamental differences in reproductive mechanisms, even among related species in the same family.

Comparison of various gonadotropin dosages is useful for determining the minimum effective eCG and hCG dosage for causing adequate follicular development and ovulation but not ovarian hyperstimulation. For low gonadotropin dosages, however, an ovulation threshold has been observed in felids. Insufficient eCG dosages produce follicles incapable of ovulation in response to an hCG stimulus.[2, 26] The recent development of fecal hormone assays for monitoring estrogen and progesterone metabolites enhances the ability to compare gonadotropin regimens (Fig. 61–6).[4–7] This noninvasive method for assessing ovarian activity has also been used to study the phenomenon of spontaneous versus induced ovulation in felids. Increased and sustained progesterone excretion as determined with fecal

TABLE 61–7. Recent Pregnancies Produced After Gonadotropin Stimulation and Laparoscopic Intrauterine Artificial Insemination in Felids

Species	Average Body Weight (kg)	Gonadotropin Dosage		Time of Ovulation After hCG (h)	Sperm Type	No. of Pregnancies	No. of Offspring	References
		PMSG (IU)	hCG (IU)					
Leopard cat *(Felis bengalensis)*	3	100	75	25–30	Fresh & frozen	2	2	20, 47
Ocelot *(Felis pardalis)*	9	500	225	~39	Fresh & frozen	2	7	42
Clouded leopard *(Neofelis nebulosa)*	15	100	75	37–40	Fresh	1	2	22, 26
Snow leopard *(Panthera uncia)*	30	600	300	~40	Fresh	1	1	39
Puma *(Felis concolor)*	35	200	100	33–40	Fresh	1	1	2
Cheetah *(Acinonyx jubatus)*	35	200	100	40–42	Fresh & frozen	9	17	23, 26, 27
Tiger *(Panthera tigris)*	250	1000	750	39–46	Fresh	1	1	8, 10

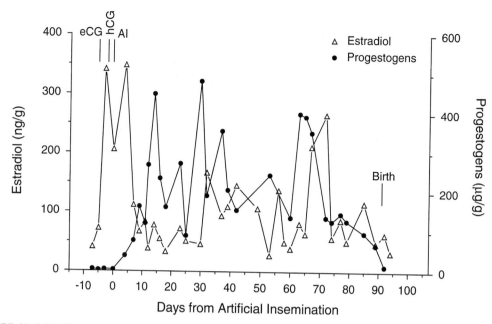

FIGURE 61–6. Profile of fecal estradiol and progestogen metabolite concentrations in a pregnant cheetah subjected to ovulation induction and laparoscopic intrauterine insemination. Female received 200 IU of eCG followed 80 hours later by 100 IU of hCG and artificial insemination (AI) 46 hours after hCG administration. (From Brown JL, Wildt DE, Wielebnowski N, et al: Reproductive activity in captive female cheetahs (*Acinonyx jubatus*) assessed by faecal steroids. J Reprod Fertil 106:337–346, 1996.)

steroid monitoring revealed that 6 of 14 (43%) clouded leopard females housed singly or with other females spontaneously ovulated.[5] In contrast, no ovulation was observed in cheetahs, indicating that this species demonstrates induced ovulation.[6]

Determination of the relative responsiveness among species to various gonadotropin dosages is necessary to identify an effective hormonal treatment for achieving pregnancies. By use of this strategy and intrauterine AI in postovulatory felids treated with eCG and hCG, offspring have been produced in the leopard cat,[47] ocelot,[42] clouded leopard,[22, 26] snow leopard,[39] puma,[2] cheetah,[23, 26] and tiger[8, 10] (see Table 61–7). Pregnancies also have resulted following intrauterine AI with frozen-thawed sperm in three felid species—leopard cat, ocelot, and cheetah. Most significantly, two cheetah litters have been produced using sperm that was collected from wild-caught males in Namibia Africa then cryopreserved and imported into the United States for use in the Cheetah Species Survival Plan program.[27] These achievements demonstrate that assisted reproduction combined with cryopreservation technology can be used in the management of endangered carnivores.

FUTURE CHALLENGES

The ability to use assisted reproduction for practical wildlife conservation requires basic research for each species. Studying basic reproductive mechanisms is the key to understanding the physiologic processes that eventually allow artificial breeding techniques to become routine. Although information in selected species

has allowed the use of assisted reproduction for enhancing propagation, further information is needed to determine factors such as the fertilizable life span of spermatozoa in the female reproductive tract, the most effective gonadotropin regimen for ovulation induction, the optimal protocol for freezing and thawing gametes, and the minimum number of spermatozoa required to produce a pregnancy. These studies will help breeding and cryopreservation strategies to be effective for long-term preservation of genetic diversity in endangered carnivores.

REFERENCES

1. Aamdal J, Andersen K, Fougner JA: Insemination with frozen semen in the blue fox. Proceedings of the 7th International Congress on Animal Reproduction and Artificial Insemination, Munich, Germany, 4:1713–1716, 1972.
2. Barone MA, Wildt DE, Byers AP, et al: Gonadotrophin dose and timing of anaesthesia for laparoscopic artificial insemination in the puma (*Felis concolor*). J Reprod Fertil 101:103–108, 1994.
3. Bowen MJ, Platz CC, Brown CD, et al: Successful artificial insemination and embryo collection in the African lion (*Panthera leo*). Proceedings of the American Association of Zoo Veterinarians, New Orleans, pp 57–59, 1982.
4. Brown JL, Wasser SK, Wildt DE, et al: Comparative aspects of steroid hormone metabolism and ovarian activity in felids, measured noninvasively in feces. Biol Reprod 51:776–786, 1994.
5. Brown JL, Wildt DE, Graham LH, et al: Natural versus chorionic gonadotropin-induced ovarian responses in the clouded leopard (*Neofelis nebulosa*) assessed by fecal steroid analysis. Biol Reprod 53:93–102, 1995.
6. Brown JL, Wildt DE, Wielebnowski N, et al: Reproductive activity in captive female cheetahs (*Acinonyx jubatus*) assessed by faecal steroids. J Reprod Fertil 106:337–346, 1996.
7. Czekala NM, Durrant BS, Callison L, et al: Fecal steroid hormone analysis as an indicator of reproductive function in the cheetah. Zoo Biol 13:119–128, 1994.

8. Donoghue AM, Byers AP, Johnston LA, et al: Timing of ovulation after gonadotropin induction and its importance to successful intrauterine insemination in the tiger (*Panthera tigris*). J Reprod Fertil 107:53–58, 1996.

9. Donoghue AM, Howard JG, Byers AP, et al: Correlation of sperm viability with gamete interaction and fertilization *in vitro* in the cheetah (*Acinonyx jubatus*). Biol Reprod 46:1047–1056, 1992.

10. Donoghue AM, Johnston LA, Armstrong DL, et al: Birth of a Siberian tiger cub (*Panthera tigris altaica*) following laparoscopic intrauterine artificial insemination. J Zoo Wildl Med 24:185–189, 1993.

11. Donoghue AM, Johnston LA, Seal US, et al: *In vitro* fertilization and embryo development *in vitro* and *in vivo* in the tiger (*Panthera tigris*). Biol Reprod 43:733–744, 1990.

12. Donoghue AM, Johnston LA, Seal US, et al: Ability of thawed tiger (*Panthera tigris*) spermatozoa to fertilize conspecific eggs and bind and penetrate domestic cat eggs *in vitro*. J Reprod Fertil 96:555–564, 1992.

13. Dresser BL, Kramer L, Reece B, et al: Induction of ovulation and successful artificial insemination in a Persian leopard (*Panthera pardus saxicolor*). Zoo Biol 1:55–57, 1982.

14. Farstad W, Hyttel P, Grondahl C, et al: Fertilization *in vitro* of oocytes matured *in vivo* in the blue fox (*Alopex lagopus*). J Reprod Fertil 47:219–226, 1993.

15. Fougner JA: Artificial insemination in fox breeding. J Reprod Fertil Suppl 39:317–323, 1989.

16. Goodrowe KL, Graham L, Mehren KG. Stimulation of ovarian activity and oocyte recovery in the caracal (*Felis caracal*) and cheetah (*Acinonyx jubatus*). J Zoo Wildl Med 22:42–48, 1991.

17. Goodrowe KL, Miller AM, Wildt DE, et al: *In vitro* fertilization of gonadotropin-stimulated leopard cats (*Felis bengalensis*) follicular oocytes. J Exp Zool 252:89–95, 1989.

18. Goodrowe KL, Wall RL, O'Brien SJ, et al: Developmental competence of domestic cat follicular oocytes after fertilization *in vitro*. Biol Reprod 39:355–372, 1988.

19. Howard JG: Semen collection and analysis in carnivores. *In* Fowler ME (ed): Zoo and Wild Animal Medicine Current Therapy, 3rd ed. Philadelphia, WB Saunders, pp 390–399, 1993.

20. Howard JG, Barone MA, Donoghue AM, et al: The effect of preovulatory anaesthesia on ovulation in laparoscopically inseminated domestic cats. J Reprod Fertil 96:175–186, 1992.

21. Howard JG, Bush M, Morton C, et al: Comparative semen cryopreservation in ferrets (*Mustela putorius furo*) and pregnancies after laparoscopic intrauterine insemination with frozen-thawed spermatozoa. J Reprod Fertil 92:109–118, 1991.

22. Howard JG, Byers AP, Brown JL, et al: Successful ovulation induction and laparoscopic intrauterine artificial insemination in the clouded leopard (*Neofelis nebulosa*). Zoo Biol 15:55–69, 1996.

23. Howard JG, Donoghue AM, Barone MA, et al: Successful induction of ovarian activity and laparoscopic intrauterine artificial insemination in the cheetah (*Acinonyx jubatus*). J Zoo Wildl Med 23:288–230, 1992.

24. Howard JG, Kwiatkowski DR, Williams ES, et al: Pregnancies in black-footed ferrets and Siberian polecats after laparoscopic artificial insemination with fresh and frozen-thawed semen [Abstract 115]. J Androl (Suppl):P-51, 1996.

25. Howard JG, Munson L, McAloose D, et al: Comparative evaluation of seminal, vaginal and rectal bacterial flora in the cheetah and domestic cat. Zoo Biol 12:81–96, 1993.

26. Howard JG, Roth TL, Byers AP, et al: Sensitivity to exogenous gonadotropins for ovulation induction and laparoscopic artificial insemination in the cheetah and clouded leopard. Biol Reprod 56:1059–1068, 1997.

27. Howard JG, Roth TL, Swanson WF, et al: Successful intercontinental genome resource banking and artificial insemination with cryopreserved sperm in cheetahs [Abstract 123]. J Androl (Suppl):P-55, 1997.

28. Johnston LA, Donoghue AM, O'Brien SJ, et al: Rescue and maturation *in vitro* of follicular oocytes collected from nondomestic felid species. Biol Reprod 45:898–906, 1991.

29. Jordan HL, Howard JG, Sellon RK, et al: Transmission of feline immunodeficiency virus in domestic cats via artificial insemination. J Virol 70:8224–8228, 1996.

30. Jordan HL, Howard JG, Tompkins WA, et al: Detection of feline immunodeficiency virus in semen from seropositive domestic cats (*Felis catus*). J Virol 69:7328–7333, 1995.

31. Miller AM, Roelke ME, Goodrowe KL, et al: Oocyte recovery, maturation and fertilization *in vitro* in the puma (*Felis concolor*). J Reprod Fertil 88:249–258, 1990.

32. Moore HDM, Bonney RC, Jones DM: Successful induced ovulation and artificial insemination in the puma (*Felis concolor*). Vet Rec 108:282–283, 1981.

33. Moore HDM, Bonney RC, Jones DM: Induction of oestrus and successful artificial insemination in the cougar, *Felis concolor*. Proceedings of the American Association of Zoo Veterinarians, Seattle, pp 141–142, 1981.

34. Moore HDM, Bush M, Celma AL, et al: Artificial insemination in the giant panda (*Ailuropoda melanoleuca*). J Zool 203:268, 1984.

35. Platz CC, Wildt DE, Seager SWJ: Pregnancy in the domestic cat after artificial insemination with previously frozen spermatozoa. J Reprod Fertil 52:279–282, 1978.

36. Pope CE, Gelwicks EJ, Wachs KB, et al: Successful interspecies transfer of embryos from the Indian desert cat (*Felis silvestris ornata*) to the domestic cat (*Felis catus*) following *in vitro* fertilization. Biol Reprod 40:61, 1989.

37. Pope CE, McRae MA, Plair BL, et al: *In vitro* and *in vivo* development of embryos produced by *in vitro* maturation (IVM) and *in vitro* fertilization (IVF) of domestic cat oocytes. Biol Reprod 52:284, 1995.

38. Reed G, Dresser B, Reece B, et al: Superovulation and artificial insemination of Bengal tigers (*Panthera tigris*) and an interspecies embryo transfer to the African lion (*Panthera leo*). Proceedings of the American Association of Zoo Veterinarians, pp 136–138, 1981.

39. Roth TL, Armstrong DL, Barrie MT, et al: Seasonal effects on ovarian responsiveness to exogenous gonadotropins and successful artificial insemination in the snow leopard (*Uncia uncia*). Reprod Fertil Dev 9:285–295, 1997.

40. Seager SWJ: Semen collection and artificial insemination in captive wild cats, wolves and bears. Proceedings of the American Association of Zoo Veterinarians, Atlanta, p 29, 1974.

41. Seager SWJ, Platz CC, Hodge W: Successful pregnancy using frozen semen in the wolf. Int Zoo Year 15:140, 1975.

42. Swanson WF, Howard JG, Roth TL, et al: Responsiveness of ovaries to exogenous gonadotrophins and laparoscopic artificial insemination with frozen-thawed spermatozoa in ocelots (*Felis pardalis*). J Reprod Fertil 106:87–94, 1996.

43. Swanson WF, Roth TL, Graham K, et al: Kinetics of the humoral immune response to multiple treatments with exogenous gonadotropins and relation to ovarian responsiveness in domestic cats. Am J Vet Res 57:302–307, 1996.

44. Swanson WF, Wolfe BA, Brown JL, et al: Pharmacokinetics and ovarian stimulatory effects of exogenous gonadotropins administered singly and in combination in the domestic cat [Abstract 530]. Biol Reprod 54 (Suppl):189, 1996.

45. Villares MC, del Campo ALG, Greenwood A, et al: Breeding and rearing a giant panda at the Madrid Zoo. *In* Klos HG, Fradrich H (eds): Proceedings of the 10th International Symposium on the Giant Panda, Bongo, Berlin, p 59, 1985.

46. Wildt DE, Bush M, Morton C, et al: Semen characteristics and testosterone profiles in ferrets kept in a long-day photoperiod, and the influence of hCG timing and sperm dilution medium on pregnancy rate after laparoscopic insemination. J Reprod Fertil 86:349–358, 1989.

47. Wildt DE, Monfort SL, Donoghue AM, et al: Embryogenesis in conservation biology—or, how to make an endangered species embryo. Theriogenology 37:161–184, 1992.

48. Wildt DE, Phillips LG, Simmons LG, et al: Seminal-endocrine characteristics of the tiger and the potential for artificial breeding. *In* Tilson RL, Seal US (eds): Tigers of the World: The Biology, Biopolitics, Management, and Conservation of an Endangered Species. Park Ridge, NJ, Noyes Publication, pp 255–279, 1987.

49. Wildt DE, Platz CP, Seager SWJ, et al: Induction of ovarian activity in the cheetah (*Acinonyx jubatus*). Biol Reprod 24:217–222, 1981.

50. Wildt DE, Pukazhenthi B, Brown JL, et al: Spermatology for understanding, managing and conserving rare species. Reprod Fertil Dev 7:811–824, 1995.

51. Wildt DE, Schiewe MC, Schmidt PM, et al: Developing animal model systems for embryo technologies in rare and endangered wildlife. Theriogenology 25:33–51, 1986.

CHAPTER 62

Gastritis in Cheetahs

RAYMUND F. WACK

Gastritis is a significant health problem in captive cheetahs (*Acinonyx jubatus*).[5] Gastritis may be acute (less
than 1 week in duration), such as occurs with dietary
indiscretion, or chronic, such as occurs with *Helicobacter*-associated gastritis. Chronic gastritis was found
in 91% of 40 cheetahs examined as part of the cheetah
Species Survival Plan (SSP) program of the American
Zoo and Aquarium Association comprehensive pathology survey.[5] Gastritis in cheetahs has been reported
from at least 16 different institutions worldwide. A
complete medical examination is often required to determine the cause and appropriate treatment.

CLINICAL SIGNS

Cheetahs with gastritis may exhibit one or more of
the following clinical signs: vomiting, hypersalivation,
weight loss, and partial or complete anorexia. The vomiting may or may not be associated with eating. Hema-
temesis and melena are seen if the gastritis includes
mucosal ulcerations.[3] It is often difficult to detect vomiting in large naturalistic exhibits because the vomitus
is frequently re-eaten or dissipates rapidly in the environment. Severe episodes of vomiting may result in
lateral recumbency or brief fainting spells. Hypersalivation and nauseous behavior are frequently seen in the
animals immediately before vomiting. With chronic
gastritis, a negative energy balance may occur, resulting
in slow progressive weight loss despite a good appetite.
As the gastritis becomes more severe, undigested food
may be seen in the feces. This is most commonly seen
when the cheetah is fed organ meats.

DIFFERENTIAL DIAGNOSIS

Potential causes for gastritis in cheetahs (as well as
domestic species) include mechanical irritation from
dietary indiscretion, ingestion of foreign bodies, and
ingestion of chemical irritants or toxins, which may
result in acute onset of vomiting. A thorough history is
important to assess the likelihood of these materials
being ingested. Trichobezoars, which are occasionally
seen on endoscopic examination of the stomach, rarely
cause clinical signs of gastritis in cheetahs. An upper
gastrointestinal obstruction, although not a direct cause

of gastritis, often manifests with vomiting as the dominant clinical sign.

A number of infectious or parasitic agents may cause
acute or chronic gastritis in cheetahs. Panleukopenia
virus, which is less common since the advent of safe
and efficacious vaccines, may cause acute gastritis and
enteritis. Ingested bacterial enterotoxins, which are often present in spoiled meat, is a frequent cause of acute
gastritis. Parasitic causes of gastritis include *Aonchotheca putorii*, *Ollulanus tricuspis*, *Physaloptera* species,
and *Spirocerca lupi*.[3]

Neoplasia, including adenocarcinoma, may cause
vomiting often as the result of pyloric outflow obstruction. Hiatal or diaphragmatic hernias may cause vomiting and gastritis as a result of obstructing normal
gastric motility. Uremia, commonly present in older
cheetahs with chronic renal failure, is a common metabolic cause of gastritis. Cheetahs with renal failure often
have oral and gastric erosions or ulcerations. Cheetahs
with moderate to severe veno-occlusive liver disease
may vomit as a result of hepatic encephalopathy.

Gastric spiral bacteria have been commonly associated with gastritis in cheetahs. Although Koch's postu-
lates have not been fulfilled and the pathogenesis of the
gastritis has yet to be determined, a number of institutions in several countries have experienced epizootic
outbreaks of gastritis in captive cheetahs.[1] Two species
of bacteria have been seen on gastric biopsy study.
Helicobacter acinonyx is most commonly associated
with chronic active gastritis, whereas *Helicobacter heilmannii* (a *Gastrospirillium*-like organism) is less often
seen and is frequently not associated with inflammation
or ulceration of the gastric mucosa. In the SSP study,
95% of the cheetahs with gastritis had gastric spiral
bacteria present on biopsy or necropsy study[5]; although
Helicobacter was seen in one case without gastritis.
Helicobacter-associated gastritis has been seen in cheetah cubs as young as 4 months of age.

DIAGNOSTIC TESTING

Cases of acute gastritis may or may not need a complete
medical examination, depending on their severity. Most
cases of dietary indiscretion and minor ingestion of
bacterial enterotoxins resolve within 24 to 48 hours
without treatment.[7] Intervention is warranted in cases of
prolonged vomiting, weakness, dehydration, decreased

mental alertness, or suspected obstructions. Depending on the management situation, the initial examination may be performed with manual restraint or with the cheetah confined to a squeeze cage. Frequently, immobilization is required for a thorough examination. In planning for the immobilization, drugs with minimal cardiovascular depression effects should be used because the metabolic status of the animal is unknown. The following anesthetic combinations have been used successfully in cheetahs with chronic gastritis: ketamine, 5 to 8 mg/kg IM, and midazolam, 0.1 mg/kg IM; tiletamine HCl and zolazepam HCl (Telazol) 2.0 mg/kg IM. Intubation and gas anesthesia with isoflurane can be used for prolonged procedures.

A complete physical examination, including an oral inspection for ulcerations, foreign bodies, or strings at the base of the tongue, ophthalmic examination including a fundic examination, palpation of the cervical esophagus and abdomen, digital rectal examination, and auscultation of the heart and lungs, is performed while the animal is immobilized. Blood should be collected (medial saphenous, cephalic, and jugular veins are commonly used sites) for a complete blood cell count and serum chemistry study, including bile acids. Particular attention should be paid to the total white blood cell count and cell type distribution to assess inflammatory response. The red blood cell count, hematocrit, and hemoglobin levels should be used to assess the presence of anemia. Serum chemistries should be used to evaluate electrolyte status, renal, and hepatic function.

A plain film radiographic examination of the abdomen is useful to visualize radiodense foreign bodies, and organ position and size. Contrast studies can be performed if indicated by the plain films. Barium should not be used in cases of suspected gastrointestinal perforations and only with caution in suspected cases of obstruction. In these cases, aqueous iodide contrast agents can be used. Ultrasound is useful to evaluate the architecture of the abdominal organs and investigate masses identified on physical examination or radiographs.

Chronic gastritis is best diagnosed by endoscopic examination of the stomach. A 24-hour fast is recommended for the animal before the examination. A 100-cm flexible endoscope (Olympus GIF XQ 10, Olympus Corporation, San Jose, CA) is sufficient to reach the proximal duodenum in most cheetahs. The entire muco-

sal surface of the stomach should be evaluated, with particular attention being paid to any hemorrhages, erosions, and ulcerations and to the appearance of the rugal folds. In severe chronic gastritis, the rugal folds may be pale, flattened, thickened, or have a cobblestone appearance. Multiple mucosal pinch biopsy specimens should be collected from all lesions identified as well as from the cardia, body, and pyloric regions. One specimen from each region should be submitted for bacterial culture (Skirrows Media, BBL Cat. No. 97793 Becton Dickerson, Cockeysville, MD) as well as for urease testing.[1] Additional mucosal pinch specimens should be submitted for histopathologic study. Silver staining (Warthin-Starry) of the biopsy specimens greatly enhances the visibility of spiral bacteria within the sample. The cheetah SSP pathologist (Linda Munson, School of Veterinary Medicine, University of California, Davis) should be consulted for standardized testing of gastric biopsy specimens.

THERAPEUTIC CONSIDERATIONS

Most cases of acute gastritis caused by dietary indiscretion resolve within 24 to 48 hours without treatment.[3] Gastric foreign bodies or obstructions should be removed endoscopically or surgically using the same technique as for domestic small animals. Gastric parasites can be treated with ivermectin or fenbendazole. Treatment may need to be repeated if re-infection cannot be prevented. Routine fecal samples should be evaluated for the presence of ova or parasites.

Dehydration and electrolyte disturbances should be treated with appropriate fluid therapy. Clinically ill cheetahs often require initial treatment with intravenous isotonic fluids supplemented with potassium as indicated by the serum chemistries. As the condition of the cheetah improves, fluid administration can be switched to subcutaneous boluses of up to 2 L BID. Metoclopramide acts on the central nervous system as an antiemetic, increases lower esophageal sphincter tone, and reduces gastric emptying time, and thus can be used to decrease vomiting in cheetahs.

Eradication of gastric spiral bacteria is difficult.[2] *H. acinonyx* is frequently associated with chronic active gastritis consisting of lymphocytic infiltration of the

TABLE 62–1. Chemotherapeutics Commonly Used in Treating Gastritis

Drug	Route	Dosage	Frequency	Comment
Amoxicillin	PO	15 mg/kg	BID to QID	Antibiotic
Fenbendazole	PO	50 mg/kg	SID 5 days	Anthelmintic[6]
Ivermectin	SQ	0.2–0.4 mg/kg	Once	Anthelmintic
Metoclopramide	PO	0.2–0.4 mg/kg	TID to QID	Antiemetic[6]
Metronidazole	PO	5–10 mg/kg	BID to QID	Antibiotic
Omeprazole	PO	0.7 mg/kg	SID	Acid inhibitor
Pepto-Bismol	PO	6–10 mg/kg	SID to QID	*Helicobacter* treatment
Sucralfate	PO	40 mg/kg	TID	Protectant
Tetracycline	PO	15 mg/kg	QID	Antibiotic

PO, per os; SQ, subcutaneously.

lamina propria, necrosis of the gastric mucosal epithelium, and dilation of the glands with necrotic debris, which becomes progressively more severe. Treatment of *Helicobacter*-associated gastritis in humans usually consists of two or more antibiotics combined with a bismuth compound and an H_2-blocker if ulcers are present (Table 62–1).[4] A clinical trial in six cheetahs using tetracycline, metronidazole, and bismuth subsalicylate per os QID for 7 days followed by bismuth subsalicylate per os SID for 1 year, controlled clinical symptoms of *H. acinonyx*–associated gastritis but did not eradicate the organism, nor did it reduce the severity of the gastritis at the 1-year posttreatment examination.[8] The treatment was effective in eradicating *H. heilmannii*. Omeprazole, a long-acting potent proton pump inhibitor, and sucralfate, a mucosal protectorant, have been useful in the symptomatic treatment of gastric ulcers in cheetahs. Amoxicillin has been substituted for tetracycline in the treatment protocol in cheetahs with glomerulonephritis, with no perceived change in efficacy.

FUTURE RESEARCH

Chronic active *Helicobacter*-associated gastritis is a significant health problem in cheetahs that requires more research to determine the pathogenesis and most effective treatment protocols. Clinical trials need to be conducted to evaluate the efficacy of combinations of chemotherapeutics. A mucosal *H. pylori* vaccine is being used in human clinical trials. Initial results suggest that the vaccine may be effective in preventing *H. pylori* infection and perhaps is efficacious as an adjunct therapy in active cases. The influence of chronic active gastritis on other chronic diseases such as glomerulosclerosis needs to be investigated.

REFERENCES

1. Eaton KA, Radin MJ, Kramer LW, et al: Epizootic gastritis associated with gastric spiral bacilli in cheetahs *Acinonyx jubatus*. Vet Pathol 30:55–63, 1993.
2. Fennerty MB: *Helicobacter pylori*. Arch Intern Med 154:721–727, 1994.
3. Johnson SE, Sherding RG, Bright RM: Diseases of the stomach. *In* Birchard SJ, Sherding RG (eds): Small Animal Practice. Philadelphia, WB Saunders, pp 655–675, 1994.
4. Marshall BJ: Treatment strategies for *Helicobacter pylori* infection. Gastroenterol Clin North Am 22:183–198, 1993.
5. Munson L: Diseases of captive cheetahs (*Acinonyx jubatus*): results of the Cheetah Research Council Pathology Survey, 1989–1992. Zoo Biology 12:105–124, 1993.
6. Plumb DC: Veterinary Drug Handbook, 2nd ed. Ames, IA, Iowa State Press, 1995.
7. Twedt DC: Diseases of the Stomach. *In* Sherding RG (ed): The Cat: Diseases and Clinical Management, 2nd ed. New York, Churchill Livingstone, pp 1181–1210, 1994.
8. Wack RF, Eaton KA, Kramer LW: Treatment of gastritis in cheetahs (*Acinonyx jubatus*). J Zoo Wild Med 28(3):260–266, 1997.

CHAPTER **63**

Veterinary Contributions to the Black-Footed Ferret Conservation Program

ELIZABETH S. WILLIAMS

E. TOM THORNE

The recovery of an endangered species such as the black-footed ferret (*Mustela nigripes*) requires expertise from a wide variety of disciplines including ecology, conservation biology, economics, sociology, physiology, epidemiology, pathology, and clinical veterinary medicine.[8] As professionals with broad training in many animal-related disciplines, veterinarians are important members of recovery teams. No recovery program can be successful without this multidisciplinary approach or without appropriate political, agency, and institutional support. The interdisciplinary nature of endangered species recovery is exemplified by the black-footed ferret

program; teamwork and individual contributions toward the goal of recovery are both critical.

Because of the impact that disease has had on black-footed ferrets, veterinary contributions to the recovery of black-footed ferrets have been of particular importance to this species. Perhaps more so than for other endangered species recovery programs, disease in black-footed ferrets played a major role in management of the original free-ranging population in planning and conducting captive propagation, and in reintroduction of the animals to the wild.

There are two integrated but separate parts of the

black-footed ferret recovery program: (1) captive propagation for maintenance of a core genetically managed population and production of animals to be released, and (2) reintroduction of captive-born black-footed ferrets to the wild. In the following discussion, veterinary contributions are addressed in the context of the overall recovery program; these contributions are also applicable to other endangered species recovery programs.

HISTORY

Black-footed ferrets lived in the great plains of North America and were found in association with prairie dogs (*Cynomys* species) upon which they depended for food and whose burrows they used as shelter. Black-footed ferrets probably were never numerous. A population was studied in South Dakota for nearly a decade until it vanished in the 1970s; the cause of the demise of the population was not known. Nine black-footed ferrets were captured from the South Dakota population by the U.S. Fish and Wildlife Service for captive propagation. Four of the ferrets died of vaccine-induced canine distemper following vaccination with a product thought to be safe for the species.[2] Propagation of black-footed ferrets was not successful, even though much basic biologic information about the species and valuable husbandry techniques were developed, greatly aiding future black-footed ferret recovery efforts.

After those attempts, black-footed ferrets were thought to be extinct in the wild until a population of animals was found near Meeteetse, WY, in the late 1970s, where a population of white-tailed prairie dogs (*Cynomys leucurus*) lived.[9, 11] The index animal was killed by a ranch dog. Necropsy by a veterinary pathologist revealed that the animal was young and healthy, suggesting the presence of reproductively active ferrets. Subsequent surveys discovered the existence of a population of animals. Over the next several years, biologists studied the natural history of black-footed ferrets via radio telemetry, snow tracking, and visual observations at night by spotlighting. These studies resulted in greatly increased knowledge of the species. Veterinarians were involved in anesthetizing animals that were captured for application of telemetry equipment, collecting biologic samples, vaccinating the animals against canine distemper, and as advocates for the animal.[10]

Because of the restricted nature of the only known population of black-footed ferrets, it quickly became apparent that a captive propagation program was needed to ensure survival of the species. In 1983, shortly after discovery of the free-ranging population, veterinary contributions to the captive propagation effort included planning facility designs, developing disease management plans, and developing husbandry protocols, as well as building agency, institutional, political, and economic support for the concept of captive propagation of black-footed ferrets.

The population of free-ranging black-footed ferrets appeared to thrive in the wild until 1985, when an epizootic of canine distemper caused loss of wild black-footed ferrets as well as loss of those that had been captured as the core of a captive propagation effort.[11, 21] The remaining free-ranging black-footed ferrets were captured, extirpating the species from the wild, and forming the basis for the current black-footed ferret population.

CAPTIVE PROPAGATION

Shortly after black-footed ferrets were captured from the wild for captive propagation, the recovery program became affiliated with the International Union for Conservation of Nature and Natural Resources and the Species Survival Plan (SSP) program of the American Zoo and Aquarium Association (AZA). A veterinarian has served as the species coordinator for black-footed ferrets since the SSP was formed. As with all SSP programs, there is a veterinary advisor to provide input to the program on animal and population health. Black-footed ferrets are currently being bred for the recovery program at seven facilities. Veterinarians are involved at all facilities in overseeing the health of the animals and participate in design and management of the local black-footed ferret captive propagation program.

Because of the exquisite susceptibility of black-footed ferrets to canine distemper and modified live virus canine distemper vaccines, it has been important to maintain the animals in isolated facilities to prevent exposure of the population to this virus. Vaccination of black-footed ferrets against canine distemper has been problematic. A killed vaccine that is used with adjuvant was developed and supplied by a research veterinarian for use in the captive population. This vaccine, as well as other vaccines, has been tested in an attempt to find an efficacious and safe vaccine.[17] Some attenuated vaccines may provide life-long protection against canine distemper but are not completely safe. Black-footed ferrets are not the only species highly susceptible to canine distemper and distemper vaccines; for this reason, a variety of vaccines that may prove to be safer and more efficacious are being tested using black-footed ferret X Siberian polecats (*Mustela eversmanni*) hybrids as surrogates.

Other diseases are important to captive black-footed ferrets and include plague caused by *Yersinia pestis*,[19] coccidiosis caused by *Eimeria furonis* and *Eimeria ictidea*,[6, 24] cryptosporidiosis,[20] toxoplasmosis,[1, 20] and neoplasia in elderly animals.[24]

Because the purpose of captive propagation is to breed as many black-footed ferrets as possible, understanding and maximizing production and weaning of kits has been an important priority for the black-footed ferret program. Using studies of the reproductive biology of female and male black-footed ferrets, veterinarians and reproductive specialists have developed techniques to effectively breed black-footed ferrets in captivity.[12, 22] By studying the black-footed ferret's vaginal cytology, changes in vulval morphology, and changes in behavior,[3, 4, 22, 23] veterinarians have characterized the estrous cycle of the animal. Artificial insemination was developed first using domestic ferrets (*Mustela putorius furo*) as surrogates,[16] then black-footed ferret X Siberian polecat hybrids, and finally black-footed ferrets.[5] These techniques have been successfully integrated into the overall management of the captive population, in particular to assist in breeding genetically important animals that have not successfully bred naturally.

Development of appropriate and safe anesthetic regimens is important to management of the captive colony of black-footed ferrets.

Anesthetic protocols have been developed using ketamine/diazepam,[10] tiletamine/zolazepam, ketamine/medetomidine, and isoflurane gas.

Additionally, understanding normal behavior of an endangered species may be very important in providing appropriate management of the animals in captivity and may contribute to successful reintroduction of captive-bred animals to the wild. Behavioral studies have contributed to better understanding of maternal behavior, food imprinting and preferences, development of predatory behavior, and play behavior.[13–15]

REINTRODUCTION

The process of reintroduction of endangered species is an interdisciplinary activity. Veterinary contributions to the reintroduction program for black-footed ferrets include participation in planning, disease control during reintroduction, consideration of animal welfare, surveillance for diseases in wild animal populations at the reintroduction site, determination of cause of death of animals that die in the wild, and direct animal care during the reintroduction process.

The planning process for reintroduction of an endangered species is a long and political process. Veterinarians have participated in the development of protocols for animal preparation for reintroduction,[13] selection of animals for reintroduction based on genetics of the population,[7] animal handling on site, establishment of protocols for monitoring animals after release, and contingency planning for disease outbreaks and significant individual animal injury.

Study of the diseases present in animals at the reintroduction sites has been important in understanding how such diseases can impact reintroduction. Sylvatic plague is an important disease of prairie dogs in many locations where black-footed ferrets are being reintroduced.[18] Surveys of coyotes (*Canis latrans*) and badgers (*Taxidea taxus*) for evidence of exposure to plague have been conducted at the reintroduction sites; seropositive animals are common in Wyoming and Montana. Long-term studies indicated that plague is endemic at these sites. Until recently, it was surmised that black-footed ferrets were resistant to plague based on research[25] and extrapolation from what was known about other carnivores, including mustelids. However, black-footed ferrets are quite susceptible to plague.[19] Thus this disease may severely impact reintroduction of black-footed ferrets in endemic areas.

Understanding dynamics of canine distemper has also been important to the reintroduction of black-footed ferrets.[18] Serologic surveillance of coyotes and badgers for evidence of exposure to canine distemper demonstrated this disease is epidemic in free-ranging populations of coyotes. Badgers, possibly because of

their behavior, may not always be exposed to canine distemper virus even in the face of an outbreak in coyotes.[18] Reintroduced vaccinated black-footed ferrets have survived outbreaks of canine distemper on several occasions,[21] although the level of this exposure to canine distemper virus was not known.

SUMMARY

Veterinary contributions have been important to the black-footed ferret conservation program both individually but perhaps more importantly as members of a team toward the goal of recovery of the species. It takes input from a wide variety of disciplines in order to reach the desired goal; and the broad-based nature of veterinary training gives veterinarians the ability to actively participate in multiple facets of endangered species recovery programs.

REFERENCES

1. Burns R, Williams ES, O'Toole D, et al: Toxoplasmosis in black-footed ferrets. Proceedings of the Annual Meeting of the American Association of Zoo Veterinarians, St. Louis, 1993.
2. Carpenter JW, Appel MJG, Erickson RC, et al: Fatal vaccine-induced canine distemper virus infection in black-footed ferrets. J Am Vet Med Assoc 169:961–964, 1976.
3. Carvalho CF, Howard J, Collins L: Captive breeding of black-footed ferrets (*Mustela nigripes*) and comparative reproductive efficiency in 1-year-old versus 2-year-old animals. J Zoo Wildl Med 22:96–106, 1991.
4. Hillman CN, Carpenter JW: Breeding biology and behavior in captive black-footed ferrets. Int Zoo Yearbook 23:186–191, 1983.
5. Howard JG, Kwiatkowski DR, Williams ES, et al: Pregnancies in black-footed ferrets and Siberian polecats after laparoscopic artificial insemination with fresh and frozen-thawed semen. J Androl Supplement P-51, Abstract 115, 1996.
6. Jolley WR, Kingston N, Williams ES, et al: Coccidia, *Giardia* sp., and a physalopteran nematode parasite from black-footed ferrets (*Mustela nigripes*) in Wyoming. J Helminthol Soc Wash 61:89–94, 1994.
7. Russell WC, Thorne ET, Oakleaf R, et al: The genetic basis of black-footed ferret reintroduction. Conservation Biology 8:263–266, 1994.
8. Seal US, Thorne ET, Bogan MA, et al (eds): Conservation Biology and the Black-Footed Ferret. New Haven, CT, Yale University Press, 1989.
9. Thorne ET, Oakleaf B: Species rescue for captive breeding: black-footed ferrets as an example. Symp Zool Soc London 62:241–261, 1991.
10. Thorne ET, Schroeder MH, Forrest SC, et al: Capture, immobilization and care of black-footed ferrets for research. *In* Anderson SH, Inkley DB (eds): Proceedings of the Black-Footed Ferret Workshop, Game and Fish Department, Cheyenne, WY, pp 9.1–9.8, 1985.
11. Thorne ET, Williams ES: Disease and endangered species: the black-footed ferret as a recent example. Conservation Biology 2:66–73, 1988.
12. Van Der Horst G, Curry PT, Kitchen RM, et al: Quantitative light and scanning electron microscopy of ferret semen. Mol Reprod Dev 30:232–240, 1991.
13. Vargas A: Ontogeny of the endangered black-footed ferret (*Mustela nigripes*) and effects of captive upbringing on predatory behavior and post-release survival. Ph.D. dissertation. University of Wyoming, 1994.
14. Vargas A, Anderson SH: The effects of diet on black-footed ferret (*Mustela nigripes*) food preference. Zoo Biol 15:105–113, 1996.
15. Vargas A, Anderson SH: Growth and physical development of captive raised black-footed ferrets (*Mustela nigripes*). Am Midland Nat 135:43–52, 1996.
16. Wildt DE, Bush M, Morton C, et al: Semen characteristics and testosterone profiles in ferrets kept in a long-day photoperiod, and the influences of hCG timing and sperm dilution medium on

pregnancy rate after laparoscopic insemination. J Reprod Fertil 86:349–358, 1989.

17. Williams ES, Anderson SL, Cavender J, et al: Vaccination of black-footed ferret (*Mustela nigripes*) x Siberian polecat (*M. eversmanni*) hybrids and domestic ferrets (*M. putorius furo*) against canine distemper. J Wildl Dis 32:417–423, 1996.

18. Williams ES, Lynn C, Welch V, et al: Survey of coyotes and badgers for disease in Shirley Basin, Wyoming in 1994. *In* Luce B, Oakleaf B, Thorne ET, et al (eds): 1994 Annual Completion Report Black-Footed Ferret Reintroduction in Shirley Basin, Wyoming. Cheyenne, WO, Game and Fish Department, pp 84–94, 1995.

19. Williams ES, Mills K, Kwiatkowski DR, et al: Plague in a black-footed ferret (*Mustela nigripes*). J Wildl Dis 30:581–585, 1994.

20. Williams ES, Thorne ET: Infectious and parasitic diseases of captive carnivores, with special emphasis on the black-footed ferret (*Mustela nigripes*). Rev Sci Tech Off Int Epiz 15:91–114, 1996.

21. Williams ES, Thorne ET, Appel MJG, et al: Canine distemper in black-footed ferrets (*Mustela nigripes*) from Wyoming. J Wildl Dis 25:385–398, 1988.

22. Williams ES, Thorne ET, Kwiatkowski DR, et al: Reproductive biology and management of black-footed ferrets (*Mustela nigripes*). Zoo Biol 10:383–398, 1991.

23. Williams ES, Thorne ET, Kwiatkowski DR, et al: Comparative vaginal cytology of the estrous cycle of black-footed ferrets (*Mustela nigripes*), Siberian polecats (*M. eversmanni*), and domestic ferrets (*M. putorius furo*). J Vet Diagn Invest 4:38–44, 1992.

24. Williams ES, Thorne ET, Kwiatkowski DR, et al: Overcoming disease problems in the black-footed ferret recovery program. Trans North Am Wildl Nat Res Conf 57:474–485, 1992.

25. Williams ES, Thorne ET, Quan TJ, et al: Experimental infection of domestic ferrets (*Mustela putorius furo*) and Siberian polecats (*Mustela eversmanni*) with *Yersinia pestis*. J Wildl Dis 27:441–445, 1991.

MARINE MAMMALS

CHAPTER 64

Diagnostic Cytology in Marine Mammal Medicine

TERRY W. CAMPBELL

DIAGNOSTIC CYTOLOGY IN PINNIPEDS, MANATEES, OTTERS, AND POLAR BEARS

Examination of cytologic samples can be a useful, inexpensive, and rapid diagnostic tool for the evaluation of the marine mammal. The materials needed for the evaluation of cytologic specimens include clean microscope slides, a proper stain, immersion oil, and a good quality light microscope. A microscope with $10\times$, $20\times$, $40\times$, and $100\times$ (oil immersion) objectives works well for this purpose. Hematologic stains, such as Wright's and new methylene blue, have become the standard for use in veterinary cytology and are easily performed in the in-house laboratory. Cytologic techniques and interpretations described for domestic mammals can be applied to marine mammals, especially pinnipeds, manatees, otters, and polar bears. Because of the unique anatomic structures of marine mammals, sample collection for cytologic specimens in cetaceans varies slightly from that for other marine mammals. Cytologic samples can be obtained by fine-needle aspiration biopsy, direct aspiration, wash techniques, thoracentesis, abdominal paracentesis, contact smears from

excised tissues or scrapings. Contact smears can also be obtained by imprinting material obtained from biopsy instruments.

The objective of the cytologist is to recognize and classify the cellular response in the specimen. The basic cellular responses include normal cellularity, inflammation, tissue hyperplasia or benign neoplasia, and malignant neoplasia. The inflammatory cells of marine mammals include neutrophils (the neutrophils of manatees have distinct eosinophilic cytoplasmic granules), eosinophils, lymphocytes, plasma cells, and macrophages. The inflammatory response is classified based on the predominant cell type being neutrophilic, mixed cell, or macrophagic inflammation. Neutrophilic inflammation is characterized by the predominance of neutrophils (i.e., 80% or greater) in the inflammatory response and is indicative of severe inflammation. The neutrophils should be evaluated for the degree of degeneration. Nondegenerate neutrophils resemble those found in peripheral blood films and may demonstrate hypersegmentation (Fig. 64–1). The presence of nondegenerate neutrophils indicates a nontoxic microenvironment for these cells. Degenerate neutrophils demonstrate varying degrees of nuclear hyalinization and swelling, karyolysis, and cytoplasmic vacuolation. Degenerate neutro-

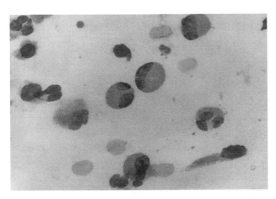

FIGURE 64–1. Nondegenerate neutrophils and neutrophilic inflammation in a nasal discharge from a West Indian manatee (*Trichecus manatus*). Note the distinct cytoplasmic granules (eosinophilic with Wright's stain) in manatee neutrophils. Original magnification, 100× (oil immersion objective).

phils reflect the presence of a toxic microenvironment, such as those caused by bacterial toxins. A mixed cell inflammatory response is represented by neutrophils and mononuclear leukocytes (i.e., lymphocytes, plasma cells, and macrophages) present in near equal numbers and suggests a less severe inflammatory response. Macrophagic inflammation can be associated with a granulomatous inflammation, a resolving neutrophilic inflammation, or a pyogranulomatous inflammation. The presence of epithelioid cells and multinucleated giant cells with varying numbers of neutrophils is suggestive of etiologies such as foreign bodies, fungi, and mycobacteria. A predominance of eosinophils is indicative of an eosinophilic inflammation and suggests an allergic response that may be associated with parasites, immune disorders, or conditions associated with mast cell degranulation.

Non-inflammatory cellular responses include tissue hyperplasia, benign neoplasia, and malignant neoplasia. A reactive population of cells may appear normal or have a slight increase in cytoplasmic basophilia. In general, benign neoplasms cannot be differentiated from normal cells or cells derived from tissue hyperplasia based on cytologic examination with Wright's or new methylene blue stains. Cells from malignant neoplasia can be differentiated from normal cells based on general, nuclear, cytoplasmic, and structural features of the cells. General features of malignant neoplasia include increased cellularity, a uniform population of cells present in an abnormal location, and a pleomorphic population of cells that appear to be related. Nuclear features of malignant cells include anisokaryosis, marked variation in nuclear to cytoplasmic ratios, abnormal chromatin patterns, large and irregular nucleoli, multiple nucleoli, multinucleation, and abnormal mitotic figures. Cytoplasmic features of malignancy include increased cytoplasmic basophilia and vacuolation. The shape and arrangement of the cells provide the structural features of malignant neoplasms and may allow the cytologist to classify the neoplasm as a carcinoma (epithelial cell origin), sarcoma (mesenchymal cell origin), discrete cell

tumor (e.g., lymphosarcoma), or a poorly differentiated neoplasm (the cells cannot be classified based on structural features).

DIAGNOSTIC CYTOLOGY IN CETACEANS

Cytology of the Blow

Blow samples for cytologic evaluation can be obtained by direct application of a sterile swab into the blow and rolling the material from the swab onto a clean microscope slide. This method usually yields a poorly cellular sample unless there is a lesion just behind the blow flap that contains a large amount of mucus or exudate. A method for routine collection of cytologic material from the blow is by voluntary exhalation onto a sterile Petri dish. This behavior can be elicited easily from cetaceans that are trained to perform other medical behaviors. It is important to allow the cetacean to blow off the water that typically pools on the blow flap before attempting to collect blow samples for cytologic study. Small flecks of mucus collected on the Petri dish can be transferred to a microscope slide by using a sterile swab. If no solid material is collected, the cellularity of the sample can be improved by suspending the sample in physiologic saline (0.5 to 1.0 ml) and concentrating the cells as is done with a wash sample (e.g., tracheal wash) using a cell-concentrating device. After air drying, the slides can be stained with Wright's stain for a permanent specimen. An alternative to this method is to collect the blow sample directly into a clean, plastic specimen container and to add new methylene blue solution to suspend the cells. The cells in the solution are transferred by pipette to a microscope slide and a coverslip is applied for microscopic examination. The advantage of this technique is that it provides a means for estimating the cellularity of the sample if the procedure is standardized, as compared to a concentrated sample in which the cellularity is increased to improve the number of cells for evaluation. Disadvantages of the new methylene blue technique are that fewer samples are available for examination, the sample does not provide a permanent specimen, and new methylene blue is less desirable than Wright's stain for cytologic examination.

The normal blow cytology of cetaceans is poorly cellular and contains primarily squamous epithelial cells, rare neutrophils or macrophages, and a small amount of noncellular debris in the background. Extracellular bacteria represented by a variety of morphologic types occur in low numbers and are often associated with the squamous epithelial cells. Large bacteria that resemble members of the Simonsiellaceae family (*Simonsiella* and *Alysiella*) appear to be a normal part of the blow flora and are not associated with inflammation (Fig. 64–2). Normal blow samples may also contain ciliate and flagellate protozoa (five different species have been observed). These protozoa are common in the blows of captive and wild-caught cetaceans. A common holotrichous ciliate protozoa (*Kyaroikeus cetarius*) is found in a variety of cetaceans (Fig. 64–3).[2] These large

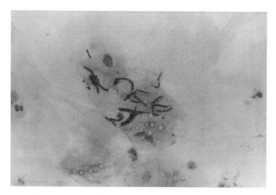

FIGURE 64–2. Large bacteria in ribbon-like chains resembling *Alysiella filiformis* bacteria associated with the surface of squamous epithelial cells in a blow sample from an Atlantic bottlenose dolphin (*Tursiops truncatus*). Original magnification, 40× (high dry objective).

(25 μm in width and 120 μm in length), rigid, cylindroid ciliates exhibit little movement on wet mounts. They stain deeply basophilic with Wright's stain, have linear rows of eosinophilic cilia, and have an eosinophilic triangular posterior podite. These protozoa are generally considered to be nonpathogenic because they are rarely associated with inflammatory responses. However, *K. cetarius* has been reported to ingest host epithelial cells and is occasionally present in high numbers and in association with a heavy mucus production and halitosis.[2] More research is needed to clarify the potential pathogenicity of this organism.

Abnormal blow cytologic findings include the presence of numerous inflammatory cells, large numbers of yeast, fungal hyphae, parasite ova or larvae, and bacterial phagocytosis by leukocytes. Numerous inflammatory cells found in a blow specimen are suggestive of an inflammatory response somewhere in the respiratory tract, most likely the upper respiratory tract or possibly the oropharynx. Leukocytic phagocytosis of bacteria is indicative of a septic inflammatory lesion. Large, yellow operculated ova of *Nasitrema*, a trematode commonly

found in the pterygoid sinus of cetaceans, may be seen in infected animals (Fig. 64–4). Large numbers of oval, narrowly based budding yeast and hyphae are indicative of a severe yeast infection (e.g., with *Candida* species). Fungal elements, such as hyphae and spores, are indicative of a mycotic etiology.

Cytology of the Trachea and Bronchi

Cytologic samples from the trachea can be obtained by performing a tracheal wash, by inserting a sterile tube through the blow, and passing it well into the trachea. Correct positioning of the tube into the trachea may require passage of the tube during exhalation. Once the tube is within the trachea, sterile saline (30 to 50 ml) is flushed through the tube and immediately aspirated back to obtain a cellular sample. Direct smears can be made from highly cellular samples, and imprints are made from mucous strands in the sample. However, in general, wash samples are poorly cellular and require a cell concentration technique to efficiently evaluate the specimen. If available, the method of choice for obtaining a tracheal or bronchial sample is with the use of a bronchoscope and biopsy or brush instruments to obtain imprints from samples taken directly from a lesion. The bronchoscope can be passed through the blow as a tracheal tube would be passed. This may require that the animal be sedated. The trachea and bronchi are lined by pseudostratified columnar ciliated epithelium and these cells, along with occasional goblet cells, are expected findings in cytologic specimens. Abnormal findings include marked numbers of neutrophils, macrophages, or lymphocytes; numerous eosinophils; yeast or fungal elements, such as spores or hyphae; and parasite ova or larvae.

Cytology of the Oral Cavity

Scrapings of the oral cavity from normal cetaceans reveal samples of variable cellularity (usually poorly to moderately cellular) that contain primarily squamous epithelial cells. Normal cytologic samples from the oral

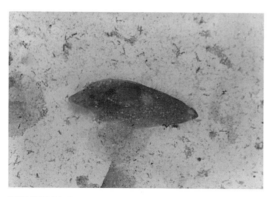

FIGURE 64–3. A large holotrichous ciliate protozoa, *Kyaroikeus cetarius*, in a blow sample from a killer whale (*Orcinus orca*). Original magnification, 40× (high dry objective).

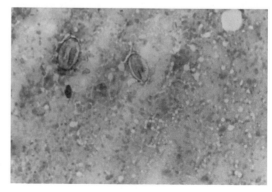

FIGURE 64–4. *Nasitrema* ova in mucus from the blow of an Atlantic bottlenose dolphin (*Tursiops truncatus*). Original magnification, 10× objective.

cavity contain a variable amount of noncellular background debris and usually low numbers of bacteria represented by a variety of morphologic types. Occasionally, cetaceans possess a white to yellow film in the oral cavity, especially noticeable in the roof of the mouth and along the margins of the mouth (chlorinated water often changes the color to green). A scraping of this material usually reveals dense sheets of cornified squamous epithelial cells that represent retention of cells that normally slough. This condition appears benign and is typically self-limiting. Abnormal cytologic findings of the oral cavity of cetaceans include large numbers of inflammatory cells that are usually associated with oral ulcerations or exudates and numerous narrowly based budding yeast as seen with candidiasis (Fig. 64–5). Lesions caused by candidiasis reveal a marked thickening of the oral epithelium.

Cytology of the Skin

The normal cytology of skin scrapings is typically poorly cellular and dependent on the force of the scraping. The sample usually yields squamous epithelial cells and, depending on the depth of the scraping, the cells vary from cornified squamous cells to less mature cells (columnar or cuboidal cells with higher nucleus-to-cytoplasm [N/C] ratios and basophilic cytoplasm). Common abnormal cytologic findings include increased numbers of leukocytes indicative of inflammation. Eosinophilic inflammation associated with skin lesions (e.g., rake marks) is suggestive of an immune response (i.e., type I hypersensitivity reaction). Numerous narrowly based budding yeast are indicative of cutaneous candidiasis. Inflammatory lesions may reveal bacterial phagocytosis in cases of septic inflammation.

Cytology of the Rectocolon

Rectocolon samples from cetaceans are collected using a sterile tube (Levine tube, Davol, Inc., Cranston, RI, which is an 18-French, 1.27-m long tube marked at

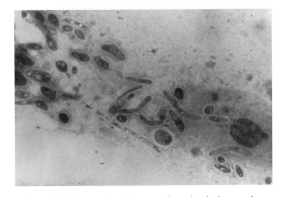

FIGURE 64–5. Scraping from an ulcerative lesion on the tongue of a killer whale (*Orcinus orca*) showing numerous yeast and developing hyphae. *Candida albicans* was isolated from the lesion. Original magnification, $100\times$ (oil immersion objective).

intervals to determine the distance) inserted into the anus and passed into the rectocolon. The liquid feces of cetaceans usually flow into the tube without the need for aspiration. Sterile saline can be used as a wash sample in the rare situation in which an adequate sample cannot be obtained in the initial passage of the tube. If aspiration is applied to the tube, excessive pressure should be avoided to prevent injury to the mucosa. Rectocolon cytologic study is indicated when abnormal feces are observed, when the animal exhibits signs of gastrointestinal disease (e.g., frequent defecations and vomiting), or as part of a routine physical examination of a cetacean. Normal samples are poorly cellular and contain squamous epithelial cells, short columnar epithelial cells (usually found in clumps as a result of traumatic exfoliation from passing the tube into the rectocolon), a few leukocytes (i.e., an average of zero to two per high-power field in an undiluted sample), and a background with a variable number of bacteria. The bacteria should be represented by a variety of morphologic types. The background also contains much noncellular debris. Some cetaceans, such as pygmy sperm whales (*Kogia breviceps*) and dwarf sperm whales (*Kogia simus*), produce a red-brown material (ink) in the colon that makes cytologic interpretation of the rectocolon sample challenging. Abnormal rectocolon cytologic findings include an increase in the number of inflammatory cells, numerous erythrocytes, many yeast cells (especially those showing hyphae formation), large numbers of bacteria represented by one morphologic type, and many bacterial rods containing swollen ends suggestive of terminal spores. A clostridial colitis is suspected when two or more rod-shaped bacteria containing clear vacuoles are found in an average oil immersion field of a thin, air-dried fecal smear. Numerous inflammatory cells, erythrocytes, and macrophages demonstrating erythrophagocytosis are associated with a severe hemorrhagic enterocolitis. A possible cause for a hemorrhagic enterocolitis is a bacterial toxin, such as clostridial toxin. The presence of erythrocytes without evidence of erythrophagocytosis or inflammation and with the presence of platelets is suggestive of peripheral blood contamination of the sample during passage of the tube. An eosinophilic inflammation associated with a rectocolon sample is suggestive of an immune-related disorder, such as an eosinophilic colitis (etiology is usually unknown) or intestinal parasitism. An eosinophilia in the hemogram is often not associated with cases of eosinophilic enterocolitis.

Cytology of the Stomach

Examination of cytologic specimens from the esophagus and stomach of a cetacean is indicated when the animal exhibits clinical signs of upper gastrointestinal disease or as part of the routine physical examination. Cetaceans with upper gastrointestinal disorders may exhibit anorexia, weight loss, vomiting, or regurgitation. Cytologic study of the stomach can be performed on fluid samples collected from a tube passed into the stomach. Fluid volume is usually adequate; however, a saline wash can be used if needed. Cetaceans can be trained to accept a gastric tube for evaluation of the gastric content as part of a routine husbandry behavior. If available, gastric endoscopy is the method of choice for obtaining gastric samples for cytologic evaluation. Endoscopy allows for direct examination of the esophagus and forestomach and for collection of samples of lesions using either a biopsy instrument or a brush passed through the instrument channel of the endoscope. The stomach of cetaceans, especially of the suborder Odontoceti (e.g., dolphins), is divided into three compartments: the forestomach, the glandular stomach (second stomach), and the pyloric stomach. The forestomach, which is a saccular extension of the distal esophagus, and the esophagus are lined with cornified, stratified squamous epithelium.[1] Cytologic samples obtained from the esophagus and forestomach contain polygonal cells with abundant light blue cytoplasm and low N/C ratio as well as keratinized anucleated squamous cells (squames). Cells from deeper layers may appear as small, round to oval cells with a small amount of dark blue cytoplasm (parabasal cells). The glandular stomach connects to the forestomach by a narrow sphincter, the true cardia. The narrow connecting channel between the glandular stomach and the duodenum is called the pyloric stomach.[1] The glandular and pyloric compartments of the cetacean stomach are lined with nonciliated simple columnar epithelium. These cells have eccentrically positioned uniformly round nuclei and pale blue cytoplasm. Although these cells may exfoliate and reflux with the gastric fluid into the forestomach, they are rarely seen in gastric samples obtained from the forestomach.

Normal cytologic findings of the esophagus and forestomach reveal a variable number of cornified and noncornified squamous epithelial cells and a marked amount of noncellular debris. Leukocytes may be present in low numbers (i.e., zero to two per high-power field). Abnormal cytologic findings include large numbers of leukocytes indicative of severe inflammation and large numbers of erythrocytes suggestive of esophageal or gastric ulcers. Usually, the gastric pH hemolyzes erythrocytes; therefore, when present, erythrocytes represent severe acute hemorrhage or they may be present with an abnormally high gastric pH. Other abnormal findings are bacterial phagocytosis indicative of septic inflammation, numerous yeast or hyphae indicative of mycotic infections, and parasite larvae or ova indicative of parasitic infestation (Fig. 64–6). Occasionally, parasite ova (e.g., *Nasitrema*) originating from the respiratory tract may be found in gastric samples.

Vaginal Cytology

Collection of samples from the vagina of a cetacean can be accomplished by passing a sterile tube (Levine tube, Davol, Inc., Cranston, RI) into the cranial vault of the vagina. Cetaceans can be trained to accept this procedure as routine husbandry behavior. Fluid for cytologic examination often flows passively into the tube, making aspiration unnecessary. If only a small quantity of fluid is obtained, it may be necessary to irrigate the vagina with small quantities of sterile saline (5 ml) to

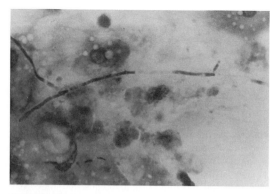

FIGURE 64–6. A brush biopsy sample obtained during an endoscopic examination of a gastric ulcer in an Atlantic bottlenose dolphin (*Tursiops truncatus*). The sample revealed numerous budding yeast, hyphae, and nondegenerate neutrophils. Original magnification, 100× (oil immersion objective).

allow aspiration of cellular material for examination. The vaginal cellularity of female cetaceans during the estrous cycle is not as distinctive as the estrous cycle of some domestic mammals (e.g., dogs and cats). Female cetaceans in estrus produce a copious flow of thick mucus that contains relatively few cells. The viscosity of the estrous vaginal fluid makes cellular evaluation difficult. Following estrus, the volume and viscosity of the mucus decreases and cytologic study shows a variable number of cornified squamous epithelial cells. Cornified squamous epithelial cells also appear in variable numbers in cytologic samples just before the stage of heavy mucous production (estrus). A small number of leukocytes, primarily nondegenerate neutrophils, appear in samples obtained 5 to 7 days following the end of heavy mucous flow. This stage most likely represents a postestrous stage (metestrus). The percentage of cornified epithelial cells at this stage is decreased and many of the cells appear as round to oval nucleated epithelial cells. The vaginal cytology of juvenile cetaceans and those in anestrus show low cellularity that consists primarily of round to oval nucleated epithelial cells. The vaginal cytologic changes in cetaceans are not as distinct as those in the dog and may not be as helpful in determining the stage of estrus for breeding purposes. The stage of heavy vaginal mucous production usually corresponds with the behavior and hormonal signs of estrus. Abnormal vaginal cytologic findings include a marked increase in leukocytes (especially those showing degenerative changes) and erythrocytes. Such a cellular response is indicative of a vaginitis or metritis.

Cytology of the Urine

Urine cytology is part of the routine urinalysis, and the interpretation is the same as that for domestic mammals. Urine can be collected by catheterization or as a free flow sample. Cetaceans can be trained to slide out of the water on their side and to urinate on command so that a free flow urine sample can be collected. They also can be trained to accept urinary catheterization. It is difficult to pass a urinary catheter in a male cetacean; therefore, urine from males is usually obtained opportunistically when they urinate while being handled out of the water. A microscopic examination of urine sediment (from 5 ml of urine) is part of the urinalysis. Normal urine contains few leukocytes (zero to three per high-power field) and erythrocytes (zero to three per high-power field). Epithelial cells also appear in small numbers in normal urine. Casts are rare in normal urine and appear as hyaline or finely granular casts when present. Bacteria are rare in normal urine and, when present, most likely represent contamination of the sample during catheterization or midstream collection. Normal cetacean urine contains a variable amount of crystals, usually amorphous phosphate crystals.

DIAGNOSTIC CYTOLOGY IN PINNIPEDS, MANATEES, OTTERS, AND POLAR BEARS

When appropriate, the following samples can be obtained from pinnipeds, manatees, otters, and polar bears

for cytologic evaluation: fine-needle aspiration of tissues or masses, imprints of excised or exposed tissues or lesions, scrapings of exposed lesions (e.g., conjuctival scrapings), abdominocentesis to evaluate abnormal fluid accumulation in the peritoneal cavity, thoracentesis to evaluate abnormal fluid accumulation in the pleural cavity, and transtracheal aspiration to obtain samples from the respiratory tract. The basic sampling techniques and cytologic interpretations for domestic animals apply to this group of animals. For example, fine-needle aspiration biopsy of an enlarged lymph node would be performed in a similar manner as described for the dog, and the cellular interpretations would be identical.

REFERENCES

1. Greenwood AG, Taylor DC, Wild D: Fibreoptic gastroscopy in dolphins. Vet Rec 102:495–497, 1978.
2. Sniezek JH, Coats DW, Small EB: *Kyaroikeus cetarius* N. G. Sp: a parasitic ciliate from the respiratory tract of odontocete cetacea. J Euk Microbiol 42 (3):260–268, 1995.

CHAPTER 65

Leptospirosis in Marine Mammals

FRANCES M. D. GULLAND

THE ORGANISM

Leptospirosis, which results from infection with the spirochete *Leptospira interrogans*, is a ubiquitous disease of humans and a wide variety of both domestic and wild animals.[4, 6] More than 250 serotypes of *L. interrogans* have been identified. All possess a common somatic antigen (lipopolysaccharide) but vary in their surface (agglutinating) antibody. Serologically distinct strains of *L. interrogans* tend to be considered as either "host-adapted," causing chronic disease and persistent infection, or "host-nonadapted," causing more acute disease.[11] In marine mammals, cases have been reported in pinnipeds but not cetaceans.[5, 9, 10, 12, 16, 18] All isolates from pinnipeds have been typed as *L. i. pomona*, which is considered to be a pig-adapted serovar.[10, 15, 18] In addition, cases of human leptospirosis have been attributed to infection with *L. pomona* contracted from California sea lions (*Zalophus californianus*) during pathologic examination,[17] and humans participating in

northern fur seal (*Callorhinus ursinus*) harvests have developed antibodies to the organism.[14]

Leptospirosis has not been previously documented in phocids. However, in 1996, three harbor seal (*Phoca vitulina richardsii*) pups housed in a rehabilitation center (The Marine Mammal Center, Sausalito, CA) showed typical clinical and hematologic signs of renal failure, and antibody titers to *Leptospira grippotyphosa* greater than 1:3200 developed. One animal died and had histologic evidence of an interstitial nephritis; two animals recovered after treatment.

EPIDEMIOLOGY

In 1970, *L. pomona* was first isolated from the kidney and urine of sea lions dying along the Oregon and California coast.[18] From 1981 to 1994, regular epizootics of leptospirosis occurred in these sea lions at 3- to 4-year intervals, mortality rates being highest in juvenile male animals during the autumn months.[10] Despite frequency of cases, the source of infection and mode of transmission of leptospirosis in marine mammals remain obscure. In most mammals, transmission is via urine from carrier animals penetrating abraded mucous membranes,[6] with urine often contaminating stagnant water sources, although indirect transmission via tick vectors is possible.[3] Leptospires are typically sensitive to extremes of pH and high salinity, so they are unlikely to persist in a marine environment outside a host animal.[6] A 7% to 15% prevalence of antibodies in juvenile northern fur seals on St. Paul Island, AL, compared to 2% prevalence of antibodies in nursing pups, suggests that exposure to infection in northern fur seal populations occurs at sea.[16] However, presence of organisms in aborted California sea lion pups in rookeries on the Channel Islands in California suggests that transmission could occur on rookeries, either transplacentally or via contact with infective urine, blood, or uterine fluids.[9, 15] The role of recovered animals as carriers is unknown.

CLINICAL SIGNS AND PATHOLOGY

Renal Disease

Leptospirosis is most commonly observed in free-living California sea lions as renal disease.[5, 10] Typical clinical signs include depression, anorexia, polydipsia, dehydration, reluctance to use the hindflippers, and, in extreme cases, vomiting, abdominal pain (demonstrated by adoption of a hunched position and holding the foreflippers over the abdomen) and muscular tremors.[5, 10] Hematologic changes include elevated blood urea nitrogen, phosphorus, globulin, sodium, and creatinine levels, and, less consistently, neutrophilia.[2, 5, 10]

Typical gross lesions on postmortem examination of affected California sea lions are marked swelling of the kidneys, loss of differentiation between renule medullae and cortices, pale tan-colored cortices, and occasionally subcapsular hemorrhages and hemorrhage at the corticomedullary junction (Fig. 65–1). In addition to renal lesions, swollen, friable livers with thick, tenacious bile

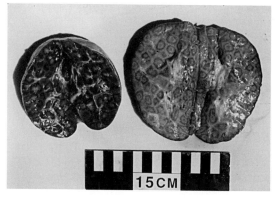

FIGURE 65–1. Normal California sea lion kidney (*left*) and one from an animal with leptospirosis (*right*). Note swollen renules and hemorrhage at the corticomedullary junction.

in the gallbladder and oral and gastric ulceration are often observed. Histologic examination usually reveals a lymphoplasmacytic interstitial nephritis.[5, 10, 12, 18] Similar pathologic findings associated with *L. pomona* infection were reported in a 13-year-old northern fur seal bull on St. Paul Island, AL.[16]

Reproductive Failure

Leptospirosis may also contribute to reproductive failure in pinnipeds. *L. pomona* has been isolated from aborted fetuses, placentas, and premature pups in California sea lion rookeries on the Channel Islands off California.[9, 15] However, high tissue levels of chlorinated hydrocarbons and polychlorinated biphenyls and a calicivirus (San Miguel sea lion virus) were also found in aborting females, leading to the suggestion that reproductive failure may be a result of interaction between pathogens and environmental contaminants.[9]

Neonatal mortality associated with *L. pomona* septicemia has been documented in northern fur seal pups on St. Paul Island.[7] Necropsy of three newborn pups revealed subcapsular hemorrhage of the kidney, free blood in the peritoneal cavity, and a friable liver with extensive capsular hemorrhage associated with *L. pomona* in the liver and kidney. This led to the suggestion that the previously named "multiple hemorrhagic perinatal complex" was acute leptospirosis, although some cases could have been a consequence of trauma.

Leptospirosis may also be endemic in Steller sea lions (*Eumetopias jubatus*) in Alaska, inasmuch as antibodies have been detected in two of six animals tested.[7]

DIAGNOSIS

Leptospires can be observed as motile organisms by direct darkfield microscopy of blood or urine from infected animals. The organisms measure 0.1 μm in diameter and 6 to 20 μm in length and consist of a helical body wound around two flagellae and covered by an external sheath.[6, 8] The tightly coiled spirals are often difficult to recognize, however, and tiny strands projecting from the surface of red blood cells or filamentous proteins in urine may be mistaken for leptospires. Detection in urine sediment and in impression smears of kidney can be enhanced using fluorescent antibody testing (FAT) of acetone-fixed smears. FAT is more sensitive than direct darkfield microscopy and can be used on frozen tissue, but its usefulness depends on the experience of the technician. Detection of leptospires in formalin-fixed tissue is best achieved by use of silver impregnation stains such as Warthin-Starry, Steinert, or Levaditis.[12, 13]

Leptospires can be cultured from blood and urine of live animals, and kidney and liver of dead animals, although isolation is often unsuccessful because of overgrowth by other bacteria.[4, 8] Leptospires may survive in blood with anticoagulant for up to 11 days. For urine, dilution at 1:10 in bovine serum albumin buffered to pH 7.0 may enhance yield. Fletcher's semisolid and EMJH (Ellinghausen-McCullough-Johnson-Harris) media are most commonly used for culture, with 5-fluorouracil often added to reduce bacterial overgrowth. Incubation is carried out at 30°C in the dark, with most isolates growing in 5 to 15 days, although some can take 4 weeks.[4, 8]

Because of the difficulties in culturing and visualizing leptospires, diagnosis of infection is often based on serologic study. Antibodies are readily detected by a macroscopic slide agglutination test. In domestic animals, a fourfold increase in titer, or an absolute titer of greater than 1:100 is considered diagnostic of infection.[8] Similar titers are probably indicative of infection in pinnipeds. However, titers to serovars other than *L. pomona* have been detected in California sea lions, and their significance is unclear.[10]

TREATMENT

California sea lions with clinical signs of renal disease and antibody titers greater than 1:3200 to *L. pomona* have successfully undergone treatment (30% chance of recovery) with tetracycline at 22 mg/kg every 8 hours or potassium penicillin G (44,000 U/kg every 12 hours) for 10 to 14 days, although whether surviving animals were persistently infected is unknown.[5] Trials with hamsters have shown dihydrostreptomycin/penicillin G at 25 mg/kg for 5 days, or oxytetracycline at 40 mg/kg, ceftiofur at 20 mg/kg, erythromycin at 10 mg/kg, ampicillin at 25 mg/kg, or tylosin at 20 mg/kg, all for 5 days, cleared infection from animals inoculated with *L. pomona*.[1]

Supportive therapy of sea lions is achieved with subcutaneous lactated Ringer's solution or 5% dextrose (100 ml/kg/day), or oral electrolyte solution by gavage. Oral aluminium hydroxide preparations (Amphojel, Wyeth Laboratories, Philadelphia, PA) at 30 to 90 mg/kg appear to assist lowering of blood phosphorous levels. Oral antacids (Maalox, Rhone-Poulenc Rorer Pharmaceuticals, Inc., Collegeville, PA) (30 to 90 mg/kg) and cimetidine (5 mg/kg) can ease discomfort of gastric ulceration.

Prophylaxis has been attempted in captive pinnipeds in aquaria using commercially available leptospira vaccines. Administration of a polyvalent killed bacterin, commercially prepared for use in cattle and swine (Lepto 5, BioCor, Inc., Omaha, NE), resulted in a decrease in the number of cases of leptospirosis seen in a colony of captive northern fur seals, with no adverse affects of vaccination noted (J. L. Dunn, personal communication, 1997). Most fur seals seroconverted after vaccination. The antibody titers to the vaccine serovars varied markedly between serovars.

REFERENCES

1. Alt DP, Bolin CA: Preliminary evaluation of antimicrobial agents for treatment of *Leptospira interrogans* serovar *pomona* infection in hamsters and swine. Am J Vet Res 57:59–62, 1996.
2. Bossart GD, Dierauf LA: Marine mammal clinical laboratory medicine. *In* Dierauf LA (ed): Handbook of Marine Mammal Medicine: Health, Disease and Rehabilitation. Boca Raton, FL, CRC Press, pp 1–52, 1990.
3. Burgdorfer W: The possible role of ticks as vectors of leptospirae. Exp Parasitol 5:571–9, 1956.
4. Collins CH, Lyne PM, Grange JM: Microbiological methods, 7th ed. Oxford, UK, Butterworth-Heinemann, 1995.
5. Dierauf LA, Vandenbroek DJ, Roletto J, et al: An epizootic of leptospirosis in California sea lions. J Am Vet Med Assoc 187:1145–1148, 1985.
6. Faine S. *Leptospira* and leptospirosis. Boca Raton, FL, CRC Press, 1993.
7. Fay FH, Dieterich RA, Shults LM, et al: Morbidity and mortality of marine mammals. *In* Environmental Assessment of the Alaskan Continental Shelf. Annual Reports of Principal Investigators for the Year Ending March 1978, Vol. 1: Mammals-Birds. Seattle: Bureau of Land Management/National Oceanic and Atmospheric Administration, pp 39–79, 1978.
8. Galton MM, Menges RW, Schotts EB, et al: Leptospirosis: epidemiology, clinical manifestations in man and animals, and methods in laboratory diagnostics [Publication No. 951]. Washington, DC, U.S. Public Health Service, 1962.
9. Gilmartin WG, Delong RL, Smith AW, et al: Premature parturition in the California sea lion. J Wildl Dis 12:104–115, 1976.
10. Gulland FMD, Koski M, Lowenstine LJ, et al: Leptospirosis in California sea lions (*Zalophus californianus*) stranded along the central California coast, 1981–1994. J Wildl Dis 32:572–580, 1996.
11. Heaty SE, Johnson R: Leptospirosis. J Am Vet Med Assoc 205:1518–1523, 1994.
12. Howard EB, Britt JO, Matsumoto GK, et al: Bacterial diseases. *In* Pathobiology of Marine Mammal Diseases, Vol. 1. Boca Raton, FL, CRC Press, pp 69–118, 1983.
13. Luna LG: Manual of histologic staining methods of the Armed Forces Institute of Pathology, 3rd ed. New York, McGraw Hill, 1968.
14. Medway W: Some bacterial and mycotic diseases of marine mammals. J Am Vet Med Assoc 177:831–834, 1980.
15. Smith AW, Brown RJ, Skilling DE, et al: *Leptospira pomona* and reproductive failure in California sea lions. J Am Vet Med Assoc 165:996–998, 1974.
16. Smith AW, Brown RJ, Skilling DE, et al: Naturally occurring leptospirosis in northern fur seals (*Callorhinus ursinus*). J Wildl Dis 13:144–147, 1977.
17. Smith AW, Vedros NA, Akers TG, et al: Hazards of disease transfer from marine to land mammals: review and recent findings. J Am Vet Med Assoc 173:1131, 1978.
18. Vedros NA, Smith AW, Schonweld J: Leptospirosis epizootic among California sea lions. Science 172:1250–1251, 1971.

CHAPTER 66

Toxicology in Marine Mammals

THOMAS J. O'SHEA

JOSEPH R. GERACI

There has been a rapid increase in interest in the potential impacts of toxic substances on marine mammals, particularly in wild populations. Although much information has been developed on the presence of persistent contaminants in wild marine mammals, there is less emphasis on developing supporting clinical or pathologic data. Furthermore, there is much uncertainty about the significance of the presence of these substances to marine mammal populations. This chapter synopsizes research and specialized knowledge regarding marine mammals and toxic contaminants. (For more information, see O'Shea, in press.[32]) A basic understanding of marine mammal biology and knowledge of the fundamentals of toxicology (particularly diagnostic aspects) are necessary adjuncts to this chapter.

ORGANOCHLORINE COMPOUNDS

Organochlorines have been widely manufactured for industry and agriculture. Millions of tons of these chemicals have been released into the environment. These compounds tend to be chemically stable and highly fat soluble, allowing them to persist in the environment, accumulate in lipids of animals, and increase in concentrations at higher levels of marine food webs. Their accumulation in marine mammals is well known; they have been identified in tissues of more than 7000 individual animals in more than 80 species, including pinnipeds, whales, dolphins, sea otters (*Enhydra lutris*), sirenians, and polar bears (*Ursus maritimus*).[32]

Organochlorines Detected in Marine Mammals

Organochlorines often found in toxicologic analyses of marine mammal samples include the insecticide dichlorodiphenyltrichloroethane (DDT) and related compounds, cyclodiene insecticides and metabolites, toxaphene, polychlorinated biphenyls (PCBs), polychlorinated dibenzofurans (PCDFs), and polychlorinated dibenzodioxins (PCDDs). DDT and metabolites dichlorodiphenyldichloroethylene (DDE) and dichlorodi-

phenyldichloroethane (DDD) were first discovered in marine mammal tissues in the 1960s and provided early evidence of what has since become widely recognized as global contamination of the marine ecosystem by organochlorines. In some areas, unusually high concentrations of DDE and related compounds have been reported in blubber of odontocete cetaceans and pinnipeds. Although the parent compound DDT is no longer in use in most developed nations, residues of DDE persist in the ecosystem and DDT is still applied as an insecticide in some developing countries. Atmospheric transport of organochlorines from tropical areas to some of the more "pristine" reaches of the globe where they subsequently accumulate in marine mammals has been well documented.[30]

Because of its high lipid content, blubber is the tissue most frequently analyzed for organochlorines. DDE concentrations in blubber are usually far higher than those of DDT or DDD, but DDE is much less generally toxic (acute toxicity to laboratory and domestic animals) than DDT or DDD. Because of an absence of controlled, detailed experimental studies, the clinical significance of residues of organochlorines in blubber remains speculative. Organochlorines have never been determined to be a cause of death in wild marine mammals. In mammals and birds, the brain is the principal tissue for diagnosing lethal levels of organochlorines; levels reported thus far in marine mammals do not approach those diagnostic of lethality in other species.[32, 33]

Aldrin, dieldrin, and endrin are cyclodiene insecticides that are more acutely toxic than DDT. Like DDT, they are neurotoxic and were in high use before restrictions were instituted in the 1970s. Dieldrin is common in blubber of marine mammals, whereas aldrin and the more toxic endrin are seldom found. The cyclodienes are found in marine mammals worldwide but nearly always at lower concentrations than ΣDDT (the sum of all detected DDT metabolites) or PCBs. Another cyclodiene found in marine mammal blubber is chlordane, a mixture of compounds and isomers that also includes heptachlor (also used as an insecticide), nonachlor, and oxychlordane. Heptachlor epoxide is the major metabolite of heptachlor found in marine mammal tissues; isomers of chlordane, oxychlordane, and nonachlor have also been reported. Toxaphene, an ag-

All material in this chapter is in the public domain, with the exception of any borrowed figures or tables.

ricultural pesticide that is banned in some countries, is a mixture of compounds technically known as chlorinated camphenes, polychlorocamphenes, and chlorinated nor-bornane derivatives. All of these organochlorines have been found in blubber of marine mammals throughout the global marine ecosystem, including polar reaches, but usually at concentrations that appear to be low from the standpoint of toxicity. Isomers of hexachloro-cyclohexane (HCH), also called lindane or benzene hexachloride (BHC), also appear in low concentrations in blubber. Other organochlorines occasionally reported in marine mammals include Kepone, mirex, endosulfan, and the fungicide hexachlorobenzene (HCB). Other or-ganohalogens, such as the polybrominated biphenyls (PBBs), are also sometimes reported.

PCBs are a mixture of up to 209 congeners and are generally found at higher concentrations than most other organochlorines. The PCBs have been used widely in industry. After their discovery as widespread contami-nants in the late 1960s, their manufacture was eventu-ally terminated. However, most of the more than 1.5 million metric tons of PCBs produced are still intact in various uses (such as in dielectric fluids in older transformers). With time and degradation, it is likely that the quantities that eventually reach the oceans will increase, as will their concentrations in marine mam-mals. PCBs are also lipophilic and are thus readily sequestered in marine food webs. However, there is wide variance among individual congeners in their tox-icity to laboratory mammals and persistence in marine mammal tissues. PCDFs, PCDDs, polychloroquater-phenyls (PCQs) and polychlorinated naphthalenes (PCNs) occur in commercial PCB mixtures as by-prod-ucts of the PCB manufacturing process. PCDDs and PCDFs are also formed as impurities in a variety of other industrial and natural combustion processes. The toxicity of the compounds is variable, however, the PCDD compound 2,3,7,8-tetrachlorodibenzo-p-dioxin (TCDD) is among the most toxic compounds known. These compounds have been detected in tissues of some marine mammals, but at concentrations thought to be of low toxicologic significance.

Methods of Analysis

Analyzing for organochlorines in marine mammal tissues is complex and expensive (high-resolution capillary gas chromatography with electron capture de-tection, combined with confirmation by mass spectrom-etry). Acceptable quality assurance procedures must be followed and well documented. Results are only as good as the sampling procedure, so every effort should be made to collect high-quality specimens.[13] Most labo-ratories report contaminant residues on the basis of mass of chemical per unit mass of tissue, which may be expressed on the basis of fresh or "wet" weight of the tissue sample, based on the weight of the sample with water removed ("dry weight"), or based on the extractable lipid components ("lipid weight"). Units of concentration are usually given as parts per million (ppm) wet weight (μg/g or mg/kg), parts per billion (ppb; ng/g or μg/kg), or parts per trillion (ppt). It

is important to keep these differences in mind when comparing results of various studies.

Interpretation of Results

Although the presence of organochlorines in marine mammal tissues is universal, there is not widespread agreement on the toxicologic significance of their pres-ence. Furthermore, much variation exists in concentra-tions of organochlorines in tissues of marine mammals. Animals from in-shore populations in heavily polluted areas have exhibited concentrations of 1000 to 2000 ppm (wet weight) or more of DDT or PCBs in blubber. More "typical" concentrations in blubber range less than 100 ppm, with many samples at 10 ppm or less, particularly in baleen whales or species from less con-taminated regions such as the open oceans or Antarctic. In comparison, during the 1960s and early 1970s, mean concentrations of ΣDDT in human adipose tissue in the United States ranged from 5 to 10 ppm.[27]

Many factors can cause the variation observed in organochlorine concentrations in marine mammals, most notably location, foods eaten, age, sex, and repro-ductive status. Fish-eating species are exposed to greater amounts of dietary organochlorines than plank-ton feeders or herbivores, and some regions are more highly polluted than others. Within a species and study area, immature animals of both sexes generally have similar organochlorine concentrations in blubber. Body burdens subsequently increase with age in males but are stable or decrease with age in mature females. This is because females transfer organochlorines to offspring during gestation and lactation (because of transfer in lipid-rich milk). The toxicologic significance of this exposure in nursing young (especially first born, which may receive largest doses) is unknown; one recent field study showed no effect on immune function in wild suckling seals.[18]

Marine mammals also have major seasonal shifts in the amounts of fat stored in blubber. In addition, indi-viduals sampled as stranded carcasses may have de-pleted lipid reserves from disease or starvation, with consequent elevations in organochlorine residue con-centrations in blubber. Time since death also alters residue concentrations in tissues. The rates at which organochlorines are either passed into the blood with lipid mobilization or are concentrated in the remaining fat are poorly known for marine mammals, but both processes occur.[2]

Effects of Organochlorines on Marine Mammals

Relationships between organochlorine exposure and toxic effects in marine mammals, especially susceptibil-ity to disease and impact on reproduction, are topics of ongoing research. It is not possible to link residue concentrations in tissues with specific effects in any straightforward, unambiguous way. Past research has suggested associations between high organochlorine concentrations in tissues and a variety of pathologic findings, but cause-and-effect relationships have not been demonstrated. This is important because diseased animals may have elevated organochlorine residues owing to starvation and mobilization of lipid reserves, old age, or lack of excretion via lactation, and these changes could obscure any toxicologic effect.

PATHOLOGY AND DISEASE

Pathologic conditions circumstantially linked with organochlorine exposure in highly polluted areas include uterine stenoses and occlusions, benign uterine tumors, adrenocortical hyperplasia, hyperkeratosis, nail deformations, skull asymmetry, and bone lesions.[7, 28] Detailed work on harbor porpoises (*Phocoena phocoena*), however, showed no relationship between organochlorine exposure and adrenal hyperplasia.[22] Studies of beluga whales (*Delphinapterus leucas*) found dead in the St. Lawrence River have revealed a seemingly high prevalence of various lesions. Because this river contains multiple contaminants, many of which are found at high levels in belugas found stranded there, linkages between pathology and contaminants have been postulated but not proven.[6, 26]

There has also been investigation into the possibility that organochlorine exposure may have contributed to the susceptibility of marine mammals during recent mass die-offs caused by morbilliviruses. This is an area of needed research and some dispute. Organochlorine concentrations in blubber of harbor seals (*Phoca vitulina*) that died in a phocine distemper virus (PDV) outbreak in Great Britain in 1988 and in those that survived, for example, showed no differences to suggest a link between death from PDV infection and organochlorine contamination.[19] Other studies have found no statistical associations between organochlorine concentrations in blubber and deaths from infectious and parasitic disease,[23] or significant differences in PCB and DDT concentrations in juvenile harbor seals collected during and before a PDV outbreak.[8] Several other studies have also failed to discover connections between disease and organochlorine contamination, including a putative association between thyroid metabolism, organochlorine contamination, and morbillivirus outbreaks. One study on harbor seals showed that the addition of PCBs to the diet did not influence susceptibility to morbillivirus challenge.[20] However, harbor seals fed diets consisting of fish contaminated with mixed organochlorines showed immunotoxic effects consistent with cellular rather than humoral responses.[12, 38] Concentrations of PCBs in blubber of some striped dolphins (*Stenella coeruleoalba*) that succumbed to a morbillivirus epidemic in the Mediterranean in the early 1990s were the highest reported in marine mammals and were significantly higher than in biopsy-sampled dolphins from the area before and after the epizootic,[3] suggesting that PCBs may have played a role in immunosuppression and susceptibility to morbillivirus. However, immunosuppression also occurs as a direct result of morbillivirus damage to lymphoid tissues, resulting in the many secondary infections characterizing recent morbillivirus epizootics in marine mammals. Morbilliviruses are virulent and historically have produced high mortality rates in immunologically naive populations of terrestrial mammals before the widespread synthesis of organochlorines.

REPRODUCTION

Organochlorines have been implicated in reproductive failure in captive harbor seals. Control and experimental females were fed fish that were low or high in PCBs and ΣDDT over a 2-year period.[36] Reproductive success was significantly lower in females fed the more contaminated fish, and failure was thought to occur at the implantation stage of pregnancy, probably because of the effects of PCBs.[36] Association of high organochlorine concentrations in blubber and impaired reproduction has also been noted in pinnipeds from the Baltic Sea and coastal southern California, regions with significant organochlorine pollution. However, female marine mammals with reproduction impaired for any reason (e.g., leptospirosis) also have higher organochlorine concentrations because they cannot excrete these chemicals through lactation, making cause-and-effect conclusions difficult.[1] There is no direct evidence for impaired reproduction caused by organochlorine exposure in cetaceans, sirenians, polar bears, or sea otters.[31, 32] Careful investigation of this topic in sea otters would be of interest, however, because PCBs can severely impair reproduction in some other mustelids.[33]

Metabolism and Biochemical Toxicity in Marine Mammals

Developing models in laboratory mammals show that certain organochlorines (especially PCBs) induce enzymes that could lead to endocrine imbalances, a possible mechanism to explain reproductive failure.[9, 37] The chief pathway investigated has involved the mixed-function oxidase (MFO) system. Cytochrome P-450 enzymes (e.g., CYP1A1) bind with oxygen and the organochlorine substrates, converting them into compounds that are more polar and subject to enhanced excretion. Some foreign compounds can function as enzyme inhibitors, inducers, or substrates, and the many interactions between different compounds and enzymes can be extremely complex. In laboratory animals, some metabolites produced from organochlorines have greater toxicity than the parent compounds. Patterns of MFO activity in liver microsomal samples have been determined for a variety of pinnipeds and cetaceans.[32] However, the significance of variability in MFO activity levels in wild marine mammals and the absence of information on relationships between organochlorine concentrations in tissues or diet and MFO activity make toxicologic interpretation of these results difficult.

The toxic equivalency factor (TEF) concept has been applied to studies of PCB contamination of marine mammals, but with caveats.[37, 39] A TEF can be calculated for a specific PCB congener based on the potency of a biologic response in relation to the response to highly toxic TCDD. The coplanar and mono-orthoplanar PCBs give the most similar responses to TCDD, but activities are generally much less pronounced. The TEF concept has been extended to include an overall estimate of the TCDD-like toxicity of the entire complex mixture of PCBs, PCDDs, and PCDFs present in marine mammal tissue samples, referred to as the total toxic equivalents, or TEQ. It is calculated as the sum of the concentration of each PCB, PCDD, or PCDF times its TEF for the sample. Although individual PCBs have much lower TEFs than the dioxins and dibenzofurans, they are usually present at much higher concentrations, and the TEQ of the mixture of contaminants in the sample may more thoroughly reflect the overall potential toxicity. However, toxic responses can be non-additive with antagonistic effects. For example, immunotoxic responses can be much less than predicted on the basis of total TEQs.[39]

Furthermore, the mixtures of PCBs found in marine mammal tissues in comparison with their prey reflects the ability of various species to metabolize specific congeners. Polar bears, for example, metabolize congeners that are particularly resistant to metabolism in some seals and cetaceans.[31] Differences among marine mammal species in relative patterns of PCB congeners in tissues make it difficult to generalize about the capacity of these animals to metabolize certain PCBs. However, knowledge about patterns of PCB metabolism in marine mammals will increase as additional studies include congener-specific analyses.

METALS

Many of the naturally occurring elements are essential chemical components of normal physiologic systems. At high exposure levels, these elements can have toxic effects, however, and some elements have no known essential role. Of particular interest in the study of toxic elements are the metals.[17] The toxic elements most studied in marine mammals are cadmium, mercury, and lead. Up to 40 trace elements have also been found in the tissues of more than 60 species of marine mammals,[32] but their possible role as toxic agents is not well understood. Generally, metals do not biomagnify in marine food webs to the extent organochlorines do. Methods for determining concentrations of toxic elements in tissues should include systematic procedures for tissue collection that prevent spurious contamination as well as acceptable quality assurance procedures. Atomic absorption spectrometry and neutron activation analysis are commonly used analytical procedures.

Cadmium

Cadmium is a nonessential element that can become an environmental contaminant through various industrial processes. Some prey species of marine mammals such as squid and certain mollusks are naturally high in cadmium. In mammals, toxic effects of cadmium exposure are mitigated by protective binding with endogenously produced metallothionein, a low molecular weight protein. Cadmium typically reaches its highest concentrations in the kidneys, although greater amounts can be found in the liver with unusually excessive exposure. Toxic effects in laboratory mammals include circulatory and nervous system disorders and testicular and renal disease. High amounts are required to produce these effects, some of which may not occur in the presence of adequate dietary zinc and selenium.

Cadmium accumulates in kidneys of marine mammals with increasing age. Concentrations of cadmium in kidneys of 500 ppm (dry weight) or more have been reported in species as diverse as narwhals (*Monodon monoceros*), Antarctic fur seals (*Arctocephalus gazella*), California sea lions (*Zalophus californianus*), northern fur seals (*Callorhinus ursinus*), ringed seals (*Phoca hispida*), and walrus (*Odobenus rosmarus*).[32] There have been no published observations demonstrating cadmium-induced disease in marine mammals. In part, this may be because of the protective action of metallothionein proteins.

Mercury

Mercury is one of the few nonessential elements that biomagnifies appreciably in marine food webs and is highly toxic to vertebrates at relatively low levels. Marine mammals, however, have biochemical mechanisms that provide tolerance to high mercury exposure in the food chain. Mercury can enter the environment from numerous human activities. Large quantities are also volatilized to the atmosphere through natural processes, and some areas such as the Arctic or Mediterranean are geologically high in mercury. Microorganisms in sediments and soils convert mercury to the methyl form, which is soluble in water and can biomagnify in the food chain.

Mercury is neurotoxic, nephrotoxic, immunotoxic, and mutagenic. Methyl mercury is readily absorbed by the gastrointestinal tract. The element accumulates in the kidneys, liver, and brain, but organ distribution and toxicity vary with the chemical form. Most mercury in marine mammal livers (which have the highest concentrations) is demethylated, despite the finding that mercury in fish prey is in the methyl form. Many of the reported mercury concentrations of elemental mercury in marine mammals are greater than levels associated with toxicity in other species, but no evidence of harm has been observed. Selenium has a protective effect against mercury toxicity; high concentrations of mercury in the liver of marine mammals are accompanied by equivalently high concentrations of selenium. Examples of extraordinarily high concentrations of mercury in livers of marine mammals (unaccompanied by reports of toxicity) include reports of more than 700 ppm (wet weight) in harbor seals and false killer whales (*Pseudorca crassidens*), more than 1000 ppm (wet weight) in gray seals (*Halichoerus grypus*) and striped dolphins, and 13,150 ppm (dry weight) in bottlenose dolphins (*Tursiops truncatus*).[32] Marine mammals that typically feed lower in the food chain, such as baleen whales and sirenians, have relatively low mercury concentrations in liver in comparison with fish-eating species. Unlike organochlorines, mercury concentrations in marine mammals are not markedly higher in males than females. The high concentrations of mercury found in some marine mammals could pose risks to people that consume organs from these animals.

Lead

Lead is a nonessential element with toxic qualities that have been recognized for centuries. Sublethal poisoning causes behavioral disorders, and chronic exposure can cause disorders of the nervous system, gastrointestinal tract, renal system (with histopathologically evident lead-based intranuclear renal inclusion bodies), and immunotoxicity. Lead exposure also interferes with the production of hemoglobin and red blood cells, and inhibition of the enzyme delta aminolevulinic acid dehydratase critical to this process is a well-known biochemical marker of lead exposure. We are unaware of any report on lead toxicity in marine mammals or of lead levels in their tissues that would be cause for concern. Most reports reveal concentrations of less than 1 ppm (wet weight) in liver, kidney, and muscle, with no consistent trend in age or sex. Marine mammals fall in line with other vertebrates in which bone is the prominent depot for long-term storage of lead. The highest concentration of lead found in any marine mammal is 61.6 ppm (wet weight) in bone of a bottlenose dolphin stranded in a region where a lead smelter was operated.[21]

OIL

Approximately 10,000 to 15,000 metric tons of petroleum enter the oceans each day, from natural seeps such as in the Santa Barbara Channel (30,000 tons/year), off-shore production activities, atmospheric deposition, river runoff, and ocean dumping. Oil from ships contribute as well, some accidentally (e.g., the *Exxon Valdez* ran aground in Alaska in 1989, spilling 11 million gallons of crude oil, which fouled nearly 1000 miles of coastline), but more by purposeful discharges of ballast and tank-washing water. (See review by Neff.[29]) Crude petroleum products—no two are alike—contain thousands of organic and few inorganic compounds. The lighter fractions, which are distilled into gasoline and other fuels, are acutely toxic; they irritate mucous membranes, inhaled vapors damage respiratory tissue, and any that are absorbed into the circulation can attack the liver, nervous system, and hematopoietic tissues. These light fractions seriously threaten an animal at the site of a fresh spill, but, because they evaporate or dissipate in a matter of hours or days, their harmful reign is short-lived. Left behind are the thick foamy emulsions that stick and spoil fur and hair and clog body openings. Eventually, the so-called "mousse" mixes with sand and debris to form tarry aggregates that sink or wash ashore, where they persist for years or decades.

Each group of marine mammals confronts oil in its own way.[14, 25] Cetaceans are entirely aquatic. Some inhabit or visit in-shore waters or ice formations that can entrain spilled oil; pelagic (open water) cetaceans are less likely to be exposed. Oil might adhere to the surface of a cetacean, although there is no firm evidence, or be inhaled with fatal results that would escape notice, but a more likely danger is that thick oil would adhere to the haired fringes of the baleen plates of a mysticete and reduce the efficiency of its giant food-strainer. There are few unequivocal reports of cetaceans being harmed by oil.

Sirenians, represented in the United States by the Florida manatee, *Trichechus manatus,* are also entirely aquatic, although they spend most of their time near shore. Manatees are intolerant of cold and, in winter, seek warm-water refuges where they converge in large numbers. A spill in such an area could be disastrous, forcing them to remain in warm oily water feeding on contaminated vegetation or to escape to clean but dangerously cold seas.

Pinnipeds, polar bears, and sea otters are amphibious and, therefore, visit beaches or ice edges where spilled oil may accumulate. Sea otters spend much time in kelp beds, which can also trap oil. These species have hair or fur that, for some, like for the sea otter, polar bear, fur seal, and some newborn phocid seals, protects against heat loss. Fouling by oil reduces or destroys this vital property, causing energy reserves to drain in the animal. This is especially true of the sea otter, which forsakes all activities, including feeding, to concentrate on grooming its spoiled fur, from which it continues to inhale and ingest toxic hydrocarbons. Sea otters are exceptionally vulnerable to the effects of spilled oil—more than 1000 fell victim to the 1989 *Exxon Valdez* spill in Prince William Sound, Alaska. There is more literature on the clinical care of oiled otters than on any other marine mammal.[15] Early management is directed toward reducing shock-induced damage to liver, kidney, gastrointestinal, and hematopoietic systems. The animal is first stabilized with fluids and antibiotics, then the job of cleaning begins. The animal is sedated and bathed with 4 to 8 L of a 1:16 solution of Dawn detergent (Procter and Gamble), rinsed using a showerhead with moderate pressure to help restore loft, and towel dried for an hour. The animal is then placed in a cage for 12 hours before being transferred to a saltwater bath. Sea otters with 20% of their body coated with oil can be successfully cleaned in this way and rehabilitated in 1 to 2 weeks.

OTHER TOXIC SUBSTANCES

The most dramatic and least ambiguous cases of known lethal poisoning of marine mammals have been due to biologic toxins produced by marine dinoflagellates, particularly during monospecific blooms. Only a small number of the marine dinoflagellates are known to produce such toxins, some of which have been described as "among the most potent nonproteinaceous lethal materials known."[40] Dinoflagellate toxins have been linked to human mortality and illness, especially after ingestion of shellfish and other seafoods that have concentrated these poisons through filter-feeding, or from food chain accumulation (as in the case of saxitoxin). Not all dinoflagellate toxins accumulate in food chains.[4] Toxic effects vary with species, exposure route, and characteristics of the toxin. Most symptoms are neurologic or gastrointestinal. Death of bottlenose dolphins and manatees has been circumstantially linked with blooms of the dinoflagellate *Ptychodiscus brevis* along the west coast of Florida.[34] This dinoflagellate was also responsible for the widely publicized manatee die-off of 1996; these animals may have been exposed through food, water, or perhaps inhalation of aerosols. Deaths caused by saxitoxins produced by the dinoflagellate *Alexandrium tamarense* have been observed in humpback whales (*Megaptera novaeangliae*) that had ingested toxin-laden fish,[16] and paralytic shellfish poisoning has been observed in sea otters.[11]

Marine mammals inhabiting urban waters are subjected to air pollutants. Carbon deposits such as those seen in humans subjected to long-term inhalation of polluted air have been found in macrophages in mediastinal lymph nodes and lung tissue of bottlenose dolphins from a metropolitan area.[35] Radionuclides have been found in marine mammals (primarily cesium-137, lead-210, potassium-40, plutonium, and americium), but none have been reported in excessive concentrations nor have any adverse effects been reported.[5, 10] The polycyclic aromatic hydrocarbons, which can stem from numerous sources but are chiefly associated with petroleum, have been found at negligible concentrations in marine mammals, with no links to toxic effects.[24] No marine mammal toxicity has been determined to be a result of contamination with organic herbicides or nonhalogenated insecticides, such as the widely used organophosphates and carbamates. In general, these compounds do not persist at high concentrations in the oceans and do not accumulate in food chains. Diagnosis of death resulting from contamination with organophosphates or carbamates requires measurement of brain acetylcholinesterase activity in relation to controls, as well as chemical confirmation of the presence of these substances in the gut. Only fresh tissues can be used for these analyses.

SUMMARY

The sight of an oil spill or even the simple knowledge of the presence of synthetic contaminants throughout the tissues and environments of such splendid wildlife as marine mammals offends human sensibilities. Some impacts, such as the *Exxon Valdez* catastrophe, are immediate and obvious: time, energy, and resources (more than $1 billion earmarked) were heavily invested in rescuing animals and in assessing and restoring the damage to the environment, with much of that attention being drawn by the suffering sea otters. Most other oceanic contaminants are not as overtly offensive and do not kill as obviously, but some may have the potential for more serious effects on populations. For various human-caused reasons, some marine mammal populations are dwindling at a rate that may mark their demise over the next few decades. Although research on the role of toxic substances in contributing to marine mammal population declines leaves many questions unanswered, efforts to abate further contamination of the oceans should be accelerated to provide future amelioration of the potential problems involved.

REFERENCES

1. Addison RF: Organochlorines and marine mammal reproduction. Can J Fish Aquat Sci 46:360–368, 1989.
2. Aguilar A: Compartmentation and reliability of sampling procedures in organochlorine pollution surveys of cetaceans. Residue Rev 95:91–114, 1985.
3. Aguilar A, Borrell A: Abnormally high polychlorinated biphenyl levels in striped dolphins (*Stenella coeruleoalba*) affected by the 1990–1992 Mediterranean epizootic. Sci Total Environ 154:237–247, 1994.
4. Anderson DM: Red tides. Sci Am 271:62–68, 1994.
5. Anderson SS, Livens FR, Singleton DL: Radionuclides in grey seals. Mar Pollut Bull 21:343–345, 1990.
6. Béland P, DeGuise S, Girard C, Lagacé A, et al: Toxic compounds and health and reproductive effects in St. Lawrence beluga whales. J Great Lakes Res 19:766–775, 1993.
7. Bergman Å, Olsson M: Pathology of Baltic grey seal and ringed seal females with special reference to adrenocortical hyperplasia: Is environmental pollution the cause of a widely distributed disease syndrome? Finn Game Res 44:47–62, 1985.
8. Blomkvist G, Roos A, Jensen S, et al: Concentrations of sDDT and PCB in seals from Swedish and Scottish waters. Ambio 21:539–545, 1992.
9. Boon JP, Oostingh I, van der Meer J, et al: A model for the bioaccumulation of chlorobiphenyl congeners in marine mammals. Eur J Pharmacol, Environ Toxicol Pharmacol Section 270:237–251, 1994.
10. Calmet, D, Woodhead D, André JM: ^{210}Pb, ^{137}Cs and ^{40}K in three species of porpoises caught in the eastern tropical Pacific Ocean. J Environ Radioact 15:153–169, 1992.
11. De Gange AR, Vacca MM: Sea otter mortality at Kodiak Island, Alaska, during summer 1987. J Mamm 70:836–838, 1989.
12. De Swart RL, Ross PS, Vos JG, et al: Impaired immunity in harbour seals (*Phoca vitulina*) exposed to bioaccumulated environmental contaminants: review of a long-term feeding study. Environ Health Perspect 104(suppl 4):823–828, 1996.
13. Geraci JR, Lounsbury VJ: Marine mammals ashore: a field guide for strandings. Galveston, TX, Texas A&M SEA Grant Publication, 1993.
14. Geraci JR, St. Aubin DJ (eds): Sea Mammals and Oil: Confronting the Risks. San Diego, Academic Press, 1990.
15. Geraci JR, Williams TD: Physiologic and toxic effects on sea otters. *In* Geraci JR, St. Aubin DJ (eds): Sea Mammals and Oil: Confronting the Risks. San Diego, Academic Press, pp 211–221, 1990.
16. Geraci JR, Anderson DM, Timperi RJ, et al: Humpback whales (*Megaptera novaeangliae*) fatally poisoned by dinoflagellate toxin. Can J Fish Aquat Sci 46:1895–1898, 1989.
17. Goyer RA: Toxic effects of metals. *In* Klaassen CD (ed): Casarett and Doull's Toxicology, The Basic Science of Poisons, 5th ed. New York, McGraw-Hill, pp 691–736, 1996.
18. Hall A, Pomeroy P, Green NK, et al: Infection, haematology and biochemistry in grey seal pups exposed to chlorinated biphenyls. Mar Environ Res 43:81–98, 1997.
19. Hall AJ, Law RJ, Wells DE, et al: Organochlorine levels in common seals (*Phoca vitulina*) which were victims and survivors of the 1988 phocine distemper epizootic. Sci Total Environ 115:145–162, 1992.
20. Harder TC, Willhaus T, Leibold W, et al: Investigations on course and outcome of phocine distemper virus infection in harbor seals (*Phoca vitulina*) exposed to polychlorinated biphenyls. J Vet Med B39:19–31, 1992.
21. Kemper C, Gibbs P, Obendorf D, et al: A review of heavy metal and organochlorine levels in marine mammals in Australia. Sci Total Environ 154:129–139, 1994.
22. Kuiken T, Höfle U, Bennett PM, et al: Adrenocortical hyperplasia, disease and chlorinated hydrocarbons in the harbour porpoise (*Phocoena phocoena*). Mar Pollut Bull 26:440–446, 1993.
23. Kuiken T, Bennett PM, Allchin CR, et al: PCB's, cause of death and body condition in harbour porpoises (*Phocoena phocoena*) from British waters. Aquat Toxicol 28:13–28, 1994.
24. Law RJ, Whinnett JA: Polycyclic aromatic hydrocarbons in muscle tissue of harbour porpoises (*Phocoena phocoena*) from UK waters. Mar Pollut Bull 24:550–553, 1992.
25. Loughlin TR (ed): Marine Mammals and the Exxon Valdez. San Diego, Academic Press, 1994.
26. Martineau D, DeGuise S, Fournier M, et al: Pathology and toxicology of beluga whales from the St. Lawrence estuary, Quebec, Canada. Past, present and future. Sci Total Environ 154:201–215, 1994.
27. Matsumura F: Toxicology of Insecticides, 2nd ed. New York, Plenum Press, 1985.

28. Mortensen P, Bergman A, Bignert A, et al: Prevalence of skull lesions in harbor seals (*Phoca vitulina*) in Swedish and Danish museum collections: 1835–1988. Ambio 21:520–524, 1992.
29. Neff JM: Composition and fate of petroleum and spill-treating agents in the marine environment. *In* Geraci JR, St. Aubin DJ (eds): Sea Mammals and Oil: Confronting the Risks. San Diego, Academic Press, pp 1–13, 1990.
30. Norstrom RJ, Muir DCG: Chlorinated hydrocarbon contaminants in arctic marine mammals. Sci Total Environ 154:107–128, 1994.
31. Norstrom RJ, Simon M, Muir DCG, et al: Organochlorine contaminants in arctic marine food chains: identification, geographical distribution and temporal trends in polar bears. Envir Sci Tech 22:1063–1071, 1988.
32. O'Shea TJ: Environmental contaminants and marine mammals. *In* Reynolds JE III, Twiss JR Jr (eds): Biology of Marine Mammals. Washington DC, Smithsonian Institution Press, in press.
33. O'Shea TJ, Brownell RL: Organochlorine and metal contaminants in baleen whales: a review and evaluation of conservation implications. Sci Total Environ 154:179–200, 1994.
34. O'Shea TJ, Rathbun GB, Bonde RK, et al: An epizootic of Florida manatees associated with a dinoflagellate bloom. Mar Mam Sci 7:165–179, 1991.
35. Rawson AJ, Anderson HF, Patton GW, et al: Anthracosis in the Atlantic bottlenose dolphin (*Tursiops truncatus*). Mar Mam Sci 7:413–416, 1991.
36. Reijnders PJH: Reproductive failure in common seals feeding on fish from polluted coastal waters. Nature 324:456–457, 1986.
37. Reijnders PJH: Toxicokinetics of chlorobiphenyls and associated physiological responses in marine mammals, with particular reference to their potential for ecotoxicological risk assessment. Sci Total Environ 154:229–236, 1994.
38. Ross P, DeSwart R, Addison R, et al: Contaminant-induced immunotoxicity in harbor seals: wildlife at risk? Toxicology 112:157–169, 1996.
39. Safe SH: Polychlorinated biphenyls (PCBs): environmental impact, biochemical and toxic responses, and implications for risk assessment. Crit Rev Toxicol 24:87–149, 1994.
40. Steidinger KA, Baden DG: Toxic marine dinoflagellates. *In* Spector DL (ed): Dinoflagellates. New York, Academic Press, pp 201–261, 1984.

CHAPTER 67

Diagnosis and Treatment of Fungal Infections in Marine Mammals

THOMAS H. REIDARSON

JAMES F. McBAIN

LESLIE M. DALTON

MICHAEL G. RINALDI

Relatively little is known concerning fungal infections in marine mammals. Since the early work by Sweeney and associates[43] that brought to light the existence of many previously undescribed fungal infections, development of new therapeutic agents has soared while the ability to make timely antemortem diagnoses has lagged. For this reason, clinicians face an immense challenge in determining the significance of a yeast or mold isolate from a clinically normal or sick animal. This chapter discusses the diagnostic challenges faced by clinicians and current therapeutic modalities.

FUNGAL DISEASES

The most common pathogenic fungi belong to an artificial taxon called the Fungi Imperfecti (asexual fungi), which includes *Aspergillus, Blastomyces, Candida, Cryptococcus, Coccidioides,* and *Histoplasma* and the class Zygomycetes (which includes *Apophysomyces, Cunninghamella, Mucor, Rhizopus,* and *Saksenaea*) as well as an unclassified fungus called *Loboa loboi,* perhaps related to *Blastomyces. Aspergillus, Candida, Cryptococcus, Fusarium,* and the Zygomycetes are opportunistic pathogens, whereas the other endemic pathogens (*Blastomyces, Coccidioides,* and *Histoplasma*) are capable of infecting healthy hosts.[39]

In humans and animals, mycoses represent only a small but often critically significant fraction of infectious diseases.[29] Table 67–1 is a compilation of fungal infections in captive and wild marine mammals examined by 79 veterinary clinicians and pathologists. In the 143 animals, 19 species of fungi were noted in 24 species of marine mammals. Forty-eight percent were stranded animals, of which 65% had an underlying illness, whereas the remaining 52% were residents of various oceanaria. Of the latter, 42% had some type of pre-existing disease, 52% were apparently healthy, and 6% percent were neonates.

TABLE 67–1. Fungal Infections in Marine Mammals

Opportunistic Fungi*	Lesion	Diagnostic Method†	Treatment/Comment	Reference
Candida albicans				
Orcinus orca	Skin, kidneys, lungs, and myocardium	Histopathology and culture	Necropsy	14
Phoca vitulina and *Callorhinus ursinus*	Nail bed and external	Histopathology and culture (3)	Povidone iodine, miconazole, clotrimazole, chlorhexidine	j
Pontoporia blainvillei	Pectoral flipper lesion	Skin scraping and culture	20 mg/kg ketoconazole BID	k
Pseudorca crassidens	Disseminated	Histopathology and culture	Necropsy	f
Tursiops truncatus	Erosive blowhole lesion	Endoscopy, cytology and immunodiffusion (3)	1.1 mg/kg fluconazole (21 days) (2)	b, o
			Desensitization (1)	s
	Tongue, blowhole	Culture and cytology (4)	10 mg/kg flucytosine TID (2 weeks)	r
			10 mg/kg fluconazole TID (2 weeks)	r
			5 mg/kg/day ketoconazole	2, c
	Mouth, bladder, kidneys	Culture and cytology	2.5 mg/kg itraconazole BID and 20 mg/kg flucytosine TID (1 year)	37
	Lung, endobronchial	Bronchoscopy and culture	2.5 mg/kg itraconazole BID (8 mo)	v
			Necropsy (2)	m
Zalophus californianus	Disseminated	Histopathology and culture	1 mg/kg itraconazole BID (2 months) (unsuccessful)	i
Other *Candida* Species				
Kogia breviceps	Blowhole lesion	Culture and cytology (*Candida parapsilosis*)	1 mg/kg fluconazole SID (1 month)	x
Tursiops truncatus	Brain/cranial sinuses	Histopathology and culture (*Candida rugosa, Candida glabrata*)	2.5 mg/kg itraconazole (11 days)	h
			5.0 mg/kg ketoconazole (12 days) (unsuccessful)	
	Disseminated	Histopathology and culture (*Candida glabrata*)	Necropsy	o, t
	Blowhole lesion	Culture and cytology (*Candida tropicalis*)	1 mg/kg fluconazole SID (1 month)	x
Tursiops truncatus gilli	Lungs, kidneys, bladder	Histopathology and culture (*Candida tropicalis*)	Necropsy	f
Zalophus californianus	Esophageal erosion	Histopathology and culture (*Candida* species)	Necropsy	f
Aspergillus fumigatus				
Arctocephalus gazello	Lungs, pericardium, lymph nodes	Histopathology and culture	Necropsy	k
Callorhinus ursinus	Flipper lesions	Culture	Necropsy	n
Cephalorhynchus commersonii	Lungs	Histopathology and culture	Necropsy	22
Lissodelphis borealis	Lungs	Histopathology and culture	Necropsy	22
Mesoplodon carlhubbsi	Lungs	Histopathology and culture	Necropsy	l
Phoca vitulina	Lungs	Histopathology and culture	Necropsy	t
Orcinus orca	Brain	Histopathology and culture (2)	Necropsy	c, v
	Tongue and lungs	Histopathology and culture	1.25 mg/kg itraconazole BID (2 weeks) (unsuccessful)	v
	Vertebral bone marrow	Biopsy with histopathology and culture	Not treated	y
Stenella coeruleoalba	Lungs and brain	Histopathology and culture (3)	Necropsy (morbillivirus positive)	9
Tursiops truncatus	Lung and endobronchial lesions	Bronchoscopy, culture, and immunodiffusion serology (3)	2.5 mg/kg itraconazole BID (approx 1 year)	e, s, 36
		Histopathology and culture (3)	Necropsy	4, 22, c
	Brain, lung, and alimentary	Histopathology and culture (3)	Necropsy	t, z
	Lungs	Histopathology and culture (29)	Necropsy	m, o, t

Table continued on following page

TABLE 67–1. Fungal Infections in Marine Mammals *Continued*

Opportunistic Fungi*	Lesion	Diagnostic Method†	Treatment/Comment	Reference
Cryptococcus neoformans				
Enhydra lutris	Lungs	Histopathology and culture	Necropsy	p
Lagenorhynchus obliquidens	Lungs, lymph nodes, spleen	Histopathology and culture	Necropsy	p
Tursiops truncatus	Lungs	Histopathology and culture	Necropsy	p
Cladophialophora bantiana				
Phocoena phocoena	Brain	Histopathology and culture	Necropsy	l
Zygomycetes				
Apophysomyces elegans				
Tursiops truncatus	Disseminated	Bronchoscopy and culture (2)	15–18 mg/kg cumulative dose Amphocil IV (12–24 days) (unsuccessful)	47
Lagenorhynchus obliquidens	Disseminated	Histopathology and culture	2.5 mg/kg itraconazole (6 days) (unsuccessful)	h
Lagenorhynchus acutus	Brain	Histopathology and culture	Necropsy	t
Saksenaea vasiformis				
Orcinus orca	Lung, uterus, and brain	Histopathology and culture	1 mg/kg itraconazole BID (3 days) (unsuccessful)	h
Other Zygomycetes				
Cystophora cristata	Disseminated	Histopathology and culture	Necropsy	c
Kogia breviceps	Pyloric stomach and local lymph nodes	Histopathology and culture	Necropsy	c
Lagenorhynchus obliquidens	Disseminated	Histopathology and culture	2.5 mg/kg itraconazole BID (4 days) (unsuccessful)	h
Orcinus orca	Brain	Histopathology and culture (2)	Necropsy	c
Phocoenoides dalli	Disseminated	Histopathology and culture	Necropsy	l
	Disseminated	Histopathology and culture	Necropsy	cc
Tursiops truncatus	Colon and mesenteric lymph nodes	Histopathology and culture	Necropsy	h
	Disseminated	Histopathology and culture (7)	Necropsy	o, z
	Hilar lymph node	Histopathology and culture	Necropsy	o
	Lungs, mandible	Biopsy and culture	2 mg/kg Amphotec IV for 2 separate treatments (unsuccessful)	aa
	Brain	Histopathology and culture (*Paecilomyces lilacinus*)	2.5 mg/kg itraconazole (9 months) (unsuccessful)	l, u
Fusarium Species				
Kogia breviceps	Skin	Histopathology and culture	Necropsy	12
Lagenorhynchus acutus	Skin	Histopathology and culture	5 mg/kg ketoconazole SID (10 days)	12
Mirounga angustirostris	All mucocutaneous junctions	Skin scraping and culture	0.5 mg/kg fluconazole BID (3 wks)	n
Phoca vitulina	Nail bed	Culture	1 mg/kg/day itraconazole (4 months)	a
	Diffuse cutaneous	Histopathology and culture	Necropsy	12
Endemic Fungi				
Blastomyces dermatitidis				
Tursiops truncatus	Disseminated	Histopathology and culture	Necropsy	5
Zalophus californianus	Disseminated	Histopathology and culture	Necropsy	q
Coccidioides immitis				
Enhydra lutris	Disseminated	Histopathology, culture, and serology (7)	Necropsy	bb, p, 46
Tursiops gilli	Disseminated	Histopathology, culture, and serology	Necropsy	v
Zalophus californianus	Lung, liver, pulmonary lymph nodes	Histopathology and culture (9)	Necropsy	11, 33, bb

TABLE 67–1. Fungal Infections in Marine Mammals *Continued*

Opportunistic Fungi*	Lesion	Diagnostic Method†	Treatment/Comment	Reference
Histoplasma capsulatum				
Tursiops truncatus gilli	Disseminated	Histopathology and culture (2)	Necropsy	c, o
Pagophilus groenlandicus	Disseminated	Histopathology and culture	Necropsy	50
Phoca groenlandica	Lung and skin	Histopathology	Necropsy	t
Pseudorca crassidens	Lung	Histopathology and culture	Necropsy	m
Loboa loboi				
Sotalia guianensis	Cutaneous	Histopathology	Necropsy	8
Tursiops truncatus	Cutaneous (melon, pectoral flipper, or disseminated)	Histopathology and electron microscopy (10)	10–16 mg/kg/day ketoconazole	2, 3, 10
			0.5 mg/kg fluconazole BID	27, 31
			1.0 mg/kg miconazole	44, c, g
			2.5 mg/kg itraconazole BID	o, w

*Non-boldface entries are the taxonomic names of the mammals that are the targets of these fungi.
†Number of animals is given in parentheses.

a. Abt D, personal communication, 1996.
b. Bigg M, personal communication, 1996.
c. Bossart G, Ewing R, personal communication, 1996.
d. Buck J, personal communication, 1996.
e. Calle P, personal communication, 1996.
f. Chen R, personal communication, 1996.
g. Cowan D, personal communication, 1996.
h. Dalton L, personal communication, 1996.
i. Dover S, personal communication, 1996.
j. Dunn L, personal communication, 1996.
k. Eyras L, personal communication, 1996.
l. Gage L, Lowenstein L, personal communication, 1996.
m. Greenwood A, Taylor D, personal communication, 1996.
n. Gulland F, personal communication, 1996.
o. Jensen E, Linnehan R, Miller G, Ridgway S, Van Bon B, personal communication, 1996.

p. Joseph B, personal communication, 1996.
q. Kapustin N, personal communication, 1996.
r. Katsumata E, personal communication, 1996.
s. Lacave G, personal communication, 1996.
t. Lipscomb T, personal communication, 1996.
u. Mathey S, personal communication, 1996.
v. McBain J, Reidarson T, personal communication, 1996.
w. Schroeder P, personal communication, 1996.
x. Stamper A, Whitaker B, personal communication, 1996.
y. Sweeney JC, personal communication, 1996.
z. Townsend F, personal communication, 1996.
aa. Walsh M, personal communication, 1996.
bb. Williams T, personal communication, 1996.
cc. Young S, personal communication, 1996.

MODES OF TRANSMISSION

Each of the fungi, except *Candida* species and *L. loboi*, is ubiquitous in certain environments. They grow as saprobes, producing mycelia and/or conidia, or they exist as yeasts constituting a part of the normal microbiota or in stool (in the case of *Cryptococcus neoformans*), which are pathogenic forms capable of producing infection. These fungi gain entry into the hosts by inhalation, trauma, or ingestion and then settle into the lungs, skin, or alimentary tract.[28] *Candida* species are the only normal fungal residents of mucous membranes, and, as such, are the only true endogenous pathogens. Buck (Buck J, personal communication, 1996) discovered *Candida albicans* and other *Candida* species in 4% to 54% of wild bottlenose dolphins (*Tursiops truncatus*) examined in Sarasota Bay from 1990 to 1992. This is comparable with what is observed in many cetaceans living in modern oceanaria.

Because fungi are poorly communicable between animals, mycoses are often endemic and rarely epidemic.[39] Except for two reported zoonotic cases involving *Blastomyces dermatitidis* and *L. loboi* in bottlenose dolphins and an Amazon dolphin,[8] infection of a host by a fungus is generally dead-end and is not contagious to other hosts or capable of becoming widespread in the species.[13, 29]

MECHANISMS OF PATHOGENESIS

After invading the alveoli of the host, the conidia of the endemic fungi (*Blastomyces, Coccidioides,* and *Histoplasma*) transform into a parasitic form and stimulate local humoral and cellular immune responses that lead to granuloma formation, caseation, fibrosis, and ultimately calcification.[48] Most infections are self-limiting and produce minimal clinical signs; however, some become blood borne and disseminate.

For a normal host, the skin and mucosa are effective barriers against invasive *Candida* organisms; however, when the barriers are broken and/or the host's defense mechanisms are impaired, local invasion and fungemia may occur. *Candida* may infect any organ; the kidneys, central nervous system, and heart valves are the most common sites of systemic invasion.[29]

Because many animals have resident *Candida* microflora, the discovery of fungus in blowhole, stomach, or stool samples may cause some confusion. Unless a thorough cytologic examination reveals evidence of local invasion (i.e., presence of budding yeast cells, pseudohyphae, and/or true hyphal elements and the presence of inflammatory cells), the fungus should be labeled a resident or contaminant, entering by way of an aerosol or accidentally being introduced at the diagnostic laboratory[21] (see Clinical Diagnostics).

Of those caused by opportunistic fungi, zygomycetous and *Aspergillus* infections are the most devastating. Zygomycetous infections begin with entry of spores through wounds or by inhalation. The spores then rapidly proliferate and aggressively invade skin or bronchial tissue causing infarction. Dissemination may occur to nearly all internal organs, followed by rapid death. In contrast, there are several forms of aspergillosis: allergic aspergillosis, chronic necrotizing aspergillosis, aspergillar fungal balls (aspergillomas), and invasive aspergillosis.[15] The first three are chronic debilitating forms, whereas the latter acts similarly to invasive zygomycosis. Finding *Aspergillus* or a zygomycete in a culture from a respiratory mucous membrane may be cause for concern. Unless there is a high clinical index of suspicion for invasion, the fungus should be considered saprobic.

Other less common diseases are caused by *Cryptococcus neoformans*, *Fusarium* species, and *L. loboi*. Cryptococcal organisms settle in the lungs, producing localized fungal balls (cryptococcomas) and occasionally extrapulmonary dissemination to the brain and meninges. *Fusarium* species are soil and plant saprobes that are capable of infecting damaged or devitalized skin, primarily causing skin disease; however, when disseminated infection occurs, mortality rates are particularly high.[23] Lobomycosis is a chronic, localized disease of the skin caused by infection with the yeast-like organism *L. loboi*. The organism has never been successfully cultured, and systemic spread has never been demonstrated.

CLINICAL FEATURES

Clinical presentations of mycotic diseases are frustratingly nonspecific, ranging from chronic to fulminating, just as with bacterial or viral disease. Fungi can affect any tissue, so unless the fungus can be identified, the origin of the disease may remain unknown.

A thorough history focusing on types and extent of previous illnesses and response to past and present treatments may give clues to the identity of the fungus. A disease that initially appears responsive to antibiotics and then apparently becomes unresponsive could be evidence of a change to a fungal etiology.

The only unique presentations are lobomycosis, which produces multifocal white crusts involving large areas of skin, and central nervous system mycoses in which animals have rapidly escalating abnormal neurologic clinical signs.

CLINICAL DIAGNOSTICS

Laboratory findings from individuals with opportunistic fungal infections often produce hematologic and biochemical changes indistinguishable from bacterial or viral infections.[7, 22, 25] An example is the individual with initial stages of zygomycosis in which laboratory findings are unremarkable until the latter stages of disease, at which time all muscle- and liver-specific enzymes escalate rapidly because of tissue infarction. On the other hand, individuals with endemic infections generally have bloodwork indicative of chronic granulomatous diseases showing persistent leukocytosis, monocytosis, eosinophilia, and hyperproteinemia with hypergammaglobulinemia; however, these features may be inconsistent.[17]

Radiography, ultrasonography, and endoscopy aid in localizing lesions.[17, 18, 26, 34, 36] The practice of culturing nasal, gastric, and stool samples has limited usefulness. In cetaceans, there appears to be very low correlation between pneumonia-causing organisms and the organisms isolated from the blowholes of the same animals. In humans, there appears to be a high correlation between bronchoalveolar lavage (BAL) isolates and pneumonia-causing organisms (J. Harrell, personal communication, 1996). Preliminary evidence suggests that the same correlation exists in dolphins. In fact, for most pulmonary mycoses listed in Table 67–1, the pathogen discovered at necropsy was not identified in antemortem blowhole samples. Therefore, BAL provides more accurate assessment of lower pulmonary disease.

Biopsy, aspiration, scrapings, and BAL are definitive diagnostic procedures. For biopsies, it is recommended to fix one piece for histopathologic study and to place another directly on the selective media (e.g., Sabouraud dextrose agar), because certain fungi, especially the Zygomycetes, may be difficult to grow from a culturette swab only and may be rendered nonviable if the tissue is ground before plating out on microbiologic media. A method for concentrating small numbers of fungi in blood, called sponin lysis and centrifugation, is the quickest procedure available with the greatest yield.[6] A negative culture does not preclude infection, as only 50% to 80% of blood cultures from proven cases of invasive candidiasis are positive. Molds are almost never recovered from blood, even in rapidly progressive, fulminating, terminal diseases.

Although serodiagnostic tests for systemic fungal diseases in humans and animals have improved over the years, most only help to corroborate physical and other diagnostic assessments. The tests with the greatest diagnostic potential are immunodiffusion, complement fixation, antigen titers, and detection of metabolic byproducts.

Immunodiffusion (ID) assays detect circulating antibodies, which are helpful in assessing exposure to a fungus. Qualitative ID measures the presence of different antibody classes (either IgM or IgG) and is reported by the number of antibody-antigen bands in a gel (or bands of identity). Quantitative tests determine the antibody titer for a specific fungal antigen. Qualitative tests may be useful with candidiasis and aspergillosis in which a change in bands of identity, from zero to one or more, is indicative of active infection, although not all investigators feel that such tests are useful. Quantitative immunodiffusion is most useful in coccidioidomycosis, in which a fourfold increase in titer over 30 days indicates an active infection and a titer of greater than 1:128 is associated with extrapulmonary dissemination.[6]

There has been considerable progress in the development of antigen-specific tests for fungal infections. The tests with the greatest potential to detect systemic candidiasis are the ones that identify metabolic by-products or secreted cell wall constituents. These materials are secreted in minute concentrations and unpredictably, however, so the tests are very unreliable.[21] In contrast, tests for wall constituents have been developed for *Histoplasma* and *Blastomyces*.[6, 40]

There are no reliable serologic tests for zygomycosis. Latex agglutination (LA) tests for cryptococcus organisms and an enzyme-linked immunosorbent assay (ELISA) antigen detection test for histoplasmosis have proven especially useful, reproducible, and accurate.[23, 49] With the exception of the cryptococcal LA test, the ELISA antigen method for histoplasmosis, and the diagnostically and prognostically useful serologic tests for coccidioidomycosis, use of serology for diagnosis of mycoses is generally dismal.

THERAPEUTICS (Table 67–2)

Various antifungal drugs have been used to treat fungal infections in marine animals. The azoles (fluconazole, Diflucan, Pfizer; itraconazole, Sporanox, Janssen Pharmaceutica; ketoconazole, Nizoral, Janssen Pharmaceutica), a microencapsulated colloidal dispersion of amphotericin B (Amphotec, Sequus Pharmaceutical, Inc.), flucytosine (Ancobon, Hoffman-LaRoche), and the combination of itraconazole and flucytosine have been used with variable success.[1, 38] Because fluconazole is water soluble and excreted in urine, it may be used in cases of renal or urinary candidiasis as well as systemic disease. Although itraconazole is effective for candidiasis, it has been directed mainly to treat *Aspergillus* infections.[42] To date, both itraconazole and the microencapsulated amphotericin B products have shown limited—but in some instances, encouraging—efficacy against Zygomycetes in humans and marine mammals.[19, 47] Experience with intravenously administered

antifungal drugs (polyenes and their lipid formulations as well as the IV form of fluconazole) is limited because of technical difficulties with administration in marine mammals.

Because itraconazole is lipophilic, tissue levels are generally higher than blood levels. Because of slow release of itraconazole, significant blood levels can persist for weeks in marine mammals after discontinuing therapy. The levels and length of release appear to be dependent on amount of blubber; however, there is some individual variation (Dalton and McBain, unpublished data). Inappetence occasionally occurs with the administration of either ketoconazole or itraconazole. Because ketoconazole appears to inhibit glucocorticoid production, it is recommended to supplement with 0.01 mg/kg of prednisolone. For itraconazole, reducing the dose generally reverses the inappetence.

Each of the azoles (although not generally an issue with fluconazole) is capable of producing 2- to 25-fold elevations of the liver-associated enzymes, asparate and alanine transaminases, and lactate dehydrogenase (LDH).[38] The patterns of LDH isoenzyme production help distinguish between enzyme induction resulting from azole administration and liver pathology. There appears to be no liver associated with itraconazole and fluconazole, in contrast to ketoconazole.[38] Furthermore, as long as drug levels persist, enzyme levels also remain elevated.

Our experience in the treatment of invasive mycoses in marine mammals has shown that fungal infections often persist if only the paradigms outlined in the medical literature are followed. Treatment must be extended beyond the apparent elimination of the fungal infection, which can be determined only by clinical reassessment of each animal. Clinical signs, cultures, and follow-up diagnostic tests assist in making the most informed decision concerning the discontinuance of therapy. Treatment of invasive fungal infections must continue past an apparent cure as indicated by a clinical, radiologic, or endoscopic disease-free state. For individuals on combination therapy containing flucytosine, both medications should be withdrawn simultaneously to prevent development of resistance. This phenomenon is

TABLE 67–2. Formulary of Antimycotic Drugs (mg/kg)

Drug	Oo	Tt	Cc	Gm	Dl	Ord	Other Pinnipeds*
Lipid formulation amphotericin B (Amphotec/ APLC)	ND	1.0–2.0 SID 2.5 g cumulative dose)	ND	ND	ND	ND	ND
Flucytosine	ND	20 TID	ND	ND	ND	ND	ND
Fluconazole	ND	2.0 BID	ND	ND	ND	ND	0.5 BID
Itraconazole	1.25 BID	2.5–5.0 BID	5.0 BID	1.25 BID	2.5 BID	1.5–2.0 SID	0.5–1.0 BID
Ketoconazole†	ND	5.0 BID	ND	ND	1.9 BID	4.4 BID	1.0 BID

*Elephant seal (*Mirounga angustirostris*), harbor seal (*Phoca vitulina*), California sea lion (*Zalophus californianus*).

†Used with low-dose prednisolone (0.01 mg/kg SID).

Oo, *Orcinus orca*, killer whale; Tt, *Tursiops truncatus*, bottlenosed dolphin; Cc, *Cephalorhynchus commersonii*, Commerson's dolphin; Gm, *Globicephala macrorhynchus*, short-finned pilot whale; Dl, *Delphinapterus leucas*, beluga whale; Ord, *Odobenus r. divergens*, walrus; ND, not done.

best illustrated with azoles and flucytosine wherein the withdrawal of the azole may lead to resistance to flucytosine.[31] Flucytosine is never used as monotherapy, because of rapid engenderment of resistance.

CONCLUSION

Most fungal infections share clinical, hematologic, and biochemical aspects of bacterial and viral infections. Clinical presentations are frustratingly nonspecific, ranging from chronic to fulminating, while laboratory findings demonstrate acute or chronic inflammation, just as with bacterial or viral diseases. Although serodiagnostic tests for systemic fungi have improved, most only help to corroborate physical and other diagnostic assessments. It is for this reason that biopsy and culture are the most definitive methods for diagnosing fungal infections, except for infection with *L. loboi,* which has never been successfully cultured.

A number of new antimycotic drugs have been introduced. These include itraconazole and fluconazole, which appear to be somewhat effective against *Aspergillus, Candida,* and the endemic fungi, and the microencapsulated lipid-bound amphotericin B products that have limited efficacy against zygomycosis. For all fungal infections, long-term therapy is necessary for a successful outcome.

Diagnostic modalities have greatly lagged behind therapeutics; however, with improvements in serodiagnostic tests for metabolic by-products and cell wall constituents as well as emerging methods involving molecular biologic techniques, the ability to make timely antemortem diagnoses should greatly improve.

Acknowledgment

This is Sea World technical contribution No. 9701-C.

REFERENCES

1. Allendoerfer R, Marquis AJ, Rinaldi MG, Graybill JR: Combined therapy with fluconazole and flucytosine in murine cryptococcal meningitis. Antimicrob Agents Chemother 35:726, 1991.
2. Bossart GD: Suspected acquired immunodeficiency in an Atlantic bottlenose dolphin with chronic-active hepatitis and lobomycosis. J Am Med Assoc 185:1413, 1984.
3. Caldwell DK, Caldwell MC, et al: Lobomycosis as a disease of the Atlantic bottlenosed dolphin, *Tursiops truncatus,* Montague (1821). Am J Trop Med Hyg 24:105, 1975.
4. Carrol JM, Jasmin AM, Caucom JN: Pulmonary aspergillosis of the bottlenose dolphin (*Tursiops truncatus*). Am J Vet Clin Pathol 2:139, 1968.
5. Cates MB, L Kaufman JH, Pletcher J, Schroeder JP: Blastomycosis in an Atlantic bottlenose dolphin. J Am Vet Med Assoc 189:1148, 1986.
6. Christin L, Sugar AM: Endemic fungal infections in patients with cancer. Infect Med 13:673, 1996.
7. Coleman JM, Hogg GG, Rosenfeld JV, Waters KD: Invasive central nervous system aspergillosis: cure with liposomal amphotericin B, itraconazole, and radical surgery—case report and review of the literature. Neurosurgery 36:858, 1995.
8. de Vries GA, Laarman JJ: A case of Lobo's disease in the dolphin *Sotalia guianensis.* Aquatic Mammals 1:28, 1973.
9. Domingo M, Visa J, Pumarola M, et al: Pathologic and immunocytochemical studies of morbillivirus infection in striped dolphins (*Stenella coeruleoalba*). Vet Pathol 29:1, 1992.

10. Dudok WH: Successful treatment in a case of lobomycosis (Lobo's disease) in *Tursiops truncatus* (mont.) at the Dolfinarium, Harderwijk. Aquatic Mammals 5:8, 1977.
11. Fauguier DA, Gulland FM, et al: Coccidioidomycosis in freeliving California sea lions (*Zalophus californianus*) in central California. J Wildl Dis 32(4):707, 1996.
12. Frasca J, Dunn JL, Cooke JC, Buck JD: Mycotic dermatitis in an Atlantic white-sided dolphin, a pygmy sperm whale, and two harbor seals. J Am Vet Med Assoc 208:727, 1996.
13. Geraci JR, Ridgway SH: On disease transmission between cetaceans and humans. Marine Mammal Science 7(2):191, 1991.
14. Griner LA: Cardiac candidiasis in a captive killer whale. Erkrankungen der Zootiere. 34. Internationalen Symposiums uber die Erkrankungen der Zoo-und Wildtiere, Santander, Spain, p 159, 1992.
15. Haque AK: Pathology of common pulmonary fungal infections. J Thorac Imaging 7:1, 1992.
16. Harley WB, Blaser MJ: Disseminated coccidioidomycosis associated with extreme eosinophilia. Clin Infect Dis 18:627, 1994.
17. Harrell JH, Reidarson TH, McBain J, Sheetz H: Bronchoscopy of the bottlenose dolphin. IAAAM Proceedings 27:33, 1996.
18. Hawkins EC, Townsend FI, Lewbart GA, et al: Bronchoalveolar lavage in a stranded bottlenose dolphin. IAAAM Proceedings 27:124, 1996.
19. Herbrecht R: The changing epidemiology of fungal infections: are the lipid forms of amphotericin B an advance? Eur J Haematol 57:12, 1996.
20. Jeraj KP, Sweeney JC: Blowhole cytology to diagnose early respiratory tract disease in bottlenose dolphins. IAAAM Proceedings 27:112, 1996.
21. Jones JM: Laboratory diagnosis of invasive candidiasis. Clin Microbiol Rev 3:32, 1990.
22. Joseph BE, Cornell LH, Simpson JG, et al: Pulmonary aspergillosis in three species of dolphin. Zoo Biology 5:301, 1986.
23. Kwon-Chung KJ, Bennett JE: Medical Mycology. Philadelphia, Lea & Febiger, pp 424–425, 1992.
24. Magaki G, Gunnels RD, Casey CW: Pulmonary cryptococcosis in an Atlantic bottlenose dolphin (*Tursiops truncatus*). Lab Anim Sci 28:603, 1978.
25. Magnussen CR: Disseminated *Candida* infection: diagnostic clues, therapeutic options. J Critical Illness 7:513, 1992.
26. McAdams HP, Rosado-de-Christenson M, Templeton PA, et al: Thoracic mycoses from opportunistic fungi: radiologic-pathologic correlation. Radiographics 15:271, 1995.
27. Migaki G, Valerio MG, et al: Lobo's disease in an Atlantic bottlenose dolphin. J Am Vet Med Assoc 159:578, 1971.
28. Muller J: Epidemiology of deep-seated, domestic mycoses. Mycoses 37(suppl 2):1, 1994.
29. Nicholls JM, Yuen KY, Tam AYC: Systemic fungal infections in neonates. J Hosp Med 49:420, 1993.
30. Nguyen MH, Peacock JE, Morris AJ, et al: The changing face of candidemia: emergence of non–*Candida albicans* species and antifungal resistance. Am J Med 100:617, 1996.
31. Poelma FG, de Vries GA, Blythe-Russell EA, Luykx HF: Lobomycosis in an Atlantic bottlenosed dolphin in the dolphinarium Harderwijk. Aquatic Mammals 2:11, 1974.
32. Presterl D, Graninger W: Efficacy and safety of fluconazole in the treatment of systemic fungal infections in pediatric patients. Multicentre study group. Eur J Clin Microbiol Infect Dis 13:347, 1994.
33. Reed RE, Migaki G, Cummings JA: Coccidioidomycosis in a California sea lion (*Zalophus californianus*). J Wildl Dis 12:372, 1972.
34. Reef VB: Ultrasonographic evaluation. *In* Beech J (ed): Equine Respiratory Diseases. Philadelphia, Lea & Febiger, pp 69–88, 1991.
35. Reidarson TH, Griner L, McBain J: Coccidioidomycosis in a bottlenose dolphin (*Tursiops gilli*). J Wildl Dis, in press.
36. Reidarson TH, McBain J, Harrell JH: The use of bronchoscopy and fungal serology to diagnose *Aspergillus fumigatus* lung infection in a bottlenose dolphin (*Tursiops truncatus*). IAAAM Proceedings 27:34, 1996.
37. Reidarson TH, McBain J: The combined use of itraconazole and flucytosine in the treatment of chronic *Candida* cystitis in a bottlenose dolphin (*Tursiops truncatus*). IAAAM Proceedings 26:13, 1995.
38. Reidarson TH, McBain J: The use of LDH isoenzymes to differentiate three medical conditions in cetaceans. IAAAM Proceedings 25:156, 1994.

39. Rippon JW: Medical Mycology. The Pathogenic Fungi and the Pathogenic Actinomycetes, 3rd ed. Philadelphia, WB Saunders, pp 3–4, 1988.
40. Soufleris AJ, Klein BS, Courtney BT, et al: Utility of anti-WI-1 serological testing in the diagnosis of blastomycosis in Wisconsin. N Engl J Med 136:1333, 1995.
41. Sparano JA, Gucalp R, Llena JF, et al: Cerebral infection complicating systemic aspergillosis in acute leukemia. J Neuro-Oncology 13:91, 1992.
42. Stevens DA, Lee JY: Analysis of compassionate use itraconazole therapy for invasive aspergillosis by the NIAID Mycoses Study Group criteria. Arch Intern Med 157:1857, 1997.
43. Sweeney JC, Migaki G, Vainik PM, Conklin RH: Systemic mycoses in marine mammals. J Am Vet Med Assoc 169:946, 1976.
44. Symmers W: A possible case of Lobo's disease acquired in Europe from a bottlenose dolphin (*Tursiops truncatus*). Bulletin de la Societe de Pathologie Exotique 76:777, 1983.
45. Thomas J, Clark G, Dall L, Willsie S: Cavitary cryptococcal pneumonia in a postpartum patient. Infect Med 12:429, 1995.
46. Thomas NJ, Pappagianis D, Creekmore LH, Duncan RM: Coccidioidomycosis in southern sea otters. Centennial Conference on Coccidioidomycosis, University of California, San Diego, p 21, 1994.
47. Townsend FI, Materese FJ, Sips DG: The use of liposomal amphotericin-B in the therapy of systemic zygomycosis. IAAAM Proceedings 27:18, 1996.
48. Walsh TJ, Mitchell TG: Dimorphic fungi causing systemic mycoses. *In* Balows A, Hausler WJ, Herrmann KL, et al (eds): Manual of Clinical Microbiology. Washington, DC, American Society for Microbiology, p 630, 1991.
49. Wheat J: Histoplasmosis in the acquired immunodeficiency syndrome. Curr Topics Med Mycol 7:7, 1996.
50. Wilson TM, Kierstead M, Long JR: Histoplasmosis in a harp seal. J Am Vet Med Assoc 165:815, 1974.

CHAPTER 68

Medical Management of Stranded Small Cetaceans

FORREST I. TOWNSEND

The phenomenon of cetacean stranding and associated issues have been addressed in numerous publications. This chapter is a guide for the medical practitioner who normally treats illness in other species, but who may be called upon to assist when a small cetacean becomes stranded. Some of the common disease conditions that may be encountered sometimes precipitate the stranding, some may result from rescue and rehabilitative efforts, and some are unrelated to the stranding but require medical intervention before the animal can be considered for release.

Live strandings are comparatively infrequent. Consequently, there are few published case histories available to serve as precedents for medical care of these animals. Some of the information in this chapter is anecdotal; much of the information is based on the care and treatment of captive cetaceans. At times, therapeutic regimens must be borrowed or adapted from those used in treating other species. Each event is unique, and medical management must be individualized to meet the demands of each case.

PREPARATION BEFORE STRANDING EVENT

Cetacean species are federally protected under the Marine Mammal Protection Act. The National Marine Fisheries Service issues permits regulating the individuals and institutions that deal with cetaceans, as well as regulating response to, and disposition of, stranded cetaceans.

Legal issues and recommended practices are frequently revised or upgraded. The veterinarian who may be involved with a stranding should keep abreast of current regulations regarding marine mammal species, the reporting of events, data and specimen collection protocols, and release criteria. For further information, see reference 7. An excellent discussion of the organization of a stranding response team and the initial response/rescue protocols can be found in reference 9.

ON-SITE ASSESSMENT

The stranded animal should be kept in the water, if possible, until transportation and equipment are on site and ready. As in all forms of rescue, the safety of the rescuers takes precedence over that of the patient, so rough water, rocky shorelines, inclement weather, sharks, impending darkness, or other conditions that pose hazards to the rescuers must be taken into account when determining when to move the animal.

It is not unusual for volunteers to become caught up in the rescue and, in their enthusiasm, place themselves or others in danger. The medical professional at the scene may be needed to provide leadership, to assess the human risk, and to control and direct the volunteers.

Concerning the animal, it is first assessed for life-threatening injuries as effectively and quickly as possible; species, sex, age (infant, juvenile, adult, older adult), and general body condition are then determined.

Species is important in determining the animal's management. In 1995 to 1996, animals of the following species were stranded alive in the United States: Atlantic bottlenose dolphin (*Tursiops truncatus*), Risso's dolphin (*Grampus griseus*), beluga whale (*Delphinapterus leucas*), pygmy sperm whales (*Kogia breviceps*), dwarf sperm whales (*Kogia simus*), false killer whales (*Pseudorca crassidens*), common dolphin (*Delphinus delphis*), white-sided dolphin (*Lagenorhynchus acutus*), spinner, spotted, and striped dolphins (*Stenella* species), harbor porpoises (*Phocoena phocoena*), pygmy killer whales (*Feresa attenuata*), pilot whales (*Globicephala* species), and rough-toothed dolphins (*Steno bredanensis*) (D. Wilkinson, personal communication, 1996).

Bottlenose dolphin generally survive the stress of handling and transport better than do deep-water species such as *Stenella*. These deep-water cetaceans tend to be more "fragile," especially when handled out of the water, so they should be evaluated and transported in water if possible.

Body condition is a good indicator of the animal's nutritional status. If the animal has not been feeding normally (suggested by apparent weight loss), it is probably dehydrated and needs fluid and electrolyte replacement therapy. The majority of water intake of cetaceans is derived from the water content of their food and the metabolic water generated by digestion and utilization of their food.[12]

As part of the initial assessment of the animal and before handling or transport, the clinician should assess the animal's mental alertness, quality and rate of respiration, and ability to maintain itself in the water (listing, sinking, inability to swim). The animal should be observed for indications of stress (Table 68–1). First arrival stranding personnel may be able to make these assessments and indicate whether the animal's condition

has changed. Often, the veterinarian is not at the stranding site and must rely on the personnel at the scene to perform and report the initial assessments.

TRANSPORT

Cetaceans should be transported head-first. Moving them tail-first can cause or exacerbate confusion and disorientation and increase stress in the animal.

Basically, there are two methods of transport: moist transport and wet transport. In moist transport, the animal is moved on foam mats, in which wet towels or sheeting are used or the animal's skin is sprayed or sponged at frequent intervals to protect the skin and reduce the risk of overheating. In a wet transport, the animal is transported in a water-filled container. Wet transport is preferred for most small cetaceans and is strongly recommended for the transport of deep-water species.

Regardless of the method of transport, the animal should be monitored for signs of overheating. The thermoregulating system of cetaceans is designed for immersion of the body, fins, and flukes in water and does not effectively transfer heat into air, so cetaceans can rapidly overheat. Ice may be used with water to provide cooling, particularly if the trip is long or the weather is hot. During long transport, periodic repositioning of the animal reduces localized overheating and helps to prevent pressure-induced avascular necrosis.

Continued observation of the animal's physical status is recommended. Emergency medications should be available because they may be required en route, and the animal should be positioned on the transport vehicle to facilitate administration of drugs.

HOLDING AREA OR REHABILITATION SITE

It is assumed that a stranded animal is ill. Most single stranded cetaceans have predisposing illnesses. Furthermore, with the discovery of cetaceans infected with morbillivirus throughout all U.S. coastal waters[5, 6] and with the attendant risk of introducing this virus to captive cetaceans, oceanaria have become less willing to accept live-stranded animals into their facilities.[1] Consequently, a sheltered holding enclosure located away from contact with other animals may be required for the short-term medical care of the animals.

In the absence of a dedicated enclosure, there are several criteria in choosing a site for a temporary holding facility. A sheltered lagoon or cove, with convenient road access, is desirable. For small cetaceans, a marine location with a sloping sandy bottom free of rocks and debris and with good tidal flushing, is ideal. The water depth should be 6 foot or less at high tide in locations with minor tidal fluctuations. Where tidal fluctuations are great, the water level should be low enough to allow access to the animal daily. Also, consideration should be given to the appropriate water temperature for the species being rehabilitated.

A holding pen can be constructed of 8- × 10-foot

TABLE 68–1. Indications of Stress in Small Cetaceans

Breath-holding; protracted holding of blowhole open; rapid, shallow, or irregular respiration; prolonged apneic episodes (normal respiratory rate is 1 to 3 per minute)

Loss of normal cardiac sinus arrhythmia (rate should be 50 to 90 beats per minute, increasing with respiration and decreasing slowly until the next inspiration)

Blank, unblinking stare; lack of visual response to movement or sound; reduced or absent palpebral reflexes

Vomiting or retching/gagging motions

Pallor of oral mucous membranes

Trembling or arching of the body, stiffening of the body*

*Arching can be a medical emergency, requiring immediate intervention. The animal should be placed quickly in the water, if possible, and provided physical support as needed. Administration of emergency drugs may help.

panels of PVC pipe to which a small mesh net is tautly lashed. Several of these panels can be tied together to form the desired size of enclosure, and the bases anchored to the bottom. Where feasible, a U-shaped pen, with the open end at the beach, allows convenient access to the animal. Where the panels must be joined to make a complete enclosure, one panel may be linked in such a way as to allow it to function as a gate. Panels of this type have the added advantage that, when they are not in use, they can be stacked and stored. Temporary portable pools have also been used.

Another requirement for the holding site is shelter for personnel and equipment. There must be a temporary or permanent kitchen facility for storage and preparation of food for the animal and availability of communication tools (such as cellular telephones or radios).

INITIAL MEDICAL ASSESSMENT

A more complete medical assessment can be accomplished in the controlled environment of the rehabilitation site. Baseline parameters should include

1. Length, girth, and weight
2. Heart rate (Tachycardia with inspiration is normal. Loss of the normal sinus arrhythmia is clinically significant.)
3. Condition of teeth, mouth, color of mucous membranes
4. External injuries, scars, parasites, skin condition, body condition

In addition, sample collection for the following tests should be performed:

1. A gastric tube should be introduced and a sample of gastric contents collected. The presence of gas, foul odor, obvious blood (either color of coffee grounds or red), and any other abnormal findings should be noted. Depending on the availability of services, the sample may be examined by routine cytopathology for the presence of red blood cells, white blood cells (WBCs), parasites or ova, and bacterial or fungal elements. Routine cultures may be performed. After the samples have been obtained, the initial fluids should be administered.
2. Blood should be drawn as soon as possible after the animal strands. This is most easily accomplished during the initial examination at the holding facility.
3. The blowhole should be swabbed for culture, cytology, or testing for presence of parasites or ova. Because the nature of the nasal passages lends itself to contamination, "blow" swab findings must not be overinterpreted.
4. If the animal's condition permits, it is also desirable to obtain a catheterized urine specimen for urinalysis (bacterial culture if indicated).

The technique for drawing cetacean blood samples is described in reference 14. The following baseline tests should be obtained:

1. Complete blood count (CBC). Dolphins normally exhibit large platelets. Electronic cell counters may read the platelets as WBCs, resulting in erroneous white cell

and platelet counts. If there is any doubt, the clinician should request that the differential and platelet counts be performed manually.
2. Reticulocyte count when anemia is present.
3. Erythrocyte sedimentation rate or, alternatively, fibrinogen level.
4. Chemistry profile and serum iron.
5. Serology. Blood samples should be sent to appropriate laboratories for infectious disease titers such as morbillivirus, herpes virus, hepatitis virus, and parvovirus.

Additional consideration should be given to other tests as warranted (e.g., serum progesterone, cortisol, and blood cultures). Extra serum and plasma should be frozen and retained for future testing.

Following the initial assessment of blood values, daily sampling is desirable for the first few days to monitor hydration and response to medication. After the first few days, assessing blood parameters every third day is adequate to monitor progress. When antibiotic and antifungal drugs are discontinued and the animal is medically stable, weekly checks of blood parameters are recommended.

Additional diagnostic testing can include ultrasonography, radiology, electrocardiography, and flexible endoscopy.

Funding for laboratory and diagnostic services, ease of access to the patient, availability of personnel, and condition of the animal must be considered in determining the types of testing and the frequency with which they are performed.

BEGINNING TREATMENT

Fluid Replacement

Dehydration is a major concern in stranded dolphins. The inability to effectively feed, secondary to illness or injury, drying and injury to the skin, wounds, fever, and reduced renal perfusion secondary to illness or injury may all contribute to dehydration.

While the gastric tube is in place during the initial examination, a 150-kg dolphin should receive 2 to 3 L of water or a mixture of half water and half pediatric electrolyte solution. Fluid administration is facilitated by gravity feeding the fluids into the animal's first gastric compartment. The use of a stomach pump is *not recommended*.

Fluids that are administered too rapidly or in greater volume than the stomach can accommodate may produce vomiting. The animal should be observed for signs of discomfort or nausea during the procedure. Before an animal vomits, it may begin to gag or exhibit exaggerated swallowing motions. If these signs are observed, fluid administration should be slowed; if the signs persist, the tube should be removed.

Electrolyte, hematocrit, and serum protein values should be obtained to evaluate hydration status; fluid volume and frequency of administration should be adjusted accordingly. When the animal begins eating, additional fluid may be given by gastric tube to maintain hydration. Small amounts of supplemental fluids may be provided by injecting food fish with water just before feeding them to the animal.

ANTIBIOTIC THERAPY

Before antibiotic therapy is begun, every effort should be made to identify pathogens and define their sensitivity to specific antibiotics. Observation and early identification of secondary pathogens (both bacterial and fungal) must continue during the course of treatment with any antibiotic.

Prophylactic administration of antibiotics is controversial. One disadvantage of antibiotic therapy is the suppression of normal flora, increasing the potential for overgrowth of opportunistic pathogenic organisms. It is not uncommon, for example, to recover *Candida* species from multiple sites (blow, gastric, feces) after even short-term antibiotic therapy. *Aspergillus* species infection may occur after prolonged use of broad-spectrum antibiotics. Some antibiotics predispose the animal to *Clostridium difficile* infection and even fatal pseudomembranous colitis.

There are equally compelling arguments in favor of prophylactic antibiotic administration. The normal bacteria encountered by ocean-going individuals may vary, both in type and concentration, from those that are encountered in lagoons, estuaries, and stranding pools. Prophylactic antibiotics can decrease the incidence of infection by these organisms. The stressful conditions surrounding stranding and rescue can alter the animal's immunocompetency. The various procedures requiring frequent handling—gastric intubation, urinary catheterization, sling placement for weighing—also increase exposure and susceptibility to bacterial infection.

Skin Protection

Sunburn, windburn, and drying can alter the integrity of the animal's skin, leaving it vulnerable to infection and producing discomfort in an already stressed animal. Materials that coat, soothe, and protect the skin may be needed during transport and in the long-term care of animals unable to swim, and who therefore have at least the blowhole and part of the head exposed for extended periods. Zinc oxide cream, or a 50/50 mixture of zinc oxide cream and A and D ointment with or without the addition of vitamin E oil, may be applied to the exposed skin to protect it from drying and sunburn. Such protective ointments may be reapplied as often as necessary to protect and soothe exposed skin.

Exposed skin surfaces may also be protected by wet sheeting or towels applied to the exposed skin. When this method of skin protection is used, the animal must not be left unattended lest the sheeting slip over the blowhole and asphyxiate the animal. Placing shading material over the pools or using a misting water spray also helps to protect the exposed skin.

Infections involving the skin should be cultured or possibly biopsied and treated with the appropriate antibiotic or antifungal medications.

Gastrointestinal Tract

Small cetaceans appear to have a propensity for development of gastric ulcers. Stranded bottlenose dolphins have a much lower incidence of gastric ulcers when compared with the off-shore species. Stranded animals undergo several stresses that can precipitate or exacerbate gastric ulcers. These ulcers range in severity from mild erosions of the mucosa to fatal perforations of the stomach. The presence of well-healed gastric ulcer scars on necropsy of wild cetaceans indicates that these ulcers may heal spontaneously.

The color of a normal gastric aspirate should be a cloudy white to clear, and gastric aspirates that appear grossly bloody or have a "coffee-grounds" appearance indicate that gastric ulcers are present. This diagnosis may be confirmed using gastric endoscopy, although often only the first gastric compartment may be visualized using gastroscopy, and ulceration may be present in the remaining gastric segments without producing any visible abnormality in the mucosa of the first gastric compartment.

Given the relatively high incidence of gastric ulceration or erosion in stranded cetaceans, a regimen of H_2-blocking agents, such as cimetidine, and coating agents, such as sucralfate, may be used initially as a prophylactic measure. Dosages for these drugs are listed in Table 68–2, although they must be adjusted for the individual.

The pH of gastric samples is useful in monitoring the response to H_2-antagonists. When frequent gastric intubation is necessary, the pH can be checked throughout the day, allowing more precise adjustment of the dosage and frequency of administration of these drugs. In the treatment of ulcer disease in humans, a pH greater than 4.0 is desirable.[3] Levels approaching neutral may interfere with digestion of fish bones, causing them to accumulate in the stomach.

The gastric aspirate should be stained with a nuclear chromatin stain (e.g., new methylene blue) and examined microscopically for WBCs, parasites, and ova. Where available, the aspirate may also be submitted to a cytopathology laboratory for evaluation of the exfoliated epithelial cells. The presence of a few WBCs in the gastric fluid is not significant, but numerous WBCs are important diagnostically, and their source needs to be determined. They can originate from an ulcer or erosion of the upper gastrointestinal tract, have been swallowed from sinus or nasal passages, or been coughed up and swallowed from upper or lower respiratory tract disease processes.

Parasitic ova or larvae are often present in gastric samples from stranded dolphins. The most commonly encountered of these are the ova of *Nasitrema* species. *Nasitrema* are common inhabitants of the sinus cavities of bottlenose dolphins, doing little apparent harm. Their presence in other species (notably *Stenella* species, *Steno* species, and *Kogia* species) is less benign. Eosinophilic meningoencephalitis may result from migration of this parasite to the brain in these species.

Yeast and fungal elements can also be identified in gastric samples, the most common being *Candida* species present in response to, among other causes, broad-spectrum antibiotic therapy. *Aspergillus* species, *Toru-*

TABLE 68–2. Emergency Drugs

Drug	Dosage	Route	Dose*
Diazepam, 5 mg/ml	1.5–0.2 mg/kg	IM	3–4 ml (15–20 mg)
Doxapram, 20 mg/ml	1.0 mg/kg	IM, IV	8–10 ml (160–200 mg)
Prednisolone sodium succinate, 100 mg/vial	1–10 mg/kg	IM, IV	1–2 vials (100–200 mg)
Epinephrine, 1 mg/ml	0.02 mg/kg	IM	2–3 ml (2–3 mg)
Furosemide, 50 mg/ml	2–4 mg/kg	IM	3–6 ml (150–300 mg)

Formulary for Stranded Cetaceans†

Antibiotics		Antimycotics	
Amikacin	7.0 mg/kg IM BID or 14.0 mg/kg SID	Itraconazole	2.5 mg/kg BID
		Ketoconazole	5.0 mg/kg BID
Amoxicillin/clavulinic acid	5–10.0 mg/kg BID	Fluconazole	2.0 mg/kg BID
Azithromycin		**Sedatives/Analgesics**	
Loading	9.6 mg/kg	Diazepam	
Subsequent	5.3 mg/kg SID	Intramuscular	0.15–0.2 mg/kg
Carbenicillin	22–44 mg/kg TID	Oral	0.2–0.3 mg/kg
Cephalexin	22.0 mg/kg TID	Demerol (meperidine)	IM 2.0 mg/kg
Cefuroxime	20.0 mg/kg BID	**Gastrointestinal Drugs**	
Ceftriaxone	20.0 mg/kg SID		
Ciprofloxacin	15–29 mg/kg BID	Ranitidine	2.0 mg/kg BID
Clindamycin	7.7–9.6 mg/kg BID	Cimetidine	4.5 mg/kg BID
Doxycycline	1.5 mg/kg BID	Sucralfate	1–2 g BID–QID
Enrofloxacin	5.0 mg/kg BID	Pepto-Bismol	Scale to human
Metronidazole	7.0 mg/kg TID	**Antiparasitals**	
Minocycline			
Loading	4.0 mg/kg	Ivermectin	200 μg/kg
Subsequent	2.0 mg/kg BID	Praziquantel	10 mg/kg (*Nasitrema*)
Ofloxacin	5.0 mg/kg BID		3 mg/kg (tapeworms)
Rifampin	2.5 mg/kg BID	Fenbendazole	11 mg/kg
Tetracycline	55–65 mg/kg BID		
Trimethoprim/sulfadiazine‡	16–22 mg/kg SID		
Vancomycin	1–1.5 mg/kg TID		

*Dose for adult bottlenose dolphin weighing 135–160 kg.
†These drugs and dosages have been used in small cetaceans; however, safety and effectiveness have not been established and clinical judgment is required.
‡This drug can cause fatal pancytopenia in cetaceans. Use the veterinary product trimethoprim/sulfadiazine (Tribrissen or Ditrim) and supplement with folic acid 10 mg BID.

lopsis species, and *Zygomyces* have also been identified in gastric samples.

If malodorous gas is noted during gastric intubation, maldigestion should be suspected. This sometimes occurs when an animal is force-fed too frequently or with excessive amounts of fish. In such a case, force-feeding should be discontinued and clear liquids should be given (to maintain hydration). Furthermore, tetracycline can be used to decrease gas-forming bacteria, and metronidazole can be administered for 48 hours to control anaerobic microbes. Once the problem has resolved, force-feeding can be resumed with smaller volumes.

Excessive gastrointestinal gas can be a serious problem. Bloat is a medical emergency that must be recognized and treated immediately by decompression via gastric intubation. Overpopulation of gas-producing bacteria (e.g., with *Clostridium* species), fermentation of food in the stomach as a result of hypomotility, overzealous administration of acid-blocking agents, obstruction, and other causes can produce life-threatening colic. Symptoms include ventral flexion of both head and tail in response to cramping or other gastrointestinal pain and flatus, or the animal may appear to be excessively buoyant and in distress.

To prevent recurrence of bloat, attempts should be made to determine the cause. Fecal culture for pathogens may be indicated. Gastric pH must be monitored to be sure adequate acid is present for digestion. Gastroscopy may be required to identify the presence of parasites, foreign objects, ulceration or erosions, or possible obstructions.

Cetacean feces are normally a thick greenish to brownish liquid that dissipates quickly in water. Excessive gas may produce feces that float before dissipation. Mucoid, stringy feces or feces that contain numerous WBCs may indicate bacterial, parasitic, or drug-related enteritis.

RESPIRATORY SYSTEM

Pulmonary diseases are common in stranded dolphins. Pneumonia is common, and the cause can be bacterial, protozoal, fungal, parasitic, or combinations of these.

Making a diagnosis of pulmonary disease is challenging because the size of the animal renders it unwieldy and special equipment is required for obtaining thoracic radiographs. Ultrasonography of the chest can be useful in diagnosing intrathoracic disease.[13] Recently, pulmonary bronchoscopy has shown promise in more accurate definitive diagnosis.[3, 4]

Occasionally, subcutaneous emphysema is a clinical problem. The excess buoyancy of the animal and difficulty with swimming and diving make diagnosis apparent. The condition may be evident when the animal is first examined or it may develop during the rehabilitative process. The condition developed peracutely in a Cuvier's beaked whale (*Ziphius cavirostris*) soon after she had been moved from one pool to another via a sling and large crane; the condition resolved within 24 hours. A dwarf sperm whale with chronic subcutaneous emphysema at postmortem examination revealed air escaping through the mediastinal tissues.

With these experiences, a possible hypothesis of subcutaneous emphysema may be that the beaching episode or the transport process results in fractures of the pulmonary bronchi that leak air into the mediastinal spaces. The air follows tissue planes anteriorly and enter the dorsal subcutaneous spaces. Cases can spontaneously resolve, as in the Cuvier's beaked whale, or, when the bronchi integrity fails to heal, the emphysema continues to be a clinical problem. The diagnosis can be confirmed with ultrasonography or radiology.

CONTINUING REHABILITATION AND TREATMENT

Diagnostic Procedures

Blood parameters should be checked daily until values indicate that it is safe to check them less frequently. The diagnostic usefulness of gastric samples is somewhat controversial, with some practitioners believing that they are of no value, whereas others believe that they are helpful.

When obtaining an elective gastric sample for diagnostic evaluation, the morning "fasting" aspiration is preferable. It is less likely to contain food particles that would obscure cellular detail and interfere with diagnostic interpretation.

Catheterized urine samples may be used to diagnose and monitor response to treatment of urinary tract infections or renalithiasis. Persistent hematuria without other abnormalities may indicate the renalithiasis. Ultrasonography of the kidneys is usually necessary for a definitive diagnosis of renalithiasis because the stones are most often radiolucent uric acid in composition. The decision to continue or discontinue monitoring urine specimens, bacterial culture sites, and so on, is based on laboratory values and clinical assessment.

Additional Diagnostic Procedures

Endoscopy

Flexible fiberoptic endoscopy is useful in examining the esophagus, the first gastric compartment, and, some-

times, the second. Visualization of gastric erosions and ulcers, foreign objects, retrieval of small foreign objects, and the collection of samples of fluid or biopsy specimens may be accomplished by gastroscopy. Examination of the fundic portion of the stomach may be difficult because it is difficult to locate and pass the scope through the sphincter between the first and second gastric compartments.

A pediatric gastroscope has been used with promising diagnostic results in bronchoscopy, including bronchoalveolar lavage, of bottlenose dolphins.[2, 4]

Electrocardiography

Electrocardiograms can be recorded from dolphins.[8] This procedure may be useful when monitoring an animal during prolonged or stressful treatment or during certain diagnostic procedures.

Diagnostic Imaging

Radiography of cetaceans is an extremely useful diagnostic procedure if done with minimal stress. Lung disease, foreign objects in the gastrointestinal tract, bone fractures, osseous spinal disease, dental disease, and pregnancy are a few of the conditions lending themselves to diagnosis by this method. As in other mammals, ultrasound examination is helpful in the diagnosis and monitoring of treatment of lung disease, liver disease, cardiac disease, and renal disease, and in visualizing the fetus in pregnancy.[11, 13]

Portable diagnostic equipment brought to the animal is preferable to transporting the animal to a facility where radiography or ultrasound examination can be performed. If transport is needed, the benefit-to-risk relationship of these procedures must be evaluated.

Support and Physical Therapy

It is not unusual for a dolphin who has stranded to be unable to maintain itself in the water, necessitating some means of support. Initially, this usually involves human volunteers physically keeping the animal afloat. Animals have been supported in this manner, 24 hours a day, for 2 weeks or more before regaining the ability to swim unaided.

As an alternative to human physical support, various types of slings may be used. These may range from typical fabric and pole transport slings to innovative wet suits that allow mobility in the pool.[15]

Regardless of what type of sling arrangement is used, the animal must be observed continuously by knowledgeable personnel who can intervene if the animal becomes entangled or turns in the sling, when asphyxiation becomes the foremost danger. Frequent checks of axillae for heat and checks of points of pressure for indications of early decubiti are essential. Pressure sores, abrasions, and even localized heat necrosis may occur if the animal is allowed to remain in the sling for too long in the same position. Furthermore, animals should be removed from the sling and "exercised" at intervals during the day.

Scoliosis can occur in wild, free-swimming dolphins, particularly those undergoing rehabilitation after stranding. One bottlenose dolphin in a long-term study appeared to do well for an extended period despite this deformity. Although dolphins can survive and maintain their vital functions while having this condition, the possibility that scoliosis may interfere with normal foraging and defense may deem the animal unsuitable for release. Some animals in whom scoliosis develops require the support of volunteers or slings, whereas others are able to remain afloat but do not swim normally. Factors that may influence the development of scoliosis are restriction of normal swimming patterns, reduced physical capacity because of wounds or illness, nutritional deficits, water quality and temperature, and possibly other factors.

Early detection and intervention may prevent scoliosis from worsening or becoming permanent. Problems with water or food quality and temperature should be addressed. If hypocalcemia is present, parenteral calcium and injection of bovine vitamin-E–selenium intramuscularly are indicated. Successful physical therapy has consisted of gently but firmly bending the tail stock both laterally and dorsoventrally several sessions a day. If the animal can swim, it may be encouraged to do so by throwing food fish in the desired direction. In several pilot whales, muscle electrostimulation has been used successfully to correct this condition.[2]

Nutrition and Fluid Maintenance

Hematocrit and total protein levels are used to assess the level of hydration, and the volume and frequency of fluid administration should be adjusted accordingly. "Normal" values of many species are not known. For example, a hematocrit of 40% in coastal bottlenose dolphin is normal but is considered low for deep water species.

Fluids may be administered by gastric tube or intraperitoneally via Teflon catheter in the severely dehydrated animal. Caution must be exercised if the intraperitoneal route is used, to avoid perforation of bowel and resulting peritonitis.

Following 24 to 48 hours of clear liquids (pediatric electrolyte solution, bottled water, or a combination of these), a gruel of ground fish may be mixed with enough of the clear liquids to produce a gruel that can be gravity fed via gastric tube. If the animal is tractable, gastric intubation and fluid administration may be accomplished with the animal suspended in the water in a sling.

The practitioner must not only adequately address the animal's hydration status but also supply the calorie and protein requirements necessary to promote healing. An adult captive bottlenose dolphin in good health requires 48 to 67 Kcal/kg/day.[10] An ill or febrile animal may require more calories and more protein per kilogram of body weight than a healthy animal, and a growing calf, juvenile, or lactating cow requires more calories, protein, and other nutrients than an adult of the same species.

In monitoring the animal's nutritional status, weight stability or gain is the most important indicator that the animal's caloric needs are being met. If weighing is not possible, successive measurements of girth (girth is measured at the leading edge of the dorsal fin) provides an indication of the trend of weight gain or loss.

A variety of vitamins and nutritional supplements are used for marine mammals. The daily intake for the stranded animal may include vitamin-B complex, 2 to 3 capsules; vitamin E, 1000 IU; vitamin B_1, 500 mg; and vitamin C, 1000 mg.

In most cases, stranded animals do not begin feeding voluntarily. These animals catch and consume live prey, so dead fish or squid may not initially be recognized as food. It is often necessary to teach and stimulate animals to feed on new food sources. Whole fish should be offered to the animal, even if it does not choose to eat. Gentle offering of small bait fish often leads to the dolphins gradually accepting hand feeding.

The process of assisted hand feeding can be initiated by placing the fish in the back of the animal's throat to stimulate the dolphin to swallow. When the animal begins to swallow as the fish touches the throat, the subsequent placement of the fish may be approximated progressively farther forward in the mouth. Shortly after the animal accepts placement of the fish in its mouth, it will begin to take fish from the hand. At this point, the dolphin may begin to eat fish thrown into the water. Standard nutrition guides for food volumes and frequency of feeding should be used.[10]

RECORD KEEPING

The care of a stranded animal is often prolonged and complex. A good record-keeping system is essential to facilitate communication between all levels of care givers, to maintain records for future reference, and for efficient medical management and retrospective evaluations of the case.

Medical Staff: SOAP Charting

Formatting the medical record into *S*ubjective observations, *O*bjective findings, *A*ssessment and differential diagnoses, and *P*lan of treatment/diagnostic studies (SOAP) charting provides a concise record facilitating veterinary staff communication. Recording of laboratory data on a multiple-entry flow sheet aids assessment of trends in those test results. Multientry flow sheets for medications and treatments may be helpful as well.

Care Giver's Records

Notes should also be recorded by the individuals observing and caring for the animal. These should include the following:

- Rate and quality of respiration
- Heart rate and presence or absence of normal sinus arrhythmia
- Medication administration—drug, dose, route, time

- Feeding records—what, when, how much, by what route, over what time period, how tolerated by the animal, any problems encountered
- Physical therapy—when, what, how long, how tolerated, any problems encountered, any changes in animal's response or level of function
- Behavioral and physical observations

Trends, as well as changes in status, should be noted. Problems encountered, suggestions for better ways to approach tasks, and necessary or desirable intrastaff communications may also be recorded in this ongoing log.

Communication Between Veterinary Staff and Volunteers or Care Givers

To reduce misinformation, a point person should be designated to speak to the media. The animal's medical progress and status should be shared with the volunteer staff on a regular basis. The volunteer care givers are better equipped to provide appropriate care if they have an understanding of the animal's status and needs. Most of the staff providing hands-on care are not involved with the medical community, nor are they familiar with medical procedures or terminology. Instructions regarding appropriate intervention and techniques can be provided, as can education concerning what changes to expect.

Expectations should be discussed with the individuals caring for the animal (especially with the naive volunteer) so as not to encourage unrealistic expectations for the animal's recovery. Most stranded cetaceans do not survive. Discussion of the animal's status and prognosis helps everyone involved to better understand the problems that may develop and to prepare for the possibility of the animal's death.

Natural Death and Euthanasia

Euthanasia is defined as the humane alternative for animals unlikely to recover from their illnesses or injury. Regardless of the circumstances, euthanasia is sometimes viewed by public and professionals alike as a failure of the rescue process. This is especially true when an animal who previously appeared to respond to treatment suffers decline to the point that euthanasia is considered. If the animal dies or is euthanized during the rehabilitation effort, it is beneficial to have a meeting of volunteers and other staff members to discuss the case. This conference gives the participants some closure and is helpful in dealing with emotionally charged issues that follow a prolonged rehabilitation attempt. Ultimately, the decision to euthanize the animal is a veterinary decision based on medical criteria.

RETURN TO THE WILD

Following successful rescue and rehabilitation, there are essentially two options for the animal: (1) reintroduction to the wild or (2) transfer to a marine mammal facility equipped to provide long-term care for the animal. The ultimate goal of rehabilitation is the reintroduction of the animal to the wild. In the past, the success in rehabilitating stranded cetaceans was so low that releasing the animal back into the wild was rarely an issue. However, rehabilitation practices have improved dramatically in recent years, making release of rehabilitated animals an important consideration.

There is considerable controversy regarding the reintroduction criteria. The National Marine Fisheries Service is publishing guidelines for the release of rehabilitated marine mammals. The following considerations should be addressed when evaluating this option.[16]

1. What is the animal's age at the time of stranding? For a number of reasons, nursing calves, in the absence of their mothers, should not be considered candidates for release.

2. Is the animal free of diseases that may endanger wild populations? Screening candidates for release for infectious diseases such as morbillivirus, herpes virus, hepatitis virus, and parvovirus is strongly recommended.

3. Can the animal be returned to its original stock or at least to a group of conspecifics.

4. Does the animal have basic survival skills—ability to swim, forage, and so on? It is unreasonable to require the animal to demonstrate *all* survival skills (normal response to predators, for example, cannot safely be demonstrated in a captive setting). However, every reasonable effort must be made to ensure that the animal has the capacity for survival before attempting release.

5. Has the animal acquired behaviors that would interfere with interaction in wild societies or reduce ability to survive once the animal has been returned to the wild?

6. Will there be provision of follow-up monitoring, with availability for recapture of the animal in case it fails to maintain itself after release?

When an animal is to be reintroduced to the wild, the National Marine Fisheries Service regional office must be notified in advance. Nonrelease determinations are made by the National Marine Fisheries Service regional offices upon recommendations of the attending veterinarian and rehabilitation staff.

Less than 3% of the bottlenose dolphin strandings reported in the last 10 years in Florida involved live animals. Fewer still survived the rehabilitation phase to either be reintroduced or remain in protective care. All of them, whether they survived or not, whether they required placement in a marine mammal facility or were successfully returned to the wild, have enhanced understanding of how to better care for the next animal to come aground.

REFERENCES

1. Bossart GD: Morbilli Virus Infection: Implications for oceanaria marine mammal stranding programs. Proceedings of the International Association of Aquatic Animal Medicine, Mystic, CT, p 50, 1995.
2. Harrell JH, Reidarson TH, McBain JF, Sheetz H: Bronchoscopy of

the bottlenose dolphin (*Tursiops truncatus*). Proceedings of the International Association of Aquatic Animal Medicine, Chattanooga, TN, p 33, 1996.

3. Haubrich WS, Schaffner F (eds): Bockus Gastroenterology, 5th ed. Philadelphia, WB Saunders, pp 458–460, 1995.
4. Hawkins EC, Townsend FI, Lewbart GA, et al: Bronchoalveolar lavage in a stranded bottlenose dolphin. Proceedings of the International Association of Aquatic Animal Medicine, Chattanooga, TN, p 124, 1996.
5. Lipscomb TP, Kennedy S, Ford BK: Morbillivirus-induced disease in an Atlantic bottlenose dolphin (*Tursiops truncatus*) from the Gulf of Mexico. J Wildl Dis 30:572–576, 1994.
6. Lipscomb TP, Kennedy S, Moffett D, et al: Mobilliviral epizootic in bottlenose dolphins of the Gulf of Mexico. J Vet Diagn Invest 8:283–290, 1996.
7. Mikota-Wells SK: Wildlife laws, regulations, and policies. *In* Fowler ME (ed): Zoo and Wild Animal Medicine: Current Therapy 3. Philadelphia, WB Saunders, pp 3–5, 1993.
8. Miller GW: Digital recording of the electrocardiogram from bottlenose dolphins (*Tursiops truncatus*). Proceedings of the International Association of Aquatic Animal Medicine, Mystic, CT, p 44, 1995.
9. Needham DJ: Cetacean strandings. *In* Fowler ME (ed): Zoo and Wild Animal Medicine: Current Therapy 3. Philadelphia, WB Saunders, pp 415–425, 1993.

10. Reddy M, Kamolnick T, Curry C, Skaar D. Energy requirements for the bottlenose dolphin (*Tursiops truncatus*) in relation to sex, age, and reproductive status. Marine Mammals: Public Display and Research 1:26–31, 1994.
11. Rhinehart, Townsend FI, Gorzelany J, Broecker S: Ultrasound-aided thoracentesis in a bottlenose dolphin. Proceedings of the International Association of Aquatic Animal Medicine, Vallejo, CA, p 175, 1994.
12. Ridgway SH (ed): Mammals of the Sea; Biology and Medicine. Springfield, IL, Charles C Thomas, pp 631–633, 1972.
13. Stone LR: Diagnostic ultrasound in marine mammals. *In* Dierauf LA (ed): Handbook of Marine Mammal Medicine. Boca Raton, FL, CRC Press, pp 235–264, 1990.
14. Sweeney JC: Blood sampling and other collection techniques in marine mammals. *In* Fowler ME (ed): Zoo and Wild Animal Medicine: Current Therapy 3. Philadelphia, WB Saunders, pp 425–428, 1993.
15. Walsh MT, Wagoner BC, Campbell TW, Rodriguez A: Use of floatation assistance devices in marine mammals: treatment and physical therapy. Proceedings of the International Association of Aquatic Animal Medicine, Mystic, CT, p 102, 1995.
16. Wells RS: Behavior, Life History, and Natural History Criteria for Release of Rehabilitated Marine Mammals. Chicago, Chicago Zoological Society, pp 2–16, 1994.

CHAPTER **69**

Hand-Rearing Techniques for Neonate Cetaceans

FORREST I. TOWNSEND

Before 1989, most efforts to save nursing cetacean calves who had been orphaned or who failed to thrive were unsuccessful. The success of the Point Defiance Zoo and Aquarium, Washington, in raising an infant harbor porpoise (*Phocoena phocoena*) set the stage for a number of successes to follow. The Gulfarium in Florida, giving around-the-clock attention to the nutritional requirements of an infant cetacean, was successful in rearing a bottlenose dolphin (*Tursiops truncatus*) calf. Because the international marine mammal community has shared information and experiences in the rescue and care of these fragile animals, there has been a dramatic improvement in survival rates.

CRITERIA FOR INTERVENTION

Immediate intervention is needed when wild calves are found stranded or when very young captive calves are orphaned. It is more difficult to decide when to intervene when a calf fails to thrive.

The first 10 days of life are critical to the survivability of cetacean calves. Normal labor and delivery of *Tursiops* usually occur within 2 hours.[6] If labor and delivery exceed this time period, the calf is more likely to experience difficulty. Most calves begin nursing within 1 to 4 hours postpartum, and they nurse four or more times per hour.[1, 6] Calves that fail to nurse or that nurse ineffectively for more than 36 hours are candidates for nutritional intervention. Delaying intervention can make the difference between failure and success in these cases.

Supplementation routine—delivery method, volume and frequency of feedings, type of supplementation—should be decided beforehand and ready to implement on short notice. Many of the supplies and formula ingredients are not readily available, so they should be acquired in advance.

There are three basic situations when intervention is required:

1. The calf that is not nursing adequately from its

mother may have nursing intake supplemented with bottle or tube feeding of formula.

2. The orphaned calf may be placed with a surrogate mother, either lactating or nonlactating, supplemented with bottle or tube feeding as required.

3. The calf may be completely formula fed. Total formula supplementation has been successful in several cases.

NUTRITION AND FEEDING

Dolphin Milk Replacement Formulas

When the decision has been made to remove a calf from its mother or when a calf is orphaned, supplementation should begin immediately. Tables 69–1 and 69–2 list the major components of dolphin milk and two successfully used dolphin calf formulas.

April Formula was named for the orphaned *Tursiops truncatus* calf rescued at an estimated 3 to 4 weeks of age and successfully raised at The Gulfarium, Fort Walton Beach, FL. Sea World Formula was developed for use at Sea World, Inc., and shared with the marine mammal community. These formulas have been used in the hand-raising of bottlenose dolphins (*Tursiops truncatus*), Risso's dolphins (*Grampus griseus*), harbor porpoises (*Phocoena phocoena*), spotted dolphins (*Sten-*

TABLE 69–1. Dolphin Milk Replacement Formulas

April Formula	Sea World Formula
Herring filets—750 ml filets with viscera	Herring filets with viscera—750 ml
MultiMilk* powder—2.5 cups	Zoological 30/55*—8 oz (225 g)
Safflower oil—50 ml	Zoological 33/40*—16 oz (450 g)
Lecithin—15 ml	Salmon oil—50 ml
Taurine—250 mg	Taurine—500 mg
Lactobacillus—3 tablets	Lactobacillus—1.5 tablets
Osteoform†—1 tablespoon	Osteoform—1 tablespoon
Pedialyte/bottled water—1100 ml	Sea World marine vitamins—one 2-pound-size tablet to every 2 pounds of formula
Multivitamins with zinc alternating with marine mammal vitamins	Heavy whipping cream—100 ml 50% Dextrose—60 ml Pedialyte/bottled water—1100 ml

Blend freshly defrosted zoo herring filets (with viscera) in a commercial blender, approximately 750 ml. Add 1100 ml Pedialyte/bottled water. Blend in milk substitute. Add salmon or safflower oil, 50% dextrose, Osteoform (powder preferred), lecithin, lactobacillus, taurine, and vitamin supplement. If using heavy whipping cream, mix in after blending other ingredients. Label formula container with date and time of preparation, refrigerate until used. Discard unused formula after 24 hours.

*Available from Pet-Ag Inc., 30 West 432, Rt. 20, Elgin, IL 60120, 1-800-323-0877.
†Available from Vetamix, Shenandoah, Iowa 51601.

TABLE 69–2. Nutritional Content of Tursiops Milk and Dolphin Formulas

	Tursiops Milk*	April Formula	Sea World Formula
Moisture g/100 g		78.4	78.4
Protein g/100 g	12.2	10.0	8.8
Fat g/100 g	29.4 ± 3.0	9.0	9.55
Ash g/100 g		1.4	1.32
Carbohydrate g/100 g	2.5 ± 0.44	1.2	1.93

*See reference 4.

ella attenuata), short-snouted spinner dolphin (*Stenella clymene*), pygmy sperm whale (*Kogia breviceps*), and *Pseudorca/Tursiops* hybrid calves. Both formulations include herring, using filets and viscera but not the larger bones of the back and skull.

Fat content is increased in both formulas by the addition of salmon oil or safflower oil. Salmon oil more closely mimics the fats in dolphin milk and is preferred; however, salmon oil may not be readily available. If a source cannot be located, safflower oil may be substituted.

A major difference in the formulas is the powdered milk substitute used in April Formula. Multimilk is a powdered milk substitute used in milk replacement for a variety of exotic species. It is composed of 55% fat, 30% protein, and a trace of carbohydrate (same formula as Zoological 30/55).

Dolphin milk contains 1% to 3% carbohydrate. The Zoological 30/55 and Zoological 33/40 in a 2:1 ratio used in Sea World Formula provides increased carbohydrates.

To increase the caloric density of Sea World Formula, heavy whipping cream is added. Historically, whipping cream has been used in most marine mammal infant milk replacement formulas. It was eliminated in April Formula out of concern that the calf would have trouble digesting lactose. In the past, the possibility of lactose intolerance was addressed by pretreating the whipping cream overnight with a lactose digesting enzyme. Dolphin milk does contain 0.5% to 1.0% lactose, so the concerns about its use may be unfounded (Tom Reiderson, personal communication, 1996). The other ingredients in the two formulas are very similar.

Levels of the amino acid taurine are considerably higher in cetacean milk, approximately 500 mg/L in killer whale (*Orcinus orca*) milk (Michael Walsh, personal communication, 1992). In veterinary medicine, taurine deficiency, particularly in cats, can affect numerous organ systems.[8] Some research suggests that taurine plays a role in immune function. Consequently, taurine has been supplemented in currently used milk substitute formulas.

DAILY CALORIC REQUIREMENTS AND DAILY WEIGHT GAIN

Understanding the nutritional management of the fragile infant cetaceans is the most important factor to success.

To calculate daily nutritional requirements, an accurate body weight of the calf and the caloric density of the formula used are necessary. Weighing the calf would seem to be an easy process, but experience indicates the contrary. When weighing a smaller calf (less than 20 to 25 kg), the calf is removed from the pool and carried to a dry handler standing on a mechanical type scale to achieve accurate results. Larger calves (greater than 25 kg) require use of a sling to accommodate their size, with holes in the bottom for water drainage. This sling is attached to a tripod or boom with a scale attached. Accurate daily or every-other-day weighing cannot be overemphasized, especially initially. These weight measurements are the foundation for assessment of the animal's status, steering the medical and nutritional direction of the case.

Analysis for caloric density of the formula being used should be obtained by a commercial laboratory.* (Approximate caloric density of the formulas are 1.5 Kcal/ml.) From these data, calf weight and caloric density of formula, a feeding schedule can be developed.

Bo Henose (*Tursiops*) and spotted (*Stenella*) dolphins require 150 to 200 Kcal/kg/day for positive weight gain. Other species, harbor porpoise (*Phocoena phocoena*) and common dolphins (*Delphinus delphis*), have substantially higher caloric requirements (250 to 300 Kcal/kg/day). And pygmy sperm whales (*Kogia breviceps*) have a lower caloric requirement (80 to 100 Kcal/kg/day). These are merely guidelines from a few previous cases. It is the calf's weight gain (or loss) that guides the proper daily amount of formula for the animal.

The following equation is used to calculate the volume of formula required for a bottlenose dolphin calf weighing 15 kg:

$$15 \text{ kg (calf weight)} \times 200 \text{ Kcal/kg/day} = 3000 \text{ kcal/day}$$

$$3000 \text{ Kcal/day} \div 1.5 \text{ Kcal/ml formula} = 2000 \text{ ml formula/day}$$

Divide milliliters of formula per day by feeding frequency to determine milliliters of volume per feeding. If the calf is bottle nursing, it often determines the amount per feeding itself. In this example, a 100-ml feed 20 times per day should be sufficient. When tube feeding, it is best to determine the maximum amounts that can safely be administered without the animal regurgitating, allowing fewer intubations per day. It is advisable to start with lower amounts, 100 to 120 ml, and gradually work toward higher amounts per feeding, warming the formula before feeding.

If the calf is suckling a bottle, it will nurse until satisfied (full), which may be considerably more than the calculated per feeding volume. Calves that nurse a bottle feed very quickly, requiring only a few seconds to consume several ounces of formula. This combination of frequent feedings and an eager, hungry calf can result in an obese calf. In both *Tursiops* and *Stenella*

species calves, daily weight gains of 0.5 kg/day were recorded. To avoid development of obesity-related disease (e.g., fatty liver), the frequency or volume of feeding was reduced, with target weight gain of 0.25 kg/day being the goal for the *Tursiops* species calf. In the smaller species (*Stenella* and *Delphinus*), 0.125 kg/day is the goal, and, in the larger species (*Pseudorca* and *Kogia*), 0.5 kg/day is recommended.

FORMULA DELIVERY METHODS

On initial presentation, calves often attempt to suckle the care givers' fingers and wet suits. If this suckling response is present, every effort should be made to deliver the formula with a nipple/bottle combination. This method reduces the serious complication of aspiration pneumonia and, in comparison to gastric intubation, significantly reduces personnel and effort required. During the early acclimation process it may be necessary to use a stomach tube to deliver the formula. An equine foal nasogastric tube works well (Kalayjian Industries Inc., 3218 E. Willow, Long Beach, CA 90806). The approximate placement of the tube can be estimated by laying the tube alongside the calf's head with the end of the tube at the tip of the tucked pectoral fin and marking the tube at the tip of the mandible with a piece of waterproof tape. The formula is gravity fed via a funnel through the gastric tube.

The suckling of the calf on an artificial nipple has to be "trained." The calf may be held with its head slightly out of the water and a finger used to initiate a suckling response. The nipple is placed over the finger, then the nipple and bottle containing formula are introduced. This process may occur quickly or may be prolonged (15 days in the *Pseudorca/Tursiops* hybrid case). Some infants (*Stenella* species and pygmy sperm whale) have not nursed the bottle at all, necessitating the formula be delivered via gastric tube. It is possible that the right combination of nipple and delivery technique has not been found in these species. In the *Tursiops* species calves, an artificial lamb's nipple proved to be a good choice. A note of caution: when a nipple has been accepted by the calf, it may be *extremely* particular about that nipple. Attempting to change to a new or slightly different nipple may result in the calf's objection to nurse.

OTHER MANAGEMENT PRACTICES

Dolphins can be conditioned to allow the use of a modified human breast pump,[5] or they can be restrained for milking purposes. This dolphin milk can be used to fortify the formula. This method was successfully used in hand rearing a *Pseudorca/Tursiops* hybrid calf in Hawaii. In this case, 600 to 800 ml/day of the calf's mother's milk was obtained with a breast pump. It may be necessary to use total formula supplementation when no surrogates are available, when surrogates do not produce milk, or when the surrogate mother becomes overprotective, interfering with hand-rearing efforts and resulting in weight loss.

---

*Available from Corning Hazelton (Covance), P.O. Box 7545, Madison, WI 53707-7545, (608) 241-4471.

FOSTER MOTHERS

Orphaned calves, when placed with a foster mother, may induce lactation. Cases have been reported in which calves introduced to nonlactating cows induced lactation in less than 10 days. Two separate orphaned calves, when placed with surrogate mothers, resulted in induced lactation.[5] Analysis of the dolphin milk soon after calves began to suckle revealed low milk fat of 6% in one cow and 10.3% in the other. After the first month, the milk fat levels increased to 22.5% and 26.5%, respectively, more closely resembling the reported values for bottlenose dolphins. Both calves were fed a supplementary milk formula to compensate for the quality and quantity of milk being produced by their foster mothers. One of the surrogate mothers had been in the collection for 24 years and had not been pregnant nor lactated during that time.

Selection of the foster mother should be done with care. In a successful case, an orphaned calf was paired with a lactating cow which had lost her own calf.[3] In a case that failed, an orphaned calf was placed in a pool with two female dolphins, one lactating and the other nonlactating, and the calf was dominated by the nonlactating cow, which would not allow the calf to nurse the lactating cow. Another case in which an orphan was placed with a cow and calf pair resulted in the orphan calf being traumatized by the cow.[7] Ideally, a solo lactating cow that has recently lost her calf is the first choice. In most situations, however, a nonlactating, nonpregnant cow is the most readily available and therefore the best choice. The timing of the introduction must be considered thoughtfully. Establishing the feeding routine for the calf before placing the foster mother with the calf is recommended.

WEANING

Timing and method of weaning the calf are important. Captive *Tursiops* species calves in a lagoon environment begin mouthing fish at 4 to 8 months of age and usually begin hand feeding at 7 to 12 months.

A *Tursiops* species calf allowed to wean on her own started eating solid fish at 8 months of age and was completely off the bottle-fed formula at 1 year of age. In this case, the formula daily totals were gradually reduced over a 3-month period. A *Tursiops* species calf "force weaned" by introducing whole fish into the mouth at 4 months of age was completely weaned by 5 months of age. The harbor porpoise began eating live bait herring at 2 months of age and was completely weaned at 3 months of age.

The method of rearing must be considered when weaning. If a surrogate cow is found and the calf is nursing without supplementation, weaning follows a more natural process. Calves that are being intubated require much more labor, compared with the calf that is voluntarily suckling a bottle, making weaning to solid food a much higher priority. Weaning the tube-fed calf also eliminates the risk of aspiration pneumonia.

With either voluntary or forced weaning, the weaning process should be gradual and carefully thought out. Body condition and weight should be checked periodically to avoid excessive deviations in either direction and to ensure adequate calories and nutrients are being consumed.

TOYS

Hand-reared calves require enormous daily human contact, often feeding 12 to 18 times per day. Placing objects, or "toys," in the pool for the calves to push around and play with is often used to enrich their environmental stimulation and to keep calves occupied when care givers are not present. Certain toys seem to have the same effect as "security blankets" for children, with the calf going to the toy when alarmed or frightened.

The combination of play with the care givers and with their toys can, however, interfere with the feeding schedule. If this becomes a problem, the toys should be removed from the pool and the calf fed at a specific "feeding station." The calf should soon be conditioned to the feeding routine. Using "time outs" in which the care giver leaves the pool area when the calf wants to play rather than nurse may be necessary. Successful nursing should be rewarded by replacing the toys in the pool and providing tactile stimulation for positive reinforcement.

PHARMACOLOGIC INTERVENTION

Frequent blood testing and monitoring complete blood counts, electrolyte balance, and organ function of the calf are recommended. Blood testing should be done twice weekly. The blood tests are often the earliest indicator of an abnormal medical condition. Treating the subclinical disease states leads to successful medical management of many conditions. In most cases, antibiotics have been administered to the calves. The most commonly used drugs are the cephalosporins and the quinolone-enrofloxacin, and many of the calves have been placed on itraconazole prophylaxis.

Neonate cetaceans are considered to derive the circulating immunoglobulins from the intestinal absorption of colostral antibodies. Failing to nurse or nursing ineffectively may result in low blood immunoglobulin levels. This lack of maternal antibodies may place the calf at greater risk for infectious disease. The availability of dolphin IgG is ideal in many of these cases, but there is difficulty in having this on hand. Doses of 20 mg of IgG in *Tursiops* species calves and 36-mg and 76-mg intravenous doses of IgG in a beluga whale (*Delphinapterus leucas*) calf[2] have been given successfully.

CONCLUSION

These cases begin full of hope, often requiring superhuman effort, a large financial investment, and great emotional involvement by the staff. Realistic expectations by the experienced staff should be related to the new and inexperienced care givers to help buffer the disappointment if the calf dies. Those who do survive help to further knowledge and understanding of these difficult yet rewarding cases.

REFERENCES

1. Cockcroft VG, Ross GJB: Observations on the early development of a captive bottlenose dolphin calf. *In* Leatherwood S, Reeves R (eds): The Bottlenose Dolphin. New York, Academic Press, pp 461–478, 1990.
2. Dalton LM, Schwertner HA, McBain JF: The use of immunoglobulin concentrate in a beluga whale calf. Proceedings of the International Association of Aquatic Animal Medicine, Chicago, p 110, 1993.
3. Kastelein RA, Dokter T, Zwart P: The suckling of a bottlenose dolphin calf (*Tursiops truncatus*) by a foster mother, and information on transverse birth bands. Aquatic Mammals 16.3:134–138, 1990.
4. Pervaiz S, Brew K. Composition of the milks of the bottlenose dolphin (*Tursiops truncatus*) and the Florida manatee (*Trichechus manatus latirostris*). Comp Biochem Physiol 84:357–360, 1986.
5. Ridgway S, Kamolinck T, Reddy M, Curry C: Orphan-induced lactation in *Tursiops* and analysis of collected milk. Marine Mammal Science 11(2):172–182, 1995.
6. Schroeder JP: Reproductive aspects of marine mammals. *In* Dierauf LA (ed): Handbook of Marine Mammal Medicine; Health, Disease, and Rehabilitation. Boca Raton, FL, CRC Press, pp 353–370, 1990.
7. Smolders J: Adoption behavior in the bottlenose dolphin. Aquatic Mammals 14.2:78–81, 1988.
8. Walsh MT, Quinton RR: Taurine levels in cetaceans, a preliminary investigation. Proceedings of the International Association of Aquatic Animal Medicine, Mystic, CT, p 115, 1995.

CHAPTER **70**

Morbillivirus Infections of Marine Mammals

PÁDRAIG J. DUIGNAN

A recent development in the field of marine mammal diseases has been the emergence of morbilliviruses as agents of mass mortality. The morbilliviruses are an antigenically related genus of single-stranded RNA viruses within the family Paramyxoviridae and, until recently, included canine distemper virus (CDV), primarily found in terrestrial carnivores, rinderpest virus (RPV), which infects cattle and other large ruminant animals, peste des petits ruminants virus (PPRV), which infects small ruminant animals, and human measles virus (MV).[3] In 1988, a series of epizootics began that resulted in the discovery of previously unknown marine mammal morbilliviruses—phocine distemper virus (PDV), porpoise morbillivirus (PMV), and dolphin morbillivirus (DMV). PDV is genetically distinct from PMV and DMV but the degree of sequence variation between the latter is so low that they may be strains of a cetacean morbillivirus.[7]

EPIZOOTIOLOGY

Epizootics

The role played by morbilliviruses in historical epizootics, such as that of Antarctic crabeater seals (*Lobodon carcinophagus*) in 1955, will likely remain speculative.[6]

However, it is more certain that a morbillivirus was responsible for a 1982 die-off among bottlenose dolphins (*Tursiops truncatus*) in Florida's Indian and Banana rivers[20] and was involved in an epizootic along the U.S. mid-Atlantic coast between 1987 and 1988 that decimated coastal migratory bottlenose dolphins.[20, 25, 45] In the latter event, emaciated carcasses washed ashore with a variety of opportunistic infections, showing evidence of intoxication by brevetoxin, a dinoflagellate neurotoxin.[25] Although no viruses were isolated, dolphins sampled at sea had morbillivirus antibodies[20, 25] and viral antigen and RNA were found in tissues.[41, 45]

The series of epizootics that resulted in the discovery of the first marine mammal morbillivirus, PDV, began in western Europe in the spring of 1988.[13, 34] In April, aborted harbor seal (*Phoca vitulina*) pups on the Danish Island of Anholt signaled the start of an event that spread rapidly through seal colonies, leaving more than 18,000 animals dead. Gray seals were also infected but relatively few died.[32, 39] A second more localized outbreak occurred in the Dutch and German Waddenzee and in northern Norway in 1989.[42]

The epizootic in western Europe was preceded in December 1987 by the deaths of thousands of Baikal seals (*Phoca sibirica*) in Siberia.[27] In this case, the culprit was a field strain of CDV that probably originated in terrestrial carnivores.[46]

Concurrent with the PDV epizootic, a number of harbor porpoises (*Phocoena phocoena*) washed ashore on the Irish coast with distemper-like lesions and, 2 years later, more were stranded with the same disease in the North Sea.[37, 38, 57] Porpoise morbillivirus was isolated on both occasions. This was soon overshadowed by events in the Mediterranean. Beginning in June 1990 and extending into 1992, DMV killed untold hundreds of striped dolphins (*Stenella coeruleoalba*) from Spain across to Greece.[1]

In the western Atlantic, recurrent epizootics occur among juvenile harbor seals wintering over on the coasts of southern New England. A morbillivirus was documented as the cause of one such event during the winter of 1991–1992.[22, 23]

Serologic Investigations

Evidence indicates that PDV did not occur in European harbor seals before 1988 and, despite equivocal serologic evidence, is not likely maintained in that population.[31, 36, 60] Looking beyond western Europe for a potential reservoir of infection, it was proposed that the harp seal (*Phoca groenlandica*) population in the White and Barents seas was a likely source.[26] Support for this hypothesis came from preliminary studies on harp seals in Greenland waters[12] and later from more extensive investigations throughout the entire harp seal range.[21, 52]

Harp seals likely play the most important role in the epizootiology of PDV in the North Atlantic and Arctic. In the Canadian Arctic, it was found that the prevalence of antibody in ringed seals (*Phoca hispida*) was higher where they are sympatric with migratory harp seals.[21] Harp seals may also act as a reservoir of infection for the less gregarious hooded seals (*Cystophora cristata*) and the relatively small Atlantic walrus (*Odobenus rosmarus rosmarus*) population, with which they are seasonally sympatric.[21, 24]

Seropositive ringed seals have been found as far west as the Mackenzie River delta,[21] but a preliminary study found no antibodies in several pinniped species from the North Pacific and Bering Sea.[49] The latter results are under review and it is thought that at least some Alaskan species have been exposed to a morbillivirus (R. Zarnke, personal communication, 1996; Duignan, unpublished data). There is no evidence that PDV has reached the large harbor seal populations on the west coasts of Canada and the United States.[23]

Along the Atlantic coast of North America, high seroprevalence of PDV over many years was found in the large gray seal population.[23] By contrast, the prevalence was significantly lower in the smaller, more fragmented, sympatric harbor seal population.[23]

In Antarctica, crabeater seals and leopard seals (*Hydrurga leptonyx*) were exposed to CDV rather than PDV.[6] In view of the threat posed to Antarctic seals by pathogens from sled dogs, the Antarctic Treaty has banned dogs from Antarctica.

Less is known about the prevalence of morbillivirus antibodies in cetaceans. Following the events in Europe, morbillivirus antibody was found in harbor porpoises, common dolphins (*Delphinus delphis*), and white-beaked dolphins (*Lagenorhynchus albirostris*) from the North Sea, and in Mediterranean striped dolphins.[57] However, no pre-epizootic samples were available. In Icelandic waters, morbillivirus antibody was not detected in several species sampled during the 1980s.[53]

Morbillivirus antibody in free-ranging bottlenose dolphins sampled in 1987 was the first indication that infection was present in cetaceans of the western Atlantic.[25] More extensive retrospective surveys found antibodies in 14 of 18 odontocete species ranging from Arctic Canada to the Gulf of Mexico as far back as 1980.[17] Among these, the pilot whales (*Globicephala* species) were identified as the most likely reservoir and possibly the cetacean equivalent of the harp seal.[18] Not only are pilot whales numerous and highly gregarious but they also interact with other species such as bottlenose dolphins in which recurrent epizootics occur.[20] Clinical morbillivirus infection has not yet been detected in cetaceans of the North Pacific, but antibodies were recently found in common dolphins stranded in California (J. Cordaro, personal communication, 1996). The Florida manatee (*Trichechus manatus latirostris*) is the only sirenian in which morbillivirus antibodies have been reported.[19]

Species Susceptibility

Based on both natural and experimental infection, harbor seals appear to be more susceptible to PDV than gray seals.[29, 39] Although the reason for this difference is unknown, it is likely determined by host-specific factors such as cell receptors for the virus, differences in antigen processing or presentation, or differences in immune responsiveness.

Serologic monitoring of harbor and gray seals during the PDV epizootics found a higher rate of seroconversion among gray seals.[10, 32] More detailed studies on moribund harbor seals showed that few had antibodies against the important external F and H glycoproteins of CDV and PDV.[51] In this regard, they were similar to dogs that develop clinical distemper.[50] However, a preliminary study using vaccinia recombinants suggested that gray seals mounted a more competent response,[8] and this was confirmed by a larger investigation using naturally infected harbor and gray seal serum and CDV antigens.[15]

Differences in immune response against morbilliviruses are also apparent between other phocids. Serologic responses in harp seals were found to be similar to those of gray seals and significantly better than those of hooded seals.[21] Thus, differences in antibody response between species may be an important determinant of morbillivirus susceptibility.

Transmission

In general, morbilliviruses are transmitted horizontally and by the respiratory route.[3] However, the presence of virus in urine, feces, saliva, and milk would not preclude other means of transmission.[39] Transplacental transmission is not yet documented for marine mammals.

Any factors that bring infected and susceptible animals into close proximity increase the likelihood of transmission. Many pinnipeds and odontocetes would seem exquisitely predisposed to morbillivirus infection because of their social behavior. Seals tend to be gregarious and form closely packed aggregations on land. Thus, contact rates are dependent not so much on the population size but on the frequency with which seals come ashore.[54] The latter varies seasonally, geographically, and with weather conditions, and it is influenced by the sex and age of the seals.[33, 54] Highly gregarious species such as harp seals may even transmit morbilliviruses when in water, and, for Arctic species, shared breathing holes in the ice or open water polynyas must pose a significant threat.[21] Aerosol transmission among odontocetes is likely mediated by synchronous breathing and explosive expiration and is dependent on social cohesiveness within pods and the frequency of interactions between pods.

For viruses that induce long-term immunity, such as the morbilliviruses, the length of the latent and infectious periods and the number of susceptible animals entering the population also affect transmission.[3, 4] Thus, species differences in life-history, behavior, and susceptibility have important effects on epizootiology.

CLINICAL SIGNS

Elevated body temperature and watery or hemorrhagic diarrhea occur in seals between 3 and 6 days after infection.[30, 57] This is followed by respiratory distress, cyanosis of mucous membranes, ocular and nasal discharge, central nervous disturbances, and weight loss.[30, 34, 57] Females infected during pregnancy are prone to abortion.[34] Weakened animals often remain ashore for extended periods, pressure necrosis of the skin develops, and the animals acquire heavy burdens of ectoparasites. Subcutaneous emphysema of the neck and thorax occurs as a sequel to lung damage, and seals have difficulty swimming and diving.[39] Neurologic disease most often manifests as depression, head tremors, convulsions, and seizures.[34]

Clinical signs are less frequently observed in free-ranging cetaceans. Infection often results in a chronic course of disease with respiratory difficulty, emaciation, abnormal behavior, and abortion.[1, 9, 25] Clinical illness in stranded pilot whales was brief, manifesting as anorexia and leukopenia.[18]

PATHOGENESIS AND PATHOLOGY

Based on experimental infection of harbor seals, the pathogenesis of PDV infection appears to be similar to that of CDV in dogs.[2] Viral replication occurs initially in the tonsil, lymph nodes, and spleen and coincides with viremia, pyrexia, and leukopenia.[30] The virus continues to replicate in lymphoid tissues but also disseminates in association with leukocytes to the skin, the mucous membranes, and the respiratory, gastrointestinal, urogenital, and central nervous systems.[30] A second

febrile period may be associated with replication in these organs.[30, 57]

Seals are generally in good body condition at necropsy with an adequate blubber layer.[34, 39] Pneumonia is the most common finding and affected lungs are edematous, fail to collapse, and may have sharply demarcated areas of consolidation in all lobes. Interlobular and subpleural emphysema frequently extends into the mediastinum and subcutis of the neck and thorax. Secondary bacterial infections often result in suppurative bronchopneumonia, and severe parasite burdens are common.[39, 48]

Affected odontocetes may be severely emaciated, with heavy burdens of ectoparasites and commensals such as barnacles and copepods attached to the skin.[14, 16] Acute and chronic ulcerative stomatitis and gingivitis may be present.[14] Pneumonia is characterized by consolidation, edema, and emphysema, but secondary bacterial or mycotic infections may cause suppurative or hemorrhagic lesions.[14, 16] Bronchial lymph nodes are generally enlarged and edematous. Leukoencephalomalacia may be evident in the brain, and secondary mycotic encephalitis may cause necrosis and hemorrhage.[14]

Histologic lesions consist of bronchointerstitial pneumonia with congestion, edema, serofibrinous exudation into alveoli, proliferation of type II pneumocytes, and formation of syncytia.[14, 16, 39, 40] Syncytia are a prominent feature of morbillivirus pneumonia in odontocetes but are less so in pinnipeds. There is necrosis of bronchial, bronchiolar, and peribronchial gland epithelium, and intracytoplasmic or intranuclear inclusions may be seen in these cells and in intra-alveolar macrophages and syncytia.[18, 22, 39]

Encephalitis is characterized by neuronal necrosis, gliosis, lymphocytic and plasmacytic perivascular cuffing, and demyelination with astrocytosis and syncytium formation.[16, 22, 39] Inclusions are found in both neurons and astrocytes. Lesions occur most commonly in the cerebrum but may be found in the cerebellum and elsewhere.[35, 39]

Lymphoid depletion is a characteristic in acute infection but less so in chronic encephalitis.[23] Syncytia are often found in depleted lymphoid tissues of cetaceans.[14] Epithelial necrosis with viral inclusions may also occur in the gastrointestinal and urinary systems and mammary gland.[11, 14, 35, 39, 40]

DIAGNOSIS

Diagnosis is based on the presence of characteristic histopathologic lesions and is supported by immunohistochemistry, immunofluorescence, or electron microscopy. Antigen-capture enzyme-linked immunosorbent assay (ELISA) may also be used on tissue homogenates,[57] and viral RNA may be demonstrated in fixed or fresh tissue using a polymerase chain reaction (PCR)-based assay.[28, 41]

Increasing antibody titers in serum are widely used to confirm clinical infection. Most laboratories use a variation of the microneutralization test to measure antibodies against the hemagglutinin (H) and the fusion (F) glycoproteins of the virus. By contrast, morbillivirus-specific ELISA tests are more likely to detect antibodies against epitopes on the neucleocapsid (N) and matrix (M) proteins and therefore do not correlate well with the neutralization tests.[5] Experimental infection studies using PDV in harbor seals have shown that virus-neutralizing antibody against the homologous virus appears as early as day 7 after infection.[30] Although there is serologic cross-reactivity between the morbilliviruses, heterologous antibody against CDV may not be detected in seals until 2 to 5 days after PDV-neutralizing antibody.[30] Furthermore, homologous antibody titers are generally higher than heterologous antibody titers.[23, 44]

Morbillivirus identification requires virus isolation and characterization. When fresh carcasses are available, a morbillivirus may be isolated from tissue homogenates in primary or secondary kidney cells.[43, 47] Alternatively, cocultivation of buffy coat leukocytes from infected animals with trypsinized Vero cells has proved successful.[56] Attempts at virus isolation from decomposed beached carcasses are generally unrewarding. However, recently developed reverse transcription-PCR techniques may be used on archival frozen or formalin-fixed tissues, making virus isolation less necessary.[41, 46]

TREATMENT AND CONTROL

There is no effective treatment for morbillivirus infection, but live attenuated vaccines are used to control infection in humans and domestic animals.[3] Whereas vaccination of free-ranging marine mammals would be logistically challenging and ethically questionable, the protection of captive animals may warrant intervention. Effective quarantine of newly arrived animals or of stranded animals under rehabilitation is essential to protect immunologically naive animals in captivity.[18]

In Europe, commercially available attenuated CDV vaccine was used to immunize stranded harbor and gray seals.[10, 36] Experimental inactivated and subunit CDV vaccines have had mixed success in protecting harbor seals.[55, 58, 59] No vaccination trials have yet been conducted on cetaceans.

REFERENCES

1. Aguilar A, Raga JA: The striped dolphin epizootic in the Mediterranean Sea. Ambio 22:524–528, 1993.
2. Appel MJG: Pathogenesis of canine distemper. Am J Vet Res 30:1167–1182, 1969.
3. Appel MJG, Gibbs EPJ, Martin SJ, et al: Morbillivirus diseases in animals and man. *In* Kurstak E, Kurstak C (eds): Comparative diagnosis of viral disease IV. New York, Academic Press, pp 235–297, 1981.
4. Anderson RM, May RM: The invasion, persistence and spread of infectious diseases within animal and plant communities. Philos Trans Royal Soc Lond B 314:533–570, 1986.
5. Barrett T, Blixenkrone-Møller M, Di Guardo G, et al: Morbilliviruses in aquatic mammals: report on round table discussion. Vet Microbiol 44:261–265, 1995.
6. Bengtson JL, Boveng P, Franzen U, et al: Antibodies to canine distemper virus in Antarctic seals. Mar Mamm Sci 7:85–87, 1991.
7. Bolt G, Blixenkrone-Møller M, Gottschlack E, et al: Nucleotide and deduced amino acid sequences of the matrix (M) and fusion (F) protein genes of cetacean morbilliviruses isolated from a porpoise and a dolphin. Virus Res 34:291–304, 1994.

8. Bostock CJ, Barrett T, Crowther JR: Characterization of the European seal morbillivirus. Vet Microbiol 23:351–360, 1990.
9. Calzada N, Lockyer CH, Aguilar A: Age and sex composition of the striped dolphin die-off in the western Mediterranean. Mar Mamm Sci 10:299–310, 1994.
10. Carter SD, Hughes DE, Taylor VJ, et al: Immune responses in common and grey seals during the seal epizootic. Sci Total Environ 115:83–91, 1992.
11. Daoust P-Y, Haines D, Thorsen J, et al: Phocine distemper in a harp seal *(Phoca groenlandica)* from the Gulf of St Lawrence, Canada. J Wildl Dis 29:114–117, 1993.
12. Dietz R, Ansen CT, Have P, et al: Clue to seal epizootic. Nature 338:627, 1989.
13. Dietz R, Heide-Jørgensen MP, Härkönen T: Mass death of harbour seals *(Phoca vitulina)* in Europe. Ambio 18:258–264, 1989.
14. Domingo M, Visa J, Pumarola M, et al: Pathologic and immunocytochemical studies of morbillivirus infection in striped dolphins *(Stenella coeruleoalba)*. Vet Pathol 29:1–10, 1992.
15. Duignan PJ, Duffy N, Rima BK, et al: Comparative antibody response in harbour and grey seals naturally infected by a morbillivirus. Vet Immunol Immunopathol 55:341–349, 1997.
16. Duignan PJ, Geraci JR, Raga JA, et al: Pathology of morbillivirus infection in striped dolphins *(Stenella coeruleoalba)* from Valencia and Murcia, Spain. Can J Vet Res 56:242–248, 1992.
17. Duignan PJ, House C, Geraci JR, et al: Morbillivirus infection in cetaceans of the western Atlantic. Vet Microbiol 44:241–249, 1995.
18. Duignan PJ, House C, Geraci JR, et al: Morbillivirus infection in two species of pilot whale *(Globicephala* sp) from the western Atlantic. Mar Mamm Sci 11:150–162, 1995.
19. Duignan PJ, House C, Walsh M, et al: Morbillivirus infection in manatees. Mar Mamm Sci 11:441–451, 1995.
20. Duignan PJ, House C, Odell DK, et al: Morbillivirus infection in bottlenose dolphins: evidence for recurrent epizootics in the western Atlantic and Gulf of Mexico. Mar Mamm Sci 12:499–515, 1996.
21. Duignan PJ, Nielsen O, House C, et al: Epizootiology of morbillivirus infection in harp, hooded, and ringed seals from the Canadian Arctic and western Atlantic. J Wildl Dis 33:7–19, 1997.
22. Duignan PJ, Sadove S, Saliki JT, et al: Phocine distemper in harbor seals *(Phoca vitulina)* from Long Island, New York. J Wildl Dis 29:465–469, 1993.
23. Duignan PJ, Saliki JT, St Aubin DJ, et al: Epizootiology of morbillivirus infection in North American harbor seals *(Phoca vitulina)* and gray seals *(Halichoerus grypus)*. J Wildl Dis 31:491–501, 1995.
24. Duignan PJ, Saliki JT, St Aubin DJ, et al: Neutralizing antibodies to phocine distemper virus in Atlantic walruses *(Odobenus rosmarus rosmarus)*. J Wildl Dis 30:90–94, 1994.
25. Geraci JR: Clinical investigation of the 1987–1988 mass mortality of bottlenose dolphins along the U.S. central and south Atlantic coast. Final report to the National Marine Fisheries Service and U.S. Navy Office of Naval Research and Marine Mammal Commission, Washington, DC, pp 4–11, 1989.
26. Goodhart CB: Did virus transfer from harp seals to common seals? Nature 336:21, 1988.
27. Grachev MA, Kumarev VP, Mamaev LV, et al: Distemper virus in Baikal seals. Nature 338:209, 1989.
28. Haas L, Subbarao SM, Harder T, et al: Detection of phocid distemper virus RNA in seal tissues using slot hybridization and the polymerase chain reaction amplification assay: genetic evidence that the virus is distinct from canine distemper virus. J Gen Virol 72:825–832, 1991.
29. Harder T, Willhaus TH, Frey HR, et al: Morbillivirus infections of seals during the 1988 epidemic in the Bay of Heligoland: transmission studies of cell culture–propagated virus in harbor seals *(Phoca vitulina)* and a grey seal *(Halichoerus grypus)*: clinical, virological and serological results. J Vet Med B 37:641–650, 1990.
30. Harder T, Willhaus T, Liebold W, et al: Investigations on course and outcome of phocine distemper virus infection in harbour seals *(Phoca vitulina)* exposed to polychlorinated biphenyls. J Vet Med B 39:19–31, 1992.
31. Harder TC, Stede M, Willhaus T, et al: Morbillivirus antibodies of maternal origin in harbour seal pups *(Phoca vitulina)*. Vet Rec 132:632–633, 1993.
32. Harwood J, Carter SD, Hughes DE, et al: Seal disease predictions. Nature 339:670, 1989.
33. Harwood J, Grenfell B: Long term risks of recurrent seal plagues. Mar Pollut Bull 21:284–287, 1990.
34. Heide-Jørgensen MP, Härkönen T, Dietz R, et al: Retrospective of the 1988 European seal epizootic. Dis Aquat Org 13:37–62, 1992.

35. Hofmeister R, Brewer E, Ernst R, et al: Distemper-like disease in harbor seals: virus isolation, further pathologic and serologic findings. J Vet Med B 35:765–769, 1988.
36. Hughes DE, Carter SD, Robinson I, et al: Anti-canine distemper virus antibodies in common and grey seals. Vet Rec 130:449–450, 1992.
37. Kennedy S, Kuiken T, Ross HM, et al: Morbillivirus infection in two common porpoises *(Phocoena phocoena)* from the coasts of England and Scotland. Vet Rec 131:286–290, 1992.
38. Kennedy S, Smyth JA, Cush PF, et al: Viral distemper now found in porpoises. Nature 336:21, 1988.
39. Kennedy S, Smyth JA, Cush P, et al: Histopathologic and immunocytochemical studies of distemper in seals. Vet Pathol 26:97–103, 1989.
40. Kennedy S, Smyth JA, Cush P, et al: Histopathologic and immunocytochemical studies of distemper in harbor porpoises. Vet Pathol 28:1–7, 1991.
41. Krafft A, Lichy JH, Lipscomb TP, et al: Postmortem diagnosis of morbillivirus infection in bottlenose dolphins *(Tursiops truncatus)* in the Atlantic and Gulf of Mexico epizootics by polymerase chain-based assay. J Wildl Dis 31:410–415, 1995.
42. Krogsrud J, Evensen O, Holt G, et al: Seal distemper in Norway in 1988 and 1989. Vet Rec 126:460–461, 1990.
43. Liess B, Frey HR, Zaghawa A: Morbilliviruses in seals: isolation and some growth characteristics in cell cultures. Dtsch Tierarztl Wochenschr 96:180–182, 1989.
44. Liess B, Frey HR, Zaghawa A, et al: Morbillivirus infection in seals *(Phoca vitulina)* during the 1988 epidemic in the Bay of Heligoland. J Vet Med B 36:601–608, 1989.
45. Lipscomb TP, Schulman FY, Moffatt D, et al: Morbilliviral disease in Atlantic dolphins *(Tursiops truncatus)* from the 1987–1988 epizootic. J Wildl Dis 30:567–571, 1994.
46. Mamaev LV, Visser IKG, Belikov SI, et al: Canine distemper in Lake Baikal seals *(Phoca sibirica)*. Vet Rec 138:437–439, 1996.
47. McCullough SJ, McNeilly F, Allan GM, et al: Isolation and characterization of a porpoise morbillivirus. Arch Virol 118:247–252, 1991.
48. Munro R, Ross H, Cornwell C, et al: Disease conditions affecting common seals *(Phoca vitulina)* around the Scottish mainland, September-November 1988. Sci Total Environ 115:67–82, 1992.
49. Osterhaus ADME, Groen J, De Vries P, et al: Canine distemper virus in seals. Nature 335:403–404, 1988.
50. Rima BK, Baczko K, Imagawa DT, et al: Humoral immune response in dogs with old dog encephalitis and chronic distemper meningo-encephalitis. J Gen Virol 68:1723–1735, 1987.
51. Rima BK, Cosby SL, Duffy N, et al: Humoral immune responses in seals infected by phocine distemper virus. Res Vet Sci 49:114–116, 1990.
52. Stuen S, Have P, Osterhaus ADME, et al: Serological investigation of virus infections in harp seals *(Phoca groenlandica)* and hooded seals *(Cystophora cristata)*. Vet Rec 134:501–503, 1994.
53. Svansson V, Arnason A, Blixenkrone-Møller M: Sero-epidemiological studies of morbillivirus infections in whales. International Whaling Commission SC/F91/F22:1–5, 1991.
54. Thompson PM, Hall AJ: Seals and epizootics—what factors might affect the severity of mass mortalities? Mamm Rev 23:149–154, 1993.
55. Van Bressem MF, De Meurichy J, Chappuis G, et al: Attempt to vaccinate orally harbour seals against phocid distemper. Vet Rec 129:362, 1991.
56. Visser IKG, Kumarev VP, Orvell C, et al: Comparison of two morbilliviruses isolated from seals during outbreaks of distemper in north west Europe and Siberia. Arch Virol 111:148–164, 1990.
57. Visser IKG, Van Bressem MF, de Zwart RL, et al: Characterization of morbilliviruses isolated from dolphins and porpoises in Europe. J Gen Virol 74:631–642, 1993.
58. Visser IKG, van de Bildt MWG, Brugge HN, et al: Vaccination of harbour seals *(Phoca vitulina)* against phocid distemper with two different inactivated canine distemper virus (CDV) vaccines. Vaccine 7:531–526, 1989.
59. Visser IKG, Vedder EJ, Van De Bildt MWG, et al: Canine distemper virus ISCOMS induce protection in harbour seals *(Phoca vitulina)* against phocid distemper but still allow subsequent infection with phocid distemper virus-1. Vaccine 10:435–438, 1992.
60. Visser IKG, Vedder VJ, Vos HW, et al: Continued presence of phocine distemper in the Dutch Wadden Sea seal population. Vet Rec 25:320–322, 1993.

CHAPTER **71**

Fetal Ultrasonography in Dolphins with Emphasis on Gestational Aging

L. RAE STONE
ROBERT L. JOHNSON
JAY C. SWEENEY
MARIA L. LEWIS

Diagnostic ultrasonography is becoming widely used as a valuable tool in the clinical assessment and management of marine mammals. It has proved to be a major advancement in clinical and research aspects of marine mammal medicine because it is safe, is noninvasive, and provides a wealth of information.[18] The uses of ultrasonography include imaging of the lungs and pleura, the reproductive organs, the bladder, kidneys, liver, spleen, and other abdominal structures, and miscellaneous soft tissues; it is used in echocardiography as well.[18] One of the most beneficial uses of ultrasonography is in the diagnosis of pregnancy and assessment of fetal viability and fetal growth.

Atlantic bottlenose dolphins (*Tursiops truncatus*) have reproduced in public display and research facilities for more than 50 years. For many years, pregnancy diagnosis was difficult because the physical signs of pregnancy in the dolphin are not always noticeable until late in gestation.[16] Current methods of early pregnancy diagnosis in dolphins can be based on persistent elevation of serum progesterone levels by radioimmunoassay[10, 15, 16] or on diagnostic ultrasonography.[18, 20] The benefits of real-time B-mode ultrasonography are that it is noninvasive, it provides an early and reliable pregnancy diagnosis, and it provides an opportunity to evaluate fetal growth, viability, and development.[18]

Diagnostic ultrasonography is used extensively in human medicine in the assessment of the fetus and pregnancy. Uses include estimations of gestational age, fetal size, and weight, assessment of fetal growth, detection of fetal abnormalities, and evaluation of fetal well-being.[1, 2] Transabdominal ultrasonography has been used widely in veterinary medicine for the diagnosis of pregnancy.[5, 6, 9, 11, 17] More recently, fetal growth charts and biophysical profiles have been developed for several species of domestic animals, including dogs, cats, and horses.[5, 9, 12, 17] Previous fetal growth charts for dolphin species, including *Tursiops,* have been based on linear regression of direct observation of the size and weight of newborn calves.[10] Some workers have used ultrasonography in the development of a fetal growth chart.[20] However, this study was hampered by limitations of the ultrasound equipment used and the relatively few data points obtained.

To develop accurate fetal growth charts that would simplify gestational aging in dolphins, four pregnant primiparous bottlenose dolphins that became pregnant at the Dolphin Quest (public display facility on the island of Hawaii) were evaluated ultrasonographically by Stone and Sweeney. In each case, numerous serial ultrasonographic evaluations were performed from 4 weeks after conception to term. At each examination, multiple fetal size parameters were evaluated, and measurements were repeated to obtain the maximal value of each parameter at each examination. After parturition, the data were analyzed in order to create fetal growth charts for each fetus.

Four live calves were delivered. On the basis of serial ultrasound examinations, perinatal complications were anticipated in two of the four deliveries. One, which was seen to be quite large (maternal/fetal disproportion), was hypoxic and died shortly after a prolonged delivery. Another, which was seen to be quite small (intrauterine growth restriction), required intensive neonatal treatment and nutritional supplementation. This calf survived and continues to develop normally.

Methods of diagnostic ultrasonography in dolphins have been previously described in detail.[18] Thorough ultrasonographic evaluation of pregnancy in dolphins requires the use of real-time transabdominal B- and M-mode ultrasonography with a 3.5-MHz sector transducer to determine fetal size, shape, and presentation; calculate fetal heart rate (FHR); observe fetal movements;

and evaluate the quantity and quality of the fetal fluids and the integrity of the uteroplacental unit.

Dolphins that are properly trained for husbandry procedures quickly become accustomed to and learn to cooperate with the ultrasonographic examination without restraint. To minimize manipulation, the pregnant dolphin should be scanned without being removed from the water if possible. Ideally, two trainers should stabilize the dolphin in the water to reduce maternal movements. The trainer at the dolphin's head maintains contact while adjusting the dolphin's position by moving the rostrum and/or pectoral fin. The trainer at the dolphin's tail supports the peduncle. Other methods of unrestrained examination include the use of slide-out behaviors or shallow water support. If the dolphin is not trained for behaviors that can be adapted to voluntary examination, the animal, in the first and second trimesters, can be removed from the water and restrained on foam pads.

Water is an excellent conducting medium for ultrasound waves; however, most ultrasound transducers are not sealed, and immersion in salt water may cause serious, expensive damage. To prevent this, the transducer must be enclosed in a watertight plastic covering. This is easily accomplished by placing a small amount of commercial ultrasound coupling gel (E-Z Scan Gel; E-Z EM Co., Westbury, NY) on the contact surface of the transducer and inverting a heavy-gauge, plastic, large animal rectal sleeve (Ag-Tek Poly Sleeve; Kane Enterprises, Sioux Falls, SD) over the transducer and its cable, taking care to avoid trapping air bubbles over the contact surface. The sleeve can be secured with elastic bands, sealing the end closest to the machine with electrical tape and being careful to avoid excessive tension on the plastic sleeve. This technique is not completely without risk, and the integrity of the sleeve should be checked frequently. Commercial transducer covers are also available (CIV-Flex Sterile Ultrasound Transducer Cover Kit, CIVCO, Kalona, IA). If the dolphin is scanned out of the water, copious amounts of ultrasound gel should be used to provide good contact to achieve optimal image quality.

Because of the extensive ventral abdominal muscle mass in dolphins, the best ultrasonographic window for the gravid uterus is generally low on either side of the lateral abdomen. It may be necessary to place the dolphin in a lateral position and scan from the "down" side to image a fetus that is in the dependent portion of the uterus.

In humans, in whom mean gestation length is 284 days (40.6 weeks) ± 23 days,[3] the gestational sac or conceptus can be imaged transabdominally as early as 4 weeks after conception.[7] Standardized measurements such as the biparietal (skull) diameter, abdominal circumference, head circumference, and femur length can be used to age the human fetus with great accuracy up to 20 weeks after conception, after which time a greater variability in size is seen around the mean as the pregnancy progresses.[8] By 26 weeks, or the third trimester of gestation, all fetal measurements become more related to the rate of fetal growth rather than gestational age, and by 30 weeks, an accurate gestational age assessment cannot be performed.[3] Current guidelines suggest that the gestational age is best determined at 8 to 10 weeks and that human high-risk pregnancies be evaluated with serial ultrasound examinations.[1, 4]

The monitoring of fetal growth in the management of human pregnancy is important because of the profound consequences that are associated with decreased growth in utero.[4] Evidence of intrauterine growth restriction (IUGR) is correlated with an increased risk for stillbirth, premature delivery, and intrapartum asphyxia. Hypocalcemia, hypoglycemia, polycythemia, meconium aspiration, intracerebral hemorrhage, and convulsions are among the neonatal complications.[4] Significant long-term effects such as reduced somatic growth, seizures, poor coordination, and mental retardation have also been reported.[4]

On the basis of serial ultrasound evaluations of four dolphin pregnancies performed from 4 weeks after conception to 1 day preparturition, measurements of fetal size were obtained and individual fetal growth rates were determined. These pregnancies lasted 48 weeks. Numerous parameters were initially evaluated. Biparietal (skull) diameter and thoracic diameter were the most consistently obtainable and repeatable and were the most reliable measurements of fetal growth.

In all of the pregnancies, the conceptus, consisting of the embryo, the yolk sac, and the developing allantois, could be visualized as early as 4 weeks. The conceptus was seen as a thin-walled fluid-filled cystic structure, which was usually round but which was sometimes irregular, measuring 3 to 4 cm in diameter. The embryo itself could be seen as a small, poorly differentiated soft tissue structure measuring approximately 1 cm (range 0.8 to 1.2 cm) in the dependent portion of the gestational sac (Fig. 71–1). By 8 weeks after conception, the thorax and skull of the fetus could be reliably identified and measured.

From 4 weeks to term, a longitudinal growth study of the four fetuses was performed. The maximal values obtained at each evaluation for biparietal diameter and thoracic diameter of each fetus were then analyzed, resulting in the development of composite fetal growth curves for these two parameters. Applying linear regression analysis, a fetal growth rate chart for biparietal

diameter and thoracic diameter by week of gestation was created (Fig. 71–2). With the collection of more data, this chart will become more refined, and an increase in sample size should decrease the standard deviation from the mean.

The biparietal diameter (BPD) is defined here as the maximal external diameter of the skull perpendicular to midline, obtained at a level where the midline of the skull can be clearly identified. This level is just above the level of the rostrum and the foramen magnum. Throughout gestation, there is a marked change in the shape of the skull. Initially, the skull appears round at all levels. Later in gestation, the skull appears oval shaped: wider than it is long in all but the uppermost levels of the cranial vault.

Thoracic diameter (TD) is defined here as the maximal lateral diameter of the thorax, measured from the outside of the rib to the outside of the rib at the level of the maximal width of the ventricles of the heart. When measuring the BPD and TD, it is critical to place the cursors exactly at the external bony margins, (i.e., excluding fetal blubber and skin) and for placement to be perpendicular to the fetal midline. Small errors in measurement can lead to underestimation or overestimation of gestational age and can obscure the diagnosis of IUGR.

The ratio of the BPD to TD can be calculated at each of the serial examinations. As seen from Figure 71–2 and in humans,[4] this ratio decreases from the first trimester to term. An abnormality of this ratio may indicate an asymmetric growth restriction that is generally associated with an increased likelihood of perinatal complications in humans.[4] Serial ultrasound evaluations of dolphin fetuses is the only way to monitor possible growth restrictions and to determine the significance of an abnormal parameter, particularly in relation to maternal weight gain.[4] Previous work with bottlenose dolphins has shown that there is a significant improvement in calf survival in the first year associated with a minimum maternal weight gain of at least 100 pounds (Jay Sweeney, personal communication, 1996). Serial ultrasound evaluations also allow the facility to make preparations for possible perinatal complications that may

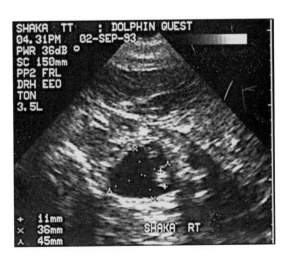

FIGURE 71–1. Dolphin embryo number 4 within gestational sac at 4 weeks' gestational age (early in the first trimester). The gestational sac may be round or irregular in shape. In this image, the embryo measures 1.1 cm and is seen on the right. The gestational sac measures 3.6 × 4.5 cm. This image was obtained with a Micro-Imager 2000 (Ausonics, Universal Medical Systems, Bedford Hills, NY), using a 3.5-MHz mechanical sector transducer at a depth of 15 cm.

Dolphin Fetal Growth Chart (BPD & TD)

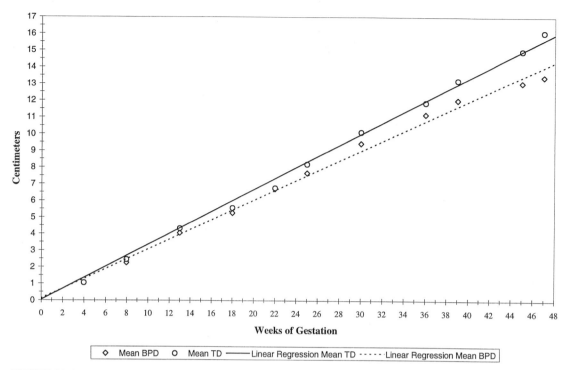

FIGURE 71–2. Dolphin fetal growth chart. Squares represent actual mean biparietal diameter (BPD); dashed lines represent linear regression of BPD data; circles represent actual mean thoracic diameter (TD); solid lines represent regression of TD data.

require intensive care and management. In Rae Stone's experience, one dolphin fetus that had a persistently abnormal BPD:TD ratio was underweight at birth and required supplementation.

Hallmarks of the first trimester (weeks 0 to 16, based on a gestation of 48 weeks) of gestation include visualization of the conceptus by 4 weeks after conception (see Fig. 71–1). Cardiac activity may be seen earlier, but, in general, organized, rhythmic cardiac activity is seen by 6 to 8 weeks after conception. Large volumes of anechoic allantoic fluid accumulate rapidly. At 4 weeks, the maximal allantoic fluid depth seen ranged from 2 to 4 cm, and by 12 weeks, the range of maximal fluid depth seen was from 8 to 19 cm. The development of such a large fluid volume may be an additional component of the countercurrent heat exchange that has been described in the dolphin uterus.[14] Later in the first trimester, the fetus shows evidence of organ differentiation. The lung, cardiac structures, liver, diaphragm, stomach, and blubber become discretely identifiable, with the dorsal and ventral musculature becoming prominent.

In the second trimester (weeks 17 to 32), there are significant ongoing growth and differentiation. However, there is a generalized increase in fetal activity and a tendency for the fetus to be oriented obliquely in relationship to the maternal long axis, making accurate fetal measurement more difficult. Some ultrasound machines are equipped with a cine recall feature that stores

up to 256 real-time frames, greatly enhancing the likelihood of obtaining good quality, accurate images even when the subject is moving. Significant increase in the TD and BPD is seen during the second trimester (Fig. 71–3). The amnion may not be discretely visible in the first or second trimester because it is relatively closely applied to the fetus. Allantoic fluid depths in this trimester range from approximately 10 to 16 cm, again influenced by fetal orientation and movement. In the first two trimesters, there is significant variability in the orientation of the fetus. The fetus may be in an anterior presentation on one examination, and then in an posterior or an oblique presentation on a subsequent examination, or even later in the same examination. FHRs can be readily evaluated in this trimester with the use of M-mode ultrasonography. The FHR should show variability of at least 15 beats per minute between resting and postactivity values (Fig. 71–4). If the heart rate does not increase significantly with exercise, fetal distress should be considered. Overall fetal activity levels are highest near the end of the second trimester.

In the third trimester, gestational aging is likely to be less accurate. It appears that, as in humans,[3] fetal size in this trimester is more highly correlated to individual fetal growth than actual gestational age (Fig. 71–5). Early in this trimester, a significant curvature of the entire fetal length develops. The fluke can be seen pointing toward the rostrum. Once the fetus assumes this curvature, the amnion may be seen as a thin mem-

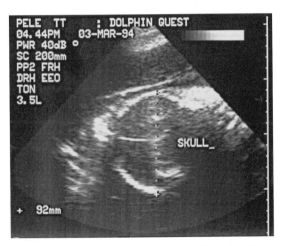

FIGURE 71–3. Dolphin fetus number 3 at 30 weeks of gestation (late in the second trimester). The skull is seen in a coronal section with a distinct midline. The skull becomes more oval (wider from side to side) as the fetus develops. The biparietal diameter measures 9.2 cm. This image was obtained with a Micro-Imager 2000 (Ausonics, Universal Medical Systems, Bedford Hills, NY), using a 3.5-MHz mechanical sector transducer at a depth of 20 cm.

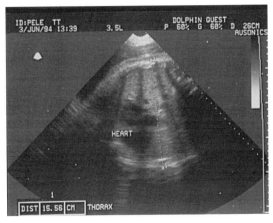

FIGURE 71–5. Dolphin fetus number 3 at 45 weeks of gestation (late in the third trimester). The thorax is seen in cross section with the dorsum of the fetus to the right of the image. Several ribs are seen casting acoustic shadows. The thoracic diameter measures 15.56 cm. This image was obtained with an Opus I (Ausonics, Universal Medical Systems, Bedford Hills, NY), using a 3.5-MHz mechanical sector transducer at a depth of 26 cm.

brane stretching from the fluke to the pectoral fin, with amniotic fluid collected within the curve. The amnion may also be occasionally seen sagging below the fetus or at its attachment to its umbilicus. The fetus may be quite active in the third trimester; however, prolonged resting phases occur in which no evidence of fetal activity is seen. As the fetus develops, breathing movements are seen by 40 to 44 weeks of gestation as discrete craniocaudal movements of the diaphragm with significant, rhythmic thoracic excursions seen in the frontal plane (Fig. 71–6).

The use of ultrasonography to evaluate the growth, viability, and development of the fetus has tremendous value to the reproductive management of cetaceans. Fetal ultrasonography, if properly used, can help predict calving dates and the possibility of perinatal complications, allowing time for planning and preparation by the animal care staff. The information gained should be considered when making husbandry decisions including appropriate social grouping and behavioral management. Fetal ultrasonography also has significant applications in the evaluations of the reproductive status of wild dolphins as a component of overall population health assessment.[19] As in other areas of research, ultrasound data collected for bottlenose dolphins may serve as a model for other cetacean species. The information in this chapter on fetal ultrasonography should be use-

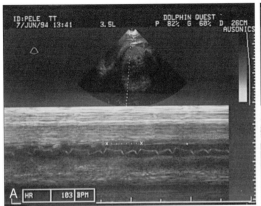

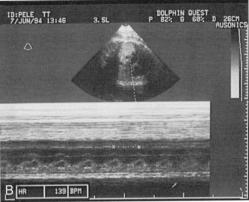

FIGURE 71–4. M-mode scans of resting and postactivity fetal heart rates in dolphin fetus number 3 at 45 weeks of gestation (late in the third trimester). Images were obtained with an Opus I (Ausonics, Universal Medical Systems, Bedford Hills, NY), using a 3.5-MHz mechanical sector transducer at a depth of 26 cm. The path of the M-mode *(bottom)* through the heart is indicated by the line seen extending through the B-mode image *(top)*. *A,* Resting FHR of 103 beats per minute. *B,* Immediate postactivity FHR of 139 beats per minute.

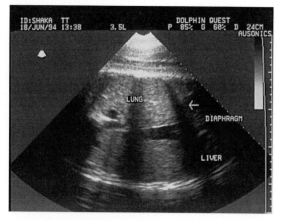

FIGURE 71–6. Dolphin fetus number 4 at 46 weeks of gestation (late in the third trimester). In this sagittal plane, the rostrum of the fetus is to the left of the image. The lung can be seen separated from the liver by the diaphragm and the caudal vena cava. In real-time, fetal breathing movements would be seen as rhythmic craniocaudal movements of the diaphragm, often associated with visible compression and expansion of the fetal thorax. This image was obtained with an Opus I (Ausonics, Universal Medical Systems, Bedford Hills, NY), using a 3.5-MHz mechanical sector transducer at a depth of 24 cm.

ful, in combination with advanced reproductive technologies, in the development of breeding programs for threatened or endangered cetacean species, or in cetacean species for which breeding programs have not yet had as much success as for bottlenose dolphins.[13]

REFERENCES

1. American College of Obstetricians and Gynecologists: Ultrasonography in Pregnancy [Technical Bulletin No. 187]. Washington, DC, American College of Obstetricians and Gynecologists, 1993.
2. Birnholz JC: Fetal behavior and condition. *In* Callen PW (ed): Ultrasound in Obstetrics and Gynecology. Philadelphia, WB Saunders, pp 159–167, 1983.
3. Bowie JD, Andreotti RF: Estimating gestational age in utero. *In* Callen PW (ed): Ultrasound in Obstetrics and Gynecology. Philadelphia, WB Saunders, pp 21–39, 1983.
4. Deter RL, Hadlock FP, Harrist RB: Evaluation of normal fetal growth and the detection of intrauterine growth retardation. *In* Callen PW (ed): Ultrasound in Obstetrics and Gynecology. Philadelphia, WB Saunders, pp 113–140, 1983.
5. Ginther OJ: Ultrasonic Imaging and Reproductive Events in the Mare. Cross Plains, WI, Equiservices, 1986.
6. Ginther OJ: Reproductive Biology of the Mare: Basic and Applied Aspects, 2nd ed. Cross Plains, WI, Equiservices, 1992.
7. Lyons EA, Levi CS: Ultrasound in the first trimester of pregnancy. *In* Callen PW (ed): Ultrasound in Obstetrics and Gynecology. Philadelphia, WB Saunders, pp 1–19, 1983.
8. National Institutes of Health Consensus Development Conference 1984. Diagnostic Imaging in Pregnancy [NIH Publication No. 84–667]. Washington, DC, U.S. Department of Health and Human Services, 1984.
9. Nyland TG, Mattoon JS: Veterinary Diagnostic Ultrasound. Philadelphia, WB Saunders, 1995.
10. Perrin WF, Reilly SB: Reproductive parameters of dolphins and small whales of the family Delphinidae. *In* Perrin WF, Brownell RL Jr, DeMaster DP (eds): Reproduction in Whales, Dolphins and Porpoises. Cambridge, MA, International Whaling Commission Special Issue 6, pp 97–133, 1984.
11. Pipers FS, Adams-Brendemuehl CS. Techniques and applications of transabdominal ultrasonography in the pregnant mare. J Am Vet Med Assoc 185:766–771, 1984.
12. Reef VB, Vaala WE, Worth LT, et al: Ultrasonographic evaluation of the fetus and intrauterine environment in healthy mares during late gestation. Vet Radiol Ultrasound 36:533–541, 1995.
13. Robeck TR, Curry BE, McBain JF, Kraemer DC: Reproductive biology of the bottlenose dolphin (*Tursiops truncatus*) and the potential application of advanced reproductive technologies. J Zoo Wildl Med 25:321–336, 1994.
14. Rommel SA, Pabst DA, McLellan WA: Functional morphology of the vascular plexuses associated with the cetacean uterus. Anat Rec 237:538–546, 1993.
15. Schroeder JP: Breeding bottlenose dolphins in captivity. *In* Leatherwood S, Reeves RR (eds): The Bottlenose Dolphin. New York, Academic Press, pp 435–446, 1990.
16. Schroeder JP: Reproductive aspects of marine mammals. *In* Dierauf LA (ed): Handbook of Marine Mammal Medicine—Health, Disease and Rehabilitation. Boca Raton, CRC Press, pp 353–369, 1990.
17. Sertich PL: Ultrasonography of the genital tract of the mare. *In* Reef VB (ed): Diagnostic Ultrasound of the Horse. Philadelphia, WB Saunders, in press.
18. Stone LR: Diagnostic ultrasound in marine mammals. *In* Dierauf LA (ed): Handbook of Marine Mammal Medicine—Health, Disease and Rehabilitation. Boca Raton, CRC Press, pp 235–264, 1990.
19. Stone LR, Rhinehart HL: Diagnostic ultrasound evaluation of wild *Tursiops truncatus* in Matagorda Bay, Texas. Marine Mammal Medicine, in press.
20. Williamson P, Gales NJ, Lister S: Use of real-time B-mode ultrasound for pregnancy diagnosis and measurement of fetal growth rate in captive bottlenose dolphins (*Tursiops truncatus*). J Reprod Fertil 88:543–548, 1990.

CHAPTER 72

Manatee Medicine

MICHAEL T. WALSH
GREGORY D. BOSSART

The order Sirenia is composed of two families: (1) the family Trichechidae, which includes the West Indian manatee (*Trichechus manatus*), the Amazonian manatee (*Trichechus inunguis*), and the West African manatee (*Trichechus senegalensis*), and (2) the family Dugongidae, which includes the dugong (*Dugong dugon*) and the extinct Steller's sea cow (*Hydrodamalis gigas*). The interested reader is referred to the book "Manatees and Dugongs" by John E. Reynolds and Daniel K. Odell[18] for more in depth information on biology and environmental relationships of these species.

Trichechus manatus has been further divided into two subspecies: the Antillean manatee (*Trichechus manatus manatus*) and the Florida manatee (*Trichechus manatus latirostris*). The Florida manatee is a herbivore that feeds on a variety of sea grasses and other aquatic plants. Although they are found along both coasts of Florida, their range is limited by cold water with portions of the population migrating to South Florida during the winter months. During warm months they may extend their range into Texas and Louisiana and up the east coast as far as the northern portions of Chesapeake Bay. One individual has been recovered as far west as Texas during the winter months.

BIOLOGIC DATA

Anatomy

Anatomically, the manatee is unique, as shown in Figure 72–1. Newborn manatees range in weight from 18 to 45 kg. They stay with their mothers for 1.5 to 2.5 years. In females the genital slit is found close to the anus; the penile opening in the male is caudal to the umbilical scar. Adult males are generally thinner than females, which may reach over 1200 kg in weight and 3.5 m in length. Average male weights are more in the range of 400 to 600 kg. The torso is tubular longitudinally but elliptical in cross section. The tail is paddle-shaped, and pelvic bones are vestigial. Front limbs are referred to as pectoral flippers and have three to four nails present. The pectoral flippers of the male are longer in proportion to body length and have a ventral Velcro-like surface, both of which are advantageous for holding the female during breeding. The skin is thick and gray to brown, depending on the age of the epidermis between sloughing episodes and the presence of algae. It is similar in texture to the skin of the elephant, with individual sparse hairs present. The mammary glands are in the axilla. The prehensile muzzle has retractable vibrissae centrally and is very tactile. The eyes are small comparatively with iris eyelids. There are no external pinnae.

Internally, the body cavities are divided longitudinally, with the lungs situated dorsally along the back. Each lung is separated into a complete hemithorax by separate hemidiaphragms. The lungs are long and flattened, extending the length of the body cavity. The heart is ventral to the lungs and located in the anterior portion of the ventral coelomic cavity anterior to the liver. The liver is not separated from the heart by the diaphragm. The stomach has one main compartment with an anterior cardiac gland, which produces digestive enzymes and acid. The proximal duodenum is enlarged and is flanked by two diverticuli. The lengthy small intestine is separated from the large intestine by a small ovoid cecum, which has two small diverticuli. Histologically, the mucosa of portions of intestinal tract is predominantly a flattened squamous epithelium.

The spleen is small and ovoid and may be multiple. The kidneys are multilobular and found caudally in the abdominal potion of the coelomic cavity beneath the caudal portion of the lungs.

Physiology

Manatees become sexually mature generally between 6 and 10 years of age; this maturity may be influenced by size as well as age. Females in estrus are often pursued and embraced by numerous males. Gestation is approximately 12 months. Manatees socialize at different periods, but females appear to seek isolation during parturition. Gross nutrient analysis of manatee milk is presented in Table 72–1. Short- and medium-chain triglycerides predominate in the fat portion, and numerous sugars are present.

Like horses, manatees are hindgut fermenters.[18]

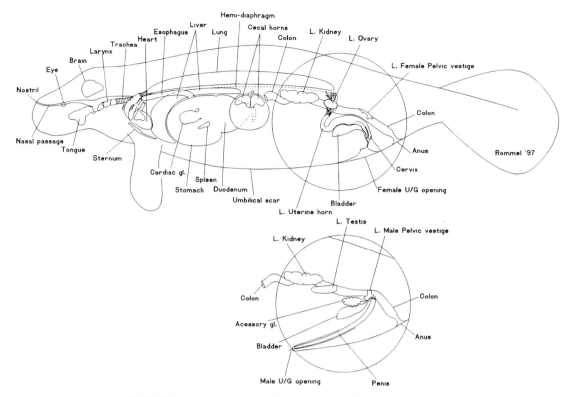

FIGURE 72–1. Artist's rendering of major organ relationships of the manatee.

They spend a large portion of their time grazing, alternating with periods of inactivity either on the surface or on the bottom of the ocean.

As a breath-holder, the manatee is capable of submerging for extended periods up to 20 minutes, although this may be quite variable. The respiratory frequency is also variable, but three or four breaths per 5-minute period are fairly typical.[19] Out of water, the respiratory rate may range from 3 to 15 breaths per 5-minute period. During rest periods, the manatee may slowly rise to the surface to breathe, then resume a resting posture. Normal heart rates average 50 and 60 beats per minute and decrease to about 30 during forced diving experiments by Scholander and Irving.[19]

In Florida, manatees generally migrate during the fall to warmer water in the south. Small populations may inhabit warm water springs during the winter, and larger groups frequent warm water discharges at power stations. Manatees prefer water temperatures greater than 20°C (68°F).

Manatees can live in fresh, brackish, or salt water environments for extended periods and in the wild move readily between both. Although most of their water source is apparently from food, there is some controversy as to whether manatees must drink from fresh water sources. It is reasonable that for some manatees, a fresh water source may be desirable during periods of illness, dehydration, or relative decreases in food intake. Fresh water exposure may also enhance turnover of skin seasonally.

TABLE 72–1. Nutritional Value of Feeds and Manatee Milk

Feed	Moisture (%)	Protein (%)	Fat (%)	Ash (%)	Carbohydrates (%)	Calories (per 100 g)
Romaine lettuce	95.6	0.9	0.04	0.6	2.9	16
Green leaf lettuce	94.8	1.1	0.1	0.8	3.2	18
Sea grass	87.0	1.8	0.2	2.5	8.5	43
Wheat (hydroponic)	87.0	2.8	0.5	0.2	9.7	60
Water lettuce	93.0	1.2	0.7	1.5	3.5	25
Water hyacinth	93.0	0.8	0.2	1.4	4.6	23
Timothy (75%) and alfalfa (25%)	6.0	8.1	2.2	7.0	76.7	354
Manatee milk*	75.0	7.5	15.5	1.0	1.0	189

*Milk from midlactation.

Husbandry

European descriptions of manatee anatomy in the 1800s were based on specimens obtained in the New World, although none actually survived the long boat trip back to Europe until 1875. Transportation mortalities appeared to be related to insufficient husbandry knowledge regarding water quality and dietary needs. Initial survivors of the voyage often died shortly after their arrival, again often compromised by diet, water quality, and temperature problems.[5, 9, 12, 13]

WATER QUALITY

Manatees in the wild spend most of their time in salt or brackish water with periods of time exposed to fresh water from springs, rivers, or runoff. Animals at zoos and aquaria are maintained permanently in salt water at one institution and predominantly in fresh water at three others in Florida. Manatees maintained exclusively in salt water (salinity, approximately 32 parts per thousand) are offered fresh water as a drinking source. No pathologic or physiologic abnormalities have been noted in two manatees maintained in these conditions for over 40 years at Miami Seaquarium. Those maintained predominantly in fresh water do show an increase in skin sloughing when moved between salt and fresh water. In addition, there appears to be an increase in corneal cloudiness in a group of animals maintained in fresh water with sun exposure and chlorine present.

Just as wild manatees are sensitive to cold water, those in captive environments do best in water ranging from 23° to 29°C (74° to 85°F). After a few days in water below 20°C (68°F), some individuals show shivering, loss of appetite, and changes in resting patterns. Alterations in immunologic parameters as evidenced by changes in lymphocyte subsets suggest that a compromised immunologic state may develop in chronically cold-stressed manatees. Temperatures greater than 31°C (88°F) may result in depression and loss of appetite in young orphans. Adult individuals can adapt to fairly high water temperatures, even greater than 32°C (90°F). Facilities should have heaters and chillers available if ambient water temperatures are outside suggested ranges.

Chlorine (less than 1 ppm) has been used as a disinfectant in some pools, usually in conjunction with ozone to promote the use of lower total chlorine levels. Filtration plants for manatees in closed environments must be substantial in comparison with those for cetaceans and pinnipeds because of the bioload produced by vegetation food use and abundant fecal production.

Space requirements based on individual physical or psychological requirements or on social needs are not well understood. Manatees have been successfully maintained in pools of varying sizes with good reproductive success at Miami Seaquarium for 40 years. The species is quite adaptable to different-sized habitats, but adequate pools should be available to accommodate shifting social structures, to separate males and females to control breeding, and for calving and nursing separately, away from other animals. A medical pool should be available with a false bottom or where the water can be drained to facilitate treatment. Minimum housing standards for marina mammals are included in the Animal Welfare Act.

NUTRITION AND FEEDING

In the wild, manatees ingest a variety of aquatic vegetation. In salt water this includes shoal grass, manatee grass (*Syringodium filiforme*), and turtle grass (*Thalassia testudinum*). Hydrilla and water hyacinth are more common food items in fresh water. The nutritional evaluation of one variety of seagrass in Table 72–1 shows that much of the caloric density is from carbohydrate sources. In captivity animals have been fed a wide variety of foods including lettuce, cabbage, hydroponic wheat and oats, vegetables such as carrots and sweet potatoes, Timothy-alfalfa hay, commercial monkey chow biscuits, and other concentrates designed for terrestrial species. Hydroponics fell out of favor because of fungal contamination during growth and clogging of filtration systems. Lettuce by itself (romaine and green leaf) has been used for extended periods but has numerous drawbacks, including poor nutritional content and expense. Overuse of dried foods such as hay mixtures could result in dehydration, and additional studies are needed to set standards for percentage of dry diet use in salt versus fresh water. Manatees maintained in fresh water often will not drink the water despite blood work changes indicating elevated serum creatinine and apparent hemoconcentration. Diets should also be designed with the prospect of future release involved. Food items that are vastly different from wild varieties such as some fruits and vegetables should not be used. In addition, animals slated for release should not be hand-fed.

A diet may incorporate 75% to 85% leafy green vegetables such as romaine and leaf lettuce, cabbage, kale, hydroponic wheat, oats, and sprouts (if available); 15% to 20% dried forage such as a Timothy-alfalfa hay (if filtration is modified to handle it); and a small percentage of vegetables (such as carrots) and concentrates such as those designed for elephants.

RESTRAINT AND HANDLING

Physical Restraint

Manatees are very powerful in the water; therefore, the key to initial restraint is removal from the wet environment. This is accomplished by draining the water from the pool and laying the animal on the bottom, using an elevating false bottom floor, or placing the animal in a stretcher in low water and removing it to a dry, padded work area. Manatees can roll on their sides and onto their backs; in these positions, the tail can be used as a powerful weapon. While a manatee is on its abdomen, a piece of foam can be placed over the tail, and one to two people can place their weight on the paddle; this limits movement for short procedures such as drawing blood, giving injections, and tube feeding. This procedure should be done with great caution by experienced personnel. As a result of their fractious nature, large manatees are rarely handled on their backs unless they are being treated for constipation or wound treatment. Animals that struggle can be placed on a restraint board to avoid injury to personnel or should be sedated. Manatees out of the water for more than a few minutes should be sprayed with water to keep the skin from drying.

Chemical Restraint

The most common drug used for sedation at Sea World is midazolam hydrochloride. At a dose of 0.045 mg/kg intramuscularly (IM), it can calm an excited manatee for approximately 60 to 90 minutes. This dose has also been used in transport to initially calm fractious, healthy animals. Movement and respiration are decreased, and the animal may appear asleep. It will, however, respond to stimuli and have an obvious palpebral reflex. Midazolam has been used in conjunction with meperidine hydrochloride at a dose up to 1 mg/kg to facilitate removal of a bony sequestrum from the radius of one manatee. Combinations of diazepam (0.066 mg/kg) with meperidine have been used at the Miami Seaquarium for removal of bony sequestra from vertebral injuries. Clinicians sedating an animal that holds its breath must pay very close attention to respiratory rate and depth, to mucous membrane color, and to responses to stimulis such as pain or to eye reflexes. Midazolam at higher doses (0.08 mg/kg) has been used to facilitate intubation for general anesthesia. The length of time until onset is up to 25 minutes. Oxygen supplementation should be available. Reversal agents are commonly used at the completion of a procedure. Flumazinil administered IM may be used to reverse the effects of diazepam and midazolam if the animal shows signs of incoordination or requires force feeding before going back into the water. If it is necessary to reverse the effects of meperidine, naloxone hydrochloride can be administered.

General anesthesia was not used in manatees until the mid-1980's.[24] This reluctance was based on the idea that manatees were voluntary breathers. Early attempts at general anesthesia in some marine mammals were inappropriate in medications, dosage, and approach, which seemed to contribute to this myth. This theory is not supported by clinical procedures and observations. Animals such as manatees or dolphins that inhale rapidly and deeply inhalations pull in volumes faster than that supplied by the average anesthesia machine. This mechanism, along with changes in rate and depth of respirations, may lead to hypoxia and hypercapnia. To augment rapid inhalation and induction, a reservoir system consisting of a modified plastic see-through, form-fitting, 5 gallon (20 L) water jug is placed over the face. The oral cavity is very small in manatees and the soft palate elongated, making access to the trachea through this route almost impossible. Once the animal is ready for intubation, an endoscope is introduced through one nostril and an elongated foal endotracheal tube with a stylet through the other. Opening of the larynx is observed endoscopically, and the endotracheal tube is inserted.

Only isoflurane has been used for general inhalation anesthesia with maintenance levels similar to those for other species. Animals should be monitored for end-tidal carbon dioxide levels, in addition to pulse oximeter and blood gases when available. Because the larynx is held open by the endotracheal tube, normal gas exchange is affected with the loss of lung expansion. To offset this, the animal should be placed on a ventilator, or, if a ventilator is not available, it must be bagged at regular intervals. Manatees left to breathe on their own are often ineffective, which again results in hypoxia and/or hypercapnia. Endotracheal tubes should be suctioned intermittently because of heavy mucus and the decreased tube size used. Dopram has been used to stimulate breathing, although placement of intravenous catheters is difficult. After the procedure, the midazolam is reversed with flumazinil on an equal-volume basis. Once the animal is awake, it is initially placed in shallow water and observed for a period of time before the water is deepened.

DIAGNOSTIC TECHNIQUES

Manatees from either wild or rehabilitating captive groups undergo diagnostic testing. As with all species, the most important initial tools are visualization, physical examination, and, when available, a history. Beyond this, the approach is similar to that for other species. Initially, a blood sample is taken from the interosseous space of the radius and ulna (Fig. 72–2). All venipuncture and injection sites are surgically scrubbed for a minimum of 2 minutes to decrease contamination from the rough skin. The middle portion of the medial surface of the pectoral flipper is cleaned, and an 18- or 20-gauge needle is inserted between the palpable medial edges of the radius and ulna. The vessels encountered are in a small plexus and are thus difficult to isolate for catheterization. If the animal is from the wild and appears emaciated or is an orphan, a reagent strip for glucose analysis is run immediately. Normal blood values are given in Table 72–2. Bossart[2] also investigated the diagnostic potential of lymphocyte phenotyping, which quantifies lymphocyte subsets, has potential correlation with immune suppression and disease response to therapy, and may provide prognostic information.

The physical examination should include an inspection for hooks in the oral cavity and may include a rectal palpation for fecal material to determine the presence of constipation and parasites. For all animals, radiographs of the torso should be taken. Interpretation is sometimes difficult because of the overlap of the respiratory and intestinal contents, but because of the unique anatomy of the manatee, this difficulty cannot be avoided.

Ultrasonography has also been used and should precede radiography if a pregnancy is likely, as evidenced by an enlarged vulva and abdominal distention. Observations from a complete examination are often affected by the gas found in a normal animal, but this technique has been used for pregnancy diagnosis, abdominal abscess evaluation, renal and bladder examination, and

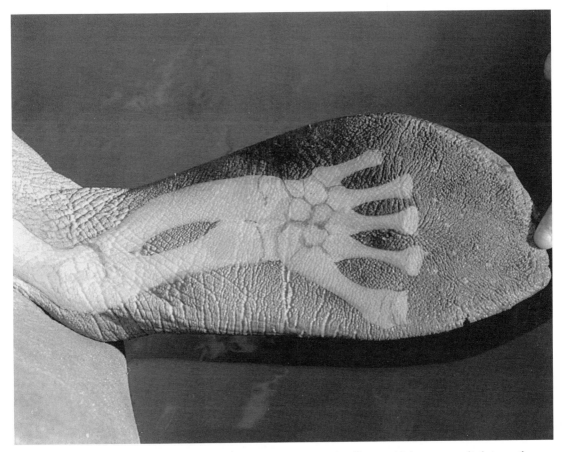

FIGURE 72–2. Bone structure of a manatee's pectoral flipper superimposed to illustrate this interosseous site between the radius and ulna used for blood sampling. The distal phalanges are not shown in this palmar view.

echocardiogram. Magnetic resonance imaging has been used on calves.

Urine collection by catheterization is extremely difficult because of the smallness of the vaginal tract, the distance of the urinary opening from the surface, and the resistance of the animal to the approach. Some success has been found in stimulating urine flow by applying pressure on the abdomen anterior to the vulva in females and posterior to the genital opening on the male. Patience is required.

In the authors' experience, endoscopic evaluation was tried in one animal to retrieve a foreign body, but general anesthesia was required. Stomach evacuation of plant material may take days, and gut transit time may range from 5 to 7 days, further complicating examination.

MEDICATION AND TREATMENT TECHNIQUES

Oral medication is usually administered by stomach tube, although some animals may take some materials voluntarily in preferred foods such as monkey chow. The crushing action of the palate and teeth does result in some drug loss into the water for some animals.

Antibiotics given orally may result in loss of normal intestinal flora, in diarrhea, and in hypermotility. As a result, the author does not recommend their use. Normal stool consistency can be reestablished by discontinuing the drug and reseeding the intestinal tract with fecal material from a normal manatee.

To avoid intestinal disturbance, most antibiotics are given in the caudal epaxial muscles. The injection site is always surgically prepared, in order to avoid contamination. The needle size is determined by the size of the animal; adults require up to a 3.5-inch, 20- to 18-gauge needle. Injections have also been given in the shoulder area, but this is discouraged because of a very small muscle mass and the potential for depositing the material in fascial planes, which could result in long-term complications. Common antibiotics used include amikacin (7 mg/kg BID IM), penicillins (penicillin G and benzathine penicillin at 22,000 U/kg), cephalosporins such as ceftrioxone (22 mg/kg SID IM), and oxytetracycline at cattle dosages. Combination antibiotic use, such as amikacin with penicillins or amikacin with ceftrioxone, have also been administered. Gentamycin has not been used because of its effect on the kidneys. Pharmacokinetic studies are needed to guide antibiotic dosages, but these are difficult to apply because of limited numbers of animals available. At present, dosages are ini-

TABLE 72–2. Values for Complete Blood Cell Count (CBC) and Serum Chemistry Profiles of 12 Healthy Florida Manatees

Test	Value
CBC	
Hemoglobin (g/dl)	10.3–12.0
Hematocrit (%)	33–38
Hematocrit/PCV (%)	32–40
RBC (10^5/mm³)	2.41–3.06
MCV (fl)	121–135
MCH (pg)	37–43
MCHC (g/dl)	30–33
RDW (%)	16.0–21.5
Platelets (10^3/mm³)	261–634
MPV (%)	5.7–7.3
NRBC/100 WBC	1–2
WBC (mm³)	4000–11,700
Bands (%)	0
Neutrophils (%)	25–64
Lymphocytes (%)	21–77
Monocytes (%)	0–18
Eosinophils (%)	0
Basophils (%)	0–1
Serum Chemistry	
Glucose (mg/dl)	56–117
BUN (mg/dl)	6.4–16
Creatinine (mg/dl)	0.4–2.1
Bilirubin total (mg/dl)	0–0.1
Cholesterol (mg/dl)	107–328
Triglycerides (mg/dl)	34–138
Total protein (g/dl)	6.8–7.3
Albumin (g/dl)	3.8–5.3
Globulin (g/dl)	1.7–3.2
Alkaline phosphate (U/L)	64–183
ALT (U/L)	6–30
AST (U/L)	5–28
GGT (U/L)	39–64
CK II (U/L)	79–302
LD (U/L)	94–372
Calcium (mg/dl)	10.1–12.2
Phosphorus (mg/dl)	3.0–8.0
Sodium (mEq/L)	142–157
Potassium (mEq/L)	4.2–6.6
Chloride (mEq/L)	90–103
CO_2 (mEq/L)	14–43
Iron (μg/dl)	59–199

PCV, packed cell volume; RBC, red blood cells; MCV, mean corpuscular volume; MCH, mean corpuscular hemoglobin; MCHC, mean corpuscular hemoglobin concentration; RDW, red blood cell distribution width; MPV, mononuclear phagocyte volume; NRBC, nucleated red blood cells; WBC, white blood cells; BUN, blood urea nitrogen; ALT, alanine aminotransferase; AST, aspartate aminotransferase; GGT, gamma-glutamyltransferase; CK, creatine kinase; LD, lactate dehydrogenase.

tially chosen on the basis of levels used in equines or cattle. Because an animal may struggle during injections, these are always given before any tube feeding.

Stomach intubation is commonly used for rehydration and nutritional supplementation. Despite the animal's size, the esophagus is relatively small. A typical equine nasogastric tube is used for intubation in adults. To avoid gastric trauma, the tube is measured by placing

it on the outside of the body to the level of the tip of the pectoral flippers, and a piece of tape is placed at the level of the mouth to verify the proper length of insertion. After multiple uses, the tube may be damaged by chewing activity, so it should be inspected before each use. Tube damage can result in leakage near the glottis, in secondary aspiration, and in ingestion of a portion of a tube. To decrease complications, the tube should be replaced as needed, or a rubber bite block can be used to protect the tube. Damage to the caudal pharynx can occur if the person performing intubation is impatient or inexperienced, so caretakers should be well trained in the procedure.

Because intravenous access is difficult to initiate or maintain, hydration is achieved by gastric intubation. The amount of water administered is determined by the state of dehydration, but the clinician should consider that a manatee may not be capable of accepting a large volume of water initially. A 320-kg manatee may require at least 2 L of water BID to improve its hydration status. For the first two treatments, only 75% of this should be administered, to ensure that there are no problems with volume or excessive reflux. The fluid is fed by gravity only. If the animal is severely dehydrated, water may be given TID, but electrolytes and packed cell volume should be closely monitored.

In cases of constipation, mineral oil may be administered at a rate of 2 to 3 mL/kg up to 1.5 L. Intestinal transit time may range from 4 to 7 days, so severely constipated animals may require more than one dose of oil. In addition, these manatees may require enemas to help move out dried fecal material. Initially, warm fresh water may be used; a 320-kg manatee should have 3 to 6 L per treatment. If the need for enemas extends beyond 2 days, saline may be substituted to avoid mucosal edema.

Nutritional supplementation in inappetent or emaciated animals is administered by gastric tube. Typically, a gruel composed of monkey chow, lettuce, and spinach is used two times per day in volumes similar to those for rehydration. The gruel is initially very thin, to allow adaptation of the stomach to the concentrate. When thickened, the gruel may be administered by stomach pump, but only after a safe volume is established. Excessive reflux of formula up the tube from a previous feeding may indicate overfeeding, although some reflux is normal because of pressure on the stomach. A manatee usually begins to eat vegetation between morning and evening feedings, but these tubings should not be discontinued until the animal's appetite is stable or adequate weight has been regained. Animals with severe weight loss, illness, skin loss, or trauma may require prolonged tube feeding to promote healing.

Extremely thin, comatose, or abnormally buoyant manatees may require support with a flotation jacket. These are constructed of wet suit material that covers the torso from flippers to the anus and can be attached with Velcro in a wrap-around manner to adapt to different body conformations. The sides should have pockets to allow addition of flotation material, such as closed cell foam, to augment flotation in manatees that require additional support. The jackets not only aid buoyancy but also can offset heat loss and maintain bandage materials. It has also been shown in the authors' experience with numerous cases that manatees that are supported will regain their appetites quicker.

DISEASE PROBLEMS

Information concerning manatee diseases is currently compiled from information on animals from the wild and from a small number of animals maintained in captivity. As a result of their endangered status, efforts are geared primarily toward recovery of injured or ill animals, rehabilitation, and their release. In addition, the Department of Environmental Protection in Florida recovers all the dead manatees found and performs complete necropsies. Mortality factors are divided into different categories, which include watercraft trauma, entanglement, gate and dam trauma, and perinatal and other natural causes. Table 72–3 lists the different disease categories for the manatees rescued at Sea World and the Miami Seaquarium, two of the three rescue and rehabilitation facilities in Florida. These groupings differ from those of previous published data[4, 6] because rehabilitation facilities compile information that includes descriptions of live animals.

Natural Illness

PERINATAL

Congenital malformations of the flipper, consisting of variations of ectrodactyly, have been reported in three cases. One manatee had bilaterally symmetric cleft hand.[25] Two other cases of ectrodactyly have been observed at Sea World. Two cases of umbilical hernia have also been observed in neonates.[6] There was mature fibrosis of the intestinal segments and covering of the coils with peritoneum without notable contamination.

Orphans make up 20% of the manatees presented to Sea World and are approaching 80% presented to Miami Seaquarium since 1993. The reasons for maternal separation are not known, nor is the time of separation. It is evident from captive observations that there are varying levels of maternal care, which may directly affect survival. Recruitment of inexperienced females into the breeding population as a result of a decreased number of experienced breeders may be a factor. In addition, numerous neonatal complications may be involved. The impact of environmental factors such as boat traffic or interference from other manatees is also unknown. Many orphans are eventually found when they are already close to death. Common symptoms associated with orphans are varying degrees of visual emaciation, metabolic exhaustion, hypoglycemia, hypothermia, constipation, foreign body ingestion, enterocolitis, and septicemia. Orphans and newborns should also be examined for signs of omphalitis and secondary peritonitis.[23] Organisms isolated from umbilical infections include *Streptococcus faecium, Plesiomonas shigelloides, Pseudomonas putrifaciens* and *putida, Escherichia coli, Morganella morganii, Acinetobacter calcoaciticus,* and *Bacteroides ureolyticus.*

Critical care techniques include a clean water source to decrease bacterial compromise, water temperatures are raised to 29.4°C, complete blood counts, serum chemistry profiles, radiographs, and fecal cultures. Dietary support has usually been based on commercial products with varying degrees of success. Initial gross analysis of manatee milk did not provide adequate insight into the differences in fatty acid and amino acid requirements. Manatee milk contains high levels of taurine and methionine, as well as short- and medium-chained fatty acids.[15] Current efforts are geared toward development of a more appropriate neonatal formula. Antibiotic use is often geared toward control of septicemia, although enterocolitis may be a major factor in mortality. Oral antibiotic use to avoid injections frequently contributes to intestinal complications. Clinically, cases of enterocolitis have been associated with infections with *Pseudomonas aeruginosa, Salmonella* species (two animals), *Clostridium difficile* (three animals) with positive toxin detected in two neonates, and *Citrobacter freundii.* A number of cases of enterocolitis may be related to nosocomial infections.

Immune system compromise also appears to be a factor, in as much as some newborns have not received colostrum. Manatee colostrum and serum immunoglobulins have been used for supplementation in newborns.

JUVENILE DISEASES

The most common reasons for presentation of juvenile manatees appears to include premature separation from the mother while still dependent on maternal care and, in young individuals just weaned inability to handle hypothermia during their first winter. Many young manatees may be in an obvious state of weight loss or

TABLE 72–3. Disease Categories of Rescued Manatees at Sea World and Miami Seaquarium

Category	Number
Human Related	
Blunt trauma	39
Propeller trauma	24
Crab trap	24
Entanglement	19
Monofilament line	8
Fish hook	2
Pipe	2
Shrimp net	1
Natural Disease	
Orphan	74
Reproductive	20
Cold stress	15
Dermatitis	12
Intestinal	6
Congenital	4
Red tide	3
Low tide entrapment	3
Septicemia	2
Pleuritis	2
Lung abscess	2

emaciation. Serum chemistry profiles often show signs of dehydration, including elevated creatinine levels. Lymphocyte phenotyping indicates that lymphocyte subsets in animals with cold shock may be affected for extended periods. Severe bacterial dermatitis may also occur in juvenile animals that are compromised by chronic cold water and emaciation. This condition has been confused with a possible etiology of chemical burns because of the extensive skin lesions. Lesions may start as pustules that erupt and ulcerate over large portions of the face, extremities, torso, and tail. Organisms isolated from abscesses have included *Staphylococcus aureus, M. morganii, Aeromonas hydrophila, Vibrio* species, *Clostridium* species, *Pseudomonas* species, *Edwardsiella tarda,* and *Yokonella* species. Skin lesions and lacerations may harbor multiple organisms, including those just listed, other anaerobes such as *Fusobacterium* species and *Bacteroides* species, and fungi such as *Mucor* species.

Treatment includes topical disinfection with a 5% Betadyne solution, parenteral antibiotics, and good water quality. Changes in salinity may also influence the bacterial component of the skin. Nutritional support by tube feeding may be necessary to meet the increased caloric needs associated with extensive damage and with maintenance and replacement of lost body condition. Constipation is also a common finding, and cold-stressed animals may require mineral oil and enemas.

ADULT MANIFESTATIONS

Natural disease problems in adults may also include complications from extended periods of cold water during the winter months. Adults metabolism appears to handle cold effects better than that of juveniles, but adults show signs of cold discomfort at temperatures less than 20°C by shivering, decreased activity, and sun bathing at the surface. As with other age groups, enterocolitis may be a mortality factor. Individual manatees may be ill with unknown primary etiologies but have numerous complicating factors such as dehydration. In addition, these animals may be constipated and inappetant. Symptoms of constipation include lack of stool production and the presence of hard, firm fecal material found on rectal examination or radiographs. Water is first given by gastric tube to treat dehydration; then mineral oil is administered orally as well as warm water enemas. The enema volume may exceed 6 L in an adult, as needed. If enemas are required for long periods, normal saline may be used to decrease the potential for intestinal edema.

Reproductive complications are also seen, constituting 8% of the cases. In the authors' experience, five females had dystocia. In three cases, the fetus was already decomposing, and the mothers were toxic and did not survive after removal of the calf. In the other cases, one calf was extracted with the mother under anesthesia, and another was removed by cesarian section. In these two cases, the mothers were released to the wild. The potential involvement of brucellosis in this species has not been documented.

Other disease processes have been reported in manatees, including intussusception,[18] dermatitis,[20] intestinal

complications, pleuritis, and lung abscesses. Other natural disease problems encountered at Sea World of Florida and at the Miami Seaquarium are listed in Table 72–3.

TOXICOSIS

Manatees are also susceptible to intoxication from blooms of marine dinoflagellates, which produce toxins that affect fish, birds, and mammals. In 1982, 37 manatees were found dead on the west coast as a result of a widespread bloom of the dinoflagellate red tide organism *Gymnodinium breve.*[17] Clinically, some animals still alive showed neurologic symptoms, including disorientation, incoordination, hyperflexion, and labored breathing. Two of the distressed animals were brought to Sea World and recovered, as did other individuals observed. In 1996, another epizootic occurred in southwest Florida, resulting in the deaths of approximately 150 manatees. In this die-off, there were substantial pathologic findings in the respiratory system, suggesting inhalation as a major contribution to the symptoms.

Manatees with neurologic symptoms were brought to Sea World in 1982 and 1995 and to Lowry Park Zoo in 1996 during problems with red tide organisms. One animal examined at Sea World exhibited dyspnea, dementia, and incoordination. Because clinicians were unable to differentiate these from symptoms of possible head trauma, the animal was treated symptomatically with steroids and a nonsteroidal anti-inflammatory drug. Perhaps of even more importance was that the animal was supported with foam to avoid inhalation of water and possible drowning. Within 12 hours, the manatee no longer showed any symptoms and was released after a few weeks of observation. Results of serologic tests for the toxin were negative. These cases show that some manatees may be exposed to levels of toxin that are reversible if caught in time before further complications are encountered.

PARASITIC

Beck and Forrester[1] listed six helminth parasites in 215 Florida manatees examined. These included one nematode (*Heterocheilus tunicatus*), one cestode (*Anoplocephala* species), and four species of trematode (*Cochleotrema cochleotrema, Chirochis fabaceus, Nudacotyle undicola,* and *Moniligerum blain*). Beck and Forrester did not find any association between intensity of infection and the cause of death. Clinically, parasite numbers are associated with some manifestations. *C. cochleotrema* organisms have been seen in high numbers in the nasopharynx and appear to be associated with chronic rhinitis and symptoms of pneumonia. Another nematode, probably *N. undicola,* was associated with a severe edematous enterocolitis in one. Manatees have not been routinely wormed unless there are complications or concerns regarding slow response to therapy or chronic intestinal complications such as diarrhea or constipation. Therapeutic agents have included fenbendazole at 10 mg/kg and ivermectin orally at 200 μg/kg. Praziquantel has been administered orally at 8 to 16 mg/kg for trematodes. The use of fenbendazole in one manatee resulted in evacuation of high numbers of trematodes. There have been no controlled studies to verify efficacy or proper dosage of these compounds.

Beck and Forrester[1] also described parasites reported in the other sirenians. *Toxoplasma gondii* has been reported in association with encephalitis in one manatee.[3] Two species of *Eimeria* (*E. nodulosa* and *E. manatus*) were detected in the intestinal tract of Florida manatees.[21] Skin parasites have included copepoda (*Harpacticus pulex*) and cirripedia (*Chelonibia manatii*). Individual manatees with chronic dermatitis may also harbor saprophytic nematodes on the skin.

VIRAL DISEASES

Investigations into viral pathogens have been relatively new. Duignan and associates[7] analyzed serum for evidence of mobillivirus in manatees and found positive results in five manatees, even though none were showing signs of an active infection. Other investigators are checking for serologic evidence of more than 20 viral and bacterial pathogens; these results are not available yet.

Human Related

Table 72–3 also lists human-related mortality factors that affect manatees. Those associated with water craft injuries are the most prevalent and also the most challenging for treatment.

PROPELLER WOUNDS

Manatees share normal feeding, calving, and resting areas with large numbers of boats along Florida's coastline. Although thought of as slow moving, a manatee will attempt to get out of the way of boats if allowed adequate time. Propeller wounds show an amazing range of injuries, from superficial abrasions to complete torso separation. Injuries are graded as mild, moderate, or severe; most manatees thus injured arrive at treatment centers with moderate to severe wounds, or else the animals would not be noticed and caught. Propeller wounds to the back may penetrate the chest cavity and are usually fatal, as a result of development of a severe pleuritis secondary to chest contamination; mortality is heavily influenced by the chronic nature of the perforation. Animals with deep laceration to the skeletal and musculature systems have a better prognosis although some may experience loss of normal mobility and suffer from chronic vertebral osteomyelitis and fistulous tracts. Recuperation is prolonged, and return to the wild is in some cases inappropriate.

Wound care is similar to that for other species. The water is maintained as clean as possible, usually including a 1-ppm level of chlorine to control secondary infections from the environment. A 3% to 8% povidone-iodine solution diluted with saline is applied to the wound two to three times a day, accompanied by debridement. The strength of the povidone-iodine solution is related to the amount of contact time available. With very short contact times the higher concentrations are more appropriate. If the wound is deep and irregular so that food material may become trapped, a water-resistant ointment such as a petroleum jelly–based triple-antibiotic ointment can be applied. Water-soluble ointments are often not retained for adequate periods of time. Custom body wraps made from wet suit material are used to protect the wound, retain the ointment, and provide buoyancy assistance. Antibiotic use is routine in such cases, as is nutritional support with tube feeding. Granulation tissue deposition is the best indicator of early nutritional and therapeutic response. Animals in which granulation occurs within a few weeks of the injury have fewer complications, especially if bone is exposed. Those in which covering of exposed bone takes 3 to 4 weeks often develop more fistulous tracts, sequestra, and secondary pleuritis. Once granulation becomes pronounced, debridement must be routine in order to avoid closure over devitalized bone or granulomatous debris in tissue crevices.[22]

Blunt Trauma

As boat speeds have increased, so has the incidence of blunt trauma. Although the injury extent is not as obvious as with propeller wounds, they can be just as devastating. The most common manifestations involve chest injuries but may also include head trauma and abdominal complications such as organ rupture or abortion. Pulmonary injuries include rib fractures (usually multiple), spinal fractures, lung perforation, pulmonary hemorrhage, and pneumothorax.

Manatees with pneumothorax are often unable to submerge, have difficulty righting themselves, are dyspneic because of damage or abnormal buoyancy, and may have a lung torsion. Radiographs should be taken to ascertain complications, and a complete blood cell counts and serum chemistry profiles should be obtained. Lung torsion appears to develop secondary to distention of the chest cavity when the animal is attempting to dive. The caudal third of the lung is normally free floating and may fold over during repeated diving attempts. If lung displacement is detected early, the manatee can be placed in a restraint and dangled head up to encourage a return of the lung to normal position. Afterward the lung is repositioned, the animal is placed in a buoyancy jacket to maintain a normal breathing position. The water can also be lowered to discourage diving, but the use of low water without buoyancy support is not recommended. Initial attempts at pneumothorax management were similar to those in terrestrial species, in which drains and valves were used, but these were found to be counterproductive for a number of reasons. Because manatees hold their breath after inspiration, the lung is under constant positive pressure. If an outlet is provided with a chest tube, the original tear is maintained by the constant drainage provided, healing is slowed, and the body rejects the tube or reacts to its presence, initiating a pleuritis after only a few weeks. Allowing the pneumothorax to be maintained promotes healing of the tear in the lung. The chest can be drained intermittently to gauge the healing response by the amount of time it takes to reinflate the chest. The time for healing without drainage ranges from 1 to 4 months, but this approach is more successful than chest tubes.

Occasionally, a subcutaneous bubble appears over the injury site, connected to the chest through a channel created by a fractured rib. In one case, this progressed to whole body subcutaneous emphysema, which when resolved still left a 30-cm bubble at the injury site. This condition has been seen in association with severe pyothorax in animals recovered from the wild. A pressure pad consisting of five layers of one inch foam padding was made in the shape of a pyramid. The base of the pyramid is larger than the elevated tissue and is kept in place by the buoyancy jacket, forcing the bubble to collapse and promoting re-adherence of the tissue. This may also avoid prolonged leakage of damaged tissue from the subcutaneous area back into the chest, which may contribute to the pleuritis.

Entanglement

The second most common traumatic injury is entanglement with monofilament line or crab trap rope. Strangulation and amputation of the pectoral flippers is the most common sequela, but the material may wrap around both arms and the axillary area. In many cases, the heavy crab trap is still attached to the rope. If found early, the damaged limb can be bandaged and amputation avoided. All limbs involved in line entanglement should be radiographed to check for possible fractures of the radius and ulna. Once cleaned and debrided, the open stricture wound is covered with a water-resistant ointment and then gauze pads. The arm is thoroughly dried and elastikon tape stirrups applied on each side of the arm as proximal to the axilla as possible. Gauze may be wrapped around the arm, followed first by a layer of Elastikon and then by a layer of waterproof adhesive tape and another layer of elastikon. To prevent unraveling, the overlapping edges of elastikon are secured with cyanoacrylate glue, and lines of glue are made longitudinally along the arm to increase the bandage's stability. Fiberglass casting material is also used when a fracture is present.

Other human-related sources of problems include waterway gate and dam injuries, entrapment in pipes and canals, ingested fish hooks, destruction of grass beds, fresh water runoff, and pollution.

The interested reader can seek further information on handling and transport in Geraci's *Marine Mammals Ashore, A Field Guide for Strandings.*

REFERENCES

1. Beck C, Forrester DJ: Helminths of the Florida manatee, *Trichechus manatus latirostris*, with a discussion and summary of the parasites of sirenians. J Parasit 74(4):628–637, 1988.

2. Bossart GD: Dolphins and West Indian manatees; morphologic characterization, correlation between healthy and disease states under free ranging and captive conditions. Ph.D. Dissertation, Florida International University, Miami, FL, 1995.

3. Buergelt CD, Bonde RK: Toxoplasmic meningoencephalitis in a West Indian manatee. J Am Vet Med Assoc 185(11):1294–1296, 1983.

4. Buergelt CD, Bonde RK, Beck CA, et al: Pathologic findings in manatees in Florida. J Am Vet Med Assoc 185(11):1331–1334, 1984.

5. Crane A: Notes on the habits of the manatees (*Manatus australis*) in captivity in the Brighton Aquarium. Proc Zool Soc Lond 30:457–460, 1881.

6. Dover S, Walsh MT, Bossart GD, et al: Congenital umbilical hernia in two neonatal manatee calves. In preparation.

7. Duignan PJ, House C, Walsh MT, et al: Morbillivirus infection in manatees. Mar Mam Sci 11(4):441–451, 1995.

8. Forrester DJ, White FH, Woodard JC, et al: Intussusception in a Florida manatee. J Wild Dis 11:566–568, 1975.

9. Garrod AH: Notes on the manatee (*Manatus americanus*) recently living in the society's garden. Trans Zool Soc Lond 10(1):137–145, 1877.

10. Geraci JR, Lounsbury VJ: Marine Mammals Ashore, A Field Guide for Strandings. Galveston, Texas A&M SEA Grant College Program Publication, 1993.

11. Irvine AB: Manatee metabolism and its influence on distribution in Florida. Zool Conserv 25:315–334, 1983.

12. Murie J: On the form and structure of the manatee (*Manatus americanus*). Trans Zool Soc Lond 8(3):127–202, 1870.

13. Murie J: Further observations on the manatee. Trans Zool Soc Lond 11(1):19–48, 1880.

14. Notes from the secretary on additions to the menagerie. Proc Zool Soc Lond:529, 1875.

15. Oftedal O, Worthy G, Walsh MT, et al: Micronutrient analysis of manatee milk. In preparation.

16. O'Shea TJ, Beck CA, Bonde RK, et al: An analysis of manatee mortality patterns in Florida, 1976–81. J Wildl Manage 49(1):1–11, 1985.

17. O'Shea TJ, Rathbun GB, Bonde RK, et al: An epizootic of Florida manatees associated with a dinoflagellate bloom. Mar Mam Sci 7(2):165–177, 1991.

18. Reynolds JE, Odell DK: Manatees and Dugongs. New York, Facts On File, 1991.

19. Scholander PF, Irving L: Experimental investigations on the respiration and diving of the Florida manatee. J Cell Comp Physiol 17(2):169–191, 1941.

20. Tabuchi K, Muku T, Satomichi T: A dermatosis in manatee. Bull Azaba Vet Coll 28:127–134, 1974.

21. Upton SJ, Odell Dk, Bossart GD, et al: Description of the oocysts of two new species of Eimeria (*Apicomplexa: Eimeridae*) from the Florida manatee, *Trichechus manatus* (*Sirenia: Trichechidae*). J Protozool 36(1):87–90, 1989.

22. Walsh MT, Bossart GD, Renner M: Traumatic injuries in manatees (*Trichechus manatus*) in Florida: categorization, diagnosis, and treatment. In preparation.

23. Walsh MT, Bossart GD, Young WG, et al: Omphalitis and peritonitis in a young West Indian manatee (*Trichechus manatus*). J Wild Dis 23(4):702–704, 1987.

24. Walsh MT, Webb A, Bailey J: Sedation and anesthesia of the Florida manatee. In preparation.

25. Watson AG, Bonde RK: Congenital malformations of the flipper in three West Indian manatees, *Trichechus manatus,* and a proposed mechanism for development of ectrodactyly and cleft hand in mammals. Clin Orthoped 202:294–301, 1986.

ELEPHANTS

CHAPTER 73

Radiographic Techniques for the Elephant Foot and Carpus

LAURIE J. GAGE

Radiography of elephant feet is a simple procedure that should be employed in any case of nonresponsive lameness. A portable equine radiographic unit with a capacity of 80 kVP and 15 mA and 8 × 10 inch (20.3 × 25.4 cm) or 14 × 17 inch (35.6 × 43.2 cm) rare earth combination 400 speed film cassettes are the only equipment needed for taking high-quality diagnostic films of elephant feet. Trained elephants may be conditioned to stand on a film cassette, allowing diagnostic films of the metacarpals and phalanges to be obtained. Elephants held in protective contact conditions may also be trained to hold a foot on a film cassette; however, the positioning of the radiographic unit medially to obtain multiple views could be a challenge. Carpal joints may also be evaluated through use of the same equipment.

An extensive review of the medical management of elephants indicated that foot disorders are one of the most common ailments observed in captive elephants.[2] Cracks in the nail or cuticle and abscesses in the sole are common and may lead to deeper infection. Severe infections in the soft tissues and nails may spread to the adjacent bones and joints of the foot, causing osteomyelitis and suppurative arthritis.[1] Radiology is useful for diagnosing osteomyelitis in the elephant foot and may also indicate prognosis when arthritis is suspected.

ANATOMY

There are five digits on the front feet of Asian and African elephants. The prominent second, third, and fourth are the weight-bearing digits, and each has three phalanges and a pair of proximal sesamoids. The first digit has two phalanges and one proximal sesamoid; the fifth digit has three phalanges and a pair of proximal sesamoids.

There are five digits on the rear feet of Asian elephants; the second, third, and fourth are prominent, and each has three phalanges and a pair of proximal sesamoids; the first and fifth digits are smaller and have one and two to three phalanges, respectively.

The number of toenails varies and does not necessarily correspond to the number of digits. Asian elephants usually have five toenails on the front feet and four toenails on the rear feet, whereas African elephants often have four toenails on the front and three or four toenails on the rear feet.

EQUIPMENT AND RADIOGRAPHIC TECHNIQUE

Diagnostic radiographs of the digits of the front and rear feet of Asian and African elephants have been

517

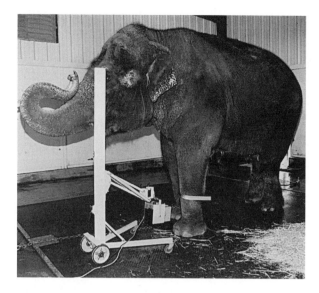

FIGURE 73–1. Positioning of the x-ray unit for an anteroposterior radiograph of the left carpal joint.

obtained with a portable equine radiographic unit. Although it has previously been stated that radiographing elephant feet requires an x-ray unit with a high milliamperage and the author has been able to take detailed films of the phalanges and metacarpal bones with a setting of 15 mA and 80 kVP with a Fischer portable x-ray unit and Agfa green-sensitive rare earth all-plastic film cassettes. The film/screen combination is 400 speed (Fig. 73–1). To obtain carpal radiographs, wide-cloth tape was used to secure a 35.6 × 43.2 cm rare earth film cassette to the limb of a well-trained elephant (see Fig. 73–6). This method has proved superior to other methods of holding the cassette because of the lengthy exposure time and the shape of the elephants' limbs. Although these films are not as detailed as those of the digits, the edges of the carpal bones can be assessed, and the joint spaces between the carpal bones can be evaluated (Fig. 73–2).

It is critical to use the correct time setting. This varies with the size of the foot and may take some trials to achieve the optimal settings for each elephant. In adult elephants, the distal phalangeal bones are thin, fragile, and attached to the toenail. They are best detailed with a 0.25- to 0.4-second setting at 80 kVP and 15 mA. Diagnostic films of the proximal and middle phalanges may be obtained through the same technique with a 0.4- to 0.7-second setting. The distal portion of the metacarpals may be radiographed with a 0.8- to 2.0-second setting, and the proximal edge of the metacarpals generally require an exposure time of 1.5 to 3.0 seconds for optimum detail. These settings have been established with the elephant standing with its foot flat on the cassette, the portable unit hand-held at an approximately 45 degree angle, and the tube head 45 cm from the surface of the foot (Fig. 73–3).

Lateral films of the metacarpals and metatarsals require time settings of 3.0 to 4.0 seconds and anterior-posterior (AP) and lateral carpal radiographs have been taken with a 4.0 second exposure. These studies require the x-ray unit set at 80 kVP and 15 mA and secured to a stand with the tube head held 45 cm from the surface of the carpus. Adequate detail may be achieved if the elephant is motionless throughout the exposure time.

Tracts caused by chronic draining wounds may be visualized and evaluated by instilling a radio opaque dye deep into the tract, plugging the opening with a cotton wad, and immediately radiographing the area.

POSITIONING OF THE RADIOGRAPHIC UNIT

Most stands designed to hold portable x-ray units are cumbersome, and although they are an acceptable aid in radiographing the foot from the lateral side, they are difficult to place under the neck of the elephant in order to obtain the correct angle for the AP views. Portable unit stands are, however, essential for obtaining adequate AP and lateral radiographs of the carpal joint because of the lengthy exposure time (see Fig. 73–1).

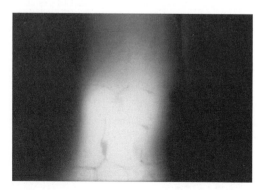

FIGURE 73–2. Radiograph of the left carpal joint.

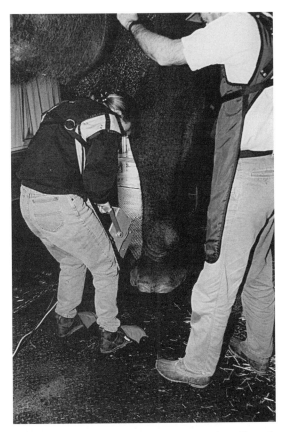

FIGURE 73–3. Positioning for an anteroposterior radiograph of the central digits of the left front foot. Note that the elephant is standing on the black film cassette.

Diagnostic films of the second, third and fourth digits may be obtained by holding the radiographic unit in an anterior position and aiming the center of the beam at the apex of the corresponding toenail and down toward the cassette at a 45 degree angle with the

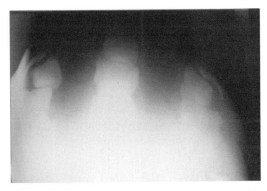

FIGURE 73–5. Dorsopalmar radiograph of the central digits of the left front foot.

elephant standing squarely on the film cassette (Fig. 73–4; see Fig. 73–3). The first digit may be radiographed by positioning the unit over the anterior medial side of the foot. This can be accomplished by standing on the opposite side of the elephant and aiming the radiographic unit over the medial nail at a 45 degree angle toward the film cassette. The fifth, or lateral, digit may be radiographed by positioning the unit over the lateral side of the foot and aiming the beam down at a 45 degree angle, centering the beam just above the apex of the lateral toenail. The medial and lateral digits are smaller and require shorter exposure time settings.

It is possible to obtain an anterior lateral oblique view of the lateral digit by directing the beam from the anterior side of the limb obliquely to a film placed posterior and lateral to the digit, and perpendicular to the ground. The medial digit may be similarly radiographed from the anterior side of the foot, aiming the beam posteriorly and medially toward the vertical cassette.

The ideal film size for taking radiographs of elephant feet and carpal joints measures 14 × 17 inch (35.6 × 43.2 cm). This size film allows AP views of two or

FIGURE 73–4. Diagram of Figure 73–1. *A,* Cone of the x-ray machine. *B,* Cassette.

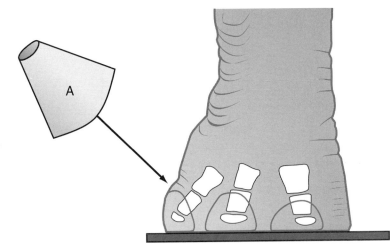

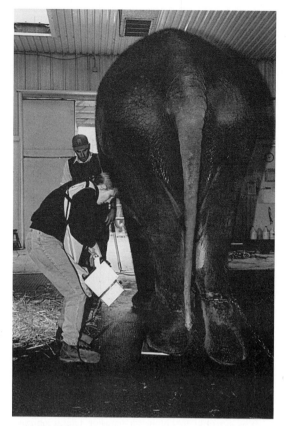

FIGURE 73–6. Positioning of the x-ray unit for a lateral radiograph of the lateral digit of the left rear foot.

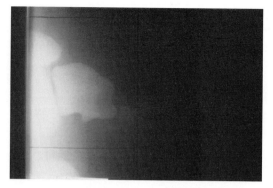

FIGURE 73–7. Radiograph of the lateral digit of the left rear foot.

three entire digits, radiographed from an anterior position (Fig. 73–5). Individual digits, especially the entire medial or lateral digits or the distal two phalanges of the larger central digits may be radiographed successfully with 8 × 10 inch (20.3 × 25.4 cm) film placed directly beneath the digit to be studied. (Figs. 73–6, 73–7).

In order to take AP foot radiographs, the plastic film cassette is placed on a flat, clean floor. A hard rubber floor surface is ideal; however, a flat concrete floor will do. Any curvature to the floor will result in damage to the film cassette. The bottom of the elephant's foot should be clean, dry, and brushed free of dirt or gravel before it is placed on the cassette. The trainer directs the elephant to place its foot directly on the film cassette. The elephant may bear full weight on the cassette without damaging it; however, this is not encouraged. The plastic intensifying film cassettes have been used in this manner to radiographically evaluate the feet of dozens of adult female Asian and African elephants. Although the author has not seen any damage to the film cassettes, the reader may wish to build a protective cassette holder. Metal screws or nails should not be used in its construction because they may obscure important features.

Care should be taken to limit the amount of metal articles such as chains or foot stands adjacent to the limb being radiographed. The author has found that even when the metal object is not in the direct path of the x-ray, it can cause significant scatter, which decreases the quality of the film.

REFERENCES

1. Fowler, ME. *In* Fowler ME (ed): Zoo and Wild Animal Medicine, 2nd ed. Philadelphia, WB Saunders, pp 448–453, 1993.
2. Mikota, SK, Sargent EL, Ranglack GS: Medical management of the elephant. West Bloomfield, Michigan, Indira Publishing House, pp 137–150, 1994.

CHAPTER 74

Calving Elephants (Normal)

MICHAEL J. SCHMIDT

MONITORING PREGNANCY

An elephant pregnancy can be diagnosed at 12 weeks by means of a weekly progesterone assay that is modified to detect the very low levels in elephants. Progesterone levels increase, then remain elevated throughout pregnancy. If progesterone is still elevated at 12 weeks, then the elephant is considered to be pregnant. Therefore, it is important to monitor progesterone on a weekly basis in all breeding female elephants.

Gestation in elephants is usually 92 weeks. In one case of twin elephants, gestation was 88 weeks; this shortened gestation is typical of twinning.

Progesterone level decreases 2 to 4 days before parturition. If this decrease in progesterone is to be used as a signal for impending parturition, daily blood samples should be collected and progesterone measured at least once every 2 days, starting a reasonable time ahead of the anticipated calving date.

ESTIMATING CALVING DATE

Calving date is best estimated using weekly progesterone measurements. Because normal gestation is 92 weeks, the calving date can be derived by extrapolating from the known breeding date that began the pregnancy.

CARE DURING PREGNANCY

The pregnant elephant should maintain exercise so that muscle tone is good at calving. Excessive supplements should not be added to the cow's diet during pregnancy. Many cow elephants have given birth normally without dietary supplements during pregnancy. Supplementation with calcium and vitamin D may be a special concern in that it has been suggested that parturient paresis may have been at least partially responsible for some cases of elephant dystocia; consultation with a nutritionist is advised.

INDICATIONS OF IMPENDING CALVING

Signs of impending calving in an elephant can be non-existent, subtle, or overt, even in the same elephant at different parturitions. About 50% of the time, cervical mucus is passed as the cervix dilates. This can be observed as a discharge of thick, ropy material. Usually, the mucous plug is passed 12 to 24 hours before parturition, correlating with the decrease in progesterone measured in the daily blood samples.

Behavioral changes before the onset of labor are not usually pronounced. "Surprise" calvings are not unusual when a cow has given no signs that calving would take place. Many elephant cows continue to eat right up until active labor begins. On occasion, colostrum drips from the mammary glands before labor, but this is not a reliable sign, because it can occur several weeks before calving. Again, the dripping of colostrum should be viewed in conjunction with daily progesterone levels to assess its significance.

ONSET OF LABOR

Elephant cows—like mares—have absolute control over the onset and continuation of labor. Therefore, it is best to avoid disturbing the cow because she may otherwise stop the calving. No persons unfamiliar to the cow elephant should be within sight or sound during calving; nor should there be visitors in the visitor area after normal visitor hours. The cow's routine should remain normal.

At the onset of labor, the cow shows signs of abdominal discomfort, including abnormal posture, restlessness, lying down and getting back up, frequent defecation, placing the trunk in the mouth, and flapping ears. Abdominal contractions are usually visible, and a bulge may appear beneath the tail and then disappear. The period of "hard labor" should last from 20 minutes to 3 or 4 hours.

During labor, it is very important to look for the rupture of the amniotic sac. This is seen as a sudden discharge of a large volume of "clear" fluid, not urine. When the amniotic sac ruptures, a time limit is established for the birth of a live calf: 12 to 24 hours. If the cow does not give birth naturally within that time period, parturition must be induced to enhance the chance of delivering a live calf. At Circus World in Florida, the longest period from the time of mucous plug passage to natural delivery of a live elephant calf was 5 days; in this case, the amniotic sac had not ruptured.

As labor progresses, the bulge under the cow's tail

521

becomes larger, and the amniotic sac often ruptures at this point. The calf is finally propelled over the pelvic brim and slides suddenly down onto the ground as it is delivered. If the amniotic sac has not already ruptured, it does so as the calf is delivered. Both anterior and posterior presentations have been observed with normal calving, but a posterior presentation is probably normal. In posterior presentation, the elephant calf's head does not have a chance to cause dystocia.

The calf should be able to get onto its feet within 30 minutes. If it takes longer, the calf is not considered to be normal. Hypoxia and hydrocephalus are two causes for a calf's being unable to stand within 30 minutes. Of five calves that did not get to their feet in the 30-minute period after birth at the Portland, Oregon, Metro Washington Park Zoo, one survived to adulthood, and the other four either died or were euthanized within 2 weeks of birth because of congenital defects.

CHAPTER 75

Dystocia in the Elephant

JOSEPH J. FOERNER

The causes of dystocia in elephants can be as varied as in other species, but the following three seem to be the most common: (1) problems in the uterus of the dam, (2) improper fetal positioning, and (3) complications resulting from fetal death.

Two types of uterine inertia appear to be frequent causes of dystocia or delayed parturition, but fortunately they have the best prognosis. Physiologic inertia can result from exhaustion of the uterine musculature or from preexisting disease of the uterus. In addition, the elephant, like the horse, can effect psychological inertia—the ability to cease labor efforts because of environmental conditions. Both conditions can prolong the labor-to-birth interval significantly. Diagnosis of either condition is difficult and mostly retrospective. If there is a delay in delivery with a positive response to treatment, this is presumptive evidence of uterine inertia.

Fetal malposition occurs less often and is more difficult to treat in elephants than in smaller mammals because of the maternal size, fetal size, and anatomic peculiarities of the cow (or female elephant). The large head of an elephant calf predisposes it to a "head-back" malposition during an anterior presentation (Fig. 75–1). The more common posterior presentation delivery eliminates the possibility of head-back problems but predisposes the calf to buttocks or breech presentation. These appear to be the most common fetal malpositions that occur in elephants (Table 75–1). Unlike domestic hoofstock, the relatively short limbs on the elephant calf rarely cause problems of fetal malposition.

Fetal death as the cause of dystocia requires further study. In the author's experience, in most cases of dystocia, the fetus has been dead and is often decom-

posing. Exactly when the fetus died is difficult to ascertain because both ultrasonography and electrocardiography have been unrewarding in determining the viability of the fetus. Whether fetal death was the cause or result of the dystocia remains a question. Often, it appears that fetal death occurs first, fetal fluids are resorbed, and the uterus contracts down on the fetus, resulting in severe unresponsive dystocia. This contraction of the uterus on the calf produces what has been called Bandl's rings and can be so severe as to cause ischemia or necrosis in the wall of the uterus.[1] Hallmarks of this

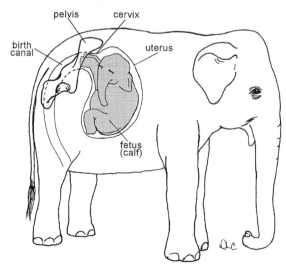

FIGURE 75–1. Fetal malposition: head-back presentation.

TABLE 75–1. Summary of Dystocia Cases

Case	Dam Age Species	Calf Sex (Weight)	Delivery Presentation	Labor to Calving Interval	Comments
1	6-Year Asian	Female (120 kg)	Posterior normal (dead)	48+ Hours	Episiotomy and mechanical traction, umbilicus around rear leg, successful delivery
2	19-Year Asian	Male (159 kg)	Posterior buttock or breech (dead, decomposing)	4 Months	Episiotomy, unsuccessful reduction, cesarean, cow died 10 days after surgery
3	32-Year Asian	Male (120 kg)	Anterior, head back (dead)	6 Days	Episiotomy, unsuccessful reduction, cesarean, cow died 19 days after surgery
4	28-Year Asian	Male (95 kg)	Posterior normal (dead)	5 Days	Episiotomy, unsuccessful reduction, cesarean, euthanized at surgery
5	25-Year Asian	Male (110 kg)	Posterior normal (live)	Approx 4 days	Psychological inertia, administered 20 IU oxytocin, live calf
6	11-Year African	Male (127 kg)	Anterior normal (dead)	4 Days	Uterine inertia, treated by acupuncture, successful delivery
7	24-Year Asian	Male (104 kg)	Posterior buttock or breech (dead, decomposing)	13 Days	Episiotomy, unsuccessful reduction, cesarean, cow died 14 days after surgery
8	30-Year Asian	Male (approx 110 kg)	Anterior normal (dead)	27 Days	Episiotomy, unable to extract fetus because of placental strangulation, euthanized
9	29-Year Asian	Twin (20 kg) sexes not determined	Unknown (dead)	Approx 4-month interval	Treated with multiple doses oxytocin, no response, 4 months later delivered macerated twins

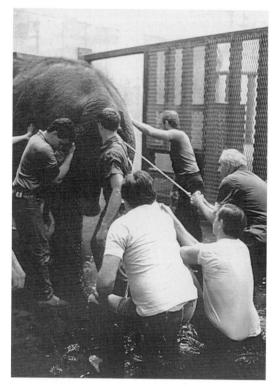

FIGURE 75–2. Traction on fetus through episiotomy.

grave situation are evidence of hard labor, absence of fetal fluid, and eventual presentation of fetal membranes.

Identifying a case of dystocia can be challenging, but several signs should lead to suspicion of dystocia. These signs include the absence of labor 30 days past the known due date and a 2- to 4-week delay after a decrease in serum progesterone levels. In addition, no delivery 24 hours after the appearance of fetal fluids, or several days after the appearance of a cervical plug, the appearance of fetal membranes, and continued nonproductive labor are all cardinal signs that dystocia is present and that medical treatment should be initiated. The lack of response to oxytocin treatment, a fetid vaginal discharge, an increase in systemic white blood cell count, and a deterioration in physical condition are all indicative of serious dystocia with a guarded prognosis for both cow and calf.

There are a few clinical procedures that assist in determining whether dystocia exists. Rectal examination can usually be performed on tractable or mildly sedated elephants; however, little information is usually gained from this procedure. Because of the large size of the animal, the clinician cannot palpate beyond the brim of the pelvis, and, unless the calf has been pushed into the pelvic canal, the position of the calf cannot be determined. If the calf's limbs have been pushed in the pelvic canal, palpation of the toes determines the direction of presentation (i.e., toes dorsal, an anterior presentation; toes ventral, a posterior presentation). Because of the length of the urogenital canal, a vaginal examination

yields little information except whether fetal membranes are present within the canal. In the elephant, endoscopy yields more information than rectal or vaginal examination and can be performed while standing. A 3-m human colonoscope is the preferred instrument. It can be inserted up the urogenital canal and directed around the brim of the pelvis for visualization of the cervix. The degree of cervical relaxation or presence of fetal membranes or fetal extremities can be visualized.

Of all diagnostic procedures, episiotomy yields the most information. It can be performed while standing on most elephants, with or without sedation. For this procedure, a local anesthetic agent is infiltrated subcutaneously just below the brim of the pelvis for a distance of approximately 30 cm. A length of 4 cm PVC pipe is inserted up the urogenital canal until it reaches the horizontal portion of the canal. The tube can then be easily palpated under the skin at the brim of the pelvis. A scalpel is used to incise through the skin and mucosa down to the PVC pipe. The incision is extended to the desired length in a vertical plane. A tubular vaginal speculum inserted through the episiotomy to the proximal end of the vagina allows direct visualization of the cervix. If the episiotomy is of adequate length, a hand can be directed through the vagina for palpation of the cervix. After the procedure, the episiotomy can be closed or left open for repeated procedures. If delayed closure of the episiotomy is desired, the edges of the wound can be freshened for primary closure or allowed to granulate closed. If the wound fistulates instead of completely closing, it can be repaired at a later date.

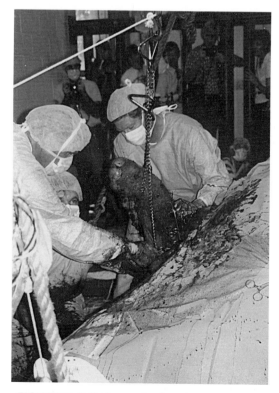

FIGURE 75–3. Fetal extraction through cesarean section.

Treatment for dystocia can be medical, manipulative, or surgical. Aside from supportive medications, oxytocin is the primary medical tool in treatment of dystocia. Uterine inertia, either physiologic or psychological, readily responds to treatment with oxytocin. As in the mare, the elephant uterus is very sensitive to the effects of oxytocin. Doses of 5 to 20 mg intravenously, with or without prior estrogenation, produce active labor contraction. The judicious use of oxytocin after cessation of labor efforts has produced delivery of a live calf in several instances (R. I. Houck, personal communication, 1989). Acupuncture was used in one case to stimulate the uterus, with successful delivery of a dead calf (Pao-chung Chen, personal communication, 1993).

Repeated doses of oxytocin after the initial dose have been unrewarding in producing a primary delivery. From a diagnostic point, the lack of productive response to oxytocin after cessation of natural labor is strong indication that a serious dystocia exists.

Manual reduction of a displaced calf is extremely difficult owing to the size of both cow and calf. The presence of a live fetus helps any reduction because movement of the calf facilitates repositioning, but this is not usually the case. After a large episiotomy incision, the position of the calf can be evaluated. If there is malposition and the uterus is contracted down on the calf, then reduction is difficult. Repulsion of the calf with a crutch device is a consideration but is very difficult to achieve because of the uterine contracture. If the calf's position is normal, traction can be used to assist delivery (Fig. 75–2). Standard obstetrical chain is not strong enough for use on an elephant calf. Heavier chains or nylon straps can be fashioned for placement on the calf's extremities or trunk. The use of these tethers along with mechanically assisted traction produces success in some cases.[2]

If none of these procedures is successful, only a few choices remain. Cesarean section is feasible (Fig. 75–3) but mechanically difficult. So far, cesarean sections have not been rewarding. The author has performed four cesarean sections, all on Asian elephants. One cow was euthanized after 8 hours of surgery because the uterus could not be accessed for secure closure. Two cows with advanced decomposition of the fetus died 7 to 10 days postoperatively as a result of diffuse necrosis of the uterus. The fourth cow died 2 weeks postoperatively as a result of renal disease and focal infarctions of the uterus. Even though these results are discouraging, early diagnosis of dystocia and determination of fetal viability would enhance the eventual results of the procedure. Conservative therapy is another alternative. The use of supportive therapy and antibiotics to prevent overwhelming sepsis from fetal decomposition has been advocated by some individuals. Several cows have been able to pass mummified fetuses at a date far beyond their due date, but these fetuses were not fully developed (N. P. Lung, personal communication, 1996). It seems unlikely that a cow would be able to macerate and pass a fully developed calf without severe sepsis developing, but this remains to be proven. Euthanasia is the only alternative remaining, but it seems a scientific waste because clinicians are only beginning to learn how to manage dystocia in elephants.

REFERENCES

1. Roberts SJ: Veterinary Obstetrics and Genital Diseases, 2nd ed. Ithaca, NY, published by author, p 231, 1971.
2. Merkt Von H, Ahlers D, Bader H, et al: Nachbehandlung und Heilungsverlauf bei einer Elefantenkuh nach Geburtshilfe durch Dammschnitt. Berl Munch Wochenschr 99:329–333, 1986.

CHAPTER **76**

Relocation of African Elephants

J. P. RAATH

The relocation of African elephants (*Loxodonta africana*), either single animals or a breeding herd, is a specialized procedure, and experts should be consulted before such a project commences. Because of the size, strength, and specific anatomic features of elephants, specialized equipment, procedures, and pharmaceutical manipulations have been developed to enable their safe handling. This equipment and technology should be studied and incorporated into the procedure. This is especially important in the relocation of free-ranging elephants.

Elephants are extremely intelligent and adaptable to most habitats or confinements where sufficient food and water is supplied. Their spatial requirements, however, must be considered when adult animals are relocated, especially if they move from a free-ranging situation to confinement.

THE EQUIPMENT

Darting Equipment

Most commercial darting systems (Dan Inject, Telinject, Capchur, Pneudart, and Paxarms) have been successfully used for the darting of elephants. Systems that deposit the drug only when the barrel of the dart hits the skin are found to be superior in pachyderms, because this results in a deep intramuscular (IM) deposition of the drugs. Darting equipment for elephants must be suitably strong and robust to withstand impact even over long distances.

The dart volume depends on the concentration of both the anesthetic and tranquilizer to be used, but a 3-ml volume fits most drug combinations and can be used for elephants of all ages.

In the Kruger National Park (KNP), a dart designed for elephant anesthesia consists of six basic components:

1. A hollow aluminum tailpiece.
2. An aluminum tube threaded on both ends, to hold volumes of 3, 4, and 7 ml.
3. A smooth, collared, or barbed aluminum needle of varying length.
4. A small circular plastic sealing ring that fits into the front end of the hollow tailpiece.
5. An asymmetric weight-plate.
6. A rubber plunger that fits snugly against the tube walls.

To charge and fill the dart, the plastic ring is fitted into the tailpiece and the tail space is filled with a 50% solution of acetic acid. The asymmetric weight-plate is fitted tightly into the ring with the off-center side protruding to the outside. The tailpiece is now ready for attachment to the tube. The tube is lubricated with a silicon gel, and the plunger is pushed through the tube to evenly spread the silicon by means of a gauge. The plunger is then placed in the tube at a set distance from the tail end. The space behind the plunger is filled with a saturated solution of sodium bicarbonate. The filled tailpiece is tightly screwed into the rear end of the tube, the two fluids now being separated by the asymmetric weight-plate. The space in front of the plunger is filled with the drug mixture, and the needle is tightly screwed on (pliers are used for extra force).

On impact, the asymmetric weight-plate topples over, allowing the acetic acid and sodium bicarbonate to mix. Carbon dioxide gas forms, which pushes the plunger forward in the tube, forcing the drug out through the needle. The advantage of this system is that it is initiated only when the body of the dart hits the skin, resulting in the required deep IM deposition of the drug. It is robust and reusable, and there is a selection of volumes.

Thicker sturdy needles with diameters of 2 to 3 mm are preferred for use in elephants. Lengths vary from 50 mm for calves to 70 mm for adults. Lumen openings on the sides of the shaft of the needle are preferred to a needle with the opening in front, because the latter can be blocked by a skin plug in the lumen as it pierces the skin. This blockage can, however, be prevented by cutting the point at a 30-degree angle and bending the tip slightly over the middle of the lumen.

Smooth needles tend to drop out soon after darting; thus all reusable darts should have collared needles. For field operations in which darts are reused, it is good practice to place the needles in a sterilizing solution overnight.

The choice of dart gun depends on the dart system used. Low-noise, adjustable air-powered rifles are preferred for all close-range darting in zoos, in bomas, or on trucks. The pressure on the air rifles must be set high enough to allow full penetration of the needle through the skin.

When darts are removed from the elephant, care must be taken to avoid contact with the anesthetic. Partially injected darts can spray the remainder of the drugs as they are removed from the elephant. If possible, darts should be inactivated before removal.

Drugs and Dosages

Many anesthetics have been used successfully for the immobilization of captive and free-ranging African elephants. The drug choice depends on the purpose of the anesthesia, the desired induction time and duration of the anesthesia, the health status and the temperament of the animal, and the necessity to fully reverse the anesthesia.

Fully reversible anesthetics are preferred for wildlife, even more so in free-ranging conditions. For this reason, opioid anesthetics are commonly used; however, they cause severe hypertension, so they are combined with the butyrophenone tranquilizer azaperone, because the peripheral vasodilation effect of this drug reduces the blood pressure.

Three preparations most commonly used for the anesthesia of elephants are etorphine hydrochloride (M99) and carfentanil and A3080 (currently used only experimentally). The dose rates currently used are given in Table 76–1. These dosages can be reduced to one quarter for animals (by 25%) in captivity. The longer wild elephants have been in captivity, the less anesthetic they require.

Carfentanil has been used at 2.1 ± 0.3 µg/kg as a single IM injection in captive elephants, resulting in recumbency in 10.1 ± 3.7 minutes. It was reversed with nalmefene, at a mean ratio for nalmefene/carfentanil of 26:1, and with diprenorphine hydrochloride, at a mean ratio for diprenorphine/carfentanil of 2.4:1. It has been stated in the literature that etorphine can be used successfully in the immobilization of adult African elephants alone or in combination with a tranquilizer or with scopolamine. When etorphine is used alone, the immobilization can be successfully reversed with M285, with reversal in 2.5 to 3.3 minutes. However, when acetylpromazine was used (15 to 25 mg total dose) in conjunction with the etorphine, all the animals took

TABLE 76–1. Dose Rates for Anesthesia in Elephants

	Shoulder Height (cm)	M99 (mg)	Carfentanil (mg)	A3080 (mg)	Azaperone (mg)
Calf	90–115	2	1	—	20
	116–140	5	3	—	50
	141–165	7	5	—	70
	166–200	9	7	—	90
Adult					
Females		12	10	—	100
Males		15	13	25–35	200

longer to stand and showed symptoms of tranquilization after getting up. No benefit could be seen with the inclusion of scopolamine (20 to 100 mg total dose); it delayed recovery time considerably.

Captive juvenile African elephants have been injected intramuscularly with a combination of xylazine (0.14 ± 0.03 µg/kg) and ketamine (1.14 ± 0.21 mg/kg). This resulted in full immobilization of 64% of the animals; the remainder were only in varying degrees of sedation. When yohimbine was administered at a dose rate of 0.13 ± 0.03 mg/kg intravenously to 86% of the immobilized animals, the mean time that the animals took to stand was 2.4 ± 1.1 minutes, mean immobilization time being 11.6 ± 6.9 minutes.

The inclusion of hyaluronidase in the dart significantly reduces the interval between darting and recumbency. Dosages between 3000 and 7500 IU per dart are recommended. As this enzyme is inactivated by heat, care must be taken to keep the drug cool and add it to the dart just before darting.

Antibiotics are administered to elephants if they are to be confined. Because of the large volumes required, these drugs are injected at several sites.

Internal parasites are more important in juveniles confined long term and can be treated with ivermectin. This is administered subcutaneously in the neck region but can result in the formation of a hard nodule.

Although external parasites occur only in extremely low numbers, the elephants are sprayed with an acaricide from a backpack sprayer. Special attention is given to the escutcheon and axilla areas. Synthetic pyrethroids have been used successfully without any side effects.

Before the anesthesia commences, care should be taken that all emergency drugs are available, accessible, and not expired. These drugs should include the antidote, cardiorespiratory stimulators, corticosteroids, nonsteroidal anti-inflammatory agents, diuretics, and a complete kit for accidental human injection.

Individual Crates

Crates for individual transportation of elephants are best constructed with a metal frame lined on the inside with wood or metal plating. Each end of a crate should have doors that open vertically or two half doors that swing to the side.

For smaller elephants, the doors can be constructed

of metal piping spaced to prevent protrusion of the head. This reduces the mass of the doors, increases ventilation, and facilitates feeding and handling of the animals. Double doors—that is, a pipe frame inner door and a solid outer door—are often used for elephants that will be crated for extended periods of time, will receive food and water, and will need cleaning. If solid doors are used on both ends, a lockable "trapdoor" should be installed in either the rear half of the roof or in the top half of the rear door. This allows for the administration of emergency drugs or tranquilizers.

The roof and floor of the crates are slatted to allow water to be poured onto the elephants and for urine and water to drain. International Air Transport Association specifications must be followed for air transportation.

Sizes of crates commonly used for the relocation of elephant calves are listed in Table 76–2.

Ideally, a crate should be constructed only if the size of the individual elephant is known. Elephants are extremely acrobatic and can turn around if the crate is too large, so crates for short-distance translocation should not be too large.

Mass Relocation Equipment

Crate size depends on the number of individuals and the size of the largest animal to be translocated. When translocating family units, the standard crate used has inside dimensions of 12 × 2.4 × 2.7 m. This is generally made by customizing a high shipping container (used for commercial shipment of food goods). For smaller numbers of animals, the principles remain the same, but the dimensions can be adjusted.

The containers are divided into two compartments separated by a vertical double-sliding door, which allows the container to be opened to its full width if

TABLE 76–2. Sizes of Crates Commonly Used for Relocation of Elephant Calves

Size of Elephant	Inside Measurements (cm) of Crate		
	Length	Width	Height
Small	200	90	190
Medium	200	110	190
Large	2500	120	220

necessary. A similar sliding door is installed immediately in front of the two rear container doors. On the sides, each compartment is fitted with two evenly spaced ventilation grids at the top, measuring 30 cm × 2 m, and three small, evenly spaced ventilation grids on floor level, measuring 20 cm × 40 cm.

Each compartment has three roof doors (80 × 100 cm), evenly spaced along the center of the container. These doors should open completely without restricting human movement along the roof. A permanent ladder should be present.

In the capture and relocation of elephant families, the elephants are walked into a trailer that allows them access to the translocation crate. It is an area where much activity takes place; therefore, it should be adequately reinforced. This crate measures 6 × 2.4 × 2.7 m (a smaller shipping container). It is fitted with sliding doors similar to those of the translocation truck but on both ends. The roof and sides are made similarly to those of the translocation crate. On the one end, the roof is reinforced, and a strong but removable pulley is installed.

In large operations, two tractors and two modified trailers are required. Each tractor is fitted with a powerful winch behind the driver's seat.

The trailers, able to incline hydraulically, are fitted with a bed of rollers 2 m wide and 4 m long. Through the use of a smooth, round pipe, the sides of the trailer are raised approximately 20 cm above the roller bed. On the front end of the roller bed, a free running pulley is attached to guide the winch cable.

Six to eight strong mats are needed for the loading of the elephants. Two sizes (6 × 2 m and 8 × 2 m) accommodate elephants of various sizes. The mats should be smooth and the ends reinforced with steel. Conveyer belting used in sugar mills is ideal for this purpose.

A loop for securing the winch cable hook should be fitted on each end in the middle of the steel enforcement. Two lengths of chain are secured to the two ends of each metal reinforcement, leaving enough chain free to allow an 80-cm-high triangle to be formed in the center point of one of these chains. Another chain that is the same length as the mat is connected. On the long sides of these mats, elongated holes are cut to act as handles for carrying the mats.

Loose Equipment

An array of equipment is required during elephant captures, especially for free-ranging elephants. This equipment includes ropes, spades, axes, cattle prodders, water carts, and buckets.

THE PROCEDURE

The muscular region of the hind limbs, the back, and shoulder muscles are considered acceptable darting sites; however, the gluteal region is preferred. To avoid subcutaneous or intradermal deposition of the drugs, care must be taken to place the dart at a right angle to the skin. When darting is performed from a helicopter, the speed of the helicopter must equal that of the elephant at the time the dart is fired. If the helicopter flies over the elephant during darting, a whiplash effect is created as the dart hits the animal, often breaking the needle of the dart.

When morphine derivatives are used, the first sign of induction seen is that the tail of the elephant is pulled in between the hind legs. This is followed by an unsteady gait and often dragging of the front feet. The movement of the trunk is reduced, the elephant stops moving, and stands with the trunk on the ground and the ears hanging forward. If undisturbed, the elephant goes into a sitting position and then rolls into lateral recumbency. Sometimes the elephant remains in the sternal sitting position.

Lateral recumbency is desirable, and elephants resting on their sternums are pushed or pulled onto their sides. Depending on the position of the legs in sternal recumbency, an elephant is rolled over by swinging the head, using the tusks for leverage. This rocking motion takes the head over the center of gravity, and by pushing on the side of the elephant, lateral recumbency can be achieved. If the legs are spread too wide and prevent pushing over by this method, a rope is secured to the base of one tusk and placed under the ear and over the neck of the animal to the opposite side. The rope is tied to a vehicle and gently pulled until the animal topples over.

With the elephant lying on its side, the top ear is flapped over the exposed eye and the trunk is straightened to facilitate breathing. Water is poured over the animal's body, particularly the ears, to control hyperthermia.

Body temperature is routinely monitored in anesthetized elephants. It averages 36°C in adults and 38.5°C in calves after herding, but it can go up to 40°C in calves herded over a long distance on hot days.

Respiration rate is easily measured with a hand held lightly over the end of the trunk. The average rate for an adult elephant is three to four respirations per minute. The respiration is usually very deep and is accompanied by snoring noises during exhalation. In calves, the respiration rate per minute varies from 16 in small calves to 8 in larger ones.

The heart rate is either read directly from the electrocardiogram or monitored by palpation of the middle ear artery on the uppermost ear. It varies according to the elephant's level of excitement, the speed and distance of the chase, and the interval between recumbency and the onset of monitoring the heart rate. The average heart rates were found to be 43 to 80 beats per minute in adults and 48 to 114 beats per minute in very small calves.

Blood oxygenation can be measured with a pulse oximeter. The probe can be clamped to the lip, tongue, vagina, or prepuce, but best results are obtained when the probe is attached to the ear. An area is prepared by gently scraping off the outside pigmented layers of the skin on both sides of the ear with a scalpel blade. Blood gas values can also be determined by collecting samples from the middle ear artery and a vein. Blood pressure is measured directly from the central ear artery or indirectly by placing a cuff around the tail of the elephant.

The level of anesthesia must be continuously monitored. Palpebral and corneal reflexes remain, and elephants have constricted pupils when sedated. Trunk movements indicate that the level of anesthesia is decreasing. Slight movements of the trunk tip are followed by a rolling up of the straightened trunk just before the first efforts to stand.

Problems During Anesthesia

Researchers have shown markedly elevated mean arterial pressure (MAP) in elephants anesthetized with opioids alone. The MAP may become so high that fluid and even blood are forced from the capillaries into the lungs. This results in massive lung edema and capillary bleeding. It is manifested by pink foam running out of the trunk of the elephant. Azaperone is added to the darts to address the problem. The amount is only a fraction of the total recommended for tranquilization of a particular-sized elephant; however, because of its vasodilatation effect, a significant reduction in the MAP is obtained. No further cases of pink foam have been observed since the addition of azaperone (at the dose rates in Table 76–1) became routine. The azaperone also has an added beneficial effect of respiratory stimulation.

"Pink foam" syndrome is life-threatening and necessitates immediate action. Treatment includes azaperone, membrane stabilizers, diuretics, and immediate reversal of anesthesia.

Although seldom seen, apnea does occur in anesthetized elephants and may be fatal. Once it is detected, treatment with respiratory stimulants such as doxapram may alleviate it. In addition, if the anesthesia is supplemented with an intravenous (IV) ketamine bolus, temporary apnea is often seen.

Elephants under anesthesia may also exhibit asynchromatic diaphragmatic flutter ("hiccups"). Treatment is not necessary; sometimes it subsides only after the antidote is administered.

On occasion, elephants lying without supervision attempt to rise as the level of anesthesia decreases. Because elephants lift their heads before they can stand, standing can be prevented by keeping the head down. This is achieved by support staff sitting on the head while anesthetic supplementation by IV administration of 20% to 25% of the initial dose, depending on the duration of anesthesia required, is administered.

Treatment of the Dart Wound

Because of the large diameter of the dart needle, the hole in the skin is a significant. The needle carries bacteria and dirt from the skin surface to the subcutaneous area. Bruising of tissue at the site of injection creates an ideal growth medium for bacteria. The thick skin of elephants does not allow for easy drainage, and large subcutaneous abscesses can form at the dart site. To counteract this, an intramammary antibiotic preparation is inserted into the dart wound.

Reversal of the Anesthesia

Good preparation reduces the duration of anesthesia. With suggested dose rates, the operator has just over an hour before the animal will attempt to rise. However, this is only a guideline, and the level of anesthesia should be monitored continuously.

The drug for reversing anesthesia is administered intravenously into an ear vein as a single bolus.

Both etorphine and A3080 can successfully be reversed with diprenorphine at three and two times the anesthetic dose, respectively. Other short-acting reversal agents that can be used are nalmefene and nalbuphine. Because of the longer half-life of carfentanil, however, a longer acting reversal agent should be used to avoid renarcotization. Naltrexone has proved to be very effective at a dose rate of 40 mg to each milligram of carfentanil used. Renarcotization was seen when this ratio was lowered to 35:1. When anesthetized animals receive additional carfentanil during the procedure, the reversal agent should be calculated according to the total number of milligrams of the anesthetic.

The normal reversal time for the opioids is 2 to 4 minutes. The elephant flips the ear back; the eye becomes alert and the pupil dilated; trunk movements commence, followed by movement of the limbs; and the elephant lifts its head and rolls sternally. The front quarters are raised first. It is not uncommon for elephants treated with diprenorphine to have slightly depressed reactions for a short time after reversal.

The Loading of Individual Animals

While laterally recumbent, the elephant calf is measured (the rump of an elephant is slightly higher that its shoulder height), and an appropriate-sized crate is selected. The crate is placed in front of the elephant in line with the front legs and as close as possible to the animal. The crate door is opened, and a strong rope or a chain covered with hose pipe is secured around the neck behind the ears of the calf. In the case of a rope, a slipknot is made approximately 1.5 m from the end; in the case of a chain, a quick-release pin should be used to secure the chain around the elephant's neck. The rope or chain is passed through the crate and through a vertical slot in the door at the far end of the crate. The short end of the rope or, in the case of a chain, a thin rope from the quick-release mechanism is passed through one of the ventilation gaps in the roof of the crate.

The center of a second rope is placed around the rump of the calf, and the two long ends of the rope are taken forward past the sides of the crate. The size of the calf determines the number of persons manning each rope and assisting on either side of the elephant's head. With all ropes secured and manned, the tranquilizer is administered, followed by the antidote to the tranquilizer into an ear vein. The top ear is flapped back, exposing the calf's eye. This allows the observers to assess the revival process as described earlier. If the interval between administration of the tranquilizer and the antidote is too long, or if the total dose of tranquilizer is given in the dart, the animal may be reluctant to stand. This may delay or jeopardize the loading process.

When the calf is standing solidly on all four legs, it is pushed, pulled, and steered into the crate. It is very important for one person to be in command and give the instructions. The loading must be conducted gently, because the animal must not stumble or be pulled onto its knees.

When the calf is standing in the crate, the rear door is closed. The neck rope or chain is removed by releasing the slipknot or quick-release mechanism and pulling the rope or chain through the hole in the door. The crate with the elephant can then be loaded.

Loading After Confinement

Confinement calms elephants down, adapts them to a feeding regimen and human presence, and familiarizes them with the crate, all of which reduce stress en route and at destination.

When a mass crate is used, it can be placed at the end of a passage in position for loading. The elephant's gate is left open by day, and it is allowed to walk up the ramp and into the crate. This is encouraged by placing food treats along the passageway and in the crate. This facilitates the loading process, inasmuch as the elephant becomes accustomed to using the passageway.

Individual crates are placed inside the confinement area with both doors removed, allowing the elephants to walk through the crates. After 3 to 4 days, one door is removed, and food treats are placed inside to encourage the animals to stand inside the crates for extended periods of time. Alternatively, one crate can be placed at the end of the passage and the same protocol as for the mass crates is followed.

Confining the elephants to their pens and depriving them of treats for 24 hours before loading makes them more suggestible to the temptation of treats at loading time. Passive luring into crates produces better results than attempting to force elephants along the passageway and into the crates. Elephants can be tranquilized at the point of loading by confining them to a section of the passageway and injecting the tranquilizer by hand.

Small elephants, as well as elephants that are well tamed, can be tranquilized with azaperone at two thirds of the capture dose. Haloperidol in combination with azaperone is used in large elephants, in wild young elephants, or when the design of the truck causes concern and a long-distance trip is anticipated. Although haloperidol has a longer effect than the short-term tranquilizers, it is not as long-lasting as in other species. The dose rates are also higher in smaller animals, as clearly shown in Figure 76–1.

When confinement is to be continued at the destination, the long-acting tranquilizer perphenazine enanthate (Trilafon) is useful (100 mg IM for calves under 1.6 m shoulder height and 200 mg IM for larger calves). Although this has been used on only a small number of elephants, a definite positive effect has been detected. The optimal dosage rate has not yet been established. If there is fighting or excessive damage to the crates, additional azaperone or haloperidol can be administered by hand or pole syringe. All animals in a compartment are tranquilized, to prevent a docile animal from being injured by more active ones. Feeding in the transport vehicle has a further calming effect on the elephants.

THE TRANSLOCATION OF FAMILY UNITS

An off-loading paddock should be constructed for the animals' initial release. The paddock is a 100 × 100 m area in which the elephants will be confined for 3 to 5 days. Dense natural vegetation for the elephants to hide in and to use as a food source must be included.

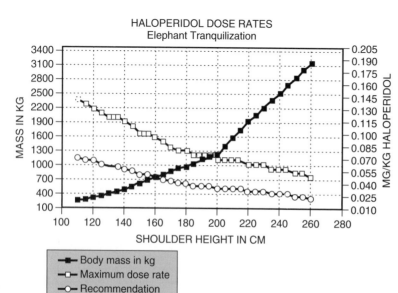

FIGURE 76–1. Haloperidol dose rates in African elephants.

The fence is the same height as the perimeter fence, but stronger. Railway lines or steel poles are placed in concrete (1 m³) every 10 m. A minimum of five steel cables, with one at ground level and then at 600-mm intervals, are strung around the camp on the inside of the poles except at the corners, where they are on the outside. This allows them to be pulled at one point, while at the same time force is placed on the planted poles when the elephants push against the fence. Normal game fencing is erected from ground level to 2.4 m high. Dropper poles are placed at 1-m intervals. The fence is electrified with three strands with the offsets to the inside, and a voltage of 6000 to 9000 V is to be maintained throughout the confinement period, even if additional generators are required. This paddock teaches the elephants to respect electricity, inasmuch as the perimeter fences do not have cables and the electrical wire is used to prevent breakouts. Although this is an expensive structure, the success of the operation depends on it.

Large trees should not be enclosed inside the fence because elephants may push them onto the fence. The off-loading ramp is placed outside the fence, to avoid confrontation with the elephants after release. It is important that the gate closing the off-loading ramp is also electrified. The off-loading ramp must be as wide and as high as the translocation truck that is used. Because the truck has doors sliding to the sides, there must not be any obstructions to the sides. The sides of the off-loading ramp leading to the paddock should be constructed of poles, set in concrete in the ramp.

Ideally, the paddock should include natural water and a mud wallow. Clean water must be available for drinking. A separate wide gate for the release of the elephants should be constructed in one corner. The paddock should be as close to the middle of the reserve or farm as possible. This will allow the animals an opportunity to become calm before coming into contact with yet another fence.

The paddock must be accessible via good roads because the transport trucks are 14 m long and 4.3 m high and make very wide turns.

The Procedure

Elephant social organization is matriarchal within bond groups and clans of related families. A basic social unit is a group of related females consisting of a mother, her young, her grown daughters, and their offspring. Herd sizes range from 2 to 24; the average is 9 to 11. Activity, direction, and rate of movement are determined by the matriarch, often recognizable as the largest cow. If disturbed, the group immediately clusters around her and follows her lead. Bulls leave the herd at the age of 12 to 20 years and thereafter never stay for long periods with any breeding herd.

Standard procedure for an elephant capture is to select a family unit of an acceptable size (5 to 16 animals). The elephants are slowly herded by helicopter to a workable area near a road, where darting commences from the helicopter. The first animal to be darted is always the matriarch, followed by the other adult cows in the group. As soon as these large animals are darted, the helicopter withdraws until these animals become recumbent. They act as an anchor for the rest of the group. The rest of the group is then darted in order of size; the smallest calves are darted last. Care is taken to identify the calf of each cow, to ensure that it is loaded with its mother.

When all animals are recumbent, the ground crew moves in, placing animals in lateral recumbency, ensuring patent airways, and cooling them down by pouring water on their ears. All darts are removed, dart wounds are treated, and the animals are sprayed with an acaricide.

The elephant mats are placed next to the adult cows, and with the use of ropes and manpower, the animals are rolled onto the mats. Each mat is folded over the elephant that lies on it, and the two ends are tied with the long chain. The tractor with the roller bed trailer is brought in front of each elephant, and the conveyer belt with the elephant is winched onto the roller bed of the tipped trailer, after which the trailer is leveled. The long chain is released for the comfort of the elephant and to ensure the that airway is not blocked.

The wake up trailer is parked against the transport truck. The tractor with the elephant backs against this trailer, and the winch cable on the tractor is extended, looped around the pulley in the front of the trailer, and attached to the loop on the mat. Thus when the winch is engaged, the mat with the elephant is slowly pulled into the trailer. Once the elephant is lying inside the trailer, the antidote to the tranquilizer is administered, and the doors are closed. As soon as the animal is standing, the sliding doors leading to the transport truck are opened, and the animal walks through into the crate on the truck. Once it is inside the crate, a combination of short- and long-acting tranquilizers is administered through the roof doors, with a pole syringe. It is important to tranquilize all large animals in one compartment of a mass crate, but the small calves should travel untranquilized. This procedure is repeated until all elephants are loaded.

To reduce the time that the animals are recumbent, two tractors and trailers are used, and the loading process continues in a production-line manner. This has reduced the average time between darting and departure to less than 20 minutes per elephant.

The very small calves are loaded first, often manually and by using a stretcher. They are followed by their mothers, and all these animals are loaded in the front compartment. The larger calves and young bulls are loaded into the rear compartment.

Transport

The route is carefully selected to ensure the shortest driving time and to avoid large cities and mountainous areas. Fuel stops are planned, and spectators are prevented from disturbing the elephants. When traveling long distances through remote areas, consideration must be given to using an escort vehicle in case of breakdown.

Plans must always be made for the worst-case scenario, and a short-range darting system, complete with darts and loading set or, alternatively, a pole syringe, should be brought. Enough drugs should be included to anesthetize all the elephants at least once. Short- and long-term tranquilizers, a powerful flashlight, a cattle prodder, a heavy caliber rifle, and a cellular phone are all essentials on the long-distance relocations.

Administrative tasks must be conducted well in advance to ensure that all necessary documents, especially in international transfers, accompany the animals en route. The destination personnel should be informed of the arrival time, and this information should be updated during the transport.

It is advisable to have three drivers on long journeys, and at least one driver should have suitable mechanical knowledge to cope with minor problems with the transport vehicle. The driving style required for some transport game also applies to elephants. Slow pull-aways and gentle stops, easy cornering, and no sudden swerving are basic principles to which to adhere.

At any time when it appears that the elephants are fighting, moving excessively, or trumpeting frequently, a stop should be made and the elephants inspected. The interval between stops should never exceed 2 hours. All animals must be physically seen during every stop (flashlights should be used at night).

Problems Encountered on Road

Elephants travel well if correctly tranquilized. The most frequent problem is an elephant lying down. Although this position is not unnatural for elephants, it is undesirable during transport because they are trampled upon and jabbed with other elephants' tusks, and it is possible for other elephants to suffocate them by standing on the recumbent animals' trunks. The recumbent animals are therefore prodded and stimulated to stand.

The drainage must be opened at every stop because urine and feces are produced en route; the latter tends to block the drainage openings, and the elephants soon stand in a pool of urine.

Fighting can occur and lead to serious injury. Again, methods of appropriate tranquilization on long journeys are important.

The Off-Loading Procedure

Approximately 30 minutes from destination, all elephants with a shoulder height higher than 2 m receive a supplemental dose of a short-acting tranquilizer such as azaperone.

Once the truck has been parked against the off-loading ramp, all gaps between the truck and the ramp should be filled with sandbags. The person in charge of the off-loading sits on the roof of the truck; from there, he or she can observe the elephants walking out, give commands for the opening of the doors, and, if necessary, prod animals through the trapdoors on the roofs. This person must, however, be careful not to be pulled from the roof, especially when large elephants leave the truck backwards.

To facilitate off-loading at night, a spotlight can be used from the roof of the truck to illuminate the pathway down the ramp, or the ramp can be lit with vehicle lights.

The rear sliding doors are opened slowly, and the elephants are allowed to walk out at their own pace. They may sniff the ground for extended periods of time before walking out. They sometimes stop just outside the truck and spray themselves with sand. As soon as the animals in the rear compartment have left the truck, the middle doors should be opened, allowing the elephants in the front compartment to leave. These doors should be opened as soon as possible to allow the family group to leave together, but opening them too soon may result in the larger cows from the front compartment trying to force their way out, injuring some of the smaller elephants.

The elephants wander slowly into the thicker parts of the confinement and almost immediately commence feeding. Should they turn around and challenge the fence or truck, they may be persuaded to leave by clapping of hands and controlled shouting. Only when the elephants have disappeared into the thickest areas of the holding pen is the gate at the bottom of the off-loading ramp closed and secured.

The amount of spectators must be kept at a minimum at the off-loading procedure. They are kept behind the truck and preferably on the back of vehicles and should remain quiet at all times. A false sense of confidence in the fence must be avoided, because the elephants can easily break it down, escape, and injure people on the outside.

Care in the temporary boma determines the success of the operation. It is important that the elephants learn to respect the electrified fence so that they do not challenge the perimeter fences of the reserve in the future.

The elephants must be disturbed as little as possible while in the temporary holding facility. The fence is inspected at least twice daily, and adequate water levels are maintained in the troughs. The elephants will break or push over some of the trees, and it must be ensured that these do not interfere with the electrified fence.

The release is a passive procedure. The large gate is opened at dawn after the elephants have been confined at least 3 days. The elephants must be left alone and allowed to leave the holding area on their own. It is not uncommon for the elephants to remain in the holding area for days after the gate has been opened, but they must never be disturbed, nor must the electric fence be switched off.

REFERENCES

1. Allen JL: Use of tolazoline as an antagonist to xylazine-ketamine-induced immobilization in African elephants. Am J Vet Res 47(4):781–783, 1986.
2. Hattingh J, Knox CM, Raath JP: Arterial blood pressure of the African elephant (*Loxodonta africana*) under etorphine anaesthesia and after remobilisation with diprenorphine. Vet Rec 135:458–460, 1994.
3. Hattingh J, Knox CM, Raath JP, Keet DF: Arterial blood pressure in anaesthetized African elephants. S Afr J Wildl Res 24(1–2):15–17, 1994.
4. Jacobson ER, Allen J, Martin H, Kollias GV: Effects of yohimbine on combined xylazine-ketamine-induced sedation and immobiliza-

tion in juvenile African elephants. J Am Vet Med Assoc 187(11):1195–1198, 1985.
5. Jacobson ER, Kollias GV, Heard DJ, Caligiuri R: Immobilization of African elephants with carfentanil and antagonism with nalmefene and diprenorphine. J Zoo Anim Med 19(1–2):1–7, 1988.
6. Kock MD, Martin RB, Kock N: Chemical immobilization of free-ranging African elephants (*Loxodonta africana*) in Zimbabwe, using etorphine (M99) mixed with hyaluronidase, and evaluation of biolog-ical data collected soon after immobilization. J Zoo Wildl Med 24(1):1–10, 1983.
7. McKenzie A: Capture and Care Manual. Pretoria, Wildlife Division Support Services and South African Veterinary Foundation, pp 484–498, 1993.
8. Wallach JD, Anderson JL: Oripavine (M.99) combinations and sol-vents for immobilization of the African elephant. J Am Vet Med Assoc 153(7):793–797, 1968.

CHAPTER 77

Antibiotic Therapy in Elephants

JOHN H. OLSEN

Like other species, elephants should be given appro-priate antibiotic regimens to achieve success in therapy. When selecting antibiotics, the clinician must evaluate the severity and location of the infection, the antibiotic sensitivities of the bacteria, the pharmacodynamics of the antibiotics, the potential toxicity of the drug, and the physical status of the animal. Antibiotic therapy in elephants can present problems because of (1) inability to reasonably estimate body weight for proper dose calculation, (2) lack of appropriate dosage information, (3) difficulties with administration of the medication, (4) volume or cost of medication needed.

BODY WEIGHT DETERMINATION

Determination of accurate body weight is desirable, but not always possible. In zoological settings, scales are becoming more available to weigh elephants. The fol-lowing weight ranges are provided as an estimate of body weights compared to average elephant sizes. Aver-age adult Asian elephant (*Elephas maximus*) cows stand 2.1 to 2.4 m high at the shoulder and weigh between 2300 and 3700 kg, whereas an average bull stands 2.4 to 2.9 m high at the shoulder and weighs from 3700 to 4500 kg. Asian bulls can reach 3.2 m at the shoulder and weigh 5500 kg, whereas cows can grow to a maxi-mum height of 2.7 m at the shoulder and weigh 4200 kg. The average height of an adult African (*Loxodonta africana*) cow is 2.3 to 2.7 m at the shoulder and average weight is 2300 to 4000 kg, whereas average African bulls can be 2.7 to 3.2 m at the shoulder and weigh 4100 to 5000 kg. Bull African elephants can reach 3.6 m in height at the shoulder and weigh 6400 kg.[31]

In addition, there are several formulas for estimating an Asian elephant's weight on the basis of various body measurements. However, varying elephant conforma-tions can present challenges. The author has tested the formulas, using measurements and weights obtained from three female Asian elephants aged 24 to 27 years old, weighing 2918 kg to 4400 kg. Some of these formulas are as follows:

1. Sreekumar and Nirmalan determined weight in Asian elephants as follows: weight (kg) $= -1010 + 0.036 \times$ (body length [from base of skull to base of tail in centimeters] $\times$ girth [behind shoulder in centimeters]).[35] Using this formula, the author found weights to be underestimated by 32.2% to 38.6%.

2. On the basis of studies on domesticated elephants in Sri Lanka, Kurt and Nettasinghe[16] generated several formulas. Determination of body weight from shoulder height is as follows: $y = -22.39 + 18.9x$, where y is the shoulder height (cm) and x is the cube root of the body weight (kg), with shoulder height measured at the withers. Using this formula, the author found that weights were underestimated by 9.0% to 27%. Ac-cording to Kurt, the shoulder height can be estimated to within 1% to 5% by measuring the circumference of one weight-bearing forefoot or footprint and multi-plying by two. In the author's test, the circumference of a weight-bearing front foot was found to be close to half the height of the back at the shoulder area (with-ers). The estimate of height was an underestimation by 1.4% to 5.8%.

3. Kurt and Nettasinghe[16] projected body weight (kg) from measurement of the chest girth as $y = -60.6 + 28.9x$, where y is the girth (cm) of the chest immedi-ately behind the elbows measured and x is the cube root of the body weight (kg). When this formula was tested, weight was overestimated by 21.2% to 52.8%.

Kurt and Nettasinghe found American circus elephants to be heavier than working elephants in Sri Lanka.

4. Hile and colleagues[13] obtained body measurements on 75 Asian elephants in North America including weight, heart girth, height at the withers, body length, and foot pad circumference. They concluded that heart girth was the best predictive factor for body weight. Hiler and colleagues developed regression equations for predicting body weight (kg) in four age classes of elephants. The first equation for all elephants aged 1 to 57 years is 18.0 × (heart girth in centimeters) − 3336 = body weight (kg). For the age class 1 to 13 years, the formula is 17.9 × (heart girth in centimeters) − 3408 = body weight (kg); in the 18- to 28-year age class, the formula is 15.5 × (heart girth in centimeters) − 2481 = body weight (kg). The 29- to 39-year-old age class formula is 19.4 × (heart girth in centimeters) − 3786 = body weight (kg) and the 40- to 57-year age class formula is 20.8 × (heart girth in centimeters) − 4249 = body weight (kg).

The average error for each of these formulas appears relatively small; however, the error range is significant, so determinations on individuals can be very inaccurate. In older (over 29 years old) animals the error range is much improved. The author tested the 18- to 28-year age class formula and the total group formula. The 18- to 28-year-old formula, based on girth, overestimated body weight by 9.2% to 35.4% and the total age class formula overestimated body weight by 16.5% to 41.7%.

More work is needed to determine formulas that will more accurately estimate body weight in elephants.

DOSAGE CALCULATION

Metabolic scaling to extrapolate drug doses from one species to another has been promoted.[34] Although useful, when pharmacokinetics information is not available, scaling must be used with caution. Numerous exceptions to scaling exist, some with potentially toxic effects.[10] Metabolic scaling seems appropriate in an elephant; however, most of the pharmacokinetic studies done on antibiotics in elephants suggest that dosage extrapolation should be done from large animal/equine doses rather than metabolic scaling.[18, 25, 32]

Furthermore, there has been little work that relates dosage requirements of African elephants to those of Asian elephants. For example, African elephants require a slightly higher initial dose of etorphine and more frequent repetition of doses than Asian elephants. Similar findings were found in another study with xylazine and etorphine in African and Asian species. The study by Page and colleagues[25] on trimethoprim-sulfamethoxazole (TMP-SMZ) included three African elephants and one Asian elephant. The limited data suggest there may be significant differences in pharmacokinetics between these species.

Several prominent elephant clinicians use the same dosage rate for both species.[14, 33] Further pharmacokinetic studies are needed.

There also may be differences in metabolism and antibiotic requirements between captive and free-ranging animals. deVos stated that carfentanil "doses for African elephants in zoos are 3/4 that of free roaming elephants."[9] Do similar differences occur with antibiotics?

Many antibiotics have not been studied at all in elephants, and clinicians must use their judgment to determine dosages. On the basis of the studies that have been done and on clinical practice, it is recommended that equine dosage rates should be the basis for dosage determination when specific dosage information is not available.

ROUTE OF ADMINISTRATION FOR SYSTEMIC ANTIBIOTICS

Antibiotic selection may depend on a number of factors such as volume, frequency, palatability, ability to mask taste, ability to safely inject on regular schedule, volume and irritability of injection, and temperament and training of the elephant.

Oral

Many elephants are not willing to eat unusual things and are adept at recognizing medication and rejecting it. Allowing the normal handlers to provide medication is usually more effective than having a veterinarian or other unfamiliar person give the medication. Often, elephants can be enticed to consume medication by hiding it in a favorite food or treat such as fruit, molasses, bread, or an ice cream cup with syrup. Microencapsulation of medication has been used to mask its taste.[33] Custom-compounded medications may also be made in different flavors. A number of antibiotics such as trimethoprim-sulfamethoxazole, sulfadimethoxine/ormetoprim (Primor, SmithKline-Beecham, Exton, PA), and enrofloxacin (Baytril, Miles Animal Health, Shawnee Mission, KS) are usually well accepted orally.

Michael Schmidt suggests that elephants can learn to accept oral medication as an alternative to injections.[33] A handler can offer oral medication. If the medication is rejected, a veterinarian immediately administers the injection. With several repetitions, the animal usually learns to take oral medications as the preferable alternative. Some tractable elephants and young elephants may be medicated by stomach tube. A speculum is placed between the molars and the tube is passed dorsal to the larynx; gentle pressure relaxes the sphincter at the posterior of the pharyngeal pouch,[31] with care being taken to ensure that the tube is placed appropriately.

Injection

Even though many elephants are well trained and can readily undergo treatment, the ability to safely inject repeated doses of medication can be a problem. Protection of the animal care staff as well as the veterinarians should be considered when giving injections. When using injectable antibiotics, it may be safer to have an elephant in a chute or squeeze apparatus for the treatment. If a chute is not available to limit mobility during the injection, the elephant can hold up one leg, or the animal can be laid down during injections. This makes it more difficult for the animal to react quickly and it may make the injections less painful because muscles are not bearing weight. Stick poles and darts can be used if necessary to administer some medications to some animals.

Intramuscular

Because the volume of antibiotic is often large, it is usually necessary to use multiple injection sites. If possible, no more than 15 to 25 ml of drug should be given at one injection site in an adult elephant, because larger doses probably prolong absorption and increase local irritation. Such irritation can be treated with an application of dimethyl sulfoxide on the skin directly over the site.[31] Murray and coworkers[21] reported giving amoxicillin injections with 30 ml of drug per site with an 18-gauge spinal needle 9 cm long. No heat or swelling was noted at the sites and the animal showed no lameness.

Recommended injection sites include the hind quarters, triceps area of the foreleg, and the neck. The skin tends to be thinner in the fore quarters than the rear quarters. Needles 3.75 cm (1.5 inches) long and 18 gauge (14 to 20 gauge) are adequate to reach the muscles in this region. Injections in the hind legs require 6.25 to 8.75 cm (2.5- to 3.5-inch) long, at least 18-gauge spinal needles with stylets, to penetrate to muscle. To minimize the tendency for abscess, the skin should be prepared with a disinfectant before injection.[31] The pain of injection can be masked by rubbing and slapping the injection site just before quickly thrusting the needle in the skin.

Intravenous

The veins in the posterior side of the ear can be used for intravenous (IV) administration of drugs. Caution should be used when irritating drugs are injected there because vascular irritation can lead to local necrosis and tissue sloughing. Dilution of drugs, use of a catheter, and slow administration can reduce this potential. The large cephalic vein on the craniomedial forelegs and the medial saphenous vein on the distal medial rear legs can also be used for IV drug therapy.[31]

Subcutaneous

Subcutaneous administration is not usually a preferred site for antibiotics because of questionable absorption. However, use of needles of insufficient length results in drugs being given at this site.

Suppository

One report describes the use of metronidazole suppositories placed in the rectum once a day to maintain adequate plasma levels.[12] This technique needs to be further investigated because there may be other opportunities to use this approach.

ANTIBIOTIC SELECTIONS

Whenever possible, selection of the antibiotic should be based on bacterial cultures and sensitivities. The pharmacodynamics of an antibiotic determines whether the drug reaches the site of infection in effective concentrations.

PHARMACOKINETIC STUDIES AND ANTIBIOTIC USAGE

There have been a number of studies on pharmacokinetics of antibiotics in elephants; however, some are of limited value because they were based on the use of one animal or used body weight estimates as the basis for dosage. This section discusses (1) pharmacokinetic studies in elephants, (2) recommendations from veterinarians experienced with elephant medicines, (3) dosages that have been used with apparent safety, and (4) problems or toxicities of certain antibiotics.

Penicillins

Penicillins are beta lactam antibiotics that inhibit the formation of bacterial cell wall and are bactericidal for growing and dividing organisms. The effective spectrum and route of administration vary with the generation of the product.

Schmidt[32] reported the use of penicillin G and amoxicillin in five Asian elephants in 1978. The dose regimen recommended is 4545 IU/kg (10,000 IU/lb) every 96 hours to treat *Bacillus anthracis, Corynebacterium diphtheriae*, streptococci, and staphylococci (non–penicillinase-producing). To treat the same organisms, the dose could also be cut in half and administered every 48 hours. To treat *Clostridia*, 4545 IU/kg every 36 hours is recommended, and the same dose every 24 hours is recommended for *Pasteurella multocida* infection.

Amoxicillin is a semisynthetic, bactericidal penicillinase-sensitive penicillin. It has less activity against gram-negative bacteria. Drug trials with dosages of 2.2 mg/kg, 6.6 mg/kg, and 11 mg/kg amoxicillin trihydrate intramuscularly (IM) were performed. The dose of 11 mg/kg produced an average maximum serum concentration of 1.567 μg/ml. The plateau level at 12 hours for this dose was 1.23 μg/ml. It appears that the serum concentration of the drug does not decrease from 12 to 24 hours, so once-a-day administration of the drug may be adequate. *Salmonella* species and *Escherichia coli* are two organisms for which amoxicillin may be used effectively.[32]

Oral administration has also been studied with 8 mg/kg ampicillin. Mean serum concentration remained above 0.06 μg/ml (the mean inhibitory concentration [MIC] for streptococcal and staphylococcal agents in the study) for more than 8 hours after administration.

The study recommends that ampicillin trihydrate be administered orally two to three times daily at the dose of 8 mg/kg to treat susceptible streptococcal and staphylococcal pathogens in foot abscesses. Although this dose may be effective against some gram-negative bacteria (e.g., sensitive strains of *P. multocida*), it would not likely be effective against *Salmonella* or *E. coli*.[30]

◆ CASE STUDIES

Case 1

A recommended treatment for Anthrax in elephants is repeated doses of penicillin at 5000 to 20,000 IU/kg body weight as well as vaccination of other exposed elephants.[31]

Case 2

Janssen and colleagues[15] reported on the treatment of *Salmonella* infection in several South African elephants. One affected animal was put on 10 g of ampicillin suspension IM twice daily as well as 100 mg of dexamethasone and 1 g of flunixin meglumine. By day 3 of treatment, the animal was essentially normal. However, a second elephant receiving similar treatment died of infection. No body weights were given, so dosage rates could not be determined.

Case 3

After the castration of a 2272-kg Asian elephant, 15 million units of aqueous potassium penicillin G was deposited in the peritoneal cavity. Twelve million units of potassium penicillin G and dihydrostreptomycin, 5 g, were given IM twice a day for 3 weeks. The elephant recovered successfully from the surgery.[11]

Case 4

In another report on the castration of elephants, 24 abdominal surgical procedures were completed successfully. Although performed using sterile technique, the procedures took place in field conditions rather then in sterile surgical suites. Each animal was given 10 mg/kg amoxicillin IM (or ampicillin as a less preferred substitute) once daily for 2 days before surgery and then for 6 days after surgery. Before closure of the peritoneum, 25 g of amoxicillin was poured into the abdominal cavity and subcutaneous tissue was sprayed with 1 g of amoxicillin.[5, 22]

Case 5

An 18-year-old, 3000-kg African elephant underwent treatment for an infected tusk with amoxicillin, 30 g SID orally for 10 days. By the seventh day of treatment, the infection appeared to be under control. Before surgical tusk removal, the animal received 25 g amoxicillin SID orally. On day 3, treatment was changed to 60 × 10^6 IU procaine penicillin IM SID for 6 days because *Corynebacterium pyogenes*

cultures were isolated and determined to be susceptible to penicillin.[2]

Tetracycline

Tetracyclines are bacteriostatic and interfere with bacterial protein synthesis. They are effective against a broad spectrum of gram-positive and some gram-negative bacteria in mammals. They are lipid soluble and are widely distributed to tissue. Oral absorption of tetracycline is generally good except in the presence of cations, such as calcium or magnesium, which chelate tetracyclines.[10, 27]

Limpoka and coworkers[17] studied the IV and IM use of oxytetracycline (OTC) in Asian elephants. OTC in aqueous 2-pyrrolidone was given IM at the dosage of 20 mg/kg. The average peak plasma concentration was 2.87 μg /ml at 2 hours and concentrations exceeding 1 μg/ml were maintained for 48 hours. Sustained blood concentrations over a 3-day period followed a single IM dose. The same dose of 20 mg/kg was given IV with average peak plasma concentration of 6.2 μg/ml at 1 hour and no OTC was detected in plasma after 60 hours.

Bush and colleagues[4] studied the use of OTC in free-ranging male African elephants. This field study was not based on body weight but used the sum of the measurements of the elephants' girth and length. This measurement was based on the body length from the base of the skull to the tail head, and the girth was twice the distance from the sternum to the dorsal midline at a point immediately posterior to the front legs. The study suggested that, with a dose of 58 mg/cm, therapeutic serum concentrations of OTC can be maintained in an adult male African elephant for 48 hours with a single IM or IV injection. The IM route may result in slightly higher and more prolonged therapeutic concentrations. However, the large volumes and the multiple injection sites required may not be tolerated by an animal that is not anesthetized. If the IV route is used, tetracyclines should be given slowly in an indwelling catheter to minimize extravascular leakage.

◆ CASE STUDY

Case 1

Several authors have reported on the unsuccessful treatment of salmonellosis with tetracycline.[6, 28] Chooi and associates discussed the treatment of a 3-year-old wild-caught female Asian elephant, for a purulent draining laceration above the carpus with 5 g long-acting tetracycline BID given twice at weekly intervals during a quarantine period. This wound resolved, but recurred weeks later when the animal died of salmonellosis.[6]

Diaminopyrimidine/Sulfonamide Combinations

Both trimethoprim and sulfonamides interfere with microbial folic acid synthesis. The combination of these two is synergistic and is effective against many gram-negative and gram-positive bacterial pathogens (excluding *Pseudomonas*). Excretion is primarily renal and the degree of hepatic metabolism varies with the species.

Photosensitization, rashes, arthritis, and hepatic disorders are side effects that have been reported in various species. Parenteral and oral preparations are readily absorbed.[10, 27]

In one study, pharmacokinetics of trimethoprim-sulfamethoxazole (TMP-SMZ) were measured after a single oral and a single IV dose of 3.7 mg/kg TMP and 18.3 mg/kg SMZ. Serum concentrations of TMP-SMZ were measured for 12 hours after IV administration and 24 hours after oral administration. In African elephants, this study showed that, following IV administration, mean terminal half-life ($t_{1/2, z}$), clearance (CL), and volume of distribution at steady state (Vd_{ss}) of TMP were 1.4 ± 0.7 hours, 856.0 ± 144.0 ml/hr/kg, and 1.1 ± 0.4 L/kg, respectively. For SMZ, these parameters were, respectively, 1.83 ± 0.06 hours, 93.6 ± 10.8 ml/hr/kg, and 0.2 ± 0.02 L/kg. After oral administration of TMP, the mean $t_{1/2, z}$ was 3.0 ± 1.1 hours, the maximum concentration (C_{max}) was 0.43 ± 0.07 µg/ml at time (t_{max}) 1.7 ± 0.6 hours, and bioavailability (F) was 61.2% ± 21.3%. For SMZ, the mean $t_{1/2, z}$ was 2.0 ± 0.3 hours, the C_{max} was 30.7 ± 2.5 µg/ml at t_{max} 3.0 ± 1.0 hours, and F was 81.7% ± 17.5%.[25]

On the basis of these findings, Page and colleagues[25] suggested that calculated absorption and elimination rates of TMP-SMZ for African elephants are comparable to those in horses. It was recommended that equine dosage rates rather than metabolic scaling be used to calculate doses for elephants. Because of the similarities in horse and elephant metabolism of TMP-SMZ, the researchers suggested that a combined dose of 22 mg/kg administered twice a day to elephants should provide an effective therapeutic response. The results in one Asian elephant differed significantly from results in African elephants,[25] so no dosage recommendations were made for that species. R. Houck, senior veterinarian for Ringling Brothers and Barnum and Bailey Circus, uses TMP-SMZ orally at the dose of 18.1 to 21.1 mg/kg SID, and, in severe infections, he doubles this dose by giving it BID (R. Houck, personal communication, 1986).[14]

Schmidt[33] has reported the regular successful use of sulfadimethoxine/ormetoprim (Primor, 1200:1000 mg of sulfadimethoxine/200 mg ormetoprim). For routine treatment, Schmidt gives 16.2 to 18.5 mg/kg BID orally on the first day, followed by 9.25 mg/kg BID for each day after that. This treatment has been given for 30 days with positive therapeutic results and no toxicity. For severe infection, this dose is increased to 23.1 to 26.4 mg/kg BID orally on the first day and the dose is decreased to 13.2 mg/kg BID orally thereafter. Treatment has been continued for 19 days before the elephant has had diarrhea, which resolved immediately after discontinuation of the medication.

Aminoglycosides

The aminoglycosides are bactericidal and interfere with bacterial protein synthesis. They must be administered parenterally because they are poorly absorbed from the gastrointestinal tract.[10, 27]

Ototoxicity and nephrotoxicity are relatively common side effects of aminoglycosides. When recommended dosage programs are followed, the resultant nephrotoxicity is usually reversible once treatment is stopped. Chronic renal disease occurs with prolonged therapy or high doses. Rapid IV administration may result in intramuscular synaptic dysfunction and paralysis.[10]

Lodwick and colleagues[18] studied the pharmacokinetics of amikacin in African elephants. They used IV injections in two female elephants and IM injections in three animals. Resultant recommendations were that 6 to 8 mg/kg IM once every 24 hours is appropriate management for elephants with bacterial infections susceptible to amikacin. The 24-hour trough level with an IM administration of 6 mg/kg in this study ranged from 1.0 to 1.4 µg/ml, whereas the trough concentration after IV dose was 0 to 3.0 µg/ml. In humans, the recommended trough for less severe infections is 1 to 4 µg/ml. An MIC of less than or equal to 4 µg/ml inhibited six pathogens in horses. The continued inhibition of bacterial growth after antibiotic exposure—the postantibiotic effect—is long for aminoglycosides, ranging from 3 to 7 hours. The blood level should not be required to exceed the MIC during the complete dosing period because of this postantibiotic effect. Trough levels that are increasing may be more predictive for nephrotoxicity than are peak levels (in humans, toxicity is associated with trough levels above 8 to 10 µg/ml).[18]

In one animal given amikacin at a dosage of 7 mg/kg IM at 24-hour intervals for 21 days, peak serum concentrations were 19.0 ± 2.8 µg/ml and the mean serum concentration at 24 hours was 1.75 ± 0.4 µg/ml. A mild reversible renal tubular insult was diagnosed based on slight elevation in serum creatinine and the presence of casts in the urine. Once the treatment was discontinued, these changes quickly resolved.[18] Several trials have indicated that horse amikacin dosages should be applied to elephants, even though pharmacokinetic parameters of amikacin were considerably different from those seen in horses.[18]

Schmidt[33] has used gentamicin sulfate 4.4 mg/kg IV (or IM) SID. When trough levels of gentamicin sulfate were measured at 24 hours, this dose level was found to keep blood levels at 1.7 to 1.8 µg/ml (trough levels for humans are recommended to be less than 2 µg/ml). The IV injection is sometimes diluted with 10% with saline.

Fluoroquinolones

The fluoroquinolones are bactericidal; they inhibit bacterial gyrase, the enzyme responsible for coiling DNA within the bacterial nucleus. These antimicrobials may cause gastrointestinal upsets and anorexia occasionally, although they are generally well tolerated. Seizures have been reported in seizure-prone animals. In young, growing animals of some species (e.g., horses, dogs, pigeons), prolonged treatment or high doses may cause permanent articular defects. Only IM preparations and tablets are available in the United States. In some countries, a water-soluble solution is available. Enrofloxacin is the only veterinary-labeled fluoroquinolone. Ciprofloxacin is labeled for human use and has an antibacterial spectrum similar to enrofloxacin, and ciprofloxacin tablets may be more water soluble than enrofloxacin. IM administration may cause some intramuscular pain and irritation at the injection site. Oral enrofloxacin is somewhat bitter and may be refused by some animals.[10, 27]

No pharmacokinetic studies on use of enrofloxacin in elephants have been published. Schmidt[33] gives 1.07 mg/kg to 1.25 mg/kg BID orally, depending on the severity of the bacterial infection. This dosage is well accepted, and elephants on treatment regimens for 2 weeks have established no toxic signs.

Houck uses 1.5 to 2.8 mg/kg enrofloxacin orally SID, depending on severity of infection (R. Houck, personal communication).[14] Monitoring blood levels of one elephant on enrofloxacin found that once-daily doses were adequate to maintain blood levels.

Cephalosporins

Cephalosporins are beta lactam antibiotics as are the penicillins. They are bactericidal for growing and dividing organisms and inhibit the formation of the bacterial cell wall. Cephalosporins are classified into first-, second-, and third-generation antibiotics. First-generation formulations generally are effective against many gram-positive and some gram-negative organisms, whereas later generation formulations usually have increased gram-negative activity with less gram-positive activity. There is a potential synergistic effect when cephalosporins are combined with aminoglycosides.[10, 27]

Third-generation agents have increased gram-negative spectrum, including effectiveness against *Pseudomonas* species, but they have variable gram-positive effect. Among cephalosporins, cefotaxime is unusual in that it penetrates the cerebrospinal fluid in effective concentrations. Cephalosporins are primarily available as parenteral formulations. The frequency of administration required for some formulations to maintain therapeutic plasma concentrations is a disadvantage. Their high therapeutic index is an advantage when animals have compromised hepatic and renal function.[10]

There are no published pharmacologic studies on cephalosporin use in elephants. Houck has used ceftiofur sodium (Naxcel) at the equine dosage rate of 2.2 to 4.4 mg/kg (R. Houck, personal communication),[14] and Schmidt has used it IM at the low end of the cattle dosage rate, 1.1 mg/kg SID. Schmidt[33] does not recommend use of cephalosporins IV because of potential toxic effects; he has used a second-generation product IV with serious renal and hepatic problems. Injections are not very painful.

Macrolides and Lincosamides

PHARMACOLOGY

Macrolides and lincosamides are bacteriostatic and interfere with bacterial protein synthesis. They are effective against gram-positive bacteria, *Pasteurella*, some mycoplasma and obligate anaerobic bacteria, and *Bordatella*. These drugs are also effective for treating infection with *Clostridia* species and *Campylobacter* species. This class of drugs includes tylosin, erythromycin, clindamycin, azithromycin, clarithromycin, and lincomycin. Some formulations are available as injectables and others are oral formulations. Usually, vomiting and gastrointestinal irritation are the only signs of toxicity.[10]

There are no published pharmocokinetic studies on macrolides and lincosamides in elephants. Erythromycin comes in a tasteless form and can be administered readily to elephants; however, in Schmidt's experience,[33] in 1 to 2 days, severe gastrointestinal upset and gut pain occur, and he does not recommend its use in elephants.

◆ CASE STUDY

Case I

Tylosin has been used in the dosage of 12 mg/kg/day IM for 5 days to treat acute mycoplasma infections in elephants. The theory is that treatment of the acute infection prevents sequelae of chronic degenerative rheumatoid arthritis. The three animals studied in the case report all recovered well without residual lameness.[27, 31]

Chloramphenicol

Chloramphenicol is bacteriostatic and interferes with bacterial protein synthesis. The spectrum of activity includes some gram-negative bacteria and many gram-positive bacteria. Both oral and parenteral forms are available; however, oral absorption can be erratic. Additionally, contact with chloramphenicol by humans carries the risk of development of blood dyscrasia. It has potential toxic side effects including reversible bone marrow depression. It is still used when penetration into the central nervous system is desired and for treating infection caused by susceptible intracellular bacteria such as *Salmonella*.[10, 27]

No pharmacokinetic study on the use of chloramphenicol was found to have been published related to its use in elephants.

◆ CASE STUDY

Case I

Wyatt[36] reports on the successful treatment of a tusk pulpitis in an African elephant. Purulent exudate was flushed with a 1:10 dilution of povidone iodine in water. *Streptococcus viridans*, a coagulase-negative *Streptococcus* species, and a gram-positive anaerobic coccus were isolated from purulent discharge. All three organisms were sensitive to chloramphenicol. The end of the open tract was sealed with a set screw and a catheter allowed flushing and filling of the cavity with 4 g of chloromycetin sodium succinate on a daily basis for 1 week.

Miscellaneous Antibiotics

◆ CASE STUDIES

Case 1

Devine and associates[8] studied the use of isoniazid (INH) in one 14-year-old Asian elephant weighing approximately 2300 kg. Blood samples were drawn for analysis at the time of dosing and each hour thereafter for 7 hours. The apparent elimination half-life for free INH is 1.62 hours and 5.78 hours for total INH. The researchers found from this limited study that a dose of 5 mg/kg/day of INH given in a single dose is adequate to achieve blood levels found to be effective for prophylactic antituberculosis therapy. In this case, no undesirable side effects occurred.

Case 2

Gulland and Carwardine[12] studied plasma metronidazole levels in an Indian elephant after rectal administration of metronidazole suppositories. The dosage rate chosen for metronidazole was 15 mg/kg/day for 10 days. This was accomplished by placing twenty-five 1-g suppositories into the elephant's rectum every 24 hours. Plasma concentrations were between 4.4 and 7.7 μg/ml during the 24-hour study period. The MIC for the human pathogens *Bacteroides* species, *Fusobacter* species, and *Clostridia* species is 0.3 to 3 μg/ml. The study showed that metronidazole suppositories can be safely and effectively used in an elephant.

COMMONLY ENCOUNTERED HEALTH CONCERNS

Local Wound/Abscess Treatment

Of 509 abscesses reported by Mikota and colleagues,[20] the most common bacterial isolate was *Staphylococcus*. Treatments occurred in 445 of these cases, with 397 cases resolving after one course of treatment. Treatments included incision and drainage, lavage, debridement, soaks, hot packs or hydrotherapy, and topical preparations and injectable antibiotics. Long-acting penicillins were the most frequently used antibiotics.

Frequently, various injuries to the body such as hook wounds, toenail or foot injuries, or abscesses and tusk abscesses require treatment. Houck's[14] most common treatment for wounds is with 1% povidone iodine solution. A fresh solution should be made daily. Schmidt[33] may use sulfur sulfadiaxine, hydrogen peroxide, triple dye, chlorhexidine gluconate solution, and Biozide powder and gel (Performance Products, Inc., St. Louis). The common systemic treatment for these abscesses is injectable amoxicillin.[14]

Leg Chain Injuries

Mikota and colleagues[20] reported on 105 leg chain injuries, with 95 of the cases being treated. Most (88.4%)

resolved successfully with one course of treatment. Common treatment was the use of nonantibiotic topical preparation such as hydrogen peroxide or povidone iodine, with these being used in 39 of the cases. In 33 cases, topical antibiotics were used.

Foot Lesions

Disorders of the feet accounted for 586 cases reported by Mikota and colleagues.[20] Most common organisms isolated were *E. coli, Pseudomonas, Klebsiella, Enterobacter, Staphylococcus, Proteus,* and *Streptococcus.* Treatments were generally aggressive and typically included debridement and curettage, lavage, and administration of topical antibiotics and nonantibiotic preparations. Eighty-two of 127 abscesses resolved with one treatment regimen; in 26 events, injectable antibiotics were used (see section on penicillins).

Tusk Injuries

Of 234 injuries to tusks reported on by McCullar,[19] injuries included chipping, cracking, or breaking. Of these, 11% of the cases had a chronic course, 69 cases resolved with no medical treatment, and 129 of 165 treated cases resolved with a first course of treatment. The most frequently administered injectable antibiotics were the long-acting penicillins or a penicillin derivative. The most commonly used topical preparation was nitrofurazone. Nonantibiotic preparations such as povidone iodine, hydrogen peroxide, and chlorhexadine were used in some cases. Other systemic antibiotics used include tetracycline, TMP-SMZ, and ampicillin. (See penicillin section, Case 3; Chloramphenicol section, Case 1; and reference 1 for further discussion.)

Temporal Gland Disorders

Rasmussen[29] reported 61 events involving temporal gland problems such as edema, swelling, abscess, and purulent discharge. Thirty-nine of these cases were treated, with 34 resolving successfully with the first treatment and five others requiring further treatment. The most common treatments included nonantibiotic topical preparations, topical antibiotics, and antibiotics instilled, flushed, or packed into the temporal gland. Systemic antibiotics were used for several animals. Of 22 cases that were not treated, 21 resolved successfully.

Diarrhea

Mikota and colleagues[20] reported on 12 cases of diarrhea that were confirmed to have bacterial origin, with the common organisms isolated including *Salmonella, E. coli, Pseudomonas,* and *Clostridia.* Eleven cases were treated, with chloramphenicol and penicillin being the most commonly used antibiotics.

Salmonellosis

Salmonellosis is a concern in elephants as well as in other species. Elephants may be asymptomatic carriers or may show signs of diarrhea, anorexia, or behavior change. Treatments include oral ampicillin and chloramphenicol for 6 days. Mikota and colleagues[20] reported on 25 cases involving salmonella infections; 16 of these were treated, 15 with antibiotics. Ten of the treated animals recovered successfully and six died.

Rheumatoid Arthritis

Even though rheumatoid arthritis in elephants is most probably caused by *Mycoplasma*, positive serology for *Mycoplasma* cannot be considered diagnostic by itself. *Mycoplasma* that can cause arthritis colonizes most animals, but arthritis does not develop in all animals. *Mycoplasma* is sensitive to lincomycin and tetracycline. In gorillas, therapy has included intermittent IV tetracycline every 2 weeks initially and then intermittently for 18 months. Oral therapy with tetracycline was continued 2.5 years, with all clinical signs not resolving until approximately 5 years.[7]

Respiratory Disease

Twenty-three cases of respiratory disease reported on by Mikota and colleagues[20] involved various minor respiratory disorders such as nasal discharge and congestion, ocular discharge, coughing, sneezing, or other respiratory sounds. Twenty cases were acute, 11 cases were treated medically, and antibiotics were given in 7 cases. The most common antibiotics used were penicillin, tetracycline, TMP-SMZ, and amoxicillin. All of the events resolved successfully.

Tuberculosis

It was discussed previously that an Asian elephant with a positive interdermal test for tuberculosis was given a dose of 5 mg/kg/day of isoniazid, which was determined to be sufficient to achieve levels known to be effective for therapy in humans. One report stated that 13 elephants were given antituberculosis drugs—isoniazid, ethambutol, or rifampin—because they had been exposed to an animal confirmed to have tuberculosis or because they reacted positive to interdermal testing. After drug therapy, six animals that had a positive reaction to mammalian old tuberculin converted to a negative status. Because of the difficulties in interpreting testing responses, the true infection status of these animals before and after treatment is uncertain.[20]

REFERENCES

1. Allen JL, Welsch B, Jacobson ER, et al: Medical and surgical management of a fractured tusk in African elephant. J Am Vet Med Assoc 185:1447–1449, 1984.
2. Briggs M, Schmidt M, Black D, et al: Extraction of an infected tusk in an adult African elephant. J Am Vet Med Assoc 192:1455–1456, 1988.
3. Burke TJ: Probable tetanus in an Asian elephant. J Zoo Anim Med 6:22–24, 1975.
4. Bush M, Raath JP, de Vos V, et al: Serum oxytetracycline levels in free-ranging male African elephants (*Loxodonta africana*) injected with a long-acting formulation. J Zoo Wild Med 27:382–385, 1996.
5. Byron HT, Olsen J, Schmidt M, et al: Abdominal surgery in three adult male Asian elephants. J Am Vet Med Assoc 187:1236–1237, 1985.
6. Chooi KF, Zahari ZZ: Samonellosis in a captive Asian elephant. J Zoo Anim Med 19:48–50, 1988.
7. Clark H: Rheumatoid arthritis. *In* Mikota SK, Sargent EL, Ranglack GS (eds): Medical Management of the Elephant. West Bloomfield, MI, Indira Publishing House, pp 151–157, 1994.
8. Devine JE, Boever WJ, Miller E: Isoniazid therapy in an Asiatic elephant (*Elephas maximus*). J Zoo Anim Med 14:130–133, 1983.
9. de Vos V: Immobilization of the African elephant. Proc Second Int Congr Vet Anesth 103:64–68, 1985.
10. Flammer K: Antimicrobial therapy. *In* Ritchie BW, Harrison GJ, Harrison LR (eds): Avian Medicine: Principles and Application. Lakeworth, FL, Wingers Publishing, pp 434–456, 1994.
11. Fowler ME: Castration of an elephant. J Zoo Anim Med 4:25–27, 1973.
12. Gulland FMV, Carwardine PC: Plasma metronidazole levels in an Indian elephant (*Elephas maximus*) after rectal administration. Vet Rec 120:440, 1987.
13. Hile ME, Hintz HF, Erb HN: Predicting body weight from body measurements in Asian elephants (*Elephas maximus*). J Zoo Wild Med 28(4):424–427, 1997.
14. Houck R: Senior Veterinarian, Ringling Brothers and Barnum and Bailey Circus, 8607 Westwood Center Drive, Vienna, Virginia, 22182, personal communication, 1986.
15. Janssen EL, Karesh WB, Cosgrove GE, et al: Salmonellosis in a herd of captive elephants. J Am Vet Med Assoc 185:1450–1451, 1984.
16. Kurt F, Nettasinghe APW: Estimation of body weight of the Ceylon elephant (*Elephas maximus*). Ceylon Vet J XVI:24–27, 1968.
17. Limpoka M, Chai-Anan P, Sirivejpandu S, et al: Plasma concentrations of oxytetracycline in elephants following intravenous and intramuscular administration of terramycin/LA injectable solution. Acta-Veterinaria-Brno 56:173–179, 1987.
18. Lodwick LJ, Dubach JM, Phillips LG, et al: Pharmacokinetics of amikacin in African elephants (*Loxodonta africana*). J Zoo Anim Med 25:367–375, 1994.
19. McCullar M: Dentistry. *In* Mikota SK, Sargent EL, Ranglack GS (eds): Medical Management of the Elephant, West Bloomfield, MI, Indira Publishing House, pp 87–94, 1994.
20. Mikota SK, Sargent EL, Ranglack GS: Medical Management of the Elephant. West Bloomfield, MI, Indira Publishing House, 1994.
21. Murray S, Bush M, Tell L: Medical management of post-partum problems in an Asian elephant (*Elephas maximus*) cow and calf. J Zoo Wild Med 27:255–258, 1986.
22. Olsen JH, Byron HT: Castration of the elephant. *In* Fowler ME (ed): Zoo and Wild Animal Medicine Current Therapy 3. Philadelphia, WB Saunders, pp 441–444, 1993.
23. Oosterhuis JE: The performance of a cesarean section on an Asian elephant (*Elephas maximus indicus*). Proceedings of the American Association of Zoo Veterinarians, South Padre Island, TX, pp 157–158, 1990.
24. Page CD: Anesthesia and chemical restraint. *In* Mikota SK, Sargent EL, Ranglack GS (eds): Medical Management of the Elephant. West Bloomfield, MI, Indira Publishing House, pp 41–49, 1994.
25. Page CD, Mautino M, Derendorf HD, et al: Comparative pharmacokinetics of trimethoprim sulfamethoxazole administered intravenously and orally to captive elephants. J Zoo Wild Med 22:409–416, 1991.
26. Page CD: Pharmacology and toxicology. *In* Mikota SK, Sargent EL, Ranglack GS (eds): Medical Management of the Elephant. West Bloomfield, MI, Indira Publishing House, pp 65–67, 1994.
27. Plumb DC: Veterinary Drug Handbook, 2nd ed. Ames, IA: Iowa State University Press, 1995.
28. Raphael BL, Clubb FJ: Atypical salmonellosis in an African elephant. Proceedings of the Annual Meeting of the American Association of Zoo Veterinarians, Scottsdale, AZ, p 57, 1988.
29. Rasmussen LEL: The sensory in communication systems. *In* Mikota SK, Sargent EL, Ranglack GS (eds): Medical Management of the Elephant. West Bloomfield, MI, Indira Publishing House, pp 207–215, 1994.
30. Rosin E, Schultz-Darken N, Perry B, et al: Pharmacokinetics of ampicillin administered orally in Asian elephants (*Elephas maximus*). J Zoo Anim Med 24:515–518, 1993.
31. Schmidt M: Elephants (Proboscidea). *In* Fowler ME (ed): Zoo and Wild Animal Medicine. Philadelphia, WB Saunders, pp 884–923, 1986.

32. Schmidt MJ: Penicillin G and amoxicillin in elephants: a study comparing dose regimens administered with serum levels achieved in healthy elephants. J Zoo Anim Med 9:127–136, 1978.
33. Schmidt MJ: Senior Research Veterinarian, Washington Park Zoo, Portland Oregon, personal communication, 1986.
34. Sedgwick CJ: Allometric scaling and emergency care: the importance of body size. *In* Fowler ME (ed): Zoo and Wild Animal Medicine Current Therapy 3. Philadelphia, WB Saunders, pp 34–37, 1993.
35. Sreekumar KP, Nirmalan G: Estimation of Body Weight in Indian Elephants *(Elephas maximus indicus)*. Vet Res Comm 13:3–9, 1989.
36. Wyatt JG: Medical treatment of pulpitis in an African elephant. J Am Vet Med Assoc 189:1193, 1986.

CHAPTER **78**

Flaccid Trunk Paralysis in Free-Ranging Elephants

NANCY D. KOCK

In December 1989, two free-ranging adult bull elephants, residents of the southern shore of Lake Kariba, Zimbabwe, were reported by game scouts from an adjacent resort to have lost control of their trunks.[5] Since that time, more than 30 elephants in the same area have been affected with what appears clinically to be ascending flaccid paralysis of the trunk. Confirmed cases have not been reported in other parts of Zimbabwe, but eight clinically similar cases were discovered in 1995 in elephants that reside, for the most part, in one region of Kruger National Park, South Africa (N. J. P. Kriek, personal communication, 1996).

All of the confirmed cases in Zimbabwe were discovered near Fothergill Island, which is not actually an island but connected to the mainland within the Matusadona National Park, which has three distinct habitats. A southern plateau with sparse high veld vegetation abuts a steep escarpment with varied riverine flora. The escarpment drops to low veld valley vegetation as the lake is approached. With the drought Zimbabwe endured during the early 1980s, the water level of the lake dropped, opening up large grassland tracts along the water's edge, adjacent to Fothergill Island. Elephants roam throughout this region and have access to a diverse variety of forage. Family groups of mature females, immature males, and juveniles forage mainly in the woodland habitats, venturing out onto the grasslands only briefly after the rains when grasses are lush. The mature bulls are semisolitary and, because they are less concerned with human activity, spend much of their time in the open grasslands near the lake's shore.

All elephants affected with trunk paralysis have been bulls, although there was one suspected case in a cow. The more secretive and high-strung nature of the females made it impossible to confirm this case. Affected bulls ranged in age from 10 to 40 years. The condition initially had the appearance of an outbreak, with the two 1989 cases being followed by another four cases 2 months later; by the end of the year, about a dozen animals were affected. New cases have been reported during the rainy season (December to February) each year since the condition was initially noticed.

The first clinical manifestation of the disease is subtle loss of prehension, involving the two opposable tips of the trunk. Later, frank atrophy of the distal trunk musculature is seen, which proceeds proximally to involve as much as three quarters of the trunk in some cases. By this time the condition is obvious from great distances, as the thinned distal trunk is no longer under control by the animal, appearing to dangle autonomously (Fig. 78–1). The changes develop slowly, over some months, during which time the animals learn to adapt to altered drinking and feeding abilities. The front feet are often used along with the more proximal, unaffected part of the trunk to scoop forage off the ground. The flaccid trunk may also be thrown over branches to bring forage into the mouth. The animals may stand deep in the lake, drinking with their mouths instead of using the trunk as a drinking straw as is normally done.

Because elephants are herbivores, they must spend great parts of the day feeding, and the trunk disability soon causes loss in body condition. When affected and unaffected animals travel together, differences in body condition are obvious (Fig. 78–2). Some animals have become emaciated and have disappeared and are presumed dead as a result of inanition. It is not known whether sensory deficits accompany the motor losses that occur in the trunk. Neither behavioral abnormalities nor other neuromuscular deficits have been apparent in any of the elephants, and affected animals do not appear

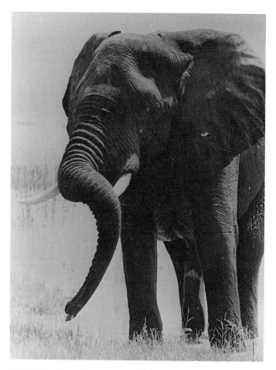

FIGURE 78–1. More than half of the distal portion of this elephant's trunk is affected by flaccid paralysis. (Photograph by Darryl Tiran.)

acute cases showed less dramatic nerve changes and more acute degenerative muscle changes. Two elephants with clinically acute cases also had degenerative neuronal changes and edema of the facial nucleus in the brain. In none of the cases have lesions been seen in other peripheral nerves or visceral organs, except for the presence of Anichkov cells in the heart. These are large cells of uncertain origin, with elongated nuclei and undulating chromatin, also referred to as *caterpillar cells.* They are thought either to function as macrophages or to indicate attempted myocyte regeneration and are found in a variety of circumstances when myocardium has been injured.[10] Complete blood counts and serum assays for total protein, albumin, globulin, creatine phosphokinase, aspartate transaminase, alanine transaminase, lactic dehydrogenase, alkaline phosphatase, gamma glutaryl transaminase, bilirubin, creatinine, and blood urea nitrogen were done on most of the elephants sampled, and all were within normal limits.[4] The only apparently significant lesions were found in the peripheral nerves of the trunk, along with what were considered secondary changes in the muscles.

Possible causes for the changes in the elephants' trunks include trauma, infectious diseases, genetically predisposed degeneration, intoxications, and nutritional deficiencies. In view of the epidemiology of the disease, trauma was ruled out. The absence of inflammation in any of the cases likely rules out infectious causes as well. Hereditary causes are difficult to document in free-ranging animals, but the Faculty of Veterinary Science of the University of Zimbabwe is investigating the degree of relatedness among the affected animals compared with unaffected animals.

Numerous plant species, some chemicals, and heavy metals have well-recognized neurotoxic properties, although agents associated with selective peripheral neuropathy are few. Chronic lead poisoning in humans can result in segmental degeneration of axons with myelin loss in nerves that supply muscles continually used in work or recreation.[1, 2, 8] Susceptibility to and signs of lead intoxication vary among species. Lead levels of 4 to 7 ppm have been found in the livers of horses with chronic fatal intoxication, whereas bovines are able to tolerate levels of 40 ppm.[2] Horses with lead poisoning may experience paresis and paralysis of the larynx and pharynx, a result of toxic damage to cranial nerves. The pathogenesis of toxicosis is obscure but protoplasmic

to be treated differently by their conspecifics. In fact, during the immobilization of one elephant, its companions tried repeatedly to assist it to rise. Game scouts familiar with the animals have reported transient improvement in the ability of some elephants to use the trunk, but none have recovered completely.

Biopsy specimens were taken from three affected elephants, and five animals were called for complete postmortem examination. The changes in all were similar, with variations consistent with temporal changes. Elephants with chronic cases tended to show neuropathy of peripheral nerves supplying the trunk, with axon and myelin loss, as well as muscle atrophy with endomysial fibrosis and compensatory muscle hypertrophy, all without inflammation (Fig. 78–3). Elephants with more

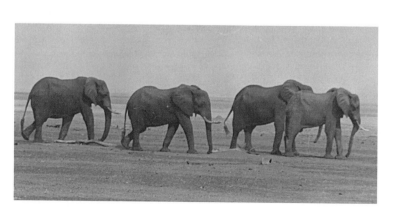

FIGURE 78–2. The leading elephant has flaccid paralysis of the trunk, evidenced by the thinness of the distal trunk in comparison with the other animals. The affected animal also has poor body condition. (Photograph by Verity Bowman.)

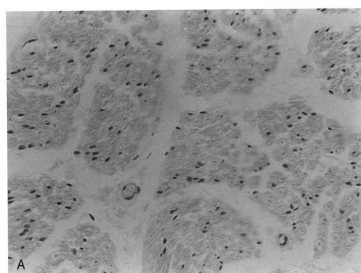

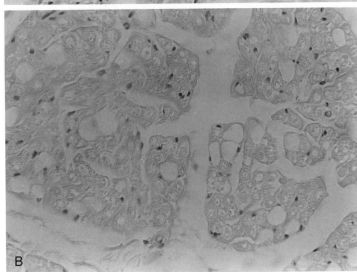

FIGURE 78–3. Photomicrograph of peripheral nerves from the trunk of a normal elephant *(A)* and one affected with flaccid trunk paralysis *(B)*. Affected nerves are largely vacuolated with axon and myelin loss. (Photograph by Nancy D. Kock.)

poisoning is suspected. Lead is obtained by ingestion, but relatively small amounts are actually absorbed because insoluble compounds are formed in the intestinal tract. The basis for the paralytic changes in horses has not been described, but it may be as in humans, in whom segmental degeneration of axons and myelin in distal motor fibers occurs.[2]

Assessment of environmental contamination with heavy metals and organochlorines was accomplished by systematic collection of water, water vegetation, terrestrial forage, silt, and soil from the southern shoreline of Lake Kariba, where both affected and unaffected animals resided. None of the levels were significant. Kidney samples from affected animals were analyzed for lead content, and levels were considered too low to be associated with intoxication. Kidney samples were examined histologically for acid-fast inclusions characteristic of lead, but such inclusions were not found. Because the disease develops slowly, however, it may be that the time of sampling or examination is crucial.

Selenium deficiency is well recognized in Zimbabwe, and because adequate levels protect against intoxication with lead and other heavy metals,[6] it is possible that a combination of deficiency and marginal toxicosis could result in clinical signs.

In view of the apparent seasonal nature of new cases, plant intoxication is considered a likely cause of flaccid trunk paralysis. Nigropallidal encephalomalacia in horses is caused by ingestion of plants of the genera *Centaurea* and *Acroptilon*, specifically *C. solstitialis* (yellow starthistle) and *A. repens* (Russian knapweed) in the United States.[3, 9] Signs become apparent after at least a month's ingestion of these thistles, which are of the family Asteraceae and which contain sesquiterpene lactones, the suspected toxic compounds. Clinically, toxicosis results in impaired ability to eat and drink owing to immobility of facial muscles; eventual death is from inanition or dehydration. Malacia is found in the pallidus and substantia nigra, often bilaterally.[9] Sesquiterpene lactones are unstable, making it unfeasible to test plant material directly (R. J. Molyneux, personal communication, 1996). Cause and effect were established with feeding trials, in which reproduction of the disease could be accomplished only in horses, which suggests a degree of species susceptibility.[9] Experimental exposure to these compounds in vitro, however, produced toxic changes irrespective of cell line or species.[9] Nigropallidal encephalomalacia has not been reported in Zimbabwe, and neither genus of the known offending plants is native to Zimbawe. Several plant species found along the southern shore of Lake Kariba are non-native, however, having been introduced from the Americas, warranting further investigation into their identification and potential toxic properties. Further investigation is also being aimed at specific identification of the plants the elephants eat. It is possible that drought conditions in southern Africa during this period may have resulted in imbalance of the ecosystem or, alternatively, that harsh conditions have caused toxic compounds to be concentrated in plants not normally toxic.

REFERENCES

1. Cotran RS, Kumar V, Robbins SL: Environmental pathology. *In* Robbins SL (ed): Pathologic Basis of Disease. London, WB Saunders, pp 492–495, 1989.
2. Jubb KVF, Huxtable CR: Lead poisoning. *In* Jubb KVF, Kennedy PC, Palmer N (eds): The Nervous System: Pathology of Domestic Animals, 4th ed, vol 1. London, Academic Press, pp 348–350, 1993.
3. Jubb KVF, Huxtable CR: Nigropallidal encephalomalacia of horses. *In* Jubb KVF, Kennedy PC, Palmer N (eds): The Nervous System: Pathology of Domestic Animals, 4th ed, vol 1. London, Academic Press, pp 344–345, 1993.
4. Kock MD, Martin R, Kock ND: Chemical immobilization of free-ranging elephants (*Loxodonta africana*) in Zimbabwe, using etorphine (M99) mixed with hyaluronidase, and evaluation of biological data collected soon after immobilization. J Zool Wildl Med 24:1–10, 1993.
5. Kock ND, Goedegebuure SA, Lane EP, et al: Flaccid paralysis of the trunk in free-ranging African elephants (*Loxodonta africana*) in Zimbabwe. J Wildl Dis 30:432–435, 1994.
6. Levander OA: Selenium. *In* Mertz W (ed): Trace elements in Human and Animal Nutrition, 5th ed, vol 2. London, Academic Press, pp 212–226, 1986.
7. Morris MA: The nervous system. *In* Robbins SL (ed): Pathologic Basis of Disease. London, WB Saunders, pp 1443–1444, 1989.
8. Polson CJ, Green MA, Lee MR: Clinical Toxicology, 3rd ed. Bath, UK, Pitman Press, pp 459–470, 1983.
9. Riopelle RJ, Stevens KL: *In vitro* neurotoxicity bioassay: neurotoxicity of sesquiterpene lactones. *In* Colagare SM, Molyneux FJ (eds): Bioactive Natural Products: Detection, Isolation, and Structural Determination. London, CRC Press, pp 457–463, 1993.
10. Robinson WF, Maxie MG: The cardiovascular system. *In* Jubb KVF, Kennedy PC, Palmer N (eds): Pathology of Domestic Animals, 4th ed, vol 1. London, Academic Press, p 30, 1993.

CHAPTER **79A**

Oral and Nasal Diseases of Elephants

ARMIN KUNTZE

Because of their protruding nature, the trunk and tusks of elephants are particularly vulnerable to trauma.

DISEASES OF THE TRUNK

The trunk is an elongation of the nose and upper lip. It is extraordinarily sensitive and highly mobile. It can be used as a strong, grasping arm for feeding and for drinking, and it can serve as a strong weapon.

Because the trunk is highly vascular, deep wounds may result in significant blood loss that can lead to shock. Immediate sedation (with xylazine) and surgical intervention to control the hemorrhage can be life-saving.[3, 8] Contusions and minor trunk lacerations can also be treated surgically. A complicating factor in suturing the trunk is its extreme mobility, which can interfere with healing; even wounds sutured with stainless steel wire frequently dehisce.[18] Superficial, nonperforating lesions of the trunk's course skin rarely undergo primary healing; instead, protrusions of granulation tissue that may be fungus-like in appearance often develop.[8, 9] This granulation tissue is often hemorrhagic and may necessitate cauterization. Attempts to shrink the granulation tissue may also include daily treatment with concentrated metacresol-sulfone solution (Lotagen) (Fig. 79A–1).

Penetrating injuries to the nasal septum at the trunk tip should be treated for several days with parenteral antibiotics. Because of the pain of such injuries, food and water intake will be restricted, and so affected elephants should be fed by hand and watered by means of a hose placed in the mouth. Lesions of the more proximal section of the trunk may be evident by nasal secretions, putrid odor on expiration, and/or stenotic sounds on inspiration. For injuries in the more proximal

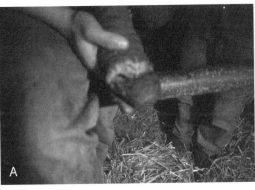

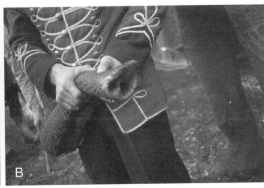

FIGURE 79A–1. *A,* Partial necrosis of the ventral aspect of the trunk in an African elephant. *B,* Eighteen months later. Now looking as Asian elephant (only one dorsal "finger").

areas of the trunk, flexible endoscopes can be used to diagnose and treat lesions.[13, 16]

DENTAL DISEASE

Elephant tusks are modified incisors that grow throughout the life of the animal. They consist mainly of dentin (ivory). In both Asian (*Elephas maximus*) and African (*Loxodonta africana*) male elephants, they can grow to a length of several meters. Among female elephants, only the African species have tusks of notable size; those of the Indian species either are not visible or extend only a short distance above the gingival line. Minor fractures or splinters of the ivory are relatively common; however, unless the pulp cavity is exposed, smoothing the sharp edges of the fragments with a grinder is sufficient treatment.[4, 17] Longitudinal tusk cracks may be stabilized with circumferential metal bands.[16, 21, 23]

Fractures that result in an exposed pulp cavity necessitate immediate treatment with topical antibiotics and, if necessary, extraction of the pulp material. The pulp canal can then be filled with calcium hydroxyapatite (beta-tricalcium-phosphate) and covered with plaster or other casting materials.[7, 14, 16, 24] If treatment of the ex-

posed pulp cavity is not addressed, ascending infections can lead to chronic pulpitis and fistulas (Figs. 79A–2, 79A–3). General malaise and/or aggressive behavior resulting from the discomfort eventually necessitate extraction of the tooth.[1, 2, 11]

Total removal of the tusk can be attempted after rupture of the periodontal ligament by rotation of the tooth. The rotation can be facilitated by placement of a metal bar drilled transversely through the tooth.[2] An alternative method has been used in seven elephants[22]: The affected teeth were cut off at the gum line, and the dental pulp was extracted with a hook. A specialized drill was used to enlarge the inner diameter of the pulp canal. With a saw, the remaining tooth is longitudinally sectioned into three or four fragments. Then, with the use of specially adapted screwdrivers and levers, the fragments are imploded into the pulp cavity and removed. The alveolar cavity is flushed with iodine and packed regularly with antibiotics. Within 4 weeks, the alveolar cavity fills with granulation tissue.

Another unique factor of elephant dentition is the structure and succession of their molars. The molars continuously move forward, and an elephant may have up to six sets during a lifetime.[5] The progression of molars proceeds faster in the mandibles than in the maxillae.[14, 15] At any time, only one complete molar is in wear in each jaw: A "set" consists of 4 molars. The

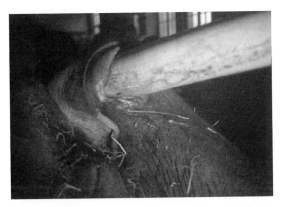

FIGURE 79A–2. Alveolitis, caused by incorrect orthodontic device.

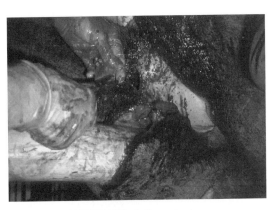

FIGURE 79A–3. Sequestrectomy.

new teeth develop in the caudal jaw and are formed of finger-like lamellae (each with its own pulp cavity) that join together to form a massive, multirooted tooth. As these teeth are formed, they move forward into full apposition, and their predecessor is displaced rostrally. The crown of the predecessor tooth is broken off in fragments, the roots are resorbed, and the tooth is eventually shed from the jaw. The tooth fragments may be spit out or swallowed and later noted in the feces. The end result is that at any one time, there is a complete molar and also portions of the incoming molar and the outgoing (preceding) molar in wear.

Abnormal mastication may be caused by malaligned or infected teeth. Coarse, poorly digested food particles may be found in the feces,[12] and emaciation may result. Excessive salivation is rarely noted, and tooth root fistulas develop only occasionally. Because obvious signs of dental disease may not be readily apparent, care must be taken to monitor an elephant's masticatory habits and body condition. On occasion, massive mechanical stress on the molars may result in alveolar fractures.[10, 20]

To prevent these complications, which may even lead to death,[6] malaligned teeth and/or tooth fragments must be extracted with hammers, chisels, and pliers.[16, 19] Extraction-induced mandibular fractures are unusual but may heal without treatment.[21] Regular flushing of the extraction site and local and parenteral antibiotics may be indicated. The natural cycle of the shedding of the molar teeth can be aided by the feeding of a hard-food diet and offering elephants wooden limbs to chew on.

REFERENCES

1. Allen JL, Welsch B, Jacobson ER, Kollias GV: Management of tusk disorders in elephants. Annual Proceedings of the American Association of Zoo Veterinarians, Louisville, KY, pp 63–64, 1984.
2. Briggs M, Schmidt M, Black D, et al: Extraction of an infected tusk in an adult African elephant. J Am Vet Med Assoc 192:1455–1456, 1988.
3. Ernst A, Romijnders J: Olifanten: Diagnose en Ziekten [in Dutch]. Vet. Thesis, University of Utrecht, 1986.
4. Fowler ME (ed): Zoo and Wild Animal Medicine. Philadelphia, WB Saunders, 1978.
5. Göltenboth R, Klös HG: Krankheiten der Zoo und Wildtiere. Berlin, Blackwell Wissenschaftsverlag, 1995.
6. Heymann H: Plötzlicher Tod eines elefanten infolge kar iöser Backzähne. Verh Erkrg Zootiere 11:119–121, 1969.
7. Jensen J: Endodontic therapy in an adult African elephant. Annual Proceedings of the American Association of Zoo Veterinarians, Scottsdale, AZ, p 5, 1985.
8. Kuntze A: Zur Chirurgie am Elefanten. Mh Vet Med 42:399–403, 1987.
9. Kuntze A: Dermatopathien bei Elefanten und deren Therapie. Klt Prax 34:405–415, 1989.
10. Kuntze A: Oronasale Krankheitsbilder bei Elefanten. Verh Erkrg Zootiere 36:337–340, 1994.
11. Lateur N, Kusse G, van der Velden M, Stolk P: Surgical management of traumatic pulpitis of the tusks in a male Indian elephant. Annual Proceedings of the American Association of Zoo Veterinarians, Scottsdale, AZ, pp 125–126, 1985.
12. Reichard TA, Ullrey DE, Roginson PT: Nutritional implications of dental problems in elephants. Annual Proceedings of the American Association of Zoo Veterinarians, New Orleans, LA, pp 73–74, 1982.
13. Rüedi D: Therapie einiger Erkrankungen bei Elefanten. Arb tagung Zootierärzte Deutschspr Raum 7:72–77, 1987.
14. Rüedi D: Zähne und Zahnbehandlung bei Elefanten. Arb tagung Zootierärzte Deutschspr Raum 9:89–95, 1989.
15. Rüedi D: Untersuchungen am Zahnwachstum von Elefanten. Arb tagung Zootierärzte Deutschspr Raum 10:61–63, 1990.
16. Rüedi D: Elefanten. In Göltenboth R, Klös HG: Krankheiten der Zoo und Wildtiere. Berlin, Blackwell Wissenschaftsverlag, pp 56–89, 1995.
17. Schmidt M: Elephants. In Fowler ME (ed): Zoo and Wild Animal Medicine. Philadelphia, WB Saunders, pp 709–752, 1978.
18. Stringer BE: Repair of a lacerated trunk in an African elephant. J Zoo Anim Med 2:12, 1971.
19. Stringer BE: The removal of a tusk in an African elephant. Annual Proceedings of the American Association of Zoo Veterinarians, Houston, TX, pp 271–272, 1972.
20. Unger KH: Tooth extraction with complications in an elephant (*Elephas maximus*). Vehr Erk Zootiere 13:235–236, 1971.
21. Wallach JD, Boever WJ: Diseases of Exotic Animals: Medical and Surgical Management. Philadelphia, WB Saunders, 1983.
22. Welsch B, Jacobson ER, Kollias GV, et al: Tusk extraction in the African elephant (*Loxodonta africana*). J Zoo Wildl Med 20(4):446–453, 1989.
23. Wiesner H, Hegel GV: Zur Stoßzahnbehandlung von Elefanten. Arb tagung Zootierärzte Deutschspr Raum 8:105, 1988.
24. Wyatt JD: Medical treatment of tusk pulpitis in an African elephant. J Am Vet Med Assoc 189:1193, 1986.

Poxvirus Infections in Elephants

ARMIN KUNTZE

Outbreaks of poxvirus infections have been observed in elephants throughout central Europe.[2, 3, 5, 6, 10, 12, 14–17, 19] Although the epidemiology of the infections, including the sources, is not definitively known, wild rodents are suspected to be the reservoirs of the cowpox-like elephant poxvirus.[4] In one case, recently vaccinated schoolchildren appeared to be the source of the infection.[5, 9] The incubation time varies from 15 to 23 days. In addition to direct elephant-to-elephant transmission of the virus, indirect transmission of the virus through contaminated food and water has also been demonstrated.[5, 9, 12, 17] The various strains of poxviruses isolated from affected elephants differ in both their genomic structures and their virulence.[1]

The clinical signs of poxvirus infection in elephants vary, probably in part because of an animal's individual resistance, its immunologic status, and possibly familial differences. Asian elephants (*Elephas maximus*) appear to be more susceptible to the infection than the African species (*Loxodonta africana*). The first clinical signs generally include difficulties in swallowing and a reduction in appetite. Other signs may include stiff movements and/or lameness of various degrees in one or more extremities. Subsequently, 1-cm to 3-cm vesicular eruptions may develop in the mucous membranes around the lips, the tongue, the tip of the trunk (Fig. 79B–1), the external aural meatus, the eyelids (Fig. 79B–2), and the perianal and perivulvar skin. After hours to several days, the vesicles may rupture, discharging a clear, bloody, or purulent fluid. After several days to weeks, the lesions are covered by crusts and then progress to unpigmented scars (Fig. 79B–3). In a few animals, there may be generalized disease, sepsis, and a fatal outcome.[5, 12, 17]

In animals that apparently have impaired resistance, possibly as a result of immunosuppression, generalized disease may develop with vesicular lesions distributed over the entire body. They may coalesce to form large, map-like ulcerations.[2, 15] Frequently, the pox lesions may extend into the corium of the nails, leading to fatal complications. In severely ill elephants, a temperature higher than 37.8°C, refusal of food and water, and marked reduction in ear and trunk movements are observed. Edema of the vulva and lower abdominal areas may indicate circulatory breakdown and a grave prognosis.

DIAGNOSIS

In addition to the characteristic nature of the lesions, diagnosis can be aided by submitting vesicular fluid or crusts for electron microscopic examination for particles (Bollinger bodies) typical of the poxvirus; for viral culture, including chicken eggs, in which alterations may be noted in the chorioallantoic membrane; and for neutralizing antibody assay.[8, 9, 14]

TREATMENT

In all cases, whether mild or severe, broad-spectrum antibiotics should be administered for 10 to 14 days. Treatments should also include intravenous treatment

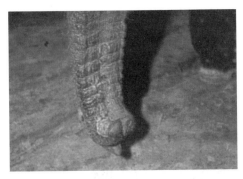

FIGURE 79B–1. Pox scabs at trunk tip.

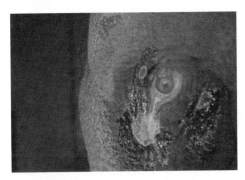

FIGURE 79B–2. Pox scabs around the eye.

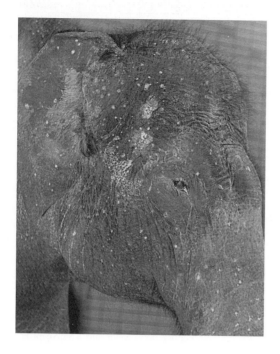

FIGURE 79B–3. Pox scars on the entire body surface in Asian elephants.

FIGURE 79B–4. Resection of under-run horn sectors. New horn near bearing surface border.

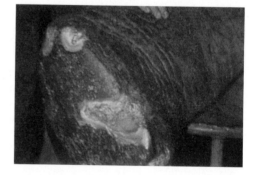

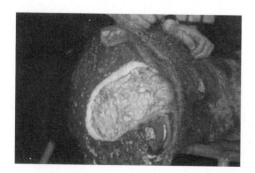

FIGURE 79B–5. Partial resection of the sole. Note granular tissue in center and new horn in periphery.

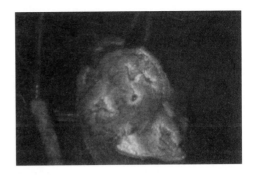

FIGURE 79B–6. 10 weeks after step-by-step resection. Most of the sole consists of yellow-brown horn.

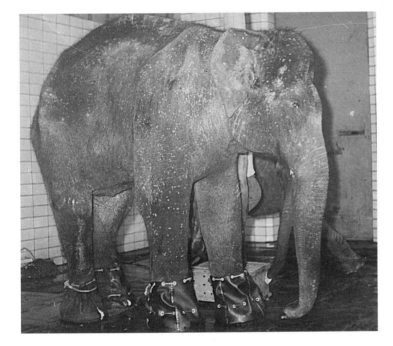

FIGURE 79B–7. Pox disease. Quadrupled exungulation: Hoof boots.

with appropriate electrolyte solutions, multivitamin (A, D_3, E) combinations, and oral supplementation with 30 to 40 g/day of ascorbic acid.

One of the most serious complications is the undermining of the nails and soles (Figs. 79B–4 to 79B–6). These areas should be opened and flushed, and drainage should be maintained. This will prevent lameness and reduce the chances that the infection will spread to other hooves. Fibrin exudates between the soles and the hooves should be removed and the cavities loosely packed, again to maintain drainage, because these actions help delay or prevent the detachment of the soles. Dressings and leather shoes can be used to protect the affected tissues (Fig. 79B–7) and assist in the recornification process, which may take 3 to 4 months to complete.[5–7]

PROPHYLAXIS

Public contact with pox-infected elephants should be restricted. In the past, animal care staff members work-

ing with infected elephants were vaccinated because cross-species transmission to humans is possible. Although protection can be achieved only by prophylactic vaccination, worldwide cessation of the smallpox vaccination program has made this option impossible.[8, 13, 17] In view of the incubation period for this disease, quarantine of new arrivals may also effectively reduce the risk of transmission to a herd.

REFERENCES

1. Baxby D, Shackleton WB, Wheeler J, Turner A: Comparison of cowpox-like viruses isolated from European zoos [Brief Report]. Arch Virol 61:337–340, 1979.
2. Gehring H, Mayer H: Vacciniapocken (Poxvirus commune) bei Zirkuselefanten. Klt Prax 17:179–181, 1972.
3. Gehring H, Mayer H: Beitrag zur Diagnostik und Bekämpfung der Pockeninfektion bei Elefanten. D Prak Tierarzt 59:100–101, 106, 1978.
4. Jacoby F: Untersuchungen zur Epidemiologie des Kuhpockenvirus in der BRD. Vet Med Diss Gießen, 1992.
5. Kuntze A: Zur Klinik der Pocken bei Asiatischen Elefanten (*Elephas maximus*). 1. Mitteilung: Pockeneinbruch und verlauf in

einer elfköpfigen Elefantenherde. Verh ber Erkrg Zootiere 16:281–289, 1974.

6. Kuntze A: Weitere Erfahrungen zur Klinik und Therapie der Pockenerkrankung beim Elefanten (*Elephas maximus*). Mh Vet Med 37:460–462, 1982.

7. Kuntze A, Bürger M, Jancke S, Töpfer I: Exungulation aller Extremitäten bei einer Elefantin im Gefolge einer Pockeninfektion. Mh Vet Med 30:703–707, 1975.

8. Kuntze A, Janetzky V: Zur Ätiologie, Serologie und Immunprophylaxe der Pocken des Asiatischen Elefanten (*Elephas maximus*). Mh Vet Med 37:496–499, 1982.

9. Kuntze A, Niemer U: Zur Klinik der Pocken bei Asiatischen Elefanten (*Elephas maximus*). 2. Mitteilung: Serologie und Epidemiologie. Verh ber Erkrg Zootiere 16:291–296, 1974.

10. Kutschmann K, Puschmann W, Rolle S: Klinische Beobachtungen bei der Elefantenpockeninfektion im Zoologischen Garten Magdeburg. Verh ber Erkrg Zootiere 33:195–201, 1991.

11. Pade K: Pockenerkrankung bei Indischen Elefanten. Klinik und Therapie. Arb tagung der Zootierärzte im Deutschspr Raum 9:127–134, 1989.

12. Pade K, Rüede D, Pilaski J, et al: Ein verlustreicher Pockenein-

bruch bei Asiatischen Elefanten (*Elephas maximus*) in einem deutschen Wanderzirkus. Verh ber Erkrg Zootiere 32:147–164, 1990.

13. Pilaski J: Beitrag zur Pockenimpfung bei Elefanten. Arb tagung der Zootierärzte im Deutschspr Raum 4:125, 1984.

14. Pilaski J, Behlert O, Höhr D: A severe case of pox disease in an Asian elephant (*Elephas maximus*) of a small travelling circus overwintering near Cologne. Proceedings of the European Association of Zoo and Wildlife Veterinarians, Rostock, pp 201–213, 1996.

15. Pilaski J, Kulka D, Neuschulz N: Ein Pockenausbruch bei Afrikanischen Elefanten (*Loxodonta africana*) in Thüringer Zoopark Erfurt. Verh ber Erkrg Zootiere 34:111–118, 1992.

16. Pilaski J, Magunna C, Hagenbeck C: Pocken bei Asiatischen Elefanten (*Elephas maximus*) im Tierpark Carl Hagenbeck Hamburg. Verh ber Erkrg Zootiere 27:437–447, 1985.

17. Potel K, Voigt A, Hiepe T, et al: Eine bösartige Haut und Schleimhauterkrankung bei Elefanten. D Zool Garten 27:1–103, 1963.

18. Rübel A: Zum Pockenimpfstoff für Elefanten. Arb tagung der Zootierärzte im Deutschspr Raum 11:104–105, 1991.

19. Rüedi D: Pockeninfektion bei Asiatischen Elefanten im Circus Barum im Früling. Arb tagung der Zootierärzte im Deutschspr Raum 9:135–139, 1989.

PERRISODACTYLIDS

CHAPTER 80

Skin Diseases of Black Rhinoceroses

LINDA MUNSON

R. ERIC MILLER

The captive population of black rhinoceroses (*Diceros bicornis*) has had persistent health problems that have impeded population growth,[9] and the most prevalent health problem has been skin disease. In the United States, nearly 50% of adult black rhinoceroses have had at least one episode of skin or oral/nasal mucosal lesions that resulted in significant morbidity and, less commonly, mortality. Although some skin conditions appear as primary disease, most episodes appear to be secondary to other major health problems, such as hepatic failure, hemolytic anemia, enteritis, pneumonia, and generalized debility. Many episodes have also been linked to stressful environmental conditions, such as transportation, introduction of new animals, or sudden cold temperatures. The relationship between skin disease and other conditions suggests that rhinoceros skin is acutely sensitive to the physiologic status of the animal and that events disrupting normal homeostasis may initiate structural and functional changes in the epidermis that result in increased fragility and poor healing. The distinctive dermatologic syndrome that accounts for the majority of lesions in captive black rhinoceroses, superficial necrolytic dermatopathy, is consistent with this concept. In contrast, skin disease in wild black rhinoceroses has been almost exclusively associated with *Stephanofilaria dinniki* infestations.

NORMAL SKIN HISTOLOGY

Black rhinoceros skin has features that most closely resemble those of human skin except for the deep collagenous dermis. Rhinoceros epidermis has prominent rete ridges and a distinct papillary dermis (Fig. 80–1). The epidermis is composed of approximately 5 to 10 layers of keratinocytes covered by several layers of cornified epithelial cells. The papillary dermis is notably less dense than the dermis below the rete ridges (reticular dermis), which is very thick (up to 2 cm) and composed of dense, interwoven collagen bundles. The skin has sparse hair with only rare, small pilosebaceous units. Evenly dispersed in the superficial reticular dermis are large, round clusters of eccrine sweat glands and prominent arterioles. These histologic characteristics suggest that black rhinoceros skin lacks the protective benefits of hair and the moisturizing effects of sebum but can rapidly disperse heat through eccrine gland secretion and abundant superficial vasculature. The epithelium of the oral and nasal mucosa is similar

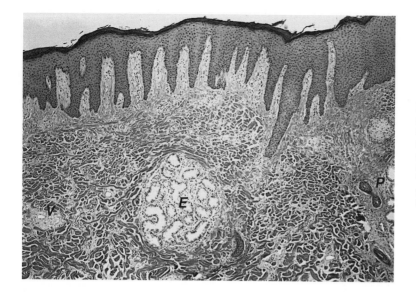

FIGURE 80–1. Histologic appearance of normal black rhinoceros skin. The reticular dermis is markedly collagenous and contains eccrine sweat glands (E) and scant pilosebaceous units (P). The epidermis is thin and has rete ridges. Hematoxylin and eosin stain; original magnification, ×400.

to the skin except that the superficial cells do not undergo cornification.

RESPONSES OF RHINOCEROS SKIN TO INJURY

Skin pustules and ulcers develop in black rhinoceroses under many circumstances, and only histopathologic study can distinguish the primary dermatologic problem. For this reason, this chapter emphasizes the histologic character of skin lesions.

Black rhinoceros skin has common responses to a variety of injuries. The skin undergoes marked epidermal hyperplasia, increasing in depth up to 30 or more layers, and rete ridges become complex and branching. Stratification of keratinocytes often becomes disorganized, and multinucleated keratinocytes appear. Altered epidermal keratinization is also common and results in dyskeratosis, parakeratosis, and hyperkeratosis. If cytokeratin immunohistochemistry or electron microscopy is not used, dyskeratotic epithelial cells may contain distinct eosinophilic keratin aggregates that can be mistaken for viral inclusions.

The papillary dermis responds to many injuries with marked neovascularization, edema, hemorrhage, and an increase in basophilic fibrillar ground substance. Hemorrhage also is common in the superficial reticular dermis, and red blood cell (RBC) exocytosis through the epithelium (which has been described as "sweating blood") results in subcorneal pooling of blood or hemorrhagic crusts. In most types of injury, dermal fibroplasia is prominent and disorganized, appearing similar to neoplasia. Neutrophils and eosinophils are the predominant inflammatory cells in most rhinoceros skin diseases, and melanophages are common in chronic inflammatory conditions because pigmentary incontinence occurs.

Ulcers, erosions, and fissures develop under many circumstances, possibly because rhinoceros skin has a relatively thin, unprotected epidermis overlying a rigid, collagenous dermis. Ulcers typically heal slowly, and the epidermis at ulcer margins can be very hyperplastic, forming large, fungating, neoplasm-like masses (pseudocarcinomatous hyperplasia). Dense granulation tissue beds form under most chronic ulcers and are often accompanied by collagen degeneration and mineralization.

SPECIFIC DERMATOLOGIC SYNDROMES

Superficial Necrolytic Dermatopathy of Black Rhinoceroses

Synonyms for this condition are mucosal and cutaneous ulcerative syndrome, hepatocutaneous syndrome, vesicular and ulcerative dermatopathy, and ulcerative skin disease. It is the most prevalent skin disease in captive black rhinoceroses and is characterized by abnormal epidermal growth, degeneration, and superficial necrosis, subsequently leading to the formation of vesicles and chronic ulcers.[11] More than 40 rhinoceroses in 21 zoological parks have been affected by this syndrome. Clinically, lesions first appear as epidermal plaques, vesicles, or pustules that subsequently erode or ulcerate. In many cases, ulcers are the first noted clinical sign and are often mistaken for abrasions when located over pressure points. The lesions are usually bilateral and relatively symmetric, located predominantly on pressure points, ear margins, coronary bands, the tip of the tail, or the lateral body surfaces. Oral or nasal mucosal lesions also occur alone or concurrently with skin lesions. Most oral lesions are on the palate or the lateral margins of the tongue or lips in contact with teeth.

The clinical course is typically one of a waxing and waning of lesions. Most rhinoceroses with lesions are anorectic and have a depressed attitude and weight loss.

Generalized weakness and unexplained lameness also accompany these lesions. Rhinoceroses with extensive skin involvement become moribund. In many rhinoceroses, serum albumin, cholesterol, and hematocrits are lower than those in unaffected wild or captive black rhinoceroses, which may reflect the direct loss of albumin and blood through the skin.

The lesions have distinctive histopathologic characteristics. Early lesions are characterized by epidermal hyperplasia, intraepithelial edema, hydropic degeneration of keratinocytes, and parakeratosis (Fig. 80–2). Vesicles or pustules form in the epidermis at sites of degeneration and edema, resulting in superficial epidermal necrosis. Ulcers subsequently occur after minimal trauma, and the ulcers expand peripherally and heal poorly. A dermal inflammatory reaction does not occur until the ulcerative stage, and it is confined to areas with exposed dermis. Secondary superficial bacterial infections are common.

The disease appears in rhinoceroses of all ages (range of 1 to 39 years) and under different management strategies, with different diets, and under different environmental conditions. The disease occurs as a primary condition or (more commonly) in association with other medical conditions, such as toxic hepatopathy, hemolytic anemia, gastrointestinal diseases, and respiratory infections. The primary disease is often associated with stress events such as sudden cold temperatures, transportation, introduction of new animals, or parturition.

This ulcerative dermatopathy has clinical and histologic features of a rare degenerative skin disease in other species, known as superficial necrolytic dermatitis (hepatocutaneous syndrome) of dogs[2, 10] and necrolytic migratory erythema of humans.[5, 6] These conditions are usually caused by hyperglucagonemia or other metabolic derangements leading to hypoaminoacidemias. The specific cause of this condition in black rhinoceroses has not been identified, although glucagon and amino acid levels have not yet been measured. The high prevalence of this syndrome exclusively in the captive population suggests a dietary deficiency or a metabolic change resulting from captivity.

Because the cause is unknown, treatment has been empiric. No treatment has consistently succeeded in reversing these lesions, and many lesions resolved without treatment. Secondary bacterial infections can be effectively controlled with topical or systemic antibiotics, topical antiseptics, moisturizing salves, and hydrotherapy. Affected rhinoceroses should be examined for underlying diseases, and management practices should be evaluated for dietary adequacy and potential stress factors. Biologic samples (from biopsies of lesions and from plasma and serum) from current cases and recording of environmental and management factors during emerging cases will contribute significantly toward establishing the cause of this condition.

Epidermal Exfoliation

Rhinoceroses sometimes exfoliate large sheets of superficial epidermis from their flanks and lateral thorax, exposing an underlying grey, shiny epidermis. Histologically, the exfoliated material is composed of multiple layers of degenerating superficial epidermis with hyperkeratosis and parakeratosis. The similarity of the epidermal changes with those of the superficial necrolytic dermatopathy and the occurrence of these two syndromes in the same rhinoceroses at different times suggests that this exfoliative syndrome is a clinical variant of superficial necrolytic dermatopathy. The syndrome has resolved without complications after topical moisturizing and antiseptic treatments.

Superficial Pustular Dermatitis

Superficial pustules and serocellular crusts commonly occur in black rhinoceros skin. Although most pustules are secondary to superficial necrolytic dermatopathy, intraepithelial pustules occur in rare cases without epithelial degeneration. Primary superficial pustular derma-

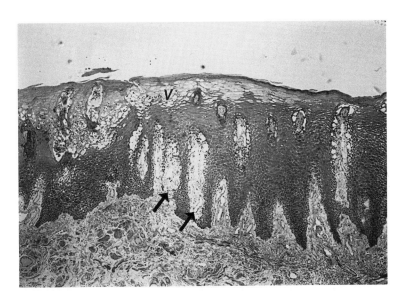

FIGURE 80–2. Black rhinoceros skin with superficial necrolytic dermatopathy. The epidermis is hyperplastic and degenerating, and intercellular edema leads to formation of an early vesicle (V). Parakeratosis also is present. The dermis has vascular dilation and proliferation (*arrows*) but lacks inflammation. Hematoxylin and eosin stain; original magnification, ×400.

titis is characterized by accumulations of neutrophils and small numbers of eosinophils in the epidermis, usually directly beneath the stratum corneum, resulting in small (1- to 2-mm) pustules (Fig. 80–3). Less commonly, transepidermal coagulative necrosis occurs in association with superficial neutrophil accumulations and colonies of bacterial cocci (*Staphylococcus* species). Dermal inflammatory reactions accompany these lesions. These lesions are similar to staphylococcal pyoderma in other species.[1] Most cases have resolved with appropriate topical or systemic antibiotic therapy.

Collagenolytic and Eosinophilic Diseases

NODULAR COLLAGEN DEGENERATION

Dermal collagen degeneration with dystrophic mineralization occurs alone or adjacent to chronic ulcers from other causes. The primary disease manifests as rapidly developing irregular plaques in the oral or nasal cavities or in the dermis. Histologically, the dermis contains discrete areas of collagen degeneration, usually with dystrophic mineralization and surrounded by aggregations of macrophages and inflammatory giant cells (Fig. 80–4). The overlying epidermis is unaffected. The cause of these lesions has not been determined, although similar lesions are seen in domestic dogs with hyperglucocorticoidism and in domestic horses with nodular collagenolytic granuloma, which are suspected to be caused by arthropod induced injury.[17] Collagen degeneration and mineralization also are a feature of eosinophilic granulomas in black rhinoceroses (see next section). Lesions of collagen degeneration have been successfully treated by excision, and untreated lesions have been described as eventually exuding chalky material.

EOSINOPHILIC DERMATITIS AND GRANULOMAS

Eosinophils are a common minor component of the dermal inflammatory response of black rhinoceroses,

but in some cases eosinophilic infiltrates predominate. Eosinophilic dermatitis is usually accompanied by eosinophilic granulomas and ulcers, most of which are associated with collagenolysis and mineralization. Most eosinophilic granulomas and ulcers occur in the oral and nasal cavities and are similar to indolent ulcers in domestic cats.[1] No parasitic or fungal agents are associated with these lesions in captive rhinoceroses, whereas in wild black rhinoceroses, eosinophilic granulomas commonly develop during bouts of stephanofilariasis.[7]

Allergic and Arthus-Like Reactions

Some rhinoceroses have manifested acute skin lesions in response to vaccinations or systemic antibiotics. One animal had small vesicles or pustules over the entire body, whereas other rhinoceroses appeared to exude blood through the skin. The pathologic basis for the hemorrhagic responses has not been determined, although vascular injury is most likely. An Arthus-like reaction (dermal vascular necrosis, thrombosis, and epithelial necrosis) has occurred in association with ulcers in other rhinoceroses, although these animals had not recently undergone systemic treatments or vaccination. However, these Arthus-like lesions also occur with frostbite, which may indicate that they are not immune mediated.

Viral Skin Diseases

A poxvirus was isolated from a rhinoceros with vesicles and pustules in a European zoo,[3, 12, 13] but no poxviral lesions have been reported in other captive and wild populations. Pox-like intracytoplasmic inclusions have been noted in the keratinocytes of captive rhinoceroses in the United States with superficial necrolytic dermatopathy, but these inclusions were determined by electron microscopy and immunohistochemistry to be composed of keratin intermediate filament aggregates. An

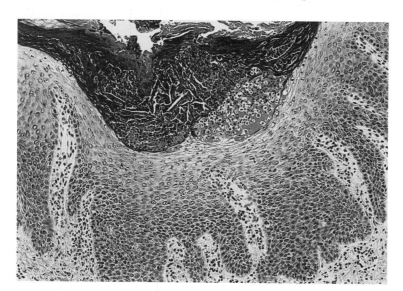

FIGURE 80–3. Black rhinoceros skin with superficial pustular dermatitis. A subcorneal pustule is present in a hyperplastic epidermis. Hematoxylin and eosin stain; original magnification, × 1000.

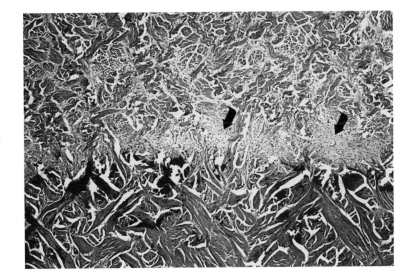

FIGURE 80–4. Black rhinoceros skin with nodular collagen degeneration. Discrete areas of degenerate and mineralized collagen in the reticular dermis are surrounded by macrophages and giant cells (*arrows*). Hematoxylin and eosin stain; original magnification, ×400.

epitheliotropic herpesvirus also has been reported in a black rhinoceros in Germany with ulcers,[8] but no herpes virus has been detected in any U.S. or wild rhinoceroses to date.

Stephanofilariasis in Wild Black Rhinoceroses

None of the aforementioned syndromes have been identified in free-ranging black rhinoceroses. However, skin ulcers associated with dermal *S. dinniki* infestations are common in southern and eastern African black rhinoceroses.[4, 7, 9, 14–16] Ulcers occur primarily on the ventral aspect of the neck and on the lateral aspect of the thorax, particularly behind the shoulder and on the back, abdomen, and forelimbs. The lesions are seasonal (occurring primarily during the summer and resolving in winter) and are markedly erythematous and pruritic,[15] in contrast to the ulcers caused by superficial necrolytic dermatopathy. Chronic ulcers from stephanofilariasis develop thick beds of granulation tissue and have marked dermal inflammatory infiltrates of eosinophils, histiocytes, inflammatory giant cells, and lymphocytes.[7, 15, 16] Stephanofilarial microfilaria and mature filarial nematodes can be identified in most lesions. Stephanofilarial dermatitis has not been identified in captive rhinoceroses, except for two cases in wild-caught rhinoceroses.[4] Transmission to other rhinoceroses in non-endemic regions is unlikely because the appropriate insect vectors[14] are not present, and anthelmintic treatments during quarantine should eliminate current infections.

REFERENCES

1. Gross TL, Ihrke PJ: Inflammatory, dysplastic, and degenerative diseases. *In* Gross TL, Ihrke PJ, Walder EJ (eds): Veterinary Dermatopathology. St. Louis, Mosby–Year Book, pp 1–326, 1992.
2. Gross TL, Song MD, Havel PJ, et al: Superficial necrolytic derma-titis (necrolytic migratory erythema) in dogs. Vet Pathol 30:75–81, 1993.
3. Grunberg W, Burtscher H: Uber eine pockenartige Krankheit beim Rhinozeros (*Diceros bicornis* L.). Zentralbl Veterinarmed Series B, Heft 6, pp 649–657, 1968.
4. Hitchins PM, Keep ME: Observations on skin lesions of the black rhinoceros (*Diceros bicornis*) in the Hluhluwe Game Reserve, Zululand. Lammergeyer 12:56–65, 1970.
5. Kasper CS: Necrolytic migratory erythema: unresolved problems in diagnosis and pathogenesis, a case report and review. Cutis 49:120–128, 1992.
6. Kasper CS, McMurry K: Necrolytic migratory erythema without glucagonoma versus canine superficial necrolytic dermatitis: is hepatic impairment a clue to pathogenesis? J Am Acad Dermatol 25:534–541, 1991.
7. Kock N, Kock MD: Skin lesions in free-ranging black rhinoceroses (*Diceros bicornis*) in Zimbabwe. J Zoo Wildl Med 21:447–452, 1990.
8. Kock RA, Garnier J: Veterinary management of three species of rhinoceroses in a zoological collection. Proceedings of an International Conference on Rhinoceros Biology and Conservation, San Diego, CA, pp 325–345, 1991.
9. Miller RE: Diseases of black rhinoceroses in captivity. Proceedings of the Symposium on Game Ranching Rhinoceroses, Onderstepoort, Republic of South Africa, University of Pretoria, pp 180–185, 1994.
10. Miller WH, Scott DW, Buerger RG, et al: Necrolytic migratory erythema in dogs: a hepatocutaneous syndrome. J Am Anim Hosp Assoc 26:573–581, 1990.
11. Munson L, Koehler JW, Wilkinson JE, et al: Vesicular and ulcerative dermatopathy resembling superficial necrolytic dermatitis in captive black rhinoceroses (*Diceros bicornis*). Vet Pathol 35:31–42, 1998.
12. Pilaski J, Schaller K, Matern K, et al: Outbreaks of pox among elephants and rhinoceroses. Verhandlungber Erkrankg Zootiere 24:257–265, 1982.
13. Pilaski J, Schaller K, Olberding P, et al: Characterization of a poxvirus isolated from white rhinoceros (*Ceratotherium s. simum*). Zentralbl Bakteriol Mikrobiol Hyg 251:440, 1982.
14. Round MC: A new species of *Stephanofilaria* in skin lesions from the black rhinoceros (*Diceros bicornis*) in Kenya. J Helminth 38:87–96, 1964.
15. Schultz KCA, Kluge EB: Dermatitis in the black rhinoceros (*Diceros bicornis*) due to filariasis. J South Afr Vet Med Assoc 31:265–269, 1960.
16. Tremlett JG: Observations on the pathology of lesions associated with *Stephanofilaria dinniki* Round 1964 from the black rhinoceros (*Diceros bicornis*). J Helminth 38:171–174, 1964.
17. Yager JA, Scott DW: The skin and appendages. *In* Jubb KVF, Kennedy PC, Palmer N (eds): Pathology of Domestic Animals, vol 1, 4th ed. New York, Academic Press, pp 531–738, 1993.

CHAPTER 81

Anesthesia of White Rhinoceroses

J. P. RAATH

White rhinoceroses *(Ceratotherium simum)* are routinely anesthetized for marking, sample collection, translocation, and treatments.

Anesthesia of white rhinoceroses is complicated by their sensitivity to opioids; reactions include hypertension, severe respiratory depression under anesthesia, and peculiar anatomic features. As each individual animal becomes more valuable, the need for further research and refining the anesthetic process becomes more important.

THE PLANNING PHASE

Ninety percent of the anesthesia effort should go into the planning phase of the procedure. Risks incurred once a rhinoceros has been darted can be minimized by good planning. A standard checklist should include drug delivery systems, anesthetic combinations, additional drugs and emergency treatments, antidotes, general equipment, and animal monitoring equipment.

Drug Delivery Systems

To ensure deep intramuscular (IM) deposition of the drugs, it is preferable to have a robust darting system in which the drug is discharged only when the collar of the dart hits the skin. The Palmer Cap Chur powder-charged darts and the Kruger National Park (KNP) aluminum acetic acid/bicarbonate darts (see Chapter 76) are effective systems. Air-powered rifles such as the

Tel-Inject or Dan-Inject systems with long needles have also been used successfully and are preferable for darting rhinoceroses in confinement. A push rod for removing darts from the barrel should be included if a rhinoceros to be darted is a different size from the one originally intended. Enough darts for the number of animals to be anesthetized, as well as extras for supplement or antidote, should be taken.

Strong needles 50 to 75 mm in length and 2 mm in diameter are recommended. If the needle opening is in front, it is suggested that the point of the needle be bent over the middle of the lumen to avoid the formation of a skin plug. A bead or collar on the needle is sufficient to prevent the darts from falling out.

Anesthetic Combinations

Many drug combinations have been used successfully in the anesthesia of white rhinoceroses. Many of the earlier drug combinations such as diethylthiambutene hydrochloride (Themalon) and 1-(1-phenylcyclohexyl)-piperidine hydrochloride (Sernyl) and scopolamine are no longer used. Drug combinations used by the Natal Parks Board of South Africa's combinations are listed in Table 81–1, and those used by the Kruger National Park (KNP) are listed in Table 81–2.

The most important goal during field anesthesia is to obtain recumbency in the shortest possible time.

Keep (1971) of the Natal Parks Board reported that although fentanyl (Janssen Pharmaceuticals) alone will anesthetize white rhinoceroses, large doses were re-

TABLE 81–1. Natal Parks Board, South Africa, Anesthetic Combinations for White Rhinoceroses

Age Group	Etorphine (mg)	Fentanyl (mg)	Hyoscine (mg)	Azaperone (mg)
Adults	3–4	—	25	—
	1–2	30	—	50–80
	3–4	—	—	50–80
Subadults	2	—	12	—
	0.5	20	—	30–40
	2	—	—	30–40
Juveniles	1	—	12	—
	0.25	12	—	15–20
	1	—	—	15–20

TABLE 81–2. Kruger National Park, South Africa, Anesthetic Combinations for White Rhinoceroses

Age Group	Etorphine (mg)	Carfentanil (mg)	Azaperone (mg)	Hyaluronidase (IU)
Adult males	5	4	50	7500
Adult females	4	3	35	7500
Subadults	3	2	20	5000
Juveniles	1.5	1	15	5000
Calves	0.5	0.5	10	3000

quired and the animals remain sensitive to noise.[8] Fentanyl was used in combination with etorphine because of fentanyl's faster action in reducing down times and preventing the animals from running too far.

In one regimen, hyoscine, a parasympatholytic drug, was included in the darts to induce temporary blindness by causing pupil dilation, with the purpose of stopping the animal sooner under free-ranging conditions. As the combinations used in Table 81–2 stop the rhinoceros in less than 4 minutes, the author does not support this practice, considering the deleterious side effects of parasympatholytic drugs.

Carfentanil (Janssen Pharmaceuticals) has been found to be slightly more potent than etorphine hydrochloride (M99, C-Vet), hence the lower dose rates.

The use of nalorphine (Lethidrone) in small doses in the dart has also been described in black rhinoceroses to counteract the respiratory depression caused by the opioids.

Xylazine (Rompun) has been used for white rhinoceros sedation and anesthesia. Dose rates of 0.48 mg/kg in combination with etorphine are suggested for free-ranging white rhinoceroses, but reluctance to stand after administration of the antidote has been noted. Excellent results have been obtained with xylazine alone at 0.25 to 0.50 mg/kg for the sedation of rhinoceroses in pens.

Under hospital or clinic conditions, rhinoceros anesthesia can be maintained with 2% isoflurane in 100% oxygen at a flow rate of 10 L per minute. For this purpose, an endotracheal tube with an inflatable cuff has to be passed, allowing an effective seal.

Additional Drugs and Emergency Treatments

All additional drugs, such as emergency drugs—for example, respiratory stimulants (Doxapram), antidotes, and antibiotics—as well as vitamin combinations and tranquilizers, must be ready and checked before darting commences. Provisions must include a complete kit to treat accidental human injection with opioids.

Antidotes

Antidotes commonly used to reverse rhinoceros anesthesia include the agonistic antagonists nalorphine and diprenorphine hydrochloride (M5050, C-Vet) and the pure antagonists naloxone (Narcan, Boots) and naltrexone.

General Equipment

Rhinoceroses, being heavy animals, are difficult to manipulate once recumbent. People handling them should always plan for the worst-case scenario and have the following necessary equipment ready:

1. Two soft cotton ropes: one long rope, approximately 30 m long, for the head and a shorter rope of 10 m for the hind foot.

2. Blindfolds and earplugs. Blindfolds can be made of towels with Velcro on the ends. Earplugs should have long strings for getting them in the rhinoceros's ears.

3. Axes. To avoid injury as the rhinoceros stands and walks, it may be necessary to remove some trees/branches around the rhinoceros before administration of the antidote.

4. Shovels. They are used to dig or fill holes on the path of a walking rhinoceros and to remove sharp stumps close to a recumbent rhinoceros.

5. Prodders. Used with discretion, they are successful in stimulating rhinoceroses to rise after administration of the partial antagonist.

6. Inflatable vehicle jacks. They have been used with great success to support rhinoceroses in lateral recumbency.

7. Two way radios: They are essential for maintaining communication between the helicopter and ground crews.

Animal Monitoring Equipment

All monitoring equipment must be in place and ready to be connected to the animal. This includes a pulse oximeter, electrocardiographic machinery, a blood pressure gauge, and a thermometer.

REQUIREMENTS FOR PHYSIOLOGIC MANIPULATIONS

Water is used to cool down rhinoceroses in extreme temperatures, and copious amounts of cold water are necessary. Oxygen supplementation can be given through a nasal catheter or endotracheal tube. It is not difficult to pass an endotracheal tube in rhinoceroses through the nose for oxygen supplementation. The diameter of this tube must be smaller than that of the trachea, and a commercial bovine stomach tube is adequate for adult white rhinoceroses. It is preferable to attach an intravenous (IV) line by using an ear vein or the large vein on the inner front leg. IV access is useful in emergencies, especially when blood pressure falls.

Personnel Requirements

It is important to have enough trained personnel who are well informed and to whom specific tasks have been designated.

Time Management

Rhinoceros anesthesia is induced in the morning, when temperatures are cool, and at the time of year that the animals are in good condition. In the field, late afternoon darting must be limited to extreme emergencies, because unforeseen circumstances can lead to working in the dark. Rhinoceroses breed all year round, and darting of heavily pregnant animals should be avoided.

Localities

Difficulties are experienced in darting in dense bush from a vehicle, between high trees from a helicopter, and on open plains when darting on foot. Natural obstacles such as cliffs, dongas, and open water pose a threat to ataxic rhinoceroses, and the animals must be steered away from these trouble areas before darting. Accessibility of the ground crew to the rhinoceros is always an important consideration.

THE PROCEDURE

The Approach

Darting from a helicopter is preferred under free-ranging conditions because continuous visual contact is possible and the helicopter can be used to chase other rhinoceroses away from the recumbent animal. When darting is done from a helicopter, both the pilot and marksman must identify the animal. They must take time to herd the animal close to the ground crew to ensure good dart placement. To avoid dart whiplash, the helicopter flies 10 to 30 m behind the animal and at the same speed as the running rhinoceros. Once the rhinoceros is darted, it is advisable to move away and steer the animal from a distance.

When darting is done from a ground vehicle, personnel must never drive directly toward the rhinoceros; rather, they should approach it in decreasing circles. Personnel should also avoid standing on the back of a pick-up truck or breaking the outline of the vehicle, and they should try to prevent bushes from scratching the vehicle or leaving on the back of the pick-up truck loose items that can make a noise. The vehicle follows the darted animal at a distance, and if contact is lost, trackers carrying blindfolds, ropes, and a two-way radio must follow it on foot.

Although white rhinoceroses appear to be very placid, they are extremely powerful and potentially dangerous. When darting is done on foot, it is sensible to have a back-up marksman with a heavy-caliber rifle. The marksman must be sure of a down-wind approach, wear sensible bush clothing, and walk softly, although white rhinoceroses, despite extremely poor eyesight, have acute senses of smell and hearing. Rhinoceroses regularly turn towards the marksman once the dart has been fired. The marksman must therefore be in a safe position and remain immobile after darting. A safe following distance must be maintained, and the ground crew is updated by a two-way radio.

Dart Site and Angle

A well-vascularized muscle area should be selected for dart placement. The darts must be placed at right angles to the skin to avoid subcutaneous deposition of the drug. Preference is given to the gluteal region from the helicopter; the neck area is often exposed in pens.

The Ataxic Phase

It is important to maintain continuous visual contact of the rhinoceros after darting. The ataxic phase is the most likely phase for physical injury; white rhinoceroses characteristically show a reduction in speed; a shortened gait, often dragging their feet, followed by a high stepping gait; standing; and sideways movement. The head is held higher. As soon as ataxia is noticed, the following distance is increased, to avoid further stimulation, and intervention is undertaken only if the animal moves to dangerous terrain.

White rhinoceroses can be stopped toward the end of this phase by allowing them to step into a rope with one hind leg, then securing the rope between the hock joint and the foot. This rope is tied to a vehicle or tree, and the animal is stopped. A blindfold is placed over the animal's eyes, and earplugs are inserted to reduce stimulation. If ataxia has not occurred by a certain set time, it is probable that the dart has malfunctioned. A second dart containing a full dose is fired if the animal shows no reaction in 8 to 10 minutes; one-third to half the dose is given if the animal is affected but does not stop or become recumbent.

Recumbency

The rhinoceros can be assisted into recumbency by pulling on the rope on the hind foot or by pushing the body. Although rhinoceroses tolerate lateral recumbency, sternal recumbency is preferred, except for heavily pregnant females, in which the fetus may elevate the pressure on the diaphragm. A rhinoceros must not be allowed to lie with its head downhill because this will also increase the pressure on the diaphragm.

Rhinoceroses also must not lie on their back legs for extended periods of time, because this results in occlusion of the blood supply and reluctance to stand after administration of the antidote. The rhinoceros's weight should be shifted from time to time during recumbency. White rhinoceroses sometimes do not become fully recumbent and maintain a dog-sitting position. This is safe for short periods, but because this position places all the weight on the hind legs, it should be avoided during long procedures.

The dart wound is treated immediately with an intramammary antibiotic preparation. It is good practice to insert a catheter into an ear vein to ensure a patent pathway into the blood stream for emergencies, and a saline solution or Ringer's lactate solution is administered.

Monitoring

It is important to keep good records of physiologic parameters for each use of anesthetics to build up sufficient baseline data allowing the determination of acceptable physiologic limits.

TEMPERATURE

A long thermometer is inserted deeply into the anus to ensure accurate measurement of body temperature. The temperature depends on the amount of activity beforehand, the environmental temperature, and the health status of the animal. Temperatures vary from 36° to 39.5°C during field capture operations.

White rhinoceroses are notorious for respiratory depression and ventilate poorly when anesthetized with morphine. Nalorphine, 10 to 15 mg IV, should be administered immediately, because this increases the rate and depth of respiration and improves blood gas values. Initial respiration rates can be as low as 3 to 4 per minute but should increase to 8 to 12 per minute after administration of nalorphine.

Pulse oximeters can be attached to the ear, after the superficial pigmented layers have been scraped off, or to skinfolds of the vulva or prepuce. Reflective probes can also be inserted into the nose to use the reading from the nasal septum. Arterial blood gas values can be determined from samples obtained from the inside ear artery, into which an 18- to 20-gauge catheter has been inserted.

Opioids cause a marked increase in rhinoceros blood pressure. This elevation is caused by increased activity of the sympathetic nervous system, evidenced by a sixfold increase in norepinephrine levels seen in horses anesthetized with etorphine. Blood pressure can be monitored by direct line in the inner ear artery or by placing a cuff around the tail. Mean arterial pressures in excess of 200 mm Hg have been routinely measured but are reduced after the administration of nalorphine.

Six white rhinoceroses darted with 2 mg of etorphine and 30 mg of fentanyl had a mean blood pressure of 183 ± 16 mm Hg, whereas six darted with 3 mg of etorphine and 25 mg of azaperone had a mean arterial pressure of 141 ± 24 mm Hg. A mean arterial pressure ranged between 280 and 210 mm Hg was recorded after a white rhinoceros was anesthetized with 2.8 mg of etorphine.

Although the blood pressure in the rhinoceros is high under anesthesia with etorphine, it may well be beneficial to the hypoxic animal. If the perfusion is decreased with the persisting low oxygen tension levels, it can be very dangerous. Thus the use of high doses of adrenergic antagonists is questionable. On the other hand, a blood pressure over 200 mm Hg can result in edema and rupture of small vasculature, causing pulmonary hemorrhage.

White rhinoceroses typically show muscle shivering or rising and stiffening of the front quarters. This can be reduced by intravenous supplementation with 10 to 15 mg of detomidine (Domosedan) or by administering small IV doses of benzodiazepine or buterophenone tranquilizers. A disadvantage of these tranquilizers is the reluctance of rhinoceroses to walk after the administration of small doses of nalorphine (see later discussion).

Monitoring depth of anesthesia in rhinoceroses can be difficult. Ear movement, respiration rate, and attempts to rise are indicators. Heart rates also increase as the level of anesthesia becomes lighter, but this may also be an indication of hypoxia.

Supplemental Doses

When supplemental doses are needed, they are administered via the catheter in the ear vein. They are 25% to 33% of the initial anesthetic dosage in the same ratio as administered in the initial dart. If the additional anesthetic is used, it is important to add it into calculations of the antidote dose. Boluses of ketamine after the use of opioids should be used with caution because they may lead to extended apneic phases.

Emergencies

Apnea is especially apparent during the early part of the procedure. Steps to avoid or counteract this are as follows: Insert catheters with an IV line. Administer nalorphine in increments of 15 mg IV or small doses of nalbuphine. Administer 10 to 20 ml of doxapram (Dopram) intravenously. Although doxapram has the immediate effect of increasing respiration rate, it has very limited effect on increasing oxygenation of the blood. If there is still little improvement, abort the operation and administer the full antidote, preferably a pure antagonist such as naltrexone.

Routine oxygen supplementation to anesthetized white rhinoceroses is indicated. A flow rate of 15 L of oxygen per minute must be maintained. If the animal was suffering from apnea and treatment was administered as described earlier, the blood oxygenation should also increase. Poor ventilation will further result in hypercapnia, which will improve only if the respiration rate and depth are increased.

If, in spite of oxygen supplementation, the blood gas values remain low, the flow rate of the oxygen can be increased and the doxapram dose repeated. Fifteen minutes of oxygen supplementation via an endotracheal tube increased the PO_2 level from 35% to 115% in one rhinoceros. A dramatic color change was also observed in the venous blood (personal unpublished data). Continued low blood oxygenation is an indication to end the procedure and administer the full antidote dose.

Low blood pressure can be caused by decreased heart rate, by decreased venous return, or by excessive peripheral vasodilation. Postural change usually rectifies the problem, but epinephrine is indicated at standard dose rates if this condition persists.

High blood pressure is reduced by the IV administration of nalorphine or by small doses (15 to 30 mg total dose) of a butyrophenone such as azaperone.

Rhinoceros body temperatures exceeding 39°C can be reduced by pouring copious amounts of water on the animal, combined with movement of air over the animal (fans or waving branches). Rhinoceroses can be covered with branches to protect them from direct sunlight, or large volumes of cold intravenous fluids or cold water enemas can be administered. If the temperature continues to rise, consideration should be given for anesthetic reversal.

If rhinoceroses recently drank water before darting, water may flow from their mouths during anesthesia. This condition may necessitate termination of the procedure, because inhalation of the water can lead to pneumonia. Care must be taken that the head is held lower than the body and the nose is pointing downwards.

Fortunately, white rhinoceroses do not generally awaken suddenly but will show prior warning signs. These include increased ear movements, curling of the tail, and increased heart rates. If the animal attempts to rise, a supplemental dose is indicated.

Reversal

Before reversal, all work on the rhinoceros must be completed and all monitoring equipment must be removed. All persons and vehicles are moved away from the rhinoceros, and the helicopter should be ready for take-off.

Heavy animals tend to compromise the arterial blood supply to the undermost muscles, and the venous draining can be completely occluded. This leads to an increase in lactate, which precipitates muscle spasms and reduces the blood flow even further. This can lead to difficulty in standing after a long recumbency. The weight of the animal should be shifted periodically during long recumbencies and the rhinoceros should be placed in lateral recumbency for 5 minutes before reversal. Rhinoceroses that are anesthetized in winter months, in poor condition, and when heavily pregnant take longer to rise than do others.

Diprenorphine at three times the etorphine dose and naltrexone at 40 times the etorphine or carfentanil dose are standard dose rates. If only nalorphine is available, a total of 250 mg is administered to an adult rhinoceros.

The antidote is administered via the catheter in the ear vein, and the ear plugs and blindfold are removed. Personnel should move clear of the animal to allow it to wake up alone and calmly. If a cow and a calf have been immobilized together, they should receive their antidotes simultaneously.

The agonistic antagonists nalorphine and diprenorphine can be used to partially or completely reverse the anesthesia in white rhinoceroses. Even after complete reversal dosages have been administered, the rhinoceroses remain docile and seminarcotized for up to 24 hours. Further administration of these antidotes does not improve this condition. Complete reversal occurs if the pure antagonists naloxone and naltrexone are used.

Sometimes it is not possible to place the transport crate close to the recumbent animal, because of habitat restrictions. It is possible to walk a white rhinoceros (up to a few kilometers) from the site of recumbency to more suitable terrain. The path toward the crate should be planned and cleared beforehand, and two persons walk ahead to remove obstacles that may jeopardize the walking rhinoceros. Walking rhinoceroses cannot negotiate sharp turns.

The middle of a 30-m rope is tied around the rhinoceros's blindfolded head. The two loose ends of approximately 15 m each are laid out in front of the rhinoceros, and four or five persons are placed on each rope to act as pullers. The rope on the hind foot must remain during this procedure to act as a brake.

Nalorphine is injected into the ear vein in 50-mg and 30-mg boluses for adults and subadults, respectively. These dosages must be adapted according to the level of anesthesia of the rhinoceros at the time of reversal. Of importance is that rhinoceroses that receive oxygen generally require less nalorphine to walk. Approximately 3 minutes should pass before the rhinoceros is stimulated to stand, by patting on the head or prodding the lip in order to raise the head. Determining whether it is necessary to administer a second bolus of nalorphine requires careful judgment. The head must raise first, and the two front legs must be extended. The rhinoceros is pulled forward until it is standing on all four legs. Still blindfolded, it will walk with an unstable gait and can be guided by lateral pulling and pushing on the horn. A steady pace must be maintained because stopping will result in recumbency.

If the rhinoceros starts running or becomes difficult to control, the brake rope is tied around a tree to stop the animal. Once the rhinoceros has calmed down, the walking can be continued. The full antidote and the tranquilizers can be administered once the rhinoceros is loaded in the crate.

POSTRECOVERY PHASE

Under free-ranging conditions, the rhinoceros is allowed to wander off undisturbed. The helicopter can be used to ensure that the reversed cow and her nonmanipulated calf are reunited. Where circumstances allow, subsequent monitoring from a distance is advised.

COMBINED ANESTHESIA OF COWS AND CALVES

If the cow and the calf are both to be anesthetized, they are darted in quick succession. The cow must be darted first, because the calf will remain with its mother and can often be darted while it is standing next to the recumbent cow. Success has been obtained by darting the cow and calf with a double-barrel dart gun. The animals should be left undisturbed, allowed to remain calmly together, and become recumbent close to each other. Problems can arise if there is a dart failure with one of the animals or if they separate during the ataxic phase, which occurs most often in dense vegetation.

Therefore, sufficient ground crew to form two teams must be available when this procedure is undertaken.

CONSIDERATIONS IN DARTING RHINOCEROSES IN CONFINEMENT

The anesthesia of a rhinoceros in a pen is far more controlled. The water trough is drained and the animals are not allowed to wallow 6 hours in advance to avoid regurgitation of water during anesthesia or even drowning during the ataxic phase.

For anesthesia in a boma, 0.25 to 0.4 mg of etorphine (M99) with 10 to 20 mg of azaperone is used if a standing immobilization is required, or 1 to 1.5 mg of etorphine (M99) and 50 mg of azaperone are used if recumbency in adults is required.

To load a rhinoceros into a crate from a pen, allow 10 to 15 minutes after darting until the animal shows a high stepping gait and the tendency to follow moving objects. A white rag tied to a long stick is waved in front of the rhinoceros and slowly moved toward the crate. The rhinoceros will follow the rag with a slow and unstable gait, toward and finally into the crate. (In a similar way, rhinoceroses can be enticed to press their heads against the pen wall when a standing anesthesia is sufficient). Once the rhinoceros is crated, the tranquilizers and antidote are administered through the trapdoor in the crate's roof. During this process, sound and movement should be limited to prevent distracting the animal.

Monitoring after reversal in the pen or crate is important for the first 12 hours to ensure that no renarcotization takes place.

REFERENCES

1. Allen JL: Immobilization of Mongolian wild horses (*Equus przewalskii przewalskii*) with carfentanil and antagonism with naltrexone. J Zoo Wildl Med 23(4):422–425, 1992.
2. Dunlop CI, et al: Temporal effects of halothane and isoflurane in laterally recumbent ventilated male horses. Am J Vet Res 48(8):1250–1255, 1987.
3. Goodman AG, Gilman LS, et al: The Pharmacological Basis of Therapeutics. New York, Macmillan, pp 485–504, 1991.
4. Hall LW, Clarke KW: Hall and Clarke Veterinary Anaesthesia, 8th ed. London, Baillière Tindall, pp 215–218, 1985.
5. Hattingh J, Knox CM, Raath JP: Blood pressure and gas composition of the white rhinoceros at capture. In press.
6. Heard DJ, Olsen JH, Stover J: Cardiopulmonary changes associated with chemical immobilization and recumbency in a white rhinoceros (*Ceratotherium simum*). J Zoo Wildl Med 23(2):197–200, 1992.
7. Jaffe RS, et al: Nalbuphine antagonism of fentanyl-induced ventilatory depression: a randomized trial. Anesthesiology 68:254–260, 1988.
8. Keep ME: Etorphine hydrochloride antagonists used in the capture of the white rhinoceros, *Ceratotherium simum simum*. Lammergeyer 13:60–68, 1971.
9. Kock MD: Use of hyaluronidase and increased etorphine (M99) doses to improve induction times and reduce capture-related stress in the chemical immobilization of the free-ranging black rhinoceros (*Diceros bicornis*) in Zimbabwe. J Zoo Wildl Med 23(2):181–188, 1992.
10. Kock MD, la Grange M, du Toit R: Chemical immobilization of free-ranging black rhinoceros (*Diceros bicornis*) using combinations of etorphine (M99), fentanyl, and xylazine. J Zoo Wildl Med 21(2):155–165, 1990.
11. LeBlanc PH, Eicker SW, Curtis M, Bechler B: Hypertension following etorphine anesthesia in a rhinoceros (*Diceros simus*). J Zoo Anim Med 18(4):141–143, 1987.
12. McKenzie A: The Capture and Care Manual. Pretoria, Wildlife Decision Support Services and South African Veterinary Foundation, pp 512–528, 1993.
13. Soma LR: Equine anesthesia: Causes of reduced oxygen and increased carbon dioxide tensions. Compend Cont Ed 2(4):57–63, 1980.
14. Taylor PM: Risks of recumbency in the anaesthetised horse. Eq Vet J 16(2):77–78, 1984.

CHAPTER 82

Tapir Medicine

DONALD L. JANSSEN
BRUCE A. RIDEOUT
MARK S. EDWARDS

The Tapiridae is an ancient family within the order Perissodactyla. Only four species of tapirs exist, all within the genus *Tapirus:* three New World species and one Old World species (Table 82–1). The majority of tapirs in captivity are Malayan and South American tapirs. Baird's tapirs are less common, and mountain tapirs are rare. In the wild, habitat loss and hunting threaten tapir populations. The South American tapir is listed in Appendix II of the Convention on International Trade in Endangered Species (CITES), and the other three species are listed in Appendix I. The mountain tapir is nearing extinction in the wild.

Tapirs range in size from 200 to 400 kg, and females are often larger than males. The Malayan tapir is the largest species, and the mountain tapir is the smallest. Individuals have lived longer than 30 years in captivity. Several authors have published reviews of the biology, husbandry, and medical problems of the Tapiridae.[2, 6, 8, 9, 11, 12] One bibliography contains citations on the medical problems and biology of Tapiridae.[5] The American Zoo and Aquarium Association (AZA) sponsors a Taxon Advisory Group and Species Survival Plans for the Tapiridae.

The internal anatomy of the tapir is analogous to those of the domestic horse and other perissodactyla. Tapirs have guttural pouches that, as in the horse, are located in the pharyngeal region, lateral to the hyoid bones. The testes are subcutaneous in the inguinal region on either side of the penis. Tapirs lack a gallbladder. Tapirs are herbivorous, and cellulose is fermented in the hindgut. The stomach is small and the cecum and colon are large, in comparison with those of ruminants. The stomach has a small squamous portion in the cardia near the gastroesophageal junction. The kidneys, like those of the horse, are not lobulated. The normal parietal and visceral pleura can be thick and prominent. Malayan tapirs, however, actually have anatomic adhesions between the lung and chest wall, like the elephant.

ANESTHESIA

Many tapirs can be habituated to being touched and scratched (Fig. 82–1). Some individuals will even lie down, allowing physical examination and venipuncture. Temperaments of individuals vary greatly, however. Caution should be exercised in working with any tapir that is being "scratched down," because tapirs can inflict serious injury with their teeth.

For chemical restraint, etorphine (10 μg/kg IM) was traditionally the injectable anesthetic most frequently used in tapirs. When etorphine became unavailable, some veterinarians chose to use carfentanil (20 μg/kg IM) alone or in combination with xylazine. Supplementation with nasal oxygen helps to maintain oxygen saturation in anesthetized tapirs. The combination of butorphanol (0.15 mg/kg IM) and an alpha$_2$-adrenergic agonist such as xylazine (0.3 mg/kg IM) or detomidine (0.05 mg/kg IM) shows promise as a new regimen to use in place of narcotic drugs. Bradycardia occurs (30 to 55 beats/minute), but relative oxygen saturation remains approximately 90% to 95%. Good relaxation generally

TABLE 82–1. Taxonomy and Distribution of *Tapirus*

Species	Commmon Names	Geographic Distribution
Tapirus indicus	Malayan, Asian, or saddleback tapir	Southern Burma, Malay Peninsula, Thailand, Sumatra
Tapirus bairdi	Central American, or Baird's tapir	Southern Mexico to Colombia and Venezuela
Tapirus pinchaque	Mountain, or wooly, tapir	Andes mountains of Colombia, Venezuela, Ecuador, Peru
Tapirus terrestris	South American, Brazilian, or lowland tapir	Amazon Basin and northern countries of South America to northern Argentina

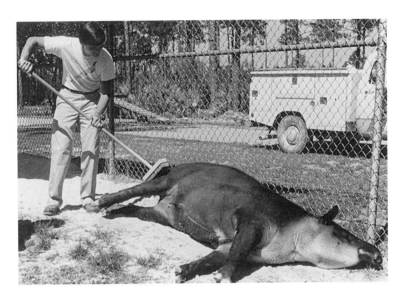

FIGURE 82–1. Tapirs can be habituated to being touched and scratched. Some individuals will even lie down, allowing minor procedures to be performed.

occurs after about 10 minutes. Ketamine (0.25 to 0.5 mg/kg IV) can be given if necessary for further restraint. The effects can be reversed with yohimbine (0.2 to 0.3 mg/kg IV) and a narcotic antagonist such as naltrexone or naloxone. Recovery is generally rapid, smooth, and complete.

Other combinations such as carfentanil/ketamine/xylazine[10] and xylazine (0.8 mg/kg IM) with azaperone (0.8 mg/kg IM) followed by ketamine (0.5 to 1.0 mg/ kg IV) have also been used successfully in tapirs. Azaperone has caused adverse reactions in horses (e.g., central nervous system excitement), and some caution may be indicated in its use with tapirs. Sedation of tapirs to ease introductions or for minor standing procedures can be accomplished with azaperone (1.0 mg/kg IM) or, less reliably, with xylazine (1.0 mg/kg IM).

CLINICAL PROCEDURES

Clinical techniques used for diagnosis and treatment in other large ungulates can be adapted for use in tapirs. Blood is readily obtained from either the medial saphenous or the carpal vein. It is common, however, for these veins to collapse or go into spasm during intravenous injections, thus necessitating multiple punctures. The jugular vein is useful for large-volume blood collection. Catheter placement is most suitable in the carpal vein distal to the carpus. The catheter is readily stabilized at that site, but long-term catheterization is difficult in a conscious adult or juvenile tapir. The carpal vein catheterization site is particularly well suited for neonates. The jugular vein can also be catheterized, but stabilization is difficult without specialized catheterization equipment. Arterial samples for blood gas determination can be obtained from the facial artery or the intermediate branch of the caudal auricular artery.

Endotracheal intubation is fairly straightforward in tapirs. Blind intubation, as in a horse, is possible with experience. Direct visualization of the larynx is not difficult with proper positioning and the use of a long laryngoscope blade. Appropriate endotracheal tube sizes are 10 to 14 mm for juveniles and 16 to 24 mm for adults. Flexible bronchoscopy can be performed via the endotracheal tube or through the nasal cavity. Tracheal washes also can be performed via the endotracheal tube or transtracheally with a through-the-needle catheter directly into the proximal portion of the trachea through the skin. These techniques, together with thoracic radiography, can be used to differentiate upper from lower respiratory tract disease.

Thoracic radiography can be a challenge in tapirs. In adult tapirs, multiple exposures to cover the entire thorax are necessary. X-ray machines with at least 300 mA capacity are needed to penetrate an adult tapir thorax. Lateral exposures, with the use of a grid, are the most useful. The feet and teeth are the other sites most frequently radiographed in tapirs.

Tuberculin testing is indicated as a preventive medicine procedure, but interpretation may be a problem. Controversy exists over the best site for testing. The cervical region is not acceptable in tapirs because the skin is too thick for reliable skin thickness measurements. Tapirs do not have a true caudal fold, but the skin around the tail is thinner and more pliable. The skin in the inguinal and axillary areas is also thin and pliable. These locations can be palpated relatively easily in a tapir that is habituated to handling.

It is important to permanently identify captive tapirs. Many tapirs receive ear injuries in their lifetimes, so ear tags or notches do not work well for identification, and tattoos are often difficult to read regardless of where they are applied. Microchip transponders, however, have been used successfully to permanently identify tapirs. The identification number can often be read without sedation. The transponder is placed either behind the left ear or between the scapulae. Adult tapirs should be anesthetized for insertion of the microchip.

CLINICAL PATHOLOGY

Analysis of hematology and clinical pathology values from Medical Animal Record Keeping System (Med-

TABLE 82–2. Hematologic Reference Values for Tapirs, from Composite MedARKS Records

Test	Malayan Tapir	Lowland Tapir	Baird's Tapir	Mountain Tapir
Hematocrit (%)	37 ± 7 (108)	39 ± 7 (166)	28 ± 10 (55)	37 ± 4 (3)
WBC count/μl	11,110 ± 6255 (115)	10,900 ± 4500 (160)	10,490 ± 3350 (61)	8122 ± 3350 (9)
Neutrophils/μl	7385 ± 5200 (111)	6608 ± 3600 (152)	6934 ± 3280 (60)	5083 ± 3900 (9)
Lymphocytes/μl	2380 ± 1350 (110)	3394 ± 1570 (155)	2941 ± 1288 (58)	2640 ± 1156 (9)
Monocytes/μl	296 ± 227 (90)	288 ± 221 (125)	157 ± 127 (36)	228 ± 195 (6)
Eosinophils/μl	140 ± 166 (67)	488 ± 421 (117)	105 ± 96 (39)	227 ± 159 (4)
Basophils/μl	34 ± 67 (44)	38 ± 51 (33)	8 ± 27 (25)	86 ± 35 (2)
Fibrinogen (mg/dl)	—	500 ± 0.0 (2)	550 ± 70 (2)	—

Values represent mean ± standard deviation (n).

ARKS) summaries showed no major differences between species of tapirs. The values followed trends similar to those of other perissodactyls, including horses. In the authors' experience, plasma fibrinogen is particularly important for evaluating the presence of inflammation in tapirs and should be included with any hematologic evaluation. The reference ranges for hematologic and serum chemical values are listed in Tables 82–2 and 82–3.

DIET AND NUTRITION

Because of the similarities of gastrointestinal tract anatomy, the domestic horse is typically used as a model for all tapir species in the development of dietary guidelines. With diets of alfalfa or timothy hay, the comparative digestibility of cellulose and hemicellulose is slightly less in tapirs than it is in horses.

Tapirs are monogastric animals with limited gastric capacity; therefore, they should be fed in such a way as to avoid overeating. Severe overeating has been implicated as a factor leading to colic, ruptured stomach, or founder in domestic horses. As a result, the authors recommend that tapirs be fed two to three times a

day or supplied food continuously if obesity is not a problem.

The diet of all perissodactyls typically includes both forages and pelleted feeds. Hay is the most common forage fed to tapirs, although browse and pasture may constitute a significant portion of the captive tapir's diet, according to the geographic location of the holding facility and the characteristics of the enclosure. Pelleted herbivore feeds, typically based on alfalfa, are most commonly fed to captive tapirs. Different pellets are formulated to be fed at different rates (e.g., complete feeds versus supplements). A herbivore pellet formulated for grazing ungulates, which contains 15% crude protein, 0.7% lysine, and 21% acid-detergent fiber dry matter basis (DMB), along with alfalfa hay (18% crude protein, 30% acid-detergent fiber [DMB]) has been successfully used for feeding all species of tapirs.

Some preliminary clinical data suggest that tapirs may have a unique metabolic requirement for copper. The mean serum copper level in samples collected from 22 captive animals representing all four species of tapirs was 0.21 μg/ml. Serum copper values above 0.7 ppm are considered normal in a horse. Dietary copper concentrations of these tapirs appear adequate, in comparison to guidelines for horses. The interaction of copper

TABLE 82–3. Biochemical Reference Values for Tapirs, from Composite MedARKS Records

Test	Malayan Tapir	Lowland Tapir	Baird's Tapir	Mountain Tapir
Sodium (mEq/L)	133 ± 4 (78)	135 ± 6 (133)	132 ± 4 (88)	138 ± 5 (5)
Potassium (mEq/L)	4.1 ± 1.1 (81)	3.6 ± 0.6 (133)	4.0 ± 0.5 (96)	3.6 ± 0.7 (7)
Chloride (mEq/L)	94 ± 6 (76)	97 ± 6 (132)	96 ± 3.9 (95)	101 ± 7 (7)
Calcium (mg/dl)	10.7 ± 1.7 (94)	10.6 ± 0.9 (137)	11.0 ± 0.9 (96)	10.5 ± 1.1 (7)
Phosphorous (mg/dl)	5.3 ± 1.6 (95)	5.3 ± 1.3 (130)	5.6 ± 1.3 (95)	5.0 ± 0.6 (7)
Blood urea nitrogen (mg/dl)	11.8 ± 5.7 (105)	8.1 ± 4.2 (147)	11.7 ± 13.2 (96)	8.1 ± 5.4 (7)
Glucose (mg/dl)	101 ± 53 (101)	109 ± 42 (141)	100 ± 30 (93)	116 ± 34 (7)
Creatinine (mg/dl)	1.8 ± 0.6 (90)	1.2 ± 0.4 (134)	1.2 ± 0.6 (94)	1.1 ± 0.4 (7)
ALT (IU/L)	10.4 ± 8.0 (70)	12.9 ± 8.8 (126)	22.8 ± 25.2 (89)	7.8 ± 2.5 (5)
AST (IU/L)	134 ± 76 (93)	83 ± 43 (142)	135 ± 102 (93)	47 ± 22 (5)
GGT (IU/L)	27 ± 10 (31)	24 ± 20 (58)	21 ± 16 (33)	—
Amylase (IU/L)	2682 ± 1819 (93)	2915 ± 1196 (20)	2520 ± 1188 (19)	—
Albumen (g/dl)	3.2 ± 0.6 (97)	3.0 ± 0.5 (115)	3.1 ± 0.6 (45)	3.2 ± 0.6 (7)
Total protein (g/dl)	7.1 ± 0.9 (99)	7.1 ± 0.8 (142)	6.7 ± 1.1 (52)	6.1 ± 0.9 (7)
Total bilirubin (mg/dl)	0.7 ± 0.4 (98)	0.8 ± 0.7 (142)	1.4 ± 1.6 (91)	3.3 ± 4.1 (7)

Values represent mean ± standard deviation (n).
ALT, alanine aminotransferase; AST, aspartate aminotransferase; GGT, gamma glutamyl transferase.

with other trace elements, including iron, zinc, sulfur, and molybdenum, may contribute to these clinically low values. The significance of these serum copper concentrations has yet to be learned. The authors have seen light-colored haircoats and repeated stillbirths in one female lowland tapir with serum copper level of 0.06 μg/ml.

NEONATAL CARE

Published information regarding the composition of maternal milk in tapirs is limited. The solid, crude protein, and ether extract concentrations are relatively higher than the same values for milk from domestic horses. The carbohydrate (lactose) fraction of tapir milk sample is lower than that of the horse.[7]

The birth weight of female Malayan tapir calves is about 10 kg. The absolute rate of growth of mother-reared calves is about 1.33 kg/day from 0 to 29 days. Solids are first consumed at 14 days (range, 8 to 19 days).[1] Transfaunation, accomplished by feeding strained feces from normal tapirs, has been useful in the authors' experience to encourage growth of normal flora in young tapirs raised in isolation.

Neonatal examinations can be useful for assessing general health and detecting the success of immunoglobulin transfer from the dam. It can be a challenge to collect blood from a struggling newborn tapir, and the jugular vein is usually the best site to try. Glutaraldehyde coagulation of serum tests for the presence of adequate immunoglobulins in tapirs. In cases in which the calf fails to nurse, it is often possible to "scratch" the female down and then place the calf on the nipple. Neonatal isoerythrolysis has been observed in a Baird's tapir.[14]

Neonatal mortality is high unless a suitable birthing environment is available. Neonatal deaths from hypothermia, trauma, drowning, and septicemia are often preventable. Males should be removed and pools drained for 1 to 3 weeks after birth. Greater effort must be directed toward solving management problems related to failure of the maternal-infant bond and toward identifying causes of stillbirths and early neonatal deaths.

CLINICAL DISORDERS

Gastrointestinal Problems

Tapirs often suffer from gastrointestinal illnesses. Chronic diarrhea may be caused by bacterial agents such as *Salmonella* and *Campylobacter* species. *Giardia* species also may cause diarrhea. Ciliates probably are normal protozoal inhabitants. Chronic cases may necessitate repeated fecal cultures and endoscopic gastrointestinal biopsies to determine a cause. An inappropriate diet (especially excessive produce) should be ruled out first in any cases of chronic diarrhea.

Colic, as in the horse, may be caused by a variety of surgical and nonsurgical problems in tapirs. Acute bacterial enterocolitis may result in colic. Intestinal ac-

cidents such as volvulus, torsion, impaction, and obstruction may result in sudden and severe colic. Sand impactions occur in tapirs. Prevention of sand impaction may include psyllium, added to the diet regularly, and addressing factors such as feeding location in relation to substrate. With colic, it is important to differentiate problems with urgent surgical solutions from those with medical solutions. Local veterinary surgeons specializing in equine colic surgery are a valuable resource for this purpose.

There have been several reports of rectal prolapse in adult tapirs. It most often occurs in Malayan tapirs. These prolapses have been successfully repaired with both internal and temporary external fixation.[13] The problem appears to be less prevalent than it was in the past. The cause is not known but is likely an inappropriate diet.

Mandibular abscesses frequently occur in tapirs and are difficult to treat. Most often they are a result of molar apical abscesses or periodontal disease. They may become a chronic problem and occasionally cause death when osteomyelitis leads to systemic disease. Treatment of these disorders is most successful when the tooth is either removed or treated endodontically. Surgical debridement of the affected bone and long-term antibiotics are also indicated.

Respiratory Disease

Nasal discharge may be an indication of upper airway disease such as bacterial rhinitis or guttural pouch infection. It may also suggest a more serious lower airway disease. Dyspnea, coughing, or stertorous breathing often indicate life-threatening disease. Diseases such as bacterial pneumonia, pulmonary tuberculosis, coccidioidomycosis, and laryngeal abscesses can cause these signs in tapirs. Bacterial causes of respiratory disease include *Streptococcus, Klebsiella, Corynebacteria, Actinomyces,* and *Fusobacterium* species.

Skin and Hoof Disease

An apparently unique skin disease of tapirs was termed *vesicular skin disease* by Finnegan and associates.[4] This disease affects tapirs in a variety of housing conditions, both indoors and outdoors. It affects males and females equally but recurs more frequently in females. The syndrome is variable but is characterized by the occurrence of lesions over the dorsal thoracic and lumbosacral regions. The lesions begin as coalescing papules and vesicles that rupture, releasing serosanguineous fluid. Histologically, early vesicles contain intact red blood cells (Fig. 82–2). Neurologic signs are often present simultaneously and include hindlimb ataxia and lameness or syncope-like episodes. The signs diminish within a few days, and the animal continues to eat normally. Approximately 1 week later, superficial skin sloughs occur, and the underlying skin heals quickly (Fig. 82–3). The cause of this syndrome remains a mystery.

Acute lameness is nearly always caused by overwearing of the foot pads. The feet of tapirs have hoof-

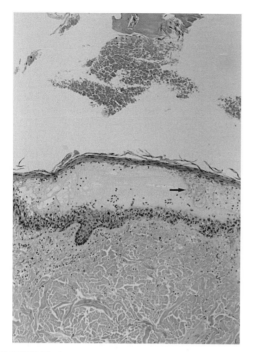

FIGURE 82–2. Skin from the dorsal thoracic region of an adult female Malayan tapir with acute onset of syncope and "blood sweats." A large intraepidermal vesicle contains serum, fibrin, erythrocytes (*arrow*), and a few neutrophils. The watery red fluid that exudes from the skin during these episodes (described as "blood sweats") consists of hemoglobin-rich serum and erythrocytes from these vesicles. Detached from the epidermal surface (*top*) is a sheet of blood and hemoglobin-rich serum, most of which is derived from ruptured vesicles.

Sudden, unexpected death in tapirs is rare but has been caused by intestinal accidents and encephalomyocarditis infection. Tapirs are not prone to fatal self-trauma, but head entrapment from enclosure hazards is a possibility in this animal group.

Chronic weight loss in tapirs should be a warning sign of serious disease. Causes of chronic weight loss in tapirs include renal failure, dental disease, tuberculosis, and chronic bacterial pneumonia. Obesity can also occur in tapirs. Tapirs are not difficult to weigh on electronic platform scales available from livestock supply distributors. Weighing tapirs routinely and objectively allows weight loss trends to be detected before serious problems result.

PATHOLOGY

There are no apparent differences in disease patterns among tapir species. Most of the neonatal deaths are stillbirths or caused by factors relating to maternal behavior (e.g., maternal neglect and trauma). In addition, aspiration pneumonia in animals being hand-reared because of maternal rejection occurs frequently. Other significant primary causes of mortality include accidental drowning, septicemia, necrotizing bacterial enteritis, cecocolonic tympany, and atresia ani.

In the adult age group, the largest proportion of mortalities is caused by gastrointestinal disease, and most of these diseases are noninfectious. Intestinal volvulus, gastric and colonic impactions, and colonic incarceration occur in tapirs. Oropharyngeal abscessation is another important problem. The syndrome appears similar to oral necrobacillosis. Acute pancreatic necrosis/

like toes in front of a soft, spongy pad adapted to a soft, spongy substrate (Fig. 82–4). Severe pad and sole ulcerations can develop when animals become overactive on a hard substrate. These periods of overactivity often occur when an animal is introduced to a new enclosure or enclosure mate. Recurrent lameness can occur with chronically ulcerated foot pads. Older animals may suffer from degenerative joint disease, but in any case of lameness, foot pad disease should first be ruled out.

Miscellaneous Conditions

Corneal cloudiness is seen frequently in tapirs, especially Malayan tapirs. The cause is unknown but probably is a combination of trauma and excessive exposure to light. The condition is sometimes associated with corneal ulceration.

Female tapirs often have a milky vaginal discharge. Tapirs normally have cloudy, chalky urine, similar to that of a horse and a rhinoceros. This cloudy fluid can be confused with signs of a vaginal or uterine disease. Genitourinary infection and neoplasia has occurred in tapirs. Urinalysis and vaginal cytologic study help determine whether an inflammatory or infectious problem exists.

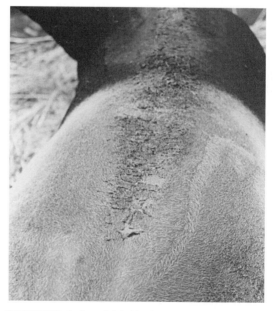

FIGURE 82–3. Superficial skin sloughs of the dorsal lumbosacral and thoracic region approximately 7 days after signs of vesicular skin disease in a Malayan tapir. (Photograph courtesy of Paul Jarand, San Diego Zoo.)

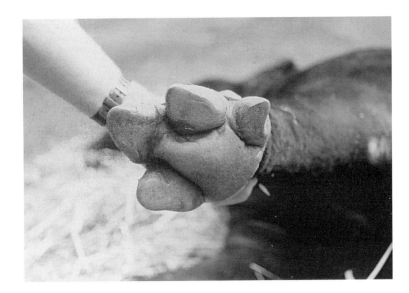

FIGURE 82–4. Sole of a normal front foot of a Malayan tapir, showing the four hoof-like toes and the soft, spongy sole. The rear foot of tapirs has three toes.

pancreatitis and eosinophilic enterocolitis have also been seen in adult tapirs.

Other significant diseases in the adult age group include *Mycobacterium bovis*–induced pneumonia, bacterial septicemia, and myocarditis caused by encephalomyocarditis virus infection.

Respiratory diseases are the most significant cause of mortality overall. The prevalence of respiratory disease is relatively uniform across the various age groups, but these diseases are uncommon in the oldest adult group. In contrast to gastrointestinal diseases, most respiratory diseases have infectious causes. Most cases are of bacterial etiology, with septicemic/embolic pneumonias predominating over bronchopneumonia. The possibility of underlying viral infection in tapir bronchopneumonia cases has not been investigated. The source of the septicemic/embolic pneumonias is not usually evident. As mentioned, pulmonary tuberculosis caused by *M. bovis* is seen sporadically in adults. Pulmonary coccidioidomycosis has also been seen but is rare. The diagnosis of respiratory disease in Malayan tapirs is often confounded by the misinterpretation of the normal pleural adhesions as evidence of pleuritis or pneumonia.

REPRODUCTION

Features of the reproductive cycle are listed in Table 82–4.

TABLE 82–4. Reproductive Features of Tapirs

Estrous cycle length	30 days[2, 9]
Estrus length	1–4 days[2]
Seasonality	None[9]
Gestation	13 months[3, 9]
Interbirth interval	14–17 months[9]
Sexual maturity	2–4 years[9]
Postpartum estrus	9–21 days[3]

Pregnancy Diagnosis

Pregnancy in tapirs may be difficult to detect through conventional means. Breedings may not be observed, and even advanced pregnancy may not be obvious. Pregnancy can be detected by means of urinary and fecal steroid analysis.[3] Transabdominal ultrasonography can been used to diagnose and monitor pregnancy in tapirs. One 11-month lowland tapir fetus had a cranial diameter measuring 6.5 cm on ultrasonography. Vulvar edema and mucoid discharge may precede parturition by 2 to 3 weeks.

Contraception

A moratorium has been placed on the breeding of *Tapirus terrestris* in North American collections. As a result, some institutions have devised methods of contraception for this species. Castration, melengestrol acetate (MGA) implants, medroxyprogesterone acetate injections (2.5 to 5.0 mg/kg), altrenogest, and porcine zona pellucida vaccine are beginning to be used in tapirs. Limited data suggest that all methods are effective except MGA implants, which are frequently rejected within 3 to 6 weeks.

REFERENCES

1. American Association of Zoo Keepers: Zoo Infant Development Notebook. Topeka, KS, American Association of Zoo Keepers, 1994.
2. Barongi RA: Husbandry and conservation of tapirs. Int Zoo Yrbk 32:7–15, 1993.
3. Brown JL, Citino SB: Endocrine profiles during the estrous cycle and pregnancy in the Baird's tapir (*Tapirus bairdi*). Zoo Biol 13:107–117, 1994.
4. Finnegan ML, Munson L, Barrett S, Calle P: Vesicular skin disease of tapirs. Proceedings of the American Association of Zoo Veterinarians, St. Louis, pp 416–417, 1993.
5. Janssen, DL, Michelet S: Bibliography for Tapiridae. San Diego, Zoological Society of San Diego, 1995.
6. Janssen DL, Rideout BA, Edwards ME: Medical management of

captive tapirs (*Tapirus* sp.). Proceedings of the American Association of Zoo Veterinarians, Puerto Vallarta, Mexico, pp 1–11, 1996.

7. Jenness R, Sloan RE: Review Article 158. Dairy Sci Abstr 32(10):599–612, 1949.
8. Kuehn G: Tapiridae. *In* Fowler ME (ed): Zoo and Wild Animal Medicine, 2nd ed. Philadelphia, WB Saunders, pp 931–934, 1986.
9. Lee AR: Management guidelines for welfare of zoo animals: Tapirs (*Tapirus* sp.). London, The Federation of Zoological Gardens of Great Britain and Ireland, 1993.
10. Miller-Edge M: Carfentanil, ketamine, xylazine combination (CKX) for immobilization of exotic ungulates: clinical experiences

in bongo *(Tragelaphus euryceros)* and mountain tapir *(Tapirus pinchaque)*. Proceedings of the Annual Meeting of the American Association of Zoo Veterinarians, Pittsburgh, pp 192–196, 1994.
11. Padilla M, Dowler RC: *Tapirus terrestris.* Mamm Sp 481:8, 1994.
12. Ramsay EC, Zainuddin Z: Infectious diseases of the rhinoceros and tapir. *In* Fowler ME (ed): Zoo and Wild Animal Medicine, 3rd ed. Philadelphia, WB Saunders, pp 459–466, 1993.
13. Satterfield W, Lester GA: Internal fixation of a chronic rectal prolapse in a Malaysian tapir. J Zoo Anim Med 5:26, 1974.
14. Wack RF, Jones AA: Suspected isoerythrolysis in two Baird's tapirs *(Tapirus bairdii).* J Zoo Wildl Med 28:285–289, 1997.

CHAPTER **83**

Rhinoceros Feeding and Nutrition

ELLEN S. DIERENFELD

Because of similarities in digestive tract morphology and digestive physiology,[1, 2] the domestic horse probably represents the most suitable nutritional model for all rhinoceros species. As such, a diet comprising good quality forage should provide primary nutrients for captive rhinoceroses, with low-energy density grain concentrate feeds used to balance identified energy, protein, mineral, or vitamins needs. General feeding guidelines as detailed in the *AZA Rhinoceros Husbandry Resource Manual*[4] appear suitable for maintenance of rhinoceroses in captivity. Until nutrient requirements are more specifically detailed for rhinoceroses, diets should be formulated according to National Research Council[12] recommendations for horses of various physiologic stages (Table 83–1).

Rhinoceros feeding behavior, however, ranges from rather unselective grazing by white rhinoceroses (*Ceratotherium simum*) to selective browsing by black rhi-

noceroses (*Diceros bicornis*), Sumatran rhinoceroses (*Dicerorhinus sumatrensis*), and greater one-horned rhinoceroses (*Rhinoceros unicornis*) on a wide diversity of plants. Whereas gastrointestinal problems contribute substantially to mortality in all captive rhinoceros species,[9] health disorders linked with possible nutrient imbalances appear limited to browsing rhinoceros species maintained on predominantly legume-based diets (either forages or concentrates, or both), at least in North America.[3, 10, 11] Thus, numerous areas of rhinoceros nutrition are currently under investigation, with implications for formulating more appropriate captive diets.

DIETARY HUSBANDRY

Rhinoceroses typically consume 1% to 3% (as-fed basis) or 1% to 2% (dry matter [DM] basis) of body mass

TABLE 83–1. Nutrient Concentrations in Total Diets for Horses and Ponies

Nutrient	Growth	Mature/ Maintenance	Pregnancy/ Lactation
Digestible energy Mcal/kg	2.45–2.90	2.0	2.25–2.60
Crude protein, %	12–15	8.0	10–13
Ca, %	0.6	0.3	0.4
P, %	0.3	0.2	0.3
Mg, %	0.1	0.1	0.1
K, %	0.3	0.3	0.4
Vitamin A, IU/kg	2000	2000	2000
Vitamin D, IU/kg	800	300	600
Vitamin E, IU/kg	80	50	80

Concentrations of Na, S, Fe, Mn, Cu, Zn, Se, I, and Co should be provided at the following levels, respectively: 0.1%, 0.15%, 50 mg/kg, 40 mg/kg, 10 mg/kg, 40 mg/kg, 0.1 mg/kg, 0.1 mg/kg, and 0.1 mg/kg.

Table to be used as a guideline in developing captive rhinoceros diets (dry matter basis, modified from reference 12).

daily. The larger, grazing rhinoceroses should be fed high-quality grass hays, whereas browsing species should be fed mixed grass: legume hays and/or a mixture of hay and less digestible browse. High-quality legume hay appears too digestible for rhinoceroses and may result in diarrhea, colic, and mineral imbalances, whereas poor quality, very fibrous hay has been implicated in torsion and impaction. Clearly, forage quality must be a prime consideration in feeding rhinoceroses. Hay and clean water should always be available; the concentrate portion of a ration should contribute no more than approximately one third of total calories, offered in at least two feedings per day for better utilization. Larger pellets (>1.0 cm diameter) can be easily manipulated and consumed by all rhinoceros species.

Particularly for the browsing rhinoceros species, the addition of fresh or frozen browse to diets may be essential to health, contributing as yet unquantified nutrients. Table 83–2 lists a number of browse species that have been successfully fed to rhinoceroses in North America. Fresh red maple (and possibly other maple species) and oak browse have been associated with hemolytic anemia in other species, as have a number of high-S containing plants including brassicas, rape, and onions. These should be avoided in rhinoceros browse.

Dietary supplements should not be necessary if rations are properly formulated. If forage is grown in an area of known mineral imbalances, hay and browse should be tested routinely for determination of mineral content to adequately address any potential problems. A possible vitamin E deficiency has been suggested but not confirmed in zoo rhinoceroses; current recommendations based on natural browse composition[6, 7] suggest that diets should contain between 150 and 200 IU of vitamin E/kg dry matter. Salt blocks should always be available.

NUTRIENTS IN FORAGES

Many of the health problems identified[10, 11] in browsing captive rhinoceroses fed legume forages may be linked to nutritional factors, as opposed to a much lower reported incidence of disease in the white or greater one-horned rhinoceroses fed primarily a grass hay–based diet. The black rhinoceros, in particular, has been shown to have unique enzyme activity that may predispose it to oxidative damage,[13] but a number of these syndromes including hemolytic anemia, ulcerative dermatitis, and encephalomalacia may also be linked with imbalances in membrane stability (fatty acids or vitamin E status) that could be nutritionally mediated. Overall, the browsing rhinoceros consumes a diet in nature that is highly lignified, poorly digested, relatively low in available protein, and marginally adequate in some minerals.

Proximate Composition

Comparison of nutrient composition in browses consumed by free-ranging black and Sumatran rhinoceroses[3] suggests that a mixture (50:50) of grass and legume forages better duplicates digestibility, hemicellulose (a potentially valuable energy source), dietary protein, and fatty acid[7, 15] profiles of native browse than either hay fed separately as a substitute forage for the browsing rhinoceros species. The soluble carbohydrate content of grass (25% of DM) compared to alfalfa (11%) hay differs considerably, which may also be important for this hindgut fermenter, although the soluble sugar content of native browses has not been quantified for comparison. Even fewer data are available to evaluate the nutritional suitability of locally available browses for feeding rhinoceros species in zoos. Palatability ranking and nutrient composition of browses consumed by rhinoceroses in zoos, with correlations to animal health and physiologic responses, have been initiated through the AZA Rhino Taxonomic Advisory Group.

Minerals

Although availability and form of minerals in dietary items significantly influence utilization by herbivores,

TABLE 83–2. North American Browse Species Eaten by Rhinoceros

Acacia farnesiana	Huisache	*Malus* species	Crabapple
Acacia roemeriana	Catclaw	*Morus alba*	White mulberry
Acer saccharum	Sugar maple	*Musa acuminata*	Banana
Alnus species	Alder	*Opuntia engelmannii*	Prickly pear
Celtis occidentalis	Hackberry	*Phaeoamerica* species	Torch ginger
Celtis pallida	Granjeno	*Phyllostachys aurea*	Golden bamboo
Condalia obovata	Brazil	*Populus alba*	White poplar
Eugenia species	Eugenia	*Prosopis juliflora*	Mesquite
Fagus granifolia	American beech	*Robinia pseudoacacia*	Black locust
Ficus benjamina	Weeping fig	*Salix babylonica*	Weeping willow
Forsythia species	Forsythia	*Salix nigra*	Black willow
Gymnocladus diocus	Kentucky coffee tree	*Viburnum* species	Fragrant honeysuckle
Hibiscus rosa	Hibiscus	*Vitis vinifera*	Grape
Liquidambar styraciflua	Sweetgum		

From Dierenfeld ES: Nutrition. *In* Fouraker M, Wagener T (eds): AZA Rhinoceros Husbandry Resource Manual. Fort Worth, Cockerell Printing Company, pp 52–53, 1996.

TABLE 83–3. Macromineral (n = 42 Species) and Trace Element (n = 39) Concentrations in Browses Eaten by Black and Sumatran (n = 44 Species) Rhinoceros Compared with Nutrient Requirements for Horses

| Component (Dry Weight Basis) | Range in Native Browses | | Equid Requirements |
	Black Rhinoceros	Sumatran Rhinoceros	
Calcium, %	0.7–6.1	0.04–6.76	0.3–0.6
Copper, mg/kg	3.0–16.1	3.4–13.3	10
Iron, mg/kg	29–215	47.9–116.0	50
Magnesium, %	0.1–0.9	0.2–1.3	0.1
Manganese, mg/kg	4.0–269	45–1940	40
Phosphorus, %	0.05–0.26	0.03–0.37	0.2–0.3
Potassium, %	0.3–2.0	0.1–6.3	0.3–0.4
Selenium, mg/kg	0.02–0.04	NA	0.1
Sodium, %	0.001–0.65	<0.01–0.45	0.1
Zinc, mg/kg	2.5–96.3	7.1–25.6	40

(Data from reference 3.)

examination of natural foodstuffs may provide some guidelines for diet development. Sodium appears limiting in native rhinoceros browses (Table 83–3), but can be obtained from natural salt licks soils or water, both of which are reportedly used by both Sumatran and black rhinoceroses. Phosphorus also appears to be limiting in natural rhinoceros browse; hypophosphatemia has been associated with hemolytic and dermatitis problems in captive black rhinoceroses,[9, 10, 13] warranting supplementation of zoo rhinoceroses with both dietary (routine) and parenteral phosphorus (in marked deficiencies). Selenium and zinc status in zoo black rhinoceroses has been suggested to be marginal based on limited blood samples,[7] and browses sampled appear to contain low levels of these nutrients in relation to equid requirements.[3] In addition, hemosiderosis, possibly linked with dietary mineral interaction, has been reported in captive but not free-ranging, black rhinoceroses.[8, 10] Iron metabolism in rhinoceroses is under investigation,[14] as is captive dietary mineral content evaluation. Mineral stressors (both deficiencies and toxicities) can impact in vivo oxidative status and should not be considered unrelated to the health syndromes noted. However, physiologic baseline data for evaluation of mineral status in the rhinoceros, or even determination of the most suitable domestic model for comparison,

have not yet been compiled, remaining a high priority research issue.

Vitamin E

The vitamin E content of native browses consumed by rhinoceroses (50 to 200 mg/kg DM)[6, 7] is considerably higher than found in most zoo-based diets without supplementation. Current recommendations for supplementation (150 to 200 IU/kg DM) derive from native forage analyses but are dependent upon the form of supplement used and should also be considered with respect to other dietary fat-soluble vitamin concentrations (see Chapter 12). Currently, no data support the hypothesis that the rhinoceros has inhibited absorption or transport mechanisms for this nutrient, but research is ongoing.

Physiologic Assessment of Status

Plasma vitamin E (measured as *d*-alpha-tocopherol) concentrations in North American zoo rhinoceroses do not differ significantly across species (Table 83–4), and mean values for the black rhinoceros have increased

TABLE 83–4. Alpha Tocopherol Concentrations in Tissues Collected from Rhinoceros Held in North American Zoological Facilities (Mean ± SD)

Tissue	Black (n)	White (n)	Greater One-Horned (n)	Sumatran (n)
Plasma (μg/ml)	0.71 ± 0.88 (224)	0.56 ± 0.49 (63)	0.69 ± 0.60 (17)	1.07 ± 0.99 (7)
Liver (μg/g wet)	19.67 ± 18.85 (21)	9.84 ± 9.11 (9)	17.75 ± 19.87 (6)	19.48 ± 1.70 (3)
Skeletal muscle (μg/g wet)	6.64 ± 5.63 (20)	4.98 ± 4.04 (8)	13.08 ± 20.39 (3)	16.57 ± 8.25 (3)
Heart (μg/g wet)	15.95 ± 14.56 (19)	11.78 ± 10.09 (8)	18.22 ± 25.57 (4)	34.71 ± 8.60 (3)
Adipose (μg/g wet)	5.41 ± 4.87 (13)	12.81 ± 12.53 (8)	5.34 ± 7.54 (4)	8.14 ± 4.13 (3)

Horse normals: plasma, 2 μg/ml; liver, 5 μg/g; muscle, 5 μg/g; adipose 25 μg/g.
Data source: Wildlife Conservation Society Nutrition Laboratory, 1997.

(from 0.2 μg/ml, n = 11) with dietary supplementation over the past several years.[3] By comparison, apparently healthy free-ranging black rhinoceroses display geographic (and presumably dietary concentration) variability, ranging from 0.23 μg/ml (Kenya, n = 7) to 0.80 μg/ml (Namibia, n = 3), but average approximately 0.6 μg/ml (n = 129 from South Africa and Zimbabwe). Plasma vitamin E concentrations in rhinoceroses are one third to one tenth lower than in other herbivores, possibly because of a lack of high-density carrier lipoproteins.[5]

Circulating concentrations of alpha tocopherol can be useful in assessing availability of vitamin E from diets; as with most biologic systems, however, coefficient of variation around a single sample should be considered plus or minus approximately 15%. In addition, storage tissue fluxes of this nutrient in response to body needs can make blood values particularly tenuous in assessing status. Tissue (liver, skeletal muscle, heart, adipose) vitamin E concentrations quantified in 39 individual rhinoceroses representing four species (see Table 83–4) provide more detail for evaluating metabolism of this nutrient both within and between species. Although widely variable, concentrations measured in liver and muscle tissues of the browsing rhinoceroses tend to be higher than those of the white rhinoceros, possibly because of higher dietary supplementation in the browsers. Normal tissue alpha tocopherol concentrations in domestic horses do not appear to provide useful comparative indicators for tissue vitamin E status in rhinoceroses, perhaps because of differences in fat storage and metabolism between the temperate-evolved horse and tropical rhinoceros. Alpha tocopherol concentrations in free-ranging rhinoceros tissues have not been measured, but may be essential to understand optimal captive animal nutrition. It is possible that antagonistic nutrients (pro-oxidant minerals, vitamins, fats) are being supplied in excess of animal requirements, leading to a necessity for elevated antioxidant vitamin supplementation in captive animals.

REFERENCES

1. Clemens ET, Maloiy GMO: The digestive physiology of three East African herbivores: the elephant, rhinoceros and hippopotamus. J Zool Lond 198:141–156, 1982.
2. Clemens ET, Maloiy GMO: Nutrient digestibility and gastrointestinal electrolyte flux in the elephant and rhinoceros. Comp Biochem Physiol 75A:653–658, 1983.
3. Dierenfeld ES: Rhinoceros nutrition: an overview with special reference to browsers. Verh ber Erkrg Zootiere 37:7–14, 1995.
4. Dierenfeld ES: Nutrition. *In* Fouraker M, Wagener T (eds): AZA Rhinoceros Husbandry Resource Manual. Fort Worth, Cockerell Printing Company, pp 52–53, 1996.
5. Dierenfeld ES, Traber MG: Vitamin E status of exotic animals compared with livestock and domestics. *In* Packer L, Fuchs J (eds): Vitamin E in Health and Disease. New York, Marcel Dekker, pp 345–370, 1992.
6. Dierenfeld ES, Du Toit R, Braselton WE: Nutrient composition of selected browses consumed by black rhinoceros (*Diceros bicornis*) in the Zambezi Valley, Zimbabwe. J Zoo Wildl Med 26:220–230, 1995.
7. Ghebremeskel K, Williams G, Brett RA, et al: Nutrient composition of plants most favoured by black rhinoceros (*Diceros bicornis*) in the wild. Comp Biochem Physiol 98A:529–534, 1991.
8. Kock N, Foggin C, Kock MD, et al: Hemosiderosis in the black rhinoceros (*Diceros bicornis*): a comparison of free-ranging and recently captured with translocated and captive animals. J Zoo Wildl Med 23:230–234, 1992.
9. Kock RA, Garnier J: Veterinary management of three species of rhinoceros in zoological collections. *In* Ryder O (ed): Rhinoceros Biology and Conservation. San Diego, pp 325–345, 1993.
10. Miller E: Health. *In* Fouraker M, Wagener T (eds): AZA Rhinoceros Husbandry Resource Manual. Fort Worth, Cockerell Printing Company, pp 41–51, 1996.
11. Miller RE: Hemolytic anemia in the black rhinoceros. *In* Fowler ME (ed): Zoo and Wild Animal Medicine, 3rd ed. Philadelphia, WB Saunders, 1993.
12. National Research Council: Nutrient Requirements of Horses, 5th ed. Washington, DC, National Academy Press, 1989.
13. Paglia DE, Miller RE, Renner SW: Is impairment of oxidant neutralization the common denominator among diverse diseases of black rhinoceroses? *In* Kirk Baer (ed): Proceedings of the Annual Meeting of the American Association of Zoo Veterinarians, Puerto Vallarta, Mexico, pp 37–41, 1996.
14. Smith JE, Chavey PS, Miller RE: Iron metabolism in black (*Diceros bicornis*) and white (*Ceratotherium simus*) rhinoceroses. J Zoo Wildl Med 26:525–531, 1995.
15. Wright JB, Brown DL, Dierenfeld ES: Omega-3 fatty acids in the nutrition of the black rhinoceros (*Diceros bicornis*) in captivity in the United States. Proceedings of the Cornell Nutrition Conference, Ithaca, NY, Cornell University, 1996.

CHAPTER 84

Infectious Diseases of Equids

LYNDSEY G. PHILLIPS, JR.

There are three groups of nondomestic equids typically maintained in zoological parks: the Przewalskii horse, the zebra, and the wild ass. Table 84–1 lists the equid species and their populations (thus representing the population at risk) held in participating zoos, according to the most current International Species Inventory System data.

RISK FACTORS

The threat of infectious disease plays a role in the populations of both captive and free-ranging nondomestic equids. The captive population is at risk through (1) contact between animals within their home institutions, (2) transfer of animals between institutions, and (3) contact with domestic equid populations in areas surrounding captive populations. The free-ranging populations are at risk from endemic disease and from contact with domestic animals. This last risk is significant in that land available to wild populations of nondomestic equids is diminishing and there is consequent encroachment of human populations and their attendant livestock on those herds. There is also the risk of transmission of disease to domestic equids from nondomestic species in captivity or the wild, or from imported wild-caught individuals.

REPORTED INFECTIOUS DISEASE

There have been few reports of infectious disease in nondomestic equids. With equids being held in many institutions internationally, reports of some causes of morbidity and mortality do not reach widespread dissemination. In addition, each incidence of illness cannot necessarily be confirmed as to exact cause. Nevertheless, it appears that infectious diseases have not had a significant impact on the health of captive populations of nondomestic equids. Table 84–2 lists the confirmed and reported cases of infectious disease in equids and lists the associated species. Most of the instances involved only one animal or fewer than five animals.

TABLE 84–1. Captive Population in International Species Inventory System, December 1995

	Males	Females
Zebra		
Equus burchelli	42	94
E. b. antiquorum	96	195
E. b. bohni	89	194
E. grevyi	136	239
E. zebra hartmannae	86	116
Asses		
E. hemionus	5	3
E. h. holdereri	29	21
E. h. kiang	2	0
E. h. kulan	40	68
E. h. onager	30	61
Horses		
E. caballus przewalskii	202	386
Total equids = 1095 males, 1084 females, + 16 unsexed		

TABLE 84–2. Published Reports of Infectious Disease in Nondomestic Equids

	Host Species
Bacterial Disease	
Yersiniosis (Nigeria)[1]	Equus burchelli
Salmonella taksory enteritis[6]	E. grevyi
Actinobacillus equui nephritis[4]	E. harmannae
Pasteurella multocida[10]	E. burchelli
Escherichia coli omphelophlebitis[6]	Zebra, Przewalskii horse
Bacillus anthracis[7]	E. burchelli, E. hartmannae
Neonatal infection[5]	E. przewalskii
Aeromonas, enterobacteria, Streptococcus	Placental
Citrobacter	Enteritis
Pseudomonas	Bronchopneumonia
Mixed bacterial infection	Omphalitis
Fungal Disease	
Coccidioides[5]	E. przewalskii
Viral Disease	
Equine herpesvirus type 1[9]	E. onager, E. burchelli
Equine herpesvirus type 1[12]	E. grevyi
Equine herpesvirus type 1[5]	E. przewalskii

NONPUBLISHED INFECTIOUS DISEASES

In the course of providing routine veterinary service within zoos, veterinarians diagnose and treat diseases that are never submitted for publication. A review of medical records from North American zoological institutions that maintain significant numbers of nondomestic equids has revealed the following confirmed disease problems. The preponderance of these cases are in neonatal or juvenile animals:

1. Salmonella polyarthritis/septicemia—*Equus grevyi* (Chicago Brookfield Zoo, M. Briggs, personal communication, 1997)
2. Tetanus (neonate)—*Equus burchelli* (National Zoological Park, Department of Pathology, D. Nichols, personal communication, 1997)
3. *Salmonella typhimurium* (juvenile, 5 months)—*E. burchelli* (National Zoological Park, Department of Pathology, D. Nichols, personal communication, 1997)
4. Beta-hemolytic streptococcus (neonate)—*E. burchelli* (National Zoological Park, Department of Pathology, D. Nichols, personal communication, 1997)

SEROLOGIC EVIDENCE OF VIRAL DISEASE

Some studies have indicated the incidence of viral disease in free-ranging equids. Positive serologic evidence was found in samples collected from zebras in free-ranging situations in South Africa, indicating exposure to or disease from the following viral agents: (1) equine encephalosis virus, (2) equine herpesvirus 1 and 4, and (3) African horsesickness (AHS). Positive serologic titers to these three agents as well as equine arteritis virus and equine influenza A (H3N8) are present in domestic horses in South Africa, but no serologic evidence of the latter two agents has been reported in zebras in South Africa.[2] No free-ranging zebra has been found to exhibit clinical disease associated with the five viral agents described. However, removal of carcasses by predators or deterioration of the carcasses in the wild make pathologic diagnosis of infection by a specific etiologic agent difficult. Table 84–2 lists the confirmed viral diseases reported in captive nondomestic equids. Infections can be inapparent or latent as evidenced by the report of an epizootic of AHS in domestic horses, mules, and donkeys in Spain that was believed to have originated from zebras imported into Spain from Namibia just before the outbreak in the domestic species.[8]

FACTORS AFFECTING SUSCEPTIBILITY TO INFECTION

A number of factors affect the susceptibility of nondomestic equids to infectious disease. Newly imported animals (from free-ranging or separate captive populations) represent two aspects of transmission of disease:

1. Naive individuals: Equids that have never been exposed to certain viruses or serotypes of bacteria that are different or nonexistent in their country or institution of origin are particularly susceptible to infection.
2. Sources of disease: Individuals or species may be possible carriers of viruses or serotypes of bacteria that are endemic to their herd of locale of origin. These organisms are not present within the captive population into which these individuals have recently been transported. This situation represents an internal risk for transmission of disease.

Pathogens from domestic livestock may infect nondomestic equids. This is possible in free-ranging animals where human land use impinges on the margins of wildlife reserves. In captive animals, pathogen exposure is from domestic livestock adjacent to zoos or in large acreage facilities such as drive-through parks. Additionally, zoos typically have domestic livestock in children's zoos or petting zoos within the boundaries of the zoological park. Without strict separation of enclosures and biosecurity practices by personnel crossing from domestic to exotic equid facilities, there is the chance of contamination from domestic species to nondomestic species. Those diseases relying on insect vectors for transmission (e.g., AHS, Potomac Valley fever) can easily cross from domestic to exotic species if the two are held in close proximity; veterinarians must be aware of the disease agents within the domestic horse population in their locale. Frequently, surveillance of the domestic horses and asses on the zoo grounds may prevent a reservoir of disease from becoming established that could allow insect vectors to become infected and transmit these diseases to the exotic equids within the zoo.

PREVENTIVE HEALTH PROGRAM

The solution for protection from infectious disease involves the establishment of a strict, well-designed preventive health program. This program exists to reduce the introduction or transmission of infectious microorganisms within and between institutions maintaining collections of nondomestic equids. It incorporates several protocols.

1. Provide quarantine—The physical facilities must be designed to handle large ungulates, be separate and distinct from the exhibit and holding quarters of the zoo's resident animals, and be staffed by personnel not contacting resident animals. All incoming animals are quarantined, regardless of origin. For the policy to be most effective, the shipping institution should conduct a thorough preshipment physical examination including appropriate serologic testing to satisfy international and state regulations and to provide assurance that an incoming animal has little likelihood of being infected with a transmissible agent. If an institution has geographically separate facilities, transfer of individual animals between those sites should be considered the same as receiving animals from outside institutions, and the quarantine period should be implemented. Strict adherence to quarantine of all incoming equid species, domestic or exotic, is necessary to prevent bringing an individual onto the zoo grounds that is infected and

may serve as a reservoir host for transmission to the resident population. Furthermore, research shows that the viremic period for some microorganisms may differ between nondomestic and domestic equids.[3]

2. Maintain a program of scheduled, periodic physical examinations on the resident herds to prevent agents from entering the herd undetected. These examinations are particularly important when different species of equids are shifted within the zoo and new contacts between herds are established, when males are transferred into female herds for breeding (particularly when the males have been kept some distance from the females and thus possibly have been exposed to a different environment and different insect populations), and when the composition of herds are changed.

3. Design a conscientious program of immunoprophylaxis that is specific for the species susceptibility and regional disease prevalence. The risk in the area should be prudently assessed and vaccines used cautiously. A thorough review of equine immunizing agents and biologics is available in current domestic animal veterinary textbooks.[11]

4. Perform serologic testing in conjunction with the physical examination program as surveillance for unknown entry of an infectious agent, discovery of a latent or chronic carrier individual, or conversion of a newly added individual. Maintain a serum bank to provide resources for convalescent studies and for epidemiologic or retrospective studies in case an infectious disease problem emerges.

5. Incorporate a program of sanitation within animal enclosures and food storage areas to prevent common or ubiquitous contaminants from accumulating and becoming health threats to equid neonates or to equids with open wounds or immune systems that are compromised because of stress, other disease, heavy parasite burdens, or poor nutrition.

6. Develop a program that is safe, feasible, and practical to control the arthropod, bird, and rodent pest populations within and surrounding the zoo, recognizing that these can be reservoirs for infectious agents.

7. Maintain current knowledge of the morbidity within the domestic horses in the regional area to provide awareness of potential diseases that could affect nondomestic equids in captive settings.

8. Remain current with the equine literature to be aware of newly recognized diseases (e.g., ehrlichiosis), of development of new diagnostic tests for previously poorly diagnosed disease conditions, or of the introduction or emergence of a disease not historically present in the region.

DOMESTIC EQUID DISEASES

Table 84–3 lists, in order of relative incidence and potential impact on health of domestic horses, potential threats from the domestic equid population.

SUMMARY

Maintenance of a low incidence of infectious disease in captive equid herds requires nonintroduction of disease

TABLE 84–3. Infectious Diseases in Domestic Equids in Order of Significance to Health of Horses*

1. Strangles (*Streptococcus equi*)
2. Influenza A 1 and 2
3. Equine herpesvirus (EHV 1 and EHV 4)
4. Rotavirus
5. *Rhodococcus equi* pneumonia
6. *Corynebacterium pseudotuberculosis* (in California only)
7. Equine protozoal myeloencephalitis (sarcocystocis)
8. Equine viral arteritis (EVA)
9. Equine infectious anemia (EIA)
10. Potomac horse fever (*Ehrlichia risticii*)
11. Salmonellosis
12. Clostridial enterocolitis (*Clostridium* species)
13. Rabies
14. Viral encephalitis (WEE, EEE)
15. Tetanus (*Clostridium tetanii*)
16. Botulism (*Clostridium botulinum*)

*Wilson D: UC Davis School of Veterinary Medicine, Department of Medicine & Epidemiology, personal communication, 1997.

through effective quarantine, vigilance through preventive health programs, cooperation between animal managers and veterinarians in decisions for animal movement and health programs, thorough prophylactic testing, rapid and accurate diagnostic testing in disease occurrences, development of reliable, specific, and sensitive diagnostic tests for nondomestic equid species, and awareness of emerging diseases and outbreaks of disease in the domestic equine population.

REFERENCES

1. Adeniyi KO, Enurah LU: Yersiniosis (*Yersinia pestis*) in a captive zebra (*Equus burchelli*). Himalayan Journal of Environment and Zoology 8(1):71–72, 1994.
2. Barnard BJH, Paweska JT: Prevalence of antibodies against some equine viruses in zebra (*Zebra burchelli*) in the Kruger National Park, 1991–1992. Onderstepoort Journal of Veterinary Research 60:175–179, 1993.
3. Barnard BJH, Bengis R, Keet D, et al: Epidemiology of African horsesickness: duration of viraemia in zebra (*Equus burchelli*). Onderstepoort Journal of Veterinary Research 61:391–393, 1994.
4. Bath GF: Nephritis associated with *Actinobacillus equuli* in the Cape mountain zebra. Koedoe 22:215–216, 1979.
5. Boyd L, Houpt KA: Przewalski's Horse: The History and Biology of an Endangered Species, 1st ed. Albany, NY, State University of New York Press, 1994.
6. Griner LA: Pathology of Zoo Animals, 1st ed. San Diego, Zoological Society of San Diego, 1983.
7. Lindeque PM, Turnbull PCB: Ecology and epidemiology of anthrax in the Etosha National Park, Namibia. Onderstepoort Journal of Veterinary Research 61:71–83, 1994.
8. Lubroth J: African horsesickness and the epizootic in Spain, 1987. Equine Practice 10(2):26–33, 1988.
9. Montali RJ, Allen GP, Bryans JT, et al: Equine herpesvirus type 1 abortion in an onager and suspected herpesvirus myelitis in a zebra. J Am Vet Med Assoc 187(11):1248–1249, 1985.
10. Okoh AEJ: An outbreak of pasteurellosis in Kano Zoo. J Wildl Dis 16(1):3–5, 1980.
11. Smith BP: Large Animal Internal Medicine, 2nd ed. St. Louis, Mosby–Year Book 1626–1642, 1996.
12. Wolff PL, Meehan TP, Basgall EJ, et al: Abortion and perinatal foal mortality associated with equine herpesvirus type 1 in a herd of Grevy's zebra. J Am Vet Med Assoc 189(9):1185–1186, 1986.

ARTIODACTYLIDS

CHAPTER 85

Use of Tranquilizers in Wild Herbivores

HYM EBEDES

J. P. RAATH

The use of wild animals has promoted game farming and game ranching as forms of sustainable utilization.[35] Game ranching in southern Africa has been stimulated by the availability of suitable natural habitats and the diversity of endemic wild animal species, together with the initiatives taken by conservationists, business personnel, and farmers.[17] Wild herbivores, including rhinoceroses and elephants, are sold at auctions or through private sales among game ranchers, dealers, and game capturers. Some animals are supplied by national and provincial conservation authorities. A high percentage of deaths that occur during this process are attributable to untreatable injuries in newly captured animals that are stressed and panic-stricken.[1, 9, 11, 22, 61, 63–65] In order to supply the game ranching industry with the thousands of animals that are required annually, special capture and tranquilization techniques have been developed to minimize stress, injuries, and mortalities.[11, 12, 14, 20, 39, 62]

The reasons for translocating wild animals vary from idealistic conservation objectives (to preserve the survival of threatened species or to re-establish certain species in habitats that they formerly occupied) to economic, recreational, and educational considerations. These include the stocking of new conservation areas, game reserves, game ranches, and zoos. In addition to the compassionate and financial reasons to prevent

mortalities and injuries in translocated wild animals, the use of tranquilizers has also been found beneficial for stress reduction in the acclimatization of wild animals to new natural environments as well as to unnatural surroundings, such as at game auctions, in quarantine for veterinary and disease surveillance, or for scientific projects.[14, 16, 18, 19, 22] The judicious use of tranquilizers in these situations has been found to reduce stress, injuries, and mortalities.[4, 32, 33, 50] Tranquilizers also facilitate the hospitalization and treatment of sick and injured animals. Translocating wild animals involves the capture by mechanical or chemical methods, transportation in a confined area, holding in temporary captivity, and the relocation and adaptation of these animals to new habitats and strange localities.[5, 8, 19, 26, 27, 29, 41, 48, 49] Practical guidelines to minimize stress during translocation procedures include a compassionate and competent approach by well-trained capture teams.[19, 21] A video, "Why Should Even One Animal Die?" is available from the Audio Visual Section, Department of Agricultural Information, Private Bag X 144, Pretoria 0001, South Africa.

Ideally, every translocation procedure should be performed as efficiently and humanely as possible and with minimal discomfort to the animals.[14, 19] Methods for reducing stress and mortalities have been previously reported.[9, 11, 20, 28, 30, 43] The successful translocation of wildlife depends on using the appropriate equipment, working with trained personnel, following basic principles, and using tranquilizers appropriately. These four points are interrelated and complementary. Specifications and basic principles for successful translocation have been documented in A. A. McKenzie's *Capture and Care Manual*[39] and others.[5–8, 15, 21, 22, 31, 40, 44–47, 51, 54–60]

"Ten commandments" have been proposed to prevent stress in mass-captured wild animals.[19] These proposals are applicable under diverse situations.

TEN COMMANDMENTS FOR PREVENTING STRESS DURING THE TRANSLOCATION OF WILD ANIMALS

1. Do not capture when it is hot, such as during the heat of the day and during the summer months.
2. Do not chase any animals too far or too fast.
3. Do not shout, scream, or swear at the animals or at personnel of the capture team.
4. Do not manhandle the animals, and always blindfold and tranquilize animals captured in nets.
5. Do not mix different breeding groups, and never mix zebra families.
6. Load and transport animals as soon as possible after the capture, and if possible, do not off-load at night.
7. Transport animals in maximum comfort, and give special attention to nonslip flooring, good ventilation, and avoidance of drafts.
8. Separate or tranquilize aggressive animals, to prevent injuries caused by fighting, hostility, and territorial behavior.
9. Alleviate stress, fear, and panic by using appropriate tranquilizers such as haloperidol, azaperone, and diazepam for short journeys and long-acting tranquilizers such as perphenazine enanthate (Trilafon LA) and zuclopenthixol acetate (Clopixol-Acuphase) for long journeys and temporary captivity.
10. Use tranquilizers correctly, to prevent overdosage and extrapyramidal symptoms.

Notwithstanding the foregoing, animals still die of stress-related causes and capture myopathy. Some capture teams seem to disregard even the most basic rules. Tranquilizers are sometimes used incorrectly and sometimes not used at all, even when their use is known to be beneficial and life-saving. The capture of heavily pregnant females and animals that have recently given birth and that are still nursing their young, must be avoided at all costs.

This paper is a subjective overview on the use of tranquilizers for the efficient translocation of wildlife.

CAPTURE

The capture methods that are used in southern Africa attempt to minimize stress and capture myopathy in animals that vary in size from a mini-antelope, such as the suni and the dik-dik, to the African elephant. Capture methods also depend on the species and the terrain on which the animals have to be captured. The following methods are used:

1. Mass capture in plastic capture corrals or bomas with the help of a helicopter.[21, 28, 31, 33, 39, 44, 45, 48] During mass capture, animals are subjected to herding, forced exercise by running from a helicopter, physical handling by humans, crowding, and confinement crates.
2. Net capture with either fixed or drop nets.[21, 39, 48]
3. Chemical immobilization, popularly known as *darting*.[5, 8, 21, 26, 27, 31, 34, 39, 49, 53, 62]
4. "Pop-up" corrals[21, 50] and "drop bomas."
5. Net guns fired from a helicopter.[42]
6. The use of spotlights to blind animals on dark, moonless nights.[2, 21]
7. Passive capture methods in which animals are trapped in an enclosed area around a watering point or artificial feeding.[21]

TRANSPORTATION

Most antelope are captured through mass capture techniques and are transported in mass crates. Transportation is stressful for all animals. Inadequate transport has resulted in a high rate of mortality, especially among sensitive species such as nyala, impala, tsessebe, and springbok.

During transportation, animals are subjected to unfamiliar surroundings, may be overcrowded, and are exposed to extremes in ambient temperature. Subnormal cold temperatures can be compounded by the chill factor. At a road speed of 80 km/hour (50 miles/hour), the chill factors, based on the ambient air temperatures, are as follows: at 10°C, the chill factor is -8°C; at 5°C, the chill factor is -15°C; and at 0°C, the chill factor is -23°C.[22, 46]

During loading and transportation, family groups become separated and excited. Some animals may suffer from injuries sustained during capture. On long journeys, animals become hungry and thirsty, and this causes increased stress. Additional stressors include proximity to humans, transportation of aggressive adult males together, crates with slippery floors, and sudden braking or excessively rough rides. Some of these problems can be addressed specifically with tranquilizers. Their use can contribute overall to the reduction of stress, injuries, and mortalities. For this reason, they should be administered as soon as possible after capture.

The basic requirements for road transportation are as follows: transport crates must be sturdily constructed, well ventilated and draft free, darkened, and equipped with dry bedding and a nonslip floor; and the transport vehicle must be roadworthy, be driven by a competent driver, and conform to the specifications recommended by the regional nature conservation authority or game association.

To reduce conflicts between animals, families or social groups should be captured and transported together, when possible. This is especially true for zebras.

In family groups it is usually necessary to tranquilize only adult animals, because their lack of activity will calm their young. However, young animals sometimes require a low dose if they become overexcited or temporarily separated from their mothers.

Adult and subadult males that show aggression toward each other should be tranquilized and transported in individual crates. If they must be kept in a group, all should be tranquilized at the same time. Untranquilized animals may become hostile and aggressive and injure the tranquilized animals.

When two captive adult males are fighting and cannot be physically separated, they should be anesthetized by darting rather than tranquilized. Tranquilizers can take too long to become effective, and the animal that becomes sedated earlier can be injured by the untranquilized animal.

TEMPORARY CAPTIVITY

Recently captured wild animals are often intractable and overanxious. Overanxiousness is seen in impala, springbok, gemsbok, and lechwe, whereas eland, kudu, and waterbuck, well known for their jumping ability, often injure themselves attempting to escape. Hartebeest, tsessebe, blesbok, black wildebeest, impala, and gemsbok display territorial and dominant tendencies and become aggressive toward conspecifics in a way that can lead to fatal injuries. When placed under restricted conditions, some captured wild animals may become aggressive and often fight and wound each other fatally.

Nonadaptation to enclosures is responsible for a significant percentage of translocation mortalities. Individual animals may not settle down in captivity and exhaust themselves by pacing or running along the sides of the enclosures and jumping into and up against the enclosure walls in numerous escape attempts. Many captured free-ranging wild animals that are confined to enclosures refuse to eat and drink, resulting in loss of condition and dehydration.[9, 61] Animals may not eat because the feed is unfamiliar or they are reluctant to drink water from unfamiliar containers.[25]

Enclosures must be spacious and constructed from durable materials with high walls that prevent injuries when animals attempt to escape. The pens must be well drained and easy to clean and must have sufficient roofing to provide shelter from the sun and inclement weather.[15, 18]

RELEASE INTO NEW HABITATS

When animals are released in new environments, they may run into fences, become lost in the bush, escape through perimeter fences and become disoriented, and be isolated from each other. Young animals may become separated from their mothers and subsequently die. Panic-stricken animals may never settle down in a specific territory. The use of tranquilizers eliminates much of this behavior.

TRANQUILIZERS

Tranquilizers that alleviate the anxieties and stresses and have a prolonged duration and safe sedative proper-

ties are recommended for reducing translocation stresses and its complications. The use of tranquilizers in wildlife translocation was originally developed in southern Africa.[4, 6, 10–14, 17, 19–21, 23, 32–34, 41, 44, 45, 50, 62]

Long-acting tranquilizers have been used since 1984 at the National Zoological Gardens, Pretoria, South Africa, where 38 captive herbivore species were treated before transportation.[20] These drugs were clearly effective and have subsequently been used successfully for translocating wildlife in other parts of Africa, Saudi Arabia, Israel, and Greenland.

The long-acting tranquilizers have also been valuable when rare and endangered wild antelope, elephants, and rhinoceroses have been transported over long distances.[14, 15, 40, 51, 52, 55]

Effect of Tranquilizers on Animals

After injection of tranquilizers, the following effects are usually observed in wild animals:

- A general calming effect (Fig. 85–1).
- Loss of interest in new and unnatural surroundings.
- Loss of fear of humans.
- Reduction of aggressive and dominant behavior.

Depending on the type of tranquilizer used, the sedative effects after a single injection can be maintained from a few hours to several days.

Short-Acting and Rapidly Acting Tranquilizers. These tranquilizers have an immediate effect and may be effective from a few to 18 hours after injection. Short-acting tranquilizers such as azaperone, diazepam, and haloperidol are in aqueous (water) solutions and are rapidly absorbed in the blood stream. They include zuclopenthixol acetate (Clopixol-Acuphase) and perphenazine enanthate (Trilafon LA).

Long-Acting Tranquilizers. These tranquilizers are effective for 3 to 7 days and longer after injection and include zuclopenthixol acetate (Lopixol) and perphenazine enanthate (Trilafon LA). Long-acting tranquilizers consist of fatty acid esters of the basic tranquilizer compounds dissolved in vegetable or medicinal oils such as sesame oil or viscoleo.[37] The prolonged sedative activity results from their slow release as the ester diffuses into tissue fluid and is absorbed and hydrolyzed in the blood with the release of the active drug. Their injection site is intramuscular (IM), never intravenous (IV).

RECOMMENDED TRANQUILIZERS

Azaperone

Azaperone has been used successfully in all the antelope species, zebras, black and white rhinoceroses, and African elephants. The sedative effect is usually seen within 10 minutes after intramuscular injection, and the duration of effect is up to 6 hours. It is a useful tranquilizer for sedating animals for short journeys.[10]

When high doses are used, animals may become heavily sedated. An advantage of azaperone over other

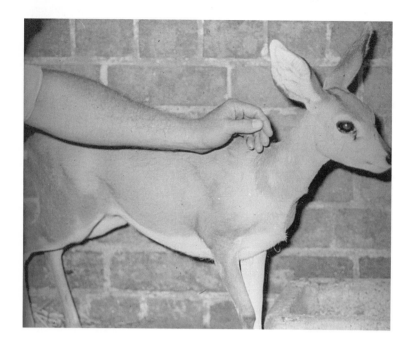

FIGURE 85–1. Wild steenbuck with fractured humerus.

tranquilizers is that it does not affect thermoregulation or the cardiovascular system.

Haloperidol

Haloperidol is a useful tranquilizer for the transportation and adaptation of wild animals to new surroundings.[2, 4, 11, 13, 17, 20, 21, 32, 33, 46] It is effective in all antelope species, African elephants, black and white rhinoceroses, and zebras. Its formulation allows IV use.

Sedation is noted within 3 to 4 minutes after IV injection and 10 to 15 minutes after IM injection. In most animals the sedative effect wears off after 16 hours. Low doses are preferable and recommended in all species.

A disadvantage of using haloperidol is that some animals may show extrapyramidal symptoms and anorexia. Restlessness has been seen in zebra, gemsbok, and impala, which may be related either to the inadvertent use of high dosages or to hypersensitivity in individual animals. Severe extrapyramidal effects have been reported in a horse.[38]

Male kudu tranquilized with haloperidol may lose their natural fear of humans and become aggressive.

Haloperidol must be also used with caution in very young and old animals because the effect may be variable and unpredictable.

Zuclopenthixol Acetate

The noticeable sedative effect starts 30 to 60 minutes after injection and may last for up to 72 hours.

Perphenazine Enanthate

The duration of the long-acting tranquilizers, such as perphenazine enanthate, appears to be dose dependent;

higher doses yield a longer period of tranquilization. Their effectiveness and duration vary from species to species and also among individual animals of the same species.

The sedative effect is usually noted from 10 to 16 hours after injection and lasts for 7 to 10 days.[12, 14, 17, 20, 22]

GUIDELINES FOR USING TRANQUILIZERS

Tranquilizers must always be used with discretion and only after consultation with an experienced wildlife veterinarian. In South Africa, tranquilizers for animal use can be obtained only from a veterinarian or purchased only with a veterinary prescription.

Overdosing must be avoided because deep sedation may interfere with feeding and drinking. Extrapyramidal side effects may result in the animal's exhausting itself and causing a disturbance to other animals in the group.

Tranquilizers should be injected immediately after capture to prevent the animals from overexerting, stressing, and injuring themselves.

Long-acting tranquilizers should be injected at the same time as the short-term, rapid-acting tranquilizers such as haloperidol or azaperone because there is a lag phase before the onset of the effects of the long-acting tranquilizer. Long-acting tranquilizers can be mixed with short-acting tranquilizers in the same syringe, despite the fact that the oil and aqueous solutions will remain separated. The short-acting tranquilizer will bridge the time until the long-acting product takes effect.

Animals that have been tranquilized should be clearly marked to avoid double dosage. Animals captured with mass-capture methods can be tranquilized with a pole syringe and strong 18- or 15-gauge needles. Animals captured in nets can be injected IM or IV with the short-acting tranquilizers if the injection can be done without delays in finding suitable veins. The jugular vein in the neck, the radial vein in the front leg, the recurrent tarsal vein in the back leg, and in some animals the ear veins are suitable for injection. When haloperidol is injected IV, the beginning of the sedative response is noted within 3 to 4 minutes after injection.

Animals that are captured in nets should preferably be blindfolded and held quietly by the handlers for about 10 minutes after the tranquilizer has been injected. This allows tranquilizers such as haloperidol sufficient time to be absorbed and reach therapeutic blood levels. Disturbance should be minimized even after the tranquilizer has become effective.

Animals injected with tranquilizers should be observed for 30 to 40 minutes so that the effect can be evaluated. By this time most of the animals should be showing signs of tranquilization.

The horns of dangerous animals must always be covered with suitable piping material before transportation, and the pipes must be removed before the animals are released at the final destination.

It is recommended that animals placed in pens for sale at live auction should be tranquilized.[16, 18]

POTENTIAL SIDE EFFECTS OF TRANQUILIZERS

Extrapyramidal Effects

Adverse reactions to tranquilization may include extrapyramidal effects such as catatonia, compulsive feeding or loss of appetite, bent neck, shivering, tremors, head swaying, pawing, and horning the ground.

Catatonia

Catatonia is a state of muscular rigidity and mental stupor. In some cases it may be caused by overdosage of a tranquilizer. In others, the animals appear to be especially sensitive to tranquilizers such as haloperidol. Animals in a catatonic state do not move and are unable to eat or drink. The condition may be fatal. In severe cases, affected animals can be treated with supportive therapy, including force-feeding foods and electrolytes by stomach tube, administration of IV fluids, and/or the injection of antiparkinsonian drugs. These drugs can include single or repeated injections of 10 to 20 mg of biperiden (Akineton) or similar antiparkinsonian drugs that are used in human medicine. Diazepam (Valium), 1 to 2 ml, has also been found to be useful for controlling symptoms.[32]

SPECIES GUIDELINES FOR TRANQUILIZERS

Table 85–1 shows doses of haloperidol and perphenazine enanthate singly or in combination for translocating wild herbivores in Southern Africa.

TABLE 85–1. Doses of Haloperidol and Perphenazine Enanthate for Some Southern African Wild Herbivores

Species	Haloperidol (mg)	Perphenazine (mg)
Black wildebeest	5–20	50–100
Blue wildebeest	10–20	50–100
Blesbok and bontebok	5–15	50–100
Cape buffalo	20–40	100–350
Cape eland	20–40	100–200
Kudu	10–20	100–200
Nyala	10–20	100–150
Impala	5–20	50–100
Red hartebeest, Lichtenstein's hartebeest, and tsessebe	5–20	50–100
Gemsbok	10–20	50–100
Roan antelope	10–20	50–200
Sable antelope	15–20	100
Springbok	5–20	25–100
Common reedbuck	5–10	50–80
Grey rhebok and mountain reedbuck	5–15	30–50
Klipspringer	5	20–30
Grey duiker, steenbok, and oribi	5–15	20–30
Suni antelope and dik-dik	5	20–30
Waterbuck	10–20	100–200
Red lechwe	10–20	50–100
Giraffe	10–30	100–250
Black rhinoceros	—*	50–200
White rhinoceros	—†	50–200
Zebra	20–30	50–100
African elephant	10–60	50–300

*Azaperone, 50 to 200 mg. †Azaperone, 100 to 400 mg.

Black Wildebeest

In the past, black wildebeest presented difficulties in transporting and maintenance. After capture, they become agitated, aggressive, and especially susceptible to capture myopathy and hyperthermia. Transport in mass crates also leads to overexcitement, hyperventilation, and hyperthermia.

Successful tranquilization has been achieved with 40 mg of azaperone in adults after mass capture in plastic bomas. Haloperidol at 20 mg per adult, 10 mg per subadult, and 5 mg per calf combined with 50 to 100 mg of perphenazine enanthate resulted in significant reduction of mortalities even with long-distance translocation.

Blue Wildebeest

Dose rates of 60 mg of azaperone for adults and 20 to 30 mg for subadults with 100 and 50 mg of perphenazine enanthate, respectively, have resulted in successful transportation and confinement of newly captured animals.

Similar good results were seen with combinations of

10 to 20 mg of haloperidol and 50 to 100 mg of perphenazine enanthate. However, two cases of extrapyramidal symptoms were seen in old cows. Uncontrollable swaying of their heads was alleviated by injection of 20 mg IM of biperiden.

Blesbok and Bontebok

Standard dose rates of haloperidol for the tranquilization of these species were 15, 12, 10, and 5 mg for adult males, adult females, juveniles, and calves, respectively. Occasionally, adult males may require low supplemental doses during long journeys.

Haloperidol and perphenazine enanthate are described in Table 85–1. Extrapyramidal symptoms and lateral recumbency have been seen when doses of 20 mg of haloperidol in adults and 15 mg of haloperidol in subadults were injected.

Cape Buffalo

Azaperone at a dose rate of 0.1 mg/kg is the recommended short-acting tranquilizer for buffalo.[52]

This can be combined with zuclopenthixol acetate at 1 mg/kg for an effective tranquilization of up to 3 days. Longer tranquilization can be achieved with perphenazine enanthate with doses of up to 300 mg per adult.

A combination of 20 to 40 mg of haloperidol and 50 to 350 mg of perphenazine enanthate was found effective for this purpose, as recommended for adult buffalo sold at auction or placed in quarantine.

Cape Eland

A combination of 80 to 100 mg of azaperone and 100 to 200 mg of perphenazine enanthate is recommended for subadult and adult elands, both for temporary confinement and for translocation (Fig. 85–2). Similar results can be obtained with 20 to 40 mg of haloperidol.

Good tranquilization with 200 mg of zuclopenthixol acetate was achieved in heavily pregnant cows.

Orphaned calves that required hand raising were injected with 50 mg of perphenazine enanthate. Repeated at 7-day intervals, this facilitated taming and bottle feeding.

Kudu

Adult kudu often do not adapt well to captive conditions. They need to be fed freshly cut branches with leaves. Injections of 10 to 20 mg of haloperidol plus 100 mg of perphenazine enanthate per adult cow and 20 mg of haloperidol plus 200 mg of perphenazine enanthate per adult bull have successfully sedated adult kudu for transportation and auctions.

Old bulls should not be confined for long times because they injure themselves in escape attempts and do not respond well to repeated doses of tranquilizer.

Tranquilized bulls may also lose the fear of humans and suddenly attack without warning. Bulls should be kept in single accommodations because they may become aggressive and fight with each other.

Nyala

Nyala are particularly shy and unpredictable animals, and the rate of mortality during translocation procedures was high before tranquilizers were used.

Because of the dense riverine terrain they usually inhabit, nyala are usually captured with nets or by hand after first being blinded with strong spotlights on dark nights.

It has become routine procedure during capture of adult nyala to inject them with 10 to 20 mg of haloperidol and 100 to 150 mg of perphenazine enanthate at the time of capture. Bulls should be tranquilized and transported separately.[46]

Nyala are usually placed in temporary captivity for 3 to 4 days after capture and then transported to destination while they are under the sedative effect of the perphenazine enanthate.

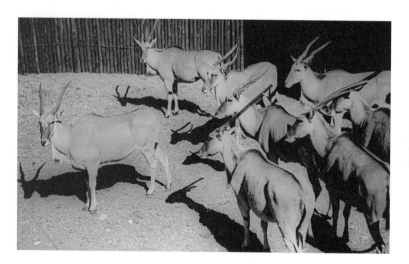

FIGURE 85–2. Wild caught Cape eland 5 days after capture and tranquilized with haloperidol and perphenazine enanthate.

Impala

Impala are usually captured in plastic corrals or nets or by some capture teams that blind them with strong spotlights on dark nights.[4]

Recently captured wild impala are excitable animals, and mortalities often occur after they have been captured and confined.[23, 32] Adults are very susceptible to stress. Adult males are aggressive under conditions of confinement and mass capture. While they are being herded by helicopter into capture corrals, they frequently attack and wound other impala. To reduce injuries and mortalities, the rams must be separated from the other animals and tranquilized immediately after capture.

Adult male impala can be translocated in mass crates after tranquilization with 15 to 20 mg of haloperidol and piping the horns with plastic or rubber pipes. Subadult males can be transported with females after tranquilization with 8 to 15 mg of haloperidol and 50 to 100 mg of perphenazine enanthate.

Extrapyramidal symptoms have been seen in adult males injected with 15 mg of haloperidol and 70 mg of perphenazine enanthate, and similar reactions were seen in some subadult males injected with 8 mg of haloperidol.

Extrapyramidal symptoms such as allotrophagia, hypertonia, torticollis, and excitement were reported in net-captured Namibian black-faced impala injected with haloperidol, 0.16 mg/kg.[32] It was speculated that these impala were sensitive to haloperidol and that the side effects were precipitated and enhanced by exertion, hyperthermia, and the rattling noise of the transportation crate.

Extrapyramidal symptoms were suppressed for short periods with injections of 5 mg of biperiden (Akineton) and 5 to 10 mg of xylazine (Rompun).[15]

Red Hartebeest, Lichtenstein's Hartebeest, and Tsessebe

Wild-caught members of these species have a poor survival rate under captive conditions.[3, 14, 22] They are prone to development of capture myopathy, and mortality rates of up to 80% have been recorded in animals translocated without tranquilization.

Under captive conditions, red hartebeest fight each other and injure themselves while attempting to escape. They also suffer from anorexia, rapidly losing condition and dying.

It is recommended that red hartebeests be tranquilized with 5 to 20 mg of haloperidol and 50 to 100 mg of perphenazine enanthate, depending on age of the animals. Zuclopenthixol acetate, 100 mg, can be used instead of perphenazine enanthate.

Standard doses of 15 to 20 mg of haloperidol for adult bulls and cows, 10 mg of haloperidol for subadults and young bulls, and 5 to 8 mg for calves have been administered immediately after capture in nets or in the plastic corrals. The same doses of tranquilizers are recommended for Lichtenstein's hartebeest and tsessebe.

High haloperidol doses (up to 40 mg in adult males) can result in extrapyramidal symptoms. These symptoms can be treated with repeated injections of 10 to 20 mg of biperiden (Akineton), injected IM, until symptoms subside.

Gemsbok

Because of their long, sharp horns and assertive behavior when cornered, gemsbok are difficult to handle and transport. As with other aggressive horned species, the horns should be covered with plastic or rubber pipes to prevent injuries. The pipes must be removed at final destination. Pipes must not be placed on the horns of young and juvenile gemsbok.

High doses of haloperidol in gemsbok cause excitement. It is recommended that the dosage of haloperidol never exceed 20 mg for adult gemsbok. Subadults can be injected with 5 to 10 mg of haloperidol or 50 to 100 mg of perphenazine. Juveniles that are together with their mothers need not be tranquilized.

Roan Antelope

Recently captured roan antelope are especially nervous and have been known to kill each other shortly after capture. Therefore, they are usually not captured with mass capture methods; instead, they are darted and transported under anesthesia.[31]

Young roan can be transported together after a period of acclimation. If they are not anesthetized, 10 to 20 mg of haloperidol or 40 mg of azaperone, combined with 150 mg of zuclopenthixol acetate or 50 to 200 mg of perphenazine enanthate, is used for the translocation and confinement of newly captured adult roan antelope.

Sable Antelope

Tranquilization protocols for sable antelope are similar to those of roan antelope, but 15 to 20 mg of haloperidol has been used successfully for shorter term tranquilization and in combination with 100 to 300 mg of zuclopenthixol acetate when longer tranquilization is required. Perphenazine enanthate, 100 mg per adult, is an excellent long-acting tranquilizer for game auctions, for confining animals for veterinary quarantine, and for long journeys.

Springbok

Springbok are difficult animals to translocate without mortalities. When captured in nets without the use of tranquilizers, the mortality rate can range from 20% to 60%. When net capture was followed by long-distance translocation, IV injection of 15 to 20 mg of haloperidol immediately after capture reduced mortality rates from 60% to 3%; a combination of 10 to 20 mg of haloperidol intravenously and 100 mg of perphenazine enanthate IM resulted in no mortalities.

In similar operations, but with confinement of 2 to 3 days before transportation (Fig. 85–3), 5 to 15 mg of

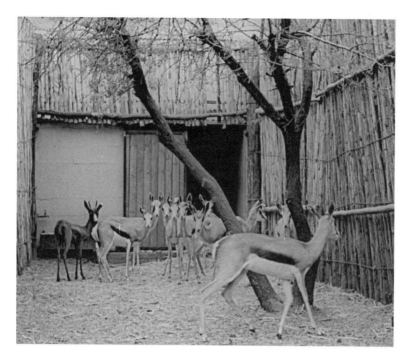

FIGURE 85–3. Wild caught springbok 3 days after capture.

haloperidol and 25 to 100 mg of perphenazine enanthate resulted in mortality rates of less than 3%.

The following doses of haloperidol are recommended for the tranquilization of springbok (Fig. 85–4): 20 mg for large rams, 12 mg for adult females, and 5 mg for subadults and lambs.

Common Reedbuck

For tranquilization, 5 to 10 mg of haloperidol and 50 to 80 mg of perphenazine enanthate are recommended. In spite of tranquilization, reedbuck do not adapt well in captivity and should be released in an appropriate habitat soon after capture.

Grey Rhebok and Mountain Reedbuck

Both species exhibit aggressive behavior towards conspecifics, and grey rhebok have sharp horns that inflict fatal wounds in conspecifics.

Haloperidol dose rates of 20, 15, 10, and 5 mg for males, females, subadults, and lambs, respectively, are recommended; 30 to 50 mg of perphenazine enanthate can be injected for confinement. They produce deep tranquilization for up to 2 days. The horns of all adult males should be piped as a precaution against injuries.

Klipspringer

A dose of 5 mg of haloperidol is recommended for adult klipspringers. This results in tranquilization of up to 20 hours. Haloperidol, 5 mg, plus perphenazine enanthate, 20 to 30 mg, is recommended for adaptation at a new habitat.

Grey Duiker, Steenbok, and Oribi

Tranquilization with 5 to 15 mg of haloperidol is recommended for adult duiker, steenbok, and oribi. This can be supplemented with 20 to 30 mg of perphenazine enanthate when longer tranquilization is required.

Dik-Dik

Haloperidol, 5 mg, has been used for translocating Damara dik-dik in Namibia. No information is available on the use of perphenazine, but it could be considered at a dose rate listed for suni antelope (next).

Suni Antelope

Haloperidol, 5 mg, plus perphenazine enanthate, 20 to 30 mg, is recommended for the transportation of adult wild-caught suni antelope. Zuclopenthixol acetate, 10 to 20 mg, can be used for adaptation of the animals to captivity.

Waterbuck

Waterbuck are difficult animals to transport and confine. They are good jumpers and will attempt to escape from an enclosure unless adequately sedated.

The recommended protocol for waterbuck is 10 to 20 mg of haloperidol with 100 to 200 mg of perphenazine enanthate or 150 mg of zuclopenthixol acetate.

Red Lechwe

See Table 85–1.

Giraffe

Short-term tranquilization is achieved with azaperone at 0.1 mg/kg.

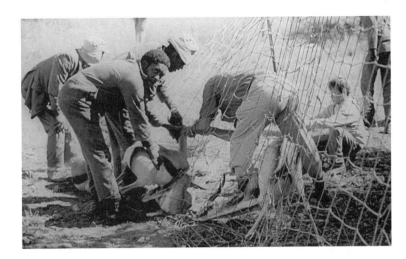

FIGURE 85–4. Injecting net-captured springbok with haloperidol.

For the transportation and confinement of adult giraffe, 10 to 30 mg of haloperidol with 100 to 250 mg of perphenazine enanthate gives optimal results. In subadults 10 to 15 mg of haloperidol and 100 to 150 mg of perphenazine enanthate is recommended.

Young giraffe quickly adapt to captivity with the use of long-acting tranquilizers such as 50 to 100 mg of perphenazine enanthate or by putting a tame adult cow in the pen with them.[24]

Black Rhinoceros

Acute and chronic stress, inappetence, aggressive behavior, breaking of horns, infections, and mortality have been reported in translocating rhinoceroses.[36] The introduction of tranquilizers into translocation procedures remarkably improved results, including fewer mortalities.[14, 34, 55, 56, 58, 59]

Azaperone is used for the short-term tranquilization of black rhinoceroses in dosage rates of 50 mg for calves and up to 200 mg for adults. Tranquilization for up to 3 days is achieved with 300 mg of zuclopenthixol acetate. Perphenazine enanthate is recommended for long-term tranquilization and taming in holding and quarantine pens at doses of 50 mg for calves, 100 mg for subadults, and 50 to 200 mg for adults.

White Rhinoceros

As with black rhinoceros, the correct use of tranquilizers can determine success or failure of transport. Doses of 100 to 400 mg of azaperone and 50 to 200 mg of perphenazine enanthate have been successfully used in subadult and adult white rhinoceroses. Dosages totaling up to 600 mg of azaperone in divided doses have been administered at 3- to 4-hour intervals to adult males to sedate them during long journeys. Detailed information on the translocation of white rhinoceroses has been recorded.[53, 54, 56, 57, 60]

Zebra

Zebras live in a family group with one mature stallion, a few mares, subadults, and foals. Bachelor groups varying from a few to 15 stallions may be found under natural conditions. Ideally, family groups should always be captured and transported together. This may, however, not always be practical with mass-capture techniques. Transport of different family groups in the same crate inevitably results in fighting, kicking, and biting.

Injecting adult zebras immediately after capture with a combination of 20 to 30 mg of haloperidol and 50 to 100 mg of perphenazine enanthate calms the animals and prevents injuries for up to 14 hours. They may remain calm for several days after arrival. Transporting zebra stallions that occur naturally in bachelor groups may present many problems and should be avoided whenever possible.

Extrapyramidal symptoms have been observed in individual yearling zebras and adult stallions injected with 30 to 40 mg of haloperidol. The symptoms were treated with injections of 20 to 60 mg of biperiden.

African Elephants

The translocation of calves, young adult bulls, and family groups is facilitated with the use of azaperone, haloperidol, and perphenazine enanthate.

It is recommended that all wild-caught adult elephants be tranquilized for transportation, to limit stress and prevent damage to the crate.

For tranquilization lasting up to 3 hours, azaperone is used. The dosage of azaperone varies from 20 mg, for animals weighing an estimated 250 kg, to 150 mg, for animals weighing up to an estimated 3000 kg. For long journeys and when tranquilization lasting up to 20 hours is required, 10 to 60 mg of haloperidol is used, and this is combined with 50 to 300 mg of perphenazine enanthate when the animals are to be confined in holding pens at destination.

For transportation from capture site to a holding pen after chemical capture, azaperone or haloperidol should be injected while the animals are still lying down and immediately before or after the antidote has been injected. This allows the animals to get onto their feet before the tranquilizer has taken full effect and facilitates loading into the crate.

When elephants are loaded from a holding pen, they should receive injections while they are in the crush immediately before they enter the crate. This allows the tranquilizer to be effective once the animals are in the crate and prevents the tranquilized animals from being reluctant to move into the crush before loading.

Elephants that are overdosed with azaperone or haloperidol stand very quietly with their ears hanging forward and the tip of the trunk lying on the ground, and they are reluctant to move.

REFERENCES

1. Basson PA, Hofmeyr JM: Mortalities associated with wildlife capture operations. *In* Young E (ed): The Capture and Care of Wild Animals. Cape Town, South Africa, Human and Rousseau, pp 151–160, 1973.
2. Bengis R: Hand capture of impala. *In* McKenzie AA (ed): The Capture and Care Manual. Pretoria, South Africa, Wildlife Decision Support Services, pp 404–406, 1993.
3. Bengis R: Care of the African buffalo, *Syncerus caffer*, in captivity. *In* McKenzie AA (ed): The Capture and Care Manual. Pretoria, South Africa, Wildlife Decision Support Services, pp 598–600, 1993.
4. Berry MPS: The tranquillization of captive hartebeest, black wildebeest and gemsbok. *In* Ebedes H (ed): The Use of Tranquillizers in Wildlife [Bulletin No. 423]. Pretoria, South Africa, Department of Agricultural Development, pp 40–43, 1992.
5. Burroughs REJ: Chemical capture of antelope. *In* McKenzie AA (ed): The Capture and Care Manual. Pretoria, South Africa, Wildlife Decision Support Services, pp 348–380, 1993.
6. Burroughs REJ: Care of antelope in captivity. *In* McKenzie AA (ed): The Capture and Care Manual. Pretoria, South Africa, Wildlife Decision Support Services, pp 440–464, 1993.
7. Burroughs REJ: Care of Burchell's zebra, *Equus burchelli*, and the mountain zebra, *Equus zebra*, in captivity. *In* McKenzie AA (ed): The Capture and Care Manual. Pretoria, South Africa, Wildlife Decision Support Services, p 631, 1993.
8. Burroughs REJ, McKenzie AA: Handling, care and loading of immobilized herbivores. *In* McKenzie AA (ed): The Capture and Care Manual. Pretoria, South Africa, Wildlife Decision Support Services, pp 184–191, 1993.
9. Clark RK, Jessup DA: Field evaluation and treatment of medical problems resulting from wildlife capture. *In* Renecker LA, Hudson RJ (eds): Wildlife Production: Conservation and Sustainable Development. Fairbanks, University of Alaska, Fairbanks, 1991.
10. Colly LP: Azaperone—a safe and well-tried tranquillizer. *In* Ebedes H (ed): The Use of Tranquillizers in Wildlife [Bulletin No. 423]. Pretoria, South Africa, Department of Agricultural Development, pp 21–22, 1992.
11. Ebedes H: Reducing translocation mortalities with tranquillizers. *In* Renecker LA, Hudson RJ (eds): Wildlife Production: Conservation and Sustainable Development. Fairbanks, University of Alaska, Fairbanks, pp 378–380, 1991.
12. Ebedes H: An introduction to long-acting neuroleptics for translocating certain South African ungulates [Manuscript]. Transvaal, South Africa, Transvaal Department of Agricultural Development, 1992.
13. Ebedes H: A note on haloperidol for translocation. *In* Ebedes H (ed): The Use of Tranquillizers in Wildlife [Bulletin No. 423]. Pretoria, South Africa, Department of Agricultural Development, pp 23–24, 1992.
14. Ebedes H: The use of long-acting tranquillizers in captive wild animals. *In* McKenzie AA (ed): The Capture and Care Manual. Pretoria, South Africa, Wildlife Decision Support Services, pp 71–99, 1993.
15. Ebedes H: Accommodation of antelope. *In* McKenzie AA (ed): The Capture and Care Manual. Pretoria, South Africa, Wildlife Decision Support Services, pp 422–439, 1993.
16. Ebedes H: Accommodation of wild animals at auctions. *In* McKenzie AA (ed): The Capture and Care Manual. Pretoria, South Africa, Wildlife Decision Support Services, pp 218–222, 1993.
17. Ebedes H: Game ranching in South Africa. *In* Fowler ME (ed): Zoo and Wild Animal Medicine: Current Therapy 3. Philadelphia, WB Saunders, pp 112–123, 1993.
18. Ebedes H: Going, going, gone—an appraisal of game auctions. *In* Van Hoven W, Ebedes H, Conroy A (eds): Wildlife ranching: A celebration of diversity. Proceedings of the 3rd International Wildlife Ranching Symposium, October 1992. Pretoria, South Africa. South African Game Organization, pp 74–80, 1994.
19. Ebedes H: Combat stress in game capture. Farmer's Weekly, p 8–12, August 11, 1995.
20. Ebedes H, Burroughs REJ: Long-acting neuroleptics in wildlife. *In* Ebedes H (ed): The Use of Tranquillizers in Wildlife [Bulletin No. 423]. Pretoria, South Africa, Department of Agricultural Development, pp 31–37, 1992.
21. Ebedes H, du Toit JG, van Rooyen J: Game capture. *In* Bothma JduP (ed): Game Ranch Management. Pretoria, South Africa, JL van Schaik, pp 271–333, 1996.
22. Ebedes H, du Toit JG, van Rooyen J: The transportation of game. *In* Bothma JduP (ed): Game Ranch Management. Pretoria, South Africa, JL van Schaik, pp 342–362, 1996.
23. Gandini GCM, Ebedes H, Burroughs REJ: The use of long-acting neuroleptics in impala, *Aepyceros melampus*. J South Afr Vet Assoc 60(4):206–207, 1989.
24. Geldenhuys L: Care of the giraffe, *Giraffa camelopardalis*, in captivity. *In* McKenzie AA (ed): The Capture and Care Manual. Pretoria, South Africa, Wildlife Decision Support Services, pp 613–614, 1993.
25. Griner LA: Pathology of Zoo Animals. San Diego, Zoological Society of San Diego, 1983.
26. Harthoorn AM: The drug immobilization of large wild herbivores other than the antelopes. *In* Young E (ed): The Capture and Care of Wild Animals. Cape Town, South Africa, Human and Rousseau, pp 51–61, 1973.
27. Harthoorn AM: The Chemical Capture of Animals. London, Baillière Tindall, 1976.
28. Harthoorn AM: The use of corrals to capture and train wild ungulates prior to translocations. Vet Rec 104:349, 1979.
29. Harthoorn AM: Physical aspects of both mechanical and chemical capture. *In* Nielsen L, Haigh JC, Fowler ME (eds): Chemical Immobilization of North American Wildlife. Milwaukee, Wisconsin Humane Society, pp 63–71, 1982.
30. Harthoorn AM: Mechanical capture as a preliminary to chemical immobilization and the use of taming and training to prevent post capture stress. *In* Nielsen L, Haigh JC, Fowler ME (eds): Chemical Immobilization of North American Wildlife. Milwaukee, Wisconsin Humane Society, pp 150–164, 1982.
31. Hofmeyr JM: Developments in the capture and airlift of roan antelope, *Hippotragus equinus equinus*, under narcosis to the Etosha National Park. Madoqua 8:37–48, 1974.
32. Hofmeyr JM: The use of haloperidol as a long-acting neuroleptic in game capture operations. J South Afr Vet Assoc 52(4):273–282, 1981.
33. Hofmeyr JM, Luchtenstein HG, Mostert PKN: Capture, handling and transport of springbok and the application of haloperidol as a long-acting tranquillizer. Madoqua 10(2):123–130, 1977.
34. Keep ME: The immobilization and tranquillization of rhino. *In* Ebedes H (ed): The Use of Tranquillizers in Wildlife [Bulletin No. 423]. Pretoria, South Africa, Department of Agricultural Development, pp 44–46, 1992.
35. Klein DR: Preface. *In* Renecker LA, Hudson RJ (eds): Wildlife Production: Conservation and Sustainable Development. Fairbanks, University of Alaska, Fairbanks, pp i–ii, 1991.
36. Kock MD: Acute and chronic stress in black rhino. *In* Ebedes H (ed): The Use of Tranquillizers in Wildlife [Bulletin No. 423]. Pretoria, South Africa, Department of Agricultural Development, p 16, 1992.
37. Lingjaerde O: Some pharmacological aspects of depot tranquillizers. Acta Psychiat Scand 246(Suppl):9–14, 1973.
38. McCrindle CME, Ebedes H, Swan GE: The use of long-acting neuroleptics, perphenazine enanthate and pipothiazine palmitate in two horses. J South Afr Vet Assoc 60(4):208–209, 1989.
39. McKenzie AA (ed): The Capture and Care Manual. Pretoria, South Africa, Wildlife Decision Support Services and the South African Veterinary Foundation, 1993.
40. Meiklejohn K: Transportation of wild animals by air. *In* McKenzie AA (ed): The Capture and Care Manual. Pretoria, South Africa, Wildlife Decision Support Services, pp 200–207, 1993.
41. Morkel P: Depot neuroleptics in roan antelope. *In* Ebedes H (ed): The Use of Tranquillizers in Wildlife [Bulletin No. 423]. Pretoria, South Africa, Department of Agricultural Development, pp 38–39, 1992.

42. Morkel P, la Grange M: Capture of antelope using the netgun. *In* McKenzie AA (ed): The Capture and Care Manual. Pretoria, South Africa, Wildlife Decision Support Services, pp 393–403, 1993.

43. Nielsen L: Definitions, considerations and guidelines for translocation of wild animals. *In* Nielsen L, Brown RD (eds): Translocation of Wild Animals. Milwaukee, Wisconsin Humane Society, Inc., and Kingsville, TX, The Caesar Kleberg Wildlife Research Institute, pp 12–51, 1988.

44. Openshaw P: Mass capture techniques. *In* McKenzie AA (ed): The Capture and Care Manual. Pretoria, South Africa, Wildlife Decision Support Services, pp 138–155, 1993.

45. Openshaw P: Mass capture of antelope, buffalo, giraffe and zebra. *In* McKenzie AA (ed): The Capture and Care Manual. Pretoria, South Africa, Wildlife Decision Support Services, pp 381–392, 1993.

46. Openshaw P: Transportation of wild herbivores. *In* McKenzie AA (ed): The Capture and Care Manual. Pretoria, South Africa, Wildlife Decision Support Services, pp 194–199, 1993.

47. Openshaw P: Transportation of antelope and zebra. *In* McKenzie AA (ed): The Capture and Care Manual. Pretoria, South Africa, Wildlife Decision Support Services, pp 407–421, 1993.

48. Pienaar Ude V: The capture and restraint of wild herbivores by mechanical methods. *In* Young E (ed): The Capture and Care of Wild Animals. Cape Town, South Africa, Human and Rousseau, pp 91–99, 1973.

49. Pienaar Ude V: The drug immobilization of antelope species. *In* Young E (ed): The Capture and Care of Wild Animals. Cape Town, South Africa, Human and Rousseau, pp 35–50, 1973.

50. Prinsloo MK, Ebedes H: The use of some long-acting neuroleptics in wildlife captured with the "pop-up corral." *In* Ebedes H (ed): The Use of Tranquillizers in Wildlife [Bulletin No. 423]. Pretoria, South Africa, Department of Agricultural Development, pp 49–51, 1992.

51. Raath JP: Transportation of wild animals by sea. *In* McKenzie AA (ed): The Capture and Care Manual. Pretoria, South Africa, Wildlife Decision Support Services, pp 208–216, 1993.

52. Raath JP: Transportation of the African elephant, *Loxodonta africana*. *In* McKenzie AA (ed): The Capture and Care Manual. Pretoria, South Africa, Wildlife Decision Support Services, pp 493–498, 1993.

53. Rogers PS: Chemical capture of the white rhinoceros, *Ceratotherium simum*. *In* McKenzie AA (ed): The Capture and Care Manual. Pretoria, South Africa, Wildlife Decision Support Services, pp 512–529, 1993.

54. Rogers PS: Transportation of the white rhinoceros, *Ceratotherium simum*. *In* McKenzie AA (ed): The Capture and Care Manual. Pretoria, South Africa, Wildlife Decision Support Services, pp 529–533, 1993.

55. Rogers PS: Transportation of the black rhinoceros, *Diceros bicornis*. *In* McKenzie AA (ed): The Capture and Care Manual. Pretoria, South Africa, Wildlife Decision Support Services, pp 556–557, 1993.

56. Rogers PS: Transportation of the rhinoceros by air or by sea. *In* McKenzie AA (ed): The Capture and Care Manual. Pretoria, South Africa, Wildlife Decision Support Services, pp 534–540, 1993.

57. Rogers PS: Care of the white rhinoceros, *Ceratotherium simum*, in captivity. *In* McKenzie AA (ed): The Capture and Care Manual. Pretoria, South Africa, Wildlife Decision Support Services, pp 546–553, 1993.

58. Rogers PS: Care of the black rhinoceros, *Diceros bicornis*, in captivity. *In* McKenzie AA (ed): The Capture and Care Manual. Pretoria, South Africa, Wildlife Decision Support Services, pp 553–556, 1993.

59. Rogers PS: Transportation and boma management of rhinos. *In* Penzhorn BL, Kriek NPJ (eds): Rhinos as game ranch animals. Onderstepoort, Republic of South Africa, South African Veterinary Association, pp 136–154, 1994.

60. Rogers PS: Care of the white rhinoceros, *Ceratotherium simum*, in captivity. *In* McKenzie AA (ed): The Capture and Care Manual. Pretoria, South Africa, Wildlife Decision Support Services, pp 558–562, 1993.

61. Spraker TR: An overview of the pathophysiology of capture myopathy and related conditions that occur at the time of capture of wild animals. *In* Nielsen L, Haigh JC, Fowler ME (eds): Chemical Immobilization of North American Wildlife. Milwaukee, Wisconsin Humane Society, pp 83–118, 1982.

62. Swan GE: Drugs used for the immobilization, capture and translocation of wild animals. *In* McKenzie AA (ed): The Capture and Care Manual. Pretoria, South Africa, Wildlife Decision Support Services, pp 2–64, 1993.

63. Young E: Muscle necrosis in captive red hartebeest *(Alcelaphus buselaphus)*. J South Afr Vet Assoc 37(1):101–103, 1966.

64. Young E: Overstraining disease (capture myopathy) in the tsessebe, *Damaliscus lunatus*, and oribi, *Ourebia ourebi*. Koedoe 15:143–144, 1972.

65. Young E, Bronkhorst PJL: Overstraining disease in game. Afr Wildl 25(2):51–52, 1971.

CHAPTER 86

Preventive Medicine Programs for Ranched Hoofstock

JAMES M. JENSEN

OVERVIEW OF GAME PRODUCTION

Game ranching is the propagation of nondomestic ungulates for agricultural or aesthetic purposes. It is a worldwide agribusiness and has had steady growth over the past half century. The United States, Canada, South Africa, the United Kingdom, Australia, New Zealand, and many other countries have growing exotic livestock industries.

Several reasons exist for the growing interest in game ranching. Ancient cultures, such as those of the

Mesopotamians, Egyptians, Chinese, and Greeks, captured and cultivated animals for aesthetic purposes and out of scientific interest. This theme has been repeated in modern history by individuals who have maintained exotic hoofstock for propagation and study. One of the most notable examples is the propagation and subsequent rescue of Pere David deer from extinction by England's Duke of Bedford. Another example is the efforts of game ranchers in South Africa in the early 1900s, which ensured the survival of blesbok (*Damaliscus dorcas phillipsi*), bontebok (*Damaliscus dorcas dorcas*), and white-tailed wildebeest (*Connochaetes gnou*).

At approximately the same time, ranchers in Texas imported exotic hoofstock such as axis deer (*Axis axis*) and nilgai (*Boselaphus tragocamelus*).[29] Their original intent was to propagate exotic animals on cattle ranch land for variety and novelty. After these species became abundant, ranchers considered hunting them for meat and sport. Information compiled by the Texas Agricultural Statistics Service summarizes exotic ungulate ranching in the state for many years, including the growth of this industry. In 1984, there were 370 exotic ungulate operations in 124 of the 254 counties in Texas. A total of 120,201 animals were maintained on ranches that encompassed 2,205,687 acres.[16] A similar survey in 1996 revealed that 1007 ranches were operating in 194 counties. The animal total had grown to 198,060 hoofstock with access to 3,107,431 acres.

Many game ranchers view exotic ungulates as ecologically viable alternatives to traditional livestock. In many habitats, indigenous wildlife may be better production animals than domestic livestock. This is often true because most domestic livestock species have evolved from temperate-region ancestors. In contrast, marginal agricultural lands of the world have historically been considered ideal sites for wildlife use. Well-conceived game ranches use animals and vegetation that are best suited for the environment. Furthermore, traditional livestock may be more susceptible to predation and disease than indigenous or introduced wild ruminants.

Many exotic ungulates are compatible with domestic livestock and can be raised along with traditional ranch animals, especially when their food preferences do not overlap significantly. Game ranch profit can be maximized when several species are raised on the same acreage. Table 86–1 lists computer programs that com-

pute the carrying capacity of land with regard to domestic and exotic livestock.

The growth in game ranching has been driven by profitability and a worldwide interest in the animal products. Trophy hunting has been an income source for game ranches for many decades, and many ranches are involved in game propagation to meet consumer demand for the lean venison that nondomestic ruminants produce. Other products such as antler "velvet" and hides have marketability and make certain species of wild ruminants more profitable.

REGULATORY MEDICINE

There is considerably less regulation of the game ranching industry in the United States than the domestic livestock industry. Two federal mandates, the Endangered Species Act and the Animal Welfare Act, do require tuberculin testing of all cervids moved interstate (unless between American Zoo and Aquarium Association [AZA]–accredited institutions). However, most regulations of the game ranching industry are invoked by individual states.[16] A survey in 1989 revealed confusion within many states about the regulation of exotic ungulates; only 13 of 50 states had applicable statutes governing nonnative deer and antelope production. Because there is a possibility of infection with contagious diseases (e.g., bovine tuberculosis, brucellosis, and bluetongue [BT]/epizootic hemorrhagic diseases [EHDs]) in herds, animal health commissions of many states have come to address exotic ruminant animals in their regulatory codes.[8] Any shipment of nondomestic livestock should not be undertaken without thorough knowledge of the regulatory medicine requirements of the states involved.

INDIVIDUAL ANIMAL MEDICINE

Animals seldom receive individual treatment in game ranching operations. However, when opportunities arise for singular procedures, it is prudent to perform preventive medicine. Occasions for individual care include during shipment of animals, during receipt of animals, and when giving attention to medical problems. De-

TABLE 86–1. Computer Programs for Carrying Capacity of Livestock and Exotic Hoofstock

Computer Program Name	System	Supplier
Exotic 3	Lotus 1-2-3	Dr. Jerry Stuth Dept. of Range Science Texas A&M University College Station, Texas 77843
Rangemaster	GW Basic	Dr. William Sheffield Route 4, No. 54 Triple Blend Road College Station, Texas 77840
Comanche Spring Ranch Reproduction Management Program	Lotus 1-2-3	Joe and Nancy Green Star Route HC 89-B55 Eden, Texas 76837

TABLE 86–2. Class III Anthelmintics Used in Nondomestic Ruminant Animals

Anthelmintic	Dosage	Comments
Albendazole	10 mg/kg body weight orally 26 mg/kg body weight orally	Broad spectrum; *Dictyocaulus viviparus* and *Fascioloides magna*
Fenbendazole	5–10 mg/kg body weight	Administer for 3 or more consecutive days; broad spectrum
Oxfendazole	4.5 mg/kg body weight	Broad spectrum
Ivermectin	0.2 mg/kg body weight orally or subcutaneously 0.5 mg/kg body weight topically	Broad spectrum

pending on the ranch facility, the animals can be controlled either with restraint devices or by chemical immobilization.

Disease prevalence can be evaluated while animals are restrained. A thorough physical examination should always be conducted on restrained animals to evaluate general health and to look for signs of contagious diseases, parasitism, or nutritional problems.

Veterinarians should target medical problems that apply to each ranch. Blood titers can be used to evaluate a number of contagious diseases. Samples can be obtained for ectoparasitic and endoparasitic examination of individual animals.

Vaccination against ungulate diseases (most commonly *Clostridium* and *Leptospira* polyvalent vaccines) can be accomplished on restrained individuals. When internal parasites are suspected, restrained animals can be given oral or injectable doses of anthelmintics (Table 86–2). Care must be taken to avoid aspiration of oral medicants when they are given to chemically immobilized animals.

The Suggested Protocol for Pre-shipment Health Screening of Antelope Species produced by the Antelope Taxon Advisory Group of the AZA is an excellent document for game ranchers to follow when working with individual animals. In addition to the procedures already mentioned for individual animals, this protocol stipulates permanent identification of the animal (ear notch, transponder, freeze brand), hoof examination and trimming, and serum banking for future reference. It also recommends supplemental testing for bovine tuberculosis (intradermal skin test), malignant catarrhal fever (serology), and Johne's disease (radiometric culture, enzyme-linked immunosorbent assay [ELISA], culture).

QUARANTINE

Quarantine facilities are seldom found on game farms and ranches, so newly arrived animals are often introduced to the existing herd. Because of infectious and parasitic disease concerns, this is a risky practice for game ranches. An ideal system has a free-standing quarantine site 50 to 100 m from the nearest herd site. It should be capable of housing animals for as long as 1 month. Quarantine periods may vary according to individual animals and the health history of their previous environment. During this period, animals are evaluated as they are for disease, mainly for tuberculosis

and parasitism. This facility should be connected by alleyways to the central herd site so that immobilization is not required to introduce them to the herd. Ideally, after their daily care, caretakers involved with the quarantined creatures should not have subsequent contact with the existing herd.

Animals can also be introduced to new dietary products and forages while in quarantine. Each new animal should be permanently identified with an ear tag, horn brand, or freeze brand before departing quarantine. Transponder implants are normally not practical for game identification on ranches or farms, so visual means of identification are much more practical.

PARASITE CONTROL

The development of a parasite control program for captive nondomestic hoofstock is discussed in Chapter 87.[19] Game farmers and ranchers readily recognize parasite control as a paramount component of a good preventive medicine program. A survey that produced responses from 96 game ranches in the United States revealed that scheduled parasite examinations and deworming were conducted at 75% of these establishments.[26a] Parasitism represented more than half of the health problems experienced by these exotic game producers. Parasite control was the most common preventive medicine program, followed by vaccination (48% of respondents) and quarantine (43%). Many general principles of parasite evaluation and treatment in domestic animals can be applied, although parasite control in game-ranched ungulates has some specific concerns. Farm- and ranch-raised ruminant animals also lack the intensive environmental management to control parasites that is often afforded captive animals.[12] Another concern is the difficulty of anthelmintic treatment when target animals are in a relatively free existence. Animals are often introduced to new parasites from other wildlife, domestic stock, or exotic ruminant hosts.

Sixty-eight zoos responded to a survey of parasite control programs used in captive wild ruminants. Members of the "antelope" group were most often listed in this survey as presenting a greater parasite control problem than other ruminant animals.[18] An evaluation of parasitism at the San Diego Wild Animal Park corroborated the findings of this survey. In this study, antelope species had significantly higher pretreatment and posttreatment parasite egg counts than other ungulate groups.[2] Although these species have not been commonly used in game harvest programs, they exist on many game ranches for breeding and aesthetic purposes. It is reasonable to consider them equally susceptible to parasitic problems in an open existence.

It is important to recognize that exotic ruminant species may harbor their own indigenous endoparasites, which can also infest traditional livestock and native wild ruminant animals. *Camelostrongylus mentulatus* and *Trichostrongylus colubriformis* are nematode parasites that are commonly seen in African antelope species. They have been identified in ranch-raised scimitar-horned oryx in central Texas and infected domestic sheep (*Ovis* species).[22] In another example, fallow deer (*Dama dama*) from Europe have introduced an abomasal worm (*Spiculopteragia asymmetrica*) to a regional population of white-tailed deer (*Odocoileus virginianus*) in the United States.[6] To prevent the transmission of new pathogenic nematodes to susceptible species, similar parasite introductions should be avoided.

Conversely, game ranchers and veterinarians should also be aware of parasites indigenous to their geographic region that can cause disease in exotic game.[33] Some of these parasites originate from domestic livestock. *Dictyocaulus viviparus*, the lungworm of cattle, is one of the most important parasites of farmed deer in New Zealand.[25] *Haemonchus* and *Cooperia* species associated with North American livestock are commonly seen in introduced ruminant species.[19] In an ironic role reversal, the plains bison (*Bison bison*), native to North America, is very susceptible to infestation by *Ostertagia ostertagi*,[24] which was introduced when European livestock was brought to the New World.

Parasites of native wild ruminants pose a similar threat to game ranching. *Fascioloides magna* is the liver fluke of white-tailed deer and elk (*Cervus canadensis*) in the eastern and Gulf Coast regions of the United States. It enjoys a well-adapted host/parasite relationship with these two native species and only causes significant disease in them when environmental conditions are severe.[32] However, cattle, sheep, goats, pigs, horses, moose (*Alces alces*), fallow deer, red deer (*Cervus elaphus*), sambar deer (*Cervus unicolor*), sika (*Cervus nippon*), and mule deer (*Odocoileus hemionus*) are affected by this parasite,[10, 31] which can cause massive liner destruction and death in these species.

Mule deer are inapparent carriers of *Elaeophora schneideri*, a vascular nematode of mule deer, and are responsible for its distribution from British Columbia to the southwestern United States. Numerous ruminant species are affected with vascular occlusion in the carotid arteries and other major vessels, and pyogranulomas, related to microfilarial infestation, are often visible. Sika deer, a common species on game ranches, are particularly susceptible to this parasite.[34]

The "meningeal worm" of white-tailed deer, *Parelaphostrongylus tenuis*, is another wildlife parasite that can potentially affect farmed game. It is found in the eastern half of North America. This organism causes destruction of central nervous system tissue as it migrates erratically in nonhost species. Many ruminant species, including fallow deer, red deer, elk, caribou (*Rangifer tarandus terraenovae*), and reindeer (*Rangifer tarandus tarandus*) can be affected. Meningeal worm infestation in fallow deer is not always fatal. They appear to be refractory to low levels of infective *P. tenuis* larvae, and immunity can possibly develop after the initial infestation.[6] Sable antelope (*Hippotragus niger*), bongo antelope (*Boocercus eurycerus*), and scimitar-horned oryx have also succumbed to cerebral nematodiasis related to *P. tenuis*.[30]

Environmental management for internal parasite control on game farms and ranches should bear close resemblance to practices in domestic livestock production.[36] Pasture rotation is one of the best environmental manipulations to reduce endoparasitism.[5] When paddocks are left ungrazed for 3 to 6 months, most free-living, infective nematode larvae are killed by sunlight.[1] Freezing temperatures and low humidity can also affect larval viability when grazing areas are rested.[11]

Another concept of pasture rotation is that weanling animals should be introduced to parasite-free pastures for their first grazing.[5] This may seem idealistic for ranch-raised wildlife because they are free-ranging and some species can calve at any time of the year (axis deer, blackbuck [*Antilope cervicapra*]). However, it is possible to remove ruminant animals from pastures for months before common calving and fawning times and then to return these herds to the same area as the offspring approach weaning. Another method of reducing the infective larvae count of a pasture is to cut the grass immediately before introducing juvenile hoofstock. An extension of this idea is to graze a pasture short with taxonomically distant species that have been dewormed before introduction. This eliminates infective larvae without introducing additional parasite concerns.[4]

Some basic points regarding fecal examination of captive hoofstock can be made. When examining a herd for parasites, aggregate fecal samples should be collected from several fresh stools.[1] Preference should be given to feces from juvenile animals as well as to stools that are poorly formed, mucoid, or have frank blood or melena. In addition, individual samples from high-risk members of a herd can provide more specific information. It is important to collect moist fecal samples and examine them immediately. If rapid examination is impossible, the samples should be placed in an airtight container and refrigerated to retard larval development of eggs.

Feces are routinely examined by direct smear and fecal flotation[19] or the Baermann simplified sedimentation technique.[1] Fecal egg counts can also be evaluated using the McMaster technique. It is useful to run fecal egg counts before and after anthelmintic treatment to evaluate the effectiveness of a drug and its delivery system.[20] Counts of more than 50 nematode eggs per gram of feces in free-ranging ungulates may indicate that anthelmintic treatment should be administered.

Anthelmintic administration is a common preventive medicine practice with regard to ranched ungulates. Four major options exist for the use of anthelmintics in controlling gastrointestinal parasites. These uses are recognized in domestic livestock medicine as (1) traditional, (2) suppressive, (3) integrated, and (4) controlled-release devices.[17] Traditional use refers to the use of deworming agents to halt clinical outbreaks of parasitism and stop deaths. This is not a preventive medicine measure. Suppressive anthelmintic therapy is the repeated dosing of a drug close to the prepatent period of internal parasites. This method interrupts reinfestation but also leads to drug resistance development by parasites. Integrated anthelmintic usage is the preferred choice for game farms and ranches. Parasite treatment is integrated with the aforementioned sound grazing management principles. These strategic treatment programs can be effective in any part of the world as long as they are based on the epidemiology of the geographic region. Controlled-release devices are the newest phase in anthelmintic therapy. These are biologic implants that can administer drugs either continuously, cyclically, or at strategic times. Their use in ranch-raised exotic ungulates is as yet untested, but their usefulness should be studied.[17]

Anthelmintics are divided into two classes based on their ability to kill immature, larval stages of nematodes. Class I worm medications kill only adult stages. Drugs in this group include thiabendazole, levamisole, and pyrantel. Class II anthelmintics kill immature and mature forms of gastrointestinal parasites. Fenbendazole, oxfendazole, albendazole, and ivermectin are commonly used therapeutic agents in this class. Because class II anthelmintics kill all developing forms of nematodes in the host, an additional 3 to 6 weeks transpires after deworming before patent infestations can recur. Integrated anthelmintic treatment should always be conducted with a class II agent.

Effective dosages of selected class II anthelmintics in nondomestic ruminant animals are listed in Table 86–2. Fenbendazole is used extensively in confined herds of wild ruminant animals and has proven to be very effective. It can produce a 98% to 100% reduction in nematode egg count when administered in the feed at a dosage of 5 mg/kg of body weight for 3 consecutive days.[21] *Trichuris* species resistant to other therapies appear to be sensitive to this regimen. Ivermectin is particularly useful against ostertagiasis and can be used on a monthly basis to intercept larval migration of *P. tenuis* before infestation of the central nervous system. Anecdotal information suggests that high doses of ivermectin (1.0 to 1.5 mg/kg) can be effective in killing larvae in the central nervous system. However, this dosage may be toxic to some ungulate species. Albendazole has a broad spectrum of activity at high doses and is effective against *Dictyocaulus viviparus* and *Fascioloides magna*.[10]

Veterinarians and game producers must be aware of the reasons for decreased anthelmintic effectiveness. Insufficient drug intake is a major problem with regard to free-roaming animals. Bait enhancement is necessary to make most anthelmintics attractive and palatable to wild ruminant animals. Corn, grain mixes, molasses licks, and mineral blocks are just a few of the vehicles used to deliver the drug. However, dominant species and aggressive individuals may consume excessive amounts of medication while other animals go unmedicated. This fact encourages the use of exclusion feeders that allow small species and juvenile animals to eat medicated food with minimal competition.[2] Decreased anthelmintic effectiveness can also be related to inap-

propriate drug selection as well as rapid reingestion of infective larvae.

Drug resistance by gastrointestinal parasites is a growing cause of decreased anthelmintic effectiveness. Benzimidazoles are most commonly reported as less effective than expected. As is well known in domestic sheep production and in antelope species,[20] when nematodes become resistant to one benzimidazole, they can display resistance to other members of this drug group without previous exposure to them. In a similar fashion, levamisole, morantel, and pyrantel are also cross-resistant anthelmintics.[4]

Annual change of anthelmintic types is probably the best approach for most infested herds. Frequent anthelmintic changes may favor multiple-resistant strains of parasites rather than eliminate the organisms. An increased frequency of anthelmintic use increases the rate at which resistance occurs in gastrointestinal nematodes. Preventive dosing on a monthly basis, for instance, is too frequent.

An in vitro assay has recently been developed for the detection of resistance of nematodes to benzimidazoles, levamisole, benzimidazole/levamisole combinations, and ivermectin/milbemycin combinations (DrenchRite, Horizon Technology Pty Limited, Roseville, New South Wales, Australia). This assay may have significant future application in parasite control programs of game farms and ranches.

Ectoparasites usually garner less attention than endoparasites in preventive medicine programs. However, they can still be causes of unthriftiness and disease transmission. Exotic ruminant species may harbor ectoparasites of native wildlife and domestic livestock, and may introduce their own indigenous ectoparasites to the regions in which they are introduced. A survey of free-ranging blackbuck in central Texas revealed three native species of ticks (*Dermacentor albipictus, Haemaphysalis leporispalustris, Amblyomma americanum*), one native louse fly (*Lipoptena mazamae*), and one native chewing louse (*Damalinia cornuta cornuta*). However, two nonnative sucking lice were also discovered (*Lignonathus cervicaprae, Lignonathus pithodes*). This was the first report of these lice in the western hemisphere.[27] *Psoroptes cuniculi*, the ear mite of rabbits and white-tailed deer, has also been reported in blackbuck in Texas. Most ectoparasites are susceptible to permethrin acaricides. These products are safe and longer acting than pyrethrin, piperonyl, and carbaryl products. Ivermectin is also fairly effective against ticks and sucking lice.

CONTAGIOUS DISEASES

Most contagious diseases of domestic livestock, including clostridial diseases, leptospirosis, brucellosis, anthrax, pasteurellosis, Johne's disease, and tuberculosis, are also found in nondomestic ruminant animals. Vaccination with polyvalent *Clostridium* vaccines is particularly important in farm-raised ruminant animals. *Clostridium perfringens* type C and D bacterin in polyvalent vaccines affords good protection against enterotoxemia.

This is particularly important in bottle-raised hoofstock that tend to be overfed and underexercised. These vaccines also stimulate immunity to clostridial diseases that may be regional in their appearance (blackleg—*Clostridium chauvoei*; malignant edema—*Clostridium septicum*). Although ruminant animals are not particularly susceptible to tetanus (*Clostridium tetani*), the presence of this bacterin in a polyvalent vaccine may also have benefits. Free-ranging hoofstock may sustain penetrating wounds in their environments as well as puncture wounds from darting. Tetanus antitoxin should routinely be given (1500 to 4500 units) to animals receiving treatment for a penetrating wound.

Leptospira species can also cause systemic disease in exotic ruminants. Addax (*Addax nasomaculatus*) deaths have resulted from leptospirosis in a confined herd. Oxytetracycline therapy and vaccination with polyvalent (5 serotype) vaccine interrupted the transmission of the disease. Vaccination for leptospirosis should similarly follow the dosage and frequency listed for comparably sized domestic livestock.

The occurrence of *Brucella abortus* in bison and elk has become a concern. They have historically become infected after cohabitation with infected cattle. No transmission has been recorded from these wild ruminants to cattle, perhaps because infected bison rarely abort. Axis deer were experimentally infected with *B. abortus* and the organism was recovered from the reproductive tracts and milk after inoculation.[7] Whenever possible, brucellosis serologic testing using the standard plate test should be used as a screening tool regarding these species.

Anthrax (*Bacillus anthracis*) is a deadly zoonotic disease that has worldwide distribution. Although outbreaks of this disease occur in the southwestern United States, vaccination of ranch-raised ungulates has not been undertaken. Inoculation could be considered in the face of outbreaks, particularly where intensive handling facilities are available.

Pasteurella haemolytica and *Pasteurella multocida* are associated with pneumonia ("shipping fever") in domestic livestock.[35] Polyvalent vaccines for these organisms are likely to be effective in exotic ruminant animals but may not be important in a preventive medicine program for ranch-raised animals. Sentinel sheep taken from an intensive farm environment displayed a decline in *P. haemolytica* titers when placed in an open environment with scimitar-horned oryx,[22] perhaps indicating that pasteurellosis is less common in extensive enclosures and that vaccination is not a high priority.

Johne's disease has been diagnosed in a diverse array of nondomestic ruminant animals. The list includes a significant number of deer, sheep, and antelope species that are represented on game farms and ranches. The infective organism, *Mycobacterium paratuberculosis*, causes emaciation, diarrhea, lymphadenopathy, and thickening of the small intestines in affected animals during a long subclinical period, during which the host sheds viable organisms in the feces. This allows many animals to be exposed before the disease is diagnosed. Circulating antibodies to this organism are not produced until late in the disease. Therefore, serologic testing is often not useful. Acid-fast staining of feces from newly arrived suspect animals is a simple and valuable diagnostic step. However, it is not an absolute indication of disease. A positive culture of *M. paratuberculosis* is absolute diagnostic proof. However, it may take 12 to 16 weeks to absolutely rule out mycobacterial growth. A faster technique is radiometric culture for Johne's organism. It is more sensitive to low numbers of organisms and provides positive results in as few as 7 days.

Additionally, a new gene probe (IDDEX Laboratories, Portland, ME), approved by the U.S. Department of Agriculture (USDA) for diagnosing Johne's disease in cattle, provides a rapid means of identifying *M. paratuberculosis*. It has 100% specificity for this organism, but it requires a large number of organisms to be shed in feces for positive results.[28] It has potential applications to nonbovine hoofstock, but supporting research should be done.

Antigen 85 complex proteins are major secretory products of actively proliferating mycobacteria. A dot blot immunobinding assay for these proteins detects mycobacterial antigens for Johne's disease and bovine tuberculosis. This test can be very effective in animals with compromised immune systems because it evaluates the presence of bacterial antigens and not host antibodies. The dot blot test has been used to identify Johne's disease in nyala (*Tragelaphus angasi*) and impala (*Aepyceros melampus*) and has shown a high correlation between test results and clinical signs.[23] Circulating antigen 85 values may eventually be used for identification of *Mycobacterium bovis*.

Bovine tuberculosis is the major contagious disease concern, and game ranches can easily become contaminated by adding an infected ruminant to the herd. In 1990 and 1991, a shipment of elk infected with *M. bovis* from a farm in the northern United States resulted in the contamination of 22 elk herds in eight states and three Canadian provinces. This prompted the USDA Animal and Plant Health Inspection Service (APHIS) to adopt single cervical tuberculin testing for cervid species. Another alarming outbreak of bovine tuberculosis was discovered in early 1995. Hunter-kill samples of a free-ranging population of white-tailed deer in northeastern Michigan indicated a 4.5% incidence of bovine tuberculosis. This represented the first epizootic of bovine tuberculosis ever recorded in free-ranging native deer in North America.[9]

The blood tuberculosis test (BTB) for *M. bovis* infection was recognized by APHIS as an ancillary test to skin testing in 1994. The BTB is a combination of two tests: one is a lymphocyte transformation test (LT) and the other is an ELISA. The LT measures the response of immune cells from each tested animal to protein isolates from *Mycobacterium avium* and *M. bovis*. It is important to have avian tuberculosis included in the LT because *M. avium* can sensitize cervids to skin testing. Mixed infections of the two organisms have also been reported. In New Zealand, 35 of 52 contaminated deer herds (67%) had both organisms present.[14] *M. avium* is primarily included in the LT to differentiate false-positive results on the intradermal cervical test. LT samples are collected in heparin tubes. The ELISA measures the serum of antibodies specific for *M. bovis* and *M. avium*. ELISA samples must be collected in serum separator tubes.

The combined BTB has a sensitivity of 95% and a specificity of 98%. It can detect bovine tuberculosis earlier and identify seriously diseased, anergic animals more effectively than conventional skin testing.[13] The BTB is an expensive test (approximately $100), making it cost prohibitive in many species of game animals. The LT is the less expensive component of the BTB (approximately $10) and can be used as a screening test that requires only one restraint episode for the animal; however, when used alone, the LT is not recognized by regulatory agencies as an acceptable bovine tuberculosis test.

A long list of pathogenic viruses can cause disease in cervids and artiodactylids. The major viral concerns of game-ranched ungulates—BT, EHD, and malignant catarrhal fever (MCF)[3]—are discussed in reference 15. Common viruses of cattle, such as bovine viral diarrhea (BVD) virus and parainfluenza 3 virus, seem to have a very low incidence of positive serology in captive hoofstock. Serologic evidence may be higher on farms and ranches where exotic ruminant animals commingle with cattle, but no significant disease transmission has been observed. Vaccination is not recommended for these viruses in nondomestic hoofstock. Vaccination for BVD with a bovine modified live virus vaccine may produce iatrogenic disease in some species.

BT and EHD are acute vascular diseases caused by similar orbiviruses. These viruses are spread by a flying arthropod vector, *Culicoides varipennis*, and outbreaks are often associated with massive *Culicoides* infestations in late summer and early fall. BT and EHD can affect wild and farm-raised white-tailed deer. BT has been diagnosed in many exotic ruminant species, some of which are currently being used in venison production (e.g., axis deer, nilgai [*Boselaphus tragocamelus*]).[18] BT is endemic in some regions of North America whereas other areas are free of the disease. This fact influences regulatory laws related to interstate and international transport of animals. In endemic regions, BT-positive animals in good health most likely have natural immunity to the disease.

SENTINEL ANIMALS

An emerging concept for monitoring infectious and parasitic diseases on game farms is the use of sentinel, or "tracer," animals. Recent research conducted on a game ranch in central Texas used weanling sheep to assess parasite load, parasite species, and infectious disease levels in a herd of scimitar-horned oryx. The sheep associated closely with the oryx herd during their stay on the ranch. After a period of 1 to 3 months, the sheep were sampled for fecal and serologic evidence of disease.[22]

In addition to sheep, cattle could also be used as sentinel animals; domestic goats are not as preferable, because, as browsers, they do less ground feeding and do not pick up as many infective nematode larvae as grazers. Exotic ruminant species could also be used, but domestic animals are usually easier to recapture and sample. Weanling sentinel animals are likely to be more susceptible to parasitism and therefore are good indicators of nematode infestation. Before introduction to the herd, the sentinel animal must be physically examined and deemed free of any signs of contagious disease; endoparasites must be eliminated by using a class II anthelmintic. Baseline serologic tests must also be done at that time. If sentinel animals are processed for meat, their carcasses can be further examined for signs of disease.

NUTRITION

Nutrition is an often overlooked facet of preventive medicine. However, it is an integral part of health management. When intensive feeding is necessary, farmers must provide all of the appropriate amounts of protein, energy, minerals, vitamins, and water for the species they are raising. In free-ranging operations, emphasis is more appropriately placed on supplementation of nutritional needs. Properly balanced nutritional supplements stimulate rumen microorganisms to work efficiently to stimulate forage intake.

Browsers are often given protein supplementation. True browsers, such as impala, eland (*Taurotragus oryx*), and white-tailed deer, consume leaves of trees, shrubs, and forbs that have significantly higher protein levels than grasses. Protein supplementation is also important to deer species during antler production. Protein requirements increase from 13% to 14% for maintenance to 16% to 20% for antler production.

Salt should always be available to ruminant animals on game farms and ranches. Exotic ruminant animals vary individually in their use of salt blocks or salt licks; however, even short-term access to salt sources can have a profound effect on the sodium status of wild ruminant animals. Salt and salt/mineral mixes might not be readily consumed by exotic hoofstock. Providing these elements, along with vitamins, in a pelletized concentrate can be a more effective delivery system. Copper deficiency is a significant nutritional disease in elk and red deer in New Zealand. Copper sulfate can be mixed into supplements so that adult animals receive approximately 100 mg/day.

If used as supplements, corn and grain mixes should be fed sparingly. Both substances can cause rumenitis and acidosis if an amount equal to 1% to 2% of the body weight is consumed in a short period of time. Grain mixes may have vitamins and minerals added, but corn does not. Corn is inexpensive in comparison to processed feed and has high energy content. However, significant feeding of corn encourages a shift of rumen microbes from forage digesters to starch digesters.

Game producers in temperate climate zones can take advantage of winter forages to supplement the energy needs of nondomestic ruminant animals. Winter rye and wheat varieties can flourish as cold-season pastures where winters are not severe. Game farmers and ranchers should be aware of the possibility of using metabolic limiters in food concentrates. Feeds are being test-marketed that prevent overeating by dominant species and aggressive individuals. Products with metabolic limiters allow self-feeders to be used for exotic rumi-nants. This potentially reduces the man-hours needed to care for these herds. Limiters may eventually be incorporated into feeds medicated with anthelmintics so that the treated feeds will be consumed by all members of the herd.

REFERENCES

1. Bird KG: Parasite control in a zoological setting. Vet Tech 8:439–444, 1987.
2. Boyce W, Allen J, Himmelwright C, et al: Implementation and evaluation of a strategic parasite control program for captive exotic ungulates. J Am Vet Med Assoc 198:1972–1976, 1991.
3. Castro AE: Applicability of virologic and serologic tests in the diagnosis of viral diseases of exotic hoofed stock. Proceedings of the Annual Meeting of the American Association of Zoo Veterinarians, South Padre Island, TX, pp 230–235, 1990.
4. Coles GC: Strategies for control of anthelmintic-resistant nematodes of ruminants. J Am Vet Med Assoc 192:330–334, 1988.
5. Craig TC, Wikse SE: Control programs for internal parasites of beef cattle. Compendium of Continuing Education for the Practicing Veterinarian 17:579–587, 1995.
6. Davidson WR, Crum JM, Blue JL, et al: Parasites, diseases and health status of sympatric populations of fallow deer and white-tailed deer in Kentucky. J Wildl Dis 21:153–159, 1985.
7. Davis DS, Heck FC, Adams LG: Experimental infection of captive axis deer with *Brucella abortus*. J Wildl Dis 20:177–179, 1984.
8. Ervin RT, Demarais S, Hughes DM: Legal status of exotic deer throughout the United States. *In* Brown RD (ed): The Biology of Deer. New York, Springer-Verlag, pp 244–252, 1992.
9. Fitzgerald SD, Sikarskie JG, Schmitt SM, et al: *Mycobacterium bovis* epidemic in free-ranging white-tailed deer. Proceedings of the Annual Meeting of the American Association of Zoo Veterinarians, East Lansing, MI, pp 474–475, 1996.
10. Foreyt WJ, Drawe DL: Efficacy of clorsulon and albendazole against *Fascioloides magna* in naturally infected white-tailed deer. J Am Vet Med Assoc 187:1187–1188, 1985.
11. Gibbs HC: Mechanisms of survival of nematode parasites with emphasis on hypobiosis. Vet Parasitol 11:25–48, 1982.
12. Gill IG, Overend DJ, Barnes LS: Parasitism in a rusa deer herd grazing irrigated pasture. Aust Vet J 63:97–98, 1986.
13. Griffin JFT, Buchan GS, Cross JP, et al: Ancillary tests in epidemiological investigations of tuberculosis in deer. Proceedings of the Deer Course for Veterinarians, University of Otago, Dunedin, New Zealand, pp 52–59, July, 1990.
14. Griffin JFT, Rodgers CR, Cross JP: Blood testing for diagnosis of TB within a national control programme. Proceedings of the Deer Course for Veterinarians, University of Otago, Dunedin, New Zealand, pp 55–65, July, 1988.
15. Haigh JC: Game farming with an emphasis on North America. *In* Fowler ME (ed): Zoo and Wild Animal Medicine Current Therapy 3. Philadelphia, WB Saunders, pp 87–100, 1993.
16. Harwell G, Robinson RM, Hughes DM, et al: Texas game ranching: overview of a new industry. Proceedings of the First International Conference on Zoological and Avian Medicine, Oahu, HI, pp 435–445, 1987.
17. Herd RP: Control strategies for ostertagiasis. Vet Parasitol 27:111–123, 1988.
18. Hoff GL, Griner LA, Trainer DO: Bluetongue virus in exotic ruminants. J Am Vet Med Assoc 163:565–567, 1973.
19. Isaza R, Courtney CH, Kollias GV: Survey of parasite control programs used in captive wild ruminants. Zoo Biol 9:385–392, 1990.
20. Isaza R, Courtney CH, Neal FC: Benzimidazole-resistant *Haemonchus contortus* in a roan antelope *Hippotragus equinus*. J Zoo Anim Med 18:96–97, 1987.
21. Janssen DL: Efficacy of fenbendazole for endoparasite control in large herds of nondomestic ruminants. J Am Vet Med Assoc 187:1189–1190, 1985.
22. Jensen JM, Craig TM: Disease and parasite surveillance of a herd of scimitar-horned oryx using domestic sheep as sentinel animals. Proceedings of the Joint Conference of AAZV/WDA/AAWV, Pittsburgh, PA, pp 129–131, 1995.
23. Mangold BJ, Raphael BL, Cook RA, et al: Detection of circulating mycobacterial antigens in *Mycobacterium paratuberculosis*-infected nondomestic ruminants. Proceedings of the Joint Conference of AAZV/WDA/AAWV, Pittsburgh, PA, pp 132–134, 1995.
24. Marley SE, Knapp SE, Rognlie MC, et al: Efficacy of ivermectin pour-on against *Ostertagia ostertagi* infection and residues in the American bison, *Bison bison*. J Wildl Dis 31:62–65, 1995.
25. Mason PC: Biology and control of lungworm in red deer. N Z J Agriculture 140(4):42–43, 1980.
26. McKellar QA: Strategic use of anthelmintics for parasitic nematodes in cattle and sheep. Vet Rec 123:483–487, 1988.
26a. Melde JM, Conner JR, Stuth JW, et al: Exotic Ungulate Production: Summary of Survey Results. College Station, TX, Texas Agricultural Experiment Station, pp 9–10, 1992.
27. Mertins JW, Schlater JL, Corn JL: Ectoparasites of the blackbuck antelope (*Antilope cervicapra*). J Wildl Dis 28:481–484, 1992.
28. Miller DX, Collins MT, Smith BB: Johne's disease in camelids: an emerging disease? Proceedings of the Annual Meeting of the American Association of Zoo Veterinarians, Puerto Vallarta, Mexico, pp 476–482, 1996.
29. Mungall EL, Sheffield WJ: Exotics on the Range—The Texas Example. College Station, TX, Texas A & M University Press, 1994.
30. Nichols DK, Montali RJ, Phillips LD, et al: *Parelaphostrongylus tenuis* in captive reindeer and sable antelope. J Am Vet Assoc 188:619–621, 1986.
31. Qureshi T, Davis DS, Drawe DL: Use of albendazole in feed to control *Fascioloides magna* infections in captive white-tailed deer (*Odocoileus virginianus*). J Wildl Dis 26:231–235, 1990.
32. Qureshi T, Craig TM, Drawe DL, et al: Efficacy of triclabendazole against fascioloidiasis (*Fascioloides magna*) in naturally infected white-tailed deer (*Odocoileus virginianus*). J Wildl Dis 25:378–383, 1989.
33. Richardson ML, Demarais S: Parasites and condition of coexisting populations of white-tailed deer and exotic deer in south-central Texas. J Wildl Dis 28:485–489, 1992.
34. Robinson RM, Jones LP, Galvin TJ, et al: Elaeophorosis in sika deer in Texas. J Wildl Dis 14:137–141, 1978.
35. Tessaro SV: Review of the diseases, parasites and miscellaneous pathological conditions of North American bison. Can Vet J 30:416–422, 1989.
36. Thomas RJ: The ecological basis of parasite control: nematodes. Vet Parasitol 11:9–24, 1982.

CHAPTER 87

Designing a Trichostrongyloid Parasite Control Program for Captive Exotic Ruminants

RAMIRO ISAZA

GEORGE V. KOLLIAS

Trichostrongyloid parasites, including *Haemonchus, Camelostrongylus, Cooperia, Ostertagia, Trichostrongylus,* and *Nematodirus* species, are a significant cause of morbidity and mortality in zoological collections.[3, 12] As a consequence, many collections use anthelmintics as the primary means of parasite control. Despite the common use of these drugs and the recognized need for routine parasite control, few reports directly address the subject of designing a parasite control program for exotic ungulates. Courtney and Kollias[6] described parasite control methods used for domestic ungulates and the possibilities of applying these techniques to exotic collections. Boyce and coworkers[3] and Mikolon and coworkers[15] subsequently applied some of these control principles and evaluated their effects in a large collection of exotic ungulates.

When designing a parasite control program it is important to realize that each collection is unique. Differences in the predominant parasite species affecting a given collection, as well as differences in climate, determine the parasite control program to be implemented. Management related factors include the variety of species of ungulates in the collection, the number of animals in each enclosure, and the nutrition of the animals. These factors may affect the level of parasitism to the point that two collections in geographically similar locations may require completely different parasite control programs. Therefore, specific recommendations for anthelmintics, dosage frequency, and parasite surveillance will not be discussed in this chapter.

Reviews have been published on the use of anthelmintics and the design of parasite control programs for domestic ungulates.[5, 17] This chapter reviews the basic principles relating to animal parasitism that are essential in designing a parasite control program, including the steps needed to design programs for collections with low, medium, and high parasite infection rates.

BASIC PRINCIPLES

Epidemiology of Trichostrongyloid Parasites

In designing an effective parasite control program, an understanding of the life cycle and epidemiology of trichostrongyloid parasites is needed. The life cycle of *Haemonchus contortus* is used to illustrate the typical trichostrongyloid parasite; detailed descriptions of specific life cycles can be found elsewhere.[1, 7] The adult *H. contortus* lives in the abomasum of the host where it feeds off blood, ultimately causing anemia in the host. Eggs produced by the adults are subsequently passed in the host's feces, where they hatch into first-stage larvae; they complete two more molts before becoming the infective third-stage larvae (L3). The L3 larvae are susceptible to climatic extremes, but they may survive on the pasture for several months until they are ingested by the host. Once ingested, they undergo another molt within the gastrointestinal tract to become the fourth-stage larvae; they can either develop into egg-laying adults or remain dormant in the host's tissue as arrested L4 (hypobiosis). The arrested larvae remain dormant for prolonged periods and thus are protected from adverse climatic conditions that kill the L3 on the pasture.

Although the life cycle of trichostrongyloid parasites appears to remain constant throughout the year, most parasite species exhibit significant fluctuations in the population with changes in environmental conditions. Differences in the weather can be used to determine the weak point in the parasite life cycle in different geographic locations. In northern climates, the cold temperatures prevent the development and survival of infective L3 larvae through the winter. In contrast, summer heat limits the survival of larvae in warmer climates. In arid environments, the seasonal variation in rainfall may become the most important climatic factor affecting survival of the infective larvae. Although climatic patterns can be used to predict parasite populations, determination of the actual epidemiology in a given collection must be achieved by serial pasture larval counts.

Types of Parasite Control Programs

There are three basic types of parasite control programs. Opportunistic treatment programs involve the use of anthelmintics only when fecal egg counts or necropsy results indicate parasite infections are occurring in the collection. In this type of program, the anthelmintics are used sporadically, so there is no attempt to suppress the underlying parasite population.

Suppressive treatment programs involve the use of anthelmintics on a regular schedule and at specific time intervals. These programs are aimed at reducing the number of adult parasites in the host and, by doing so, keeping the infection at a subclinical level.

Strategic or tactical treatment programs are based on an understanding of parasite epidemiology to determine the most efficacious use of anthelmintics. The rationale of strategic anthelmintic use is to decrease the adult parasite population at critical times of the year, thus limiting the number of infective L3 larvae in the enclosure. In this type of program, several anthelmintic treatments, in rapid succession, may be given during a particular season and no treatments may be given in subsequent seasons.

Anthelmintic Resistance

Anthelmintic resistance has been defined as a "heritable change in the ability of individual parasites to survive the recommended therapeutic dose of an anthelmintic drug."[16] This becomes evident when previously effective anthelmintic treatments fail to prevent clinical disease. Resistance to all classes of anthelmintics has been reported in domestic animals, and resistance to benzimidazoles has been documented in exotic ungulates.[10, 11] Recommendations for limiting the development of anthelmintic resistance include reducing the use of anthelmintics, ensuring correct application of the anthelmintics, and rotating anthelmintic medications.[4] Many of the most common parasite control practices used in exotic ungulate collections are similar to those that have led to resistance in domestic ungulates.[9] When designing a parasite control program, it must be assumed that development of anthelmintic resistance may occur; overuse of anthelmintics is probably the most important factor in development of resistance.

Identification of Nonparasitic Diseases

Nonparasite-related factors that may be influencing the health of the herd should be investigated. Steps taken to improve nutrition and overall health of the herd decrease the effects of parasitism in the collection. For example, poorly nourished animals tend to show more apparent clinical illness than well-nourished animals exposed to the same parasite loads. Similarly, infectious diseases in the herd should be considered; malabsorption associated with Johne's disease, causing weight loss and diarrhea, may be confused with clinical evidence of parasitic disease and potentiate the effects of parasitism.

Management Considerations in an Integrated Parasite Control Program

Historically, anthelmintics have been used as the principal tool for parasite control in exotic ungulate collections and other methods of decreasing parasite transmission have been largely ignored. Management decisions can both directly and indirectly influence parasite infection rates, and an integrated parasite control program that considers management factors along with anthelmintic use is more effective for parasite control than drugs alone.

A popular management tool used in domestic ruminant animals is pasture rotation in a "treat and move" method. In this system, the susceptible animals are given anthelmintics and then moved to a new pasture. The contaminated pasture is then left ungrazed for a period of time, allowing the infective larvae to die off. By using continual pasture rotation, the herd is not exposed to larval contaminated pastures and consequently there is a decreased need for anthelmintics. Although this is a simple method of decreasing larval contamination in the pasture, the limitations of exhibit space in most exotic ruminant collections make this an impractical strategy.

Another means of decreasing the larval concentration in the pasture is by changing the exhibit substrate. Parasite eggs survive best in warm, moist, protected areas, so survival time on sand, clay, and concrete is shortened because of heat exposure, desiccation, and direct sunlight. In a collection where parasites are a major problem, changing the substrate of the exhibit from a grass pasture to clay or dirt may greatly decrease the parasite population. Conversely, irrigation of an exhibit to provide a more lush grass substrate can result in increased numbers of infective larvae.

Pasture or exhibit hygiene can be an important parasite control tool. The number of infective larvae on the pasture can be decreased by regular removal of the feces from the pasture.[8] Manual removal of the feces is impractical in large exhibits or very large collections, but it is often a viable alternative in small exhibits. In large collections, pasture vacuuming machines, designed for horse pastures, may be considered as a method of providing pasture hygiene.[8]

The number of animals in an enclosure is an important factor in determining the concentration of infective larvae on the pasture. Often, exotic ruminant collections have high stocking rates when compared to domestic ungulates. Removal of some of the animals from an exhibit can often help to reduce parasite exposure.

In domestic ungulates, species differences in susceptibility to parasitic disease have been well documented.

Goats appear to have the weakest immunity, followed by sheep and cattle.[13] Although never documented, some species of exotic ungulates are suspected of being more susceptible to parasites than others. Some collection managers have anecdotally observed that desert-adapted antelope species appear to be more susceptible to parasitic infections than other antelope. Given this concern, segregation of the susceptible species should be considered, allowing the susceptible animals to receive more intense treatment or to be removed from the collection.

Maintaining good quarantine protocols is a valuable tool for preventing the introduction of new parasite species or parasite strains into the collection. Ideally, new animals should test negative for parasites before shipment. Once at the new facility, multiple fecal tests should be performed during the quarantine process. Consideration should be given to routine treatment of all animals for parasites during the quarantine period, regardless of the fecal examination results.

STEPS IN DESIGNING A PARASITE CONTROL PROGRAM

Determine the Important Parasite Species

An exotic ungulate herd may be host to a variety of parasite species, only a small number of which may be of clinical significance. Although only trichostrongyloid parasites are discussed here, other parasitic infections should be identified and controlled in the population. To determine the clinically important trichostrongyloid parasite species in the collection, a series of comprehensive fecal examinations and larval cultures should be performed on a significant portion of the ungulate population. The collection manager should also review previous necropsy reports and clinical records from the collection, paying particular attention to parasite-related diseases. Previous parasite control programs should also be carefully reviewed. Finally, during this investigational phase, there should be a necropsy protocol that includes parasite collection and definitive identification and quantitative measurements of any parasites identified. When the aforementioned information is gathered, the collection manager should be able to determine the most important parasite species in the collection, as well as the magnitude of the parasite problem.

Select an Anthelmintic

Descriptions of available anthelmintics and recommended dosages have been published elsewhere.[5] The modern anthelmintics effective against trichostrongyloid parasites can be grouped into four classes: (1) the benzimidazoles and probenzimidazoles, (2) the macrolide endectocides (ivermectin, moxidectin, and doramectin), (3) the membrane depolarizers that include both imidothiazoles (levamisole) and the tetrahydropyrimidines (pyrantel and morantel), and (4) the organophosphates. Drug selections should be based on practical considerations such as host species, drug availability, antiparasitic spectrum, relative toxicity, palatability, volume of dosage, and route of administration. Once a prospective drug is selected, its effectiveness should be tested using the fecal egg count reduction test. In this test, feces from a small group of animals is collected before and 14 days after anthelmintic treatment. Both samples are tested using a quantitative fecal examination and compared. To consider an anthelmintic efficacious, fecal egg reduction should be at least 90%.[14] Routine testing of drugs before use in the overall control program not only decreases the use of ineffective drugs but also tests the safety of the selected dose; it can be used as a method for detection of development of anthelmintic resistance.

Select the Anthelmintic Dosage

Most of the currently available anthelmintics have a wide margin of safety, and the common practice of using dosages recommended for domestic ungulates in exotic species has not been associated with overt toxicity. Ideally, dosage recommendations should be made from clinical trials in exotic ruminant species; however, such studies are limited, forcing the extrapolation of data from dosages meant for domestic animals. These dosages may be based on the false assumption that the pharmacokinetics between ruminant species are similar. This was not the case when the pharmacokinetics of oxfendazole was compared between sheep and goats.[2] Anthelmintic dosages formulated for domestic animals should therefore be used with some degree of caution in exotic ungulates.

Determine the Optimal Route of Administration

In drugs marketed for use in domestic animals, the assumption is made that the animals can be dosed individually and accurately at regular intervals. However, most exotic ruminant animals cannot be handled on an individual or regular basis. Treatment programs requiring individual manipulation of the animals via immobilization or physical restraint are often associated with injuries to the animals. As a result, oral drenches or pour-on applications of anthelmintics are impractical. Injectable anthelmintics can be given to unrestrained animals with projectile darts; however, a parasite control program based on regular darting is impractical for most large herds.

Given the difficulties of individual dosing, the most common method of anthelmintic administration in exotic ungulate collections is by placing the drug in or on the feed.[9] Anthelmintics can be "top dressed" onto the feed or commercially milled into the diet. The advantages of top dressing are that it is simple and inexpensive, and it allows for variation of the dosage. The disadvantages are that drugs given by this method are often distributed unevenly in the food, the palatability of the mixtures may be poor, and dominant animals may eat more than their share, whereas the subordinate animals may be underdosed. The advantages of custom milling are that milled products offer a better distribution of the anthelmintic and often are more palatable to the animals, but it is expensive, so this method is often cost prohibitive in all but the largest collections.

Determine the Frequency of Anthelmintic Application and Anthelmintic Rotation

The type of parasite control program (opportunistic, suppressive, or strategic) and the severity of the parasite load are the important factors in determining the frequency of anthelmintic administration. In collections with heavy parasite infections, opportunistic and suppressive treatment programs result in very high treatment frequency. As the frequency is increased, the potential for development of anthelmintic resistance also increases until the anthelmintic program fails. Strategic treatment programs reduce this problem by limiting the number of anthelmintic applications.

Anthelmintic rotation is an important key in decreasing anthelmintic resistance. When selecting a new anthelmintic, it is important to select a drug from a different class because side-resistance within drug classes has been well documented.[4] Most parasite control programs in exotic animal collections use anthelmintics in the benzimidazole and macrolide endectocide classes, suggesting that the occurrence of resistance within these drug classes may become a common problem.[9, 10] Frequency of anthelmintic rotation is controversial, with a wide range of recommendations being made. Because frequent drug rotation has been shown to increase selection for anthelmintic resistance, current recommendations in domestic animals involve the use of an effective drug for a full year, then selection of a new drug from a different class the following year.[4, 7]

Evaluate the Parasite Control Program

The final step in designing a parasite control program is surveillance of the herd to monitor the effectiveness of the implemented program. The primary method of surveillance consists of performing regular fecal examinations from the herd. In most situations, quantitative flotation tests, such as the MacMaster's technique, are preferred over simple fecal flotation tests. These quantitative data can be used to measure relative changes in fecal egg production over time. Ideally, every animal in the collection is routinely tested; in large collections, however, this may be impractical. In these situations, a random sampling from a portion of the population is often used for surveillance. In conjunction with the fecal sampling program, necropsies should be performed on all dead herd members. This is a method of measuring both the effectiveness of the program and of periodically monitoring that the primary pathogenic parasite species have not changed.

Detection of decreasing program effectiveness or failure necessitates a reevaluation of the entire program. Although anthelmintic resistance is often considered first, other factors such as inappropriate drug dosage or application, rapid reinfection due to heavy pasture contamination, or host-related problems should first be corrected. If anthelmintic resistance is suspected, a fecal egg count reduction test may be the simplest method for confirming resistance.

EXAMPLES OF PARASITE CONTROL PROGRAMS BASED ON PARASITE LOADS

Light Parasite Load

In some collections, parasite infection and clinical disease is rare. In these situations, the most important aspect of the parasite control program is establishment of a surveillance program for detection of any parasitic infections. A typical program consists of periodic (semiannual) fecal flotation tests, with anthelmintic treatment being given only when infections are detected. Management considerations should be focused on identifying factors in the collection that are responsible for the low parasite population and preservation of those favorable conditions. An important component of this program is a strict quarantine protocol that is designed to limit the introduction of new strains or species of parasites to the herd.

Moderate Parasite Load

In collections with moderate parasite loads, parasitic infection is common, but clinical disease is relatively rare. In this situation, the goal of the parasite control program is to minimize the occurrence of clinical disease. Generally, anthelmintics are administered in a suppressive type program. An emphasis should be on a surveillance program that monitors the relative parasite population over time as well as the effects of the anthelmintic treatments. Quantitative fecal examinations collected at regular intervals are performed, and data should be reviewed regularly to help determine whether the parasite population is changing. The aim of management should be to decrease factors that tend to promote parasite transmission.

Severe Parasite Load

In a heavy parasite load in which the incidence of clinical disease is common, there is an absolute need for anthelmintic treatments to prevent animal death. Significant resources are often needed to design and implement a parasite control program, and the services of a parasitologist may be cost effective in these instances. A consultant can help with definitive identification of the pathogenic parasite species, provide advanced studies of epidemiologic factors, and evaluate the climatic factors that impact parasite transmission in the collection. The routine use of quantitative fecal flotation tests is limited in herds with severe parasite loads because most animals consistently shed large numbers of parasites in their feces. Efforts should instead be aimed at determining the epidemiology of the parasite population and implementing a strategic parasite control program.

Because of the potential limitations of overreliance on anthelmintics, attention should be given to management practices that help limit the parasite population. In addition to pasture hygiene and reducing host stocking rates, aggressive steps should also be considered. Elimination of grass from enclosures greatly facilitates pasture hygiene, but it may not be done for aesthetic reasons. Segregation of the collection into groups of animals with similar sensitivity to parasitic infections may also be a viable tool. In some collections, a particular species in a mixed species herd may be consistently affected by severe parasitism; removal of the susceptible animals from the herd may be necessary.

REFERENCES

 1. Anderson N, Dash KM, Donald AD, et al: Epidemiology and control of nematode infections. *In* Donald AD, Southcott WH, Dineen JD (eds): The Epidemiology and Control of Gastrointestinal Parasites of Sheep in Australia. Melbourne, Commonwealth Scientific Industrial Research Organization, Division of Animal Health, pp 24–51, 1978.
 2. Bogan J, Benoit E, Delatour P: Pharmacokinetics of oxfendazole in goats, a comparison with sheep. J Vet Pharmacol Therap 10:305–309, 1987.
 3. Boyce W, Allen J, Himmelwright C, et al: Implementation and evaluation of a strategic parasite control program for captive exotic ungulates. J Am Vet Med Assoc 198:1972–1976, 1991.
 4. Coles GC: Strategies for control of anthelmintic-resistant nematodes for ruminants. J Am Vet Med Assoc 192:330–334, 1988.
 5. Corwin RM: Anthelmintic therapy. *In* Howard JL (ed): Current Veterinary Therapy 3, Food Animal Practice. Philadelphia, WB Saunders, pp 47–51, 1993.
 6. Courtney CH, Kollias GV: Management concepts for control of endoparasitism in exotic ungulates. Avian/Exotic Practice 2:13–17, 1985.
 7. Craig TM: Epidemiology and control of gastrointestinal nematodes and cestodes in small ruminants. Vet Clin North Am Food Anim Pract 2:367–372, 1986.
 8. Herd RP: Equine parasite control—solutions to anthelmintic associated problems. Equine Vet Educ 2:86–91, 1990.
 9. Isaza R, Courtney CH, Kollias GV: Survey of parasite control programs in captive wild ruminants. Zoo Biol 9:385–392, 1990.
10. Isaza R, Courtney CH, Kollias GV: The prevalence of benzimidazole-resistant trichostrongyloid nematodes in antelope collections in Florida. J Zoo Wildl Med 26:260–264, 1995.
11. Isaza R, Courtney CH, Neal FC: Benzimidazole resistant Haemonchus contortus in roan antelope (*Hippotragus equinus*). J Zoo Anim Med 18:96–97, 1987.
12. Kaneene JB, Taylor RF, Sikarskie JG, et al: Disease patterns in the Detroit Zoo: a study of the mammalian population from 1973 through 1983. J Am Vet Med Assoc 187:1166–1169, 1985.
13. Le Jambre LF, Royal WM: A comparison of worm burdens in grazing Merino sheep and Angora goats. Aust Vet J 52:181–183, 1976.
14. McKenna PB: The detection of anthelmintic resistance by the fecal egg count reduction test: an examination of some of the factors affecting performance and interpretation. N Z Vet J 38:142–147, 1990.
15. Mikolon AB, Boyce WM, Allen, et al: Epidemiology and control of nematode parasites in a collection of captive exotic ungulates. J Zoo Anim Med 25:500–510, 1994.
16. Taylor MA, Hunt KR: Anthelminthic drug resistance in the United Kingdom. Vet Rec 125:143–147, 1989.
17. Uhlinger CA, Brumbaugh GW: Parasite control programs. *In* Smith BP (ed): Large Animal Internal Medicine. St. Louis, CV Mosby, pp 1513–1528, 1990.

CHAPTER 88

Embryo Transfer and Semen Technology from Cattle Applied to Nondomestic Artiodactylids

C. EARLE POPE

NAIDA M. LOSKUTOFF

In both humans and domestic livestock, tremendous advances have been made in the development and application of assisted reproductive biotechnology.[9] The principal components of this technology are artificial insemination (AI) and embryo transfer, but maximal utility requires the incorporation of auxiliary techniques such as manipulation and control of the ovarian cycle and ovulation, stimulation of follicular development, gamete cryopreservation, and in vitro embryo production methods. The potential value of applying such technology to the preservation of endangered nondomestic artiodactylids is enormous. This chapter discusses the current status of AI and in vivo production of embryos as well as the emerging field of in vitro embryogenesis, including in vitro oocyte maturation, fertilization, and culture.

ESTROUS CYCLE SYNCHRONIZATION

An essential element of assisted reproduction biotechnology is the use of exogenous hormones to control the timing of the estrous cycle and ovulation. Factors necessary for successful cycle regulation in domestic livestock are well defined and are based on intensive management practices that maximize productivity. In contrast, the combination of a more extensive management and lack of knowledge of reproductive processes in nondomestic artiodactylids presents unique challenges in implementing these protocols. In general, cycle control is based on (1) treatment with a luteolytic dose of prostaglandin f$_2\alpha$ (or analogs), (2) progestogen administration, or (3) a combination of the two. The prostaglandin method is attractive because it involves minimal treatment and stress; however, progestogens are more effective in seasonally polyestrous species,[23, 44, 49] especially if the effort includes modification of the breeding season.

Because of the economic importance of cervids, methods of estrous cycle control have been most thoroughly studied in them. The situation is unique because these farmed cervids are being managed as domestic animals. Therefore, they are conditioned to the handling required for using progestogens as vaginal pessaries incorporating medroxyprogesterone acetate (MAP), as intravaginal controlled internal releasing devices (CIDR) containing progesterone, or as ear implants of norgestomet. The most widely used progestogen delivery system is insertion of CIDR devices[29] for 11 to 12 days in red deer (*Cervus elaphus*)[6] and the wapiti[43] or for 14 days in fallow deer (*Dama dama*)[70] and the endangered Eld's deer (*Cervus eldi thamin*).[68]

Only two New World species of Camelidae are considered as nondomestic, the guanaco (*Lama guanicoe*) and vicuna (*Lama vicugna*). New world camelids are induced ovulators with nonseasonal ovarian activity, and ovulation can be synchronized by mating, injection of human chorionic gonadotropin (hCG), or gonadotropin-releasing hormone (GnRH), alone or after norgestomet implantation.[13, 20]

Except in the North American bison (*Bison bison*), minimal information is available on artificial control of the reproductive cycle of nondomestic Bovidae, in part because there is no economic incentive. Accordingly, efforts at applying artificial breeding methods to bison have shown that both prostaglandins and norgestomet ear implants can be used for estrous synchronization during the breeding season.[23] Comparing the two methods in Wood bison (*Bison bison athabascae*) revealed that most were in behavioral estrus within 5 days, but frequently failed to ovulate.[66]

In comparison, most scimitar-horned oryxes (*Oryx dammah*) ovulated following gonadotropin treatment and estrous synchronization using either prostaglandin injections or MAP pessary treatment, but fewer than half showed overt signs of estrus.[83] The use of the CIDR intravaginal device containing the quantity of progesterone (P$_4$, 0.375 g) used in small domestic ungulates failed to maintain blood P$_4$ at levels similar to that produced by the corpus luteum in the scimitar-horned oryx.[71] Previously, AI was performed successfully in scimitar-horned oryxes after insertion of CIDR devices containing the same quantity of P$_4$ for 13 days.[35] For cycle synchronization in suni (*Neotragus moschtus zeluensis*), one of the smallest antelope, 15-day insertions of vaginal sponges containing 20 mg MAP with replacement of the first one after 8 days with a fresh sponge was more effective than insertion of a single sponge for 11 days.[61] In wild cattle, two prostaglandin injections at an 11-day interval resulted in consistent occurrence of ovulation within 2 to 4 days after the second injection in the banteng (*Bos javanicus*),[3] but, in gaur (*Bos gaurus*), estrus was observed in only half of the cows within 5 days.[37] Prostaglandins were also used to synchronize estrus in superovulated gaur donor cows[77, 88] with only partial success.

Efforts at interspecies embryo transfer to domestic goats (*Capra hircus*) or sheep (*Ovis aries*) from nondomestic species have used some form of progestogen, as a subcutaneous Silastic implant of progesterone in mouflon (*Ovis musimon*),[18] MAP vaginal pessaries in Dall's sheep (*Ovis dalli dalli*, 60 mg),[17] vaginal CIDR devices in Armenian red sheep (*Ovis orientalis*),[32] or fluorogestone acetate (FGA, 45 mg) sponges in Spanish Ibex (*Capra pyrenaica*).[31]

Synchronization of estrus in reticulated giraffes (*Giraffa camelopardalis reticulate*) has been achieved following insertion, while the animal is manually restrained, of a progesterone-releasing intravaginal device for 12 days, oral administration of altrenogest for 10 days,[19] or multiple injections of prostaglandin at 9-day intervals.[33]

ARTIFICIAL INSEMINATION

AI is a relatively simple assisted reproduction technique but prerequisites to successful application include characterization of the reproductive cycle and development of methods of estrous cycle control. A particularly good example of this is the success with which AI has been implemented for commercial production of red deer and fallow deer. Offspring have also been obtained from AI with fresh or frozen/thawed semen in other Cervidae, including silka deer (*Cervus nippon*),[94] reindeer (*Rangifer tarandus*),[24] chital deer (*Axis axis*),[72] and white-tailed deer (*Odocoileus virginianus*).[42, 65] A low dose of equine chorionic gonadotropin (eCG) given at progestogen withdrawal in red deer improves synchrony of estrus and ovulation, and improves subsequent fertility.[30] Semen is deposited laparoscopically at a fixed time ranging from 55 (red deer),[43] 60 (sika deer),[94] or 65 to 70 hours (fallow deer)[5] after progestogen withdrawal, with conception rates ranging from 51% to 80%. The techniques were used successfully in endangered Eld's deer to produce offspring following insemination with frozen/thawed spermatozoa at 70 hours after CIDR removal.[68]

As additional information about the reproductive

cycles of nondomestic Bovidae is gained, the species-specific differences must be incorporated into these procedures. For example, the estrous cycle of the scimitar-horned oryx was recently reported to be 24.4 days,[85] compared to the 21-day estrous cycle of domestic cattle. In contrast, the 16.9-day estrous cycle of the blackbuck (*Antilope cervicapra*)[46] is approximately half the length of the addax (*Addax nasomaculatus*) estrous cycle (32.3 days).[4] Captive management systems are seldom conducive to sample collection and physical restraint; therefore, procedures such as AI frequently must be done under general anesthesia. However, gaur and addax calves have been born after transcervical AI with frozen/thawed semen during mechanical[37] or manual[21] restraint, respectively. Transvaginal intrauterine insemination of 11 anesthetized blackbuck females with fresh (n = 8) or frozen/thawed (n = 3) semen produced six calves, including one from frozen semen.[46] Transcervical insemination of four mature scimitar-horned oryx females with frozen/thawed semen while under anesthesia at 54 hours after removal of CIDR devices resulted in the birth of two calves.[35] Laparoscopic intrauterine insemination of suni antelope with fresh or frozen/thawed semen (two each) following progestogen sponge removal was not successful, but a pregnancy was diagnosed after transcervical insemination of two females with frozen/thawed semen.[79] AI with fresh semen has been successfully applied in Speke's gazelle (*Gazella spekei*).[11]

An offspring was born to a reticulated giraffe after AI with extended semen stored at 4°C. Five intracervical inseminations were done every 12 hours during physical restraint in a hydraulic chute, beginning 12 hours after the last prostaglandin injection.[33]

Primarily because of problems associated with semen collection and storage, AI has not been widely used in New World camelids. Offspring have been obtained using fresh, but not frozen/thawed, semen.[20] Semen can be collected either by electroejaculation or artificial vagina; the latter technique is more desirable because anesthesia is not required and, therefore, is more repeatable.[15, 58]

RECOVERY AND TRANSFER OF IN VIVO DERIVED EMBRYOS

Procedures used for applying embryo technology to nondomestic ungulates are also based on those used in domestic animals; however, they are also complicated by management systems designed for minimal contact. Thus, with the exception of domestically managed Cervidea, it is difficult to attain the required accessibility without compromising the animals and, consequently, the results obtained.[83]

Ovarian Stimulation with Exogenous Gonadotropins

For farmed Cervidae, the most widely used method for hormonal stimulation of follicular development of donor hinds consists of multiple injections of ovine follicle stimulating hormone (oFSH) beginning 72 hours before CIDR device removal and an injection of 100 IU (fallow deer) or 200 IU eCG (red deer) at the first or last oFSH injection. An oFSH dose-response (0.25 to 1.00 units) study in red deer and fallow deer revealed similar ovulatory responses with the optimal number of corpora lutea (CL) in each species produced from the 0.5 unit dose (9.5 ± 6.3 and 9.6 ± 7.5, respectively).[29] However, Pere David's deer (*Elaphurus davidianus*) produced fewer ovulations (3.8 ± 1.2) than red deer (10.8 ± 3.8) after similar treatment.[1] Multiple ovulations were induced in half of the white-tailed deer given 1000 IU eCG after synchronization with MAP pessaries or a midcycle prostaglandin injection.[91]

In reticulated giraffes, eCG administered in doses ranging from 2000 to 4000 IU on day 10 after insertion of progesterone-releasing intravaginal devices for 12 days produced an average of two to three CL.[19]

In the North American bison, several trials have reported an average of 3.6 to 4.2 ovulations after a total of 34 mg porcine FSH (FSH-P) was administered in a decreasing dose for 4 days in conjunction with a norgestomet ear implant.[23] Bison do not adapt to the increased handling required with the multiple injection FSH protocol; therefore, a single injection of eCG has been advocated as a less stressful alternative.

Mouflon ewes (n = 21) injected with 800 to 1200 IU eCG after subcutaneous delivery of progesterone for 14 days responded with an average of 3.6 to 10.3 CL, but no embryos were recovered if more than 1000 IU eCG was used.[18] Similarly, Dall's sheep donors (n = 4) administered 1200 IU eCG during treatment with MAP sponges produced multiple CL, but few transferrable embryos.[17] Subsequently, donors administered 20 mg FSH-P over 3 days starting on day 12 after sponge insertion produced an average of 4.6 CL and most embryos recovered were transferable. Four Armenian red sheep embryo donors given a total of 22.5 mg FSH-P for 3 days starting on day 9 after intravaginal CIDR device insertion produced a total of 37 ovulations, although CL in two females were prematurely regressing at 5 days after breeding.[32] To avoid multiple injections, Spanish ibexes were subcutaneously implanted with micro-osmotic pumps containing 9 mg oFSH 2 days before removal of progestogen sponges. One group was naturally mated and the others were laparoscopically inseminated with frozen semen. Although the average ovulation rate was similar for each group, 5.9 and 5.2, respectively, fertilization and embryo recovery rates were higher following natural mating.

Attempts at superovulation in the gaur have not resulted in a consistently satisfactory ovarian response nor in estrus induction necessary for natural breeding. In one study, four females were administered an injection of 2000 or 2500 IU eCG or 50 mg FSH-P over 5 days. Embryos were only recovered on two occasions from one female, five blastocysts from the first and eight blastocysts from 12 embryos on the second recovery.[88] Ova/embryos were recovered from 5 of 10 uterine flushes in three females after treatment with 45 to 60 mg FSH-P over 5 days.[76] In the nonsuccessful attempts,

CL were not palpable and the failure was attributed to lack of ovarian response.

Most antelope ovarian stimulation trials have involved scimitar-horned oryx, bongo *(Tragelaphus eurycerus)*, and common eland *(Tragelaphus oryx)*. Of 33 scimitar-horned oryxes administered eCG (2000 IU) or FSH-P (50 mg total over 5 days), 25 responded with at least 1 CL. The average ovulation rate was higher after FSH treatment (4.6) than after eCG (2.7). In a second trial using the same females, most of them ovulated but there was no difference in CL between the two gonadotropins, despite doubling the eCG dose. Bongo and eland females administered eCG produced fewer CL (1.4 and 1.0, respectively) than after treatment with multiple FSH injections (4.6 and 10.6, respectively).[83] Ovulatory responses as measured by number of ova/embryos nonsurgically recovered from mated females of four species of antelope following treatment with FSH or eCG (eland only) are outlined in Table 88–1 (Pope and Dresser, unpublished data). More ova/embryos were recovered from the larger species (eland and bongo) than the smaller ones. In suni antelope, average ovulation rate was slightly higher when a total of 3.75 mg FSH-P was injected over 3 days after a 15-day estrous synchronization protocol than after 2.25 to 8.25 mg doses of FSH-P for 4 days after 11-day use of intravaginal sponges, 6.6 and 1.7 to 5.5, respectively.[61]

Embryo Recovery and Transfer

The method of embryo recovery and transfer is largely dictated by animal size and reproductive tract anatomy, particularly the cervix. The techniques used for transcervical uterine access in domestic cattle can be applied to wild cattle, bison, camelids, and the larger species of African antelope; however, other approaches or equipment are usually required for Cervidae and small Bovidae. Either laparoscopy or transcervical passage of small, stiff catheters with visual or digital guidance[53] can be used to avoid surgical exteriorization of the uterus.

In farmed Cervidae, embryo recovery and pregnancy rates are comparable to those obtained in domestic cattle, although embryo recovery requires laparotomy and transfers are done by laparotomy or laparoscopy. Embryo recovery rates range from 30% to less than 50% in fallow deer[48, 69] to 65% in red deer.[29] Large-scale transfer of fresh and frozen red deer embryos has resulted in pregnancy rates of 61% to 70%.[22, 29] Whether transferred to the oviduct on day 3 or to the uterus on day 6,[48] pregnancy rates following transfer of fresh embryos in fallow deer were approximately 55%. When clenbuterol was administered to fallow deer recipients to reduce uterine turgidity, the pregnancy rate after laparoscopic transfer was 57% for fresh and 26% for frozen embryos.[69]

The first nondomestic artiodactylid births from interspecies embryo transfers were mouflon lambs born to domestic sheep recipients.[18] Ten mouflon embryos at the 4-cell to 32-cell stages were transferred on day 3 to the uterus of 10 domestic sheep. Of the five that were at least 16-cell embryos, three resulted in pregnancy and two went to term. Intraspecific embryo transfer has been successful in Dall's sheep but, of nine domestic ewes pregnant at 18 days after receiving Dall's sheep embryos, none were able to maintain the pregnancy to term.[17] The only interspecific pregnancies occurred in domestic ewes that had previously been recipients of Dall's sheep embryos. Armenian red sheep lambs were born after laparoscopic uterine transfer of in vivo and in vitro derived embryos to Rambouillet ewes.[32]

Embryo transfer has been successfully demonstrated in several species of nondomestic Bovidae, albeit with less efficiency than in their domestic counterparts. There is interest in its commercial application in bison, but pregnancy and calving rates are usually lower than in domestic cattle.[23] Bison producers would prefer to transfer bison embryos into domestic cow recipients. A

TABLE 88–1. Nonsurgical Embryo Recovery in Four Species of Antelope by the Center for Reproduction of Endangered Wildlife, Cincinnati Zoological and Botanical Garden, Cincinnati, Ohio, 1982–1993

Species	Location	Gonadotropin* Type/Dose	No. of Donors	Embryo Recoveries Total†	Embryo Recoveries Rec emb‡	Ova/Embryos Total	Ova/Embryos Embryos	Embryos Mean	Embryos Range
Bongo	LAZ	FSH/40–50 mg	6	11	7	41	25	1.6	0–6
Eland	CZ	eCG/1800 IU	2	2	2	13	9	4.5	3–6
Eland	CZ	eCG/2500 IU	5	7	3	11	10	1.4	0–6
Eland	CZ	FSH/50 mg	10	22	10	123	86	3.9	0–22
Eland	CMF	FSH/50 mg	6	17	9	76	73	4.3	0–17
Scimitar horned oryx	KI	FSH/30–50 mg	7	25	11	23	19	0.76	0–4
Yellow-backed duiker	CZ	FSH/25–37 mg	4	11	3	5	5	0.45	0–2

LAZ, Los Angeles Zoo; CZ, Cincinnati Zoo; CMF, Cincinnati Mast Farm; KI, King's Island
*Estrous synchronization = 2 prostaglandin (or analog) injections 10–13 days apart
†Total = total embryo recovery procedures.
‡Rec Emb = total number of embryos recovered.

few pregnancies have resulted, but abortions invariably occur by 120 days of gestation.

In banteng and gaur, calves have been produced by interspecies transfer of embryos into domestic cattle (*Bos taurus*) recipients. The first gaur calf was born after induction of parturition at 10 months following transfer by standing laparotomy of four nonsurgically recovered blastocysts. Three recipients were diagnosed as pregnant at 60 days, but two aborted, one at 4 months and the other at 9.5 months after transfer.[88] The second gaur calf was a healthy male born unassisted to a Holstein cow at 10 months of gestation after nonsurgical recovery of three blastocysts and one morula and transcervical transfer to four recipients.[77] Transfer of frozen/thawed gaur embryos into Holstein or gaur recipients has not been successful. Two banteng calves were born from four pregnancies established in domestic heifers after nonsurgical transfer of nine embryos.[93]

Intraspecies embryo transfer has been used successfully to produce calves in four species of antelope—common eland,[54] bongo,[27] scimitar-horned oryx,[78, 84] and suni.[62] Additionally, interspecies transfer of bongo embryos into four common eland recipients resulted in the birth of a live female calf.[27] A summary of the embryo transfer trials conducted in common eland and bongo from 1982–1987 at the Cincinnati Zoo is given in Table 88–2. Common eland calves were born after intraspecies transfer of fresh,[54] frozen/thawed,[25] and demiembryos.[36] Gestation length of common eland calves ranged from 271 to 278 days as compared to 285 and 290 days for bongo calves after interspecific and intraspecific embryo transfer, respectively.

In the mid-1970s, a South American camelid cria (alpaca, *Lama pacos*) was born after embryo transfer, and commercial interest is dramatically increasing.[20] The first llama (*Lama glama*) offspring was born after two blastocysts, nonsurgically recovered from one of two donors, were nonsurgically transferred to two recipients. One gave birth to a live male cria.[92] In one of the largest trials, after superovulation of llama donors with eCG and induction of ovulation with hCG or GnRH,

the average zygote recovery rate with nonsurgical collection was 1.3 to 2.3.[12] Two crias were born after nonsurgical transfer of 15 embryos to 11 recipients. The pregnancies occurred in recipients induced to ovulate with GnRH, but none were produced in llamas given hCG or progestogen ear implants. The highest pregnancy rate reported to date is five pregnancies, with four carried to term, following transcervical transfer of eight llama and four guanaco embryos to 10 llama recipients.[13] At least one of the births was from interspecies transfer of guanaco embryos to llama recipients.

The first successful interspecies embryo transfer in the *Capra* genus was recently reported.[31] Embryos from the eight-cell stage to compacted morulae were surgically recovered from Spanish Ibex donors. A total of 22 embryos were transferred to 11 domestic goats, and two Spanish Ibex kids were born to two of them. The low pregnancy rate was thought to be due to placental incompatibility.

In miniature Lanya (*Sus scrofa*), an endangered breed of pigs native to Taiwan, embryos were intraspecifically transferred to domestic Duroc and Landrace recipients.[95] Most of the 13 Duroc recipient sows did not return to estrus within 25 days after transfer, but only three farrowed (23%). All six Landrace recipients were diagnosed as pregnant, yet none farrowed. In contrast, when an average of 9.6 Lanya embryos were transferred to six Lanyu recipients, five farrowed an average of 5.3 live piglets per litter.

IN VITRO EMBRYO PRODUCTION

One of the most powerful reproductive technologies currently available for ungulate species is embryo production by in vitro oocyte maturation (IVM) and fertilization (IVF). For domestic livestock, an advantage is a decrease in the generation interval by collecting oocytes from prepubertal animals,[28] overcoming infertility,[59] increasing reproductive potential of pregnant ani-

TABLE 88–2. Embryo Transfer in Bongo and Common Eland Antelope by the Center for Reproduction of Endangered Wildlife, Cincinnati Zoological and Botanical Garden, Cincinnati, Ohio, 1982–1987

Donor Species	Recipient Species	Embryo Type	No. Embryos*	No. Recipients†	No. Calves	Sex	Gestation, Days	Ref.
Eland	Eland	Fresh	3	3	1	Female	271	54
Bongo	Eland	Fresh‡	4	4	1	Female	285	27
Bongo	Bongo	Fresh‡	1	1	1	Female	290	27
Bongo	Eland	Frozen	7§	6	0	—	—	—
Eland	Eland	Frozen[trial 1]	6	6	1‖	Female	274	54
Eland	Eland	Frozen[trial 2]	5	5	1	Female	278	25
Eland	Domestic cow	Fresh	5	5	0	—	—	26
Eland	Eland	Demi¶	10.5 demi	6	1	Male	275	36

*Morvulae/blastocysts
†2× prostaglandin (or analog)
‡9 to 14 hours after recovery
§Fair/poor at recovery
‖Stillborn
¶Bisected

mals,[82] and assisting in propagation of rare or endangered domesticated breeds.[87] For conservation efforts, probably the single most important outcome of this technology is the capacity for salvaging genetic material and producing offspring from animals postmortem.[96] Furthermore, owing to the inconsistent results at in vivo embryo recovery directly from nondomestic ungulates, in vitro embryo production offers the potential for producing more embryos, which is further enhanced by the reduced numbers of viable spermatozoa needed to achieve fertilization in vitro compared to AI or natural breeding.

Spermatozoa Recovery and Cryopreservation

It has been demonstrated that the viability and fertilizing capacity of spermatozoa are maintained for extended periods after death in a variety of ungulate species. Live offspring have been obtained from caudal epididymal spermatozoa recovered 40 hours postmortem in mouflon sheep.[34] As determined by overall progressive spermatozoa motility, viable caudal epididymal spermatozoa were recovered after refrigerating testicles at 4°C for 2 days in Burchell's zebra (*Equus burchelli*), 4 days in red hartebeest (*Alcelaphus buselaphus*) and eland, and up to 5 days in African buffalo (*Syncerus caffer*).[10] Caudal epididymal spermatozoa have been recovered and successfully cryopreserved from several African antelope species,[60, 63] African buffalo,[86] and reticulated giraffes.[50]

Because of the relative infancy of assisted reproductive technology, evidence for the long-term survival of cryopreserved spermatozoa does not exceed 40 years.[57] However, it has been formally estimated that biologic specimens (e.g., embryos and spermatozoa) cryopreserved in liquid nitrogen may remain viable more than 3000 years.[67]

Oocyte Maturation and Fertilization in Vitro

Since offspring were first born after transferring embryos derived from oocytes matured and fertilized in vitro in domestic ruminants (reviewed in reference 14), modifications of these procedures have been applied successfully for producing offspring in nondomestic ungulates, including Armenian red sheep,[32] water buffalo (*Bubalus bubalis*),[64] gaur,[2, 51] red deer,[8] and llamas.[20] In addition, uterine stage embryos have been produced in a variety of African antelope species,[60] African buffalo,[86] klipspringer (*Oreotragus oreotragus*),[80] reindeer,[55] reticulated giraffes,[50] and the wapiti.[75]

Most reports on oocyte maturation in vitro in nondomestic ungulates have described procedures for oocytes recovered postmortem. More recently, techniques have been developed in domestic cattle[74] and goats[40] for transvaginal ultrasound-guided follicular aspiration. These have been successfully applied for the safe and repeatable recovery of oocytes from live donors in several African antelope species and African buffalo,[60] gaur,[2] llamas,[16] and water buffalo.[73]

Effective IVF protocols developed for domestic ruminant animals are generally applicable to an assortment of nondomestic ruminant species. Fertilization by spermatozoa microinjection (reviewed in reference 47) is a relatively new biotechnique that offers considerable promise as a method of enhancing in vitro embryo production by using killed[39] or immature testicular spermatozoa.[38]

Embryo Culture and Development In Vitro

There are excellent reviews on the requirements for oocyte IVM and IVF and culture of preimplantation mammalian embryos.[7, 41, 89] For domestic cattle, commercial units have reported similar results in embryo production efficiencies: development rates from starting oocytes to the morula-blastocyst stages (32 to >100 cells) typically range from 12% to 20%.[52] Pregnancy rates following transfer of in vitro derived embryos have been higher for fresh than for frozen/thawed embryos (45% to 60% versus 30% to 40%).[45, 59]

Although the developmental competency of in vitro produced embryos has been demonstrated by the production of normal calves, in vitro generated embryos clearly differ in many respects from in vivo derived embryos.[45, 81] Comprehensive studies have shown a higher incidence of problems associated with domestic calves[56] and lambs[90] produced from in vitro derived embryos, including abnormally large birth weight, dystocic parturition, perinatal mortality, and congenital abnormalities. Although it is not known what part of the in vitro culture process is responsible for these disturbances, it is certain that continued research with domestic livestock will contribute to improved protocols for minimizing such problems and increasing efficiency of in vitro embryo production.

REFERENCES

1. Argo CMcG, Jabbour HN, Goddard PJ, et al: Superovulation in red deer (*Cervus elaphus*) and Pere David's deer (*Elaphurus davidianus*), and fertilization rates following artificial insemination with Pere David's deer semen. J Reprod Fertil 100:629–636, 1994.
2. Armstrong DL, Looney CR, Lindsey BR, et al: Transvaginal egg retrieval and in vitro embryo production in gaur (*Bos gaurus*) with establishment of interspecies pregnancy [Abstract]. Theriogenology 43:162, 1995.
3. Asa CS: Synchronization of ovulation in banteng (*Bos javanicus*). Proceedings of the Society of Theriogenology, San Diego, CA, pp 351–352, 1991.
4. Asa CS, Houston EW, Fischer MT, et al: Ovulatory cycles and anovulatory periods in the addax (*Addax nasomaculatus*). J Reprod Fertil 107:119–124, 1996.
5. Asher GW, Kraemer DC, Magyar SJ, et al: Intrauterine insemination of farmed fallow deer (*Dama dama*) with frozen-thawed semen via laparoscopy. Theriogenology 34:569–577, 1990.
6. Asher GW, Fisher MW, Fennessy PF, et al: Oestrous synchronization, semen collection and artificial insemination of farmed red deer (*Cervus elaphus*) and fallow deer (*Dama dama*). Anim Reprod Sci 33:241–265, 1993.
7. Bavister BD: Culture of preimplantation embryos: facts and artifacts. Human Reprod Update 1:91–148, 1995.
8. Berg DK, Asher GW, Pugh PA, et al: Pregnancies following the transfer of in vitro matured and fertilized red deer (*Cervus elaphus*) oocytes [Abstract]. Theriogenology 43:166, 1995.
9. Betteridge KJ, Rieger D: Embryo transfer and related techniques in

domestic animals, and their implications for human medicine. Human Reprod 8:147–167, 1993.

10. Bezuidenhout C, Fourie F, Meintjes M, et al: Comparative epididymal sperm cell motility of African ungulate and equid game species stored at 4°C [Abstract]. Theriogenology 43:167, 1995.

11. Boever W, Knox D, Merilan PC, et al: Estrus induction and artificial insemination with successful pregnancy in Speke's gazelle. Proceedings of the 9th International Congress of Animal Reproduction and Artificial Insemination, Madrid, Spain, pp 565–569, 1980.

12. Bourke DA, Adam CL, Kyle CE, et al: Superovulation and embryo transfer in the llama. Proceedings of the 1st International Camel Conference, Newmarket, UK, pp 183–185, 1992.

13. Bourke DA, Kyle CE, McEvoy TG, et al: Superovulatory responses to eCG in llamas (*Lama glama*). Theriogenology 44:255–268, 1995.

14. Brackett BG: In vitro fertilization in farm animals. *In* Lauria A, Gandolfi F (eds): Embryonic Development and Manipulation in Animal Production: Trends in Research and Applications. London, Portland Press, pp 59–76, 1992.

15. Bravo PW: Reproductive physiology of the male camelid. Vet Clin North Am 10:259–264, 1994.

16. Brogliatti GM, Palasz AT, Adams GP: Ultrasound-guided transvaginal follicle aspiration and oocyte collection in llamas (*Lama glama*) [Abstract]. Theriogenology 45:249, 1996.

17. Buckrell BC, Gartley CJ, Mehren KG, et al: Failure to maintain interspecific pregnancy after transfer of Dall's sheep embryos to domestic ewes. J Reprod Fertil 90:387–394, 1990.

18. Bunch TD, Foote WC, Whitaker B: Interspecies ovum transfer to propagate wild sheep. J Wildl Management 41:726–730, 1977.

19. Calle PP, Loskutoff NM, Threlfal WR, et al: Estrous synchronization and superovulation induction in the giraffe. Proceedings of the 1st International Conference on Zoological and Avian Medicine, Turtle Bay, HI, pp 389–390, 1987.

20. Del Campo MR, Del Campo CH, Adams GP, et al: The application of new reproductive technologies to South American camelids. Theriogenology 43:21–30, 1995.

21. Densmore MA, Bowen MJ, Magyar SJ, et al: Artificial insemination with frozen, thawed semen and pregnancy diagnosis in addax (*Addax nasomaculatus*). Zoo Biol 6:21–29, 1987.

22. Dixon TE, Hunter JW, Beatson NS: Pregnancies following the export of frozen red deer embryos from New Zealand to Australia [Abstract]. Theriogenology 35:193, 1991.

23. Dorn CG: Application of reproductive technologies in North American bison (*Bison bison*). Theriogenology 43:13–20, 1995.

24. Dott H, Utsi MNP: Artificial insemination of reindeer (*Rangifer tarandus*). J Zool Lond 170:505–508, 1973.

25. Dresser BL, Kramer L, Dahlausen RD, et al: Cryopreservation followed by successful transfer of African eland antelope (*Tragelaphus oryx*) embryos. Proceedings of the 10th International Congress of Animal Reproduction and Artificial Insemination, Urbana, IL, pp 191–193, 1984.

26. Dresser BL, Kramer L, Pope CE, et al: Superovulation of African eland (*Taurotragus oryx*) and interspecies embryo transfer to Holstein cattle [Abstract]. Theriogenology 17:86, 1982.

27. Dresser BL, Pope CE, Kramer L, et al: Birth of bongo antelope (*Tragelaphus euryceros*) to eland antelope (*Tragelaphus oryx*) and cryopreservation of bongo embryos [Abstract]. Theriogenology 23:190, 1985.

28. Duby RT, Damiani P, Looney CR, et al: Prepubertal calves as oocyte donors: promises and problems. Theriogenology 45:121–130, 1996.

29. Fennessy PF, Asher GW, Beatson NS, et al: Embryo transfer in deer. Theriogenology 41:133–138, 1994.

30. Fennessy PF, CG Mackintosh, GH Shackell: Artificial insemination of farmed red deer (*Cervus elaphus*). Anim Prod 51:613–621, 1989.

31. Fernandez-Arias A, Folch J, Alabart JL, et al: Successful interspecific embryo transfer between Spanish Ibex (*Capra pyrenaica*) and domestic goat (*Capra hircus*) using micro- osmotic pumps for FSH administration [Abstract]. Theriogenology 45:247, 1996.

32. Flores-Foxworth G, Coonrod SA, Moreno JF, et al: Interspecific transfer of IVM IVF-derived red sheep (*Ovis orientalis gmelini*) embryos to domestic sheep (*Ovis aries*). Theriogenology 44:681–690, 1995.

33. Foxworth B, Robeck T, Foxworth G. et al: The successful development of artificial insemination technology in the reticulated giraffe (*Giraffa camelopardalis reticulata*) with subsequent birth of a live offspring. Proceedings of the American Association of Zoological Parks and Aquariums, Omaha NE, pp 275–277, 1993.

34. Garde J, Perez S, Aguado MJ, et al: Live birth of hybrid (*O. musimon x O. aries*) lambs following intrauterine insemination in domestic sheep with Mouflon semen obtained 40 hours postmortem [Abstract]. Theriogenology 43:218, 1995.

35. Garland P, Frazer L, Sanderson N, et al: Artificial insemination of scimitar-horned oryx at Orana Park with frozen semen from Metro Toronto Zoo. Symposia Zool Soc London 64:37–43, 1992.

36. Gelwicks EJ, Pope CE, Gillespie DE, et al: Embryo collection, splitting and transfer in the common eland (*Tragelaphus oryx*) [Abstract]. Theriogenology 31:196, 1989.

37. Godfrey RW, Lunstra DD, French JA, et al: Estrous synchronization in the gaur (*Bos gaurus*): behavior and fertility to artificial insemination after prostaglandin treatment. Zoo Biol 10:35–41, 1990.

38. Goto K, Kinoshita A, Nakanishi Y, et al: Blastocyst formation following intracytoplasmic injection of in vivo or in vitro derived spermatids into bovine oocytes [Abstract]. Theriogenology 45:301, 1996.

39. Goto K, Kinoshita A, Takuma Y, et al: Fertilization of bovine oocytes by the injection of immobilized, killed spermatozoa. Vet Rec 127:517–520, 1990.

40. Graff KJ, Meintjes M, Paul JB, et al: Ultrasound-guided transvaginal oocyte recovery from FSH-treated goats for IVF [Abstract]. Theriogenology 43:223, 1995.

41. Greve T, Madison V: In vitro fertilization in cattle: a review. Reprod Nutr Dev 31:147–157, 1991.

42. Haigh JC: Artificial insemination of two white-tailed deer. J Am Vet Assoc 18:146–147, 1984.

43. Haigh JC, Bowen G: Artificial insemination of red deer (*Cervus elaphus*) with frozen-thawed wapiti semen. J Reprod Fertil 93:119–123, 1991.

44. Haigh JC, Cranfield M, Sasser RG: Estrus synchronization and pregnancy diagnosis in red deer. J Zoo Anim Med 19:202–207, 1988.

45. Hasler JF, Henderson WB, Hurtgen PJ, et al: Production, freezing and transfer of bovine IVF embryos and subsequent calving results. Theriogenology 43:141–152, 1995.

46. Holt WV, Moore DM, North RD, et al: Hormonal and behavioural detection of oestrus in blackbuck, *Antilope cervicapra*, and successful artificial insemination with fresh and frozen semen. J Reprod Fertil 82:717–725, 1988.

47. Iritani A, Utsumi K, Hosoi Y: Fertilization by assisted micromanipulation of gametes. *In* Lauria A, Gandolfi F (eds): Embryonic Development and Manipulation in Animal Production: Trends in Research and Applications. London, Portland Press, pp 51–57, 1992.

48. Jabbour HN, Marshall VS, Agro CmcG: Successful embryo transfer following artificial insemination of superovulated fallow deer (*Dama dama*). Reprod Fertil Dev 6:181–185, 1994.

49. Jabbour HN, Veldhuizen FA, Green G, et al: Endocrine responses and conception rates in fallow deer (*Dama dama*) following oestrous synchronization and cervical insemination with fresh or frozen-thawed spermatozoa. J Reprod Fertil 98:495–502, 1993.

50. Johnston LA, Loskutoff NM: Embryo technology in domestic cattle and its application to endangered species conservation. Proceedings of the American Association of Zoo Veterinarians, St. Louis, MO, pp 270–272, 1993.

51. Johnston LA, Parrish JJ, Monson R, et al: Oocyte maturation, fertilization and embryo development in vitro and in vivo in the gaur (*Bos gaurus*). J Reprod Fertil 100:131–136, 1994.

52. Keefer CL: Update on bovine in vitro embryo production. Embryo Transfer Newsletter, International Embryo Transfer Society 13:8–12, 1995.

53. Kraemer DC: Embryo collection and transfer in small ruminants. Theriogenology 31:141–148, 1989.

54. Kramer L, Dresser BL, Pope CE, et al: The nonsurgical transfer of frozen-thawed eland (*Tragelaphus oryx*) embryos. Proceedings of the American Association of Zoo Veterinarians, Tampa, FL, pp 129–131, 1983.

55. Krogenaes A, Ropstad E, Thomassen R, et al: In vitro maturation and fertilization of oocytes from Norwegian semi-domestic reindeer (*Rangifer tarandus*). Theriogenology 41:371–377, 1994.

56. Kruip ThAM, den Daas JHG: In vitro produced and cloned embryos: effects on pregnancy, parturition and offspring. Theriogenology 47:43–52, 1997.

57. Leibo SP, Semple EM, Kroetsch TG: In vitro fertilization of oocytes by 37 year old cryopreserved bovine spermatozoa. Theriogenology 42:1257–1262, 1994.

58. Lichtenwaner AB, Woods GL, Weber JA: Seminal collection, sem-

inal characteristics and pattern of ejaculation in llamas. Theriogenology 46:293–305, 1996.

59. Looney CR, Lindsey BR, Gonseth CL, et al: Commercial aspects of oocyte retrieval and in vitro fertilization (IVF) for embryo production in problem cows. Theriogenology 41:67–72, 1994.

60. Loskutoff NM, Bartels P, Meintjes M, et al: Assisted reproductive technologies in nondomestic ungulates: a model approach to preserving and managing genetic diversity. Theriogenology 43:3–12, 1995.

61. Loskutoff NM, Raphael BL, Nemac LA, et al: Reproductive anatomy, manipulation of ovarian activity and non-surgical embryo recovery in suni (*Neotragus moschatus zuluensis*). J Reprod Fertil 88:521–532, 1990.

62. Loskutoff NM, Raphael BL, Wolfe BA, et al: Embryo transfer in small antelope. Proceedings of the Society of Theriogenology, San Diego, CA, pp 341–342, 1991.

63. Loskutoff NM, Simmons HA, Goulding M, et al: Species and individual variations in cryoprotectant toxicities and freezing resistances of epididymal sperm from African antelope. Anim Reprod Sci 42:527–535, 1996.

64. Madan ML, Singla SK, Chauhan MB, et al: In vitro production and transfer of embryos in buffaloes. Theriogenology 41:139–143, 1994.

65. Magyar SJ, Biediger T, Hodges C, et al: A method of artificial insemination in captive white-tailed deer (*Odocoileus virginianus*). Theriogenology 31:1075–1080, 1989.

66. Matsuda DM, Bellem AC, Gartley CJ, et al: Endocrine and behavioral events of estrous cyclicity and synchronization in Wood bison (*Bison bison athabascae*). Theriogenology 45:1429–1411, 1996.

67. Mazur P: Freezing and low-temperature storage of living cells. *In* Muhlbock O (ed): Basic Aspects of Freeze Preservation of Mouse Strains. Stuttgart, Gustav Fischer Verlag, pp 1–12, 1976.

68. Monfort SL, Asher GW, Wildt DE, et al: Successful intrauterine insemination of Eld's deer (*Cervus eldi thamin*) with frozen-thawed spermatozoa. J Reprod Fertil 99:459–465, 1993.

69. Morrow CJ, Asher GW, Berg DK, et al: Embryo transfer in fallow deer (*Dama dama*): superovulation, embryo recovery and laparoscopic transfer of fresh and cryopreserved embryos. Theriogenology 42:579–590, 1994.

70. Morrow CJ, Asher GW, Macmillan KL: Oestrous synchronisation in farmed fallow deer (*Dama dama*): effects of season, treatment duration and the male on the efficacy of the intravaginal CIDR device. Anim Reprod Sci 37:159–174, 1995.

71. Morrow CJ, Monfort SL: Endocrine responses to exogenous progestogen and prostaglandin administration in the scimitar-horned oryx. Proceedings of the Annual Meeting of the American Association of Zoo Veterinarians, East Lansing, MI, pp 369–373, 1995.

72. Mylrea GE, English AW, Mulley RC, et al: Artificial insemination of farmed chital deer. *In* Brown RD (ed): The Biology of Deer. New York, Springer-Verlag, pp 334–337, 1991.

73. Pavasuthipaisit K, Holyoak RG, Tocharus C, et al: Repeated transvaginal follicular aspiration in swamp buffalo [Abstract]. Theriogenology 43:295, 1995.

74. Pieterse MC, Kappen KA, Kruip ThAM, et al: Aspiration of bovine oocytes during transvaginal ultrasound scanning of the ovaries. Theriogenology 30:751–762, 1988.

75. Pollard J, Bringans MJ, Buckrell B: In vitro production of wapiti and red deer (*Cervus elaphus*) embryos [Abstract]. Theriogenology 43:301, 1995.

76. Pope CE, Dresser BL: Development of assisted reproduction techniques in nondomestic bovids and felids. Proceedings of the Society of Theriogenology, San Diego, CA, pp 334–337, 1991.

77. Pope CE, Dresser BL, Kuehn G, et al: Live birth of a gaur (*Bos gaurus*) calf following nonsurgical embryo transfer to a Holstein (*Bos taurus*) recipient [Abstract]. Theriogenology 29:289, 1988.

78. Pope CE, Gelwicks EJ, Burton M, et al: Nonsurgical embryo transfer in the scimitar-horned oryx (*Oryx dammah*): birth of a live offspring. Zoo Biol 10:43–51, 1991.

79. Raphael BL, Loskutoff NM, Howard JG, et al: Embryo transfer and artificial insemination in suni (*Neotragus moschatus zuluensis*) [Abstract]. Theriogenology 31:244, 1989.

80. Raphael BL, Loskutoff NM, Huntress SL, et al: Post-mortem recovery, in vitro maturation and fertilization of klipspringer (*Oreotragus oreotragus*) ovarian oocytes. J Zoo Wildl Med 22:115–118, 1991.

81. Reinders JMC, Wurth YA, Kruip ThAM: From embryo to calf after transfer of in vitro produced bovine embryos [Abstract]. Theriogenology 43:306, 1995.

82. Ryan DP, Blakewood EG, Swanson WF, et al: Using hormone-treated pregnant cows as a potential source of oocytes for in vitro fertilization. Theriogenology 40:1039–1055, 1993.

83. Schiewe MC, Bush M, Phillips LG, et al: Comparative aspects of estrus synchronization, ovulation induction and embryo cryopreservation in the scimitar-horned oryx, bongo, eland and greater kudu. J Exp Zool 258:75–88, 1991.

84. Schmidt DL: Nonsurgical embryo transfer in scimitar-horned oryx. Proceedings of the Annual Meeting of the American Association of Zoo Veterinarians, Chicago, IL, pp 10–11, 1986.

85. Shaw HJ, Green DI, Sainsbury AW, et al: Monitoring ovarian function in scimitar-horned oryx (*Oryx dammah*) by measurement of fecal 20α-progestogen metabolites. Zoo Biol 14:239–250, 1995.

86. Shaw DG, Kidson A, van Schalkwyk JO, et al: In vitro production of African buffalo (*Syncerus caffer*) embryos derived from follicular oocytes and epididymal sperm [Abstract]. Theriogenology 43:322, 1995.

87. Solti L, Machaty Z, Barandi Z, et al: IVF embryos of known parental origin from the endangered Hungarian grey cattle breed [Abstract]. Theriogenology 37:301, 1992.

88. Stover J, Evans J: Interspecies embryo transfer from gaur (*Bos gaurus*) to domestic holstein cattle (*Bos taurus*) at the New York Zoological Park. Proceedings of the 10th International Congress of Animal Production and Artificial Insemination, Vol II, Urbana, IL, pp 243–245, 1984.

89. Thompson JG: Defining the requirements for bovine embryo culture. Theriogenology 45:27–40, 1996.

90. Walker SK, Hartwich KM, Seamark RF: The production of unusually large offspring following embryo manipulation: concepts and challenges. Theriogenology 45:111–120, 1996.

91. Waldhalm SJ, Jacobson HA, Dhungel SK, et al: Embryo transfer in the white-tailed deer: a reproductive model for endangered deer species of the world. Theriogenology 31:437–450, 1989.

92. Wiepz DW, Chapman RJ: Non-surgical embryo transfer and live birth in a llama. Theriogenology 24:251–257, 1985.

93. Wiesner VH, Lampetr WW, Rietschel W: Experience from nonsurgical embryo transfer from banteng to domestic cattle [In German]. Int Symp Erkrank Zootiere Brno, Czechoslovakia, pp 99–102, 1984.

94. Willard ST, Hughes DM Jr, Bringans M, et al: Artificial insemination, hybridization and pregnancy detection in silka deer (*Cervus nippon*). Theriogenology 46:779–789, 1996.

95. Wu MC: Survival and coat colour modulation of endangered miniature Lanyu pig embryos transferred into Landrace and Duroc sows [Abstract]. Theriogenology 41:339, 1994.

96. Xu KP, Hill B, Betteridge KJ: Application of in vitro fertilization techniques to obtain calves from valuable cows after slaughter. Vet Rec 130:204–206, 1992.

Rotavirus and Coronavirus Infections in Nondomestic Ruminants

SCOTT B. CITINO

Rotaviruses and coronaviruses have been incriminated as causes of diarrheal disease in numerous mammalian species, including humans[2, 8, 10, 12, 21, 26, 32, 36, 37] and are considered the most common viruses involved in the neonatal calf diarrhea syndrome.[1, 20] Both viruses are distributed worldwide and appear to be ubiquitous in cattle populations.[9, 19, 24] Even though there are few reports, discussions with zoo and wildlife veterinarians suggest that rotaviruses and coronaviruses are also commonly involved in diarrheal disease of captive, nondomestic ruminant animals.[8]

Rotavirus was mentioned as one cause of diarrhea in hand-raised, neonatal exotic ruminant animals in a large zoo nursery.[16] Overcrowding and colostrum deprivation were considered to be contributing factors in those cases. Another zoo nursery reported an outbreak of pneumoenteric disease in neonatal hoofstock associated with a rotavirus antigenically related to bovine rotavirus and an encapsulated *Escherichia coli*.[10] This outbreak affected impala (*Aepyceros melampus*), addax (*Addax nasomaculatus*), Thomson's gazelle (*Gazella thomsoni*), and Grant's gazelle (*Gazella subgutterosa*) and had a mortality rate of 50%. Rotavirus was also reported as a cause of diarrhea and death in recently captured neonatal pronghorn antelope (*Antilocapra americana*)[21] and as a cause of uncomplicated diarrhea in captive, adult bongo antelope (*Tragelaphus eurycerus*).[13] A study to determine the prevalence of rotavirus in normal and diarrheic stool using a commercial enzyme-linked immunosorbent assay (ELISA) found rotavirus in 20 of 35 (57%) animals of 15 exotic animal species.[2] Most of the animals included in this study were younger than 2 weeks old and included addax, lowland nyala (*Tragelaphus angasi*), saiga (*Saiga tatarica*), white-tailed gnu (*Connochaetes gnou*), greater kudu (*Tragelaphus strepsiceros*), sitatunga (*Tragelaphus spekei*), Grant's gazelle (*Gazella granti roosevelti*), sable antelope (*Hippotragus niger niger*), and kob (*Kobus kob leucotis*). Rotavirus has been associated with diarrhea in both adult and neonatal okapi (*Okapia johnstoni*) housed in several facilities in North America with severe, complicated cases seen in a few neonates.[8] Rotavirus has also been detected by electron microscopy in the diarrheic stool of both hand-raised and mother-raised calves of the following species: gerenuk

(*Litocranius walleri*), lowland nyala, greater kudu, giant eland (*Taurotragus derbianus gigas*), and reticulated giraffe (*Giraffa camelopardalis reticulata*) at a private conservation center.[8]

Besides being recognized as a common causative agent of calf diarrhea, bovine coronavirus has been incriminated by several researchers as the causative agent for winter dysentery, an acute diarrheal disease of adult cattle.[1, 14, 23, 26] A winter outbreak of diarrheal disease was reported in several species of adult, nondomestic ruminant animals in a zoo collection.[13] This outbreak was reminiscent of winter dysentery in cattle, and the only potential pathogen found in stool from the affected animals was coronavirus. Species involved in this outbreak were gemsbok (*Oryx gazella*), bongo antelope, dama gazelle (*Gazella dama*), slender-horned gazelle (*Gazella leptoceros*), banteng (*Bos javanicus*), axis deer (*Cerus axis*), blackbuck (*Antilope cervicapra*), and pronghorn antelope. Similarly, acute outbreaks of diarrhea, associated with a coronavirus, have occasionally occurred during the cooler months of the year at a private conservation center and have affected subadults to adults of the following species: giant eland, bongo antelope, okapi, lowland nyala, gerenuk, Kafue Flats lechwe (*Kobus leche kafuensis*), and Nile lechwe (*Kobus megaceros*).[8]

With very little published information or ongoing scientific research regarding rotaviruses and coronaviruses in nondomestic ruminant animals, continuing discussion must rely heavily on published information about bovine rotavirus and coronavirus.

THE VIRUSES

Enteric diarrheagenic viruses are categorized as either type 1 or type 2 viruses according to their sites of replication within the intestinal tract.[28] Type 1 viruses infect villous epithelial cells and generally do not cause systemic infections. Type 2 viruses infect primarily crypt enterocytes and intestinal lymphoid cells and usually cause systemic infections. Rotaviruses and coronaviruses are both classified as type 1 enteric viruses and share common physiochemical and biologic characteristics.[28] Both viruses are stable at low pH (3 to 4) and to proteolytic enzymes, allowing them to survive and function in the gastrointestinal environment, and they are heat labile, which partially explains their peak occurrence in winter months.[28, 29]

Rotavirus is the name for a genus within the family Reoviridae and is derived from the Latin word for wheel, *rota*, because complete virions appear as little wheels, having a wide hub with short spokes and a thin, clearly defined circular rim when viewed by electron microscopy.[11] Rotaviruses are non-enveloped viruses with a diameter of 65 to 70 nm and with a double-stranded RNA genome of 11 segments surrounded by a double capsid.[12] The outer capsid layer appears to be necessary for infectivity.[12] Because of their segmented genome, rotaviruses can mutate by genetic recombination.[33] Rotaviruses contain a common group antigen located in the virus core and type-specific neutralization antigens present in the outer shell of the virion.[7, 12, 31] Serogroup A rotaviruses are the most common rotaviruses infecting humans and animals.[32, 37] Group A rotaviruses possess two major type-specific neutralization antigens in the outer capsid layer.[32] Classification of group A rotavirus serotypes has been based primarily on the specificity of the VP7 neutralization antigen (G serotypes) and to a limited extent on the VP4 neutralization antigen (P serotypes).[17] A total of 14 G serotypes have been described to date.[17] Serotypes can be further characterized by genome electropherotyping.[33] Rotavirus synthesis and maturation occur within the cytoplasm of enterocytes with formation of small granular inclusions. Mature virions are usually found in endoplasmic vesicles. Because of their non-enveloped nature, rotaviruses are relatively resistant to lipid solvents and are long-lived in many environments.[18]

Bovine rotavirus (BRV) was first recovered from diarrheic calves in Nebraska in 1969. It was initially referred to as neonatal calf diarrhea virus, Nebraska calf diarrhea virus, reo-like virus, or reovirus-like agent. Most bovine rotaviruses belong to serogroup A and are of subgroup 1 classification.[19, 20] Serotypic diversity exists among BRV, with serotypes G1, G2, G3, G6, G8, G10, and G11 being reported for cattle.[17] There is serotypic similarity between bovine and human rotaviruses, with serotypes G1, G6, G8, and G10 also being reported for humans, which suggests possible zoonotic potential for some BRV serotypes.[17] Studies using electropherotyping have shown substantial genomic diversity of bovine group A rotaviruses recovered from diarrheic calves within a small defined region of the United States.[19, 33] Virulence variation has been identified among different isolates of BRV, and some isolates replicate without clinical signs in nonimmune calves.[3, 4, 15] Non–group A rotaviruses are occasionally seen by electron microscopy in diarrheic stool of calves and have been designated as group B rotaviruses, atypical rotaviruses, or pararotaviruses.[7] Group B rotaviruses are a much more common cause of diarrhea in lambs.[20]

Little to no research has occurred regarding group, serotype, and electropherotype determination of rotavirus isolates from nondomestic ruminant animals. In four reports of rotavirus infection in nondomestic ruminants, the rotavirus responsible was classified as a group A rotavirus by ELISA, immunofluorescence, or immunoelectron microscopy.[2, 10, 13, 21] Atypical rotaviruses were present in diarrheic stool from gerenuk calves and adult okapi on several different occasions at a private conservation center, suggesting that non–group A or atypical rotaviruses may play a more significant role in diarrheal diseases of nondomestic ruminant animals.[8]

Coronavirus is the name given to viruses within the family Coronaviridae and is derived from the Latin word for garland or fringe, *corona*. Coronaviruses are pleomorphic to spherical enveloped viruses ranging from 80 to 160 nm in diameter and have a distinct appearance when examined by electron microscopy.[11] The virus envelope appears as a distinct pair of electron dense shells from which the spike (S) glycoproteins radiate to form a fringe of surface projections called peplomers.[9] These petal-shaped peplomers are about 20 nm long and lie external to a second fringe of shorter projections formed by the hemagglutinin-esterase (HE) glycoproteins.[9] Both types of projections may be lost during sample storage and preparation.[9, 30] The coronavirus genome consists of a single strand of nonsegmented RNA of positive sense.[26] Coronavirus particles possess four major structural proteins: the nucleocapsid protein (N), the integral membrane glycoprotein (M), the spike glycoprotein (S), and the hemagglutinin-esterase glycoprotein (HE).[25]

Coronaviruses belong to five distinct antigenic groups that share within a group common antigens detected by immunologic assays. Bovine coronavirus (BCV) belongs to group 2 of the Coronaviridae family along with hemagglutinating encephalomyelitis virus of swine and human respiratory coronavirus OC43.[25] Two reports suggest possible transmission of coronaviruses between calves and humans, suggesting a possible zoonotic potential for BCV.[28] BCV does not cross-react antigenically with other enteropathogenic coronaviruses (i.e., transmissible gastroenteritis virus, porcine epidemic diarrhea virus, canine coronavirus, equine coronavirus, turkey coronavirus, and feline enteric coronavirus).[28] To date, BCV isolates all belong to a single serotype in that polyclonal sera study has only detected minor antigenic variations.[9, 25] Studies with monoclonal antibodies have detected variations in the N, S, and HE proteins of BCV isolates.[9] Some isolates also vary in their physicochemical properties as well as in their ability to produce cytopathic effects in cell culture.[9] The biologic behavior of isolates also varies (e.g., between calf diarrhea isolates and winter dysentery isolates).[9, 23] Immunologic and genomic characterization of coronavirus isolates from nondomestic ruminant animals has not been reported; however, it has been postulated that BCV can infect or exist in all ruminating animals.[13]

BCV attaches to receptors on enterocyte membranes via the S and HE glycoproteins.[9] The virus enters cells by direct fusion of the virus envelope with the plasma membrane of the cell or by endocytosis followed by fusion of the virus envelope with the endocytic vesicle membrane. BCV replication then occurs entirely within the cell cytoplasm. Infective virions are released through normal cell secretory mechanisms from intact cells or by lysis of dying cells.

EPIZOOTIOLOGY

Diarrhea is considered the most important disease of young calves in both dairy and beef herds and causes significant economic losses from morbidity, mortality, treatment costs, and poor growth of the animals.[19] Within captive collections of nondomestic ruminant animals, diarrhea is also a common disease manifestation in calves and results in significant morbidity and mortality. Rotavirus and coronavirus are considered the most common viruses involved in calf diarrhea, and both are thought to have worldwide distributions.[1, 9, 24]

BRV and BCV are transmitted most commonly by the fecal-oral route, resulting in direct infection of villous epithelial cells via the luminal surface.[28] The more labile enveloped enteric viruses such as BCV may undergo initial replication in the oropharynx with delivery of massive doses of virus to the small intestine.[9, 28] BCV also infects the respiratory tract of calves and adult cattle, so aerosol transmission may also occur.[9] Rotaviruses also survive well airborne, but the role of air as a vehicle for spread of infection remains to be shown.[29] Both viruses are shed in large numbers in the stool of infected animals and are highly contagious with fomite transmission (e.g., from feed, bedding, equipment, and people) occurring readily and rapidly. Rotaviruses are generally shed in the stool of newly infected animals for a period of 5 to 8 days.[32] Human rotavirus in fecal material can survive for prolonged periods on several types of materials commonly found in institutions and domestic environments.[29] The stability of rotaviruses is influenced by environmental factors such as relative humidity, temperature, and type of surface contaminated.[29] Survival of rotaviruses is longer on nonporous surfaces at lower temperatures and lower humidity.[29] Rotavirus survival on porous surfaces is variable. High relative humidity is detrimental to rotavirus survival at ambient temperatures.[29] BCV appears to prefer a cool, moist environment.[9] Both BRV and BCV outbreaks are more prevalent during winter months, which may reflect the enhanced capacity of these viruses to survive under cool conditions. Overcrowding and confinement appear to be contributive management factors in rotavirus outbreaks in both domestic and nondomestic ruminant calves, possibly because of stress-related effects on immunity and ease of transmission under these conditions.[8, 16, 20, 24]

BRV generally causes diarrhea in calves 4 to 14 days old, but it can also be a problem in younger and older calves.[20] Some strains of rotavirus cause disease in all age groups, some infect all ages but cause disease only in the young, and other strains infect the young without disease.[4] Morbidity during BRV outbreaks in cattle herds can reach 100% and mortality rate may range from 0% to 50%.[2, 24] BCV can cause problems in calves of all ages but is a particular problem in calves 4 to 30 days of age.[20] The incubation period for these viruses can be as short as 14 to 48 hours. The outcome of infection by these viruses most likely involves several factors, including the immune status of the animal at the time of infection, the virulence of the infecting virus strain, and the age of the infected animal.[4] Experience with rotavirus and coronavirus infection in nondo-

mestic ruminant calves suggests that rotavirus most commonly infects very young calves and calves that are immunologically compromised, whereas coronavirus tends to infect older calves ($\geq$30 days) after maternal and lactogenic antibody levels have significantly waned.[8] It is not uncommon to have dual infections in calves with both viruses or co-infections with other pathogens such as enterotoxigenic *E. coli*, which can greatly alter the severity of infection.[20, 35]

Most adult cattle worldwide are seropositive for antibodies to BRV and BCV, confirming the endemicity of these viruses.[9, 28] BCV has been detected in the feces of a high proportion of clinically normal adult cows despite the presence of specific antibodies in the serum and feces.[9] Consequently, it is likely that adult cattle, which are persistently infected with these viruses, act as an initial source of infection for susceptible calves. Studies of rotaviral pathogenesis under field conditions suggest that the dam may shed virus near parturition and, thus, serve as a source of virus for susceptible neonates.[27] Persistent infections or carrier states develop in calves as well, consequently maintaining the viruses in the environment.[9, 27]

Neonatal infections may thus occur at birth or shortly after, and the infections remain subclinical as long as adequate levels of colostral, milk, or serum antibodies persist.[28] Because most of these viral infections occur in calves younger than 3 weeks of age, passive lactogenic immunity within the gut lumen plays an important role in protection.[9, 27, 28] Effective lactogenic immunity against enteropathogenic viral infections has been shown to be contingent on the frequent ingestion of colostrum or milk containing adequate levels of protective antibodies.[9, 27, 28] The age susceptibility of calves to these enteropathogenic viruses may be related to the dramatic decline in milk antibody titers during week 1 postpartum.[27] Enteric infections in young calves and lambs may be modulated by local transient protection provided by reverse transport of serum IgG_1 antibodies back into the small intestine.[27, 28] Depending on a number of poorly understood variables, infected calves may then begin shedding virus with or without accompanying disease. Whereas active protective immunity from subclinical infections may develop in most animals that are infected while receiving passive immunity, other animals may remain susceptible to subsequent infection, becoming a source of virus for additional animals.[27]

In nondomestic ruminant calves, diarrheal disease caused by rotavirus has been a particular problem in young calves being hand-raised in nursery settings.[2, 8, 10, 16, 21] Many of these calves are hypogammaglobulinemic because of failure of transfer of passive immunity, and they receive formulas that lack lactogenic immunoglobulins, making them highly susceptible to infection.[8] The close confinement of most nurseries allows enteric viruses to spread easily between highly susceptible animals. New calves are frequently introduced into nursery populations, and calves of different ages and species are housed in close proximity, increasing the likelihood of virus introduction and maintenance in the nursery setting.

Winter dysentery is thought to be caused by BCV

in adult cattle.[1, 9, 23, 26] This disease is most common during the winter months and is characterized by rapid spread with a high morbidity rate (50% to 100%) but a low mortality rate (1% to 2%).[9] The duration of clinical disease in affected herds ranges from a few days to several weeks.[23] Spread is facilitated by close confinement during winter months and the enhanced survivability of BCV and, thus, higher levels of environmental contamination at cooler temperatures.[9, 23] Cows that are pregnant, recently calved, or lactating are most severely affected. Usually, there is little to no illness among calves during an outbreak.[23] Herds with a previous history of winter dysentery are more likely to suffer further outbreaks of disease, suggesting the presence of persistently infected or carrier animals.[23] Recurrences of winter dysentery outbreaks generally occur at 1- to 5-year intervals in cattle herds, which implies the development of short-term immunity.[23] Winter dysentery–like outbreaks have occurred in captive collections of nondomestic ruminant animals with rapid spread within and apparent spread between species.[8, 13]

CLINICAL SIGNS

The primary clinical sign associated with rotavirus and coronavirus infections in calves is diarrhea. This diarrhea is acute in nature, and the severity of diarrhea depends on the viral strain involved, numerous environmental influences, and the immune status of the affected calf (passive, active, and local lactogenic). The duration and severity of illness as well as the mortality rate also appear to be related to the type and severity of secondary infections or co-infections that develop in calves infected with rotavirus or coronavirus.[20, 35] First signs of infection are mild to complete anorexia, mild to moderate fever, and a change to a lighter fecal coloration. In nursing calves, a yellowish, watery diarrhea then develops. The amount of feces produced is a good indicator of the severity of disease.[4] Other clinical signs that can be seen in more severe cases include depression, dullness, salivation, dehydration, collapse, and death. Because coronaviruses produce more widespread illness than rotaviruses, they are more likely to produce a more severe diarrhea of longer duration.[28] Because coronavirus also infects the colonic mucosa, signs of colitis such as straining and passage of mucus and blood in feces may be seen. Coronavirus also causes mild upper respiratory clinical signs such as rhinitis, sneezing, and coughing in domestic and nondomestic ruminant animals.[9, 13] BCV may also predispose calves to more severe secondary lower respiratory tract infections with associated clinical signs.[9] Pneumoenteric clinical signs were also reported from nondomestic ruminant calves infected with rotavirus in a zoo nursery.[10]

Winter dysentery associated with BCV is characterized by acute onset of often profuse, dark, foul-smelling, and often blood-tinged diarrhea accompanied by variable depression and anorexia.[14] Weight loss is often evident, caused by dehydration and loss of rumenal fill.[14] The duration of clinical signs ranges from a few days to several weeks in large herds.[23] Nasolacrimal discharge or coughing may also been seen.[23] In dairy cattle, a dramatic decrease in milk production may occur, and production may not return to normal for months. Similar clinical signs have been seen in nondomestic ruminant herds experiencing winter dysentery–like disease associated with coronavirus.[8, 13]

PATHOLOGY

Gross pathology associated with BRV and BCV infections can be variable, depending on the severity of secondary and co-infections. Uncomplicated cases of BRV and BCV infection generally show minimal gross pathology. There may be increased volume of fluid-like digesta within the small and large intestine and a lack of formed fecal material in the distal colon and rectum. The small or large intestine may show diffuse to patchy or segmental mucosal hyperemia, congestion, or petechiation.[22, 25] Cases of BCV infection may show increased evidence of colonic hemorrhage with blood-tinged or mucoid digesta present within the colon.[20] Hyperemia or petechiation of the nasal and tracheal mucosa and variable degrees of pulmonary edema or congestion may be seen in cases of BCV infection.[9, 20] Mesenteric lymphadenopathy with congestion or edema may or may not be present in BRV and BCV infections.

Type 1 enteropathogenic viruses such as BRV and BCV invade mature villous enterocytes on the intestinal surface, and the enterocytes are killed and sloughed as the viruses replicate within them.[15, 28] This desquamation of villous enterocytes leads to varying degrees of villous atrophy. Principal microscopic lesions of BRV and BCV infection include variable degrees of exfoliation, disarrangement, and vacuolization of enterocytes, enterocyte metaplasia, and villous atrophy with clubbing, truncation, and fusion of villi.[3, 9, 12, 15, 22, 24, 28, 35] A decrease in the number of goblet cells tends to accompany these other mucosal changes. An increase in the relative density of connective tissue and lymphoid cells may be seen in the lamina propria of the villi. Other and more severe lesions may be seen when secondary or co-infections with other pathogens occur.[20, 35]

BRV and BCV differ in their sites of replication, both horizontal and vertical, within the gastrointestinal tract. Rotaviruses primarily infect enterocytes on the apical half of the villi (the more enzymatically mature cells), producing a milder, transient diarrhea, whereas coronaviruses infect enterocytes throughout the length of the villi, producing more severe villous atrophy and clinical signs.[28] Rotaviruses generally replicate and cause villous atrophy in the distal half of the small intestine, whereas coronaviruses cause an almost continuous infection of enterocytes throughout the distal small intestine and colon.[28] Within the colon, coronavirus causes atrophy or desquamation of the colonic ridges with metaplasia of colonic ridge epithelial cells.[9] Cases of BCV-associated winter dysentery have also exhibited focal degeneration and necrosis of colonic crypt epithelium.[23] Rotavirus and coronavirus infections tend to be self-limiting because, once susceptible mature enterocytes have been destroyed, there are no further target cells for viral invasion. Although infections with rotavirus and coronavirus tend to be short-lived, it takes time for villi to repair through replication and migration of epithelial cells from the crypts, which prolongs clinical signs. The turnover and repair rate of villous epithelium is slower in neonatal calves than in adult ruminant animals, making calves more susceptible to severe disease from these viruses.[28] It has been shown that different strains of rotavirus preferentially infect different sections of the small intestine and that rotavirus virulence is associated with extensive spread of infection throughout the small intestine with preferential colonization of the proximal small intestine.[3, 4, 15] BCV also invades and replicates in epithelial cells of the nasal cavity and trachea, and, in some cases, the lung can also be involved, with subsequent development of interstitial pneumonia.[9, 20]

The ultimate effect of BRV and BCV infections is a decreased absorptive capacity of the intestine caused by loss of surface area and the increased presence of immature enterocytes.[9, 20, 28] The immature enterocytes are also less enzymatically active, leading to decreased digestive capacity.[9] This decreased absorptive and digestive capacity of the gut allows nutrients such as lactose to accumulate, producing an osmotic diarrhea with loss of water and electrolytes. In severe infections, diarrhea can lead to severe dehydration, electrolyte imbalance, metabolic acidosis, hypoglycemia, and resultant death.

DIAGNOSIS

Difficulties in the clinical diagnosis of infectious enteritis arise from frequent nonspecific clinical signs and lesions, the presence of asymptomatic infections, the involvement of multiple agents, and the interaction of intrinsic and extrinsic factors that predispose the host to infection. It is important to remember that the detection of a virus in normal or diarrheic stool does not, by itself, qualify it as a cause of enteritis and that it is common to find more than one potential pathogen in cases of enteritis. Consequently, determination of the causes of diarrheal disease requires careful screening for all known causative agents together with thorough epidemiologic and pathologic investigation where possible.

Transmission electron microscopy (TEM) has been instrumental in the initial detection and identification of many of the enteropathogenic viruses from stool samples, and it remains the "gold standard" assay used for identification of fecal rotaviruses and coronaviruses by many research and diagnostic laboratories.[1, 11, 34] TEM has the potential for rapid diagnosis (within 24 hours), permits detection of novel enteric viruses, permits simultaneous detection of multiple viruses, and is done relatively inexpensively at many reference laboratories. TEM, however, suffers from lack of sensitivity in that 10^6 viral particles per gram of feces must be present for detection.[11] Problems also arise when a virus has a pleomorphic morphology or an uncharacteristic shape or size, or the sample is contaminated with virus-like particles such as cellular membranes, ribosomes, cellular organelles, and bacteriophages.[1, 11, 20] There can sometimes be problems identifying coronaviruses by TEM, because they may not always exhibit a typical morphologic appearance.[1, 20] Fresh specimens that are refrigerated but not frozen should be shipped to diagnostic laboratories for TEM. Improper handling of specimens, such as repeated freezing and thawing, can alter virus morphology (loss of peplomers in coronaviruses) and compromise the identification of a virus. Immunoelectron microscopy (IEM) using group-specific antibodies for BRV or BCV can greatly increase the sensitivity and specificity of electron microscopy.[1, 9] Although not suitable for large-scale screening of specimens, IEM can prove indispensable for identification of selected or doubtful specimens or for verifying results of other tests.[1]

In many laboratories, ELISAs are the most practical method for screening large numbers of fecal samples for BRV and BCV.[1, 19, 30] A number of comparative studies with feces have shown that ELISA and TEM give similar results when searching for specific pathogens; agreement between these two methods varies from 65% to 100%.[20] ELISAs are very sensitive but fail to detect virus if it is already complexed to host antibody or if the ELISA antibody does not recognize the virus.[20] Commercial rotavirus ELISAs use antibody directed against common group-specific internal capsid antigens, and all are specific for group A rotaviruses only.[20] All group A rotaviruses including BRV can be detected in fecal samples by commercial ELISA systems such as Rotazyme (Abbott Laboratories, Diagnostic Division, Abbott Park, IL, 60064) used to diagnose human rotavirus.[2, 32, 37] Commercial ELISAs have been successfully used to detect group A rotavirus in the stool of nondomestic ruminant animals.[2, 8] Rapid, single-test ELISA systems such as Abbott Test Pack Rotavirus (Abbott Laboratories, Diagnostic Division, Abbott Park, IL 60064) can be useful in clinical zoological medicine settings for in-house diagnosis of group A rotaviruses.[8] Rapid latex agglutination slide tests are also available commercially for diagnosis of group A rotaviruses in the clinical setting. Group B or atypical rotaviruses carry a different group antigen, so viruses in this group cannot be identified by present commercial ELISA systems.[20] Atypical rotaviruses may be a more prominent cause of diarrheal disease in nondomestic ruminant animals than in cattle, so care should be taken when using the commercial ELISA systems in the zoological setting.[8] ELISAs that use specific monoclonal antibodies have been shown to be sensitive and specific for detection of BCV in feces and are widely used for screening fecal samples in diagnostic laboratories.[9, 30]

Histopathologic study often supports the diagnosis of viral enteritis but does not, in itself, allow a definitive diagnosis. Fluorescent antibody (FA) testing of intestinal sections for BRV and BCV can be useful to confirm a diagnosis.[20] FA testing of postmortem or antemortem nasal scrapings or swabs can be helpful in the diagnosis of BCV respiratory infections.[9] Intestinal sections, scrapings, or swabs should be shipped cold but not frozen to a reference laboratory for this procedure. It is also helpful to collect intestinal contents from necropsy specimens and have them tested by EM or ELISA for the presence of rotaviruses and coronaviruses.[8]

Because of the difficulty or inability to propagate many of the fastidious enteropathogenic viruses, virus isolation by cell culture is rarely used as a diagnostic test for infectious diarrheal disease.[20, 28] This has often hampered the study of these viruses. New molecular genetic techniques such as the polymerase chain reaction (PCR) are emerging for diagnosis and study of enteric viruses.[17] PCR is a rapid and extremely sensitive assay that can quickly differentiate between different strains or mutants of a virus. These emerging molecular genetic techniques will undoubtedly play an important role in the future study of rotaviruses and coronaviruses of nondomestic ruminant animals.

TREATMENT

Because there are no specific treatments for rotavirus and coronavirus infections, therapy is primarily supportive in nature. Secondary or co-infections are common, so when these are detected, they must be treated specifically. The intensiveness and length of therapy usually depends on the severity of the diarrheal disease and on the age and immunologic status of the animal.

Calves with diarrheal disease generally require more intensive and long-term treatment than adult animals. Initial therapy involves correction of dehydration, hypoglycemia, and electrolyte and acid-base imbalances with oral or intravenous fluid therapy. Calves should be kept warm and stress should be minimized. Plasma transfusions are frequently helpful in calves with infectious diarrheal disease because many have failure of passive transfer of maternal antibodies and are hypoproteinemic.[8] Plasma transfusions improve the immune status of the sick calf as well as its osmotic homeostasis. Frozen plasma banks are useful for this purpose in facilities that propagate large numbers of nondomestic ruminant animals.[8] If secondary bacterial infections or sepsis is evident in the diarrheic calf, aggressive and specific antibiotic therapy must be used to control the infection quickly. In sick calves receiving broad-spectrum antibiotic therapy, gastrointestinal *Candida* species infections should be watched for closely. The use of H_2-receptor antagonists, gastric proton pump inhibitors, and sucralfate may be useful in calves of species prone to abomasal ulceration. When bloody or mucoid diarrhea is evident, intestinal protectants such as bismuth subsalicylate or Kaopectate can be helpful. Sick calves have high caloric requirements, and calves with extensive villous atrophy can have protracted malabsorption. Consequently, nutritional support of diarrheic calves is often paramount for therapeutic success. Calves with mild to moderate enteritis can often be continued on full-strength or diluted milk-based formulas with lactase added, but formulas given per os in calves with severe malabsorption exacerbate the disease. Calves with severe malabsorption caused by viral enteritis often benefit greatly from total enteral nutrition (TEN), using elemental diets that do not require digestion and that are easily absorbed, or total or partial parenteral nutrition (TPN or PPN).

Malabsorption tends to be short-lived and less severe in adult ruminant animals with rotaviral or coronaviral enteritis, so less intensive or no treatment may be required. Adult ruminant animals often drink large amounts of oral electrolyte replacement solutions when dehydrated, so these should be offered free-choice along with water. Environmental and other stressors should be reduced or eliminated. Because most adult ruminant animals will continue eating during viral enteritis, nutritional support is generally not needed. If secondary infections occur and animals show a more severe or protracted illness, specific antibiotic therapy may be needed.

PREVENTION AND CONTROL

Immunity against rotaviruses and coronaviruses must be directed toward protection of the susceptible intestinal epithelial cell through the presence of adequate levels of specific antibodies in the gut lumen.[9, 28] Serum antibodies appear to be of less value in protection against these viruses.[28] In calves, local immunity is passively acquired from the dam in the form of antibodies ingested in the colostrum and milk. The predominant antibody in colostrum and milk is IgG_1, which is unique to ruminants and which is largely derived from serum by a selective transport mechanism in the ruminant mammary gland.[27] The level of lactogenic antibodies is very high at parturition but then declines rapidly and is almost nonexistent at 1 week postpartum.[28] There is a high correlation between colostrum rotavirus antibody titers, the amount of colostrum fed, and protection against experimental rotavirus challenge.[27] As little as 40 ml (total) of high-rotavirus-titered colostrum fed BID to calves completely protected them against both diarrhea and virus shedding when challenged.[27] The daily feeding of fresh or frozen colostrum supplements from immunized cows to calves should provide effective passive immunity against rotavirus and coronavirus for the duration of colostrum feeding.[9, 27, 28] Reducing the number of animals occupying the nursery and inclusion of bovine colostrum at 10% of the daily ration for the first 3 weeks of life markedly reduced morbidity and death resulting from neonatal diarrhea in hand-raised exotic ruminant animals in a large zoo nursery.[16] If bovine colostrum is used in neonatal nondomestic ruminant animals, extreme care must be exercised to prevent introduction of serious pathogens through the colostrum (e.g., *Mycobacterium paratuberculosis*).[8] The feeding of commercial bovine colostral supplements to nondomestic ruminant calves as part of the daily ration may also be beneficial for prevention of rotavirus and coronavirus infections.[8] Feeding serum or plasma with each feeding has also been helpful in preventing rotavirus infections in at-risk nondomestic ruminant calves.[8] Serum or plasma can be collected and banked frozen from adult ruminant animals that have previously been vaccinated against or exposed to rotavirus, and fed to calves at 4.5 ml/kg/day.

The duration of passive immunity in calves is prolonged by re-secretion of absorbed colostral IgG_1 antibodies back into the gut lumen and by adherence of immunoglobulins to the surface of enterocytes.[9, 27] The transport of serum IgG_1 into the intestine has been reported in both sheep and cattle.[27] Additionally, high serum immunoglobulin concentrations correlate with the absence of diarrhea in young calves.[27] Consequently, calves with low serum immunoglobulin levels resulting from failure of passive transfer should benefit from homologous plasma transfusion by having a reduced incidence of infectious diarrheal disease.

A modified-live virus vaccine (Calf Guard, Pfizer Animal Health, Exton, PA 19341) and a killed virus vaccine (Scourguard 3[K], Pfizer Animal Health, Exton, PA 19341) vaccine are commercially available for prevention of BRV and BCV infections in calves. The efficacy of both of these vaccines for prevention of BRV and BCV infections under typical field conditions has been seriously questioned by authorities.[5, 20] Both vaccines contain only one group A BRV serotype fraction, so both vaccines are ineffective in eliciting antibodies against group B or atypical rotaviruses[5] and may not necessarily protect against challenge with other strains.[5, 20, 31] The efficacy of these vaccines for prevention of winter dysentery in adult ruminant animals is unknown.

Calf Guard must be given to calves immediately after birth and before they suckle colostrum to prevent maternal antibodies from neutralizing the vaccine viruses.[5] This is impractical in many cases in captive collections of nondomestic ruminant animals because such early disturbances often disturb maternal-calf bonding and lead to calf rejection or trauma.[8] The vaccine viruses can potentially be shed in the feces, which can interfere with diagnostics and control programs.[2, 34] There is also the potential danger of the modified-live viruses in Calf Guard not being attenuated enough for some highly susceptible species and actually causing disease or reverting back to a more virulent form and spreading through a collection. It has also been shown that the resistance induced by vaccination with Calf Guard is easily overwhelmed by exposure to the large amounts of virus shed by naturally infected calves.[5] Calf Guard can also be given intramuscularly to periparturient cows; however, it has been shown to be inefficient in increasing colostral and lactogenic antibodies for protection of calves.[5, 20, 27] Vaccination with Calf Guard has been reported as being safe and somewhat efficacious on two occasions in collections of nondomestic hoofstock.[10, 13]

Scourguard 3(K) is given intramuscularly as directed to pregnant cows before parturition to increase BRV and BCV colostral and lactogenic antibodies for protection of calves. This vaccine can also be used to boost humoral and secretory antibodies for protection against BRV and BCV infections in older ruminant animals. Because this is a killed virus vaccine, problems are frequently encountered in inducing high titers of local secretory IgA antibodies, cell-mediated immune responses are often poor, and the duration of immunity is often short-lived.[25] Scourguard 3(K) has been used with some success in okapis and giraffes to prevent calfhood rotaviral infections by giving intramuscular injections of the vaccine to pregnant dams at 4 and 2 weeks before anticipated parturition and then intramuscular injections to calves at 4, 8, and 12 weeks of age.[8] Scourguard 3(K) has induced moderate to severe muscular swelling, edema, and pain in a few adult okapis after multiple vaccinations.[8]

Experimental, high-titer rotavirus vaccines containing Freund's incomplete adjuvant or other oil-based adjuvants appear to stimulate much higher and longer-lasting lactogenic antibody titers than commercial vaccines.[6, 20, 27, 28] Consequently, the production and use of high-titer, autogenous rotavirus or coronavirus vaccines with Freund's incomplete adjuvant may be beneficial in some collections of nondomestic hoofstock in which rotavirus or coronavirus infections are a significant problem.

Isolation, sanitation, stress-reduction, and common sense can all play important roles in controlling and preventing the spread of rotavirus and coronavirus infections. Isolation of outbreaks in herds or nursery settings using rigid quarantine standards is difficult but can be effective. Keepers should use common sense and be instructed on how to prevent fomite transmission of rotaviruses and coronaviruses between herds. Removal and isolation of diarrheic calves from nurseries reduces contamination and viral spread. Having several nursery areas and using an "all in, all out" philosophy can reduce and control infectious diarrheal disease. Housing calves in single age-groups, eliminating overcrowding, and reducing interspecies contact in nurseries can reduce stress and viral exposure. Use of outdoor, movable calf hutch systems have greatly reduced transmission of infectious disease in commercial dairy calf operations and could be adapted for use with nondomestic ruminant calves.[20] Keeping nurseries warm reduces rotavirus and coronavirus survival in the environment. Humidifying the air in nurseries also reduces rotavirus survivability.[29] Proper nursery ventilation helps prevent aerosol spread of coronaviruses. Good, proper, and frequent sanitation, cleaning, and hygiene are essential components of disease prevention and control.[18, 20] Surfaces and materials used in nurseries should be easily cleaned and disinfected. Rotaviruses, being non-enveloped, are relatively resistant to disinfectants, whereas the enveloped coronaviruses are less resistant.[18, 20] The phenolic disinfectants are highly effective against rotaviruses, are not inactivated by organic material, but are highly toxic and irritating.[18, 20] Hypochlorite and quaternary ammoniums are only moderately effective against rotavirus, and hypochlorite is easily inactivated by organic material. Biguamides (e.g., chlorhexidine) and iodophors are not effective against rotavirus.

REFERENCES

1. Athanassious R, Marsolais G, Assaf R, et al: Detection of bovine coronavirus and type A rotavirus in neonatal calf diarrhea and winter dysentery of cattle in Quebec: evaluation of three diagnostic methods. Can Vet J 35:163–169, 1994.
2. Baumeister BM, Castro AE, McGuire-Rodgers SJ, et al: Detection and control of rotavirus infections in zoo animals. J Am Vet Med Assoc 183(11):1252–1254, 1983.
3. Bridger JC, Hall GA, Parsons KR: A study of the basis of virulence variation of bovine rotaviruses. Vet Microbiol 33:169–174, 1992.
4. Bridger JC, Pocock DH: Variation in virulence of bovine rotaviruses. J Hyg Camb 96:257–264, 1986.
5. Brumbaugh GW, Hjerpe CA: The use of biologics in the prevention of infectious diseases: neonatal enteric disease vaccines. *In* Smith RP (ed): Large Animal Internal Medicine. St. Louis, CV Mosby, pp 1508–1512, 1990.
6. Castrucci G, Ferrari M, Angelillo V, et al: Field evaluation of the efficacy of Romovac 50, a new inactivated, adjuvanted bovine

rotavirus vaccine. Comp Immun Microbiol Infect Dis 16(3):235–239, 1993.

7. Chasey D, Davies P: Atypical rotaviruses in pigs and cattle. Vet Rec 114:16–17, 1984.

8. Citino SB: Unpublished data, 1997.

9. Clark MA: Bovine Coronaviruses. Br Vet J 149(1):51–70, 1993.

10. Eugster AK, Strother J, Hartfiel DA: Rotavirus (reovirus-like) infection of neonatal ruminants in a zoo nursery. J Wildl Dis 14:351–354, 1978.

11. Flewett TH: Electron microscopy in the diagnosis of infectious diarrhea. J Am Vet Med Assoc 173(1):538–543, 1978.

12. Flewett TH, Woode GN: The rotaviruses. Arch Virol 57:1–23, 1978.

13. Gillespie D, Ellis AC, Rowe-Rossmanith SE, et al: Winter dysentery: Rotavirus and coronavirus infection in hoofstock. Proceedings of the Annual Meeting of the American Association of Zoo Veterinarians, Pittsburgh, PA, pp 393–397, 1994.

14. Guard C: Winter dysentery in cattle. *In* Smith RP (ed): Large animal internal medicine, St. Louis, CV Mosby, pp 816–818, 1990.

15. Hall GA, Bridger JC, Parsons KR, et al: Variation in rotavirus virulence: a comparison of pathogenesis in calves between two rotaviruses of different virulence. Vet Pathol 30:223–233, 1993.

16. Heuschele WP, Janssen DL: Etiology and prevention of neonatal diarrhea in hand-raised exotic ruminants. Proceedings of the Annual Meeting of the American Association of Zoo Veterinarians, Louisville, KY, p 67, 1984.

17. Hussein HA, Parwani AV, Rosen BI, et al: Detection of rotavirus serotypes G1, G2, G3, and G11 in feces of diarrheic calves by using polymerase chain reaction-derived cDNA probes. J Clin Microbiol 31:2491–2496, 1993.

18. Jones RL, Brumbaugh GW: Disinfectants and control of environmental contamination. *In* Smith RP (ed): Large Animal Internal Medicine. St. Louis, CV Mosby, pp 1468–1477, 1990.

19. Lucchelli A, Lance DE, Bartlett PB, et al: Prevalence of bovine group A rotavirus shedding among dairy calves in Ohio. Am J Vet Res 53(2):169–174, 1992.

20. Naylor JM: Diarrhea in neonatal ruminants. *In* Smith RP (ed): Large Animal Internal Medicine. St. Louis, CV Mosby, pp 348–367, 1990.

21. Reed DE, Daley CA, Shave HJ: Reovirus-like agent associated with neonatal diarrhea in pronghorn antelope. J Wildl Dis 12:488–491, 1976.

22. Reynolds DJ, Hall GA, Debney TG, et al: Pathology of natural rotavirus infection in clinically normal calves. Res Vet Sci 38:264–269, 1985.

23. Saif LJ: A review of evidence implicating bovine coronavirus in the etiology of winter dysentery in cows: an enigma resolved? Cornell Vet 80(4):303–311, 1990.

24. Saif LJ: Bovine rotavirus. *In* Castro AE, Heuschele WP (eds): Diagnostic Veterinary Virology: A Practitioner's Guide. Baltimore, Williams & Wilkins, pp 126–130, 1991.

25. Saif LJ: Coronavirus immunogens. Vet Microbiol 37:285–297, 1993.

26. Saif LJ, Heckert RA: Enteropathogenic coronaviruses. *In* Saif LJ, Theil KW (eds): Viral Diarrheas of Man and Animals. Boca Raton, FL, CRC Press, pp 185–252, 1990.

27. Saif LJ, Redman DR, Smith KL, et al: Passive immunity to bovine rotavirus in newborn calves fed colostrum supplements from immunized or nonimmunized cows. Infect Immunol 41(3):1118–1131, 1983.

28. Saif LJ, Smith L: Enteric viral infections of calves and passive immunity. J Dairy Sci 68:206–228, 1985.

29. Sattar SA, Lloyd-Evans N, Springthorpe VS: Institutional outbreaks of rotavirus diarrhoea: potential role of fomites and environmental surfaces as vehicles for virus transmission. J Hyg Camb 96:277–289, 1986.

30. Smith DR, Tsunemitsu H, Heckert RA, et al: Evaluation of two antigen-capture ELISAs using polyclonal and monoclonal antibodies for the detection of bovine coronavirus. J Vet Diagn Invest 8:99–105, 1996.

31. Snodgrass DR, Ojeh CK, Campbell I, et al: Bovine rotavirus serotypes and their significance for immunization. J Clin Microbiol 20(3):342–346, 1984.

32. Theil KW: Group A rotaviruses. *In* Saif LJ, Theil KW (eds): Viral Diarrheas of Man and Animals. Boca Raton, FL, CRC Press, pp 36–72, 1990.

33. Theil KW, McCloskey CM: Molecular epidemiology and subgroup determination of bovine group A rotaviruses associated with diarrhea in dairy and beef cattle. J Clin Microbiol 27(1):126–131, 1989.

34. Theil KW, McCloskey CM: Rotavirus shedding in feces of gnotobiotic calves orally inoculated with a commercial rotavirus-coronavirus vaccine. J Vet Diagn Invest 7:427–432, 1995.

35. Torres-Medina A: Effect of combined rotavirus and *Escherichia coli* in neonatal gnotobiotic calves. Am J Vet Res 45(4):643–651, 1984.

36. Tzipori S, Caple IW: Isolation of a rotavirus from deer. Vet Rec 99:298, 1976.

37. Yolken RH, Barbour B, Wyatt RG, et al: Enzyme-linked immunosorbent assay for identification of rotaviruses from different animal species. Science 201:259–262, 1978.

CHAPTER 90

Paratuberculosis in Zoo Animals

ELIZABETH J. B. MANNING
MICHAEL T. COLLINS

Paratuberculosis, also known as Johne's disease, is a fatal, contagious gastrointestinal disease of ruminants. This disease develops slowly and its management in a zoological park can be troublesome. The depopulation strategy sometimes chosen by a dairy producer with a high prevalence of the disease in a milking herd is neither an agreeable nor serviceable option for a herd of endangered livestock. In addition to the genetic loss, the public's response to the eradication can be another complicating factor.

Surveillance of this disease is difficult because clinical signs can be subtle and appear late in the disease process. Markers for diagnosis (e.g., antibody production, fecal shedding of the organism) show up months to years following infection, after which they can wax and wane. The majority of infected animals are themselves infectious but go undiagnosed. The full impact of herd infection can be aggravated both by the years that can pass before emaciated animals are detected and by the dispersion of animals (and the infection) to other collections through breeding exchanges and sale.

Recent speculation about a link between *M. paratuberculosis* and Crohn's disease, a human inflammatory bowel condition, has raised concerns of a perceived, if not real, public health risk.[8] Because small ruminant animals are susceptible to infection by *M. paratuberculosis* and are a frequent choice for "petting zoos," they are of particular concern for a possible zoonotic risk.

As with so many preventable problems, the prevention is much more effective than attempting a cure. In fact, for Johne's disease, there is no cure. There are no reports of an economically feasible and clinically effective therapeutic protocol.[11] It is critical, therefore, to establish a workable surveillance plan for each collection to prevent introduction of the disease or limit spread of existing infection.

ORGANISM AND TRANSMISSION

The agent causing Johne's disease—*Mycobacterium paratuberculosis*—is a hardy, acid-fast, gram-positive staining, rod-shaped bacterium. Since much of its DNA mirrors the DNA structure of *Mycobacterium avium*, the organism is also known as *M. avium* subspecies *paratuberculosis*. The two mycobacteria are not the same, however, and methods exist to distinguish between them. The organism causing Johne's disease is characterized by a ribosomal insertion sequence (IS900) that is detectable by genetic probes[14] and by phenotypic characteristics such as a slow growth rate and dependence on a growth factor (mycobactin) for in vitro cultivation.

It is assumed that transmission of *Mycobacterium paratuberculosis* in all species follows the pattern described in cattle.[6] Young animals are the most susceptible, although adults can be infected in some circumstances. The fecal-oral transmission route accounts for the majority of infections. Ingestion of contaminated milk or colostrum is another infection route for young stock. In utero infection has been documented in sheep, cows, and goats and may occur in other species as well.[13] Transplacental infection is more likely to occur when the dam is in the final stages of clinical disease.

HOST RANGE

All hoofstock are candidates for paratuberculosis. Although primarily affecting ruminant animals, Johne's disease has also been reported in pseudoruminants (camelids), rabbits, and primates.[3, 7, 9, 12] Under experimental conditions, mice, pigs, hamsters, and chickens have been successfully infected with *M. paratuberculo-*

sis. Even though different strains of the organism are cultured from different species, cross-species infection by most, if not all, strains of *M. paratuberculosis* is likely.

CLINICAL SIGNS AND PATHOLOGY

Much of the information on the clinical and pathologic presentation of paratuberculosis is based on the disease as it develops in bovids: infection as a calf, a subclinical phase that can last for years, eventual emaciation, and death. Whereas many of these aspects are comparable across species, distinct species differences do exist. For instance, the onset of clinical signs can occur at younger ages in sheep, goats, deer, and camelids than is common in cattle.

M. paratuberculosis infection should be considered in any "unthrifty" appearing ungulate. Chronic weight loss and a scruffy hair coat in the face of a continued good appetite are the most common clinical signs of Johne's disease. In cattle, chronic diarrhea is common, whereas, in other species, diarrhea may be absent or intermittent. The clinical signs of paratuberculosis are essentially the same as those observed with intestinal parasitism, that is, the animal remains alert and responsive but can appear depressed and increasingly weak during the latter stages of the disease. Except for hypoproteinemia in some cases, there are few abnormalities in either clinical chemistry or hematologic values.[5]

Gross lesions reflect the diffuse granulomatous intestinal inflammation and emaciation that characterize the disease. Classic (i.e., bovine) lesions include variably severe thickening and corrugation of the mucosal layer of the small intestine (predominantly the ileum and jejunum), edema, and enlargement of mesenteric lymph nodes and corded lymphatics. These lesions may not be seen in other zoological ruminants. For example, the distal small intestine may appear normal in goats, deer, and elk. In those species, serous atrophy of fat may be observed as may excessive pericardial, abdominal, and thoracic fluid, which may reflect the hypoproteinemia. Lesion severity is a function of the stage of the disease—disseminated infection in late stage clinical disease can be seen as granulomatous lesions throughout and beyond the gastrointestinal viscera.

Histologically, the intestinal submucosa is infiltrated with epithelioid macrophages and multinucleate giant cells. Numerous short intracellular rods are exhibited with Ziehl-Neelsen staining. (In sheep in particular, a paucibacillary form of paratuberculosis has been described. The predominant infiltrating cells are lymphocytes, and a few acid-fast rods are noted.)[1] Lymphatic channels can also be filled with macrophages containing *M. paratuberculosis*. Lymph nodes can undergo caseous necrosis and sometimes mineralization, a finding similar to that found with *Mycobacterium bovis* and *M. avium* infection in cervids. Further diagnostics (culture of tissue or gene probes) may be necessary to distinguish the infecting organism in these animals.

DETECTION METHODS

There are a number of accurate and cost-effective methods available to the zoo community for surveillance and detection of animals with Johne's disease. Rather than relying on one method, application of a number of techniques greatly improves the effectiveness of a Johne's disease control program. As in any disease control program, reliable animal identification systems and accurate record keeping are critical to managing this disease.

Clinical Assessment

Animal care staff should be taught about the disease and trained to notice subtle changes. Has the animal been eating well yet ribs and spine appear or feel more prominent? Have episodes of loose stool been recorded? Regular monitoring for these simple but telling signs can improve detection of infected animals. Cases of Johne's disease in a zoological setting are often masked by coexisting parasite problems, treatment of which can produce a temporary clinical improvement that confounds Johne's disease diagnosis.

Necropsy Screens

Individual animals should be scrutinized to strengthen herd surveillance. On every necropsy, especially for ungulates, lesions compatible with Johne's disease should be sought, even if the immediate cause of death is known. Because Johne's disease develops so slowly in many species, other more acute conditions may arise simultaneously. Culture of tissue harboring suspicious lesions should accompany histologic examination with acid-fast staining. In herd (elk, goat, cattle) infections evaluated by the authors, culture of tissues was more effective at detecting the organism in some herds, whereas, in other case studies, paratuberculosis was confirmed more often by histologic study.

Feral and wild inhabitants of zoo premises can also be sources of infection. Free-ranging white tail deer, tule elk, bighorn sheep, and rabbits have all been infected by *M. paratuberculosis* and may serve as reservoirs of the disease (see Chapter 91).[4]

Direct Smear/Touch Press

Ziehl-Neelsen staining of either a direct fecal smear or a touch press of biopsy samples can occasionally reveal the large clumps of short, red mycobacterial rods. This method is easy, swift, and inexpensive, but it is neither sensitive nor definitive.

Serologic Detection

It is thought that most animals eventually produce antibodies in response to infection by *M. paratuberculosis*. This humoral response is not protective and is a futile attempt by the immune system to fight the disease. It is likely that animals have been shedding the infective organism in their feces and milk long before they mount an antibody response. Three serologic assays have been used to detect antibodies to *M. paratuberculosis* in cattle, goats, and sheep[2]; however, none of these have been validated for use in other zoological ruminant animals. The three assays are (1) complement fixation (CF), (2) agar gel immunodiffusion (AGID), and (3) enzyme-linked immunosorbent assay (ELISA). The sensitivity of the assays is a function of the stage of disease when the animal is sampled. Species-specific ELISAs exist for cattle and goats; camelid and cervid assays will soon be available. For an animal of any species showing clinical signs of Johne's disease, the AGID may be used as a "rule-in" test. Given the low sensitivity of the assay in subclinical animals and the uncertainty about its accuracy in nondomestic species, negative results cannot rule out a diagnosis of Johne's disease.

Bacteriologic Culture

The culture method is useful for fecal, tissue, soil, compost, and water samples. Animals that are the greatest threat to the rest of the collection can be detected by bacteriologic culture. Animals shed *M. paratuberculosis* in their feces onto the premises, and infective organisms have been recovered from soil a year after contamination. Animals shedding the organism are also more likely to infect their offspring through contaminated milk and in utero transmission.

Isolation of *M. paratuberculosis* is 100% specific for a diagnosis of Johne's disease as long as isolates are tested for IS900, the genetic marker distinguishing *M. paratuberculosis* from other closely related mycobacteria. However, detection of "pass-through" organisms, that is, simple oral ingestion and direct excretion of the organism without true infection and replication in the gastrointestinal tract, is a possible but rare occurrence.

The greatest disadvantage of this diagnostic method is that it is slow, relying on the protracted growth cycle of the organism. The generation time for *M. paratuberculosis* is 2 days, and 3 to 4 months is required to generate the sufficient number of organisms that can be seen as a colony on an agar slant by conventional culture methods. The radiometric culture method is faster, but its radioisotope-based method of growth detection still takes from 4 to 7 weeks.

To maximize the diagnostic value of the culture technique, the testing laboratory should be consulted for the best methods for sample collection and handling. Collection of 3 g (approximately 1 tablespoon) of fecal material directly from the rectum is recommended. Decontaminating the sample with HPC (hexadecylpyridinium chloride) at the time of sample collection can decrease problems with overgrowth of normal microflora while the sample is in transit to the laboratory.

Biopsy

For exceptionally valuable animals (e.g., for bull studs or for valuable animals in zoological parks), surgical confirmation of a positive culture or serologic test result is often desired. Biopsy specimens can be collected with minimal risk. The samples most likely to harbor the organism are the ileum (a full-thickness section should be sampled) and a mesenteric lymph node (an enlarged node should be sampled). Enough tissue should be collected (at least 2 cm × 1 cm) to be divided for both culture and histologic study. Rectal biopsies are not sufficiently sensitive to merit their use.

Genetic Probe

Detection of the unique insertion sequence (IS900) by PCR amplification is a fast way to confirm that an animal is shedding *M. paratuberculosis.*[10] The specificity of this probe is 100%, but it has a high detection limit; an organism count of at least 10^4 per gram of sample is needed. (Both conventional and radiometric culture methods are more sensitive than the probe.)

SUGGESTED TESTING PROTOCOLS

Confirmation of a Clinical Diagnosis

When clinical signs compatible with Johne's disease are observed, the *M. paratuberculosis* organism or the animal's immunological response to infection must then be detected. The choice of detection method is influenced by available resources (time as well as money), animal species, and Johne's disease prevalence. For most situations, fecal culture is the best choice to confirm clinical suspicion. Submission of 2 to 3 ml of serum for an AGID or ELISA may also be useful for faster verification of the diagnosis in animals with clinical signs consistent with Johne's disease.

If clinical diagnosis is confirmed, further steps are necessary because Johne's disease in a single animal is a herd problem. Once a diagnosis is made, other members of the herd, the animal's offspring, and the exhibit should be examined for routes of infection. Possible routes include the source of colostrum/milk for hand-reared infants, the exposure of young stock to adult manure (including water sources) in the exhibit, and fecal contamination of feed bunks. An annual fecal culture screen of all adult animals in the exhibit should be considered. The infected animal should be euthanatized or at least isolated and its offspring should be evaluated as well.

Control Program

Johne's disease should always be on the list of differential diagnoses for a thin animal. The ramifications of missing the diagnosis in a herd of exotic hoofstock can be severe, so the expense of ruling it out must be accepted. If there is any possibility of Johne's disease (based on clinical assessment, exposure, or test results), *early detection of infectious animals is critical.* Regular

(annual) screening of adult animals over a period of years is necessary to reveal and eliminate a herd infection. For optimal fecal culture screens, three samples should be collected over the period of 1 week. This schedule improves the likelihood of recovering organisms from animals shedding *M. paratuberculosis* intermittently. Picking up samples from a clean stall or pen floor from animals held for a short time or from the ground in the exhibit itself is acceptable for animals that cannot easily be penned and handled. To minimize testing costs, albeit with some reduction in test sensitivity, fecal samples for culture can be pooled (with a maximum of 3 animals per pool), followed by an individual retest of each animal from samples that are positive. The pooling of equal amounts of feces, by weight, should be done by the testing laboratory. Control of disease transmission should include the following:

1. Keeping up proper sanitation of exhibits, including removal and composting of feces
2. Teaching keeper and veterinary staff members the clinical signs of Johne's disease
3. Performing necropsy screens
4. Giving milk and colostrum from Johne's disease–free sources to hand-reared neonates
5. Testing herds annually, testing animals with compatible clinical signs, and culling or isolating animals that test positive for *M. paratuberculosis* infection.

Sale/Exchange

At many zoos, three negative fecal cultures must be collected some weeks apart before animals are accepted into quarantine at the new site. While in quarantine, an additional fecal culture should be obtained, preferably a sample collected immediately after shipment to the new facility, because it is thought that an animal is more likely to shed the organism when stressed. Testing requirements for export are as specified by the receiving country; the U.S. Department of Agriculture has not detailed Johne's disease testing requirements for the import of exotic hoofstock.

TREATMENT

There is no cure for Johne's disease. Disease in animals of high genetic value has been treated to suppress the debilitating effects of *M. paratuberculosis* infection long enough to rescue offspring at birth or to collect germ cells. (While *M. paratuberculosis* has been isolated from semen and reproductive organs and can survive freezing and sample processing, its presence in germ plasm is not thought to be infective.) Treatment protocols developed for cattle are expensive, inconvenient, long term, and palliative only. The drugs most often used were chosen for their ability to affect intracellular organisms such as *M. paratuberculosis* and include isoniazid, rifampin, streptomycin, amikacin, kanamycin, clofazimine, and dapsone. A discussion of dosages and their efficacy can be found in reference 11.

Studies assessing the teratogenic risks of treatment have not been completed.

CONCLUSION

Because *M. paratuberculosis* is an obligate intracellular parasite, it is possible to eradicate Johne's disease. The zoo community, including all hoofstock suppliers to zoos, would benefit from plans that identify and control the infection and prevent the disease from becoming an even greater threat to endangered hoofstock.

REFERENCES

1. Clarke CJ, Patterson IAP, Armstrong KE, et al: Comparison of the absorbed ELISA and agar gel immunodiffusion with clinicopathological findings in ovine clinical paratuberculosis. Vet Rec 139:618–21, 1996.
2. Collins MT: Diagnosis of paratuberculosis. Paratuberculosis (Johne's disease). Vet Clin North Am Food Anim Pract 12(2):357–371, 1996.
3. Greig A, Stevenson K, Perez V, et al: Paratuberculosis in wild rabbits *(Orcyctolagus cuniculus)*. Vet Rec 140:141–143, 1997.
4. Jessup DA, Abbas B, Behymer D: Paratuberculosis in tule elk in California. J Am Vet Med Assoc 179:1252–1254, 1981.
5. Jones DG, Kay JM: Serum biochemistry and the diagnosis of Johne's disease (paratuberculosis) in sheep. Vet Rec 139:498–499, 1996.
6. Lepper AWD: The aetiology and pathogenesis of Johne's disease. *In* Milner AR, Wood PR (eds): Johne's Disease. East Melbourne, Australia, Commonwealth Scientific and Industrial Research Organization. 1992.
7. McClure HM, Chiodini RJ, Anderson DC, et al: *Mycobacterium paratuberculosis* infection in a colony of stump tail macaques *(Macaca artoides)*. J Infect Dis 155:1011–1019, 1987.
8. Mishna D, Katsel P, Brown ST, Gilberts ECAM, et al: On the etiology of Crohn's disease. Proc Natl Acad Sci USA 93:9816–9820, 1996.
9. Ridge SE, Harkin JT, Badman RT, et al: Johne's disease in alpacas *(Lama pacos)* in Australia. Aust Vet J 72:150–153, 1995.
10. Sockett DC, Carr DJ, Collins MT: Evaluation of conventional and radiometric fecal culture and a commercial DNA probe for diagnosis of *Mycobacterium paratuberculosis* infections in cattle. Can J Vet Res 56:148–152, 1992.
11. St Jean G: Treatment of clinical paratuberculosis in cattle. Paratuberculosis (Johne's disease). Vet Clin North Am Food Anim Pract 12(2):417–430, 1996.
12. Steinberg H: Johne's disease *(Mycobacterium paratuberculosis)* in a Jemela topi *(Damaliscus lunatus jimela)*. J Zoo Anim Med 19(1–2):33–41, 1981.
13. Sweeney RW, Whitlock RH, Rosenberger AE. *Mycobacterium paratuberculosis* isolated from fetuses of infected cows not manifesting signs of the disease. Am J Vet Res 53:477–480, 1992.
14. Vary PH, Andersen PR, Green E, et al: Use of highly specific DNA probes and the polymerase chain reaction to detect *Mycobacterium paratuberculosis* in Johne's disease. J Clin Microbiol 30:166–171, 1992.

CHAPTER **91**

Paratuberculosis in Free-Ranging Wildlife in North America

DAVID A. JESSUP
ELIZABETH S. WILLIAMS

HISTORY

Paratuberculosis (Johne's disease), caused by *Mycobacterium paratuberculosis* (*Mycobacterium avium* subspecies *paratuberculosis*), is an infectious bacterial disease of livestock that may be transmitted to captive and free-ranging wildlife.[4, 28] This disease is rare in free-ranging wildlife. Clinical disease has been diagnosed only in Rocky Mountain bighorn sheep (*Ovis canadensis canadensis*) from a few herds in Colorado and Wyoming,[32] in Rocky Mountain goats (*Oreamnos americanus*) in Colorado,[32] and in tule elk (*Cervis elaphus nannodes*) at one national seashore in California.[14] *M. paratuberculosis* has been cultured from the feces, collected at Point Reyes National Seashore in California, of clinically normal free-ranging fallow deer (*Dama dama*) and axis deer (*Axis axis*).[17] Similarly, *M. paratuberculosis* has been cultured from feces of white-tailed (*Odocoileus virginianus*) deer sharing pastures with cattle in Ohio and New York.[3, 18] However, even though clinical paratuberculosis is rare, its presence in free-ranging herds may cause serious and unique problems for the management of affected populations.

In free-ranging wild ruminants, paratuberculosis was first diagnosed in bighorn sheep in the Grant–Mount Evans herds in Colorado in 1972 and in sympatric mountain goats in 1978. The origin of the disease has never been determined, but there is ample evidence that these wild bovid populations are capable of maintaining the infection. One or two clinical cases of paratuberculosis are recognized each year, which suggests a clinical incidence of approximately 1%; known annual mortality from 1977 to 1981 was 1.3%. Actual mortality from paratuberculosis is not known but has been estimated[27] to be as high as 5%; this may be an overestimate. Prevalence of subclinical infection is also not known, but of 24 bighorn sheep sampled from the Grant–Mount Evans herds, 14 (58%) had either clinical or subclinical paratuberculosis, diagnosed at necropsy. This suggests a relatively high rate of subclinical infection in the herd. However, surveillance efforts within these herds, including use of fecal culture, serologic profiles, and histopathology, did not identify any infected animals (M. W. Miller, unpublished data, 1997).

The options for management of paratuberculosis infected herds are limited. Neither bighorn nor mountain goats are used for relocation because of fear of transplanting paratuberculosis along with them. Mountain goats are of more concern because they may be more likely to spread paratuberculosis from the endemic area to other bighorn and mountain goat populations. Mountain goats move greater distances during periods of dispersal and are more exploratory than bighorn. Management objectives for these herds are to decrease their density to reduce the likelihood of dispersal to paratuberculosis-free herds. Hunting strategies, including harvest of either sex and of younger animals have been instituted. However, the objectives for management of these herds have not always been consistent. For example, these bighorn sheep have been treated for lungworms even though growth of the herd was not desirable.

Paratuberculosis was diagnosed in a single ram from the Laramie Range in Wyoming. This emaciated animal was found dead and decomposed; *M. paratuberculosis* was cultured from the mesenteric lymph nodes. The animal was from a low-density and relatively low-elevation bighorn sheep herd. The disease does not appear to have persisted in this herd, inasmuch as no additional clinical cases have been recognized since 1983; although specific surveys have never been conducted.

In March 1978, 14 tule elk were relocated to the Point Reyes National Seashore in California. Despite agreements to the contrary, cattle had not been removed from the fenced northern peninsula of the National Seashore onto which the elk were released, although that was accomplished several months later. Malnutrition and copper deficiency affected the elk during their first 2 years at Point Reyes.[12] Two calves born in March 1978 and one calf born in March 1979 manifested severe clinical signs of paratuberculosis in the 12 to 18 months after birth. These animals were removed from the herd for necropsy in 1980 and 1981. One additional animal showing signs of diarrhea and emaciation was removed in 1985 and another in 1987. Both of these elk were 4 years old (born in 1981 and 1983, respectively), both had a thickened and rugose ileum and enlarged mesenteric lymph nodes filled with acid-fast bacteria, and cultures from both yielded positive findings for *M. paratuberculosis*. Although periodically since that time a small number of elk have been re-

ported to have prolonged diarrhea or signs of straining during defecation, no additional clinical cases have been diagnosed in tule elk. A fecal plot survey at Point Reyes was conducted in 1993 with radiometrically enhanced culture to identify infected animals; 4% of the 100 samples were identified as positive.[7] The elk population at Point Reyes has not been hunted or routinely culled (except for a very few clinically affected animals) and in 1996 numbered approximately 400 animals.

Paratuberculosis has a wide host range and has caused several chronic, very difficult-to-manage, multispecies infections in North American zoological and wild animal parks and is also a significant problem in commercial game farms and ranches worldwide.[9, 11, 16] Severe, rapidly progressing cases of paratuberculosis in young (1- to 2-year-old) ranch-raised fallow deer were reported in New York.[22] This herd had been assembled from a single source 3 years previously, and some older adults were in poor condition. Diagnosis was based on serologic tests (agar gel immunodiffusion [AGID]), histopathology, and fecal and ileocecal junction cultures (positivity for *M. paratuberculosis* was confirmed by IS900 probe). Granulomatous lesions in the thoracic lymph nodes and lungs of heavily infected individuals were indistinguishable from those caused by *M. bovis*. Pulmonary granulomas caused by paratuberculosis have been reported in experimentally infected mule deer (*Odocoileus hemionus*).[31] Cases of paratuberculosis in ranch-raised red deer in Canada have been reported to occur under circumstances that could have resulted in exposure of hundreds of other red deer to infected feces.[20] Paratuberculosis has also been reported to be a chronic problem in farmed red deer in Ireland.[16]

PATHOGENESIS

The etiologic agent of paratuberculosis, *M. paratuberculosis*, is typical of mycobacteria in its degree of environmental resistance.[15] It survives desiccation but is susceptible to ultraviolet light and to heat. The organism may remain infectious on pastures under favorable conditions for approximately 1 year.

Paratuberculosis is transmitted primarily through ingestion of bacteria shed in feces. However, the bacteria have been recovered from milk, and congenital infection of domestic calves has been reported. The organism has been isolated from the uterus and a fetus of a clinically affected bighorn ewe.[27] The relative importance of congenital infection in free-ranging species is unknown. Young animals in contaminated environments are most susceptible to infection. Under experimental conditions, as few as 1000 bacteria may establish an infection in domestic lambs. This appears to be the situation faced by calves born to cow elk at Point Reyes, inasmuch as only they and not adult animals manifested clinical infections. The relatively limited range of tule elk on contaminated pastures at Point Reyes, in an area known to have conditions favorable for persistence of the bacteria, probably ensures that many elk are exposed to the organism. Exposure of bighorn sheep is probably through traditional bedding areas, which may predispose the bighorn to fecal-oral

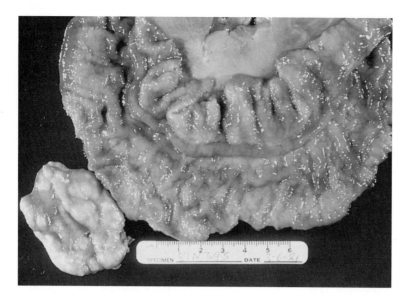

FIGURE 91–1. Section of ileum and mesenteric lymph node from tule elk with paratuberculosis. Note the thickened, rugose nature of the mucosa and the proliferative and swollen appearance of the lymph node.

transmission of the organism, even though they are not constrained by fences or limited range.

Ingested bacteria proliferate within the distal portions of the small intestine, spiral colon, and colon and within their draining lymphoid structures. On occasion, the organism may be found in tissues distant from the digestive tract, especially in the liver and the lungs. The bacteria elicit a granulomatous inflammatory response, which may result in thickening of the intestinal wall, enlargement of regional lymph nodes (Fig. 91–1), and thickening and possibly blockage of afferent lymphatic vessels (Fig. 91–2). The inflammatory reaction results in significant disruption of intestinal function; fluids and nutrients are not absorbed normally, and this results in chronic watery diarrhea, usually excreted without straining. Emaciation and other signs of malabsorption

and malnutrition follow. Dissemination to the liver and other vital organs may eventually occur. As in domestic species, many wild animals may be subclinically infected, with limited proliferation of bacteria. However, these animals may shed the organism at low levels, contributing to environmental contamination, and may insidiously serve to transmit the infection into previously uninfected herds.

Paratuberculosis is a chronic disease. Incubation periods are variable but usually many months to years in duration. Clinical disease appears to be more common in yearling and young adult wild ruminants than in domestic species. The most common clinical signs in wild ruminants are loss of body condition to a state of emaciation (Fig. 91–3), hypoproteinemia, intermandibular edema, and diarrhea.[4, 21, 28] Duration of diarrhea may be variable; in bighorn sheep, emaciation was the most prominent sign, and diarrhea occurred only in the last few months of life. In deer, hypoproteinemia and intermandibular edema may be the only signs.[21] The chronicity of disease and loss of body condition may adversely influence the growth of antlers or horns. Once clinical

FIGURE 91–2. Section of distal ileum from a tule elk with paratuberculosis. Note the thickened and chorded afferent lymphatic vessels and edema along the mesenteric attachment.

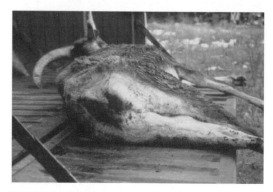

FIGURE 91–3. This free-ranging bighorn sheep died of paratuberculosis but showed only signs of emaciation and general ill thrift until shortly before death.

manifestations are evident, paratuberculosis is invariably fatal. There is no effective therapy or treatment for paratuberculosis in free-ranging wild ruminants. Vaccinations are being investigated for use in domestic species, but none have been tested in wildlife.

DIAGNOSIS

The gross lesions of paratuberculosis are variable. Animals with severe clinical disease may not have severe lesions. Well-developed gross lesions include thickened and folded walls of the distal small intestine, enlarged pale or mineralized lymph nodes, subserosal and mesenteric edema, and thickening and cording of mesenteric lymphatic vessels. Microscopic lesions are primarily those of a multifocal or diffuse granulomatous inflammation.[30] Lesions are prominent in organs with gross abnormalities, but they may also be observed in grossly normal organs, including the tonsils, multiple lymph nodes, the spleen, the liver, and the lungs. Presence of giant cells is variable. Foci of necrosis and mineralization may be present and are more common in wild ruminants than in cattle.

Acid-fast stains are useful for diagnosis; in some severely affected animals essentially all phagocytic cells are filled with bacteria. Truant's auramine-rhodamine technique for mycobacteria may also be useful for diagnosis[28] (Fig. 91–4). More recently, immunohistochemistry has been employed for detection of mycobacterial antigens in tissues.[25]

A presumptive diagnosis of paratuberculosis can be reached by finding clumps of acid-fast organisms, sometimes within sloughed cells, in fecal smears from live animals that are emaciated and/or have diarrhea. Stains of fecal smears or tissue impressions may not detect subclinical carriers or animals with clinical disease that are not shedding large numbers of organisms. A culture of feces or tissues (mesenteric lymph nodes, ileocecal junction) is the most sensitive way to reach a definitive diagnosis. Traditional culture is performed on a mycobactin-enriched (i.e., Harold's egg yolk) media and may take 6 to 12 weeks. Improvements in techniques, culture media, detection of growth, and identification of organisms have decreased the time necessary to make a diagnosis.[2, 6, 8, 26] A commercial polymerase chain reaction test to detect mycobacteria in feces developed for use on cattle may provide results much more rapidly than culture, but it has higher potential for false-positive and false-negative results.[24] It is important to remember that subclinically affected animals may shed organisms only intermittently and at low levels, and thus their true carrier status may not be detected by tests of feces for presence of *M. paratuberculosis*.

Many serologic tests have been developed in an attempt to diagnose paratuberculosis. None are ideal, and none are reliable in subclinical stages of the disease. None have been extensively tested in wild ruminants; therefore, sensitivity and specificity for most species are not known. Enzyme-linked immunosorbent assay (ELISA) is probably the most useful for clinically affected animals.[1, 5, 18, 23] Radioimmunoassay (RIA),[17] complement fixation,[29] and AGID tests[10] have been used with some success. Comparison of an ELISA, a complement-fixation test, and an AGID test revealed the ELISA to be most sensitive in herds of cattle in which paratuberculosis persists.[24] In a high percentage of subclinically affected cattle from which paratuberculosis was isolated at necropsy, mycobacterial antibodies are not detectable in sera. Therefore, ELISA and other serologic tests are of limited value in detecting cattle in early stages of infection or those shedding small numbers of organisms.[24] This is certainly likely to be true in free-ranging wildlife as well.

Diagnostic tests for mycobacteriosis based on cell-mediated immunity have also been developed[13, 29] but are of limited practical value in free-ranging wild species. A test for production of gamma-interferon has been developed for diagnosis of subclinical paratuberculosis[19] but has not yet been tested in nondomestic species.

MANAGEMENT

Paratuberculosis is difficult to control in captive animals, and in free-ranging wildlife, control efforts have not been systematically evaluated. In captivity, clinically affected animals can be culled, available diagnostic tests can be used (even if they are not perfect), neonates can be raised in clean environments, and appropriate sanitation and disinfection can be used to assist in control of paratuberculosis. These techniques are not practical in free-ranging populations. Management is complicated by the chronicity of the disease, by environmental resistance of the causative organism, and by lack of efficacious diagnostic tests. A small number of clinically infected tule elk were shot in California, and hunting seasons were used in Colorado to check population growth; however, neither of these approaches were consistently applied or evaluated for effect on disease prevalence over time. Even with culling of affected individual tule elk, the apparent prevalence of infection declined only to at least 4% of the herd approximately 15 years later.[7] The marginal to deficient copper levels of tule elk may be a predisposing

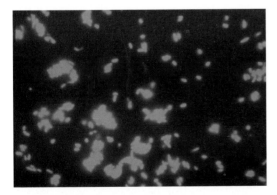

FIGURE 91–4. The Truant's auramine-rhodamine technique can help to identify acid-fast organisms in tissues in which they are not abundant enough to be appreciated by more traditional acid-fast staining techniques.

factor in their susceptibility to paratuberculosis. Paratuberculosis was still present in bighorn in Colorado more than 20 years after its discovery.

Prevention of paratuberculosis infection or of the establishment of disease in free-ranging populations is extremely important. This is particularly true where and when wildlife populations are overabundant and where game farm wildlife or infected livestock may mix with free-ranging wildlife. However, in the few populations of affected free-ranging wildlife, paratuberculosis has not appeared to spread widely or rapidly, and unless infected animals are moved, it may be self-limiting. Infected wild animals or herds in which paratuberculosis is endemic should not be relocated. Shipment of infected captive wildlife between ranches or zoos is strongly discouraged. The relatively low infectivity of the organism and low yearly mortality rates make it unlikely that a wild animal population could be severely affected from the point of view of animal numbers; however, constraints on the management of infected herds are significant. Individual infected animals may show decreased productivity and physical condition and could be predisposed to predation. Feces and carcasses of infected animals should be treated as infectious waste. All applicable state and federal laws and policies for livestock should serve as bases for wildlife and exotic animal management decisions.

REFERENCES

1. Burnside DM, Rowley BO: Evaluation of an enzyme-linked immunosorbent assay for diagnosis of paratuberculosis in goats. Am J Vet Res 55:465–466, 1994.
2. Challans JA, Stevenson K, Reid HW, et al: A rapid method for the extraction and detection of *Mycobacterium avium* subspecies *paratuberculosis* from clinical specimens. Vet Rec 134:95–96, 1994.
3. Chiodini RJ, Kruiningen HJV: Eastern white-tailed deer as a reservoir of ruminant paratuberculosis. J Am Vet Med Assoc 182:168, 1983.
4. Chiodini RJ, Kruiningen HJV, Merkal R: Ruminant paratuberculosis (Johne's disease): the current status and future prospects. Cornell Vet 74:218–262, 1984.
5. Collins MT, Kenefick KB, Sockett DC, et al: Enhanced radiometric detection of *Mycobacterium paratuberculosis* by using filter-concentrated bovine fecal specimens. J Clin Microbiol 28:2514–2519, 1990.
6. Collins MT, Sockett DC, Ridge S: Evaluation of a commercial enzyme-linked immunosorbent assay for Johne's disease. J Clin Microbiol 29:272–276, 1991.
7. Cook W, Cornish TE, Shideler S, et al: Evidence of *Mycobacterium paratuberculosis* in the feces of tule elk from Point Reyes National Park. J Wildl Dis 33:635–637, 1997.
8. Cousins DV, Evans RJ, Francis BR: Use of BACTEC radiometric culture method and polymerase chain reaction for the rapid screening of faeces and tissues for *Mycobacterium paratuberculosis*. Aust Vet J 72:458–462, 1995.
9. deLisle GW, Yates GF, Collins DM: Paratuberculosis in farmed deer: case reports and DNA characterization of isolates of *Mycobacterium paratuberculosis*. J Vet Diagn Invest 5:567–571, 1993.
10. Dubash K, Shulaw WP, Bech-Nielsen S, et al: Evaluation of an agar gel immunodiffusion test kit for detection of antibodies to *Mycobacterium paratuberculosis* in sheep. J Am Vet Med Assoc 208:401–403, 1996.
11. Fawcett AR, Goddard PJ, McKelvey WAC, et al: Johne's disease in a herd of farmed red deer. Vet Rec 136:165–169, 1995.
12. Gogan PJP, Jessup DA, Akeson M: Copper deficiency in tule elk at Point Reyes, California. J Range Manage 42(3):233–238, 1989.
13. Hutchings DL, Wilson SH: Evaluation of lymphocyte stimulation tests for diagnosis of bovine tuberculosis in elk (*Cervus elaphus*). Am J Vet Res 56:27–33, 1995.
14. Jessup DA, Abbas B, Behymer D: Paratuberculosis in tule elk in California. J Am Vet Med Assoc 179:1252, 1981.
15. Mitscherlich E, Marth EH: Microbial Survival in the Environment. New York, Springer-Verlag, 1984.
16. Power SB, Haagsma J, Smyth DP: Paratuberculosis in red deer (*Cervus elaphus*) in Ireland. Vet Rec 132:213–216, 1993.
17. Reimann H, Zaman MR, Ruppaner R, et al: Paratuberculosis in cattle and free-living exotic deer. J Am Vet Med Assoc 174:841–843, 1979.
18. Shulaw WP, Gordon WP, Bech-Nielsen S, et al: Evidence of paratuberculosis in Ohio's white-tailed deer as determined by an enzyme-linked immunosorbent assay. Am J Vet Res 47:2539–2542, 1986.
19. Stabel JR: Production of gamma-interferon by peripheral blood mononuclear cells: an important diagnostic tool for detection of subclinical paratuberculosis. J Vet Diagn Invest 8:345–350, 1996.
20. Starke RKA: Paratuberculosis (Johne's disease) in a captive wapiti. *In* Renecker LA, Hudson RJ (eds): Wildlife Production: Conservation and Sustainable Development [Alaska Fairbanks Educational Series misc. pub. 91–6]. Fairbanks, University of Alaska, Fairbanks, pp 435–437, 1991.
21. Stehman SM: Paratuberculosis in small ruminants, deer, and South American camelids. Vet Clin North Am Food Anim Pract 12(2):441–455, 1996.
22. Stehman SM, Rossiter C, Shin S, Lein DH: Severe paratuberculosis in a farmed fallow deer herd. *In* Proceedings of the American Association of Veterinary Laboratory Diagnosticians, Reno, NV, p 44, 1995.
23. Sweeney RW, Whitlock RH, Buckley CL: Evaluation of a commercial enzyme-linked immunosorbent assay for the diagnosis of paratuberculosis in dairy cattle. J Vet Diagn Invest 7:288–293, 1995.
24. Thoen CO, Haagsma J: Molecular techniques in the diagnosis and control of paratuberculosis in cattle. J Am Vet Med Assoc 209(4):734–737, 1996.
25. Thorsen OF, Falk, K, Evensen O: Comparison of immunohistochemistry, acid fast staining and cultivation for detection of *Mycobacterium paratuberculosis*. J Vet Diagn Invest 6:195–199, 1994.
26. Thorsen OF, Olsaker I: Distribution and hybridization patterns of the insertion element IS900 in clinical isolation of *Mycobacterium paratuberculosis*. Vet Microbiol 40:293–303, 1994.
27. Williams ES: Spontaneous and experimental infection of wild ruminants with *Mycobacterium paratuberculosis*. PhD dissertation, Colorado State University, Fort Collins, 1981.
28. Williams ES: Paratuberculosis (Johne's disease). *In* Thorne ET, Kingston N, Jolley WR, et al (eds): Diseases of Wyoming Wildlife, 2nd ed. Cheyenne, Wyoming Game and Fish Department, pp 91–94, 1982.
29. Williams ES, Demartini JC, Snyder SP: Lymphocyte blastogenesis, complement fixation, and fecal culture as diagnostic tests in North American wild ruminants and domestic sheep. Am J Vet Res 46:2317, 1985.
30. Williams ES, Snyder SP, Martin KL: Experimental infection of some North American wild ruminants and domestic sheep with *Mycobacterium paratuberculosis*: clinical and bacteriological findings. J Wildl Dis 19:185, 1983.
31. Williams ES, Snyder SP, Martin KL: Pathology of spontaneous and experimental infection of North American wild ruminants with *Mycobacterium paratuberculosis*. Vet Pathol 20:274, 1983.
32. Williams ES, Spraker TR, Schoonveld GS: Paratuberculosis (Johne's disease) in bighorn sheep and Rocky Mountain goats in Colorado. J Wildl Dis 15:221–227, 1979.

CHAPTER 92

Brucellosis Caused by *Brucella abortus* in Free-Ranging North American Artiodactylids

DAVID L. HUNTER

TERRY J. KREEGER

Brucellosis is a highly contagious bacterial disease of both animals and humans recognized since the 19th century. Several species of the genus *Brucella* are recognized, including *Brucella abortus, Brucella suis, Brucella canis, Brucella melitensis, Brucella neotomae*, and *Brucella ovis*. Species susceptible to brucellosis vary from artiodactylids and perissodactylids to rodentia and carnivora. This chapter discusses brucellosis caused by *B. abortus* in free-ranging artiodactylids (even-toed ungulates) with particular emphasis on brucellosis in North American wildlife.

MICROBIOLOGY AND TAXONOMY

Brucella species are small, gram-negative, nonmotile, non–spore-forming rods that can be isolated on a variety of media, such as tryptose agar, incubated in 10% CO_2 at 37°C. Smooth, light greenish-blue colonies with central beige coloration that are 1.5 to 2.0 mm in diameter are visible in 3 days. The various species and biovars can be identified by their ability to grow on media containing basic fuschin, thionin, thionin blue, penicillin, and erythritol.[25]

The current taxonomic scheme recognizes eight biotypes (biovars) of *B. abortus*, although at least 22 have been reported. *B. abortus* type 1 is probably the most common isolate from North American wildlife.[49, 56] There is evidence that the progenitor organism for all *Brucella* species was *B. abortus* type 2.[30] Molecular biology techniques, such as polymerase chain reaction, provide additional epidemiologic tools to trace sources of infection among populations and between species.

PATHOGENESIS AND PATHOLOGY

Brucellae are facultative intracellular parasites causing chronic disease that usually persists for life. Within a population, the organism causes high morbidity and low mortality rates in adults, but mortality rate may be high in offspring of a recently infected herd. Regardless of the route of transmission, the organisms must attach to and penetrate the epithelial lining of the membranes of the conjunctival, oral, pharyngeal, intestinal, respiratory, vaginal, or preputial mucosa.[16] Invasion of the submucosal epithelium evokes an inflammatory response characterized by phagocytosis of brucellae by polymorphonuclear leukocytes (PMNs) or macrophages. However, some of these organisms survive and multiply intracellularly.[36] Brucellae that survive the submucosal defenses are transported, probably within the phagocytes, to regional lymph nodes via lymphatic drainage. Infected lymph nodes enlarge as a result of lymphoid and reticuloendothelial hyperplasia and infiltration of inflammatory cells. Failure to destroy *B. abortus* in the lymph node results in persistent infection and eventual escape of the organism into the blood.[16]

Phagocytized brucellae are protected from humoral and cellular bactericidal mechanisms during bacteremia. During this phase, brucellae may localize in lymphoid tissue, mammary gland, reproductive tract or glands, bones, joints, eyes, and sometimes brain.[16] It is thought that infection of both the male and female reproductive tract is due to a specific tropism of brucellae to tissues having a high concentration of erythritol.[23]

Infection of the female reproductive tract results in abortion as a result of (1) placentitis causing impaired delivery of oxygen and nutrients to the fetus, (2) brucellae endotoxins, or (3) fetal stress resulting in increased cortisol, decreased progesterone, and increased prostaglandins ($PGF2_{\alpha[ay2]}$) resulting in premature delivery.[16] Also seen with infection are retained placentas and metritis accompanied by excessive vaginal discharge. Fetuses delivered near term often are stillborn or fail to thrive because of overwhelming brucellae infection.[50, 57] Infection of the male reproductive tract can cause necrotizing orchitis and epididymitis of one or both testicles,[57] seminal vesiculitis, or prostatitis.[16] Brucellae in bone and synovial membranes cause bursitis or hygromas[50] and, in the renal cortex, cause focal nonsuppurative interstitial nephritis.[16]

Researchers have identified a gene (natural resistance associated macrophage protein gene, or NRAMP) associated with resistance to intracellular (phagocytized) brucellae. There are two forms of the gene: sensitive and resistant. Of the three to four alleles found in elk and bison, one or two have been associated with resistance. Those artiodactylids with resistant forms of the gene show no signs of infection or disease when challenged with virulent *B. abortus*. This gene has been found in 12% to 15% of free-ranging bison and elk tested. This resistance factor may become a monitoring tool when assessing the disease in free-ranging animals.

TRANSMISSION

The most common route of transmission is thought to be oral as a result of licking or ingestion of infected fetuses, placentae, fetal fluids, or vaginal exudates.[50] Such transmission can be exacerbated under conditions that artificially congregate infected and susceptible animals, such as winter feedgrounds. Species such as elk normally prefer to calve in isolation, but they may abort while still congregated on feedgrounds.[19, 52] Under feedground conditions, it is not uncommon for other elk to lick, mouth, or even consume aborted fetuses that are not their own.[50] Although males can potentially transmit brucellosis through contaminated semen,[40] this is not thought to play an important role in natural venereal transmission.[50]

Under cool, moist conditions, brucellae can persist up to 100 days in the environment, and transmission may occur when animals graze on infected pasture or consume other feedstuffs and water supplies contaminated by discharges or fetal membranes.[2, 58]

Evidence of *B. abortus* has been found in a large number of carnivores including foxes (*Vulpes vulpes,*[10, 26] *Urocyon cinereoargenteu*[43]), coyotes (*Canis latrans*[11]), black-backed jackals (*Canis mesomelas*), spotted hyena (*Crocuta crocuta*), and wild hunting dogs (*Lycaon pictus*[42]). Davis and coworkers[12] infected coyotes with *B. abortus*, strain 2308 by feeding them inoculated beef. The infected coyotes secondarily transmitted *B. abortus* to pregnant cattle, resulting in infection and abortion. Thus, under experimental conditions, carnivores can become infected with and transmit *B. abortus*. Transmission from a scavenger back to a susceptible ungulate has not been shown to constitute a significant role in the wild. Nonetheless, these scavengers could serve as sentinel animals for the presence of brucellosis.[13]

The role of shedding viable organisms in the urine and feces in the transmission of brucellosis is unknown, but environmental contamination via calf elk feces was not considered important by Thorne and colleagues.[50] Domestic dogs (*Canis lupus familiaris*), and presumably related wild canids, are susceptible to infection with *B. abortus* and they can disseminate organisms in their urine and feces.[57] Again, however, there is no evidence that such environmental shedding by carnivores contributes to the maintenance of brucellosis in the wild.

DIAGNOSIS

A presumptive diagnosis of brucellosis in wild animals can be made through a variety of serologic tests. None of these tests, however, has been validated for such species. Morton and coworkers[34] correlated serologic tests with known brucellosis infections in elk. Using standard plate agglutination (SPT), buffered *Brucella* antigen rapid card (BBA), rivanol (Riv), and complement fixation (CFT) serologic tests, they found that combinations of any two of the four tests had close agreement in concurrently identifying infected elk. Currently, the Wyoming Game and Fish Department (WGFD) considers a nonvaccinated elk to be positive if there are reactions on any two tests, but that if only one test was used, the criteria would be (1) positive at 1:100 dilution on the SPT, (2) positive BBA, (3) positive at greater than or equal to 1:25 dilution on the Riv, or (4) 2+ reading at a 1:20 dilution on the CFT (S. Pistono, personal communication, 1996).

Definitive diagnosis of infection can only be made by culturing the causal organism from tissues or blood. Blood cultures are usually rewarding only within the first few weeks following exposure. Tissues for culturing include but are not limited to mandibular, parotid, retropharyngeal, suprapharyngeal, mediastinal, bronchial, prescapular, mesenteric, hepatic, external iliac, internal iliac, popliteal, and supramammary lymph nodes; synovial and cerebrospinal fluid; lungs; spleen; liver; kidney; ileum; rectum; urine; feces; uterus; cervix; vagina; mammary; testes; epididymis; seminal vesicle; ampullae; prostate; bone marrow; and muscle.

TREATMENT

Treatment of brucellosis in animals is generally unsatisfactory. Antibiotics such as sulfonamides, tetracyclines, and streptomycin alone or in combination may be partially successful, but these cannot be relied upon to clear the disease.[2, 57] There is little or no information on the efficacy of such regimens in wildlife.

PREVENTION AND CONTROL

In domestic cattle, brucellosis can be controlled with an effective vaccination program or eradicated using a test and slaughter program.[2] Some researchers speculate that the same processes may be applicable to free-ranging wildlife; however, little data exist to confirm this hypothesis. Theoretically, an intensive vaccination program could eliminate infection within a population if no immigration of infected animals occurred. This could happen even if less than 100% of the population was vaccinated because of a decreased probability that an unvaccinated animal will contract the infection.[24] Intensive, persistent vaccination programs have succeeded in eliminating brucellosis from cattle herds without test and slaughter.[35] However, the likelihood of vaccinating a significant portion of an elusive, free-ranging population is probably low. Successful vaccination of a population is a function of (1) the percent of animals within the population that can be located, (2) the percent of those animals located that actually receive the vaccine, and (3) the efficacy of the vaccine. These probabilities are multiplicative. For example, in an optimistic scenario, if 90% of a population could be located and a vaccine that was 90% efficacious could be delivered to 90% of those animals, only 73% (.90 × .90 × .90 = 0.73) of the population would be protected.

Brucellosis vaccines are comprised of living mutant *Brucella* organisms that infect the host, but which are less pathogenic than the parent while providing prolonged immunity. Two licensed brucellosis vaccines of importance are *B. abortus* strain 19 (S19) and strain RB51 (SRB51). Strain 19 has been used for decades in cattle; however, it induces production of antibodies to the lipopolysaccharide (LPS) O side chain that are detected in some serologic tests.[47] Thus, differentiation between infection and vaccination is obfuscated. Strain RB51 is a laboratory-derived rough mutant of virulent *B. abortus* strain 2308. It lacks most of the antigenic LPS O side chain[44] and it does not give false-positive results in particle concentration fluorescence immunoassay, card, tube agglutination, or complement fixation tests.[46] Because of this, SRB51 has become the preferred vaccine for cattle.

BRUCELLOSIS IN NORTH AMERICAN WILDLIFE

Brucellosis is a worldwide disease of ungulates, carnivores, and rodents (see reviews in references 15, 32, and 57). The presence of this disease in many of these wild populations apparently does not unduly constrain population growth nor interfere with domestic animal production. However, Waghela and Karstad[55] reported that 30% of African buffalo (*Syncerus caffer*) in Kenya were tested positive for brucellosis and stated that, because of this high seropositivity, shared grazing and watering with cattle must be considered in any control program. Likewise, in Canada and the United States, brucellosis in free-ranging wildlife potentially creates a conflict with federal government programs to eradicate the disease in all its forms.

Serologic evidence of brucellosis in North American wildlife was first reported in 1917 when bison (*Bison bison*) in Yellowstone National Park (YNP) were observed aborting.[31] In 1930, *B. abortus* was isolated from the testes of a bison from the National Bison Range (NBR) in Montana.[9] Extensive testing in the 1930s from both YNP and NBR indicated that more than 50% of bulls, steers, and cows reacted positively to the tube agglutination test.[54] In Alberta, Canada, serologic evidence ranging from 16%[33] to 42% seropositivity was found in bison from Elk Island National Park and 31.2% from Wood Buffalo National Park.[8]

The first serologic evidence of brucellosis in elk was found in 1932 when 13 of 67 serum samples from YNP were positive or suspect on the tube agglutination test.[41] Subsequently, seropositive samples were found in elk from Canada (25 of 221),[8] Colorado (11 of 3833),[1] and Utah (3 of 113).[29] In an extensive serologic survey in Wyoming, Thorne and colleagues[49] found 31% of 1165

elk positive by defined criteria, and *B. abortus* type 1 was isolated from 17 of 45 necropsied elk. McCorquadale and DiGiacomo[27] summarized serologic surveys for *B. abortus* in North American elk in 1985 and found that 446 (6.1%) of 7267 elk tested were classified as positive reactors.

Brucellosis appears to be highly pathogenic to moose (*Alces alces*). The first case in moose was described in 1942 when *B. abortus* was isolated from a moribund moose from Minnesota.[17] *B. abortus* was also isolated from a female moose that died in Montana in 1953.[22] In both these cases, serum agglutination titers were quite high (1:50,000 and 1:20,000, respectively). Surveys for brucellosis in moose found 9 of 44 positive in Montana,[22] 0 of 124 positive in Alberta (although two other obviously sick moose were destroyed and found to be strongly positive),[8] 0 of 104 in British Columbia,[21] 0 of 44 in Alberta,[59] 1 of 39 in Alaska,[60] and 0 of 208 from Quebec.[3] It has been postulated that brucellosis in moose is usually fatal, thus explaining the low seropositivity rate in these surveys.[49]

Neither white-tailed (*Odocoileus virginianus*) nor mule deer (*Odocoileus hemionus*) are considered significant reservoirs of brucellosis. More deer have been surveyed than any other species. From more than 25,000 deer in more than 50 serologic surveys conducted in 29 states, only 46 (0.18%) reacted positively to a variety of tests.[15] Additionally, *B. abortus* has been isolated only once from white-tailed deer.[7]

Pronghorn (*Antilocapra americana*) also do not appear to be significant hosts for brucellosis. In surveys conducted in Wyoming, North Dakota, Arizona, Idaho, Nebraska, Alberta, and Saskatchewan, no reactors were found in a total of 774 samples.[15] In Colorado, a total of 5272 pronghorn were evaluated by the plate agglutination test, with only one reactor at the 1:50 dilution.[1]

Wild sheep are not a significant reservoir for bovine brucellosis. Of 52 bighorn sheep (*Ovis canadensis*) tested in Arizona and Alberta, no reactors were found.[15, 59] Three (4%) of 73 Dall's sheep (*Ovis dalli dalli*) in Alaska were found to be positive.[18]

Brucellosis in caribou and reindeer (*Rangifer tarandus*) and muskox (*Ovibos moschatus*) is a significant circumpolar disease (rangiferian brucellosis), whose causative agent has been identified as *B. suis* type 4 (see reviews in references 15 and 48; see also Chapter 93).

CONTROL AND ERADICATION OF BRUCELLOSIS IN WILDLIFE

Brucellosis is endemic in bison and elk in the ecosystem encompassing YNP, Grand Teton National Park (GTNP), and surrounding areas in Wyoming, Montana, and Idaho (greater Yellowstone area [GYA])[51, 56] as well as in Wood Buffalo National Park in Alberta.[5] Brucellosis was probably introduced into these wildlife populations from domestic cattle. At the beginning of the 20th century, bison were often held in semidomesticated, ranch-like conditions to increase their numbers before being released into the nationals parks.[53] For economic and health purposes, a cooperative state and federal brucellosis eradication program (Cooperative Brucellosis Eradication Program) began in 1934 with the goal of controlling, then eliminating, brucellosis from the United States by the end of 1998. Most states have since been classified as brucellosis-free. The presence of brucellosis in wildlife creates a conflict with the goal of eradication.

To address this problem, state and federal agencies formed the Greater Yellowstone Interagency Brucellosis Committee (GYIBC) to protect and sustain the existing free-ranging elk and bison populations in the GYA while protecting the public interests and economic viability of the livestock industry in the states of Wyoming, Montana, and Idaho. The mission of the GYIBC is to facilitate the development and implementation of brucellosis management plans for elk and bison, and their habitat, in the GYA. One of the 10 objectives of the GYIBC is to plan for the elimination of brucellosis from the GYA by the year 2010.

There are more than 95,000 elk and more than 3000 bison in the GYA.[53] Elk have extensive annual migrations throughout the GYA between summer and winter ranges. To a lesser degree, bison also migrate out of YNP in search of forage during winter. These migrations potentially cause elk and bison to commingle with domestic cattle. In addition, there are private inholdings, within GTNP where cattle graze in and amongst resident and migrating elk and bison.

It is theoretically possible for elk or bison to transmit brucellosis to cattle under the aforementioned conditions. Under captive conditions, both infected elk[51] and bison[13] can transmit brucellosis to susceptible cattle. Also, the rate of seropositivity can be as high as 77% in bison[56] and 50% in elk using winter feedgrounds.[20] Up to 70% of elk[51] and 67% of bison[13] lose their first calf when infected with *B. abortus*. Considering elk and bison population sizes, their rates of exposure, potential infective materials (fetuses, tissues) available in the environment, and commingling of wildlife and cattle, there is a degree of risk, albeit unknown, that susceptible cattle could contract brucellosis from wildlife.

There are several management alternatives that bear consideration in addressing the conflict between potentially infected wildlife and susceptible cattle (Table 92–1). Eradication of all elk and bison within the GYA is probably socially, ecologically, politically, and economically unacceptable. Capturing, testing, and slaughtering all bison testing positive for brucellosis is potentially feasible, but fraught with difficulties. First, certain segments of society would be rigorously opposed to such action and would attempt through legal and political means to prevent such action. Second, even if all the bison could be captured and tested, it is possible that some infected animals would test negative,[6] be released, and serve as a potential source of infection to other bison. Third, bison test and slaughter would be fruitless if brucellosis was not concomitantly cleared in elk as well. And it is widely accepted that capturing and testing upwards of 100,000 elk loosely scattered throughout the GYA would be virtually impossible.

Large-scale vaccination of elk and bison is also potentially feasible, although models have indicated that eradication through vaccination alone is unlikely.[39] The WGFD vaccinates thousands of elk on feedgrounds

TABLE 92–1. Alternative Solutions to the Conflict Between Brucellosis in Wildlife and Domestic Cattle in the Greater Yellowstone Area

1. Eradicate all elk and bison within the greater Yellowstone area (GYA).
2. Test all bison and elk and slaughter those testing positive for brucellosis.
3. Intensively vaccinate all elk and bison for brucellosis.
4. Vaccinate elk and bison, followed by test and slaughter.
5. Eliminate feedgrounds to decrease transmission of brucellosis.
6. Create suitable winter habitat as an alternative to feedgrounds.
7. Vaccinate cattle within the GYA.
8. Eliminate all cattle grazing within the GYA.
9. Abandon the Cooperative Brucellosis Eradication Program.
10. Manage the risk of disease transmission between wildlife and cattle.

with a reduced-dose S19 vaccine delivered remotely by biobullet[20] and a significant decrease in seropositivity has been documented.[45] Although bison do not congregate on feedgrounds to the degree that elk do, large-scale vaccination would be potentially feasible given their relatively low numbers, large size and sightability, and known ranges and movements.[28] Currently, however, no suitable vaccine has been found for bison. Strain 19 vaccination of pregnant bison caused 58% abortion, persistent antibody titers, and chronic S19 infection, although the vaccine was efficacious in preventing infection or abortion caused by field strain *B. abortus*.[14] Strain RB51 also causes abortion in pregnant bison, but the abortifacient potential appears to be less than that of S19.[38] Vaccination of bison calves with RB51 is being conducted, which may prove as efficacious as calfhood vaccination of cattle[4] and would circumvent problems associated with adult vaccination. Strain RB51 appears to persist longer in lymph nodes than does S19 in bison calves, although lymph node lesions were similar.[37]

Vaccination of cattle within the GYA is feasible, practical, and achievable. However, the goal of the Cooperative Brucellosis Eradication Program to eradicate brucellosis would not be achieved, and funding for such a program would have to be established. Besides the actual vaccination of cattle, a program of brucellosis monitoring would have to be implemented and maintained in perpetuity. Elimination of cattle grazing on public lands within the GYA would reduce, but not eliminate, contact between potentially infected wildlife and cattle. Loss of public grazing would result in the termination of many ranch operations. This would result in sale of highly desirable lands to developers who would break up the holdings into smaller parcels, causing large-scale loss of wildlife habitat. In the long run, replacing ranches with intensive human development would be more detrimental to the ecosystem of the GYA than perhaps any other proposed alternative to the problem.

The rate of seropositivity of elk using winter feed-grounds is much higher than of elk using natural winter range (37%[20] versus 2%, respectively; S. Smith, unpublished data, 1997), but closing winter feedgrounds abruptly would be catastrophic for elk. Hungry elk would depredate cattle feedlots and hay stackyards, causing extensive damage and increasing contact with cattle.[53] Many elk would starve, resulting in widespread public criticism and legal actions. As an alternative, the WGFD has engaged in programs to improve natural winter habitat, to modify feedground operation, and to develop alternative damage control methods. These actions reduce both the number of elk and the length of time elk use feedgrounds in order to decrease the opportunities for transmission of brucellosis among elk.[53] Such programs are effective, but they are long term and costly.

Abandoning the Cooperative Brucellosis Eradication Program is unlikely, but it may be the best answer when combined with risk management. Cooperating agencies can certainly eliminate brucellosis from domestic animals and, having achieved that goal, may wish to simply declare victory. Models are currently being developed that will attempt to assess the risk of cattle contracting brucellosis from wildlife (Kreeger, unpublished data, 1998). It may turn out that the solution to the problem is a combination of many of the alternatives posed in (see Table 92–1). That is, by reducing the number and duration of elk on feedgrounds, by reducing seroprevalence through vaccination of elk and bison, by vaccinating cattle, and by reducing some grazing on selected public lands, the probability of transmission would be reduced significantly and to an acceptable degree.

REFERENCES

1. Adrian WJ, Keiss R: Survey of Colorado's wild ruminants for serologic titers to brucellosis and leptospirosis. J Wildl Dis 13:429–431, 1977.
2. Blood DC, Radostits OM: Veterinary Medicine, 7th ed. London, Baillière Tindall, 1990.
3. Bourque M, Higgins R: Serologic studies on brucellosis, leptospirosis and tularemia in moose (*Alces alces*) in Quebec. J Wildl Dis 20:95–99, 1984.
4. Cheville NF, Olsen SC, Jensen AE et al: Effects of age at vaccination on efficacy of *Brucella abortus* S51 to protect cattle against brucellosis. Am J Vet Res 57:1153–1155, 1996.
5. Choquette LPE, Broughton E, Cousineau JG, et al: Parasites and diseases in Canada: IV. Serologic survey for brucellosis in northern Canada. J Wildl Dis 14:329–332, 1978.
6. Cordes DO, Carter ME: Persistence of *Brucella abortus* infection in six herds of cattle under brucellosis eradication. N Z Vet J 27:255–259, 1979.
7. Corey RR, Paulissen LJ, Swartz D: Prevalence of Brucellae in the wildlife of Arkansas. Wildl Dis 36:(WD-63–2), 1964.
8. Corner AH, Connell R: Brucellosis in bison, elk, and moose in Elk Island National Park, Alberta, Canada. Can J Comp Med 22:9–20, 1958.
9. Creech GT: *Brucella abortus* infection in a male bison. North Am Vet 11:35–36, 1930.
10. Davies G, Ockey JH, Lloyd HG: Isolation of *Brucella abortus* from a fox (*Vulpes vulpes*). State Vet J 28:250, 1973.
11. Davis DS, Boer WJ, Mims JP et al: *Brucella abortus* in coyotes: I. A serological and bacteriologic survey in eastern Texas. J Wildl Dis 15:367–372, 1979.
12. Davis DS, Heck FC, Williams JD, et al: Interspecific transmission of *Brucella abortus* from experimentally infected coyotes (*Canis lupus*) to parturient cattle. J Wildl Dis 24:533–537, 1988.
13. Davis DS, Templeton JW, Ficht TA, et al: *Brucella abortus* in captive bison: I. Serology, bacteriology, pathogenesis, and transmission to cattle. J Wildl Dis 26:360–371, 1990.
14. Davis DS, Templeton JW, Ficht TA, et al: *Brucella abortus* in bison: II. Evaluation of strain 19 vaccination of pregnant cows. J Wildl Dis 27:258–264, 1991.
15. Davis DS: Brucellosis in wildlife. *In* Nielsen K, Duncan JR (eds): Animal Brucellosis. Boca Raton, FL, CRC Press, pp 321–334, 1990.
16. Enright FM: The pathogenesis and pathobiology of *Brucella* infection in domestic animals. *In* Nielsen K, Duncan JR (eds): Animal Brucellosis. Boca Raton, FL, CRC Press, pp 301–320, 1990.
17. Fenstermacher R, Olson OW: Further studies of diseases affecting moose. Cornell Vet 32:241–254, 1942.
18. Foreyt WJ, Smith TC, Evermann JF, et al: Hematologic, serum chemistry, and serologic values of Dall's sheep (*Ovis dalli dalli*) in Alaska. J Wildl Dis 19:136–139, 1983.
19. Herriges JD, Thorne ET, Anderson SL, et al: Vaccination of elk in Wyoming with reduced dose strain 19 *Brucella*: controlled studies and ballistic implant field trials. Proceedings of the 93rd Annual Meeting of the U.S. Animal Health Association, Las Vegas, NV, pp 640–655, 1989.
20. Herriges JD, Thorne ET, Anderson SL: Brucellosis vaccination of free-ranging elk (*Cervus elaphus*) on western Wyoming feedgrounds. *In* Brown RD (ed): The Biology of Deer. New York, Springer-Verlag, 1991.
21. Hudson M, Child KN, Halter DF, et al: Brucellosis in moose (*Alces alces*). A serological survey in an open range cattle area of north central British Columbia recently infected with bovine brucellosis. Can Vet J 21:47–49, 1980.
22. Jellison WL, Fishel CW, Cheatum EL: Brucellosis in a moose, *Alces americanus*. J Wildl Management 17:217–218, 1953.
23. Keppie J, Williams AE, Witt K, et al: The role of erythritol in tissue localization of the Brucellae. Br J Exp Pathol 46:104, 1965.
24. May RM: Vaccination programmes and herd immunity. Nature 300:481–483, 1982.
25. Mayfield JE, Bantle JA, Ewalt DR, et al: Detection of *Brucella* cells and cell components. *In* Nielsen K, Duncan JR (eds): Animal Brucellosis. Boca Raton, FL, CRC Press, pp 97–120, 1990.
26. McCaughey WJ: Brucellosis in wildlife. Symp Zool Soc London 24:99, 1968.
27. McCorquadale SM, DiGiacomo RF: The role of wild North American ungulates in the epidemiology of bovine brucellosis: a review. J Wildl Dis 21:351–357, 1985.
28. Meagher M: The bison of Yellowstone National Park. National Park Service Scientific Monthly Series No. 1, pp 70–72, 1973.
29. Merrell CL, Wright DN: A serologic survey of mule deer and elk in Utah. J Wildl Dis 14:471–478, 1978.
30. Meyer M: Current concepts in the taxonomy of the genus *Brucella*. *In* Nielsen K, Duncan JR (eds): Animal Brucellosis. Boca Raton, FL, CRC Press, pp 1–17, 1990.
31. Mohler JR: Pathological division, abortion disease. Annual Report of the U.S. Department of Agriculture. pp 105–106, 1917.
32. Moore CG, Schnurrenberger PR: A review of naturally occurring *Brucella abortus* infections in wild mammals. J Am Vet Med Assoc 179:1105–112, 1981.
33. Moore T: A survey of buffalo and elk herds to determine the extent of brucella infection. Can J Comp Med Vet Sci 11:131, 1947.
34. Morton JK, Thorne ET, Thomas GM: Brucellosis in elk: III. Serologic evaluation. J Wildl Dis 17:23–31, 1981.
35. Nicoletti P: The efficacy of Strain 19 vaccination in reducing brucellosis in large dairy herds. Calif Vet 9:35–36, 1981.
36. Nicoletti P, Winter AJ: The immune response to B. abortus: the cell-mediated response to infections. *In* Nielsen K, Duncan JR (eds): Animal Brucellosis. Boca Raton, FL, CRC Press, pp 83–95, 1990.
37. Olsen SC, Cheville NF, Kunkle RA, et al: Bacterial survival, lymph node pathology, and serological responses of bison (*Bison bison*) vaccinated with *Brucella abortus* strain RB51 or strain 19. J Wildl Dis 33:146–151, 1997.
38. Palmer MV, Olsen SC, Gilsdorf MJ, et al: Abortion and placentitis in pregnant bison (*Bison bison*) induced by the vaccine candidate, *Brucella abortus* strain RB51. Am J Vet Res 57:1604–1607, 1996.
39. Peterson MJ, Grant WE, Davis DS: Bison-brucellosis management: simulation of alternative strategies. J Wildl Management 55:205–213, 1991.
40. Rankin JEF: *Brucella abortus* in bulls: a study of 12 naturally infected cases. Vet Rec 77:132–135, 1965.

41. Rush WM: Bang's disease in Yellowstone National Park buffalo and elk herds. J Mammal 13:371–372, 1932.
42. Sachs R, Staak C: Evidence of brucellosis in antelopes of the Serengeti. Vet Rec 79:857, 1966.
43. Scanlan CM, Pidgeon GL Sawngo LJ, et al: Experimental infection of gray foxes *Urocyon cinereoargenteus* with *Brucella abortus*. J Wildl Dis 20:27–30, 1984.
44. Schurig GG, Roop RM, Bagchi T, et al: Biological properties of RB51: a stable rough strain of *Brucella abortus*. Vet Microbiol 28:171–188, 1991.
45. Smith S, Thorne ET, Anderson-Pistono S, et al: Efficacy of brucellosis vaccination of free-ranging elk in the greater Yellowstone area: the first 10 years. Proceedings of the 45th Annual Wildlife Disease Association Conference, Fairbanks, AK, p 20, 1996.
46. Stevens MG, Hennager SG, Olsen SC, et al: Serologic responses in diagnostic tests for brucellosis in cattle vaccinated with *Brucella abortus* 19 or RB51. J Clin Microbiol 32:1065–1066, 1994.
47. Stevens MG, Olsen SC, Cheville NF: Comparative analysis of immune responses in cattle vaccinated with *Brucella abortus* strain 19 or strain RB51. Vet Immunol Immunopathol 44:223–235, 1995.
48. Tessaro SV, Forbes LB: *Brucella suis* biotype 4: a case of granulomatous nephritis in a barren ground caribou (*Rangifer tarandus groenlandicus L.*) with a review of the distribution of rangeriine brucellosis in Canada. J Wildl Dis 22:479–483, 1986.
49. Thorne ET, Morton JK, Thomas GM: Brucellosis in elk: I. Serologic and bacteriologic survey in Wyoming. J Wildl Dis 14:74–81, 1978.
50. Thorne ET, Morton JK, Blunt FM, et al: Brucellosis in elk: II. Clinical effects and means of transmission as determined through artificial infections. J Wildl Dis 14:280–291, 1978.
51. Thorne ET, Morton JK, Ray WC: Brucellosis, its effect and impact on elk in western Wyoming. *In* Boyce MS, Hayden-Wing LO (eds): North American Elk: Ecology, Behavior and Management. Laramie, WO, University of Wyoming, 1979.
52. Thorne ET, Herriges JD, Reese AD: Bovine brucellosis in elk: conflicts in the greater Yellowstone area. Proceedings of the Symposium on Elk Vulnerability, Bozeman, MT, pp 296–303, 1991.
53. Thorne ET, Herriges JD: Brucellosis, wildlife and conflicts in the greater Yellowstone area. Transactions of the 57th North American Wildlife National Research Conference, pp 453–465, 1992.
54. Tuunicliff EA, Marsh H: Bang's disease in bison and elk in Yellowstone National Park and on the National Bison Range. J Am Vet Med Assoc 86:745–752, 1935.
55. Waghela S, Karstad L: Antibodies to *Brucella* spp, among blue wildebeest and African buffalo in Kenya. J Wildl Dis 22:189–192, 1986.
56. Williams ES, Thorne ET, Anderson SL, et al: Brucellosis in free-ranging bison (*Bison bison*) from Teton County, Wyoming. J Wildl Dis 29:118–122, 1993.
57. Witter JF: Brucellosis. *In* Davis JW, Karstad LH, Trainer DO (eds): Infectious Diseases of Wild Mammals, 2nd ed. Ames, Iowa State University Press, pp 280–287, 1981.
58. Wray C: Survival and spread of pathogenic bacteria of veterinary importance within the environment. Vet Bull 45:543-548, 1975.
59. Zarnke R, Yuill TM: Serologic survey for selected microbial agents in mammals from Alberta, 1976. J Wildl Dis 17:453–461, 1981.
60. Zarnke RL: Serologic survey for selected microbial pathogens in Alaskan wildlife. J Wildl Dis 19:324-329, 1983.

CHAPTER **93**

Brucella suis Biovar 4 Infection in Free-Ranging Artiodactylids

ROBERT A. DIETERICH

Brucellosis was diagnosed in humans in Alaska as early as 1939, with 49 cases being recorded between that year and 1953. During that period, it was believed that these cases were attributable to unpasteurized milk or contact with cattle or swine. It was not until 1963 that isolates from caribou were found to be the same species of *Brucella* (*Brucella suis* biovar 4) as was isolated from humans in Alaska and Canada. *B. suis* biovar 4 has been known to infect reindeer, caribou, and humans in the former Soviet Union for a number of years.[1, 3] It is not known whether the disease was introduced into Alaska with the importation of reindeer from Siberia in the late 1800s or whether it has been present since prehistoric times. *B. suis* biovar 4 is considered a distinct subspecies of *Brucella* based on differences in its biochemical reactions and antigenic structure. The common serologic tests used to diagnose brucellosis in domestic animals are currently being used successfully in reindeer and caribou with slight modifications in the interpretation of significant titer levels. In reindeer, a combination of the card, plate, and complement fixation tests appears to be the best battery of serologic tests to detect infected animals. False-positive reactions occur, but the number of false-negative reactions in animals is reduced using this technique.

In 1964, approximately 20% of the residents of Fort Yukon and Arctic Village, AK, had positive titers for brucellosis as determined by the rapid slide test. In a serologic study of seven villages from 1962–1964, 11% of 763 individuals tested had evidence of past *Brucella* infection. It was also reported that eight clinical cases occurred from 1962–1964 in Eskimos having frequent contact with reindeer or caribou in northern Alaska. No cases were diagnosed at that time among individuals living outside that area. Additional cases of brucellosis have been diagnosed in humans associating with caribou and reindeer in arctic and subarctic areas of North America since that time, but the numbers have not been great.

Following the detection of brucellosis in reindeer and caribou, evidence of the disease was also found in Alaskan grizzly bears, wolves, red and arctic foxes, sled dogs, and arctic ground squirrels that come into contact or feed upon tissues of reindeer and caribou.[4] Brucellosis caused by *B. suis* biovar 4 has rarely been reported in moose and muskox. Limited studies have indicated that moose may be highly susceptible to brucellosis, and it has been postulated that infected moose may die within a short period of time and, thus, are removed from any population being sampled. Further research is needed before any conclusion can be reached. Serologic testing of reindeer and caribou over the past 30 years has revealed a varying pattern of infection, ranging from up to a 30% prevalence in herds at times and commonly cycling to a much lower level as immunity increases and infection decreases. This cycle appears to be repeated on an irregular basis.

TRANSMISSION AND PATHOGENESIS

Brucella have an affinity for the male and female reproductive organs, and the major impact on herd health occurs because of abortion and sterility. Brucellosis causes abortion, retained placentae, and impaired health in female reindeer and caribou. In males, infection of the seminal vesicles, ampullae, testicles, and epididymides is seen. In both males and females, there can be swelling of the joints and associated lameness.[2] It is believed that the primary spread of the disease is by contact with infective uterine discharges following abortion. Abortion in reindeer appears to occur 1 to 2 months before normal calving time.[5] Calves can also be born alive but weak and die within a few days. Other calves born to infected females can survive but possibly

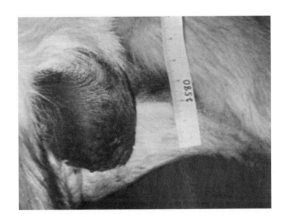

FIGURE 93–1. Enlarged testicles of a caribou infected with brucellosis.

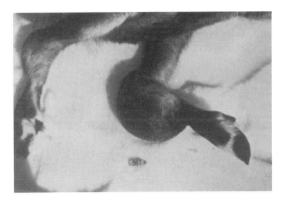

FIGURE 93–2. Swollen, fluid-filled carpal joint of a reindeer infected with brucellosis. Swelling on the right carpus is extreme; animals infected with brucellosis that exhibit swollen joints usually resemble the smaller, left carpus.

become carriers of the disease. It appears that female reindeer commonly abort when initially infected, but produce viable calves in following years. As infection progresses, osteoarthritis, abscesses, and other signs of the disease appear. It is estimated that approximately 5% of serologically positive reindeer have clinically visible signs, such as swollen testicles (Fig. 93–1), enlarged carpal or fetlock joints (Fig. 93–2), and draining abscesses, which are recognizable from a distance. Abscesses containing an odorless, thick, light-green purulent material are often found. Abscessed testicles as large as 12 to 20 cm in diameter have been observed. Other males may have a swollen epididymis, which can only be detected by palpation or necropsy. Abscesses are also found in mammary glands, other reproductive organs, liver, kidney, and abdominal cavity, or as subcutaneous enlargements.

The importance of brucellosis in reindeer and caribou appears to be substantial. It is a disuease of low mortality rate and of moderate morbidity for adult animals. The occasional observer of a herd is not impressed with the impact of the disease because few animals are seen in obvious distress. The actual impact is seen in herd reproductive success, which is difficult to assess in free-ranging populations. Other factors, such as climate, nutrition, and predation, all affect population numbers, but it is difficult to assess the influence of each factor in groups of animals that are only occasionally observed.

A killed homologous vaccine has been developed by the University of Alaska and used in Alaskan free-ranging reindeer herds. The prevalence of brucellosis in vaccinated herds decreases, but reinfection from non-vaccinated animals has been a problem. Newer vaccines are being tested that elicit a serologic response distinguishable from that of an infected animal.

REFERENCES

1. Brody JA, Huntley B, Overfield TM, et al: Studies of human brucellosis in Alaska. J Infect Dis 116:263–269, 1966.

2. Dieterich RA: Brucellosis. *In* Dieterich RA (ed): Alaskan Wildlife Diseases. Fairbanks, AK, University of Alaska, pp 53–58, 1981.
3. Meyer ME: Identification and virulence studies of *Brucella* strains isolated from Eskimos and reindeer in Alaska, Canada and Russia. Am J Vet Res 37:353–358, 1966.
4. Neiland KA: Further observations in rangiferine brucellosis in Alaskan carnivores. J Wildl Dis 11:45–52, 1975.
5. Rausch RL: Brucellosis in reindeer, *Rangifer tarandus* L., inoculated experimentally with *Brucella suis* type 4. Can J Microbiol 24:129–135, 1978.

CHAPTER **94**

Contraception in Artiodactylids, Using Porcine Zona Pellucida Vaccination

IRWIN K. M. LIU

JOHN W. TURNER

JAY F. KIRKPATRICK

The successful use of porcine zona pellucida (PZP) as a contraceptive vaccine was first demonstrated in the domestic equid (*Equus caballus*). The results obtained from field and experimental trials from this species laid the foundation for the application of PZP immunocontraception in artiodactylids. The investigation in equids demonstrated the effectiveness of the vaccine using a two-inoculation protocol consisting of homogenized PZP as the antigen, with the incorporation of Freund's complete adjuvant in the first inoculation and incomplete adjuvant in the second inoculation as immunizing agent.[4, 7] Experimental data in the equid described the dynamics of antibody response resulting from immunization and its relation to the ability of mares to be protected from conceiving at following matings. In addition, reversibility of the contraceptive effect following diminishing antibody titers, its safe use in pregnant mares, and the continuation of cyclicity with acceptance of the stallion was demonstrated. Further indications from studies in the equid suggested that the antibodies produced as a result of the inoculations exerted their effect at the level of the oocytes, whereby zona receptors to spermatozoa, present on the surface of the oocytes, are being blocked, thus preventing spermatozoa penetration into the oocyte and subsequent fertilization.

In artiodactylia, experimental design to obtain detailed physiologic data as a result of PZP immunization is limited because of the physiologic stresses and high risks for injury associated with physical or chemical restraint of the animals. In particular, frequent and repeated blood collections for determining the dynamics of antibody titers following inoculations, albeit important, can involve major risks.

APPLICATION IN CAPTIVE AND FREE-ROAMING DEER

Successful PZP contraception in artiodactylids was first demonstrated in captive deer (*Odocoileus virginianus*).[10] In this investigation, eight does were given three inoculations of PZP administered remotely with a dart gun, 3 weeks apart. As a result of these inoculations, none of the PZP-treated does produced fawns compared with seven control does that yielded a live fawn rate of 86%. Even though antibody response was not determined in this study, it clearly demonstrated the potential effectiveness of the immunogen as a contraceptive agent for this species. Because populations of white-tailed deer were increasing and because, in some urban areas, parks, and preserves, hunting or killing of excess populations of deer was prohibited, contraception with PZP appeared to be an attractive alternative to population control and management. As a result, further studies on captive and free-roaming deer were performed. In one recent investigation,[11] 53 captive white-tailed deer were studied under three different treatment protocols: (1) three PZP inoculations administered 3 weeks apart, (2) two PZP inoculations administered 3 weeks apart, and (3) one PZP inoculation consisting of continuous release vehicles including an osmotic pump or microspheres (biodegradable lactide and glycolide polymers). The results of this study confirmed the effectiveness of PZP as an immunocontraceptive in this species when at least two inoculations were administered to the does before the mating season. In this investigation, no does administered the two- and three-inoculation protocols produced fawns during a treatment year. In comparison, the fawning rate for control does was 93.8%. Even though there appeared to be some contraceptive effect elicited on does receiving only one inoculation with sustained release vehicles, the overall contraceptive effectiveness (80%) was not as significant compared with the two- and three-inoculation protocols (100%). This study further demonstrated that, in all does given PZP, antibody responses developed to the inoculum 4 to 6 weeks after the treatment, regardless of the number of inoculations (Table 94–1). The antibody levels generated represent a significantly elevated increase in antibody titer and is far more than what is believed by the investigators to be the contraceptive titer (>50% of positive reference serum) in this species. The duration of antibodies generated persisted for at least 32 to 40 weeks after inoculation in most does. The protective titers remained elevated for up to at least 64 weeks in two of the four does tested and in those receiving the two-inoculation protocol. Antibody titers for the remaining does in this study were not available. The persistence of antibody titers for such extended periods without additional inoculations in the two does tested is unexplained. Reversibility of the contraceptive effect of the inoculations was substantiated, however, when a majority of the does inoculated became pregnant in subsequent breeding seasons and produced fawns.

Field trials on captive and free-ranging deer have also been carried out in other locations within the eastern and midwestern United States, with approximately 250 does being inoculated with differing formulations of the PZP inoculum.[6] The successful application of PZP was confirmed in these field trials using one- and two-inoculation protocols, with one-inoculation protocols also comprising vehicles for sustained antigen release (osmotic pumps and microspheres). Logistically and economically, the advantage of achieving a slightly lower contraception rate within a breeding season through one inoculation is better than achieving an overall higher conception rate with the administration

of two inoculations to each free-ranging wildlife animal. Although the differences in antibody response, duration of immunity, and contraception between one- and two-inoculation protocols were anticipated before each study, single inoculation protocols were included in the field trials to determine the effectiveness of contraception, if any. The results achieved using single injections of PZP (with or without osmotic pumps and biodegradable microspheres) throughout one breeding season, although moderately effective (70%), did not achieve the contraception rates equal to that of the two-inoculation protocols (100%) in most of the field studies in deer.

In all of the field studies, a limited number of ovaries have been examined from inoculated deer that were accidentally killed. Preliminary evidence indicates that pathologic effects on ovarian tissue have not been detected as a result of PZP inoculations. The continued use of PZP as an immunocontraceptive agent is encouraging. However, the design and release of PZP via a one-inoculation protocol to maintain contraceptive effect in wildlife through one breeding season needs improvement. In addition, the long-term side effects, if any, following yearly PZP inoculations require further investigation.

APPLICATION IN EXOTIC ARTIODACTYLIDS

Application of PZP immunocontraception in other artiodactylids has also taken place in captive zoo animals.[6] Increased reproductive successes of many species of animals within zoos have resulted in "overcrowded" populations. Translocation of excess animals to their natural habitat is not always feasible, nor is translocation to other zoos. In addition to overcrowding factors, animals whose genetic traits are not desirable have also been subjected to contraceptive studies. Among many agents used for contraception purposes, PZP may have

TABLE 94–1. Anti-PZP Antibody Titers During One Breeding Season in Captive White-Tailed Does Given PZP Contraceptive Vaccine*

		Anti-PZP Antibody Titers (% of Positive Reference Serum)†			
		Prevaccination Baseline‡ (Week 0)	Prebreeding Season (Weeks 4–6)		Postbreeding Season§ (Weeks 32–40)	
Experiment	No. of Does Tested		$\bar{x}$	SE	$\bar{x}$	SE
3-Injection	4	<8	102.1	1.2	72.7	15.7
2-Injection	4	<8	100.0	0.0	92.0	5.2
1-Injection/pump	3	<8	76.3	7.2	69.5	11.8
1-Injection/microspheres	4	<8	53.7	15.5	19.1	4.3
Control‖	2	<8	<8		<8	

*Does were treated in October–November; fawning occurred the following summer.
†Positive reference serum, designated as 100%, was the average value of maximal titers achieved in six PZP-treated does that did not produce fawns.
‡Placebo-treated does from 2-injection experiment.
§All values were below the lower limit of detection.
‖No differences between prebreeding and postbreeding season titers in any treatment group, based on analysis of variance with repeated measures, $p < 0.05$.

an important role to play in contraception in zoos. Although the numbers of animals representing each species have been few (5 to 15), of at least 68 different species of animals in which PZP was used, contraception was successful in three families (Cervidae, Bovidae, and Capridae) of artiodactyla (Table 94–2). The number of blood samples obtained for antibody detection following PZP inoculations in zoo animals has been limited by constrained policies for blood collections; however, of those available, the antibody levels in species (except fallow deer) of the artiodactylids are equivalent to those found in free-roaming and captive white-tailed deer. Reasons for poor antibody response to PZP inoculations and the resulting ineffectiveness in contraception in fallow deer (eight does fawned out of 10 vaccinated does) are unknown.

The use of PZP as a means of contraception in artiodactylids continues to provide results that make this mode of contraception a potentially attractive alternative to population control in this and other wildlife animal species. Current immunocontraception strategies using PZP are directed only at populations of animals in which hunting or killing as a means of culling is prohibited.

ADVANTAGES OF IMMUNOCONTRACEPTION

The advantages of using PZP as an immunocontraceptive agent over other available contraceptive agents are compelling. The effectiveness of PZP as an immunocontraceptive agent covers a broad range of animal species. Although PZP cross-reactivity studies are limited to a few animal species, it appears that macromolecules within the zona pellucida are highly conserved across species. Thus, PZP is highly tissue specific but not species specific.[3] The safety of PZP in pregnant mares is documented, but further studies are necessary to evaluate its safety in pregnant artiodactylids. The effects of PZP are reversible, in that antibodies generated as a result of inoculations eventually decay if the animal is not re-inoculated, thus diminishing protection against pregnancy. There is convincing evidence that there are threshold levels of antibodies that correlate with contraception and that this level varies according to the animal species inoculated. So, the mere presence of antibodies does not necessarily indicate protection against fertilization. Once antibodies decay to levels below the threshold, fertilization resumes. PZP can be delivered remotely with a darting rifle, making it unnecessary for highly stressful, physical restraint of the animal for inoculation purposes. Immunocontraception with PZP in the herd animals investigated does not disrupt the social behavior nor does it disrupt the band integrity. Most importantly, PZP and the antibodies generated as a result of an inoculation are not passed on to other wildlife species during scavenging of carcasses.

DISADVANTAGES OF IMMUNOCONTRACEPTION

One disadvantage of immunocontraception with PZP is the use of Freund's adjuvant in wildlife. It results in seroconversion to *Mycobacterium tuberculosis* antigen and cross-reactivity with active infections of *M. tuberculosis* and potentially other mycobacterial agents. Attempts to incorporate alternative adjuvants with PZP vaccines are being investigated.[1] There is also conclusive evidence of development of ovarian malfunction following the use of PZP in laboratory animals studied—the canine species and nonhuman primates.[2, 8, 9, 12] The primary side effects were the disruption of folliculogenesis and oocyte atresia. In a small number of ovaries obtained from both inoculated equids and Cervidae, evidence of short-term effects on ovarian function caused by PZP inoculations has not been found nor is there evidence of histologic abnormalities associated with the use of PZP.[6, 7] The disparity in side effects

TABLE 94–2. Captive Exotic Zoo Artiodactylids Inoculated with Porcine Zona Pellucida

Family	Common Name	Contracepted	Not Contracepted	Results Pending
Bovidae	North American bison	3	2	1
	Bangteng	2	0	2
	Siberian ibex	16	0	—
	Greater kudu	6	0	8
	Water buck	4	1	2
	Impala	3	0	—
Cervidae	Barasingha	1	0	2
	Axis deer	3	2	—
	Muntjac deer	2	0	—
	Sika deer	9	1	—
	Roosevelt elk	7	1	—
	Sambar deer	9	1	—
	White-tailed deer	5	0	8
Caprinae	Himalayan tahr	6	0	9
	Rocky Mountain big horn sheep	3	0	3
	Rocky Mountain goat	2	0	8
	West Caucasian tahr	6	0	—
Giraffidae	Reticulated giraffe	4	2	—

found in other mammalian species studied may be related to the amount of antigen used for each inoculum.[2] Indeed, following long-term use of PZP immunizations (5 to 6 years of annual inoculations), ovarian function ceases temporarily in the equid.[5] While the cause of impaired ovarian function is not understood, cessation of yearly inoculations allows for resumption of ovarian function in the equid. Investigations of long-term effects of PZP immunization in artiodactylids is not available. Other criticisms directed against PZP immunocontraception include the extension of breeding activity outside of the natural mating season and concerns of the survival of newborns born late in the season as a result of this procedure.

For immunocontraception of wildlife, a single inoculation program that ensures contraception for one or two mating seasons is most desirable. The incorporation of various forms of matrices with PZP agents is being investigated in continuous or controlled release patterns to achieve effectiveness following single inoculations of PZP. Preliminary evidence of matrix-incorporated PZP inoculations in a field study of a small number of inoculated horses (28) indicates that the method can be applied to large-scale field studies in wildlife and that the method shows promise of being as successful as the standard two-inoculation protocol. In this investigation, 2 of 28 mares were tentatively determined to be pregnant by microtiter enzyme immunoassays for estrone conjugates and nonspecific progesterone metabolites of feces collected 8 months after a single inoculation of PZP containing Freund's adjuvant and the controlled-release matrix.

REFERENCES

1. Dunbar BS, Lo C, Powell J, et al: Use of a synthetic adjuvant for the immunization of baboons with denatured and deglycosylated pig zona pellucida proteins. Fertil Steril 52:311-318, 1989.
2. Gulyas BJ, Gwatkin RBL, Yuan LC: Active immunization of cynomolgus monkeys (*Macaca fascicularis*) with porcine zonae pellucidae. Gamete Res 4:299–307, 1983.
3. Henderson CJ, Hulme MJ, Aitken RJ: Contraceptive potential of antibodies to the zona pellucida. J Reprod Fertil 83;325–343, 1988.
4. Kirkpatrick JF, Liu IKM, Turner JW: Remotely delivered immunocontraception in feral horses. Wildlife Society Bulletin 18:326–330, 1990.
5. Kirkpatrick JF, Naugle R, Liu IKM, et al: Effects of seven consecutive years of porcine zona pellucida contraception on ovarian function in feral mares. Biology of Reproduction Monograph Series 1: Equine Reproduction VI:411–413, 1995.
6. Kirkpatrick JF, Turner JW, Liu IKM, et al: Applications of pig zona pellucida immunocontraception to wildlife fertility control. J Reprod Fertil Suppl 50:183–189, 1996.
7. Liu IKM, Bernoco M, Feldman M: Contraception in mares heteroimmunized with pig zona pellucida. J Reprod Fertil 85:19–29, 1989.
8. Mahi-Brown CA, Yanagimachi R, Hoffman J, et al: Fertility control in the bitch by active immunization with porcine zonae pellucidae: use of different adjuvants and patterns of estradiol and progesterone levels on estrous cycles. Biol Reprod 32:761–772, 1985.
9. Skinner SM, Mills T, Kirchick HJ, et al: Immunization with zona pellucida proteins results in abnormal ovarian follicular differentiation and inhibition of gonadotropin-induced steroid secretion. Endocrinology 115:2418–2432, 1984.
10. Turner JW, Liu IKM, Kirkpatrick JF: Remotely delivered immunocontraception of captive white-tailed deer. J Wildl Management 56:154–157, 1992.
11. Turner JW, Kirkpatrick JF, Liu IKM: Effectiveness, reversibility and serum antibody titers associated with immunocontraception in white-tailed deer. J Wildl Management 60:45–51, 1996.
12. Wood DM, Liu C, Dunbar BS: Effect of alloimmunization and heteroimmunization with zonae pellcidae on fertility in rabbits. Biol Reprod 25:439–450, 1981.

CHAPTER 95

Parelaphostrongylus tenuis and *Elaphostrongylus cervi* in Free-Ranging Artiodactylids

LORA RICKARD BALLWEBER

Throughout the world, the capture and translocation of free-ranging wild ungulates not only has become a common wildlife management tool but also is an essential component of game farming and ranching. Translocation of wildlife has been used to restock historic ranges, supplement dwindling populations, and reduce undesirably high densities of wildlife in urban areas.[45] Among the many issues associated with translocation events are concerns that introduced animals do not carry diseases or parasites that could establish new endemic foci and thereby endanger indigenous species. Within the Cervidae, ample historical evidence shows that long-range translocation of animals has introduced parasites into new areas.[31, 43, 50]

The genus *Parelaphostrongylus* contains three species restricted primarily to North American cervids.[6] *P. tenuis* (commonly called meningeal or brain worm) occurs in the cranium of white-tailed deer (*Odocoileus virginianus*) that inhabit eastern North America. *P. odocoilei* is located in muscles of mule and black-tailed deer (*Odocoileus hemionus*) and woodland caribou (*Rangifer tarandus*) in western North America. This parasite is also the only species of the genus found in a bovid host, the mountain goat (*Oreamnos americanus*).[39] *P. andersoni* is also located in muscles of white-tailed deer and woodland and barren-ground caribou and is found in scattered foci in eastern and western North America. Phylogenetic analysis indicates these parasites probably cospeciated with Nearctic deer and may explain the limited geographic distribution of the genus.[12]

Until the 1990s, the taxonomic status of species in the closely related genus *Elaphostrongylus* has been disputed. Studies of experimental and natural infections aimed at issues of host specificity and pathogenicity have been greatly confused by the uncertainty of identification and taxonomic status of this genus. Current morphologic data, supported by cross-transmission experiments, indicates that the genus *Elaphostrongylus* is composed of three fairly host-specific species.[21, 25, 48, 49] These nematodes are associated with loose connective tissue of the central nervous system (CNS) and the muscle fasciae of their hosts. Based on identification of adult nematodes, *E. cervi* (= *E. panticola*) parasitizes red deer (*Cervus elaphus*), sika deer (*Cervus nippon*), and roe deer (*Capreolus capreolus*). *E. rangiferi* parasitizes reindeer and caribou, and *E. alces* parasitizes moose (*Alces alces*). Historically, these nematodes have been restricted to areas of the Palearctic.[21, 29, 48] However, *E. cervi* and *E. rangiferi* (reported as *E. cervi*) have been introduced into New Zealand and Newfoundland, respectively, through the importation of infected hosts.[11, 31]

The risk of introducing pathogenic parasites into nonendemic regions is real. This risk, coupled with potential negative impacts on indigenous fauna, forms the basis for regulations that forbid the importation of specific groups of animals. For example, cervids from countries where *E. cervi* is endemic have been prohibited from entering Canada.[20] Within countries, some wildlife management agencies prohibit importation of white-tailed deer from *P. tenuis*–endemic areas in an attempt to prevent the spread of this nematode. This chapter focuses on the biology of *P. tenuis* and *E. cervi* in cervid hosts, emphasizes their effects on aberrant hosts, and summarizes available information on translocational events and ecologic implications of each.

PARELAPHOSTRONGYLUS TENUIS

Biology in White-Tailed Deer

P. tenuis is a generally benign nematode of the CNS of white-tailed deer. The life cycle is indirect, requiring both definitive and intermediate hosts. Adults are found in the subdural space and venous sinuses of the cranium. Eggs may be found on the meninges, but those deposited in the venous circulation are transported to the heart and lungs. The eggs lodge in the lungs where they are incorporated into granulomas. First-stage larvae (L1) develop and hatch from the eggs, move into the alveoli, and are coughed up, swallowed, and excreted out with the feces.[2, 3] L1, which have a prominent dorsal spine, are found only in the mucus that coats the outside of the fecal pellet and have been shown to be resistent to drying and freezing.[30, 47] Continued larval development requires an intermediate host, which can be one of a variety of terrestrial gastropods.[6, 8] L1 penetrate the gastropod foot and molt twice to become the infective third-stage larvae (L3). The time required for L3 development within the gastropod varies with environmental conditions. Larval development ceases in estivating snails but resumes when snail activity increases. Infective larvae are capable of overwintering in the intermediate host.[6]

Deer become infected by ingesting gastropods containing infective L3. Larvae are freed from the snail tissue by digestion, penetrate the abomasal wall, and migrate across the peritoneal cavity, gaining access to the vertebral canal probably by following lumbar nerves.[9] An estimated 10 days is required for the larvae to complete this migration, after which they invade the neural parenchyma of all regions of the spinal cord. Larval development, primarily in the dorsal horns of gray matter, continues and the fourth-stage larvae (L4) are present by day 25. Developing larvae leave the neural tissue, beginning around day 25, and migrate to the subdural space. By about day 40, most larvae are present in the subdural space, where L4 molt to the immature adult stage. Nematodes mature and migrate to the cranium. Some nematodes remain in the subdural space; others invade cranial venous sinuses.[2, 3] The prepatent period has been reported as 82 to 91 days[6] but may be somewhat inversely related to the number of ingested larvae.[44]

Clinical disease attributable to *P. tenuis* in naturally infected adult white-tailed deer or in experimentally infected fawns has been rarely reported.[1, 3, 17, 38] Lack of apparent disease in face of neurologic invasion has been attributed to the manner in which the larvae reside within the neuropil. Lesions associated with developing larvae are relatively minor.[3] Larvae are generally uncoiled, located in cell-free tunnels in the dorsal horns of the gray matter. Little reaction of, or cellular infiltration in, adjacent tissue is observed; rather, compressed neural tissue surrounds the tunnels. In white matter, scattered single myelin sheath degeneration is a common finding. Foreign-body reactions around pieces of cuticle and hemorrhages associated with larval migration out of the spinal cord are sometimes found. The neural parenchyma quickly assumes a normal appearance after the larvae have left. Lesions associated with adult nematodes in the cranium are equally unremarkable.[8]

Eggs transported to lungs form isolated occlusions that eventually become embedded in fibrous nodules. Nodules may be found in any area of lung. Once larvae have hatched and entered alveoli, foreign-body reaction occurs around the remains of eggshells. Congestion, hemorrhages, and eosinophilic and lymphocytic infiltrates are common in areas of lung that contain eggs, larvae, and eggshells. Alveoli may also collapse and disappear, with subsequent fibrosis of the region. Although not observed under field conditions, respiratory signs as a result of these changes may be the most significant feature associated with meningeal worm presence in naturally infected white-tailed deer.[8]

The only reliable method for diagnosing infections with *P. tenuis* is recovery and identification of nematodes from the CNS. The presence of nematode eggs or larvae in the meninges and venous sinuses is suggestive of infection.[8] Recovery of dorsal-spined L1 in the lungs or feces is also suggestive of infection but is not conclusive evidence. Several nematodes that infect cervids have dorsal-spined larvae in their lungs that are indistinguishable from *P. tenuis*, including species of *Elaphostrongylus* and *Varestrongylus*.[24, 40] Likewise, the presence of dorsal-spined larvae in feces is not conclusive evidence of infection. Compounding the difficulty of identifying the L1, the reliability of fecal examination techniques has been questioned.[32, 52] The Baermann technique is a reasonably effective method for recovering nematode larvae from feces; however, larvae must be present to be detected. Intermittent shedding can result in patent infections going undetected, despite repeated sampling. Diagnosing infections by identification of L3 derived from the artificial infection of gastropods with L1 recovered from deer has been proposed. Although the L3 of species of *Parelaphostrongylus* may be distinguishable,[10] this is not a viable option in most cases. An even less viable suggestion is to artificially infect white-tailed deer fawns to determine the prepatent period. Should patency not be achieved before 3 months, a provisional diagnosis of *P. tenuis* could be made. However, recovery of adults would still be necessary for confirmation.

There is no practical method for controlling *P. tenuis* in wild populations of white-tailed deer. Control of gastropod intermediate hosts is not feasible, particularly on a large scale, nor is control of the nematode in the definitive hosts. Aside from the impracticality of treating wild herds, no treatment is available that can kill or eliminate nematodes once they reside in the CNS.[27]

Biology in Wild Ungulates

Numerous wild, semidomesticated and domesticated ungulates have been shown to be susceptible to infection with *P. tenuis*[5, 8, 22]; however, the previously accepted role of meningeal worms in the ecology of cervids is being questioned. The early phase of the *P. tenuis* life cycle in aberrant hosts parallels that in the white-tailed deer, but development in the CNS tends to produce neurologic signs that can result in death. The severity of the signs is related to several factors, including the tendency of the larvae to be unusually active in the neural tissue, inflicting considerable damage, and the failure of some larvae to leave the neural tissue, resulting in damage as the nematode grows and migrates. Other factors include the tendency of some of the nematodes to invade and damage the ependymal canal and reinvasion of the spinal cord or brain after maturation in the subdural space.[8]

MOOSE

"Moose sickness," a neurologic disorder of free-ranging moose, was documented well before *P. tenuis* was identified as the causal agent.[8] A variety of neurologic signs occur, including lumbar weakness, ataxia, torticollis, blindness, paresis, paraplegia, and death. Moose most likely acquire infection through ingestion of infected gastropods when feeding on shrubs or forbs.[22]

Although the clinical signs and associated mortality of moose sickness can be dramatic, ample evidence suggests that moose may survive infection and shed larvae in the feces. No evidence indicates, however, that the parasite can maintain itself in populations of moose when white-tailed deer are absent.

CARIBOU AND REINDEER

P. tenuis has been demonstrated to be highly pathogenic to woodland caribou under both experimental and natural conditions. In addition to the signs described for moose, exophthalmos is a consistent finding. The failure of introduced caribou to survive on a game reserve and in a national park concurrently inhabited by white-tailed deer has been attributed to cerebrospinal parelaphostrongylosis. Although small numbers of larvae have been found in feces of infected caribou, the extreme susceptibility of caribou makes it unlikely that the parasite would establish itself in caribou populations. Acquisition of infected gastropods may be more likely by caribou than other cervids because of their feeding habits.[4, 8]

WAPITI AND RED DEER

As for moose, neurologic disease had been noted in wapiti for many years before it was linked to *P. tenuis*. Signs include depression, listlessness, and progressive weakness of the hind quarters. In experimental infections, signs have persisted for as short as 2 days or as long as 56 days before resolution or death. Not all wapiti infected with meningeal worm die.[7, 45] It appears that severity of clinical signs, resolution of clinical signs, and death are dose dependent.[45] Fatal neurologic disease developed in all 13 calves given 125, 200, or 300 larvae. Larvae were detected in the feces and lungs of two of the calves (prepatent period 78 and 105 days after exposure). Six of eight calves given 25 or 75 larvae experienced moderate to severe neurologic disease. Two became severely debilitated, which necessitated euthanasia, but the other four recovered. Two of the eight did not exhibit clinical signs. Seven of the eight calves became patent 83 to 165 days after exposure (median, 91 days). Larval shedding was variable and intermittent. All 5 calves exposed to 15 larvae survived without having neurologic signs, and no larvae were detected in their feces. It can be assumed that infections of *P. tenuis* in wapiti does not automatically translate into death of the host. The role of wapiti in sustaining populations of *P. tenuis* or in possible translocation of the parasite is unknown.

MULE AND BLACK-TAILED DEER

Fatal parelaphostrongylosis, characterized by lameness, posterior weakness and ataxia, and progressive neurologic deterioration, has been experimentally produced in mule deer. Although remission of signs was common, neurologic problems did return, culminating in paralysis and fatalities. Only one of nine deer showed mild signs, which disappeared. Larvae were not found in any of the deer.[51]

Naturally occurring neurologic disease resulting from *P. tenuis* has been reported in black-tailed deer and experimentally produced in a black-tailed × white-tailed hybrid. Failure of black-tailed deer to survive when introduced into an endemic area was attributed to infections with this parasite.[33]

FALLOW DEER

Clinical neurologic disease and death of fallow deer infected with *P. tenuis* have been reported. The pathogenesis of experimental infection differed from other cervids in that infective larvae apparently penetrate the intestinal tract rather than the abomasum. Doses of 125 and 150 larvae quickly resulted in fatal peritonitis and colitis, lesions not observed in other cervids. The severe damage was most likely associated with the large number of larvae that penetrated the gut wall and crossed the peritoneal cavity. Young fallow deer are apparently unable to limit this phase of the nematode migration, which allows larvae in doses as small as 25 to reach the CNS. At all levels of infection, neurologic disorders and death resulted.[41]

These results experimentally demonstrating mortality in fallow deer apparently conflict with field data, which indicate that some animals survive infection. In one area where fallow deer and infected white-tailed deer are sympatric, the impact of *P. tenuis* on fallow deer populations was considered to be much less devastating than reported for other cervids.[34] Evidence exists of a substantial immune response within the CNS against the nematode, suggesting that an innate immunity occurs in fallow deer. Protection against fewer numbers of larvae, such as may be expected to be encountered in many field situations, may occur, allowing survival of fallow deer in an enzootic area.[15, 41] There is no evidence that fallow deer play any role in the maintenance or transmission of *P. tenuis* in an enzootic area.

Implications

RANGE EXPANSION AND TRANSLOCATION

Because *P. tenuis* can cause mortality in other North American cervids, the distribution of the parasite is particularly important to wildlife managers. Concern centers on the potential for translocating and establish-

ing the parasite in nonendemic regions as a result of either natural range expansion or translocation of infected hosts. Numerous surveys documenting the distribution of the parasite have been conducted[8, 14] and indicate a discontinuous distribution in which there are areas where the parasite is locally abundant and areas in which it is absent. The discontinuous distribution appears to be associated with certain major soil types, although other major environmental attributes (physiographic provinces, forest types, and land use patterns) have a similar spatial distribution. Consequently, whether the observed association with soil type reflects inherent soild properties, other environmental attributes, or a combination thereof, is not known. The level (i.e., larval survival, gastropod population dynamics, cervid population dynamics) at which these factors are acting and, therefore, what constitutes the barrier to generalized distribution, are also unknown.

It is debatable whether *P. tenuis* is expanding its range as has been previously suggested. Natural range expansion has been proposed as a mechanism by which infected white-tailed deer could spread the parasite through aspen parklands and extend to the foothills of the Rocky Mountains in Canada.[8] Evidence is insufficient to indicate that *P. tenuis* is expanding its range, however.[14, 18] In the southeastern United States, the area for which the most detailed information is available, survey results do not indicate that the parasite has expanded its range since its distribution was described earlier.[14]

Evidence indicating that translocation events have resulted in establishment of new endemic foci is also lacking. A single infected white-tailed deer was found in Florida in 1968 and was thought to be a result of the introduction of infected deer from Wisconsin. Examination of numerous additional deer since that time has not revealed more infected animals, indicating that the parasite did not become established or spread in the area.[14] Efforts to restock white-tailed deer within Oklahoma moved deer from areas where the prevalence of the parasite varied between 53% and 80% into areas where the parasite did not exist. Even with the presence of potentially susceptible molluscan hosts, there is no evidence the parasite survived in the new areas.[28] Recently, however, a focus of infection in white-tailed deer was identified on Wassaw Island, Georgia.[16] Circumstantial evidence—including the absence of *P. tenuis* along the southeastern coast from North Carolina to Louisiana and the prevalence of the parasite in Pennsylvania, where some of the deer were reputed to have originated as the island was restocked—was interpreted as confirmation that *P. tenuis* can be spread to nonendemic sites through translocation of infected hosts.[16]

ECOLOGIC EFFECTS OF MENINGEAL WORM

The hypothesis that *P. tenuis* prevents overlapping distributions of white-tailed deer and other cervids (particularly caribou and moose) and could be responsible for negative changes in cervid population numbers arose from the observations that other cervids succumb to infections. As such, the hypothesis has gained acceptance and has been cited by many in discussion of moose population regulation and reintroduction attempts of other species.[22, 37] White-tailed deer populations did increase at the northern extent of their range during the first 40 years of this century at the same time moose populations declined, contributing circumstantial evidence that *P. tenuis* was limiting moose populations. More recently, however, moose numbers in some areas (Maine) began to increase, and both moose and deer populations are thriving. Additionally, reports have been made of sympatric populations of moose and white-tailed deer, fallow deer and white-tailed deer, and wapiti and white-tailed deer in which meningeal worm infection is present.[15, 22, 42] These findings appear to contradict the doctrine that cervid populations will not thrive in the presence of sympatric white-tailed deer populations with a high prevalence of the parasite.

Several explanations have been offered as to why these populations may coexist. One possibility is that a decline in the prevalence of *P. tenuis* in the white-tailed deer population has occurred over time, which decreases the opportunity for moose to encounter infected gastropods. Studies in Maine, however, showed essentially no change in prevalence in white-tailed deer between 1968–1970 and 1988–1989. The interpretation has been that moose were being subjected to equivalent levels of exposure. This is true only as long as the gastropod populations have not changed. However, reductions in density of infected gastropods as a result of climatic effects such as acid rain and forestry practices such as clear cutting could decrease potential exposure of cervid hosts. Again this is not supported by the data.[22]

Ecologic separation between white-tailed deer and other cervids as a result of different habitat use patterns has been proposed as another possible explanation. For instance, sympatric populations of white-tailed deer and wapiti occur in an area of Oklahoma endemic for meningeal worm. Wapiti were found to spend most of their time in meadows and open fields, where gastropods were relatively scarce. In contrast, white-tailed deer spent most of their time in forested areas, where most gastropods were found.[42] In another example, moose and white-tailed deer were shown to select different habitats during winter. Because parasite transmission does not occur at this time, however, ecologic separation during winter months would not be expected to influence transmission.[22] Yet, in other areas, little overlap in habitats during the May-June period and no overlap in the July-August period (optimal transmission periods) supports the theory that ecologic separation reduces transmission to moose. It has been suggested that moose could exist and prosper in the presence of heavily infected white-tailed deer if refugia were available, permitting little contact with infected white-tailed deer and gastropods.[22]

The importance of *P. tenuis* as a primary mortality factor influencing population dynamics is being questioned.[13, 23, 35, 36, 46, 53] Some question whether the available evidence actually indicates *P. tenuis* caused significant declines in cervid populations. Arguments that the same data that generated this hypothesis cannot be used to prove the hypothesis cast doubt on whether evidence exists that *P. tenuis* caused significant declines in cervid populations.[35, 36] Recent data generated by separate studies designed to investigate this question conflict. Some results do not support the theory,[53] whereas others, although inconclusive, could not rule out meningeal worm infection as a factor in reductions of moose populations.[46] Nevertheless, the latter authors advise caution in applying evidence for significant effects of the parasite at the individual level to the populational level.

ELAPHOSTRONGYLUS CERVI

Biology in Red Deer

E. cervi was described from nematodes found in the intermuscular fascia of red deer in Scotland. The life cycle is indirect, requiring terrestrial gastropods as intermediate hosts. Adults are usually found coiled in the connective tissue between muscle bundles or associated with the CNS. Female nematodes lay eggs that either hatch near the sites where the adults reside or are transported by the circulatory system to the lungs and hatch there. L1 move into alveolar spaces and are coughed up, swallowed, and excreted in the feces. The L1, which also have a prominent dorsal spine, are resistant to drying and can tolerate changing climatic conditions, surviving for more than 2 years outside of a host. Continued development requires that the larvae actively penetrate the foot of a suitable gastropod intermediate host. Two molts occur, and the L3 stage is reached in 27 to 50 days, depending on temperature, infection level, and species of mollusk. Infective larvae can survive in the intermediate host for up to 2 years with no loss of infectivity to the definitive host. Deer become infected by ingesting gastropods that contain infective L3. Larvae are freed from the snail tissue by digestion, penetrate the gastrointestinal tract, and travel to the final site where they mature. Experimentally, the prepatent period varies from 86 to 206 days. Shorter prepatent periods are associated with higher numbers of ingested L3. Adult *E. cervi* are long-lived, producing eggs for up to 6 years.[6, 20, 31]

The migration route the larvae take to the final site is not known for *E. cervi*. Involvement of the CNS in the migratory route has been recently demonstrated for the closely related nematode. *E. rangiferi*, in which maturation occurs in the CNS with subsequent migration occurs in the CNS with subsequent migration to skeletal musculature, where it reproduces. Direct migration to skeletal musculature could not be ruled out, and the route of migration from the gut to the CNS could not be identified.[26] Involvement of the CNS during the migratory phase of *E. cervi* may be indicated by recovery of these nematodes from neural tissue of infected animals.[6, 29]

Although deaths have been reported in marals (*Cervus elaphus sibiricus*) infected with *E. cervi*, concurrent neurologic infection with *Setaria altaica* combined with other pathogenic gastrointestinal nematodes does not allow for unequivocal proof that death was due to *E. cervi*.[6] Rather, it appears that natural infections of *E.*

cervi in red deer and wapiti are normally clinically silent. In New Zealand, natural infections in farmed deer are usually light and have not resulted in overt signs of disease. In central Europe, where *E. cervi* has been reported as one of the most common endoparasites of red deer, no nervous signs have been reported despite the association of the parasite with the CNS. Inflammatory proliferative lesions caused by eggs and larvae have been seen in the lungs, resulting in a mild, diffuse interstitial pneumonia. Hemorrhages in the muscles in proximity to the nematodes have also been detected, which can require trimming and result in downgrading or condemnation of carcasses of animals in commercial production.[6, 31]

Clinical reactions to infections with *E. cervi* have been divided into three categories: (1) an acute disease characterized by hindlimb paralysis, (2) a chronic disease with nonspecific signs of not doing well, and (3) a type of pneumonia associated with larvae in the lungs. This generalization was based primarily on reactions observed in marals with multiple nematodes (see earlier) or in reindeer.[20, 31] In light of current *Elaphostrongylus* taxonomy, this generalization must be considered incorrect. Of the three, only pulmonary lesions are associated with *E. cervi*.

The only reliable method for diagnosing infections with *E. cervi* is recovery and identification of nematodes. The L1 are indistinguishable from those of several other genera of nematodes infecting cervids, including *Parelaphostrongylus* and *Varestrongylus*.[24, 40] In addition to the difficulty associated with identification of L1, reliability of fecal examination techniques has been questioned.[20, 31] As for *Parelaphostrongylus* species, the Baermann technique is used to recover larvae from feces. However, intermittent shedding of larvae, the long and variable prepatent period, and the ability of anthelmintics to suppress larval output have been cited as possible factors limiting the usefulness of the Baermann assay.[20]

There is no practical method for controlling *E. cervi* in wild populations of red deer for the same reasons as cited for *P. tenuis*. In addition, definitive control through anthelmintic intervention has not been successful in farmed animals.[31]

Biology in Other Ungulates and Implications

Among the species of *Elaphostrongylus*, a certain degree of host specificity has been reported for *E. cervi* and *E. alces* but not *E. rangiferi*. Several reports exist in the literature that link *E. cervi* in reindeer with clinical signs and death.[31] These reports are actually associated with *E. rangiferi* rather than *E. cervi*, however. Experimental transmission of *E. cervi* to fallow deer has been reported, but again the species involved was *E. rangiferi* not *E. cervi*.[11]

Little is known about the biology of *E. cervi* in other ungulates. The only other host known in which this parasite can complete its life cycle is sika deer.[29] Experiments attempting to transmit *E. cervi* from red deer to reindeer failed,[24] and the species has not been found in

fallow deer in endemic areas.[31] Experimental transmission to sheep also failed, and natural transmission to sheep, goats and cattle has not occurred.[29] Consequently, it appears this parasite has little impact on other ungulates, even in areas in which it has been introduced.

The potential impact of translocation of *E. cervi* into North America was examined in a study in which two mule deer fawns were exposed to relatively large numbers (102 and 406) of infective L3.[19] The L1 were derived from red deer recently moved from New Zealand into Canada. The L3 developed in two species of North American mollusks and were infective to the red deer control animal, which showed no clinical signs of infection. Clinical signs were evident in the mule deer, however, although not until 104 days after exposure. Initial bilateral incoordination in the hind legs progressed until euthanasia was required 128 and 151 days after exposure. The mule deer that received 406 larvae survived longer. This fawn also passed L1 intermittently in the feces beginning on day 121. The second fawn had L1 in rectal feces at the time of euthanasia (day 128). Consequently, because (1) wapiti can serve as definitive hosts,[31] (2) mule deer can serve as definitive hosts, (3) appropriate intermediate hosts are available for establishment of the parasite in North America, (4) debilitating disease was produced in the two mule deer, and (5) fecal examinations are unreliable in detecting infections, the translocation of red deer from *E. cervi*–endemic areas into North America has been discouraged.

SUMMARY

It is clear that *P. tenuis* can cause neurologic disease and death in cervids. Unequivocal evidence for a direct inverse relation between the parasite in white-tailed deer and numbers of cervids (particularly moose) is lacking, however.[22] Indeed, analyses have indicated that reintroduction of moose and caribou to range occupied by infected white-tailed deer need not automatically be presumed to fail as a result of the presence of the parasite.[37, 46] In addition, evidence that the parasite is expanding its range or has been translocated into nonendemic sites is still lacking, despite 30 years of study. It is evident, however, that *E. cervi* has established new endemic foci as a direct result of the transportation of infected hosts. That this parasite does not apparently cause disease in wapiti, which can serve as definitive hosts, indicates that it could become established in North America should it be accidently imported. In that event, available evidence may be interpreted to indicate it would have minimal effect on caribou (unable to infect reindeer) but may adversely effect mule deer (death when exposed to high numbers of larvae). Data are insufficient, however, to make predictions of the actual impact *E. cervi* may have on North American cervids.

REFERENCES

1. Alibasoglu M, Krader DC, Dunne HW: Cerebral nematodiasis in Pennsylvania deer (*Odocoileus virginianus*). Cornell Vet 51:431–441, 1961.

2. Anderson RC: The incidence, development, and experimental transmission of *Pneumostrongylus tenuis* (Dougherty) (Metastrongyloidea: Protostrongylidae) of the meninges of the white-tailed deer (*Odocoileus virginianus borealis*) in Ontario. Can J Zool 41:775–792, 1963.

3. Anderson RC: The development of *Pneumostrongylus tenuis* in the central nervous system of white-tailed deer. Pathol Vet 2:360–379, 1965.

4. Anderson RC: Neurologic disease in reindeer (*Rangifer tarandus tarandus*) introduced into Ontario. Can J Zool 49:159–166, 1971.

5. Anderson RC: The ecological relationships of meningeal worm and native cervids in North America. J Wildl Dis 8:304–310, 1972.

6. Anderson RC: Nematode parasites of vertebrates: their development and transmission. Cambridge, UK, Cambridge University Press, 1992.

7. Anderson RC, Lankester MW, Strelive UR: Further experimental studies of *Pneumostrongylus tenuis* in cervids. Can J Zool 44:851–861, 1966.

8. Anderson RC, Prestwood AK: Lungworms. *In* Davidson WR, Hayes FA, Nettles VF, et al (eds): Diseases and parasites of white-tailed deer [Misc. Publ. No. 7]. Tallahassee, Tall Timbers Research Station, pp 266–317, 1981.

9. Anderson RC, Strelive UR: The penetration of *Pneumostrongylus tenuis* into the tissues of white-tailed deer. Can J Zool 45:285–289, 1967.

10. Ballantyne RJ, Samuel WM: Diagnostic morphology of the third-stage larvae of three species of *Parelaphostrongylus* (Nematoda: Metastrongyloidea). J Parasitol 70:601–604, 1984.

11. Carreno RA, Lankester MW: Additional information on the morphology of the Elaphostrongylinae (Nematoda: Protostrongylidae) of North American Cervidae. Can J Zool 71:592–600, 1993.

12. Carreno RA, Lankester MW: A re-evaluation of the phylogeny of *Parelaphostrongylus* Boev & Schulz, 1950 (Nematoda: Protostrongylidae). Systemat Parasitol 28:145–151, 1994.

13. Cole GF: Alternative hypotheses on ecological effects of meningeal parasite (*Parelaphostrongylus tenuis*). J Minn Acad Sci 47:8–10, 1981.

14. Comer JA, Davidson WR, Prestwood AK, et al: An update on the distribution of *Parelaphostrongylus tenuis* in the southeastern United States. J Wildl Dis 27:348–354.

15. Davidson WR, Crum JM, Blue JL, et al: Parasites, diseases, and health status of sympatric populations of fallow deer and white-tailed deer in Kentucky. J Wildl Dis 21:153–159, 1985.

16. Davidson WR, Doster GL, Freeman RC: *Parelaphostrongylus tenuis* on Wassaw Island, Georgia: a result of translocating white-tailed deer. J Wildl Dis 32:701–703, 1996.

17. Eckroade RJ, Zu Rhein GM, Foreyt W: Meningeal worm invasion of the brain of a naturally infected white-tailed deer. J Wildl Dis 6:430–436, 1970.

18. Foreyt WJ, Compton BB: Survey for meningeal worm (*Parelaphostrongylus tenuis*) and ear mites in white-tailed deer from northern Idaho. J Wildl Dis 27:716–718, 1991.

19. Gajadhar AA, Tessaro SV: Susceptibility of mule deer (*Odocoileus hemionus*) and two species of North American molluscs to *Elaphostrongylus cervi* (Nematoda: Metastrongyloidea). J Parasitol 81:593–596, 1995.

20. Gajadhar AA, Tessaro SV, Yates WDG: Diagnosis of *Elaphostrongylus cervi* infection in New Zealand red deer (*Cervus elaphus*) quarantined in Canada, and experimental determination of a new extended prepatent period. Can Vet J 35:433–437, 1994.

21. Gibbons LM, Halvorsen O, Stuve G: Revision of the genus *Elaphostrongylus* Cameron (Nematoda: Metastrongyloidea) with particular reference to species of the genus occurring in Norwegian cervids. Zool Scripta 20:15–26, 1991.

22. Gibbs HC: Meningeal worm infection in deer and moose. Maine Nat 2:71–80, 1994.

23. Gilbert FF: Retroductive logic and the effects of meningeal worms: a comment. J Wildl Manage 56:614–616, 1992.

24. Gray JB, Samuel WM, Shostak AW, et al: *Varestrongylus alpenae* (Nematoda: Metastrongyloidea) in white-tailed deer (*Odocoileus virginianus*) of Saskatchewan. Can J Zool 63:1449–1454, 1985.

25. Halvorsen O, Skorping A, Bye K: Experimental infection of reindeer with *Elaphostrongylus* (Nematoda: Protostrongylidae) originating from reindeer, red deer, and moose. Can J Zool 67:1200–1202, 1989.

26. Hemmingsen W, Halvorsen O, Skorping A: Migration of adult *Elaphostrongylus rangiferi* (Nematoda: Protostrongylidae) from the spinal subdural space to the muscles of reindeer (*Rangifer tarandus*). J Parasitol 79:728–732, 1993.

27. Kocan AA: The use of ivermectin in the treatment and prevention of infection with *Parelaphostrongylus tenuis* (Dougherty) (Nematoda: Metastrongyloidea) in white-tailed deer (*Odocoileus virginianus* Zimmermann). J Wildl Dis 21:454–455, 1985.

28. Kocan AA, Shaw MG, Waldrup KA, et al: Distribution of *Parelaphostrongylus tenuis* (Nematoda: Metastrongyloidea) in white-tailed deer from Oklahoma. J Wildl Dis 18:457–460, 1982.

29. Kontrimavichus VL, Delyamure SL, Boev SN: Osnovy Nematodologii, Tom XXVI, Metastrongiloidei Domashnikh i Dikikh Zhivotnykh. (Translated by A.K. Dhote, Oxonian Press Pvt, New Delhi, 1985.) Moscow, Nauka Publishers, 1976.

30. Lankester MW, Anderson RC: Gastropods as intermediate hosts of *Pneumostrongylus tenuis* Dougherty of white-tailed deer. Can J Zool 46:373–383, 1968.

31. Mason PC: *Elaphostrongylus cervi*—a review. Surveillance 16:3–10, 1989.

32. McCollough MA, Pollard KA: *Parelaphostrongylus tenuis* in Maine moose and the possible influence of faulty Baermann procedures. J Wildl Dis 29:156–158, 1993.

33. Nettles VF, Prestwood AK, Nichols RG, et al: Meningeal worm-induced neurologic disease in black-tailed deer. J Wildl Dis 13:137–143, 1977.

34. Nettles VF, Prestwood AK, Smith RD: Cerebrospinal parelaphostrongylosis in fallow deer. J Wildl Dis 13:440–444, 1977.

35. Nudds TD: Retroductive logic in retrospect: the ecological effects of meningeal worms. J Wildl Manage 54:396–402, 1990.

36. Nudds TD: Retroductive logic and the effects of meningeal worms: a reply. J Wildl Manage 56:617–619, 1992.

37. Pitt WC, Jordan PA: A survey of the nematode parasite *Parelaphostrongylus tenuis* in the white-tailed deer, *Odocoileus virginianus*, in a region proposed for caribou, *Rangifer tarandus caribou*, reintroduction in Minnesota. Can Field Nat 108:341–346, 1994.

38. Prestwood AK: Neurologic disease in a white-tailed deer massively infected with meningeal worm (*Pneumostrongylus tenuis*). J Wildl Dis 6:84–86, 1970.

39. Pybus MJ, Foreyt WJ, Samuel WM: Natural infections of *Parelaphostrongylus odocoilei* (Nematoda: Protostrongylidae) in several hosts and locations. Proc Helminthol Soc Wash 51:338–340, 1984.

40. Pybus MJ, Samuel WM: Nematode muscleworm from white-tailed deer of southeastern British Columbia. J Wildl Manage 45:537–542, 1981.

41. Pybus MJ, Samuel WM, Welch DA, et al: Mortality of fallow deer (*Dama dama*) experimentally-infected with meningeal worm, *Parelaphostrongylus tenuis*. J Wildl Dis 28:95–101, 1992.

42. Raskevitz RF, Kocan AA, Shaw JH: Gastropod availability and habitat utilization by wapiti and white-tailed deer sympatric on range enzootic for meningeal worm. J Wildl Dis 27:92–101, 1991.

43. Rickard LG, Hoberg EP, Allen NM, et al: *Spiculopteragia spiculoptera* and *S. asymmetrica* (Nematoda: Trichostrongyloidea) from red deer (*Cervus elaphus*) in Texas. J Wildl Dis 29:512–515, 1993.

44. Rickard LG, Smith BB, Gentz EJ, et al: Experimentally induced meningeal worm (*Parelaphostrongylus tenuis*) infection in the llama (*Lama glama*): clinical evaluation and implications for parasite translocation. J Zoo Wildl Med 25:390–402, 1994.

45. Samuel WM, Pybus MJ, Welch DA, et al: Elk as a potential host for meningeal worm: implications for translocation. J Wildl Manage 56:629–639, 1992.

46. Schmitz OJ, Nudds TD: Parasite-mediated competition in deer and moose: how strong is the effect of meningeal worm on moose? Ecol Appl 4:91–103, 1994.

47. Shostak AW, Samuel WM: Moisture and temperature effects on survival and infectivity of first-stage larvae of *Parelaphostrongylus odocoilei* and *P. tenuis* (Nematoda: Metastrongyloidea). J Parasit 70:261–269, 1984.

48. Steen M, Chabaud AG, Rehbinder C: Species of the genus *Elaphostrongylus* parasite of Swedish cervidae: a description of *E. alces* n. sp. Ann Parasitol Hum Comp 64:134–142, 1989.

49. Steen M, Johansson C: *Elaphostrongylus* spp. from Scandinavian cervidae—a scanning electron microscope study (SEM). Rangifer 1:39–46, 1990.

50. Suarez VH, Busetti MR, Fort MC, et al: *Spiculopteragia spiculoptera*, *S. asymmetrica* and *Ostertagia leptospicularis* from *Cervus elaphus* in La Pampa, Argentina. Vet Parasitol 40:165–168, 1991.

51. Tyler GV, Hibler CP, Prestwood AK: Experimental infection of mule deer with *Parelaphostrongylus tenuis*. J Wildl Dis 16:533–540, 1980.

52. Welch DA, Pybus MJ, Samuel WM, et al: Reliability of fecal examination for detecting infections of meningeal worm in elk. Wild Soc Bull 19:326–331, 1991.

53. Whitlaw HA, Lankester MW: A retrospective evaluation of the effects of parelaphostrongylosis on moose populations. Can J Zool 71:1–7, 1994.

CHAPTER **96**

Anesthesia for Captive Nile Hippopotamus

MICHAEL R. LOOMIS

EDWARD C. RAMSAY

The Nile hippopotamus (*Hippopotamus amphibius*) presents several anesthesia challenges.[2] Preplanning can increase the possibility of a positive outcome. A review of Nile hippopotamus anesthesia has been published and should be referred to for detailed information.[4]

PREANESTHESIA PLANNING

Because of the aquatic nature of Nile hippopotamuses and their propensity to seek refuge in water when threatened, drowning is a major concern during anesthesia.[1] It is imperative to block access to pools and moats before delivery of anesthetic agents. The large bulk of Nile hippopotamuses presents additional problems. Once anesthetized, the animals are difficult to move. The area of anesthesia induction should be chosen to eliminate corners and maximize working space around the animal. Ideally, the area should be padded. If possible, a forklift, crane, or winch should be available to move the animal if it becomes recumbent in a position that can compromise respiration. The subcutaneous blubber layer poses several challenges, including the potential for the development of hyperthermia and the difficulty of intramuscular injection of anesthetics and venipuncture delivery of drugs or collection of blood. Ice and cold water should be available in case the animal becomes hyperthermic. Prevention of hyperthermia is important because it is difficult to lower the core temperature with ice or cold water once the animal becomes overheated. Anesthetic procedures should be planned during the coolest part of the day and performed in shade. Peripheral veins can occasionally be seen on the pinna or on the foreleg. When the animal is in lateral recumbency, a vein can sometimes be seen on the medial side of the nondependent foreleg.

Fasting for 24 to 48 hours and restricting water intake for 12 to 24 hours before anesthesia reduces the possibility of regurgitation and aspiration during recumbency.

ANESTHETIC INDUCTION

In North American zoos, the anesthetic agent of choice for the Nile hippopotamus is etorphine hydrochloride. The dose varies from 2 to 6 mg intramuscularly in an adult animal.[4] The lower doses are used in animals that are thin or otherwise debilitated. Acetylpromazine or xylazine are occasionally used in conjunction with etorphine. If used, a dose of xylazine of 100 mg intramuscularly can be given either with the etorphine or 20 minutes earlier. Acetylpromazine is given as a component of Immobilon. Drugs should be delivered in an area with a thin subcutaneous fat layer. The most often used site for delivery of anesthetic agents is in the neck just caudal to the ear. A needle length of 64 mm is generally adequate for intramuscular delivery in this area. Anesthetic induction time varies widely but is generally longer than experienced with other artiodactyls routinely anesthetized with etorphine. Induction times average 30 minutes, but induction times of 60 minutes or longer have been reported. Additional doses of etorphine should not be delivered until 60 minutes after the initial dose. Supplemental doses of etorphine should be based on the degree of anesthesia attained with the first dose. The long and inconsistent induction times are probably related to the degree of success of intramuscular injection. Anesthetic reversal can be accomplished with diprenorphine at two to three times the total dose of etorphine or naltrexone at 100 times the total dose of etorphine. If reversal agents are given intramuscularly, naltrexone appears to produce more rapid reversal than diprenorphine. If xylazine is used, it should be reversed with yohimbine at the dose rate of 0.1 mg/kg.

In general, the first sign of anesthetic effect is hypermetria. The animal may begin to sweat profusely and may vocalize. It should be remembered that Nile hippopotamus sweat is red tinged. As the effect of the anesthetic deepens, the animal may assume a dog-sitting position. Depending on the procedure planned, it may be possible to cross tie the head and begin the procedure at this point. Cutting teeth and other nonpainful procedures can usually begin at this stage. For long or painful procedures, intubation and maintenance on isoflurane is recommended.

MANAGEMENT DURING ANESTHESIA

Endotracheal tubes, oxygen, doxapram, and reversal agents—in addition to standard anesthetic emergency drugs—should be available during the procedure. A 24- to 30-mm endotracheal tube is required for an adult Nile hippopotamus. After a bite block has been positioned in the mouth, the tube is placed by manually palpating the glottis and inserting the tube. Delivery of oxygen at flow rates up to 15 L/min and intermittent positive-pressure ventilation at a rate of 5 breaths/min can greatly improve oxygen saturation. Doxapram can be given at a total dose of 100 to 400 mg either intravenously or intramuscularly for bradypnea or apnea.

A report in the literature states that atropine and other parasympatholytic agents are contraindicated in Nile hippopotamuses because they block the sweating reflex and lead to fatal hyperthermia.[3] One author (M.R.L.) routinely uses atropine during anesthesia of Nile hippopotamuses and has noticed improved heart rates without hyperthermia.

Bradypnea, cyanosis, and apnea are the most frequently encountered complications during anesthesia. Hemoglobin saturation, electrocardiogram pattern, respiratory rate, and heart rate should be closely monitored during anesthesia. Reducing the recumbency time to a minimum is important in avoiding complications. Nasal insufflation with oxygen can be initiated when the animal is in a sitting position and should be continued throughout the procedure. If the animal's airway becomes obstructed, which is usually expressed by snoring, placing a bite block in the mouth and retracting the tongue as far cranially as possible may alleviate the obstruction. Although limited hemoglobin saturation data are available for anesthetized Nile hippopotamuses, it appears that oxygen saturation, especially in recumbent animals, is low (55%–79%).[4] Intubation and delivery of intermittent positive-pressure ventilation with high oxygen flow rates may be required to raise hemoglobin saturation.

REFERENCES

1. Henwood R, Kemp M: The capture and translocation of hippopotamus by means of chemical immobilization. Lammergeyer 40:30–38, 1989.
2. Jarofke D: Hippopotamidae (hippopotamus). *In* Fowler ME (ed): Zoo and Wild Animal Medicine, 3rd ed. Philadelphia, WB Saunders, pp 523–524, 1993.
3. Pienaar UDeV: The field immobilization and capture of hippopotamus (*Hippopotamus amphibius* Linnaeus) in the aquatic environment. Koedoe 10:149–157, 1967.
4. Ramsay E, Loomis M, Mehren K, et al: Chemical restraint of the Nile hippopotamus (*Hippopotamus amphibius*) in captivity. J Zoo Wildl Med, in press.

CHAPTER **97**

Anesthesia for Nondomestic Suids

PAUL P. CALLE

PATRICK J. MORRIS

All suids are artiodactylids in the suborder Suiformes, which includes the Suidae and Tayassuidae families. The Suidae comprise nine Old World species. The red-river hog (*Potamochoerus porcus*) is also known as the bush pig, African bush pig, African water hog, and African river hog. Babirusa (*Babyrousa babyrussa*) are characterized by their upturned maxillary tusks, which grow through the nasal bone and erupt through the skin without entering the oral cavity. Male warthogs (*Phacochoerus aethiopicus*) have large tusks and prominent facial warts. The giant forest hog (*Hylochoerus meinertzhageni*) has not frequently been maintained in captivity. The genus *Sus* includes five species: pygmy hog (*Sus salvanius*), Javan warty pig (*Sus verrucosus*), bearded pig (*Sus barbatus*), Celebes wild pig (*Sus celebensis*), and the wild boar (*Sus scrofa*), from which all domesticated and feral varieties (including Vietnamese pot-bellied pigs) are derived.[11–13, 37, 38]

The Tayassuidae consist of three peccary species, all found in the New World: collared peccary (*Tayassu tajacu*), white-lipped peccary (*Tayassu pecari*), and Chacoan peccary (*Catagonus wagneri*).[8, 12, 13, 37, 38]

All suids are omnivores with powerful compact bodies, large heads, short legs, a tough skin with limited sebaceous and sweat glands, and a thick layer of subcutaneous fat. Nondomestic suids range in size from 6 to 275 kg, have prominent tusk-like canines (larger in males) with which they can inflict significant wounds, and a characteristic strong snout ending in a flexible cartilaginous disc that is used for rooting. Several species have prominent facial warts with no bony core, and most are sparsely haired. Except for peccaries, all suids are sexually dimorphic with males being larger than females. Suids are intelligent but excitable. Importation of nondomestic suids into the United States from countries with endemic foot-and-mouth disease, rinderpest, or African swine fever is regulated. Because African nondomestic suids can be asymptomatically infected with African swine fever virus, it is only recently that their importation into the United States has been allowed at all. Species more commonly exhibited in the United States include warthogs, babirusa, red-river hogs, and both collared and white-lipped peccaries.[8, 11, 12, 13, 37, 38]

GENERAL ANESTHESIA PRINCIPLES

Domestic Swine

Because of their physiologic, anatomic, and pathologic similarities to humans, domestic swine are commonly used in biomedical research for investigations of organ transplantations, cardiovascular and cardiopulmonary research, skin grafting, and wound healing.[2] Many anesthetic protocols for laboratory, agricultural, and pet swine involve either intravenous (IV) or inhalant induction, which are not practical in nondomestic suids.[5, 18, 20, 28, 35, 36] Local and regional analgesia are also commonly used in domestic swine for cesarean section and minor surgical procedures.[5, 20, 31] However, these techniques are not usually practiced for nondomestic suids. Exceptions might include either analgesia for painful conditions or postoperative regional anesthesia following immobilization of a nondomestic suid. Cutaneous fentanyl patches (50 μg/hour every 48 to 72 hours) (Duragesic; Janssen Pharmaceutica) for analgesia have been used in both domestic swine[28] and babirusa.

Reviews of the pharmacology of anesthetic agents and their application to suids and suid anesthetic emergency procedures are discussed in references 5, 24, 28, and 35. Intramuscular (IM) protocols for premedication, sedation, and anesthesia of domestic swine are most pertinent for application to zoological species and are summarized in Table 97–1.[4–7, 18, 28, 35]

TABLE 97–1. Premedication, Anesthetic, and Reversal Drug Doses for Domestic Pigs

Drug	Dose*
Premedication	
Atropine	0.044–0.088
Sedation	
Acepromazine	0.11–0.22
Azaperone	1.25–8
Diazepam	5.5–8.5
Droperidol-fentanyl	1 ml/13.6 kg
Midazolam	1
Anesthesia	
Tiletamine-zolazepam	4.4–6
Tiletamine-zolazepam	4.4–6
+ ketamine	+ 2.2
Tiletamine-zolazepam	4.4–6
+ xylazine	+ 1.1–4.4
Tiletamine-zolazepam	4.4–6
+ xylazine	+ 2.2
+ ketamine	+ 2.2
Reversal	
Yohimbine	0.3 IV
Tolazoline	2.2 IV

*Doses are mg/kg IM unless otherwise indicated.
(Data from references 4, 5, 20, 21, 22, 28, 32, 34, 35.)

Domestic swine are frequently premedicated to decrease total anesthetic drug needed, ease induction, provide analgesia, and promote smooth recovery.[4, 5, 28] Anticholinergics (atropine [Large Animal Atropine; Vedco, Inc.]) are frequently administered to decrease salivation and prevent vagal-induced bradycardia. Commonly used agents include acepromazine (Acepromazine; Vedco, Inc.), azaperone (Stresnil, Mallinckrodt Veterinary), diazepam (Diazepam, Steris Laboratories), or droperidol-fentanyl (Innovar-Vet; Mallinckrodt Veterinary).[4, 5, 28, 35] Midazolam (Versed; Roche Pharmaceuticals, Inc.) induces sedation within 5 minutes, deep sedation lasts for 20 minutes, and recovery to normal occurs within 1 hour. Mildly decreased heart and respiratory rates, with normal cardiovascular function, occurs.[32] Reversal can be accomplished with flumazenil (Romazicon; Roche Laboratories). Sedation resulting from administration of xylazine alone is variable and only marginally effective, with inadequate analgesia even at dose levels that result in adverse cardiovascular effects.[15] Swine may differ in the number or type of alpha$_2$-adrenergic receptors, the physiologic response to receptor stimulation, or both.[15] Because swine are so resistant to the effects of xylazine, it should be used only when combined with other agents.[6, 15, 28]

With or without premedication, anesthesia can be induced in domestic swine with any one of innumerable injectable anesthetic protocols.[4, 5, 7, 18, 26, 28, 35, 36] Swine are more resistant to the effects of opioids and alpha$_2$-adrenergic agonists, and they are more sensitive to benzodiazepines than are other species.[6, 15, 28] Tiletamine-zolazepam (Telazol; Fort Dodge Laboratories, Inc.) alone, or in combination with either xylazine (Cervizine; Wildlife Pharmaceuticals) or xylazine and ketamine (Ketamine; Phoenix Scientific, Inc.), are popular drug combinations that lend themselves well to use in nondomestic suids.[4, 5, 21, 22, 28, 34, 35] Tiletamine-zolazepam is a combination of the dissociative anesthetic tiletamine (an arylcycloalkylamine) and the benzodiazepine derivative zolazepam. This combination results in rapid immobilization with good muscle relaxation and is effective with a small volume. It is best to combine tiletamine-zolazepam with other agents such as the alpha$_2$-adrenergic agonist xylazine, which improves muscle relaxation and analgesia, and smoothes recovery.[5, 21, 22, 28, 34]

IM doses of tiletamine-zolazepam reconstituted with xylazine or ketamine are stable for 2 weeks, provide decreased injection volumes, and provide rapid smooth induction to sternal recumbency within 1 to 2 minutes and lateral recumbency within 5 minutes. Swine are left undisturbed for 5 minutes after immobilization before they are approached. Animals do not become excited, and they can be manipulated for 30 to 60 minutes. These drug combinations provide stable cardiac and respiratory function, good muscle relaxation, short-term analgesia for mildly invasive procedures, and, with most xylazine combinations, the ability to intubate. Ventral rotation of the eye and loss of palpebral reflex reflect an analgesic plane; nystagmus and a return of ocular position and palpebral reflex occur as the analgesic plane is lost. With some drug combinations, pigs are able to ambulate with moderate ataxia 60 to 100 minutes after drug administration. The addition of xylazine to the combination enhances its sedative and analgesic effects, reduces the possibility of potential adverse CNS responses to dissociative anesthetics, and prevents excessive salivation. This probably results from xylazine sedation's masking the CNS stimulatory effects of tiletamine or ketamine as the sedative effects of zolazepam wear off. When tiletamine-zolazepam is used alone, or in combination with ketamine, recoveries are often rough, with the pig demonstrating paddling, vocalizations, unsuccessful attempts to rise, and hyperthermia. Side effects are reduced and recovery is markedly smoother when xylazine is incorporated. Addition of ketamine to tiletamine-zolazepam/xylazine combinations did not enhance analgesia or prove beneficial. Even when pigs were not fasted, no adverse consequences were encountered.[21, 22, 34] Residual zolazepam is responsible for extended recoveries. Prolonged hindlimb paresis and ataxia with tiletamine-zolazepam anesthesia has been reversed with flumazenil.[35] Yohimbine (Antagonil; Wildlife Laboratories, Inc.) and tolazoline (Priscoline; Ciba) have been used to reverse the sedative effects of xylazine (see Table 97–1).[20, 35]

Continuous IV infusion of propofol (Diprivan Injection; Zeneca Pharmaceuticals) has been used for anesthesia in both domestic swine and Vietnamese pot-bellied pigs.[28, 35] Although a useful adjunct to anesthesia of nondomestic suids, apnea may occur and result in the need to use ventilatory support.[28]

Domestic swine are generally fasted for 24 hours and water is withheld for 4 hours before inhalant anesthesia is given to decrease the potential for gastrointestinal, respiratory, or circulatory complications.[5, 28, 35] Isoflurane (Forane; Ohmeda) is the preferred anesthetic agent, but halothane (Halothane; Fort Dodge Laboratories), methoxyflurane (Metofane; Mallinckrodt Veterinary), and other agents have also been used. Inhalant anesthetic agents can be delivered by mask, catheterization or intubation of nares, or endotracheal intubation.[5, 28, 32, 35] Intubation can be difficult because of the limited ability to open the mouth, the long oral cavity, and a mobile larynx that is prone to laryngospasm. Despite this, intubation can be accomplished with adequate sedation, good positioning with the head and neck extended, an elongated laryngoscope blade, and topical lidocaine (Cetacaine; Cetylite Industries, Inc.).[5, 6, 18, 28, 35, 38] The endotracheal tube may be passed directly or a stylet may be placed in the trachea and the endotracheal tube advanced over the stylet.[5, 18, 28] Upon entering the tracheal lumen, the endotracheal tube should be directed ventrally and then rotated 180 degrees. Placing an endotracheal tube over an endoscope, passing the endoscope into the tracheal lumen, and then advancing the endotracheal tube and removing the endoscope is also effective when the laryngeal opening is difficult to visualize. The endotracheal tube should not be secured by wrapping tape or gauze around the muzzle because swine are obligate nasal breathers and passive congestion of nasal passages may occur, resulting in airway obstruction after extubation.[28] Prolonged dorsal recumbency should be avoided because increased pressure on the thoracic cavity can compromise cardiorespiratory function.[35] Anesthetic monitoring should include continuous heart and respiratory rates, and core body temperatures. For extended procedures, electrocardiogram (often with alligator clip leads attached to small gauge needles placed subcutaneously), blood pressure (via a cuff placed on the metatarsus), and pulse oximetry (probes can be placed on the tongue, eyelid, lip of the vulva, or rectally) can be included. In addition, respiratory support and intravenous fluids should be provided.[28] The animal should be well padded for the duration of the procedure and monitored closely, especially for airway obstruction, during the recovery period.[28]

In most suids, the thick subcutaneous adipose layer and limited sebaceous and sweat glands, as well as the proportionally small lung capacity, results in heat retention.[4, 13, 38] This can be exacerbated by drug-induced respiratory depression.[4] Environmental and body temperature should be monitored during anesthesia. Malignant hyperthermia is a heritable myopathy of domestic swine, resulting in exaggerated and prolonged muscle contraction. Clinically, the disorder is characterized by hyperthermia, tachycardia, tachypnea, muscle rigidity, metabolic acidosis, hyperkalemia, hyperglycemia, and elevated lactate and creatine kinase levels. The condition can be induced by exposure to a wide range of stressors, including environmental factors and either injectable or inhalant anesthetics. Treatment consists of efforts to decrease body temperature, administration of bicarbonate, cessation of anesthesia, and administration of dantrolene (Dantrium; Norwich Eaton Pharmaceuticals, Inc.) (1 to 5 mg/kg IV). Although malignant hyperthermia is common in agricultural swine, there is only one report of a suspected case in a Vietnamese pot-bellied pig and none in nondomestic suids. A commercial DNA-based blood test is available for diagnosis.[9, 28, 35]

Vietnamese pot-bellied pigs have become popular pets. There are a number of protocols for sedation and anesthesia of these animals Table 97–2.[6, 18] Premedication with anticholinergics such as atropine or glycopyrrolate (Robinul; A. H. Robins Co.) IM, IV, or subcutaneously (SQ) 30 minutes before induction is recommended to decrease salivary secretions as well as gastric and intestinal motility, to reduce the risk of vomiting, and to minimize bradycardia.[6] Sedation can be accomplished with IM acepromazine, azaperone, droperidol (Inapsine; Janssen Pharmaceutica, Inc.), or diazepam.[6] Anesthesia can be induced with isoflurane administered by mask or IM ketamine and acepromazine; ketamine and xylazine; azaperone; tiletamine-zolazepam; tiletamine-zolazepam and xylazine; or ketamine with xylazine and butorphanol (Torbugesic; Fort Dodge Laboratories, Inc.).[6, 10, 18, 27] In addition, a drug combination of atropine, detomidine (Dormosedan, Pfizer Inc.), butorphanol, and midazolam mixed together in one syringe and given IM provides smooth induction with excellent muscle relaxation, which can be rapidly reversed with IV naloxone (Narcan, Dupont

Pharma) and yohimbine. Flumazenil can also be given if necessary (P. J. Morris, unpublished data, 1996). Isoflurane is most commonly used for inhalant anesthesia.[6, 18] Pot-bellied pigs have anatomic features similar to larger swine, and procedures for intubation are similar.[18]

Nondomestic Suids

Nondomestic suid chemical restraint protocols generally are used to provide sufficient sedation and relaxation for physical examination (including oropharyngeal examination and intubation), venipuncture or intravenous catheter placement, administration of injectable medications, minor wound care, short distance transport without crating, and weight determination. Ideally, it is desirable to reverse chemical restraint with appropriate antagonists. Although many of the drugs and drug combinations discussed in this section are useful, there is no such thing as a safe anesthetic protocol; rather, anesthetic protocols must be safely implemented. This can be achieved only by a thorough knowledge of the individual drugs and combined effects of the agents discussed. For further information on the pharmacology of the drugs discussed, refer to references 5, 19, 24, 27, 28, 32, and 35.

Manual restraint can be performed for smaller nondomestic suids, but, because of their excitable nature, strength, and sharp tusks, it can be stressful and dangerous for both the suid and personnel.[13, 23, 38] Although restraint of captive babirusa in Indonesia is routinely accomplished by netting and manual restraint (P. Kalk, personnel communication, 1997), and free-ranging collared peccaries have been caught and restrained by netting,[12] fatal human injuries have occurred during attempted manual restraint of suids.[23] Chemical restraint is most commonly used in zoological settings.

Chemical restraint is most commonly achieved with an agent administered IM by projectile dart or pole syringe.[38] Immobilization agents for nondomestic suids include ketamine (10 to 30 mg/kg)[3, 14, 19, 23, 25, 38]; a combination of tiletamine-zolazepam (2 to 32 mg/kg)[1, 16] or tiletamine-zolazepam (2.0 to 4.0 mg/kg) and xylazine (4.4 mg/kg)[29]; phencyclidine (0.7 to 3.0 mg/kg) and promazine (Promazine, Fort Dodge Laboratories, Inc.) (0.7 to 3.0 mg/kg)[38]; etorphine (1.0 to 6.0 mg/adult or 0.02 to 0.04 mg/kg)[13, 38]; and azaperone (2.0 to 14.0 mg/kg) alone or azaperone (10 mg/kg) combined with fentanyl (Sublimaze; Janssen Pharmaceutica, Inc.) (0.33 mg/kg).[23] Although atropine (0.044 mg/kg) has sometimes been administered to control excessive salivation,[38] we do not administer it routinely.

Although a 24-hour fast before sedation or anesthesia of domestic swine is generally recommended,[6, 28] unfasted domestic swine have been immobilized with combinations of xylazine, ketamine, and tiletamine-zolazepam without vomiting or other adverse effects.[21, 22] When possible, nondomestic suids should be fasted for 12 to 18 hours before immobilization. Caution must be exercised, however, to ensure that fasted suids do not consume bedding material as a substitute for the food that has been withheld.

TABLE 97–2. Premedication, Anesthetic, and Reversal Drug Doses for Vietnamese Pot-Bellied Pigs*

Drug	Dose
Premedication	
Atropine	0.04 IV, IM, SQ
Glycopyrrolate	0.005–0.01 IV, IM, SQ
Sedation	
Acepromazine	0.03–1.1
Azaperone	0.25–2
Droperidol	0.1–0.4
Diazepam	0.5–8.5
Anesthesia	
Ketamine	10–20
+ acepromazine	+ 0.05–0.5
Ketamine	5–20
+ xylazine	+ 1–2
Azaperone	2–8
Tiletamine-zolazepam	4–6
Tiletamine-zolazepam	6
+ xylazine	+ 2.2
Ketamine	11
+ xylazine	+ 2
+ butorphanol	+ 0.22
Atropine	0.06
+ detomidine	+ 0.125
+ butorphanol	+ 0.3
+ midazolam	+ 0.3
Reversal	
Naloxone	4 mg total dose IV
Yohimbine	0.3 IV
Flumazenil	1 mg/10–15 mg midazolam

*Doses are mg/kg IM unless otherwise indicated.
(Data from references 6, 10, 18, 27, and P. J. Morris, personal communication, 1996.)

Sufficient pressure must be used when darting and the needle must be of an appropriate length (1.8 to 2.0 cm) to penetrate the thick skin and subcutaneous fat for IM injection.[6, 28, 38] The best anesthetic effect is achieved by a well-placed IM injection, generally in the middle of the semimembranosus, semitendinosus, and gluteal muscles[22, 26] or in the dorsal prescapular or cervical region. Some species such as warthogs have less subcutaneous fat. Drug leakage from injection sites frequently complicates drug administration and can result in suboptimal drug effect.

In general, the immobilized suid should be isolated to prevent conspecific trauma or stimulation during induction. An exception would be if an animal becomes excited when isolated, in which case a companion should be present until sedation is sufficient to allow the companion to be shifted out of the enclosure. During induction and recovery, a substrate with adequate traction and a well-bedded enclosure is necessary to prevent slipping or splaying and to lessen the chances of inadvertent injury. Induction and recovery are generally smoother in a quiet, undisturbed, dimly lit environment.[28] In addition, the suid can be placed in a well-bedded crate for recovery. Because of their excitable nature, disturbances during either induction or recovery can result in the animal partially overcoming drug effects, compromising the anesthetic plane, and attempting to ambulate when still ataxic, with the potential for injury.

Anesthesia can be prolonged or deepened by supplemental doses of injectable agents administered either IV or IM or by the administration of halothane or isoflurane by face mask, catheterization or intubation of nares, or endotracheal intubation.[6] Smooth, rapid induction and an ability to reverse sedation at the termination of the procedure are desirable.

Anesthesia should be monitored by noting mucous membrane color, heart and respiratory rates, body temperature, thoracic auscultation, and pulse oximetry.[1] Pulse oximeter probes are most commonly placed on the tongue or ear, although they can also be placed against the hard palate, on the mandibular or maxillary gingiva, on the coronary band, intrarectally, or on the vulvar lip. Supplemental oxygen can be readily administered by nasal catheter.

Blood sampling of both domestic swine[6, 28, 33] and collared peccary[25] has been reported from the anterior vena cava, ear veins, and orbital venous sinus. In addition, the saphenous vein is easily accessible in the collared peccary.[25] Additional sites used in swine include the jugular, femoral, and cephalic veins; ear or tail vessels; and cardiac puncture.[6, 12, 28, 33] Vessels in the tail, ear, or superficial veins on the medial surfaces of the forelimbs and hindlimbs may be accessed in some species or individuals. The authors recommend cephalic and saphenous venipuncture for nondomestic suids and avoid anterior vena cava puncture, cardiocentesis, or orbital venous sinus sampling because of the potential for complications.

KETAMINE

Captive collared peccaries given 20 mg/kg IM ketamine were immobilized in 10 to 12 minutes. Although physiologic monitoring demonstrated statistically significant decreases in body temperature, total serum protein, albumin, cholesterol, calcium, and alanine aminotransferase, and increases in aspartate aminotransferase, inorganic phosphorus, and testosterone, these physiologic alterations did not have adverse health effects on the animals.[19] Peccaries immobilized with ketamine (15 to 25 mg/kg IM) were sedated for 72 minutes and experienced smooth, although somewhat prolonged (122 minutes) recoveries with the only significant complication consisting of heat stress with deaths in hot weather.[14]

TILETAMINE-ZOLAZEPAM

Overall, the combination of tiletamine and zolazepam provides adequate chemical restraint for suids. After a single IM dose of 2 to 5 mg/kg, induction is relatively smooth and results in stable immobilization for the duration of maximum anesthetic effects. Usually, sedation is sufficient to conduct routine procedures but access to the oropharynx can be difficult because of increased jaw muscle tone. Duration of effect is variable, but most cases recover quickly (able to stand within an hour) after a single dose. At higher doses, however, adverse recovery phenomena increase, especially when doses exceed 3 mg/kg. Adverse reactions include prolonged recovery with or without hyperkinesis, which can be especially dangerous if hyperthermia and its metabolic sequelae occur. In addition, hyperkinesis can result in trauma and airway obstruction by abnormal positioning or accumulation of secretions or blood. Administration of midazolam (0.3 to 0.5 mg/kg, IV or IM) is usually effective in controlling these adverse reactions. Rather than titrating anesthesia with repeated injections of tiletamine-zolazepam, it is better to administer other adjuncts to maintain sedation/anesthesia and minimize the risk of adverse effects of residual tiletamine. Combination of tiletamine-zolazepam with an alpha$_2$-adrenergic compound (xylazine, detomidine, or medetomidine [Domitor; Pfizer Animal Health]), ketamine, a benzodiazepine (diazepam or midazolam), propofol, or an inhalant agent (isoflurane or desflurane [Suprane; Ohmeda]) greatly minimizes these recovery problems.

Captive Chacoan peccaries immobilized with tiletamine-zolazepam IM at a combined drug dose of 2.18 mg/kg had an induction time of 7.6 minutes. Induction and recovery were smooth, good muscle relaxation was attained, reflexes (palpebral, corneal, and swallowing) were maintained, and no adverse effects or complications were noted. Recovery (when the animals stood) ranged from 90 to 240 minutes. The peccaries were ataxic with dulled mentation, however, and a normal behavior was not attained for 6 to 8 hours after immobilization.[1]

Semicaptive white-lipped peccaries and free-ranging white-lipped and collared peccaries have been immobilized with 1 to 9 mg/kg tiletamine-zolazepam IM, occasionally supplemented with either ketamine or diazepam and at times reversed with flumazenil. Doses less than 2 mg/kg resulted in light sedation adequate for blood sampling and ear tagging, whereas doses greater than

5 mg/kg resulted in deep sedation or anesthesia with prolonged recoveries. Doses in the range of 2 to 3 mg/kg resulted in good relaxation, heavy sedation or light anesthesia for approximately 1 hour, and smooth recovery. Slightly higher doses (3 to 5 mg/kg) resulted in a deeper anesthetic plane but longer recoveries. High doses have generally been used to allow more rapid induction in free-ranging situations. Blood samples have been obtained from these animals by cephalic, saphenous, or jugular venipuncture (W. Karesh and M. Stetter, personal communication, 1997). Tiletamine-zolazepam (2.2 mg/kg) has also been successfully used in captive collared peccaries.[1]

Sedation of a babirusa with 5.3 mg/kg tiletamine-zolazepam IM, followed by intubation and halothane anesthesia, has been reported.[30]

TILETAMINE-ZOLAZEPAM AND XYLAZINE

Babirusa have been successfully immobilized by premedication with xylazine (1 to 2 mg/kg IM) followed in approximately 20 minutes with tiletamine-zolazepam (1 to 3.5 mg/kg IM). This combination is inexpensive and small dart volumes (<3 ml for each drug) are possible. In most cases, animals are fasted for 12 hours before immobilization. This protocol results in smooth induction, analgesia, and muscle relaxation sufficient for minor procedures. Xylazine premedication produces sedation, ataxia, and, in some cases, recumbency within 10 minutes. It is important to leave babirusa undisturbed during the premedication period to allow maximal sedative effects. It is generally possible to handle babirusa within 10 minutes of tiletamine-zolazepam administration. Excessive salivation has not been observed.

Appropriate physiologic monitoring should be conducted. In general, minimal cardiovascular changes are observed, although some animals receiving high xylazine doses can exhibit moderate bradycardia. Supplemental 100% oxygen is generally administered by nasal catheter. Anesthetic plane can be deepened or prolonged with supplemental ketamine (1.5 to 2.5 mg/kg IV or IM) or inhalant isoflurane administered by mask. Doses of xylazine and tiletamine-zolazepam used are inversely related, with high initial xylazine doses lowering the tiletamine-zolazepam requirement. The xylazine can reverse with yohimbine (0.1 to 0.3 mg/kg IV or IM[6, 28]) resulting in a rapid increase in respiratory rate and depth and arousal. Flumazenil can also be used to reverse zolazepam (1 mg flumazenil/20 mg zolazepam IV or IM) if necessary. To minimize hyperkinesis from residual tiletamine, reversal should be performed at least 20 minutes after administration of tiletamine-zolazepam. Animals are generally ambulatory in 30 to 45 minutes.

BUTORPHANOL COMBINATIONS

A combination of butorphanol (0.3 to 0.4 mg/kg), detomidine (0.06 to 0.125 mg/kg), and midazolam (0.3 to 0.4 mg/kg) mixed together and administered IM has been used successfully in Vietnamese pot-bellied pigs, red river hogs, warthogs, babirusa, bearded pigs, and European wild boars (P. J. Morris, unpublished data,

1996). This combination results in rapid induction to recumbent sedation 2 to 10 minutes after IM injection. The rate of induction in most cases is dependent on the injection site, the animal's arousal state, and completeness of administration. Immobilization is characterized by excellent relaxation, including the jaw muscles, allowing oropharyngeal examination and fair to good analgesia. P. J. Morris has used xylazine at 2 to 3 mg/kg as a substitute for detomidine, and tiletamine-zolazepam at a combined dose of 0.6 mg/kg as a substitute for midazolam in selected species (red river hogs, bearded pigs, Vietnamese pot-bellied pigs, European wild boars) with good results. However, there have been occasional prolonged recoveries typical of tiletamine-zolazepam residual activity. Using these substitutions, in most cases, the injection volume easily falls within the 3-ml dart limit.

Consistent side effects include bradycardia and associated hypotension, likely secondary to detomidine-induced increases in peripheral vascular resistance. The combination of bradycardia and hypotension can result in poor oximetry values. In these cases, administration of small doses of atropine (0.02 to 0.04 mg/kg) IV usually results in partial reversal of the bradycardia and more reliable oximetry values. Recumbency, bradypnea, and costal muscular relaxation can also contribute to hypoxemia. Hypoxemia can be easily remedied by administering 100% oxygen via nasal cannula into one nostril at a flow rate of 4 to 8 L/minute. During prolonged procedures (>1 hour), hypercapnea and respiratory acidosis can develop if animals are not intubated. Minor acidosis observed during shorter procedures appears to resolve spontaneously when pharmacologic antagonists are administered.

The combination can be antagonized by administering yohimbine (0.3 mg/kg), naltrexone (Naltrexone; Wildlife Laboratories, Inc.) (5 mg/kg), and flumazenil (0.03 to 0.04 mg/kg or at a ratio of roughly 1:10 to 1:15 mg flumazenil:mg midazolam). Flumazenil is not typically required to achieve recovery to standing sedation. The antagonists are routinely mixed into one syringe and administered IV. Most animals recover to standing posture in 2 to 10 minutes following antagonist administration. Typically, animals wander slowly and aimlessly for 10 to 15 minutes following recovery to ambulation, followed by a slow return to normalcy within an hour after standing. Cases have been observed in which animals were aroused after administration of antagonists as if no residual sedative were present. Conversely, animals have remained sedated after administration of sedative antagonists. In all of the latter cases, the addition of flumazenil has resulted in prompt arousal, suggesting that the midazolam component was responsible for the delay.

The advantages of this combination are rapid induction, good relaxation, and rapid arousal and recovery. Disadvantages are bradycardia and hypoxemia, both of which are easily dealt with. In addition, midazolam is prepared in 1- and 5-mg/ml solutions for injection. This dilute form results in larger than desired injection volumes. For example, a 60-kg animal typically requires a total volume of injection of 7 ml or more. Additionally, this protocol is more costly than other available protocols. This combination is not recommended for field procedures because of its slower induction time, larger delivery volumes, and higher cost. However, for pet swine and captive suids requiring relaxation for intubation, and for rapid arousal from anesthesia, this combination works well.

Two categories emerge when using butorphanol combinations in suids: easily immobilized/sensitive species and difficult to immobilize/resistant species. Red river hogs, Vietnamese pot-bellied pigs, and babirusa are predictably easy to immobilize with this combination. This may be related to the fact that all three species are readily tamed in captivity. For these species, the lower range of suggested dosages for butorphanol combinations seems to work well. Bearded pigs, warthogs, and European wild boars usually require doses at the high end of the suggested dose range. European wild boars are especially resistant to these drugs, usually requiring one or more supplemental doses of midazolam at 0.3 mg/kg IM or IV during induction to render these animals immobile. When supplemental doses of midazolam are used, it should be remembered that additional flumazenil may be necessary to antagonize the total cumulative dose of midazolam given, which adds to the expense of the procedure. In all cases the administration of the antagonists should result in a standing posture in less than 10 minutes.

INHALANT ANESTHESIA

The preferred inhalant anesthetic agent is isoflurane, but halothane can also be used. Inhalant anesthesia can be used as a primary agent in neonatal, small, tame, or debilitated suids. Most commonly, inhalant anesthetics are used to deepen or prolong anesthesia after the animal is immobilized with an injectable agent.[30] Inhalant agents are most commonly administered by face mask or intubation or by catheterization of nares. This can be performed in the field with a portable anesthesia machine or an oxygen cylinder connected to an anesthetic vaporizer. Endotracheal intubation is conducted similarly to that for domestic suids.

DISCUSSION

Etorphine and carfentanil (Carfentanil; Wildlife Laboratories, Inc.) have been used for sedation of both domestic[5] and nondomestic suids,[13, 38] and, although their effects can be reversed, their use is not recommended. Respiratory depression, muscle rigidity, hyperthermia, and renarcotization can occur.[5, 28] Swine are more susceptible to renarcotization than most artiodactylids because they have abundant fat stores, and renarcotization has been observed in wild boar.[17]

IM ketamine or tiletamine-zolazepam have been used most often for sedation and anesthesia of nondomestic suids. Although ketamine results in a rapid induction with minimal cardiovascular or respiratory depression, disadvantages reported in either domestic swine[4, 26] or peccaries[14] include excessive salivation, prolonged recovery, or postanesthetic excitement. Either ketamine or tiletamine-zolazepam when given alone

provide poor muscle relaxation and frequently result in rough recoveries, especially when given IM.[4, 6, 28]

Another disadvantage of both tiletamine-zolazepam and ketamine is the inability to reverse sedation. More effective is the administration of xylazine as a premedication or of alpha$_2$-adrenergic agonists (xylazine, detomidine, or medetomidine) as coadministered adjuncts, to decrease the ketamine or tiletamine-zolazepam requirement. The sedative effects of zolazepam and xylazine can then be reversed by administration of flumazenil and yohimbine, allowing more rapid reversal than would otherwise occur.

Butorphanol-based combinations, although more expensive, provide rapid smooth induction and excellent muscle relaxation. Resulting bradycardia, hypotension, or hypoxemia can be readily controlled with atropine and oxygen supplementation when necessary. Immobilization can be rapidly reversed by the administration of naltrexone, yohimbine, and flumazenil.

Our preferred anesthetic protocols are either premedication with xylazine followed by administration of tiletamine-zolazepam or butorphanol-based combinations incorporating detomidine, midazolam, xylazine, or tiletamine-zolazepam. These combinations are effective with a drug volume that fits in a small dart. They have proven to be safe with smooth induction, excellent muscle relaxation including the ability to intubate, sufficient duration for transportation or moderate length procedures, and analgesia adequate for mildly invasive procedures. Both protocols are reversible with combinations of yohimbine, flumazenil, or naltrexone, and are characterized by smooth, rapid recovery. The safety, utility, and convenience of these drug combinations have advanced and enhanced the ability to provide high-quality medical and surgical care for nondomestic suids maintained in zoological collections.

Acknowledgment

The authors would like to thank Dr. Stephanie James for review and analysis of babirusa anesthesia records at the Wildlife Conservation Park/Bronx Zoo, Bronx, New York.

REFERENCES

1. Allen JL: Immobilization of giant Chacoan peccaries (*Catagonus wagneri*) with a tiletamine hydrochloride/zolazepam hydrochloride combination. J Wildl Dis 28(3):499–501, 1992.
2. Almond GW: Research applications using pigs. Vet Clin North Am Food Anim Pract 12(3):707–716, 1996.
3. Beck CC: VETALAR (ketamine hydrochloride). A unique cataleptoid anesthetic agent for multispecies usage. J Zoo Anim Med 7(3):11–38, 1976.
4. Benson GJ, Thurmon JC: Anesthesia of swine under field conditions. J Am Vet Med Assoc 174(6):594–596, 1979.
5. Bolin SR, Runnels LJ, Bane DP: Chemical restraint and anesthesia. *In* Leman AD (ed): Diseases of Swine, 7th ed. Ames IA, Iowa State University Press, pp 933–942, 1992.
6. Braun WF, Casteel SW: Potbellied pigs, miniature porcine pets. Vet Clin North Am Small Anim Pract 23(6):1149–1177, 1993.
7. Breese CE, Dodman NH: Xylazine-ketamine-oxymorphone: an injectable anesthetic combination in swine. J Am Vet Med Assoc 184(2):182–183, 1984.
8. Castellanos H: Peccaries. *In* Macdonald D (ed): The Encyclopedia of Mammals. New York, Facts on File Publications, pp 504–505, 1984.

9. Claxton-Gill MS, Cornick-Seahorn JL, Gamboa JC, Boatright BS: Suspected malignant hyperthermia syndrome in a miniature pot-bellied pig anesthetized with isoflurane. J Am Vet Med Assoc 203(10):1434–1436, 1993.

10. Clifford DH: Preanesthesia, anesthesia, analgesia, and euthanasia. *In* Fox JG, Cohen BJ, Loew FM (eds): Laboratory Animal Medicine ACLAM Series. New York, Academic Press, pp 527–562, 1984.

11. Cumming DHM: Wild Pigs and boars. *In* Macdonald D (ed): The Encyclopedia of Mammals. New York, Facts on File Publications, pp 500–503, 1984.

12. Fowler ME: Wild Swine and peccaries. *In* Fowler ME (ed): Zoo and Wild Animal Medicine, Current Therapy 3. Philadelphia, WB Saunders, pp 513–522, 1993.

13. Fowler ME, Boever WJ: Superfamily Suidoidae. *In* Fowler ME (ed): Zoo and Wild Animal Medicine, 2nd ed. Philadelphia, WB Saunders, pp 964–967, 1986.

14. Gallagher JF, Lochmiller RL, Grant WE: Immobilization of collared peccaries with ketamine hydrochloride. J Wildl Management 49(2):356–357, 1985.

15. Gomez de Segura IA, Tendillo FJ, Mascias A, et al: Actions of xylazine in young swine. Am J Vet Res 58(1):99–102, 1997.

16. Gray CW, Bush M, Beck CC: Clinical experience using CI-744 in chemical restraint and anesthesia of exotic specimens. J Zoo Anim Med 5(4):12–21, 1974.

17. Haigh JC: Opioids in zoological medicine. J Zoo Anim Med 21(4):391–413, 1990.

18. Heard DJ: Principles and techniques of anesthesia and analgesia for exotic practice. Vet Clin North Am Small Anim Pract 23(6):1301–1327, 1993.

19. Hellgren EC, Lochmiller RL, Amoss MS, Grant WE: Endocrine and metabolic responses of the collared peccary (*Tayassu tajacu*) to immobilization with ketamine hydrochloride. J Wildl Dis 21(4):417–425, 1985.

20. Ko JCH, Thurmon JC, Benson GJ, et al: A new drug combination for use in porcine cesarean sections. Vet Med 88:466–472, 1993.

21. Ko JCH, Williams BL, Rogers ER, et al: Increasing xylazine dose-enhanced anesthetic properties of telazol-xylazine combination in swine. Lab Anim Sci 45(3):290–294, 1995.

22. Ko JCH, Williams BL, Smith VL, et al: Comparison of telazol, telazol-ketamine, telazol-xylazine, and telazol-ketamine-xylazine as chemical restraint and anesthetic induction combination in swine. Lab Anim Sci 43(5):476–480, 1993.

23. Kohn A: Pigs. *In* Klos HG, Lang EM (eds): Handbook of Zoo Medicine. New York, Van Nostrand Reinhold, pp 205–208, 1982.

24. Kruse-Elliott KT: Management and emergency intervention during anesthesia. Vet Clin North Am Food Anim Pract 12(3):563–578, 1996.

25. Lochmiller RL, Hellgren LEC, Robinson RM, Grant WE: Techniques for collecting blood from collared peccaries, *Dicotyles tajacu* (L.). J Wildl Dis 20(1):47–50, 1984.

26. Loscher W, Ganter M, Fassbender CP: Correlation between drug and metabolite concentrations in plasma and anesthetic action of ketamine in swine. Am J Vet Res 51(3):391–398, 1990.

27. Lumb WV, Jones EW: Veterinary Anesthesia. Philadelphia, Lea and Febiger, 1984.

28. Moon PF, Smith LJ: General anesthetic techniques in swine. Vet Clin North Am Food Anim Pract 12(3):663–691, 1996.

29. New JC, Delozier K, Barton CE, et al: A serologic survey of selected viral and bacterial diseases of European wild hogs, Great Smoky Mountains National Park, USA. J Wildl Dis 30(1):103–106, 1994.

30. Schaftenaar W: Treatment of a fractured tusk in a male babirusa (*Babyrousa babyrussa*) using a polyoxymethylene bolt. J Zoo Wildl Med 22(3):364–366, 1991.

31. Skarda RT: Local and regional anesthesia in ruminants and swine. Vet Clin North Am Food Anim Pract 12(3):579–626, 1996.

32. Smith AC, Zellner JL, Spinale FG, Swindle MM: Sedative and cardiovascular effects of midazolam in swine. Lab Anim Sci 41(2):157–162, 1991.

33. Straw BE, Meuten DJ: Physical examination. *In* Leman AD, Straw BE, Mengeling WL, et al (eds): Diseases of Swine, 7th ed. Ames, IA, Iowa State University Press, pp 793–807, 1992.

34. Thurman JC, Benson GJ, Tranquilli WJ, et al: The anesthetic and analgesic effects of telazol and xylazine in pigs: evaluating clinical trials. Vet Med 83:841–845, 1988.

35. Tranquilli WJ, Grimm KA: Pharmacology of drugs used for anesthesia and sedation. Vet Clin North Am Food Anim Pract 12(3):501–529, 1996.

36. Vainio OM, Bloor BC, Kim C: Cardiovascular effects of a ketamine-medetomidine combination that produces deep sedation in Yucatan mini swine. Lab Anim Sci 42(6):582–588, 1992.

37. Walker EP, Warnick F, Lange KI, et al: Mammals of the World, Vol II. Baltimore, The Johns Hopkins Press, 1964.

38. Wallach JD, Boever WJ: Disease of Exotic Animals. Philadelphia, WB Saunders, 1983.

CHAPTER 98

Okapi Medicine and Surgery

BONNIE L. RAPHAEL

Okapi (*Okapia johnstoni*), in the family Giraffidae, are native to the rain forests of northeastern Zaire. Although there may be as many as 100,000 free-ranging animals, their existence is threatened by limited distribution and increasing levels of human disturbance. Only 485 okapi have been maintained in the United States and Europe since they were first discovered by non-Africans in the early 20th century. One hundred and ninety animals have been born in captivity since 1970 and, as of December 1995, the total world captive population was 92 animals.[7, 16]

Adult weights range from 250 to 350 kg for females and 200 to 290 kg for males. Only males have horns; the horns are covered with haired skin unless they are traumatized. Free-ranging females occupy home ranges of 1.9 to 5.1 km^2 and males are somewhat nomadic. Males may travel up to 9 km per day and have home ranges up to 10 square kilometers.[11] Free-ranging males enter a female's territory and travel with her during estrus, but it is uncommon for adult males to be found near females at other times. They may visit multiple female home ranges over the course of a year.

REPRODUCTION

Estrous cycles are 14.5 to 15 days in length and estrus lasts approximately 18 hours.[5] Multiple matings during estrus are normal, although mating can occur at other times including during pregnancy. Gestation length ranges from 14.5 to 15 months with an average of 440 days.[4] Estrus occurs 1 to 3 weeks postpartum,[21] followed by an apparent lactational anestrus for 2 to 8 months. Females reach sexual maturity at 1.5 to 2 years of age, but most do not conceive until they are 3 to 4 years old. Fecundity in females drops dramatically at 15 to 17 years of age, although healthy calves have been born to females as old as 26 years. Male okapi typically are fertile until age 24 years.

Before 1982, one of the obstacles to effective okapi breeding programs was the inability to accurately determine pregnancy. Since then, the reproductive physiology of female okapi has been well characterized using urinary hormone analysis, and both normal and abnormal estrous cycles and gestations have been characterized.[5] Fecal progestogen levels,[21] transabdominal ultrasonography, and measurements of body weight changes[8] have been used to diagnose pregnancy. Pregnant female okapi body weight typically increases by 13%, with the greatest gains occurring between 100 and 200 days of gestation.

Parturition in okapi averages 3 to 4 hours.[1] Dystocias caused by posterior presentation or uterine inertia have been successfully resolved using manual manipulation and extraction of calves following xylazine-induced standing tranquilization of the female.[5] Obesity in females may contribute to dystocia and, in at least one case, was associated with ketosis. Postparturient hypocalcemia has also occurred.

One of the most common causes of okapi infertility is behavioral interactions that result in poor acceptance of the male by females. Breeding behavior in some males may be aggressive. Females may display submissive behavior by lying in lateral recumbency while the male circles her, pawing and nudging or raking her with his horns. Additionally, anestrus and infertility in females has been associated with stressors such as transport or environmental factors. In captivity, males that are continuously housed with females may be a cause of stress or trauma because of their excessive pursuit of the female. In aged females, irregular cycles and subsequent infertility often develop. Reproductive disorders reported in at least two males include paraphimosis and preputial strictures, resulting in the need for surgical intervention.

PEDIATRICS AND NEONATAL DISORDERS

Okapi calf weights range from 14 to 30 kg and are typically 7% to 8% of the dam's nonpregnant body weight. Calves are usually able to stand within 30 minutes of birth.[1, 2, 15] Calves born on substrates with poor traction or with pre-existing weaknesses may not be able to rise. Normal healthy calves first attempt to nurse within 40 minutes of birth and are successful within 1 to 2 hours. During the first 3 days of life, calves nurse an average of twice per hour. Once they establish typical nesting behavior, the frequency is reduced.[1, 2, 15] Infrasound studies have demonstrated that calves communicate with their dams to initiate nursing, even if they are not in visual contact.[14]

Calves begin to eat solid food at approximately 21 days of age, with rumination starting at 42 days[4] and weaning at 6 months. Calves double their body weight in 4 weeks and triple it by 7 weeks. Normally, spontaneous defecation does not take place until 30 to 70 days of age. At that time, meconium is found with the pelleted feces, indicating that the calf has retained feces for the entire time. Early defecation is usually associated with medical problems.[2, 19] Fecal bacterial flora of nursing calves is primarily gram-positive bacteria as opposed to the more gram-negative flora in adults.[4]

Okapi calves do not thermoregulate well until 51 to 60 days of age.[2] External ambient temperatures have been significantly and positively correlated with body temperature in okapi calves in the first 2 months of life. Normal rectal temperatures vary from 37.0° to 39.2°C, with an average of 38°C from birth to 90 days of age.

Maternal Neglect and Trauma

The neonatal mortality rate of okapi in North America is approximately 30%.[8, 13, 16] Factors contributing to this high rate include infection, inbreeding, trauma, abortions, and stillbirths. Inadequate maternal care may lead to failure to nurse and consequently failure of passive antibody transfer. Maternal trauma immediately after calving has been seen most commonly in primiparous females. Calves up to 4 months of age have been attacked by their dams, resulting in fractured long bones, fractured mandibles, and fatal injuries. The attacks may be precipitated by external disturbances such as loud noises or disturbances by people, but occasionally they have been the result of an exaggerated maternal response to a calf's behavior. Maternal overgrooming has caused loss of tail tips in some young animals. One female had the habit of excessive grooming of her calf's tail. A protective jacket was constructed for the calf, which allowed it to remain with the dam without exposing it to further trauma. Occasionally, excessive perineal grooming, including licking the inside of the rectum, has resulted in rectal strictures and stenosis, requiring local treatment or surgical repair in several calves.[10, 12]

Infectious Diseases

Diarrheal diseases can cause severe problems in neonates. A virus morphologically similar to rotavirus has been identified via electron microscopy in calves with severe diarrhea.[19] At least one calf died as a result of a coronavirus-like enteritis with villus atrophy and a secondary *Escherichia coli* infection. Supportive therapy, consisting of oral electrolyte solutions, intravenous (IV) fluids, and vitamins is recommended in severe cases. Parenteral antibiotics are often administered to preclude opportunistic bacterial infections.

Navel ill, polyarthritis, meningitis, bacterial and viral pneumonia, septicemia, enterotoxemia, coliform enteritis, fungal pneumonia, and fungal meningoencephalitis have also caused morbidity and mortality in young okapi.[3, 7, 10, 12, 16, 18, 20] Calves born subsequent to dystocia have had associated problems such as pneumonia, presumably resulting from inhalation of placental fluids. A 1-month-old calf that died of trauma inflicted by its dam also had subclinical nephritis, and fluorescent antibody staining of the kidney was positive for *Leptospira* species.

MUSCULOSKELETAL DISORDERS

The primary reason for chemical immobilizations of both female and male okapi is for hooftrimming. Free-ranging okapi walk many miles per day on varied terrain, so causes of overgrown hooves are probably related to lack of wear on appropriate substrate and differences in hoof quality between captive and wild okapi. The constant wearing of hooves is limited in a captive environment, particularly where animals are housed indoors during cold weather. Older animals may also move less, leading to hoof overgrowth. Because of reluctance to anesthetize pregnant or lactating females, there may be prolonged intervals between which hoof trimming can be accomplished. Overgrown hooves place excessive strain on flexor tendons and can result in conformation stresses, leading to permanent deformities or arthritis.

Two female okapi that were offspring of mother-son matings had severe posterior locomotor problems manifested as cow-hocks and laxity of flexor tendons. Although not documented, the cause was thought to involve marginal vitamin and mineral nutrition, improper substrate, and inbreeding. One of the females produced normal offspring.

Miscellaneous musculoskeletal disorders that have been seen include greenstick fracture of a metacarpal bone in a 5-month-old animal, valgus rotation of the forelimbs in two animals (one of which was successfully surgically corrected), and fractures of long bones.

DIGESTIVE DISORDERS

Infectious

Rotavirus-like particles have been found via transmission electron microscopy in numerous cases of diarrhea in both adults and neonates.[20] Uncomplicated cases consist of anorexia or clumped to liquid feces for 24 to 48 hours. Rotavirus was the cause of death in one 10-month-old animal.[16] Coronavirus-like particles have been documented in the clumped feces of at least one adult male (rotavirus and coronavirus in nondomestic hoofstock is discussed further in Chapter 89).

Mandibular abscesses caused by *Actinomyces* species and other bacteria are not uncommon and are treated with debridement and antibiotics. *Mycobacterium paratuberculosis* was the cause of death in one animal.[16]

Mechanical

The okapi dental formula is 0/3,0/1,3/3,3/3 (total 32).[4] Abnormal tooth wear, particularly in older animals, leads to difficult or poor mastication with subsequent loss of body condition. Feces from affected animals may contain fibers that are longer and coarser than normal. Floating or filing teeth to remove points and irregular surfaces is usually curative.

Phytobezoars and trichobezoars have been documented at necropsy in several animals. They have been found in the reticulum and in the small intestines, resulting in anorexia, obstructions, colic, and death. If an animal has a tendency to groom excessively or if hair is found in the feces, the animal should be given mineral oil (1 L/day per os) or other gastrointestinal lubricant to enhance passage of hair before formation of bezoars. Occasionally, a trichobezoar has been regurgitated. Uncomplicated constipation caused by other factors is encountered occasionally and is treated similarly.

Death has also resulted from sudden change in diet with subsequent colic, cecal dilatation and torsion, and spiral colon obstruction.[7, 12]

Parasitic

When there were greater numbers of wild caught okapi in the captive population internal parasites were of major significance.[3] Nematodes, trematodes, and cestodes were encountered regularly. In captivity, parasites are no longer a significant cause of morbidity or mortality. Deworming agents used on okapi at standard ruminant doses include ivermectin, mebendazole, fenbendazole, levamisole, and thibendazole.[17]

INFECTIOUS DISEASES

It should be assumed that okapi are susceptible to any infectious diseases that occur in artiodactyla. Bacterial diseases including tuberculosis, salmonellosis, and actinomycosis can affect any system and may cause pneumonia, enteritis, meningitis, septicemia, and other syndromes.[3, 7, 10, 12, 16, 18–20]

Fungal meningitis has been documented in two juvenile okapi in California, and *Aspergillus* pneumonia was found in two calves in Europe.[16] Pox virus was documented in okapi in Europe,[12, 18] but has not been seen clinically recently. Two young okapi died subsequent to contracting the disease, presumably because of the effects of dehydration and inanition.

DERMATOLOGIC CONDITIONS

Hair loss is primarily associated with overgrooming. It can occur with erythema and inflammation or as noninflamed alopecia. Because okapi are fastidious groomers, they lick their coats clean when foreign material is present. This trait can be used to advantage for administering medications, by pouring them on the backs where the animal will lick it off.

PREVENTIVE MEDICAL PROCEDURES

Neonatal examinations of okapi during the first 12 to 48 hours of life is recommended. The calf should receive a physical examination, treatment of umbilicus with iodine, collection of blood for determination of passive transfer of antibodies, complete blood count, and total solids, glucose, and genetic studies. Vitamin E (1.5 to 2 IU/kg) injections are routinely administered at that time. An *E. coli* bacterin (Genecol 99; Schering-Plough) has been used safely if coliform enteritis is a concern. Calves can be vaccinated with that product per os during the first 12 hours of life.

Vaccination of pregnant females with a killed rotacorona viral (ScourGuard 3; SmithKline Beecham) vaccine is recommended in collections in which the organisms has been detected. The dam is vaccinated twice at 3- to 4-week intervals, followed by one vaccination given 4 to 6 weeks prepartum.

Other vaccinations that are administered include tetanus toxoid, polyvalent clostridium, rhinopnuemonitis, and rabies.[17] Parasite prevention and monitoring is recommended on a twice yearly basis, with appropriate treatment as indicated.

CLINICAL PATHOLOGY

In Giraffidae, the only significant difference in serum chemistries and vitamins from Bovidae are low cholesterol and low alpha-tocopherol.[9] Although not necessarily clinically relevant, these low levels may become important if vitamins in the diet are limited.

Urine of adult okapi is alkaline (pH 7.5 to 8.5); however, that of nursing calves is acidic (pH 6.0). The specific gravity ranges from SG 1.006 to 1.025 in normal animals.[4]

RESTRAINT

Complications secondary to anesthesia are the most significant single cause of death for adult okapi.[16]

Standing tranquilization using intramuscular (IM) xylazine (Cervizine, Wildlife Pharmaceuticals) (60 to 225 mg total dose, 1 to 1.3 mg/kg) is useful for procedures such as venipuncture, radiographs, dystocias, and physical examination.[5, 6, 17] Most animals remain standing and may walk slowly around a stall. Stimulation or excessive restraint may result in the animal overriding the effects of the xylazine. Some animals may still kick while tranquilized. Reversal with yohimbine (Antagonil, Wildlife Laboratories)(0.16 mg/kg IM or IV) or tolazoline (Priscoline, Ciba-Geigy Corporation, Greensboro,

NC) (0.49 mg/kg IM or IV) is incomplete. The experimental alpha$_2$-antagonist RX821002 (5 mg total dose for an adult IV) provides the most complete reversal of sedation.[6, 17]

Complete chemical immobilization of okapi is most often achieved using an opiate with or without xylazine. When xylazine is administered approximately 30 minutes before carfentanil (Carfentanil; Wildlife Pharmaceuticals) a dose of 110 to 130 μg/kg IM (total adult dose of 25 to 30 mg) xylazine and 2.7 to 2.9 μg/kg carfentanil (total adult dose of 0.55 to 0.8 mg) has been used. If xylazine and carfentanil are used in the same dart, an average of 65 to 90 μg/kg (15 to 25 mg total adult dose) xylazine and 4 to 6 μg/kg (0.75 to 2.0 mg total adult dose) carfentanil is used.[6] The latter dose may result in faster but "stormier" inductions. For reversal of carfentanil, naltrexone (Naltrexone HCl; Wildlife Pharmaceuticals) is administered IM at a rate of 100 mg naltrexone per 1.0 mg carfentanil used. Time of injection of antagonist to standing is 2 to 3 minutes.

Etorphine hydrochloride (M99; Wildlife Pharmaceuticals) at a rate of 4 to 4.5 mg (total dose) with 48 to 55 mg xylazine (total dose) IM has been used. Regurgitation, regardless of pre-immobilization fasting, has occurred with this regimen. Diprenorphine at a rate of 2 mg diprenorphine per milligram etorphine provides reversal, but renarcotization has been seen when using this antagonist.[6, 17]

Medetomidine (Domitor; Pfizer Animal Health) (60 to 90 μg/kg) IM in combination with ketamine (Ketaset, Ft. Dodge) (1 to 3 mg/kg) IM induces a smooth deep sedation in 10 to 15 minutes. Once the animal becomes recumbent, it should be left undisturbed for a few minutes before approaching it. Animals typically remain sternal, muscles are relaxed, and respirations are regular. Reversal using atipamizole at the rate of 5 mg per milligram of medetomidine results in the animal standing in 5 to 8 minutes (W. Schaftenaar, personal communication, 1995).[22]

Haloperidol (Haldol; McNeil Pharmaceutical) (15 mg) IV has been used in a male, resulting in very mild calming effects seen for 1 to 2 days. It has also been used in a female to allow a calf to nurse. Azaperone (Stressnil, Mallinckrodt Co. (50 mg) IM resulted in mild tranquilization in one female for 1 hour.[6, 17]

MISCELLANEOUS CONDITIONS

Blood transfusions have been successfully performed in okapi.[20] One okapi is reported to have died after ingestion of cherry leaves. In the United States, animals that die at greater than 20 years of age are noted to have geriatric conditions such as nephritis. Umbilical hernias have been successfully repaired surgically in calves.

Acknowledgment

As the veterinary advisor for the okapi SSP, I would like to acknowledge the efforts of all veterinarians who have worked on okapi. They have shared their professional experiences via surveys, informal meetings, proceedings, conversations, and participation in MedARKS and the okapi SSP and EEP, and thus to this chapter and to improved veterinary care of these special animals.

REFERENCES

1. Bennett CL, Lindsey S: Preliminary findings on the behavioural budgeting of two okapi calves during the first six months of life. American Association of Zoological Parks and Aquariums Regional Proceedings, Wheeling, WV, pp 751–758, 1989.
2. Bennett CL, Lindsey S: Some notes on the physiological and behavioural ontogeny of okapi (*Okapia johnstoni*) calves. Zoo Biology 11(6):433–442, 1992.
3. Bernirschke K: General survey of okapi pathology. Acta Zoologica et Pathologica Antverpiensia 71:63–78, 1978.
4. Bodmer RE, Rabb GB: *Okapia johnstoni. In* Mammalian Species No. 422. Mammalian Species 422:1–8, 1992.
5. Calle PP, Raphael BL, Loskutoff NM: Giraffid reproduction. *In* Fowler ME (ed): Zoo and Wild Animal Medicine, Current Therapy 3. Philadelphia, WB Saunders, pp 549–554, 1993.
6. Citino S: Okapi anesthesia data—White Oak Conservation Center/ Epulu data. *In* Lukas J (ed): Okapi Metapopulation Workshop. White Oak Conservation Center, Yulee, FL, 1996.
7. De Bois H, Van Puijenbroeck B: The Stud-book of the okapi: the Inventory and World Management Plan. Zoo Anvers. 56(4):62–65 1991.
8. De Bois H, Vercammen P, Immens P, et al: Evolution of body weight in pregnant okapis (*Okapia johnstoni).* Acta Zoologica et Pathologica Antverpiensia 82:29–34, 1992.
9. Dierenfeld E. Nutrition session data and summary. *In* Lukas J (ed): Okapi Metapopulation Workshop. White Oak Conservation Center, Yulee, FL, 1996.
10. Griner LAL: Pathology of Zoo Animals. San Diego, Zoological Society of San Diego, pp 507–510, 1983.
11. Hart JA, Hart TB: Ranging and feeding behavior of okapi (*Okapia*

johnstoni) in the Ituri forest of Zaire: food limitation in a rain-forest herbivore? Symp Zool Soc London 61:31–50, 1989.
12. Klos HG, Lang EM: Handbook of Zoo Medicine, Diseases and Treatment of Wild Animals in Zoos, Game Parks, Circuses and Private Collections. New York, Van Nostrand Reinhold, pp 247–256, 1982.
13. Lacey RC, Leus K, Petric A, et al: An overview of the genetic status of the captive populations of okapi. *In* Lukas J (ed): Okapi Metapopulation Workshop. White Oak Conservation Center, Yulee, FL, 1996.
14. Lindsey S, Bennett CL, Pritchard JK, Fried JJ: Functional Analysis of infrasound in the okapi (*Okapia johnstoni*): Mother-infant communication. Proceedings of the Annual Conference of the American Association of Zoological Parks and Aquariums, Omaha, NB, pp 299–305, 1993.
15. Lindsey S, Bennett C, Pyle E, et al: Calf management and the collection of physiological data for okapi (*Okapia johnstoni*). Int Zoo Yearbook 33:263–268, 1994.
16. Leus K, Van Puijenbroeck B: Okapi (*Okapi johnstoni*) International Studbook. Antwerp, Belgium, Royal Zoological Society of Antwerp, 1995.
17. MedARKS Library Reference Disc. Okapi Anesthesia Data, 1995.
18. Pilaski J, Rosen A, Darai G: Comparative analysis of the genomes of orthopoxviruses isolated from elephant (*Elaphas maximus*), rhinoceros (*Ceratotherium simum*), and okapi (*Okapi johnstoni*) by restriction enzymes. Arch Virol 88:135–142, 1986.
19. Raphael BL, Sneed L, Ott-Joslin J: Rotavirus-like infection associated with diarrhea in okapi. J Am Vet Med Assoc 189(9):1183–1184, 1986.
20. Raphael BL: Neonatal illness characterized by dermatitis, hyperthermia and anemia in an okapi. Acta Zoologica et Pathologica Antverpiensia 80:43–52, 1988.
21. Schwarzenberger F, Patzl M, Francke R, et al: Fecal progestagen evaluations to monitor the estrous cycle and pregnancy in the okapi (*Okapia johnstoni*). Zoo Biol 12:549–559, 1993.

CHAPTER **99**

Mycobacterium bovis Infection of Cervids: Diagnosis, Treatment, and Control

ROBERT A. COOK

The first evidence of the existence of *Mycobacteria* species was documented in the bones of Neolithic humans dating from approximately 8000 years ago.[52] The mammalian tubercle bacilli *Mycobacterium bovis* can cause disease in a great many mammals.[49] The family Cervidae is comprised of 17 genera and 38 species, which inhabit North America, South America, Eurasia, many associated continental islands, and northern Africa. In addition, wild populations of deer have been introduced into regions where the family did not natu-

rally occur.[37] Many species of cervid are maintained in zoological parks and many are listed in the International Union for the Conservation of Nature, Red List of Threatened Animals as endangered. All members of the Cervidae family are susceptible to mycobacterial infection and therefore great vigilance should be exercised in preventing the outbreak of this potentially life-threatening disease. The insidious nature of the organism, the difficulties confronted in diagnosis, treatment, and prevention, and the zoonotic characteristics of the infection make disease caused by infection with *M. bovis* of major concern to the zoo and wildlife health community.[6]

ETIOLOGY

The tuberculosis complex is comprised of four species: *Mycobacterium tuberculosis, M. bovis, Mycobacterium africanum,* and *Mycobacterium microti.* Typically, these organisms are slow growing and may not appear on Löwenstein-Jensen culture media for up to 8 weeks.[47] Microscopically, the organism appears as a slender rod, 0.2 to 0.6 μm in diameter and 1.5 to 3 μm in length. Forms on culture may vary from coccoid to filamentous. The Ziehl-Neelsen or the Kinyoun staining techniques with carbol fuchsin are the most commonly used methods for demonstrating the acid-fast nature of the organisms. Typically, mycobacteria grow aerobically at 37°C. The addition of sodium pyruvate to media enhances the growth of *M. bovis.* In recent years, DNA species-specific probes have been shown to provide a more rapid method of speciation versus the standard biochemical differentiation testing.

INCIDENCE OF *M. BOVIS* IN FARMED, ZOO, AND FREE-RANGING CERVIDS

Tuberculosis has been documented to occur in a number of species of Cervidae, including white tail deer (*Odocoileus virginianus*), fallow deer (*Dama dama*), roe (*Capreolus capreolus*), axis deer (*axis*), sika deer (*Cervus nippon*), and red deer (*Cervus elaphus*), also referred to as the wapiti or elk.[5] In the United States in 1969, a zoo collection was exposed to *M. bovis* via an infected herd of axis deer.[13] In 1974, an outbreak of *M. bovis* infection occurred in a herd of 130 sika and fallow deer in southern California.[23] In 1981, there was a major outbreak in Cervidae involving a cluster of farmed herds in South Dakota. The cervids were believed to have transferred the *M. bovis* infection to bison (*Bison bison*).[10] Infected bison were traced to 25 states. In 1984, 24 infected bison herds were discovered in 10 states, seven of which were accredited tuberculosis-free states. The source of this outbreak was believed to be bison exposed to *M. bovis*-infected farmed elk. The elk had been purchased by a rancher from a small managerie/farm in Iowa. These cervid-associated outbreaks were not believed to significantly impact the United States livestock industry until 1991 when bovine tuberculosis was confirmed in a United States captive elk herd epidemiologically linked with an infected Canadian elk herd.[10] This prompted the closing of the Canadian border to llamas (*Lama glama*) and cervids from the United States, which negatively impacted both of these budding livestock industries. In 1992, an episode was reported in a captive elk herd in Colorado[35] and in a captive herd of sika deer in Illinois.[36]

Worldwide, bovine tuberculosis in Cervidae has been reported from multiple sites, including free-ranging deer in Ireland[9] and Taiwan,[58] in captive axis deer in India,[45] in fallow deer in Australia,[42] and in sika deer in Japan.[22] The widespread occurrence of tuberculosis in cattle and farm-raised deer in New Zealand led to the creation of the BTB test.[16] The wild possum (*Tichosurus vulpecula*) is the source of the disease spread into the New Zealand hoofstock.[31]

There is great concern that *M. bovis* will become active in free-ranging deer in the United States. In 1995, it was reported in free-ranging mule deer (*Odocoileus hemionus*) in Montana[39]; however, a 3-year survey for bovine tuberculosis in hunter-killed free-ranging elk in northwestern Wyoming revealed no acid-fast bacteria on microscopic evaluation of representative lymph nodes.[57]

DIAGNOSTIC TESTS AND PATHOLOGIC EXAMINATION

There is no 100% reliable antemortem test for the detection of *M. bovis* infection in Cervidae. The most definitive diagnostic test available is the growth of *M. bovis* organisms on mycobacterial culture media. However, in the living animal, it is oftentimes difficult to acquire the appropriate specimens for culture. Even in cases of known acid-fast positive postmortem tissues, the organism has failed to grow in appropriate media under optimal conditions. The most appropriate strategy, therefore, is to develop a battery of diagnostic tests which together with the clinical herd history can provide an indication of the mycobacterial status of the group.

Diagnostic Tests

Appropriate pretreatment tests for tuberculosis include cell-mediated immunologic tests and serologic tests. Proper interpretation of these diagnostic tests can be confused by infection with related mycobacteria such as those of the *M. avium* complex.[1, 27, 46]

CELL-MEDIATED IMMUNOLOGIC TESTS

The intradermal tuberculin test is the standard test for the detection of tuberculosis in hoofstock greater than 6 months of age. It relies on the intradermal injection of mycobacterial antigens. Two to 3 days following injection of a previously exposed animal, a characteristic inflammatory response usually occurs that includes erythema, swelling, and induration at the site.[30] Two types of tuberculin preparations are in use. Old tuberculin (OT) is made from concentrated heat-sterilized culture filtrates of mycobacteria.[26] OT is a crude preparation and may produce more nonspecific inflammatory responses.[2] The second type of tuberculin is purified protein derivative (PPD) prepared as the protein precipitant fraction of OT from cultures of *M. bovis* (bovine PPD) and *M. avium* (avian PPD).[55]

The immune response to the intradermal tuberculin test depends on the prior antigen exposure followed by lymphocyte differentiation; therefore, there is a varying length of time after infection when the immune response cannot be detected. As the *M. bovis* infection grows, so too does the antigenic stimulation, resulting in an increased intensity of response. In addition to lack of antigenic stimulation, there are a number of other causes of poor immune responses. Differential gene expression during the course of infection might affect which antigens are recognized by the immune system.[59] Biological variability, possibly genetically based, may lead to differences in the antigens that are recognized by different classes, species, or breeds of animals.[38] Other pathophysiological processes that alter immune function, such as viral infections of lymphoid tissues, environmental toxins specific for lymphocytes, stress, and immune-modulating therapy, can also alter response to the test. Anergy is sometimes observed in mycobacteria infected hosts which lose responsiveness to a particular antigen. False-negative tuberculin tests can also be the result of a loss of product activity because of improper storage, handling, contamination, or operator errors in administration.

Nonspecific or cross-reactive false-positive responses may result from previous immune stimulation by non–*M. bovis* mycobacterial antigens or from cross-reaction from antigens that nonmycobacterial organisms such as *Nocardia* species may have in common with *M. bovis*.

Single Cervical Tuberculin Test

The single cervical tuberculin test (SCT) is an intradermal skin test of the caudal tail fold that was developed for domestic cattle as a method for monitoring the incidence of *M. bovis* in herds of unknown status.[55] The caudal tail fold proved to be a less sensitive site for response to tuberculin in cervids and the cervical neck region was selected as the optimal site. The SCT is the official U.S. Department of Agriculture (USDA) tuberculin test for routine use in individual cervids, and herds of cervids where the tuberculosis status is unknown. A study of the SCT in Tasmanian fallow deer demonstrated that, with a reactor response set at 1 mm or more, 25 of 34 deer tested did not react to the skin test, giving a specificity of 73.5%. With the reactor response set at 2 mm or greater, the specificity of the test was 100%.[32] It is administered by the intradermal injection of 0.1 ml (5000 tuberculin units) of USDA PPD bovis tuberculin in the midcervical region. The test is read by visual observation and palpation in 72 hours (plus or minus 6 hours) following injection. In the United States, the test is only legally administered by a state, federal, or designated accredited veterinarian.

Comparative Cervical Tuberculin Test

In the United States, the comparative cervical tuberculin test (CCT) is administered by the intradermal injection of biologically balanced bovine PPD and avian PPD tuberculin at separate sites in the midcervical area to determine the probable presence of bovine tuberculosis, by comparing the response of the two tuberculins 72 hours (plus or minus 6 hours) following injection. This test is administered only by an approved state or federal veterinarian.[54] All responses are measured to the nearest 0.5 mm and interpreted as follows:

- Animals having a response to bovine PPD of less than 1 mm are classified negative.
- Animals whose response to bovine PPD is 1 mm through 2 mm and whose response is equal to or greater than the response to the avian PPD are classified as suspects.
- Animals whose response to bovine PPD is greater than 2 mm but equal to the response to avian PPD are classified as suspects, except when the testing veterinarian judges the animal to be a reactor.
- Animals meeting the criteria for suspect classification on two successive CCTs are classified as reactors.
- Animals having a response to bovine PPD that is greater than 2 mm and at least 0.5 mm greater than the avian PPD response are classified as reactors.

The CCT was evaluated in cervids naturally exposed to mycobacteria and the test exhibited a high degree of sensitivity (84%) and specificity (80%) in detecting infected animals but a low level of accuracy (57%) in differentiating *M. bovis* infections from infections caused by *M. avium* and other Runyon groups III and IV mycobacteria.[24]

IN VITRO IMMUNODIAGNOSTIC ASSAYS

M. bovis infection induces a humoral immune response; however, there can be a markedly prolonged latent period during which no antibody response is detected. The antibody response is proportional to the antigenic load circulating in the animal. Often, the granulomatous nature of the infection may hide a significant antigenic load until the organism breaks out of the sequestered lesion. Therefore, tests that measure antibody response cannot replace tests that detect cell-mediated immunity but rather should be performed as complementary diagnostic assays.

Lymphocyte Transformation Test

The lymphocyte transformation test (LT) has also been referred to as the lymphocyte blastogenic test or lymphocyte stimulation test. It is performed on a heparinized blood sample from which lymphocytes are separated via differential centrifugation. This mononuclear cell fraction is challenged with antigens and incubated for 3 to 5 days, at which time the cultures are pulsed with a radioisotope-labeled nucleotide.[29] Following further incubation, the cells are harvested and the incorporation of the radioisotope is measured. Elevated incorporation of the marker indicates blastogenesis. Cells that have been previously challenged with antigen in the host begin proliferating in response to the presence of the antigen. In one study of 433 blood samples collected from elk in *M. bovis*-infected herds, it was shown that using a comparative LT of *M. bovis* PPD and *M. paratuberculosis* PPD yielded a sensitivity of 76% with confidence limits of 63% to 85% and specificity of 77% with confidence limits of 72% to 81%.

This study also indicated that the LT identified different elk than did other *M. bovis* isolation tests.[21]

Enzyme-Linked Immunosorbent Assay (ELISA)

Enzyme-linked immunosorbent assay (ELISA) is a primary binding test that can be used to detect and quantitate either antibody or antigen. The label-antigen ELISA is most commonly used in mycobacterial testing. The mycobacterial antigen is bound to the plate before testing. The antibody to be tested is added, followed, after washing, by labeled antigen. The antibody binds to the labeled antigen on the plate and further procedures indicate the degree of antibody binding. The ELISA has been used as a supplemental test for the detection of antimycobacterial antibodies in sera from certain exotic species exposed to clinically significant mycobacteria.[50, 51] The use of purified antigen preparations extracted from virulent mycobacterial strains using deoxycholate or potassium chloride provides improved specificity.[48]

A five-antigen ELISA was tested on 12 cervid herds, five of which were thought to be infected. The specificity was 78.6% and the sensitivity was 70.0%. The results suggested that the five-antigen ELISA would not be a good test for tuberculosis if used alone. However, when results of the ELISA and tuberculin skin test were interpreted in parallel, sensitivity of the combination was greater than sensitivity of either test alone.[15] The ELISA has become an important component of the blood tuberculosis test (BTB).

Blood Tuberculosis Test

The BTB was developed as an ancillary test to clarify the status of skin test–positive deer, with nonspecific sensitization following exposure to saprophytic mycobacteria.[8, 19, 53] It is a series of assays which includes measurement of the relative levels of LT of deer mononuclear cells cultured with avian or bovine tuberculin (PPD). In addition, an ELISA was developed that measures antibody specific for mycobacterial antigens. This assay has been shown to be of special value in the identification of false skin test reactors harboring tuberculosis.[18] Another set of components are the soluble inflammatory proteins. These are used as markers of disease, and both plasma viscosity and haptoglobin have a high predictive value in identifying animals with proliferative tuberculosis. The results of the LT, ELISA, and soluble inflammatory protein assays are combined to produce the BTB. It is expressed as a diagnostic radial plot that can identify nondiseased, diseased, and immune deer. The composite BTB has a sensitivity of greater than 95% and a specificity of greater than 98% for diagnosis of *M. bovis* in Cervidae.[17, 19] The methodology, originally developed in New Zealand, has been acquired for use in the United States.

Gamma Interferon Assay

When lymphocytes respond to antigen, they produce a number of intercellular messenger molecules termed lymphokines, in addition to going through transforma-

tion. The detection of specific messenger lymphokines may help differentiate nonspecific lymphocyte transformation from antigen-specific stimulation and may therefore yield a more accurate in vitro assessment of the cell-mediated immune response.[29] A sandwich ELISA gamma interferon test was developed in Australia for the detection of bovine tuberculosis in cattle. This method uses monoclonal antibodies in a sandwich ELISA to detect the release of gamma interferon as a response to PPD stimulation in a whole-blood culture.[44] The lymphocytes must remain viable and functional to properly release the lymphokines on stimulation; therefore, it is important that the blood sample be handled gently and be quickly brought to the laboratory for analysis.[29] This test is specific for bovine gamma interferon and has not been proven to detect deer gamma interferon.[44]

Ag85 Dot Blot Immunoassay

Antigen 85 (Ag85) complex proteins are major secretory products of actively proliferating mycobacteria in vitro. These fibronectin-binding proteins have been detected in serum from human patients with active tuberculosis, suggesting that the presence of circulating Ag85 proteins may correlate with active mycobacterial infection. Diluted serum samples and Ag85 standards are blotted to nitrocellulose. Ag85 is detected by dot immunobinding using mouse monoclonal anti-*M. bovis* Ag85. Blots are developed using horseradish peroxidase-conjugated goat antimouse immunoglobulin and luminescent substrate. Luminescence is detected by standard x-ray film. Ag85 levels in serum are assessed by comparison with purified *M. bovis* Ag85 standards. The dot blot immunobinding assay detects mycobacterial antigens, not antibodies produced in response to these antigens, and therefore is not dependent on the immunocompetency of the host.[34] The test is relatively new and is as yet unproven. It appears to offer the potential of early, rapid, antemortem diagnosis of *M. bovis* infection in nondomestic animal species.

MAKING THE DIAGNOSIS

At preshipment, there is often a need to look at the *M. bovis* status of individuals rather than a herd. An animal that responds to the SCT must undergo further diagnostic tests to best assess its tuberculosis status. Suspects on the SCT may be retested by either the CCT or the BTB. The CCT may be applied within 10 days following the SCT injection or after 90 days. If the CCT is applied within 10 days of the SCT, the opposite side of the neck must be used. The sample for the BTB is obtained after 12 days and optimally before 30 days after the SCT injection. An animal that is positive to either the CCT or BTB is classified as a reactor. A suspect to the SCT may be necropsied in lieu of retesting by supplemental tests and, if there is no evidence of *M. bovis* infection by culture or histopathologic study (including study of selected specimens submitted from animals having no gross lesions indicative of tuberculosis), the animal is thought to be negative for tuberculosis.[54]

Pathology and Herd History

Identification, medical, and necropsy records must be maintained on all animals within the herd. In order to establish a verifiable herd history, all individuals that die, for whatever reason, should be thoroughly evaluated via a complete postmortem examination. Postmortem inspection, histopathologic study, and culture are all necessary components in verifying bovine tuberculosis in cervids. In one study of a captive herd of wapiti infected with bovine tuberculosis, it was found that the lungs and retropharyngeal lymph nodes were the most frequently affected sites.[41] An abattoir study of tuberculosis in a herd of farmed elk found that lesions were predominantly suppurative rather than caseous and mineralization was less evident than in tuberculosis lesions in cattle. The lesions occurred predominantly in lymph nodes and lungs.[56] A study of gross pathology in elk found that, in the 73 animals examined, gross lesions were most often found in the lung (48 animals), retropharyngeal lymph nodes (36 animals), mesenteric lymph nodes (35 animals), and mediastinal lymph nodes (16 animals).[43]

A comparative histopathologic study of a number of cervid species noted that elk usually had scattered peripheral mineralization rather than central mineralization and lesions contained more neutrophils and fewer giant cells than did bovine lesions. Fallow deer lesions contained more giant cells but were otherwise indistinguishable from elk lesions. Sika deer lesions had more giant cells and fewer neutrophils than did lesions from cattle or other cervid species, and sika deer giant cells were larger and contained more nuclei than did giant cells in the other species.[40]

THERAPEUTICS

There are three situations in which treatment of an individual or a herd of cervids might be contemplated:

1. A positive animal is confirmed on necropsy and the contact group is negative on all immunodiagnostic assays including the SCT.
2. A positive animal is confirmed on necropsy and the contact group is positive on one or a number of immunodiagnostic tests.
3. An individual or group of individuals within a herd are found to be positive on one or a number of immunodiagnostic tests including the SCT and CCT but no animals have been confirmed at necropsy or via culture.

The decision to give treatment to a reactor individual or herd, or to treat a confirmed *M. bovis* infection in a herd should be based on the following:

- An evaluation of the severity of disease in affected individuals. Overwhelming infection increases the risk of spread to other populations within the facilities and to personnel.
- The ability to isolate the affected individual or herd.
- The ability to treat the individual or herd.

- The ability to follow a prolonged course of treatment.
- The value of the animal to its species.
- If an organism is isolated, its specific sensitivity to the antimycobacterial drugs.
- The ability to protect humans who must work with the affected animals.
- The ability to achieve and maintain therapeutic levels of the desired antimycobacterial drugs.

In the United States, all cervid herds in which reactor animals have been identified are quarantined. Cervid herds in which *M. bovis* is confirmed must remain under quarantine, if not depopulated, and must pass three consecutive whole-herd SCTs. The BTB may be used, if it is used simultaneously with a whole-herd SCT. The effects of quarantine and restricted movement of animals must be considered before lengthy treatment is undertaken. The ability of some of the antimycobacterial drugs to clear the rumen and achieve therapeutic circulating levels must be verified via pharmacokinetic trials of the animals in question.

Chemotherapy has been successful in selected exotic hoofstock when multiple drug therapy was used for 9 to 12 months.[4, 14] The traditional three-drug regimen has included isoniazid, rifampin, and ethambutol. However, if possible, the choice of drug therapy should be based on the sensitivities of the mycobacterial isolate.

VACCINATION

The live attenuated strain of *M. bovis*—bacillus Calmette-Guérin (BCG)—has been used as a vaccine against *M. tuberculosis* and *Mycobacterium leprae* in children. The efficacy of the vaccine has been questioned both because of its reported failure to protect some human populations and because it precipitates a delayed type hypersensitivity response to intradermal skin test challenges. This negates the use of the intradermal skin test as a screening method for tuberculosis infection in the vaccinated population. In known noninfected deer, the BCG vaccine administered in an oil adjuvant induced strong LT and ELISA responses.[20] A Russian study of BCG vaccine in farmed marals (*Cervus elaphus maral*) demonstrated protection from infection for 6 months after two 20-mg doses were given at 2-month intervals.[33]

The use of BCG vaccination to prevent *M. bovis* infection does not appear to provide a lasting or predictable protection. Its use would also confound required testing for the interstate movement of cervids within the United States. It is therefore not recommended. However, with the re-emergence of tuberculosis as a worldwide disease of concern for both animals and humans, there has occurred a renewed interest in the development of efficacious vaccines. The ability to isolate specific petides, such as Ag85, may at some point yield mycobacterial specific immunoprotection from infection.[25]

REGULATORY CONTROL MEASURES IN THE UNITED STATES

On May 15, 1994, the USDA Animal and Plant Health Inspection Service finalized the Uniform Methods and Rules for Tuberculosis Eradication in Cervidae.[54] It outlines the minimum requirements to control and eradicate tuberculosis in farm- or ranch-raised cervids (deer, elk, and moose). These minimum standards do not and have not precluded the adoption of more stringent standards by state regulatory agencies. The rules include testing criteria, interstate or movement requirements, identification of reactors, quarantine procedures, disposition of responders, methods of achieving tuberculosis-free herd status, and disinfection procedures.

Cervids maintained in American Zoo and Aquarium Association (AZA) accredited facilities are exempt from the federal requirements when moving between accredited member facilities. Any other movement from AZA accredited member facilities must comply with all federal requirements. State and federal regulations are subject to change. Regulatory officials should always be consulted for the most recent information.

ZOONOTIC IMPLICATIONS

The World Health Organization estimates that worldwide cases of tuberculosis in humans will reach 11.9 million in the year 2005, an increase of 57.6% from 1995.[11] In addition, the prevalence of multidrug-resistant tuberculosis is increasing globally.[7] Furthermore, there is a growing number of humans with human immunodeficiency virus who may become immunocompromised. All these factors considered, it is important to protect humans who come in contact with cervids with indications of mycobacterial disease.

An outbreak of *M. bovis* in domesticated elk in Alberta, Canada, exposed more than 446 humans to the disease. Eighty-one people had positive skin tests, with one case of active *M. bovis* infection diagnosed via sputum culture.[12] Two herds of deer and elk were depopulated at a slaughter facility in Ontario, where 104 workers were exposed and 17 people had positive skin tests.[28]

DISEASE CONTROL MEASURES

Disinfection

When an *M. bovis* case is suspected, the facility should be thoroughly cleaned and decontaminated using a 2% cresylic compound or a derivative of phenol such as sodium orthophenylphenate. When possible, the premises should be disinfected twice, at 14- to 21-day intervals, before it is repopulated.[52] When the substrate is natural, the challenges of disinfection are much greater. A pH greater than 9 inhibits most bacteria. Lime (CaO) soaked in water produces $Ca(OH)_2$ calcium hydroxide and can be used to disinfect large natural areas under the guidance of a federal veterinarian.

Sanitation and Hygiene

All workers must be advised of the risks of working with animals suspected of or determined to be infected with *M. bovis*. Eating, smoking, or otherwise performing activities that can increase the potential for human contamination should be restricted. Depending on the level of risk, coveralls or disposable overgarments should be worn, such that all materials can be shed and properly disinfected following the procedure. Proper respiratory protection should be worn at all times in the form of an approved reusable respirator or approved disposable type N95 particulate respirator. The disposable mask type respirators, which are necessarily tight, are more comfortable for extended wear when personnel must clean facilities or handle animals on a repeated basis. Before using respirator masks, the personnel must be trained by the employer in proper respirator use. OSHA standard 29 CFR 1910.134(e)(5) requires that the wearer be fit tested, usually via the saccharin qualitative fit test. Waterproof, nonporous gloves and footwear, either disposable or reusable, should be worn at all times. Reusable gloves and footwear must be completely disinfected in an approved solution following each use.

Testing Staff

Methods of evaluating staff for exposure to mycobacterial infection should be performed for the health of the employee, to protect the animals that the employee may contact, and to act as a means of surveillance for the animal collection. At a zoo, it is advisable to consult with an infectious disease or disease control physician to evaluate potential exposure and outline methods for human evaluation. A Mantoux test[3] (intracutaneous administration of 5 units of PPD tuberculin) should be considered as part of a pre-employment or new employee examination. Thereafter, yearly Mantoux intradermal skin testing is recommended. When personnel have a history of BCG vaccination, then the intradermal skin test is invalid and those individuals should be evaluated via a chest radiograph. Following an outbreak of *M. bovis* infection, all contact employees should be evaluated via a Mantoux intradermal skin test as soon as possible and again 3 months following resolution and decontamination of the facility.

REFERENCES

1. Arora BM: A case of avian tuberculosis in spotted deer. World Animal Review 77(4):53–55, 1993.
2. Benoit CA, Beschin M, Desmecht P, et al: Delayed hypersensitivity reactions by the mycobacterial antigen A60 and cutaneous testing in tuberculosis. Med Microbiol Immunol 178:105–112, 1989.
3. Bloch AB: Screening for tuberculosis and tuberculosis infection in high-risk populations. Recommendations of the Advisory Council for the Elimination of Tuberculosis. MMWR Morb Mortal Wkly Rep 44(RR-11):18–34, 1995.
4. Bush M, Montali RJ, Phillips LG, et al: Bovine tuberculosis in a bactrian camel herd: clinical, therapeutic, and pathologic findings. J Zoo Wildl Med 21:171–179, 1990.
5. Cook RA: Tuberculosis in cervidae. An Informational Guide for Veterinarians of AAZPA Accredited Zoos. American Association of Zoo Veterinarians Infectious Disease Reviews, 1992.

6. Cook RA: Review and update on USDA cervid TB regulations and their effects on AAZPA accredited zoos. Proceedings of the Annual Meeting of the American Association of Zoo Veterinarians, St. Louis, pp 232–235, 1993.

7. Dey AB, Nagarkar K: Multi drug resistant tuberculosis. Trop Gastroenterol 16(2):92–100, 1995.

8. Diagnosis of TB by Blood Testing. Dunedin North, New Zealand, The Deer Research Laboratory, 1992.

9. Dodd K: Tuberculosis in free-living deer. Vet Rec 115(23):592–593, 1984.

10. Essey M: Status of the state-federal bovine tuberculosis eradication program; FY 1991. Proceedings of the 95th Annual Meeting of the U.S. Animal Health Association, Reno, NV, pp 515–525, 1995.

11. Exner-Freisfeld H: Reappearance of tuberculosis, risks and consequences. Gesundheitswesen 57(12):798–805, 1995.

12. Fanning A, Edwards S: *Mycobacterium bovis* infection in human beings in contact with elk (*Cervus elaphus)* in Alberta, Canada. Lancet 338(8777):1253–1255, 1991.

13. Fowler ME: Clinical experiences with tuberculosis in zoo hoofed stock. *In* Montali RJ (ed): Mycobacterial Infections of Zoo Animals. Washington, DC, Smithsonian Institution Press, pp 179–184, 1978.

14. Fowler ME: Treating giraffes with isoniazid. *In* Montali RJ (ed): Mycobacterial Infections of Zoo Animals. Washington, DC, Smithsonian Institution Press, pp 185–188, 1978.

15. Gaborick CM, Salman MD, Ellis RP, et al: Evaluation of a five-antigen ELISA for diagnosis of tuberculosis in cattle and cervidae. J Am Vet Med Assoc 209(5):962–966, 1996.

16. Griffin JFT: Tuberculosis, its diagnosis, management, and control within New Zealand deer herds. *In* Proceedings of the 14th Annual Meeting of the New Zealand Deer Farmers Association, Invercargill, New Zealand, 1989.

17. Griffin JFT, Buchan GS: Aetiology, pathogenesis and diagnosis of *Mycobacterium bovis* in deer. Vet Microbiol 40(1–2):193–205, 1994.

18. Griffin JFT, Cross JP, Buchan GS: Laboratory assays for the diagnosis of tuberculosis in farmed red deer (*Cervus elaphus*). *In* The Biology of Deer. Proceedings of the International Symposium on the Biology of Deer, Mississippi State University, MS. New York, Springer-Verlag, pp 130–135, 1992.

19. Griffin JFT, Cross JP, Chinn DN, et al: Diagnosis of tuberculosis due to *Mycobacterium bovis* in New Zealand red deer (*Cervus elaphus*) using a composite blood test and antibody assays. N Z Vet J 42(5):173–179, 1994.

20. Griffin JF, Hesketh JB, Mackintosh CG, et al: BCG vaccination in deer: distinctions between delayed type hypersensitivity and laboratory parameters of immunity. Immunol Cell Biol 71(Pt 6):559–770, 1993.

21. Hutchings DL, Wilson SH: Evaluation of lymphocyte stimulation tests for diagnosis of bovine tuberculosis in elk (*Cervus elaphus*). Am J Vet Res 56(1):27–33, 1995.

22. Itoh R, Kagabu Y, Itoh F: *Mycobacterium bovis* infection in a herd of Japanese shika deer (*Cervus nippon*). J Vet Med Sci 54(4):803–804, 1992.

23. Kollias GV: Clinical and pathological features of mycobacterial infections in sika and fallow deer. *In* Montali RJ (ed): Mycobacterial Diseases of Zoo Animals. Washington, DC, Smithsonian Institution Press, pp 173–177, 1978.

24. Kollias GV, Thoen CO, Fowler ME: Evaluation of comparative cervical tuberculin skin testing in cervids naturally exposed to mycobacteria. J Am Vet Med Assoc 181(11):1257–1262, 1982.

25. Leo SC, Lopes JD, Patarroyo ME: Immunological and functional characterization of proteins of the *Mycobacterium tuberculosis* antigen 85 complex using synthetic peptides. J Gen Microbiol Vol 139(Pt 7):1543–1549, 1993.

26. Lepper AWD, Corner LA: Naturally occurring mycobacterioses of animals. *In* Ratledge C, Stanford J (eds): The Biology of the Mycobacteria, Vol 2, Immunological and Environmental Aspects. London, Academic Press, pp 417–521, 1983.

27. Lisle GW de, Joyce MA, Yates GF, et al: Mycobacterium avium infection in a farmed deer herd. N Z Vet J 43(1):1–3, 1995.

28. Liss GM, Wong L, Kittle DC, et al: Occupational exposure to *Mycobacterium bovis* infection in deer and elk in Ontario. Can J Public Health 85(5):326–9, 1994.

29. Livestock Disease Eradication. Evaluation of the Cooperative State–Federal Bovine Tuberculosis Eradication Program. National Research Council. Washington, DC, National Academy Press, p 31, 1994.

30. Livestock Disease Eradication. Evaluation of the Cooperative State–Federal Bovine Tuberculosis Eradication Program. National Research Council. Washington, DC, National Academy Press, pp 22–23, 1994.

31. Livingstone PG: Tuberculosis in New Zealand—current status and control policies. Surveillance (Wellington) 19(1):14–18, 1992.

32. Lloyd-Webb EC, Campbell PH, Witt DJ: The specificity of the single cervical intradermal tuberculosis test in a population of Tasmanian fallow deer putatively free of bovine tuberculosis. Prev Vet Med 21(4):347–353, 1995.

33. Lunitsyn VG, Guslavskii II, Ognev SI, et al: BCG vaccine to control tuberculosis among farmed marals (*Cervus elaphus maral*). Veterinariya (Moskva) 9:31–33, 1990.

34. Mangold JM, Raphael BL, Cook RA, et al: Detection of circulating mycobacterial antigens. *In Mycobacterium paratuberculosis*-infected nondomestic ruminants. Proceedings of the Joint Conference of the American Association of Zoo Veterinarians, Wildlife Disease Association, and the American Association of Wildlife Veterinarians, East Lansing, MI, pp 132–134, 1995.

35. Miller MW, Seidel JW, Malmsbury TL: Depopulating a bovine tuberculosis-infected captive elk herd in Colorado: logistics and public relations. Proceedings of the Annual Meeting of the American Association of Zoo Veterinarians, Oakland, CA, p 94, 1992.

36. Mirsky ML, Morton D, Piehl JW, et al: *Mycobacterium bovis* infection in a captive herd of sika deer. J Am Vet Med Assoc 200(10):1540–1542, 1992.

37. Nowak RM, Paradiso JL: Walker's Mammals of the World, 4th ed. Baltimore, The Johns Hopkins University Press, pp 1198–1199, 1983.

38. Pritchard DG: A century of bovine tuberculosis 1888–1988: conquest and controversy. J Comp Pathol 99:357–399, 1988.

39. Rhyan JC, Aune K, Hood B, et al: Bovine tuberculosis in a free-ranging mule deer (*Odocoileus hemionus*) from Montana. J Wildl Dis 31(3):432–435, 1995.

40. Rhyan JC, Saari DA: A comparative study of the histopathologic features of bovine tuberculosis in cattle, fallow deer (*Dama dama*), sika deer (*Cervus nippon*), red deer and elk (*Cervus elaphus*). Vet Pathol 32(3):215–220, 1995.

41. Rhyan JC, Saari DA, Williams ES, et al: Gross and microscopic lesions of naturally occurring tuberculosis in a captive herd of wapiti (*Cervus elaphus nelsoni*) in Colorado. J Vet Diagn Invest 4(4):428–433, 1992.

42. Robinson RC, Phillips PH, Stevens G, et al: An outbreak of *Mycobacterium bovis* infection in fallow deer (*Dama dama*). Aust Vet J 66(7):195–197, 1989.

43. Rohonczy EB, Balachandran AV, Dukes TW, et al: A comparison of gross pathology, histopathology, and mycobacterial culture for the diagnosis of tuberculosis in elk (*Cervus elaphus*). Can J Vet Res 60(2):108–114, 1996.

44. Rothel JS, Jones SL, Corner LA, et al: A sandwich enzyme immunoassay for bovine interferon-gamma and its use for the detection of tuberculosis in cattle. Aust Vet J 67(4):134–137, 1990.

45. Shah NM, Lalita Kaul, Chandel BS, et al: A note on tuberculosis in captive spotted deer (*Axis axis*). Indian Vet J 69(10):965–966, 1992.

46. Shiau JR, Lee SH, Yang YH, et al: Evaluation of comparative tuberculin skin test and isolation of mycobacteria in deer naturally exposed to mycobacteria in Taiwan. J Chin Soc Vet Sci 14(2):121–126, 1988.

47. Thoen CO: Mycobacterium. *In* Carter GR, Cole JR (eds): Diagnostic Procedures in Veterinary Bacteriology and Mycology. San Diego, Academic Press, pp 287–298, 1990.

48. Thoen CO: Tuberculosis and other mycobacterial diseases in captive wild animals. *In* Fowler ME (ed): Zoo and Wild Animal Medicine, Current Therapy 3. Philadelphia, WB Saunders, pp 45–49, 1993.

49. Thoen CO, Karlson AG, Grimes EM: *Mycobacterium tuberculosis* complex. *In* Kubica GP, Wayne LG (eds): The Mycobacteria, A Sourcebook. New York, Marcel Dekker, pp 1209–1235, 1984.

50. Thoen CO, Mills K, Hopkins MP: Enzyme-linked protein A: an enzyme-linked immunosorbent assay reagent for detecting antibodies in tuberculous exotic animals. Am J Vet Res 40:833–835, 1980.

51. Thoen CO, Temple RMS, Johnson LW: An evaluation of certain diagnostic tests for detecting some immune responses in llamas exposed to *Mycobacterium bovis*. Proceedings of the 92nd Annual Meeting of the U.S. Animal Health Association, Little Rock, AR, p 524, 1988.

52. Thoen CO, Williams DE: Tuberculosis, tuberculoidoses, and other mycobacterial infections. *In* Beran GW (ed): Handbook of Zoonoses, 2nd ed. Boca Raton, FL, CRC Press, pp 41–59, 1994.

53. Tuberculin Testing of Deer. Animal Health Division, Ministry of Agriculture and Fisheries, Wellington, New Zealand, undated.
54. U.S. Department of Agriculture. Tuberculosis eradication in cervidae. Uniform Methods and Rules Effective May 15, 1994. [Animal and Plant Health Inspection Service 91-45-001]. Washington, DC, U.S. Department of Agriculture, 1994.
55. U.S. Department of Agriculture. Bovine Tuberculosis Eradication. Uniform Methods and Rules. Effective January 4, 1982. Washington, DC, U.S. Department of Agriculture, 1982.
56. Whiting TL, Tessaro SV: An abattoir study of tuberculosis in a herd of farmed elk. Can Vet J 35(8):497–501, 1994.
57. Williams ES, Smith SG, Meyer RM, et al: Three-year survey for bovine tuberculosis in hunter-killed free-ranging elk (*Cervus elaphus nelsoni*) in northwestern Wyoming. Proceedings of the 92nd Annual Meeting of the U.S. Animal Health Association, Reno, NV, pp 631–637, 1995.
58. Wu Y-H: Etiological and pathological studies on dead deer in southern Taiwan. J Chin Soc Vet Sci 14(2):113–120, 1988.
59. Young DB, Mehlert A: Serology of mycobacteria: characterization of antigens recognized by monoclonal antibodies. Rev Infect Dis 11:431–435, 1989.

CHAPTER **100**

The Use of Chutes for Ungulate Restraint

J. C. HAIGH

Techniques for the physical restraint of ungulates are exceedingly ancient. The early Syrians developed sophisticated trapping devices for antelope about 11,000 years ago.[14] In Scandinavia, reindeer (*Rangifer tarandus*) have been physically restrained for hundreds of years,[1] and the Neutral Iroquois had developed handling systems for white-tailed deer (*Odocoileus virginianus*) that were first reported by Champlain in 1611 AD.[15] Except in a few cases, such handling systems were designed for capture and killing rather than husbandry.

Historically, zoos were either managed with little or no direct handling or they were handled in ways that involved risks to both their handlers and themselves. The advent of remote drug delivery systems and, soon afterward, the development of potent immobilizing agents with high margins of safety allowed wildlife managers and zoo personnel to handle virtually all the species of exotic ungulates that were held in zoological collections. However, there has been an increasing realization that methods of physical restraint may provide suitable alternatives for many routine procedures.

A major driving force behind the development of handling systems has been the emergence of the game ranching industry, particularly the growth of deer farming and bison (*Bison bison*) ranching. On these commercial operations, the use of drugs for routine restraint is not practical. The costs and risk factors associated with the drugs, the time taken when using them, the legal restrictions involved for the user, the concern over tissue residues in products destined for the food chain, and the increasingly complex national and international disease testing protocols have all played a role in the move toward improved methods of physical restraint. Furthermore, the hematologic or chemical results of blood samples may be different when drugs, as opposed to physical restraint, are used.

Habituation is a critical factor in the handling of most species. It markedly reduces stress on animals. Habituation should also include the human handlers to the operation. Additionally, some people are better able to handle animals than others, and a quiet temperament and good "stockmanship" are essential.[5, 6] Negative experiences for animals in a handling system create agitation that persists over time, whereas gentle handling ensures that animals are calmer and easier to handle on future occasions.[7–9, 12]

There are marked differences in the way that various species react to being handled, and operators must learn from experience. For some species, the use of a blindfold during physical restraint may reduce struggling. There are also differences among individuals of a given species, which may be ascribed to genetic makeup or previous negative experience of which the current caretaker is unaware.

BASIC REQUIREMENTS

Basic requirements for handling systems are summarized in Table 100–1.[2, 6, 12] Although these basic tenets are optimum, all the chutes described herein have been built as portable units for use in zoos or on game farms. Scales are easily incorporated into handling systems and provide valuable information on animal condition.

TABLE 100–1. Basic Components of Handling Systems for Ungulates

Paddocks or pens	Strategic gates allow easy exit.
Alleyways	Paddock or pens can be connected by alleyways to allow movement to a central handling area. Animals baulk and return in alleyways that are too straight for too long a section. Corners or baffles can be incorporated.
Visual reminders	As animals come under pressure near yards, sight boards or shade netting can be added to alley fences to ensure that animals do not test wire.
Sorting yards	Holding and sorting yards can play a useful role in management of large groups. Some species can be drafted in such yards.
Gates	In paddocks or large pens, gates should be placed to form funnel effects.
Catwalks	Catwalks are advocated by some authors, but they may not always be needed.
Holding pens	Holding pens can be set up before handling chutes so that logical progression of animals can be maintained. A system of sliding and swinging gates provides maximum safety for both handlers and animals.
Dark and light	For some species, variable light regimens are essential for safe handling.
Tubs and half-tubs	These are suitable for some species.
Chutes	Designs vary.
Exit	The ability to draft and direct animals to specific locations is a considerable asset.

Many designs were tested in the early days of deer farming in both New Zealand and the United Kingdom, and the most economical and practical have been retained. Further developments occurred in North America; particularly, the growth of wapiti (*Cervus elaphus*) and white-tailed deer farming has spawned new designs that have made handling of these species a routine matter involving minimal risk to both animals and personnel.[11] Two such designs are shown in Figures 100–1 and 100–2 and one is shown in use (Fig. 100–3).

There are many designs of pens and chutes that work well. Some are constructed inside sheds, where low lighting can help reduce stress on the animals. For fallow deer (*Dama dama*), white-tailed deer, mule deer (*Odocoileus hemionus*), and axis deer (*Axis axis*), the use of dark and light, using dimmer switches, is essential for success. If the lights are on in the shed, the animals are a danger to themselves and their handlers because they make athletic and apparently random leaps. With these species, an entirely dark room quiets the deer and allows a handler to safely enter. For example, fallow deer and white-tailed deer can be efficiently drafted by a handler working amongst them if the pen is dark. The animals move out of such an area into a chute or another pen that is lighted. It is likely that other fractious ungulates will be found to respond to similar designs and the use of light as a physical restraint is tested on a growing number of species.

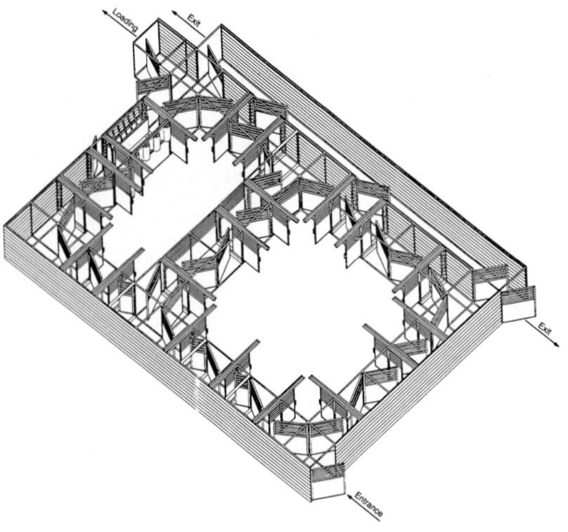

Some authors have reported that animals may quickly learn the weak points of a handling system and exploit them,[10, 17] and the ability to modify such design faults is important. The modular system illustrated in Figure 100–1 allows modifications without major reconstruction.

FIGURE 100–1. Perspective of the layout of a handling system designed for a large-scale wapiti farm. (Courtesy of John Cameron, Safe Side Systems, Winfield, Alberta, Canada.)

HANDLING CHUTES

There are several types of chutes or squeezes. They generally fall into one of the following three categories: drop floor, box, and mechanical/hydraulic squeeze systems. However, many types of box chutes have mechanical squeezes. Some chutes are portable and can be moved from site to site within a facility or, on wheels, from location to location.

Drop Floor Chutes

Drop floor chutes are popular, especially for smaller hoofed stock (Figs. 100–4, 100–5). They have been developed from sheep handling systems in which it was recognized that an animal, suspended by hip and shoulder and held off its feet, would cease to struggle.

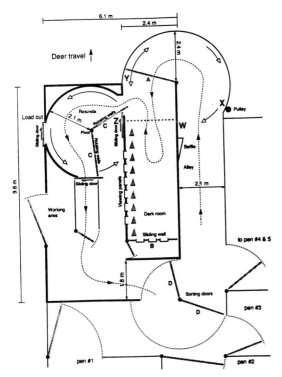

FIGURE 100–2. Sorting area and handling shed for white-tailed deer farm. Lights in the shed are controlled by rheostat switches. The direction of movement for animals is indicated by the fine dotted line and closed arrows. Open arrows with solid shafts indicate the movement of swinging gates. Shaded arrows without shafts indicate the movement of the sliding wall. (From Haigh JC, Friesen RW: A handling system for white-tailed deer [*Odocoileus virginianus*]. J Zoo Wildl Med 26:321–326, 1995.)

Among smaller deer, drop floor chutes have been particularly used for red deer, fallow deer, white-tailed deer, and axis deer.[3, 4, 13, 12] A drop floor chute has been used by Russian wapiti producers for at least 100 years,[12] but, in most locales, other systems are now in more common use.

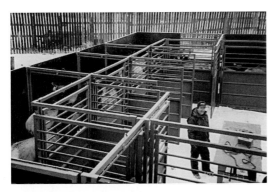

FIGURE 100–3. Aerial view of a wapiti handling system in use. (Photograph by Donna Costley, NV Elk, Bateman, Saskatchewan, Canada.)

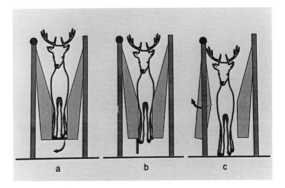

FIGURE 100–4. Diagram of a basic drop floor chute in operation. *A*, The animal enters when the floor is up. *B*, The floor is tripped by a handler-operated side lever. *C*, The animal is released when the side wall is allowed to swing out of the way.

Drop floor chutes allow access from below for hoof care, and, because the animal cannot obtain leverage or move backward or forward, they allow access to head and hind end for a variety of manipulations (Fig. 100–5).

Hundreds of accident-free restraint events have taken place at both the St. Louis Zoological Park and the Fossil Rim Wildlife Center. More than 1000 procedures involving addax (*Addax nasomaculatus*) have

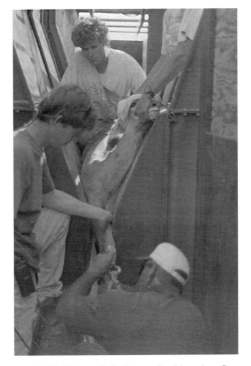

FIGURE 100–5. Juvenile kudu restrained in a drop floor chute. A tuberculin test has been administered in the mid-cervical region (note the black felt-tip marker ring identifying the site), and a handler is attending to an overgrown hoof. (Photograph by Matt Read.)

been completed at the former, and, at the latter, 289 procedures involving 13 species were conducted in 14 months.[17] Similarly, at the San Diego Wild Animal Park, a drop floor chute has been used as an alternative to chemical restraint.[16] At the Western Plains Zoo in Dubbo, Australia, a drop floor chute is routinely used for vaccination and contraceptive treatment of a large herd of Indian blackbuck (*Antilope cervicapra*) (Blyde, personal communication, 1994–1995). It has been estimated that several thousand procedures have been carried out with zoological specimens using drop floor chutes.[2]

A modification of the drop floor chute that reduces struggling and improves restraint is the addition of a back-press that can be applied just over the withers after the floor has been dropped out. Some species (e.g., rusa deer [*Cervus timorensis*]) struggle unduly in a drop floor chute unless a back-press is applied.

A corollary to the drop floor chute has been in use for deer restraint in China. It involves the use of belly bands that lift the animal off the ground, achieving the same calming effect as a dropped floor.

However, drop floor chutes are not suitable for all species. For instance, it was found that scimitar horned oryx (*Oryx dammah*) panicked when the floor suddenly dropped and would even turn upside down.[17] Most larger bovids are handled in other ways.

Box Chutes

Box chutes are usually of simple design and need to be custom built to suit a particular species. They may have access panels that allow work to be carried out. Early handling systems for wapiti in Canada consisted of this type of chute, and they are still used for some procedures. A simple type of box chute consists of the use of one wall of a rectangular pen that is hinged part way along one side and can be swung to meet the opposite wall. It allows access for sample collection, tuberculosis testing, and even artificial insemination through a rear panel.

Tubs for animal handling are well known in the cattle industry and can easily be built for other species of ungulates. They can also be adapted as box chutes. However, if both walls of a tub are rotated off a single central pole, problems with the triangular shape will be encountered. This disadvantage can be overcome either by building a rotating wall with an angle joint or by constructing the system as a half-tub, in which the walls rotate from offset posts and create a chute if placed in parallel.

An innovative padded side-opening box chute that can be rotated around a horizontal axis to allow access for hoof trimming has been developed at the Orana Park Zoo in New Zealand.[17] A smaller tiltable chute has also been developed at the Forestry Farm Zoo in Saskatoon, Saskatchewan, Canada.

A remarkable exercise in habituation and restraint of Nyala (*Tragelaphus angassii*) at the Denver Zoological Gardens has been reported. After a 3-month period of positive reinforcement with food treats, a group of these animals could be individually held in a box chute and palpated; blood samples could even be collected.[9]

Giraffe can also be habituated to specially designed box chutes, many of which consist only of rails, without solid sides. I have treated foot-rot in a giraffe over a period of several days by offering food at the front of a chute in which a warm water and Epsom salts mixture was incorporated in a depression. Similarly, black rhinoceros (*Diceros bicornis*) can be habituated to transport crates that double as chutes in which they can receive treatment within 3 or 4 days of capture.

Mechanical and Hydraulic Chutes

Mechanical and hydraulic squeezes and chutes are seen on many game farms and in a growing number of zoos. They are particularly valuable for larger, robust species. For example, a hydraulic chute has been in use for many years for elephant restraint at the Henry Doorly Zoo in Omaha, Nebraska. On the other hand, custom built chutes also work well for smaller specimens such as white-tailed deer.[10, 18]

Commercial cattle chutes with head gates have been used for a variety of large bovids, but they are not always suitable for cervids and many antelopes because species of these groups have lighter builds and longer, thinner necks. The animals can easily be damaged if held by the neck.

For bison and the very large bovids such as gaur (*Bos gaurus*), special mechanical chutes have been developed. An important feature of bison chutes is the so-called crash gate. This is a heavy duty gate that is placed about 45 cm in front of the head gate. When bison are handled, the head gate should be closed until the animal has entered the chute and settled somewhat. At this point, the head gate can be opened and the animal usually moves forward and hits the crash gate, at which time the head gate must be quickly closed. It is virtually impossible to catch a bison in a head gate unless a crash gate is present to stop its forward motion (Fig. 100–6).

The latest type of chute to emerge in the game farming industry has been the hydraulic chute, which has walls that move in and out and up and down. Some models also have walls that allow for adjustment of angle to suit individual species or situations. In many hydraulic chutes, the walls are contoured to fit the

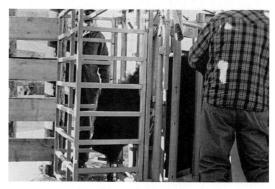

FIGURE 100–6. Custom designed bison chute showing the crash gate. (Photograph by Jerry Haigh.)

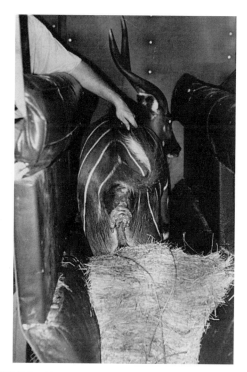

FIGURE 100–7. Bongo with a vaginal prolapse in a hydraulic chute. This animal had been habituated to the chute over several months of treatment and no longer needed the walls to be applied with pressure. (Photograph by White Oaks Conservation Center, Yulee, FL.)

general body shape of an ungulate, and most have some form of padding (Fig. 100–7). Virtually all such chutes are built with panels in the side walls that allow access for sample collection and a variety of treatments. Hydraulic chutes must be used with caution. Death from anoxia resulting from excessive pressure on the thorax has occurred. Animals that struggle unduly should be released, at least temporarily, and pressure release valves should be incorporated into the lines to prevent overzealous application (Fig. 100–8).

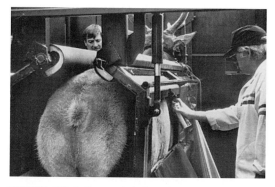

FIGURE 100–8. Rear-angled view of a wapiti in a hydraulic chute showing contouring of walls and side opening panels. The rear door has been left open to permit photography. (Photograph by Jerry Haigh.)

Hydraulic chutes have been used with success in several zoos and on a few bison ranches. They are widely used for red deer, although drop floor chutes are also in common use for this species. Hydraulic chutes are considered to be the industry standard for wapiti.

EXITS

The last part, or exit, of the handling system is often ignored. It must be designed with some sort of ability to herd animals after they are through the chute. Gates and yards can be set up so that animals can be directed to desired locations (see Fig. 100–1). Again, as animals leave the squeeze, it is important for them to know their way around. If they have been given the chance to familiarize themselves with the set-up, they will move unconcernedly through gates and along alleyways.

CONCLUSION

The basic tenets of handling consist of an understanding of the importance of training for both the animals and the personnel. It is probably true to say that these components have about equal value.

Alleyways, corners, visual reminders, sorting yards, dividing gates, tubs, chutes, and squeezes make up the physical structures. People and animals familiar with their surroundings, and knowing their objectives, make up the active parts. Routine handling of animals has become an integral part of deer farming and bison ranching operations and, in some cases, has become the norm in zoological collections for other species as well.

REFERENCES

1. Baskin LM: Herding. *In* Hudson RJ, Drew K, Baskin LM (eds): Wildlife Production Systems. New York, Cambridge University Press, pp 187–196, 1989.
2. Blumer ES, deMaar TW. Manual restraint systems for the management of non-domestic hoofstock. Proceedings of the American Association of Zoo Veterinarians, St. Louis, pp 156–159, 1993.
3. English AW: Management strategies for farmed chital deer. *In* Brown RD (ed): The Biology of Deer. New York, Springer-Verlag, pp 189–196, 1992.
4. Fletcher J: Handling farmed deer. Practice January:30–37, 1995.
5. Grandin T: Animal handling. *In* Price EO (ed): Veterinary Clinics of North America: Food Animal Practice. Farm Animal Behavior, 3rd ed. Philadelphia, WB Saunders, pp 323–338, 1987.
6. Grandin T:. Behavioral principles of animal handling. The Professional Animal Scientist 5:1–10, 1989.
7. Grandin T: Behavioral agitation during handling of cattle is persistent over time. Appl Anim Behav Sci 36:1–9, 1993.
8. Grandin T: The effect of previous experiences on livestock behavior during handling. Agri-Practice 14:15–20, 1993.
9. Grandin T, Rooney MB, Phillips M, et al: Conditioning of nyala (*Tragelphus angasi*) to blood sampling in a crate with positive reinforcement. Zoo Biol 14:261–273, 1995.
10. Haigh JC: Game farming, with an emphasis on North America. *In* Fowler ME (ed): Zoo and Wild Animal Medicine. Current Therapy 3. Philadelphia, WB Saunders, pp 87–101, 1993.
11. Haigh JC, Friesen RW: A handling system for white-tailed deer (*Odocoileus virginianus*). J Zoo Wildl Med 26:321–326, 1995.
12. Haigh JC, Hudson RJ: Farming Wapiti and Red Deer. St. Louis, Mosby–Year Book, 1993.
13. Langridge M: Establishing a fallow deer farm: basic principles. *In* Asher GW, Langridge M (eds): Progressive Fallow Farming. Auckland, New Zealand, Ministry of Agriculture and Fisheries, pp

Auckland, New Zealand, Ministry of Agriculture and Fisheries, pp 17–28, 1992.

14. Legge AJ, Rowley-Conwy PA: Gazelle killing in Stone Age Syria. Sci Am 257:88–95, 1987.

15. Noble WC, Crerar JEM: Management of white-tailed deer by the Neutral Iroquois A.D. 999–1651. Archaeozoologica 6:19–70, 1993.

16. Petrovsky A, Blue A: "Drop-Chute" hoofstock restraint as an alternative to chemical immobilization at the San Diego Wild Animal Park. Animal Keepers Forum 23:643–650, 1996.

17. Read BW, Williams B, Christman J: Restraint devices for management and research procedures for ungulates. Int Zoo Yearbook 32:148–154, 1993.

18. Schmitt SM, Cooley TM, Schrader LD, et al: A squeeze chute to restrain captive deer. Wildl Soc Bull 11:387–389, 1983.

CHAPTER 101

Scrapie-Like Spongiform Encephalopathies (Prion Diseases) in Nondomesticated Species

JAMES K. KIRKWOOD

ANDREW A. CUNNINGHAM

Scrapie-like spongiform encephalopathies (SEs) are chronic diseases characterized by long incubation periods followed by development of clinical signs associated with progressive loss of central nervous function. Aspects of their etiology and transmission remain obscure and no specific treatments are available.

Before 1980, naturally occurring scrapie-like SEs had been recognized in four species: in sheep and goats[11] as the widespread disease of scrapie; in humans as kuru in Papua, New Guinea, as Creutzfeldt-Jakob disease (CJD), which occurs worldwide, as Gerstmann-Sträussler-Schenker syndrome (GSS), and as fatal familial insomnia (FFI); and in minks (*Mustela vison*) as transmissible mink encephalopathy (TME) in the United States.[12] Since then, however, such transmissible encephalopathies have been diagnosed in a growing number of other species. An SE has been found to be the cause of chronic wasting disease (CWD) in captive mule deer (*Odocoileus hemionus*)[45] and Rocky Mountain elk (*Cervus elaphus*)[46] in the United States, and, recently, 44 cases of the disease have been reported in free-living individuals of these species and in white-tailed deer (*Odocoileus virginianus*) in north central Colorado.[37] An SE assumed to be scrapie has been diagnosed in mouflon (*Ovis musimon*) in the United Kingdom.[48] In association with the bovine spongiform encephalopathy (BSE) epidemic in domestic cattle in Europe,[3, 43] SEs have been diagnosed in more than 60 domestic cats[5, 30] and in a total of 25 individuals of 10 species of zoo animals in or from Great Britain. The latter were all from the families Bovidae and Felidae, and comprise the following: one nyala (*Tragelaphus angasi*), five eland (*Taurotragus oryx*), six greater kudu (*Tragelaphus strepsiceros*), one gemsbok (*Oryx gazella*), one Arabian oryx (*Oryx leucoryx*), one scimitar-horned oryx (*Oryx dammah*), four cheetah (*Acinonyx jubatus*), three puma (*Felis concolor*), two ocelot (*Felis pardalis*), and one tiger (*Panthera tigris*).[23–25, 27] The ages of birth and death of the British zoo animal cases thought to be associated with the BSE epidemic are shown in Figure 101–1 (bovids other than greater kudu), Figure 101–2 (greater kudu), and Figure 101–3 (felids). Furthermore, some of these SEs have been experimentally transmitted to a range of other species. For example, BSE has been transmitted experimentally by parenteral inoculation to mouse, sheep, goat, pig, common marmoset (*Callithrix jacchus*), and mink and to five of these species via the oral route.[5]

Several cases of SE were reported in white tigers that died at the Bristol Zoo, United Kingdom, during the 1970s,[20] but it was subsequently considered that this differed from scrapie-like SEs largely because the disease was not shown to be transmissible to a range of mammalian species.[5] An SE, which likewise may not be scrapie-like (but possibly of nutritional or toxic etiology), has been reported in three ostriches (*Struthio camelus*) in Germany.[35]

Because SEs between which there is no known association (e.g., kuru and scrapie) occur in at least two (man and sheep) of the relatively small number of

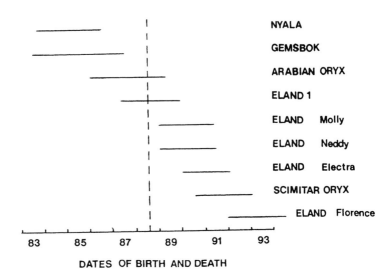

FIGURE 101–1. Birth and death dates for the cases of scrapie-like spongiform encephalopathy (SE) thought to have been caused by the bovine SE agent in captive wild bovids (other than greater kudu; see Fig. 101–2) in zoos in Great Britain.[29] From the pattern of the epidemic in cattle, it is known that the ban on the inclusion of ruminant-derived protein in ruminant feeds did not become fully effective until many months after it was imposed (dotted line) and the possibility that continued foodborne exposure was the cause of the cases shown that were born after this date cannot be absolutely ruled out.

animals in which such diseases would be likely to have been detected (man and the species in his direct care), it is perhaps not unlikely that these diseases occur, albeit maybe at a low incidence, in many other species.[24]

EPIZOOTIOLOGY

There is growing evidence in support of the hypothesis that scrapie and the scrapie-like SEs are caused by the presence of abnormal, protease-resistant forms (PrP^{sc}) of a protein (PrP) that is normally coded for and expressed in the central nervous system (CNS) and other tissues of a wide range of species.[7] It is thought that these abnormal forms occur through post-translational differences in tertiary structure. These "prions" may

arise spontaneously, as appears to be the case in CJD, which affects about one person per million, and in other human familial forms in which much higher incidences are associated with particular mutations to the PrP gene.[33] However, on entering the CNS of other susceptible animals following ingestion or by experimental or iatrogenic inoculation, some of these agents can promote the production of PrP^{sc}, thus inducing disease in these new hosts. Epidemics then may be triggered when susceptible animals are exposed to agent-containing tissues from a spontaneously arising case and may be sustained if further transmission occurs via the oral (or perhaps other) route. Epidemics of kuru in humans and BSE in cattle and other species appear to fit this model, but the original sources of the agents of these diseases are unknown.

Knowledge of rates and routes of transmission in

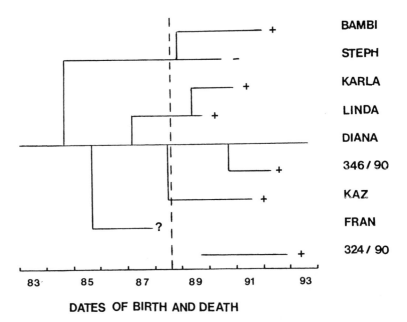

FIGURE 101–2. The temporal and familial relationships of cases of scrapie-like spongiform encephalopathy (SE) in greater kudu at the Zoological Society of London. The dotted line shows the date of the ban (July, 1988) on the inclusion of ruminant-derived protein in ruminant feeds (see Fig. 101–1). +, SE-positive, − SE-negative, ?, animals that may have had the disease based on clinical signs. Diana was euthanized in May 1995 and was SE-negative. (From Kirkwood JK, Cunningham AA: Epidemiological observations on spongiform encephalopathies in captive wild animals in the British Isles. Vet Rec 135:301, 1994.)

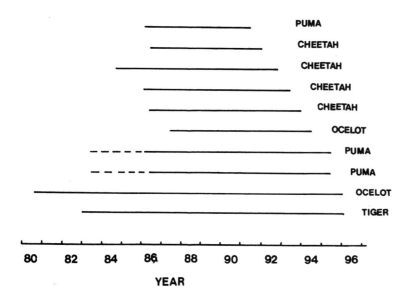

FIGURE 101–3. Birth and death dates for the cases of scrapie-like spongiform encephalopathy (SE) thought to have been caused by the bovine SE (BSE) agent in captive wild felids at or from zoos in Great Britain. It is thought that these animals probably acquired the disease from eating tissues from cattle carcasses that were unfit for human consumption. In 1991, a ban was imposed on feeding "specified offals" (tissues that may contain the BSE agent) from any cattle older than 6 months of age.[2] The dotted lines reflect that the precise dates of birth of two of the pumas were unknown.

these diseases is incomplete. Although debate continues, it is thought that scrapie is naturally transmissible among susceptible sheep and goats via exposure to placenta and fetal fluids from infected individuals.[5] Analyses of the pattern of the BSE epidemic have provided evidence that about 10% of calves from cattle with BSE acquire the disease by maternal transmission in some way,[3] although this hypothesis and the strength of the case for maternal transmission in other species have been questioned.[32] It is thought that CWD may be naturally transmissible in deer.[47] The pattern of cases of BSE in greater kudu (*Tragelaphus strepsiceros*) at the Zoological Society of London and in some other zoo antelope suggested that, after the disease had initially entered the populations via contaminated feed, animal to animal transmission might have occurred subsequently.[10, 24] However, it has proved impossible to absolutely rule out the possibility that continuing foodborne exposure was the cause.[27] It is thought that CJD and TME are not naturally transmissible either horizontally or vertically.

It is known that there is great variation between species in the ease with which prion diseases can be experimentally transmitted between them and that susceptibility varies in an unpredictable way. The pattern of incidence of SEs in zoo animals associated with exposure to the BSE agent suggests variation in susceptibility between species because cases have occurred in far fewer species than are thought to have been exposed. Furthermore, variation in incidence between zoo species has tended not to correlate with the numbers of individuals thought to have been at risk.[24, 27] The relatively large number of cases occurring in greater kudu, cheetahs, and pumas associated with BSE in Great Britain suggest, for example, that these species may be particularly susceptible to the BSE agent. However, no firm conclusions can be drawn because it is possible that the observed patterns of variation in incidence were due to variation in incubation period or intensity of exposure.

The incubation periods of prion diseases are long and are known, in mice and sheep, to be influenced by genotype.[16] In field cases, it may not be possible to determine incubation periods precisely because dates of exposure are usually unknown, but age at death can provide some indication. Among the species affected by BSE via the oral route, there is evidence of considerable variation in incubation period between species (Table 101–1). It might be expected that variation in incubation period between species could be related to metabolic rate, because pathogenesis is associated with a build-up of protease-resistant protein and because rates of protein synthesis and turnover parallel rates of metabolism between species.[39] However, although there is evidence that the incubation period is longer in felids than bovids, a clear body weight (and thus metabolic rate) effect is not apparent (Fig. 101–4).

CLINICAL SIGNS

The clinical signs of the prion diseases reflect progressive loss of aspects of CNS function and show some differences between species and with the nature of the agent in accordance with the distribution of lesions. Typically, signs have an insidious onset and relatively slow progression (weeks to months) and include ataxia, abnormal posture and head and ear carriage, fine muscle tremors and myoclonus, abnormal activity patterns, wasting, hyperesthesia and anxiety, nibbling of the tail base, decreased rumination, excessive lip movements, and head and flank rubbing.[24, 26, 45, 46] However, the picture is variable; for example, wasting is not a consistent finding. In some cases, clinical signs appear to have much more sudden onset and to progress rapidly (days). The disease cannot be differentiated, on the basis of clinical signs, from some other diseases of the CNS, and differential diagnoses include metabolic diseases (ketosis), cerebrocortical necrosis, CNS neoplasia, congenital CNS dysplasias, CNS infections (e.g., rabies,

TABLE 101–1. Species Variation in Age at Death in Animals that Died with Spongiform Encephalopathies (SE) Thought to Be Caused by Ingestion of the Bovine SE Agent

| | Age at Death (months) | |
Species	Means or Ranges	Youngest Recorded
Muridae		
Laboratory mouse *Mus domesticus*[4]	14–17 (n = 10)	14
Felidae		
Puma (*Felis concolor*)	62 (n = 1)	62
Ocelot (*Felis pardalis*)	135 (n = 2)	84
Domestic cat (*Felis catus*)[30]	78 ± 38.5 (n = 5)	54
Cheetah (*Acinonyx jubatus*)	82 ± 18.5 (n = 4)	55
Tiger (*Panthera tigris*)	156 (n = 1)	156
Bovidae		
Eland (*Taurotragus oryx*)	28 ± 3.0 (n = 3)	24
Nyala (*Tragelaphus angasi*)	33 (n = 1)	33
Greater kudu (*Tragelaphus strepsiceros*)	31 ± 9.0 (n = 4)	19
Domestic cattle *Bos domesticus*[42]	30–96 (many)	30
Scimitar-horned oryx (*Oryx dammah*)	30 (n = 1)	30
Gemsbok (*Oryx gazella*)	48 (n = 1)	48
Arabian oryx (*Oryx leucoryx*)	38 (n = 1)	38

(Data from Figures 101–1, 101–2, 101–3.)

listeriosis, toxoplasmosis), hepatic encephalopathy, and cranial trauma.[18]

DIAGNOSIS

Provisional diagnosis of the disease, based on the absence of other explanations for suspicious clinical signs (and especially if there is a history of exposure to potentially infectious tissues) cannot be confirmed during life (except by brain or, in some cases, lymphoid tissue biopsy). However, proteins that appear to be specific markers of the disease have been detected recently in cerebrospinal fluid of cattle with BSE and this

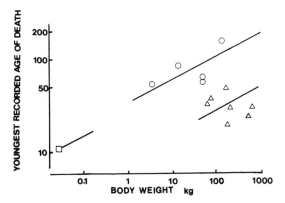

FIGURE 101–4. Youngest recorded age at death (months) in cases of SE in the species of bovids (triangles) and felids (circles) and the laboratory mouse (square) that were known or thought to have acquired the agent of bovine spongiform encephalopathy via the oral route plotted in relation to adult body weight. The lines show the mean minimum age (months) at death per $kg^{0.25}$ for the bovids, the felids, and the mouse.

may offer a route to antemortem diagnosis.[19] At present, diagnosis depends on detection of characteristic histopathologic changes in the CNS and tests for the presence of the abnormal, protease-resistant form of the PrP protein. These include detection of scrapie-associated fibrils (an ultrastructural manifestation of PrP^{sc}) by electron microscopic examination of detergent extracts of brain[15, 28, 34, 42] and immunostaining and immunoblotting techniques for the detection of PrP^{sc}.[34] The latter may also offer a means to diagnosis before death through detection of PrP^{sc} in lymphoid tissue biopsies in species in which infectivity can occur in this tissue (sheep and goats). Further confirmation and information about "strain" type can be obtained by inoculation of brain homogenates into panels of mice of various genotypes because it has been found that different prion diseases produce characteristic patterns of variation in incubation period and lesion distribution in these panels.[6, 17] Recently, it has also been shown that strains can be distinguished by physicochemical properties of PrP^{sc}.[7]

Guidelines on postmortem tissue sampling for the diagnosis of SEs in zoo animals have been published by Cunningham and Wells.[9]

TREATMENT

No treatment is available to arrest or slow the progression of the disease nor is any in prospect. Euthanasia is indicated to limit suffering.

PATHOLOGY

There are no specific gross lesions. Wasting and signs of trauma secondary to ataxia may be apparent. Histopathologic changes are limited to the CNS and comprise vacuolation of neuronal perikarya and neurites, neuronal degeneration and loss, gliosis (mainly astrocytic), and amyloidosis.[42] The distribution of lesions varies between the prion diseases and with species (and strains) of hosts.[41]

PREVENTION

In at least a proportion of the prion diseases of humans, especially when there are abnormalities of the PrP gene, prion disease appears to arise spontaneously. It seems possible that such spontaneous cases may also arise in other species and there is currently no prospect of preventing this. More significant epidemics occur through widespread ingestion of infectious tissues and it is appropriate to direct efforts to minimizing such risk. Transmission from live animals incubating the disease is also thought to play a role in some cases, and there may be a carrier state in animals that outlive the incubation period of the disease. It is pertinent, therefore, to consider which species might be susceptible, which tissues might contain infectivity, and by what route infection might occur. As discussed, prion diseases have been diagnosed in a wide range of mammals and it is not unlikely that all mammals and possibly other taxa are potentially susceptible to these types of disease.

The most infectious tissue from animals with prion disease is CNS tissue, but infectivity has been demonstrated also (by inoculation of homogenates intracranially into mice) in spleen, lymph nodes, placenta, and fetal fluids from sheep with scrapie; in distal ileum from cattle with BSE[40]; and in spleen, lymph nodes, thymus, and salivary gland in mice.[22] Furthermore, CJD has been iatrogenically transmitted. There is, therefore, some evidence that the tissue distribution of the agent may vary between species or with the nature of the agent. Even though it is likely that CNS tissues will contain the greatest concentration and thus pose the greatest risks, the possibility of more widespread tissue distribution should be considered.

A small number of iatrogenic cases of CJD have occurred in humans following dura mater transplants, corneal graft, brain surgery (using contaminated instruments), and treatment with human growth hormone or gonadotrophin prepared from pituitaries collected postmortem.[1, 36] Transplants and inoculations involving potentially infected materials are thus a potential source of infection. Larger scale epidemics (e.g., BSE in cattle, TME in mink, and kuru in humans) have occurred through ingestion of contaminated tissues, and prevention of this is a crucial part of control of these diseases. Although not all prion diseases may present a threat to other species (e.g., there is no evidence that ingestion of any tissue from scrapie-infected sheep causes disease in humans or carnivores), clearly some can; therefore, in the zoo context, it is probably simplest and safest to recommend that no tissues from any animal that might have a prion disease be used as food or as an ingredient in the feed of any species. The approach to the control of the BSE epidemic in cattle in Great Britain has been to prevent potentially contaminated tissues from being fed back to cattle or other ruminants[29] and it seems likely that the exclusion of ruminant-derived protein from ungulate feeds is largely responsible for the observed decline and hopefully disappearance of the cases in zoo hoofstock (Fig. 101–5). In 1990, a further order[2] was passed prohibiting the inclusion of "specified offals" (tissues that could contain infectivity) from cattle older than 6 months in the food of any animal. It is hoped that this will, likewise, lead to the disappearance of cases in zoo felids (see Fig. 101–5). However, it is expected that such a disappearance will take longer than for bovids because of the longer incubation periods in felids.

The agents of prion disease are extremely resistant to deactivation and can, for example, survive in formalin-fixed tissues or autoclaving at 138°C for more than 1 hour.[1, 38] These agents are not significantly affected by the majority of chemical disinfectants. Repeat cycles of high-temperature autoclaving are the method of choice for decontamination, but if this is not possible, 1-hour treatment with sodium hypochlorite at 20,000 ppm available chlorine is recommended.[2] It is possible that the infectivity remains in contaminated soil for long periods. The possible role of environmental contamination in the epidemiology of prion diseases is unknown, but it has been suggested as a factor in the epidemiology of scrapie[21] and CWD.[47]

If transmissible SEs are detected in new host species, from the disease control perspective, it would be prudent to assume that CNS and possibly other tissues might cause disease through ingestion or iatrogenic inoculation into other animals. The possibility that the disease could be naturally transmissible vertically or horizontally should be seriously considered. The occurrence of vertical or horizontal transmission could result in the disease being sustained (becoming endemic) in the population, which appears to be the case in scrapie and possibly in CWD. In view of the great importance

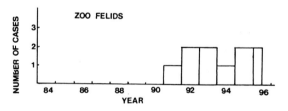

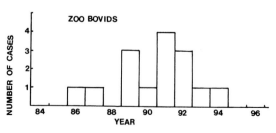

FIGURE 101–5. Temporal variation in the annual incidence of cases of scrapie-like spongiform encephalopathy (SE) thought to have been caused by the bovine SE agent in captive wild felids and bovids at or from zoos in Great Britain.

of individuals of rare and endangered species maintained in zoos and the need for great care not to introduce or spread infections among them that might compromise their potential contributions to world gene pools, it has been suggested that no animals that may have been exposed to the agent of BSE or their offspring or in contacts should be used for reintroductions, and that translocations to other collections should not be undertaken without careful consideration of the risks.[8, 24] It would seem appropriate to extend this level of caution in the control of any prion disease unless detailed knowledge is available of the epidemiology of particular cases suggesting otherwise.

RISKS TO HUMAN HEALTH FROM PRION DISEASES OF ANIMALS

No cases of human SEs have been recognized to be associated with exposure to animals or the tissues of animals affected by scrapie, TME, or CWD. However, there is great concern and growing evidence[7] that the BSE agent, acquired through consumption of infected tissues of affected cattle, may be the cause of "new variant" CJD cases reported recently in Britain.[44] (As of December 1996, the number of confirmed cases was 15.) This emphasizes the need for special care when handling potentially infectious tissues from animals suspected to have died of prion disease. Although there is no evidence for any form of direct transmission from clinical cases or animals incubating the disease that could present a risk to human health, it is always prudent to observe high standards of hygiene in the handling of animals.[1, 13] Occupational guidance notes for veterinarians involved in postmortem or research work with BSE-infected animals have been provided by the UK Health and Safety Executive.[14] Further guidance notes on handling infected animals and recommendations on the laboratory handling of infected tissues are provided by the Advisory Committee on Dangerous Pathogens.[1]

Acknowledgments

Information on the cases of spongiform encephalopathies in zoo animals in Great Britain was collected from the literature and from discussions with many veterinary and curatorial colleagues to whom we are most grateful.

REFERENCES

1. Advisory Committee on Dangerous Pathogens: Precautions for Working with Human and Animal Spongiform Encephalopathies. London, Her Majesty's Stationery Office, 1994.
2. Amendment Order: Bovine Spongiform Encephalopathy (No. 2). Statutory Instrument No. 1930. London, Her Majesty's Stationery Office, 1990.
3. Anderson RM, Donnelly CA, Ferguson NM, et al: Transmission dynamics and epidemiology of BSE in British cattle. Nature 382:779–788, 1996.
4. Barlow RM, Middleton DJ: Oral transmission of BSE to mice. *In* Bradley R, Savey M, Marchant B (eds): Sub-Acute Spongiform Encephalopathies. Dordrecht, Kluwer Academic Publishers, pp 33–39, 1991.
5. Bradley R: Bovine spongiform encephalopathy distribution and update on some transmission and decontamination studies. *In* Gibbs CJ Jr (ed): Bovine Spongiform Encephalopathy: The BSE Dilemma. New York, Springer-Verlag, pp 11–27, 1996.
6. Bruce ME, Chree A, McConnell I, et al: Transmission of bovine spongiform encephalopathy and scrapie to mice: strain variation and species barrier. Philos Trans R Soc Lond B 343:405–411, 1994.
7. Collinge J, Sidle KCL, Meads J, et al: Molecular analysis of prion strain variation and the aetiology of new variant, CJD. Nature 383:685–690, 1996.
8. Cunningham AA: Bovine spongiform encephalopathy and British zoos. J Zoo Wildl Med 11:605–634, 1991.
9. Cunningham AA, Wells GAH: Samples to be taken for the detection of spongiform encephalopathy in zoo animals. Br Vet Zool Soc Newsletter Summer 1996:27–29, 1996.
10. Cunningham AA, Wells GAH, Scott AC, et al: Transmissible spongiform encephalopathy in greater kudu (*Tragelaphus strepsiceros*). Vet Rec 132:68, 1993.
11. Dickinson AG: Scrapie in sheep and goats. *In* Kimberlin RH (ed): Slow Virus Diseases of Animals and Man. Amsterdam, North Holland, pp 209–241, 1976.
12. Hartsough GR, Burger D: Encephalopathy of mink. I. Epizootiological and clinical observations. J Infect Dis 115:387–392, 1965.
13. Health and Safety Executive: Occupational Health Risks from Cattle [HSE Information Sheet No. 19]. London, Her Majesty's Stationery Office, 1996.
14. Health and Safety Executive: Bovine Spongiform Encephalopathy: Background and General Occupational Guidance. London, Health and Safety Executive Books, 1996.
15. Hope J, Reekie LJD, Hunter N, et al: Fibrils from brains of cows with new cattle disease contain scrapie-associated protein. Nature 336:390–392, 1988.
16. Hunter N, Foster JD, Hope J: Natural scrapie in British sheep: breeds, ages and PrP gene polymorphisms. Vet Rec 130:389–392, 1992.
17. Jeffrey M, Scott JR, Williams A, et al: Ultrastructural features of spongiform encephalopathy transmitted to mice from three species of bovidae. Acta Neuropathol 84:559–569, 1992.
18. Jeffrey M, Simmons MM, Wells GAH: Observations on the differential diagnosis of bovine spongiform encephalopathy in Great Britain. *In* Bradley R, Marchant B (eds): Transmissible Spongiform Encephalopathies. Brussels, European Commission, Directorate General for Agriculture, pp 347–358, 1993.
19. Jones VT, Martin TC, Keyes P, et al: Protein markers in cerebrospinal fluid from BSE-affected cattle. Vet Rec 139:360–363, 1996.
20. Kelly DF, Pearson H, Wright AI, et al: Morbidity in captive white tigers. *In* Montali RJ, Migaki G (eds): The Comparative Pathology of Zoo Animals. Washington, DC, Smithsonian Institution Press, pp 183–188, 1979.
21. Kimberlin RH: Unconventional 'slow' viruses. *In* Parker MT, Collier LH (eds): Topley and Wilson's Principles of Bacteriology, Virology and Immunity, 8th ed. London, Edward Arnold, pp 671–693, 1990.
22. Kimberlin RH, Walker A: Pathogenesis of experimental scrapie. *In* Novel Infectious Agents and the Central Nervous System. (Ciba Foundation Symposium 135). Chichester, Wiley, pp 37–62, 1988.
23. Kirkwood JK: Occurrence of spongiform encephalopathies in zoo animals. Abstracts of the Conference on Transmitting Prions: BSE, CJD and other TSEs. London, Royal College of Pathologists, July 4, 1996.
24. Kirkwood JK, Cunningham AA: Epidemiological observations on spongiform encephalopathies in captive wild animals in the British Isles. Vet Rec 135:296–303, 1994.
25. Kirkwood JK, Cunningham AA: Patterns of incidence of spongiform encephalopathy in captive wild animals in the British Isles. Proceedings of the Wildlife Disease Association (European Division) Symposium, Paris, p 28, November 22–24, 1994.
26. Kirkwood JK, Cunningham AA, Austin AR, et al: Spongiform encephalopathy in a greater kudu Tragelaphus strepsiceros introduced into an affected group. Vet Rec 134:167–168, 1994.
27. Kirkwood JK, Cunningham AA, Flach EJ, et al: Spongiform encephalopathy in another captive cheetah (*Acinonyx jubatus*): evidence for variation in susceptibility between species? J Zoo Wildl Med 26:577–582, 1995.
28. Merz PA, Rohwer RG, Kascsak K, et al: Infection-specific particle from the unconventional slow virus diseases. Science 225:437–440, 1984.

29. Order: The Bovine Spongiform Encephalopathy Order 1988, Statutory Instrument No. 1039. London, Her Majesty's Stationery Office, 1988.

30. Pearson GR, Wyatt JM, Gruffydd-Jones TJ, et al: Feline spongiform encephalopathy: fibril and PrP studies. Vet Rec 131:307–310, 1992.

31. Prusiner SB, Hadlow WJ: Slow transmissible diseases of the nervous system. New York, Academic Press, 1979.

32. Ridley RM, Baker HF: No maternal transmission? Nature 384:7, 1996.

33. Ridley RM, Baker HF, Poulter M, et al: Genetics of human transmissible dementia. *In* Bradley R, Savey M, Marchant B (eds): Subacute Spongiform Encephalopathies. Dordrecht, Kluwer Academic Publishers, pp 203–214, 1991.

34. Scott AC, Wells GAH, Stack MJ, et al: Bovine spongiform encephalopathy: detection and quantitation of fibrils, fibril protein (PrP) and vacuolation in brain. Vet Microbiol 23:295–304, 1990.

35. Schoon H-A, Brunckhorst D, Pohlenz J: Beitrag zur neuropathologie beim rothalsstrauss (*Struthio camelus*)—spongiforme enzephalopathie. Verhandlungs bericht des 33 Internationalen Symposiums uber die Erkrankungen der Zoo- und Wildtiere 33:309–314, 1991.

36. Spongiform Encephalopathy Advisory Committee: Transmissible Spongiform Encephalopathies: A Summary of Present Knowledge and Research. London, Her Majesty's Stationery Office, 1995.

37. Spraker TR: Spongiform encephalopathy in free-ranging cervids in Colorado. Proceedings of the American Association of Zoo Veterinarians, Wildlife Diseases Association, and American Association of Wildlife Veterinarians Joint Conference, East Lansing, MI, p 515, 1995.

38. Taylor DM, Fraser H, McConnell I, et al: Decontamination studies with the agents of bovine spongiform encephalopathy and scrapie. Arch Virol 139:313–326, 1994.

39. Webster AJF: Bioenergetics, bioengineering and growth. Anim Prod 48:249–269, 1989.

40. Wells GAH, Dawson M, Hawkins SAC, et al: Infectivity in ileum of cattle challenged orally with bovine spongiform encephalopathy. Vet Rec 135:40–54, 1994.

41. Wells GAH, Hawkins SAC, Cunningham AA, et al: Comparative pathology of the new transmissible spongiform encephalopathies. *In* Bradley R, Marchant B (eds): Transmissible Spongiform Encephalopathies, Brussels, European Commission, Directorate General for Agriculture, pp 327–345, 1993.

42. Wells GAH, McGill IS: Recently described scrapie-like encephalopathies of animals: case definitions. Res Vet Sci 53:1–10, 1992.

43. Wilesmith JW, Wells GAH, Cranwell M: Bovine spongiform encephalopathy: epidemiological studies. Vet Rec 123:638–644, 1988.

44. Will RG, Ironside JW, Zeidler M, et al: Variant of Creutzfeldt-Jakob disease in the UK. Lancet 347:921–925, 1996.

45. Williams ES, Young S: Chronic wasting disease of captive mule deer: a spongiform encephalopathy. J Wildl Dis 16:89–98, 1980.

46. Williams ES, Young S: Spongiform encephalopathy of Rocky Mountain elk. J Wildl Dis 18:465–471, 1982.

47. Williams ES, Young S: Spongiform encephalopathies in Cervidae. Rev Sci Tech Off Int Epiz 11:551–567, 1992.

48. Wood JLN, Lund LJ, Done SH: The natural occurrence of scrapie in mouflon. Vet Rec 130:25–27, 1992.

CHAPTER **102**

Medical Management of Duikers

MICHELLE WILLETTE FRAHM

In comparison to other mammals with the distribution and biomass of duiker antelope, little is known about this subfamily, and still less has been published. This is due in large part to their secretive nature and forest habitat. The papers that have been issued have come from relatively few sources or have been limited in their scope. Popular topics involving duikers include South African rain forest ecology, human and wild animal interactions, diet preferences of free-ranging animals, and parasites of free-ranging animals, especially those with zoonotic potential. This chapter is a summary of materials concerning duikers with anecdotal information from several United States institutions that maintain duikers.

TAXONOMY AND DISTRIBUTION

Native to Africa, duikers belong to the family Bovidae, subfamily Cephalophinae and comprise two genera, a dozen or so species, and more than 70 subspecies. The name "duiker" comes from the Afrikaans word *duik*, which means dive, and refers to the animal's habit of plunging—high speed, head down—into dense vegetation when frightened.[11] The duikers are primitive antelope and are thought to have diverged early in bovid evolution, thereby retaining many early characteristics.[13] The cytogenetic relationship of duikers to other members of the family Bovidae have been examined.[32] There is some disagreement about what constitutes a species versus a subspecies.[42]

The common, or gray, duiker (*Sylvicapra grimmia*) is the only representative of its genus. Only male common duikers have horns. This species is more adaptable, has a greater range of dispersal, and is unique among duikers in preferring brush habitat.

All other duiker species belong to the genus *Cephalophus*. The species of this genus have much more limited distributions because of their more specialized habitat requirements. All reside in portions of the rain forest belt; many species are sympatric. Three species are referred to as "giants"—the Jentink's duiker (*Cephalophus jentinkii*), the yellow-backed duiker (*Cephalophus sylvicultor*), and the Abbot's duiker (*Cephalophus spadix*).

CONSERVATION

Only one species, the Aders' duiker (*Cephalophus adersi*), is endangered, but several more species (the Jentink's duiker, the Abbot's duiker, and the zebra duiker [*Cephalophus zebra*]) are vulnerable, and numerous additional species are conservation dependent or near threatened.[19] The Convention on International Trade in Endangered Species of Wild Fauna and Flora (CITES) lists the Jentink's duiker as Appendix I and the bay duiker (*Cephalophus dorsalis*), the blue duiker (*Cephalophus monticola* and *C. m. maxwelli**), the Ogilby's duiker (*Cephalophus ogilbyi*), the yellow-backed duiker, and the zebra duiker as Appendix II.[41]

The number of at-risk species can be expected to increase as more populations come under pressure. The reasons are familiar: habitat destruction for fuel and agricultural development, low animal population densities, and the bushmeat trade, which is highly commercialized and provides a significant amount of animal protein and income to the local inhabitants.[1, 11] The ever increasing dependence on bushmeat to support large rural communities has prompted the investigation of the use of common duikers in game ranching.[16]

In captivity, the International Species Inventory System (ISIS) lists approximately 442 individuals of nine species in 44 institutions.[20] The blue duiker, the common duiker, the yellow-backed duiker, the bay duiker, and the red duiker (*Cephalophus natalensis*) are the species most commonly held and bred. The Jentink's duiker is currently kept in only one institution (Gladys Porter Zoo, Brownsville, TX) and without additional animals or genetic material, their future is limited; the zebra duiker is currently held in only two institutions.

CAPTIVE MANAGEMENT

Husbandry

Relatively few institutions have maintained large numbers or species of duikers. The Chipangali Duiker Research and Breeding Centre (Bulawayo, Zimbabwe), Edinburgh Zoo—Scottish National Zoo (Edinburgh, Scotland), Societé Royale de Zoologie d'Anvers-Antwerp (Antwerp, Belgium), Pretoria National Zoologic Gardens, South Africa (Pretoria, South Africa), San Diego Zoo (San Diego, CA), and NYZS Wildlife Conservation Society (Bronx, NY) currently house major collections. In the past, the Pennsylvania State University Deer and Duiker Research Facility (University Park, PA), kept more than 100 blue duikers, and, at one time, the Gladys Porter Zoo kept more than 30 specimens of six species.[44]

*The Maxwell's duiker (previously *Cephalophus maxwelli*) is now generally recognized as a subspecies of the blue duiker (*Cephalophus monticola*).[42]

Several reports on captive management have been published.[13, 24, 30] In describing duikers, adjectives such as shy, wary, and elusive are usually followed by warnings such as fractious, explosive, and unpredictable. Duikers are best maintained in captivity in small, dimly lit indoor quarters and large, heavily planted outside enclosures that are situated well away from the public; flooring should be nonskid and provide good footing. These animals have a strong flight response but quickly hide if given the opportunity. If there is no such opportunity, the animals continue to flee, into moats and walls, until exhausted.

Duikers have acute auditory, olfactory, and visual faculties. Activity patterns vary and species are diurnal, crepuscular, or nocturnal. In the wild, duikers are generally solitary or found in pairs associated with subadult offspring; some species may be more social[38] and the blue duiker may be monogamous.[24] Males are territorial and combative with each other, they can be contentious with females in estrus, and are frequently hostile with calves; short lengths of hose can be placed over the horns of particularly aggressive individuals.

Duikers are best transported in darkened, enclosed, individual crates or portable dog kennels. The crate should be high enough for the animal to stand but not high enough to allow for jumping.[26] Tranquilization of particularly high-strung individuals should be considered. These crates also work well for maintaining individuals short term when circumstances require frequent handling (C. Miller, personal communication, 1996).

Longevity in the giant duikers appears to be 10 to 15 years, although some individuals have lived to be 19 to 21 years. Longevity in the smaller species of duikers is reported to be 10 to 12 years.[42]

Feeding and Nutrition

Much interest has been generated in the area of feeding and nutrition (W. C. Sadler, Mazuri Feeds, personal communication, 1996; S. Crissey, Nutritional Advisor, Antelope TAG, personal communication, 1996) because it is one of the most unique and least understood aspects of captive management. Simultaneously browsers and frugivores and occasionally carnivorous, duikers are considered concentrate selectors. There is also some variation in diet between species.[38] Free-ranging animals routinely consume fruit (majority of diet), seeds, fallen leaves, tubers, roots, bark, insects, termites, lizards, mice, and other small rodents. They have even been seen stalking, killing, and eating small birds.[42]

Duikers are described as primitive ruminants with significant cecal fiber fermentation. Numerous ruminal and cecal adaptations facilitate a quick turnover of food and a high fermentation rate; a mean transit time of 42.2 ± 6.4 hours has been recorded for a Maxwell's duiker.[10] Published articles concerning duiker nutrition have primarily focused on diet selection and preferences of free-ranging animals. Several digestive studies on captive duikers have also been published.[2, 3, 10, 14] In one feeding trial, neutral-detergent fiber (insoluble fiber) consumption averaged 34.2% of dry matter (DM), whereas crude protein consumption averaged 16.1% of

DM. Apparent DM digestion was 73% in Maxwell's duikers but was significantly lower in bay duikers (67%). Critical information regarding the chemical composition of natural diets and seasonal variation in nutritional requirements or food preferences is lacking to aid in the formulation of captive diets.[10] Papers on mineral metabolism[36, 37] and hindgut volatile fatty acid production[7, 8, 15] have also been written. Nutrient requirements have not been determined but Roeder and colleagues[36] suggest that a calcium:phosphorus ratio of 0.5%:0.4% appears to be the best suited for the blue duiker. Diets should contain vitamin E at a level of 200 IU/kg DM.[10]

It has been reported that common duikers rarely drink water[38]; however, this has not been the observation in captive giant duikers (J. Stones, personal communication, 1996).

In captivity, duikers are generally fed a base concentrate diet supplemented with a variety of fruits and vegetables and alfalfa hay; mineral blocks are supplied as needed. Additional menu items include dog chow, rabbit pellets, pig starter, bread, fresh browse, dried egg and dairy products, and vitamins. There have been numerous anecdotal reports of "nutritional" problems in duikers, including calcium/phosphorus imbalances, copper deficiencies, urolithiasis, and "wasting syndromes." However, there have been no systematic investigations of these presumed dietary induced maladies. Copper deficiency has been diagnosed several times, primarily in the smaller species including the bay, the black (*Cephalophus niger*), and the zebra duikers. Clinical signs include weight loss, despite an excellent appetite; a rough, dull, or sparse hair coat; a wide, pendulous abdomen; soft, dog-like stools; and general debilitation.[13]

A diagnosis is made based on clinical signs, on hematologic and chemistry results including anemia (red blood cell count [RBC] 4 to 6 $\times$ 10^6, normal 7.94 $\times$ 10^6; hematocrit [Hct] 20% to 30%, normal 40%) and hypocupremia (0.00 to 0.3 ppm, normal 0.7 to 2.0 ppm), and response to treatment.

Therapies have included copper supplementation in the form of intravenous (IV) injections (product unavailable) and oral bolusing. An oral copper oxide product (Copasure 12.5, Schering-Plough Animal Health, Kenilworth, NJ, 07033) was administered manually at a rate of 1 bolus (12.5 g)/duiker (weight range 11.34 to 16.78 kg). Blood copper levels increased an average of 10-fold within 1 month; one animal's blood copper level increased from 0.04 to 1.12 ppm. Normal copper blood levels were maintained for at least 1 year in at least one individual (author's unpublished data, 1994). This same product administered at a much lower dose in zebra duikers failed to produce a clinical response (M. Campbell, personal communication, 1994). Karesh and coworkers[22] found differences in plasma copper levels among free-ranging species (mean 0.65 to 1.18 ppm), which may reflect variation in dietary composition, absorption, or metabolism. In addition, copper levels were significantly lower in animals that were positive for trichurids.

Several veterinarians recount case histories of a "duiker wasting syndrome." Clinical signs range in severity between institutions and between individuals: poor hair coats and variable fecal consistency, fluid-filled, distended rumens, or cachexia and emaciation (C. Miller, personal communication, 1996; M. Campbell, personal communication, 1996). Even though these problems are especially prevalent in the smaller species of duikers, they have occurred in both Jentink's and yellow-backed duikers (H. Weston, personal communication, 1996, and J. Stones, personal communication, 1996). In some instances, these conditions have been responsive to changing the base concentrate to a browser diet (Mazuri Bovine Browser Breeder Diet Number 5653, PMI Feeds Incorporated, St. Louis, MO, 63144) (B. Gonzales, personal communication, 1992). It is not known whether these cases are related to a copper deficiency or whether these clinical signs represent one or more unrelated health problems, nutritional or otherwise.

At one zoo, there was improvement in the overall appearance of bay duikers and a decrease in the calf mortality rate with the inadvertent introduction of meat and poultry chicks into the diet. These items were apparently routinely "stolen" from the hornbills placed into the exhibit.[30]

At least one institution has had recurrent problems with urolithiasis in bay duikers. This problem has been substantially diminished by feeding a base concentrate containing ammonium chloride (Shepherd's Choice 15, Countrymark Cooperative, Incorporated, Indianapolis, IN, 46204) along with salted, grated carrots. A calculus was analyzed as 20% calcium oxalate, 20% calcium phosphate, 30% uric acid, and 30% ammonium acid urate (C. Bonner, personal communication, 1995); another calculus was composed solely of uric acid (C. Miller, personal communication, 1996).

Reproduction and Neonatology

REPRODUCTION

The estrous cycle in duikers appears to be about 1 month in length and is not seasonal.[13] Male duikers can be insistent with females, driving them, licking the female's perineum, and occasionally striking them with a foreleg or goring them with their horns. Copulation is brief. When not in estrus, the female generally runs away or lies down where the male cannot approach her rump.[13, 24] Calving intervals in duikers have been published as 235 days in red duikers, 265 days in blue duikers, and 399 days in yellow-backed duikers.[24, 38] One institution reports calving intervals as 268 days in bay duikers and 321 days in both the Jentink's and the yellow-backed duikers (J. Stones, personal communication, 1996). Because these intervals substantially exceed the presumed gestation periods, females may go through a postpartum anestrus or several periods of nonfertile estrous before becoming pregnant.[24]

Duikers produce a single calf, generally carried in the right uterine horn[38]; young are born throughout the year.

Published gestation lengths for the smaller duiker species vary widely from 126 days in a black duiker[13] to 191 days in the common duiker to 196 to 210 days in the blue duiker and the red duiker[6, 38] to possibly 255 to 270 days in the bay duiker.[42] Boehner and colleagues[6] noted considerable variation in the gestation lengths of blue duikers and proposed that male courtship of pregnant females may account for these discrepancies. Sexual maturity in these species is reported as generally less than 1 year but occasionally up to 18 months.[42]

There is only one reported gestation length in a giant duiker species, that of 151 days in a yellow-backed duiker.[13] An assisted reproduction pregnancy in a yellow-backed duiker that resulted in the birth of twins had a gestation length of 206 days. Although the female calves were substantially smaller than normal (1.85 kg; average 4.8 kg) and failed to survive, they appeared to be well developed, indicating that they were close to term (author's unpublished data, 1993). Sexual maturity probably occurs at a later age in the giant duikers. At the Gladys Porter Zoo, the youngest age at which a female has given birth is 2 years 5 months and the youngest age at which a male has sired offspring is 3 years 1 months, minus the gestation length (J. Stones, personal communication, 1996).

Two research projects in assisted reproduction in giant duikers have been undertaken[23, 31] (B. Foxworth, unpublished data, 1993). The study done by Pope and coworkers[31] involved two yellow-backed duikers and was conducted to develop a nonsurgical embryo collection technique. Prostaglandin injections were used for synchronization of estrus and follicle-stimulating hormone (FSH) injections were used to induce superovulation. No overt estrous behavior was observed and no ovarian observations were performed to document a response to FSH. Transcervical catheterization was used for uterine flushes. Although two embryos were collected from one female, there were no other successful collections.

A second study was undertaken at the Gladys Porter Zoo using both yellow-backed and Jentink's duikers in an effort to develop the techniques necessary for artificial insemination, interspecies embryo transfer, and the introduction of unrelated germ plasm into captive populations. Synchronization of estrus was accomplished using a combination of a controlled internal drug release (CIDR Type G, Harvey, Hamilton, New Zealand) progesterone implant, and prostaglandin injections. Superovulation was accomplished with FSH and pregnant mare serum gonadotropin injections. Transcervical catheterization of the uterus was performed for the uterine flushes. No embryos were collected. Laparoscopic evaluation demonstrated that the protocol did result in synchronization of estrus and yielded normal appearing corpora lutea, although follicular recruitment was poor. Transrectal ultrasonography proved useful for pregnancy detection, uterine evaluation, ovarian evaluation, and in monitoring uterine flushing.

As an adjunct to this investigation, determination of the estrous cycle, ovulation, and pregnancy based on the urinary hormone metabolite pregnanediol-3-glucuronide (PdG) was attempted, but this assay has yet to be successful.

Semen evaluations were also conducted. Initial attempts at semen collection by electroejaculation under manual restraint yielded poor results, probably because of the overall stress on the animal. Good erections were not achieved, although small samples could be collected. Electroejaculation under gas anesthesia also produced poor results. Although a good erection and extension of the penis was achieved, the sample was frequently contaminated with urine. Chemical immobilization with carfentanil and ketamine yielded the best semen results. Sample volumes ranged from 0.2 to 1.2 ml and contained 10 to 20 $\times$ 10[6] spermatozoa/ml (B. Foxworth, unpublished data, 1993).

NEONATOLOGY

Pregnancy in duikers is not always apparent, especially among the giant duikers. Distention of the udder (two inguinal mammae), a swollen vulva, and movements of the calf may be noted within 5 to 7 days of parturition.[24] Duiker calves are generally delivered quickly, easily, and in private. For the first few weeks, the calves stay hidden, only interacting with their dams during short nursing bouts. The milk composition of blue duiker milk and milk intake by blue duiker calves has been determined.[39, 40] Gross milk composition averaged 27.5% total solids, 12.2% fat, 9.8% crude protein, 3.8% lactose, and contained 178.6 kcal/100 g milk. Calves consumed 61, 76, 75, 64, 55, 46, and 31 g of milk/day when measured at weekly intervals from day 4 to day 53 postpartum.

Healthy calves require little medical attention beyond routine neonatal examinations. The glutaraldehyde coagulation test is a reliable indicator of passive transfer of colostral immunoglobulins. Elevated gamma-glutamyltransferase (GGT) and total protein values in young neonates may also be useful indicators of colostral intake. Neonatal blue duikers exhibit a microcytic hypochromic anemia at 2 to 4 weeks of age, possibly associated with hypoferremia and hyperphosphatemia. Serum enzyme activities are also elevated in the neonate, similar to the conditions observed in domestic animals.[35]

At birth, the deciduous incisors and lower canines of common duikers are either partially or fully erupted and the upper and lower premolars are just starting to erupt. The deciduous dentition is i 0/3 c 0/1 d 3/3 = 20. The first permanent tooth to erupt is the first lower molar, which appears within 2 to 3 months of birth. The second lower molar erupts at 8.5 to 10 months, the third at about 17 to 23 months. The permanent premolars appear at about 26 to 48 months and the incisors and canine teeth at about 60 months and older.[38, 43]

Calves grow rapidly and should double their birth weight, attaining at least 18% of adult weight, by 1 month of age.[24, 38] One institution reports that, although the calves do generally double their birth weight by 1 month of age, this weight represents only 15% of adult weight in Jentink's duiker and 5% to 10% of adult weight in yellow-backed duikers (J. Stones, personal communication, 1996). Calves from dams in their fourth or greater lactation consume more milk and gain weight more rapidly than calves from younger dams. Average daily weight gain (21 g/day in blue duikers) is greatest for the first 2 weeks after birth.[39, 40]

Calves are readily hand-reared for a variety of medical reasons including failure to thrive, maternal illness, and maternal rejection, or for management reasons such as to maximize a single female's reproduction or to make individuals more tractable and less fractious as adults. In management cases, calves should be left with their dams for 12 to 24 hours to allow for adequate colostrum consumption. A nursing test should be performed as part of the neonatal examination. Calves with sufficient colostral intake can be started on a dilute whole cow's milk formula at 10% to 20% of body weight per 24 hours, divided into equal feedings every 4 hours.

Healthy calves are generally "pulled" in the late afternoon and allowed to fast overnight to improve acceptance of the artificial nipple and formula. Concentration and volume are gradually increased and frequency of feedings decreased. Calves with inadequate colostral intake can be started on a dilute colostrum substitute at the same rate. Alternatively, plasma transfusions (dosed at 20 ml/kg IV) or whole blood transfusions (dosed at 2.2 ml/kg/1% increase in packed cell volume [PCV] with equal amounts of 0.9% NaCl IV) can be administered; usually the sire is used as a donor. Diarrhea is not uncommon in either case and generally resolves with time or with oral transfaunation from adult feces or commercially available products.

Water, hay, and concentrates are normally introduced at 1 to 2 months of age. Calves are generally raised with other hoofstock and given wide exposure to human caretakers. In most cases, this process results in calmer individuals; no deleterious effects on introduction or breeding propensities have been noted.

Duiker calves have been hand-reared at numerous institutions with minimal problems; goat's milk and powdered milk have also been used as replacement formulas[24] (C. Miller, personal communication, 1996; M. Campbell, personal communication, 1996).

Neonatal medical problems generally involve hypoglycemia, septicemia, or parental trauma. Severe hypoglycemia is a reliable prognostic indicator of immediate or impending poor health; rarely is it a transient, preprandial phenomenon.

Jentink's duikers in captivity are moderately inbred and the dams aged; in numerous calves, neonatal septicemia has developed, resulting in septic arthritis, hematogenous eye infections leading to blindness, pneumonia, and peritonitis. These illnesses are treated aggressively with IV fluids, antibiotics, blood transfusions, and joint and ocular therapy; the survival rate is 30%.

Parental trauma usually results when the sire is not removed before an impending birth or when an occasional primiparous dam inflicts injury. Two zoos have reported maternal aggression after a calf was returned following a neonatal examination (C. Miller, personal communication, 1996; M. Kinsey, personal communication, 1996).

Congenital abnormalities include luxated scapulohumeral joints bilaterally, uterine aplasia, and microphthalmia in yellow-backed duikers (C. Miller, personal communication, 1996).

ANESTHESIA AND RESTRAINT
Manual Restraint

Duikers can be restrained by either physical or chemical means. Physical restraint may be used to facilitate ad-

ministration of chemical restraint, or as the sole restraint agent for minor, rapid procedures. Animals must initially be netted or driven into a small, solid, heavily bedded stall; night quarters work well. This method is easier with smaller species, but even the giant duikers can be physically restrained with proper technique. Some individuals may be too fractious for manual restraint or, in the case of a giant duiker, too aggressive for keeper safety.

Duikers vocalize, kick, gore, and even attempt to bite, and precautions including wearing proper clothing, gloves, and shoes should be taken to avoid keeper injury. A small bale of hay may be carried and used to deflect the horns of larger species.

Once caught, the animal should be secured in lateral recumbency and quickly sedated or processed. Afterward, the animal should be released into another small, heavily bedded, darkened stall; in most cases, the animal immediately settles down, as long as there is no additional visual or auditory stimulation.

Chemical Restraint

Several chemical restraint protocols for tranquilization or immobilization of free-ranging or captive duikers have been published (Tables 102–1 and 102–2).[4, 5, 13, 18, 26]

IMMOBILIZATION

Gladys Porter Zoo currently maintains bay duikers, yellow-backed duikers, and Jentink's duikers. The bay duikers are usually manually restrained and immobilized with isoflurane via facemask. Several chemical restraint protocols have been used for the giant duikers, depending on circumstances. All injectable protocols have resulted, at some time, in effects ranging from excellent anesthesia to anesthetic death.

Regurgitation is the leading anesthetic complication; animals should be intubated as soon as possible and care should be taken to minimize movement of the animal. Withholding food and water for 24 to 48 hours seems to have little effect on the incidence of regurgitation but it is generally practiced nonetheless. Roeder and colleagues[37] stated that blue duikers fasted for 18 hours (food) and 6 hours (water) had ingesta in their forestomachs, although in a reduced quantity. Animals remained adequately hydrated as reflected by normoproteinemia and PCV values as compared to unfasted duikers. To minimize anesthetic complications during assisted reproduction attempts, giant duikers were manually restrained and masked down with isoflurane. Even though this was by far the safest anesthetic protocol, this method does have some drawbacks including cost, the necessity of moving a large animal anesthesia machine around the zoo, and stress to the duikers and their keepers because manual restraint is still required. And, whereas this method provided excellent relaxation for procedures in the female, it yielded poor electroejaculation results. A preanesthetic tranquilizer should be considered with this immobilization protocol.

Overall, there appear to be fewer anesthetic complications with etorphine than with carfentanil, with the

TABLE 102–1. Immobilization Protocols for Duiker Species

Duiker Species	kg	Etorphine	Fentanyl	Ketamine	Xylazine	Medetomidine	Zoletil*	Azaperone	Reversal
Cephalophus monticola	4–10		0.3–0.5 mg/kg +		0.4–0.8 mg/kg[4]				Narcotic reversal
			2–3 mg +	75 mg +	1–2 mg[26]		25 mg[26]	5 mg[26]	Narcotic reversal
		0.03 mg/kg +		2.2 mg/kg +	0.4–0.8 µg/kg[4]	190 µg/kg			Narcotic reversal Atipamazole 0.95 mg/kg; 1/2 IV + 1/2 IM[4]
Cephalophus m. maxwelli	4–10	0.5 mg[13]							Narcotic reversal
Cephalophus natalensis	11–13	0.5 mg OR	5 mg +					5 mg[26]	Narcotic reversal
Sylvicapra grimmia	10–20			100 mg +	3 mg[26]		70 mg[26]		
				2.2 mg/kg +		190 µg/kg			Atipamazole 0.95 mg/kg; 1/2 IV + 1/2 IM[4]
		0.5–1.0 mg OR	8–10 mg +	13.1 mg/kg +	16.4 mg/kg[5] 1–2 mg OR 5 mg[26]			20 mg[26]	Narcotic reversal
				100 mg +			110–140 mg[26]		Narcotic reversal
Syvicapra grimmia		0.02 mg/kg[26] 0.3–0.6 mg[26]	5–7 mg[26]		1–2 mg OR 15 mg[26]			20 mg[26]	Narcotic reversal
		0.5–1.0 mg OR	8–10 mg +	100 mg +	5 mg[26]			25 mg[26]	Narcotic reversal
Cephalophus dorsalis	15 kg	0.75–1.25 mg[13]					6–8 mg/kg[26]		Narcotic reversal
Cephalophus niger	15–20	1–2 mg[13]							Narcotic reversal
Cephalophus zebra	15–20	0.75–1.0 mg[13]							Narcotic reversal

Note some doses are in mg/kg and some are in total dose; note also that each line may be a drug combination of one narcotic or another plus one neuroleptic or another.
All doses are intramuscular unless otherwise indicated.
*Zoletil, Palmvet Services, Rynfield 1514, Republic of South Africa.

TABLE 102–2. Gladys Porter Zoo Immobilization Protocols for Giant Duiker Species

Duiker Species	kg	Etorphine	Carfentanil	Xylazine	Ketamine	Acepromazine	Diprenorphine	Naltrexone	Yohimbine
C. jentinkii OR	70	4–6 mg +		20–30 mg		8–10 mg	8–12 mg IV		5 mg IV
C. sylvicultor	80	3.0 mg +	1–2 mg	10–15 mg	100 mg IV if required for intubation		6.0 mg IV	100 mg/l mg carfentanil; 1/4 IV + 3/4 SQ	10 mg IV

Note that each line is a drug combination.
All doses are intramuscular unless otherwise indicated.

highest percentage of complications related to the use of IV carfentanil in manually restrained duikers—even at very low doses of the narcotic.

TRANQUILIZATION

Haloperidol is the tranquilizer of choice for duikers, with dosages ranging from 0.25 to 0.75 mg/kg, 3 to 5 mg/animal for smaller species, 5.0 to 7.5 mg/animal for mid size species, and 10 to 20 mg/animal for giant duiker species.[18, 26] The drug is generally administered IV to animals before their removal from capture nets; effects are noted within 5 minutes. Higher doses may induce sternal recumbency and drowsiness, but usually no pronounced soporific effects. Extrapyramidal effects such as chewing, licking, and pica may occur, but are usually transitory. Therapeutic levels are generally maintained for at least 12 hours. Auditory and visual stimuli as well as prior chemical immobilizing agents may influence the degree of neuroleptic effect.[18]

The long-acting tranquilizer perphenazine has been used alone at a dose of 25 to 50 mg/animal in free-ranging blue duiker, red duiker, and common duiker, and at lower doses in combination with haloperidol. Azaperone has also been used in the common duiker at 10 to 20 mg/animal[26] and 0.5 to 1.0 mg/kg, and in the yellow-backed duiker at 0.8 to 1.0 mg/kg (C. Miller, personal communication, 1996).

MEDICINE

Biological Data

Baseline physiological data for "at rest" duikers has not been determined. Values obtained from blue duikers under ketamine/medetomidine anesthesia were temperature of 39.4°C, heart rate of 83.3 beats/minute, and respiratory rate of 36.3 respirations/minute.[4]

ANATOMY

With so many species of duikers, there are considerable physical variations among them. The smallest is the 4-kg blue duiker, the largest is the yellow-backed duiker, which can weigh up to 80 kg. Females are typically larger than males. In contrast to captive individuals, free-ranging bay duikers were considerably heavier (23.5 kg versus 15 kg); the blue duikers averaged 4.5 kg. The average weights of an additional three midsize species of free-ranging duikers has also been determined.[22] The horns are short, straight, and point backwards; both males and females sport horns (except among the common duiker). Pelage colors include hues of gray, blue, red, brown, and black; some species are solid colored, others have shadings, patches, or stripes; the skin is tough. Duikers have short legs in relation to body size, are higher and wider in the rear quarters, and are well muscled overall; the giant duikers are powerful and formidable.

The position and number of glands for scent marking vary with species and include preorbital, maxillary, pedal, and inguinal.

The adult dentition is I 0/3, C 0/1, P 3/3, M 3/3 = 32.[38] The rumen is a small, simple, sacculated S-shaped tube, densely papillated with highly vascular, fungiform papillae; the ostia are large and the pillars weak. The omasum is reduced in size, having few leaflets with horny papillae; it is thought to serve a filtration function.[15] Duikers do not possess a gallbladder.

CLINICAL PATHOLOGY

The International Species Inventory System (ISIS) lists normal blood values compiled for five species of captive duikers[21] (Tables 102–3 and 102–4). In addition, papers have been published with comparative blood values for captive blue duikers by age group,[35] captive common versus blue duikers,[5] and a comprehensive health assessment of five species of free-ranging duikers.[22]

In general, duikers exhibit a 20% to 30% neutrophil:70% to 80% lymphocyte ratio similar to other ruminants; erythrocyte values and indices are most similar to those of equine species. Platelet counts vary widely. In general, they appear to be elevated in comparison with those of other hoofstock, often two or three times higher; this is especially true in abnormal individuals (T. Hermann, personal communication, 1996). With few exceptions, duikers have serum/plasma biochemical, vitamin, and mineral levels similar to those of domesticated ruminants.[35] Roeder and coworkers[35] reported that significant differences in hematologic and serum biochemical values do exist among neonatal, juvenile, and adult male and female blue duikers. The differences in electrolytes, glucose levels, and lipid products between young and adult duikers appear to be associated with dietary intake and rumen maturity; no reasons were put forth for the variety of hematology and chemistry differences between adult male and female duikers.

Roeder and colleagues[35] also reported higher inorganic phosphorus (Pi) levels (10.4 mg/dl) and lower calcium (Ca) levels (9.3 mg/dl) in blue duikers than in domestic ruminants. Blue duikers (and possibly other duiker species) may be unique in their serum electrolyte homeostasis. Diet appears to influence the mechanisms controlling circulating levels of serum Ca and Pi as well as acid-base balance. Adult male blue duikers respond to levels of dietary Ca, Pi, and other minerals with altered serum and or urinary concentrations of these elements. Unlike domestic ruminants, blue duiker serum Pi levels are affected by Ca intake and their serum Ca concentration is not decreased by increasing Pi intake. Volumetric urine clearance data may be valuable in this species to help understand Ca and Pi homeostasis and dietary balance of minerals.[36, 37]

In a comprehensive health assessment of five free-ranging duiker species, Karesh and colleagues[22] reported higher PCV values (range 48.3% to 57.1%), lower total solids (range 6.1 to 7.4 g/dl), and higher glucose levels (range 162.4 to 211.2 mg/dl) than had been previously published; also noted were lower cholesterol levels (range 97.9 to 113.1 mg/dl) but the ratio of tocopherol to cholesterol remained in the normal 1.0 to 3.0 range. In addition, mean Pi levels were lower (range 7.2 to 9.4 mg/dl) and Ca levels (range 10.5 to

TABLE 102–3. Hematology and Serum Chemistry Values for Captive Duiker Species[21]

Parameter	Units	*Cephalophus dorsalis* Mean SD (n)	*Cephalophus maxwelli* Mean SD (n)	*Cephalophus monticola* Mean SD (n)	*Cephlaophus niger* Mean SD (n)
Red blood cells	$\times 10^6/\mu l$	7.94 ± 1.93 (30)	10.42 ± 3.46 (44)	10.66 ± 2.15 (11)	7.50 ± 0.00 (1)
Hematocrit	%	40.2 ± 8.7 (77)	40.3 ± 10.1 (64)	41.6 ± 8.2 (20)	39.8 ± 11.3 (4)
Hemaglobin	g/dl	14.1 ± 2.6 (60)	14.7 ± 3.3 (59)	13.5 ± 2.4 (17)	12.7 ± 6.1 (2)
MCH	pg	16.8 ± 44 (29)	14.7 ± 4.0 (43)	12.8 ± 1.4 (11)	11.2 ± 0.0 (1)
MCHC	g/dl	34.1 ± 2.8 (59)	35.9 ± 4.8 (58)	33.0 ± 5.0 (17)	34.1 ± 4.2 (2)
MCV	fl	49.3 ± 13.0 (30)	40.6 ± 8.00 (43)	38.0 ± 5.0 (11)	36.0 ± 0.0 (1)
Erythrocyte sedimentation rate	mm/hour	2 ± 1 (3)		1 ± 1 (2)	
White blood cells	$\times 10^3/\mu l$	8.016 ± 3.288 (59)	4.939 ± 2.672 (49)	5.758 ± 3.129 (21)	5.487 ± 1.551 (3)
Neutrophils	$\times 10^3/\mu l$	2.844 ± 2.086 (54)	2.020 ± 1.924 (42)	2.466 ± 1.940 (20)	2.553 ± 1.159 (3)
Bands	$\times 10^3/\mu l$	0.742 ± 1.292 (4)	0.170 ± 0.308 (5)	0.035 ± 0.000 (1)	
Lymphocytes	$\times 10^3/\mu l$	4.480 ± 2.175 (54)	2.808 ± 1.677 (42)	3.018 ± 1.679 (20)	2.840 ± 0.520 (3)
Monocytes	$\times 10^3/\mu l$	0.389 ± 0.482 (41)	0.246 ± 0.343 (27)	0.559 ± 0.548 (16)	0.137 ± 0.016 (2)
Eosinophils	$\times 10^3/\mu l$	0.254 ± 0.285 (25)	0.164 ± 0.262 (10)	0.101 ± 0.040 (3)	
Basophils	$\times 10^3/\mu l$	0.068 ± 0.046 (5)	0.024 ± 0.035 (5)		
Nucleated RBC	/100 WBC	3 ± 0 (1)	2 ± 0 (1)		0 ± 0 (1)
Reticulocytes	%			0.1 ± 0.0 (2)	
Platelets	$\times 10^3/\mu l$	457 ± 317 (8)	957 ± 856 (10)	631 ± 131 (3)	
Fibrinogen	mg/dl	300 ± 141 (2)		100 ± 0 (1)	
Glucose	mg/dl	102 ± 47 (57)	110 ± 57 (43)	107 ± 89 (14)	87 ± 27 (4)
Blood urea nitrogen	mg/dl	31 ± 11 (55)	30 ± 8 (41)	28 ± 13 (16)	28 ± 21 (4)
Creatinine	mg/dl	1.4 ± 0.3 (54)	1.5 ± 0.5 (35)	0.8 ± 0.4 (15)	1.1 ± 0.2 (3)
Uric acid	mg/dl	0.9 ± 0.8 (22)	0.2 ± 0.2 (17)	0.0 ± 0.1 (9)	0.2 ± 0.0 (1)
Calcium	mg/dl	9.8 ± 1.0 (56)	9.9 ± 1.8 (40)	9.1 ± 0.7 (14)	10.5 ± 0.6 (3)
Phosphorus	mg/dl	9.1 ± 2.3 (54)	10.0 ± 2.7 (40)	9.6 ± 2.9 (14)	11.6 ± 1.6 (3)
Sodium	mEq/L	143 ± 6 (51)	151 ± 7 (35)	146 ± 3 (14)	149 ± 10 (3)
Potassium	mEq/L	5.4 ± 1.1 (51)	6.3 ± 1.9 (37)	6.0 ± 1.6 (14)	8.3 ± 2.6 (3)
Chloride	mEq/L	101 ± 5 (48)	109 ± 5 (34)	101 ± 5 (14)	108 ± 1 (3)
Iron	μg/dl	154 ± 81 (9)	194 ± 151 (4)	271 ± 56 (2)	
TIBC	μg/dl	400.3 ± 26.6 (3)†			
Magnesium	mg/dl	3.95 ± 0.43 (8)	2.10 ± 0.00 (1)	2.70 ± 0.00 (1)	
Copper	ppm	0.626 ± 0.564 (11)†			
Molybdenum	mg/L	16.20 ± 12.45 (2)†			
Zinc	mg/L	1.160 ± 0.000 (1)†			

11.5 mg/dl) were higher than values reported for captive duikers and more within the range of reported normal values for domestic bovines. As discussed, this could be diet related and implies that the diets of captive animals are not providing levels of calcium and phosphorus that are biologically equivalent to those in the diets of their free-ranging counterparts. Other plasma mineral concentrations fell within normal ranges for domestic ruminant animals except for magnesium (range 3.8 to 4.4 mg/dl), which was greater than expected; it was also higher than the ISIS means for magnesium, except in the bay duiker.

Roeder and coworkers[35] reported that blue duikers urinate frequently and have highly concentrated urine.

Infectious Disease

PARASITIC DISEASES

Published reports of external, internal, and hemoparasites of free-ranging duikers comprise the vast majority of literature review abstracts. It should be assumed that duiker species are susceptible to the same nematode, cestode, and trematode parasites as other Bovidae species and perhaps other families as well. Karesh and associates[22] found 34% of free-ranging duikers sampled positive for parasites or parasite ova in their feces; coccidia and strongyles were the most prevalent. Ticks were found only on rare occasion. There was no correlation between an animal's general condition and the presence of parasitic ova. Despite the apparent good physical condition of all the animals in this study, there were significant differences in mean hematology values, and serum chemistry, enzyme, mineral, and vitamins levels in parasite positive individuals. These abnormalities included higher total protein and immunoglobulin levels in animals with strongyles, lower total solids in animals with trichurids and coccidia, lower copper levels in animals with trichurids, lower alpha-tocopherol and cholesterol ratios in animals with coccidia, and a higher percentage of eosinophils and a lower percentage of lymphocytes in animals with strongyles.

TABLE 102–3. Hematology and Serum Chemistry Values for Captive Duiker Species *Continued*

Parameter	Units	*Cephalophus dorsalis* Mean SD (n)	*Cephalophus maxwelli* Mean SD (n)	*Cephalophus monticola* Mean SD (n)	*Cephlaophus niger* Mean SD (n)
Cholesterol	mg/dl	122 ± 35 (44)	117 ± 34 (41)	157 ± 39 (14)	92 ± 28 (3)
Trigly	mg/dl	33 ± 23 (20)	41 ± 34 (14)	123 ± 227 (8)	64 ± 0 (1)
T Protein	g/dl	8.5 ± 1.0 (50)	7.9 ± 1.5 (38)	6.9 ± 0.7 (15)	7.1 ± 2.4 (3)
Albumin	g/dl	3.8 ± 0.6 (49)	3.7 ± 0.9 (30)	3.4 ± 0.6 (9)	3.2 ± 1.1 (3)
Globulin	g/dl	4.6 ± 1.2 (48)	4.1 ± 1.6 (30)	3.4 ± 1.0 (9)	4.0 ± 1.3 (3)
AST (SGOT)	IU/L	134 ± 71 (55)	171 ± 158 (35)	159 ± 108 (15)	185 ± 39 (3)
ALT (SGPT)	IU/L	18 ± 8 (46)	61 ± 116 (39)	21 ± 9 (12)	19 ± 1 (3)
T Bilirubin	mg/dl	0.3 ± 0.4 (51)	0.4 ± 0.4 (36)	0.2 ± 0.1 (14)	0.8 ± 0.9 (3)
D Bilirubin	mg/dl	0.1 ± 0.1 (29)	0.0 ± 0.1 (9)	0.1 ± 0.1 (7)	0.5 ± 0.7 (3)
I Bilirubin	mg/dl	0.2 ± 0.1 (29)	0.2 ± 0.1 (9)	0.1 ± 0.1 (7)	0.3 ± 0.2 (3)
GGT	IU/L	94 ± 30 (25)	79 ± 82 (8)	42 ± 11 (8)	167 ± 59 (3)
Lipase	U/L	10 ± 0 (1)			111 ± 22 (3)
Amylase	U/L	112 ± 156 (20)	450 ± 26 (3)	157 ± 85 (7)	
ALK PHOS	IU/L	984 ± 828 (52)	570 ± 571 (43)	349 ± 347 (15)	693 ± 897 (3)
LDH	IU/L	569 ± 289 (35)	806 ± 1248 (35)	717 ± 717 (10)	205 ± 0 (1)
CPK	IU/L	588 ± 297 (26)	278 ± 345 (17)	375 ± 151 (8)	266 ± 5 (3)
Osmolality	mOsm/L	294 ± 10 (12)	302 ± 16 (2)		
Anion gap		26.50 ± 10.61 (2)†			
CO_2	mmol/L	18.0 ± 7.0 (9)	15.9 ± 6.9 (15)	17.0 ± 5.6 (2)	14.7 ± 7.0 (3)
HCO_3	mmol/L			11.0 ± 0 (1)	
Cortisol	μg/dl	3.9 ± 1.8 (7)			
CORT (POST)*	μg/dl	5.450 ± 0.354 (2)†			
ENDOG ACTH	pg/ml	755.3 (7)†			
ACTH (POST)*	pg/ml	6992.0 (6)†			
Total T_4	μg/dl	1.9 ± 1.3 (4)			
Free T_4	ng/dl	16.23 ± 1.10 (4)†			
T_3 (RIA)	ng/dl	1.175 ± 0.263 (4)†			
Retinol	μg/dl	0.932 ± 0.212 (5)†			
α-Tocopherol	μg/ml	2.230 ± 0.633 (7)†			

ACTH, adrenocorticotropic hormone (POST, postadministration of the ACTH); ALK PHOS, alkaline phosphatase; ALT, alanine aminotransferase (SGPT, serum glutamic pyruvate transaminase); AST, aspartate aminotransferase (SGOT, serum glutamic-oxaloacetic transaminase); CORT, cortisol; CPK, creatine phosphokinase; ENDOG, endogenous; GGT, gamma glutamyltransferase; LDH, lactate dehydrogenase; MCH, mean corpuscular hemoglobin; MCHC, mean corpuscular hemoglobin concentration; MCV, mean corpuscular volume; RBC, red blood cell; TIBC, total iron binding capacity; Trigly, triglyceride.

*ACTH Stimulation Test; results obtained 2 hours after administration of ACTH.

†Values from Gladys Porter Zoo.

From International Species Inventory System: MedARKS ISIS Physiologic Data. Apple Valley, ISIS, 1996.

Parasites usually present few problems for captive individuals, although serious illness has been attributed to both coccidiosis and intestinal nematodiasis; positive animals should be treated with routine antiparasitics.[13]

Besnoitiosis of the reproductive tract of a captive born blue duiker was noted as an incidental necropsy finding. This benign condition was in sharp contrast to the severe orchitis, epididymitis, and infertility caused by besnoitiosis in cattle.[17] Verminous pneumonia in common duikers has been reported. The nematodes were similar to *Muellerius capillaris*, but a definitive identification was not possible.[29]

BACTERIAL AND VIRAL DISEASES

As with parasites, it should be assumed that duikers are susceptible to a wide variety of bacterial and viral agents; frequently these infections may be nonpathologic. Wild duiker species were found to have positive antibody titers for leptospirosis, bluetongue virus, infectious bovine rhinotracheitis, and epizootic hemorrhagic disease; serologic tests for foot-and-mouth disease, rinderpest, bovine viral diarrhea, brucellosis, and anaplasmosis were negative. Once again, significant differences in mean hematology values and in serum chemistry, enzyme, mineral, and vitamins levels were seen between serologically positive and negative individuals.[22] Other researchers have reported duikers positive for brucellosis[28] and anaplasmosis.[25]

Leptospirosis may deserve some further attention because of its prevalence (26% of the free-ranging population), zoonotic potential, and a possible leptospirosis related abortion in a bay duiker at the Wildlife Conservation Park/Bronx Zoo.[22]

There have been several reports of viral and bacterial diseases in captive duiker species. A red-flanked duiker (*Cephalophus rufilatus*) died of malignant catarrhal fever. Clinical signs included diarrhea, ataxia, and recumbency.[27] A presumed outbreak of viral encephalomyelitis occurred in giant duikers. Clinical signs included

TABLE 102–4. Hematology and Serum Chemistry Values for Captive Giant Duiker Species

Parameter	Units	*Cephalophus sylvicultor* Mean SD (n)	*Cephalophus jentinkii* Mean SD (n)
Red blood cells	$\times 10^6/\mu l$	8.56 ± 2.07 (34)	
Hematocrit	%	41.5 ± 8.3 (86)	41.2 ± 7.1 (31)
Hemoglobin	g/dl	13.5 ± 2.6 (36)	
MCH	pg	16.2 ± 2.1 (34)	
MCHC	g/dl	35.7 ± 2.5 (35)	
MCV	fl	44.6 ± 4.8 (33)	
White blood cells	$\times 10^3/\mu l$	7.099 ± 3.410 (79)	5.821 ± 2.023 (28)
Neutrophils	$\times 10^3/\mu l$	3.134 ± 1.535 (73)	2.254 ± 1.321 (28)
Bands	$\times 10^3/\mu l$	0.065 ± 0.130 (27)	0.225 ± 0.258 (3)
Lymphocytes	$\times 10^3/\mu l$	3.366 ± 1.700 (73)	3.297 ± 1.465 (28)
Monocytes	$\times 10^3/\mu l$	0.201 ± 0.160 (53)	0.203 ± 0.138 (25)
Eosinophils	$\times 10^3/\mu l$	0.128 ± 0.177 (48)	0.156 ± 0.075 (12)
Basophils	$\times 10^3/\mu l$	0.043 ± 0.069 (28)	
Nucleated RBCs	/100 WBC	0 ± 0 (12)	1 ± 1 (2)
Reticulocytes	%	0.0 ± 0.0 (1)	
Platelets	$\times 10^3/\mu l$	899 ± 598 (6)	
Fibrinogen	mg/dl	317 ± 117 (6)	
Glucose	mg/dl	94 ± 43 (53)	74 ± 37 (11)
Blood urea nitrogen	mg/dl	28 ± 9 (50)	31 ± 17 (11)
Creatinine	mg/dl	1.3 ± 0.3 (49)	2.1 ± 0.5 (11)
Uric acid	mg/dl	0.1 ± 0.2 (18)	0.2 ± 0.0 (1)
Calcium	mg/dl	9.3 ± 1.0 (50)	9.7 ± 1.6 (11)
Phosphorus	mg/dl	8.4 ± 1.8 (47)	9.5 ± 2.0 (11)
Sodium	mEq/L	141 ± 5 (43)	145 ± 3 (2)
Potassium	mEq/L	4.9 ± 1.0 (44)	4.9 ± 0.4 (2)
Chloride	mEq/L	100 ± 4 (43)	107 ± 5 (2)
Iron	$\mu g/dl$	123 ± 60 (13)	25 ± 16 (2)
Magnesium	mg/dl	3.40 ± 0.98 (5)	3.52 ± 0.48 (9)
Copper	ppm	0.425 ± 0.306 (6)*	1.030 ± 0.515 (4)*
Molybdenum	mg/L	51.00 ± 0.00 (1)*	
Cholesterol	mg/dl	114 ± 38 (41)	45 ± 0 (2)
Trigly	mg/dl	40 ± 45 (17)	11 ± 1 (2)
T Protein	g/dl	7.5 ± 1.1 (45)	7.7 ± 2.3 (11)
Albumin	g/dl	3.5 ± 0.7 (35)	2.9 ± 0.7 (11)
Globulin	g/dl	4.0 ± 1.1 (35)	4.8 ± 1.9 (11)
AST (SGOT)	IU/L	222 ± 244 (50)	155 ± 42 (11)
ALT (SGPT)	IU/L	19 ± 10 (44)	16 ± 4 (2)
T Bilirubin	mg/dl	0.5 ± 0.4 (47)	0.5 ± 0.6 (11)
D Bilirubin	mg/dl	0.3 ± 0.2 (3)	
I Bilirubin	mg/dl	0.1 ± 0.1 (3)	
GGT	IU/L	85 ± 28 (22)	106 ± 11 (10)
Amylase	U/L	162 ± 79 (10)	37 ± 0 (1)
ALK PHOS	IU/L	658 ± 427 (47)	691 ± 1095 (11)
LDH	IU/L	640 ± 516 (38)	722 ± 569 (11)
CPK	IU/L	530 ± 351 (29)	508 ± 287 (9)
Osmolality	mOsm/L	295 ± 5 (2)	
Anion gap			20.50 ± 4.95 (2)*
CO_2	mmol/L	23.4 ± 5.6 (18)	22.5 ± 2.1 (2)
HCO_3	mmol/L	27.0 ± 2.7 (5)	
Total T_4	$\mu g/dl$	14.0 ± 0.0 (1)	
T_3 (RIA)	ng/dl	5.8 ± 0.0 (1)	
Retinol	$\mu g/dl$	0.519 ± 0.116 (7)*	0.445 ± 0.276 (2)*
α-Tocopherol	$\mu g/ml$	1.488 ± 0.580 (9)*	1.700 ± 0.221 (4)*

ALK PHOS, alkaline phosphatase; ALT, alanine aminotransferase (SGPT, serum glutamic pyruvate transaminase); AST, aspartate aminotransferase (SGOT, serum glutamic oxaloacetic transaminase); CPK, creatine phosphokinase; GGT, gamma glutamyltransferase; LDH, lactate dehydrogenase; MCH, mean corpuscular hemoglobin; MCHC, mean corpuscular hemoglobin concentration; MCV mean corpuscular volume; RBC, red blood cell; Trigly, triglyceride.

*Values from Gladys Porter Zoo.

From International Species Inventory System: MedARKS ISIS Physiologic Data. Apple Valley, MN 1996.

anorexia, rough hair coat, mild diarrhea, and a progressively severe ataxia; individuals became comatose before death. Some laboratory results implicated Venezuelan equine encephalitis (VEE).[12] Since that incident, all duikers in the institution have been vaccinated with a three-way equine encephalitis product. A recent spate of clinical cases involving possible neurologic disease at that same institution (Gladys Porter Zoo) prompted an investigation of serologic titers in two serially vaccinated animals. One yellow-backed male had clinical signs of a head-tilt and ataxia, which stabilized (but did not completely resolve) after several weeks. The Western equine encephalomyelitis (WEE) titer was positive at 1:20 and was considered not significant; titers to VEE and Eastern equine encephalitis (EEE) were negative. A second animal had severe, peracute ataxia. Titers to all three viruses were negative. This individual died within 48 hours, and no cause of death was determined on gross necropsy or histopathologic study (author, unpublished data, 1995).

Two papers have been published involving subcutaneous abscesses in duikers. *Actinomyces pyogenes* was isolated from a subcutaneous abscess (anatomic site not listed) and a foot abscess in two yellow-backed duikers in the first report.[45] *Fusobacterium necrophorum*, *Actinomyces pyogenes*, *Bacteroides* species and other bacteria were isolated from 12 blue duikers in the second report.[34] In many cases, abscesses appear sterile on cytology and fail to grow an organism in culture. It is unclear whether these are sterile abscesses or infections resulting from fastidious or anaerobic bacteria. Once opened and drained, they rarely recur. They do not occur in locations used for vaccinations.

Roeder and coworkers[34] reported that facial soft tissues and mandibles were the tissues most often affected; tissues within the oral cavity were not affected initially. A unique aspect of this infection was the presence of nondestructive mandibular proliferation. Total protein and globulin levels were elevated in all individuals; some showed a neutrophilic leukocytosis or shifts in the lymphocyte:neutrophil ratio above or below the usual 70:30 range. This epizootic appeared to be related to the introduction of infected carrier animals brought from another institution, coarse feed texture, and masticatory behavior. Although most infections are considered endogenous in origin, carrier animals have been implicated in the introduction of pathogenic bacteria to previously naive animals. Most duikers in this herd chewed in a clockwise motion, leaving most of the food on the right side of the oral cavity. This observation correlated with a pattern of predominantly right sided facial abscesses. Treatment consisted of antibiotic therapy and local debridement, flushing with antibacterial solutions, and drain placement. Septicemia developed in one animal, which died. Abscesses were resolved in the remaining animals, but the mandibular proliferation appeared to be permanent. In addition to nondestructive mandibular proliferation, mandibular osteomyelitis (classic "lumpy jaw") is a common problem in duikers. Several institutions report problems of this nature in their collection (C. Miller, personal communication, 1996; C. Bonner, personal communication, 1996; M. Campbell, personal communication, 1996; personal ob-

servation). In cases of malalignment of the dental arcade, malocclusion, or mandibular osteomyelitis, oral surgery with tooth extraction should be considered.

Antibiotic usage should be based on culture and sensitivity. Oral trimethoprim-sulfamethoxazole dosed on an equine schedule has proven anectodally to be an effective antibiotic regimen for sensitive organisms; tilmicosin has also proven effective at a bovine dose and has the added advantage of an every 72 hours dosing schedule (M. Campbell, personal communication, 1996). Salmonellosis was responsible for the death of a bay duiker at one institution (C. Miller, personal communication, 1996). Pneumonia appears to be a common cause of death. Antibiotics should be used long-term but the benefits must be weighed against the stress and hazards of administration.

Non-Infectious Disease

Common non-infectious problems that occur at multiple institutions include exhibit mate trauma, such as with male-female or parental-calf interactions, overgrown hooves, and self-trauma. Wounds, abrasions, luxations, and fractures frequently result from an exaggerated flight response. Acral lick dermatitis is common as duikers frequently "worry" a wound, often enlarging it and impeding healing. Chronic renal disease seems to be a common necropsy finding, especially in aged individuals. Several incidents of possible adrenal exhaustion have occurred in bay duikers. Clinical presentation was one of acute, generalized paresis or recumbency. Clinical pathology usually indicated hypoglycemia (25 mg/dl; normal 102 mg/dl) and an abnormal Na:K ratio (20:1; normal 26.5:1). Cases readily responded to fluid therapy with 0.9% NaCl and 5% dextrose. Serum electrolyte values improved within a few days. Experimental adrenocorticotropic hormone (ACTH) stimulation tests were performed. Serum cortisol and endogenous ACTH were measured before and 2 hours after administration of 2.2 U/kg of ACTH (H.P. Acthar Gel, Armour Pharmaceutical, Collegeville, PA, 19426). Cortisol levels generally increased twofold to threefold (see Table 102–3). Results were inconclusive (author, unpublished data, 1994).

Two case reports involving duikers have been published. The first involved an otitis in a blue duiker[33] and the second, surgical correction of bilateral laryngeal paralysis in a yellow-backed duiker.[9] Treatment of the laryngeal paralysis included the use of a temporary laryngostomy.

Preventive Medicine

Preventive medicine protocols generally include neonatal examinations, periodic fecal parasitology examinations, immunizations, and necropsies. Optimally, annual physical examinations could be performed but must be weighed against the anesthetic and accidental injury risks. All opportunistic examinations should include diagnostic tests to monitor the aforementioned health problems.

NEONATAL EXAMINATION

Examinations should be performed within 12 to 24 hours of birth and minimally include physical examination and weight, blood collection for hematology, assessment of colostral immunoglobulin absorption, glucose, and GGT, prophylactic administration of an iron supplement and a vitamin E supplement, treatment of the umbilicus if required, application of ophthalmic ointment, and placement of permanent identification.

Additional follow-up examinations, biweekly or monthly, can also be performed, especially with hand-reared individuals.

FECAL PARASITOLOGY

Routine fecal flotations should be performed biannually and more often in heavily contaminated exhibits, problem herds, or individuals.

IMMUNIZATION

Vaccination guidelines are those for Bovidae, modified as needed for local disease prevalences. A killed virus rabies vaccine should be included in endemic areas. Duikers should also be vaccinated for the equine encephalitides because these species may be susceptible to the viruses. Although at least two vaccinated individuals failed to build a titer, this situation should be investigated further before the recommendation is withdrawn; serologic tests are currently ongoing (personal observation, 1996). In several individuals, sterile abscesses have developed at the site of seven- or eight-way clostridial vaccines. This has not been a problem when using two-way clostridial vaccines (Fermicon CD/T, Bio-Ceutic Division/Boehringer, Ingelheim Animal Health, Inc., St. Joseph, MO, 64506).

NECROPSY

Necropsies should be performed in all cases with appropriate additional diagnostic tests.

Acknowledgments

I would like to thank the veterinarians who took the time from their busy schedules to discuss duiker medicine with me. I would also like to thank Teri Hermann, R.V.T., Diana Lucio, Registrar, and Jerry Stones, General Curator, for their assistance in gathering the required information and their patience as I put it together. Lastly, I also thank Colette Hairston-Adams, Curator of Herpetology, Dave Martin, Reptile Keeper, Leo Garrett, Computer Support, and Julie Pomerantz, Cornell College of Veterinary Medicine, Class of 1997, for their editorial expertise.

REFERENCES

1. Anadu PA, Elamah PO, Oates JF: The bushmeat trade in southwestern Nigeria: a case study. Human Ecology 16(2):199–208, 1988.
2. Arman P, Hopcraft D: Nutritional studies on East African herbivores. 1. Digestibilities of dry matter, crude fibre and crude protein in antelope, cattle and sheep. Br J Nutr 33(2):255–264, 1975.
3. Arman P, Hopcraft D, McDonald I: Nutritional studies on East African herbivores. 2. Losses of nitrogen in the faeces. Br J Nutr 33(2):265–276, 1975.
4. Bailey TA, Baker CA, Nicholls PK, et al: Reversible anesthesia of the blue duiker (*Cephalophus monticola*) with medetomidine and ketamine. J Zoo Wildl Med 26(2):237–239, 1995.
5. Bailey TA, Baker CA, Nicholls PK, et al: Blood values for captive grey duiker (*Sylvicapra grimmia*) and blue duiker (*Cephalophus monticola*). J Zoo Wildl Med 26(3):387–391, 1995.
6. Boehner J, Volger K, Hendrichs H: Breeding dates of blue duikers. Z Saeugetierkd 49(5):306–314, 1984.
7. Boomker EA: Volatile fatty acid production in the grey duiker, *Sylvicapra grimmia*. Symposium on Herbivore Nutrition in the Subtropics and Tropics. S Afr J Anim Sci 13(1):33–35, 1983.
8. Boomker EA: Rumen gas composition, fermentation rates and carbohydrate digestion in the grey duiker, *Sylvicapra grimmia*. S Afr J Wildl Res 14(4):123–126, 1984.
9. Burton MS, Gillespie DS, Robertson JT: Surgical correction of bilateral laryngeal paralysis in a yellow-backed duiker (*Cephalophus sylvicultor*). J Zoo Wildl Med 20(2):203–206, 1989.
10. Conklin-Brittain NL, Dierenfeld ES: Small ruminants: digestive capacity, differences among four species weighing less than 20 kg. Zoo Biol 15:481–490, 1996.
11. Emanoil M (ed): Encyclopedia of Endangered Species. Detroit, Gale Research Inc., pp 373–376, 1994.
12. Farst DD, Thomas WD: An outbreak of viral encephalomyelitis in Artiodactyla. Proceedings of the American Association of Zoo Veterinarians, Columbus, OH, pp 240–241, 1973.
13. Farst DD, Thompson DP, Stones GA, et al: Maintenance and breeding of duikers. *Cephalophus* spp. at Gladys Porter Zoo, Brownsville. Int Zoo Yearbook 20:93–99, 1980.
14. Faurie AS, Perrin MR: Diet selection and utilization in blue duikers (*Cephalophus monticola*) and red duikers (*Cephalophus natalensis*). Rev de Zool Afr 107(4):287–299, 1993.
15. Faurie AS, Perrin MR: Rumen morphology and volatile fatty acid production in the blue duiker (*Cephalophus monticola*) and the red duiker (*Cephalophus natalensis*). Fuer Saeugetierkunde 60(2):73–84, 1995.
16. Feron EM: New food sources, conservation of biodiversity and sustainable development: can unconventional animal species contribute to feeding the world? Biodiversity and Conservation 4:233–240, 1995.
17. Foley GL, Anderson WI, Steinberg H: Besnoitoisis of the reproductive tract of a blue duiker (*Cephalophus monticola*). Vet Parasitol 36(1–2):157–163, 1990.
18. Hofmeyr JM: The use of haloperidol as a long-acting neuroleptic in game capture operations. J S Afr Vet Assoc 52(4):273–282, 1981.
19. International Union for the Conservation of Nature (IUCN) 1996: IUCN, Red List of Threatened Animals. Gland, Switzerland, IUCN-The World Conservation Union, 1996.
20. International Species Information System: ISIS Mammal Abstract, as of 30 June 1996. Apple Valley, MN, ISIS, 1996, pp 222–224.
21. International Species Inventory System. MedARKS ISIS Physiologic Data. Apple Valley, MN, ISIS, 1996.
22. Karesh WB, Hart JA, Hart TB, et al: Health evaluation of five sympatric duiker species (*Cephalophus* spp). J Zoo Wildl Med 26(4):485–502, 1995.
23. Kramer DC: Embryo collection and transfer in small ruminants. Theriogenology 31(1):141–148, 1989.
24. Kranz KR, Lumpkin S: Notes on the yellow-backed duiker *Cephalophus sylvicultor* in captivity with comments on its natural history. Int Zoo Yearbook 22:232–240, 1982.
25. Kuttler KL: Anaplasma infections in wild and domestic ruminants: a review. J Wildl Dis 20(1):12–20, 1984.
26. McKenzie AA (ed): The Capture and Care Manual. Capture, Care, Accommodation and Transportation of Wild African Animals. Pretoria, South Africa, Wildlife Decision Support Services and The South African Veterinary Foundation, 1993.
27. Meteyer CU, Gonzales BJ, Heuschele WP, et al: Epidemiologic and pathologic aspects of an epizootic of malignant catarrhal fever in exotic hoofstock. J Wildl Dis 25(2):280–286, 1989.
28. Moore CG, Schunurrenberger PR: A review of naturally occurring *Brucella abortus* infections in wild mammals. J Am Vet Med Assoc 179(11):1105–1112, 1981.
29. Pandey GS: Verminous pneumonia in common duiker (*Sylvicapra grimmia*) in Zambia. Bulletin of Animal Health and Production in Africa 38(3):329–330, 1990.

30. Pinger C: The captive breeding and management of the black-backed duiker at the Memphis Zoo. Proceedings of the 20th National Conference of the American Association of Zoo Keepers, Atlanta, 1993.

31. Pope CE, Dresser BL, Kramer LW, et al: Nonsurgical embryo recovery in the yellow-backed duiker (*Cephalophus sylvicultor*)—a preliminary report [2: Paper No. 184]. Proceedings of the 11th International Congress on Animal Reproduction and Artificial Insemination, Dublin, Ireland, 1988.

32. Robinson TJ, Wilson V, Gallagher DJ, et al: Chromosomal evolution in duiker antelope (Cephalophinae, Bovidae)—karyotype comparisons, fluorescence in situ hybridization and rampant X chromosome variation. Cytogenet Cell Genet 73(1–2):116–122, 1996.

33. Roeder BL: What is your diagnosis? J Am Vet Med Assoc 193(10):1319–1320, 1988.

34. Roeder BL, Chengappa MM, Lechtenberg KF, et al: *Fusobacterium necrophorum* and *Actinomyces pyogenes* associated facial and mandibular abscesses in blue duiker. J Wildl Dis 25(3):370–377, 1989.

35. Roeder BL, Loop GC, Johnson JE: Comparative hematologic and serum chemistry values for neonatal, juvenile, and adult blue duiker (*Cephalophus monticola bicolor*). J Zoo Wildl Med 21(4):433–446, 1990.

36. Roeder BL, Varga GA, Wideman RF Jr: Effect of dietary calcium and phosphorus on mineral metabolism and acid-base balance in blue duiker antelopes. Small Ruminant Research 5:93–107, 1991.

37. Roeder BL, Wideman RF Jr, Varga GA: Effects of varied dietary calcium and phosphorus on renal function of male blue duiker antelope. Small Ruminant Research 11:17–32, 1993.

38. Skinner JD, Smithers RHN: The mammals of the Southern African Subregion. Pretoria, South Africa, University of Pretoria, pp 634–642, 1990.

39. Taylor BA, Varga GA, Whitsel TJ, et al: Composition of blue duiker (*Cephalophus monticola*) milk and milk intake by the calf. Small Ruminant Research 3(6):551–560, 1990.

40. Taylor BA, Varga GA, Whitsel TJ: Lactation in the blue duiker (*Cephalophus monticola*): milk composition and calf milk intake. J Dairy Sci 71(suppl 1):292, 1988.

41. U.S. Fish and Wildlife Service: Appendices I, II and III to the Convention on International Trade in Endangered Species of Wild Fauna and Flora. Washington, DC, U.S. Fish and Wildlife Service, Department of the Interior, 1995.

42. Walther RF: Duikers and dwarf antelopes. *In* Grzimek B (ed): Encyclopedia of Mammals, 5. New York, McGraw-Hill, pp 325–343, 1990.

43. Wilson VJ, Schmidt JL, Hanks J: Age determination and body growth of the common duiker *Sylvicapra grimmia* (Mammalia). J Zool 202(pt 2):283–297, 1984.

44. Wilson VJ, Wilson BLP (eds): The Pan African Decade of *Cephalophus* Research (1985–1994). Nature-et-Faune (FAO-PNUE) 4(3):24–30, 1988.

45. Zulty JC, Montali RJ: *Actinomyces pyogenes* infection in exotic Bovidae and Cervidae: 17 cases (1978–1986). J Zoo Anim Med 19(1–2):30–32, 1988.

CHAPTER **103**

Capture and Handling of Mountain Sheep and Goats

DAVID A. JESSUP

In North America, bighorn sheep (*Ovis canadensis*), Dall sheep (*Ovis dalli*), and Rocky Mountain goats (*Oreamnos americanus*) are managed as important aesthetic resources, as game animals, or as specially protected species depending on population status and state and federal laws. As such, they are often captured for translocation and restocking, or for sampling, marking, and subsequent population research.[2, 10] Free-ranging nonnative wild sheep and goats include mouflon (*Ovis musimon*), aoudad or Barbary (*Ammotragus lervia*), and ibex (*Capra ibex*), which live in parts of New Mexico and are loosely confined on large game ranches in Texas. A wide variety of wild sheep can be found in zoos, private collections, and game parks and game farms. The term "wild sheep and goats" includes both North American native and exotic wild species, but may also include feral domesticated species such as Corsican and Barbados sheep. For those reasons, the term mountain sheep and goats, which generally excludes feral

species, is used in this chapter when that exclusion is implied. In general, mountain sheep and goats raised in captivity can be tamed and habituated such that only rarely should they have to be captured from out of large areas or remotely injected with immobilization drugs. In zoos, facility design and feeding of mountain sheep and goats into chutes, paddocks, or stalls has reduced the need to dart or net animals. Habituation to feed and human presence also facilitates darting and trapping of free-ranging mountain sheep and goats.

Although mountain sheep and goats have impressive and usually curled horns, essentially all species elude predators and attempts to capture them by flight, usually into very steep terrain. Free-ranging bighorn sheep survive only where they have access to vast areas of undisturbed and precipitous terrain. Although they can accelerate rapidly and can negotiate perilous terrain, wild sheep do not appear to be able to sustain prolonged efforts to flee without suffering hyperthermia and metabolic disturbances. These attributes make them a challenge to capture and handle. Methods for remote delivery of drugs and medications to mountain sheep and goats that avoid the necessity of capturing them are discussed in reference 9.

North American natives killed or captured these animals for consumption in ways not dissimilar to those still in use for live capture. Bighorn sheep or mountain goats were driven into nets woven of native grasses (of a size and shape very similar to modern drive nets) erected along narrow escape trails in mountain passes by tribes in northwestern North America. Southwestern native peoples ambushed desert bighorn at water holes in summer, using arrows instead of dart guns. Although pioneers usually used rifles to kill bighorn for food, some early efforts were made to capture bighorn sheep alive. Around 1900, Will Frakes used modified leg hold traps with gaps filed into them to catch bighorn sheep by the hoof; he would then tie the sheep to a ramada post by the horns and slowly tame it.

Early efforts by game managers in North America to capture bighorn sheep involved baiting or driving them into heavily built corral traps or darting them from Korean War–vintage light helicopters. Mortality rates of 10% to 25% were common in the 1960s. In zoo and wildlife practice, drugs were used with poor success when only succinylcholine or phencyclidine and/or xylazine were the only drugs available.[23, 24] Subsequently, etorphine combined with a tranquilizer or alpha-adrenergic sedative proved to be much more effective.[23] In the 1970s and early 1980s, drop nets and drive nets were used effectively to physically capture bighorn sheep and mountain goats. Capture by these methods seldom resulted in greater than 5% acute mortality rate, but capture myopathy was consistently a problem seen in mountain sheep and goats captured by all methods.[13] By the mid-1980s, darting with carfentanil and xylazine,[12] xylazine,[16] or ketamine and xylazine,[3] and net gunning[8, 14, 18] came into use. Current practice when mountain sheep or goats must be immobilized or captured is to dart the animal over bait, to place bait under a drop net, or to net-gun the animal.

CAPTURE OF FREE-RANGING MOUNTAIN SHEEP AND GOATS

The development and evolution of capture techniques for mountain sheep and mountain goats have advanced in parallel for these species and are discussed together. Mountain sheep in more northerly climates that suffer seasonal food deprivation can be more easily trained to bait than can desert-adapted species. Baits such as salt, alfalfa hay, and fermented apple pomace have been used to induce animals to enter corrals or even crates.[13, 24] The door is usually connected to an interior trip line and closed by gravity. Fermented apple pomace has proven particularly effective with Rocky Mountain bighorn (*Ovis canadensis canadensis*). Mountain goats are most often attracted to salt. Baiting requires many hours of preparation and can be undone by unpredictable weather or predators near the trap site. There may be a

small return in captured animals for the investment of time, and it is difficult to preselect the individual animals for relocation or research, possibly capturing the hungriest or most dominant animals. However, where bighorn sheep have been habituated to bait and where crews are practiced with this technique, it has been used to capture many bighorn sheep and mountain goats with minimal expense and loss of animal life.

By extending fence wings from an existing corral trap, drive or wing traps have also been constructed to capture bighorn sheep. Because bighorn sheep do not herd well, this technique has seldom proved successful and has historically resulted in high mortality rates from physical injury and myopathy.[13] This method of capture is seldom used.

Habituation to feed or apple pulp is also the first step in drop net capture (Fig. 103–1). Open areas allow more animals to come under the net and there is some ability to select the number and composition of animals to be captured. Initially, mountain sheep to be drop netted are calm and do not show signs of stress. When the net comes down, this attitude changes quickly.[18] One of the most serious errors that can be made in drop net capture of mountain sheep or goats is to drop the net on more animals than can be quickly and efficiently handled. If bighorn sheep are allowed to struggle for more than 10 or 15 minutes, even when the ambient temperature is low, they may become hyperthermic and suffer capture myopathy.[18] If adult animals, especially large rams, are captured along with females and young animals, the smaller animals tend to get injured in the melee. For these reasons, it is important not to drop the net on too many animals and to have at least 1.5 to 2 people available per animal (i.e., at least 30 people immediately available to handle 20 bighorn sheep). Water can be used as bait in desert climates. Rocket nets have also been used but appear to have few if any advantages over drop nets. They require an explosives expert, the noise creates great panic and stress, and the rockets and leading edge of the net have greater potential to kill or maim.

One hundred foot sections of 10- to 14-inch stretch mesh net have been erected in a number of configurations across escape routes, and mountain sheep and goats have been driven into them (Fig. 103–2), usually with a helicopter.[13] If the nets are camouflaged (dark in sage brush and rocky areas, white in snow) and the animal does not see the net until too late, then this technique can be quite effective. Drive nets must be properly erected and manned to reduce potential for escape. Usually, three to five animals are captured per drive. These nets require a crew of about a dozen people and are not too selective, but they are portable and adaptable to many types of terrain.

A net firing gun, which is usually hand held but is occasionally mounted on helicopter skid, developed for red deer capture in New Zealand, has been effective in the capture of free-ranging mountain sheep and goats in most types of terrain (Fig. 103–3).[14] This method is used extensively in the desert Southwest where animal populations are scattered over vast areas and are difficult or impossible to habituate to bait.[8] The net is fired over and in front of the fleeing animal at relatively

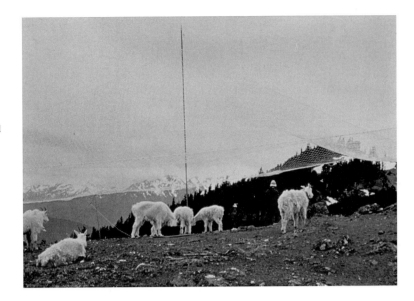

FIGURE 103–1. These Rocky Mountain goats have been attracted to salt licks beneath this drop net. When a complement of animals suitable for relocation are present, the net will be triggered. (Photograph courtesy of Olympic National Park, Washington.)

close range (7 to 10 m) to tangle it. A forest canopy can limit helicopter approach to the ground, thus limiting the effectiveness of this technique. In dense vegetation, the net may not entangle the animal, but low vegetation helps catch the trailing weights and stops the animal rapidly. When snow covers the ground, the weights may not tangle the animal. Very steep terrain and cliff faces must be avoided. One key to success is to keep the time interval between sighting the animal and capturing it as short as possible to avoid exertional stress. Efficiently extricating the tangled animal from the net requires experience. The capture team should carry a full complement of sampling and treatment equipment in backpacks to allow on-site treatment and release of stressed individuals. When capture teams are well trained, this method is one of the safest and most cost effective for free-ranging desert bighorn sheep.[14]

When mountain sheep and goats are captured by physical means, they must be firmly but carefully restrained.[13] Mountain sheep usually cease struggling if their legs are bound with leather hobbles and their eyes are covered, and they are subsequently handled quietly and gently. When black Spandex cloth eye covers are used, it may require several minutes for the animal's eyes to adjust to sunlight upon release. Eyes are often rinsed out with ophthalmic eye wash solutions and may be treated with bland antibiotic eye ointment. Mountain goats may fight restraints and hooks with their very sharp horns. Sections of rubber hosing should be applied to protect the handler and other animals (Fig. 103–4). Mountain sheep horns are not pointed or usually used as weapons by submissive animals (although adult males will attempt to batter any threatening individual), and they can actually provide good leverage

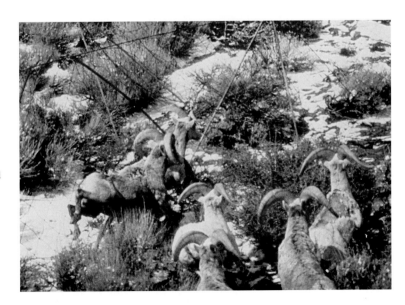

FIGURE 103–2. This group of California bighorn rams have been driven for less than a mile by a helicopter and will tangle in the drive net in front of them. They must be quickly subdued, monitored for capture stress, and triaged. (Photograph courtesy of Landells Aviation.)

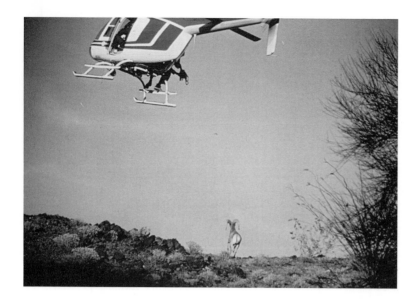

FIGURE 103–3. The distance and angle between this desert bighorn and the helicopter are perfect for a net gun shot over the animal. In this type of terrain, most animals tangle and are stopped immediately. (Photograph courtesy of Dr. Mike Kock.)

for restraint. Care must be taken not to pull off the horn sheath of young animals. Mountain sheep and goats can be carried upright by three people, one holding and restraining the head and the other two on opposite sides forming a "fireman's carry" with hands locked beneath the axilla and the groin. Heavy weave plastic mesh bags

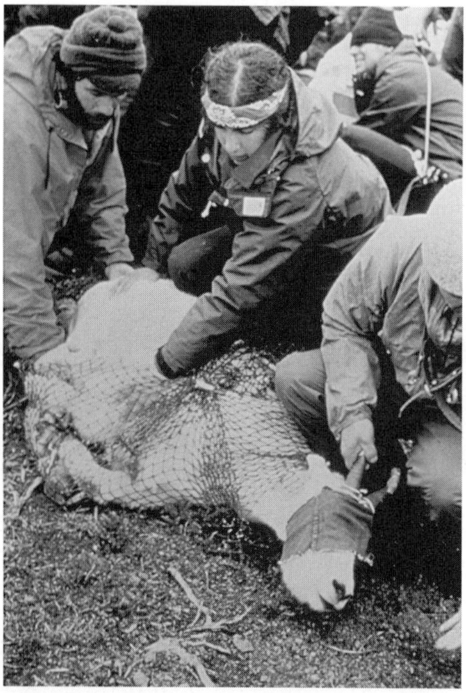

FIGURE 103–4. This Rocky Mountain goat has been hobbled, is confined in a net bag, and an eye cover is applied. Note the sections of rubber hose over the horns to protect against the sharp-tipped horns and hooking behavior of this species. (Photograph courtesy of Olympic National Park, Washington.)

large enough to hold adult mountain sheep and goats work well for air transport, as well as for restraining animals in such a way that they can be cooled and monitored easily. They also provide for easy carrying on the ground. Air transport of mountain sheep upside down suspended by their hobbled legs, as practiced by some professional capture operators, is inappropriate and unnecessary.

CHEMICAL IMMOBILIZATION OR SEDATION OF FREE-RANGING MOUNTAIN SHEEP OR GOATS

The greatest problems associated with the darting of free-ranging mountain sheep and goats are due to misplaced darts or partial injection, capture stress and myopathy, and falls and other accidents that occur during the 5- to 10-minute period between darting and immobilization. Free-ranging bighorn sheep have been chemically immobilized using etorphine (2.5 to 4 mg) and acepromazine (10 mg) per adult animal, or etorphine (3.5 to 3.75 mg) and xylazine (20 to 50 mg) per adult animal.[22] Carfentanil (0.044 mg/kg) and xylazine (0.2 mg.kg) has also been effective for immobilization of free-ranging desert bighorn sheep.[12] With carfentanil, immobilization is more rapid and relaxation more complete than with etorphine. Net gun capture has largely replaced helicopter darting of desert bighorn sheep with narcotics. Efforts to capture Dall sheep in Alaska with etorphine and acepromazine has sometimes been successful. In one mountain range, 2.5 mg etorphine and 7.5 mg acepromazine per adult animal was very effective; in a second mountain range, doses had to be doubled to be effective, immobilizations were often incomplete, and deaths were excessive.[21]

Etorphine (4 to 5 mg) per adult animal has been used to capture free-ranging mountain goats in Alaska.[23]

In the 1980s, mountain goats in Olympic National Park were captured for relocation and to reduce environmental impacts of this nonnative species by a variety of methods including drop netting, drive netting, and net gunning. However, chemical immobilization with carfentanil at 0.035 mg/kg (2.7 mg/adult) proved to be more flexible and applicable to remote populations. The extremely steep terrain and snow fields, the remote nature of the operation, and animal behavior made darting with relatively high doses of rapid-acting narcotics preferable to net gunning. Over a 3-year period, as animal numbers were reduced and animals were found in progressively more inhospitable terrain, there was an increase in mortality rate to 8.75% in 1988 and to 19% in 1989. Human safety and animal mortality considerations finally forced the abandonment of these efforts.

Researchers in Canada found that they could effectively immobilize Rocky Mountain bighorn sheep with ketamine and xylazine when they darted them from a helicopter.[3] Subsequently, darting from a blind over the bait, they immobilized 124 bighorn sheep using xylazine alone at 70 to 130 mg per lamb, 250 mg per adult female, and 360 mg per adult male.[16] Females hand injected in box traps required significantly less xylazine to produce field immobilization than females that were darted. Idazoxan at 0.1 mg/kg administered intravenously was effective when used for reversal.[16] Four deaths (3% of the total) occurred before idazoxan was available. Much lower doses of xylazine (30 mg/44-kg adult animal, mean dosage 0.71 mg/kg) have been used to sedate desert bighorn sheep captured by physical means for holding or relocation.[15]

Diazepam given intramuscularly (IM), at 10 mg/adult desert bighorn sheep has also been used for sedation.

If xylazine, detomidine, or medetomidine is used to sedate mountain sheep or goats, there are some apparent species differences in response to reversal agents. Desert bighorn sheep sedated with low doses of xylazine respond to yohimbine at a mean dose of 0.21 mg/kg[15] and are alert and able to flee, but Barbary sheep do not appear to respond to this or higher doses of yohimbine. Both idazoxan and atipamezole appear to be more effective than yohimbine, with the latter being both the most potent and specific known alpha-adrenergic antagonist. Atipamezole should be used to reverse the effects of medetomidine sedation in mountain sheep or goats.

CHEMICAL IMMOBILIZATION OF CAPTIVE WILD SHEEP AND GOATS

Although properly designed chutes and runs and physical restraint should eliminate the need for routine darting in most game farm, ranch, and zoo situations, anesthesia of wild sheep and goat species for surgical procedures or immobilizations of large or fractious individuals can be accomplished using a number of drugs and combinations. Markhors (*Capra falconeri*) have been chemically immobilized using mean doses of 69 μg/kg medetomidine and 1.6 mg/kg ketamine.[6] They showed adequate muscular relaxation; most clinical,

hematologic, and serum chemical parameters remained within physiologic limits; and there was a significant increase in serum glucose and a decrease in heart rate and temperature. Complete reversal was achieved using approximately 300 μg/kg atipamezole given by various routes.[6] When this drug combination was compared to immobilization with etorphine and acepromazine, it was observed that the etorphine combination resulted in incomplete immobilization and myorelaxation as well as decreased respiratory rate and depth, but these signs as well as alterations in hematology and serum chemistry parameters were relatively insignificant.[6]

Adult male and female aoudad have been successfully immobilized with 1.5 to 3 mg carfentanil mixed with 5 to 10 mg ketamine and 5 to 10 mg xylazine.[22] Adult markhor have been immobilized with 1.5 to 2 mg carfentanil with 5 to 20 mg ketamine and 5 to 20 mg xylazine.[22] Similarly, adult Siberian ibex have been immobilized with 1.5 to 2 mg carfentanil with 20 mg ketamine and 20 mg xylazine.[22]

There have been several reports of efforts to evaluate the physiologic effects of narcotics (etorphine and carfentanil) on domestic goats (*Capra capra*), presumably in an effort to better understand effects on rare exotic wild sheep and goats.[4, 5] When these drugs were given IM at the same doses (5, 10, 20, and 40 μg/kg), both caused rapid catatonic immobilization, neck and limb hyperextension, and occasional vocalization and bruxation.[5] Immobilization was more rapid with carfentanil, and etorphine caused more struggling. Both drugs increased systemic and left ventricular end-diastolic pressures, total peripheral resistance, left atrial, and pulmonary O_2 content and hemoglobin concentration. They decreased respiratory and heart rates and $Paco_2$.[5] Neither drug had significant effects on cardiac output, aortic flow, rate-pressure product, or oxygen consumption. Etorphine (20 μg/kg) given IV resulted in immobilization in 2.5 minutes and recovery to standing in 2 hours without a reversal agent, but the goats were not really able to flee until 4 hours later.[4] Carfentanil (20 μg/kg) given under the same conditions resulted in somnolence at 2 hours, continued recumbency at 4 hours, standing depression and ataxia at 8 hours, and return to normal behavior by 24 hours. Thus, it appears that immobilizing dosages of carfentanil have a considerably longer half-life in goat species. This work suggests that care should be taken to ensure that sufficiently long-lasting narcotic reversal agents such as naltrexone or nalmefene are used, especially in free-ranging mountain sheep or goats.

EVALUATION OF CAPTURE TECHNIQUES

In the early 1980s after one particularly disastrous capture attempt, the California Department of Fish and Game undertook to evaluate the various methods being used to capture free-ranging bighorn sheep in the western United States. The captures of a total of 634 animals by drop net (n = 158), drive net (n = 249), chemical immobilization (n = 90), and net gun (n = 137) were evaluated for indicators of exertional stress and myopathy,[19] for capture-associated morbidity and mortality,[18] and for postcapture outcome.[17] Biologic parameters affected by capture stress included core body temperature, respiration rate, cortisol, glucose, potassium, creatine phosphokinase (CPK), serum glutamic oxaloacetic transaminase, and white blood cell count.[19] For this comparison, capture stress was defined as a body temperature of more than 42.2°C and evidence of shock, or prolonged helicopter pursuit resulting in open-mouthed breathing or excessive struggling.[17] In these studies, the use of drop nets to capture bighorn sheep resulted in a 2% mortality rate from capture myopathy and a 1% mortality rate from physical injury, and 15% of animals captured were stressed.[18] Of bighorn sheep captured in drive nets, 3% died of capture myopathy, 1% died of physical injury, and 16% were stressed.[18] Chemical immobilization resulted in a 2% capture myopathy mortality rate and a 6% mortality rate from physical injury, and 19% of bighorn sheep were stressed.[18] Net gun capture caused no capture myopathy deaths, 2% of bighorn sheep died of physical injuries, and 11% were stressed.[18] Drop net and net gun capture caused the least physiologic change associated with capture stress and myopathy. Follow-up studies confirmed that stressed animals had poorer survival rates than animals whose parameters fell within "normal" limits, but also suggested that postcapture survival of net-gunned bighorn sheep might be more problematic than initial evaluation suggested.[17] Since this work, advances in net gun capture and improved handling and treatment methods have resulted in reduction of the capture-associated mortality rate to about 1%, with more than 600 additional bighorn sheep being captured.

BLOOD GAS AND STRESS LEVELS IN DESERT BIGHORN SHEEP

Based on studies by Kock and coworkers[17–19] and further field observations, an attempt was made to define a threshold for capture stress to allow triage and determination of which animals needed intensive care during large-scale capture operations. Hematology, serum chemistry, blood gas parameters, and catecholamines were evaluated in 47 otherwise normal free-ranging desert bighorn sheep captured by net gunning.[20] Rectal temperatures were somewhat elevated (37.8° to 42.2°C), but respiratory and heart rates were not sufficiently elevated to suggest aggressive treatment was necessary. Serum CPK and glucose were within normal limits. Venous blood measured within minutes of capture showed severe metabolic acidosis (mean base deficit, 23 mEq/L) with no evidence of respiratory acidosis (mean Po_2 8.0 mm Hg, mean Pco_2 3.7 mm Hg). There were moderate elevations in plasma epinephrine, norepinephrine, and dopamine, reflecting moderate exertional stress similar to that seen in racing greyhounds after brief strenuous exercise.[20] All animals recovered from this capture stress and appeared to adapt well during follow-up studies using radiotelemetry. This study confirms previous observations that there is a capture stress threshold, below which normal physiologic homeostatic adaptation mechanisms allow stressed bighorn sheep to recover without aggressive medical treatment.

Free-ranging mountain goats appear to be very susceptible to capture myopathy. Any prolonged struggling or excessive exertion may result in muscle damage and necrosis. Blood selenium levels in many of these animals were low when compared with domestic goats and bighorn sheep and may have contributed to the problem.

ROUTINE AND INTENSIVE TREATMENT

All mountain sheep and goats that are captured and held or relocated, or that have punctures or noticeable injuries should receive injectable long-acting antibiotics. Most of the organisms cultured from wounds and abscesses in mountain sheep are still sensitive to penicillins and tetracyclines. Tetanus toxoid and multivalent clostridial bacterins are also commonly used. In California, vitamin E and selenium are given routinely. Anthelminthics or other location-, population-, or operation-specific treatments, or those required for relocation may also be given.[1, 13] Most of the disease problems associated with capture and relocation of wild sheep have been published in the previous edition of this book.[2, 10, 11]

Wild sheep or goats with a temperature of more than 42.2°C (107°F), respirations of more than 75 per minute, and/or heart rate of more than 200 per minute should be given intensive treatment for capture stress/myopathy with cooling baths, balanced intravenous fluids, anti-inflammatory drugs (I prefer prednisolone sodium succinate), vitamin and mineral supplements, and possibly intraperitoneal (IP) bicarbonate.[1, 10, 13]

SUMMARY

Although there has been some controversy as to what the "best" way is to capture mountain sheep,[8] the many variables that must be considered make the answer to that question, "it depends on where you are and what you want to do with them." For most situations where captive-reared wild sheep need to be handled for examination, vaccination, worming, hoof trimming, and blood sampling, physical restraint is adequate. Chemical immobilization of captive and free-ranging mountain sheep and goats can be achieved with a variety of drugs and combinations of drugs. The optimal method for capturing free-ranging mountain sheep or goats at one location for treatment, marking, or later study may be very different from the method required to capture more than 20 animals a day for herd relocation. Terrain, weather, mobility, capture team skills, cost effectiveness, and other factors as well as potential animal and human safety considerations must be taken into account. If they are blindfolded, hobbled, or bagged, and are handled quickly and quietly, wild sheep, and to a lesser degree wild goats, become passive. Quick, quiet, and efficient handling or short distance relocation can be accomplished without sedation or anesthesia. In summary, capture of free-ranging animals requires either manipulating them to come to bait where they can be captured by physical means (usually a drop net) or by brief pursuit and tangling them with a gun-fired net. Baiting also facilitates darting of free-ranging mountain sheep and goats. Mortality rate associated with capture and handling of mountain sheep and goats should not routinely exceed 1%.

REFERENCES

1. Clark RK, Jessup DA: Field evaluation and treatment of medical problems resulting from wildlife capture. *In* Renecker LA, Hudson R (eds): Wildlife Production: Conservation and Sustainable Development. Fairbanks, AL, University of Alaska, Fairbanks Press, p 381–386, 1991.
2. Clark RK, Jessup DA, Weaver RA: Relocation of bighorn sheep within California. Proceedings of the American Association of Wildlife Veterinarians, Toronto, Ontario, Canada, pp 121–129, 1988.
3. Festa-Bianchet M, Jorgenson JT: Use of xylazine and ketamine to immobilize bighorn sheep in Alberta. J Wildl Management 49:162–165, 1985.
4. Heard DJ, Kollias GV, Caliguiri R, Conigliaro J: Comparative cardiovascular effects of intravenous etorphine and carfentanil in domestic goats. Proceedings of the American Association of Zoo Veterinarians, Greensboro, NC, pp 9–10, 1989.
5. Heard DJ, Nichols WW, Buss D, Kollias GV: Comparative cardiopulmonary effects of intramuscularly administered etorphine and carfentanil in goats. Am J Vet Res 57(1):87–96, 1996.
6. Jalanka HH: Evaluation of medetomidine and ketamine induced immobilization in markhors (*Capra falconeri megaceros*) and reversal by atipamezole. J Zoo Wildl Med 19(3):95–105, 1988.
7. Jalanka HH: Chemical restraint and reversal in captive markhors (*Capra falconeri megaceros*): a comparison of two methods. J Zoo Wildl Med 20(4):413–422, 1989.
8. Jessup DA: On capturing bighorn sheep. J Wildl Dis 28(3):512–513, 1992.
9. Jessup DA: Remote treatment and monitoring of wildlife. *In* Fowler ME (ed): Zoo and Wild Animal Medicine, Current Therapy 3. Philadelphia, WB Saunders, pp 499–504, 1993.
10. Jessup DA: Translocation of wildlife. *In* Fowler ME (ed): Zoo and Wild Animal Medicine, Current Therapy 3. Philadelphia, WB Saunders, pp 493–499, 1993.
11. Jessup DA, Boyce WM: Diseases of wild sheep. *In* Fowler ME (ed): Zoo and Wild Animal Medicine, Current Therapy 3. Philadelphia, WB Saunders, pp 554–560, 1993.
12. Jessup DA, Clark WE, Jones KR, et al: Immobilization of free-ranging desert bighorn sheep, tule elk and wild horses, using carfentanil and xylazine: reversal with naloxone. J Am Vet Med Assoc 187(11):1253–1254, 1985.
13. Jessup DA, Clark WE, Mohr RC: Capture of bighorn sheep: management recommendations. California Department of Fish and Game Wildlife Management Branch, Sacramento, CA, Administrative Report 84–1:33, 1994.
14. Jessup DA, Clark RK, Weaver RA, Kock MD: Safety and cost-effectiveness of net-gun capture of desert bighorn sheep. J Zoo Anim Med 19(4):208–213, 1988.
15. Jessup DA, Jones KR, Mohr R, Kucera T: Yohimbine antagonism to xylazine in free-ranging mule deer and desert bighorn sheep. J Am Vet Med Assoc 187(11):1251–1252, 1985.
16. Jorgenson JT, Sampson J, Festa-Bianchet M: Field immobilization of bighorn sheep with xylazine hydrochloride and reversal with idazoxan. J Wildl Dis 26:522–527, 1990.
17. Kock MD, Clark RK, Franti CE, et al: Effects of capture on biological parameters in free-ranging bighorn sheep: evaluation of normal, stressed and mortality outcomes and documentation of postcapture survival. J Wildl Dis 23(4):652–662, 1987.
18. Kock MD, Jessup DA, Clark RK, et al: Capture methods in five subspecies of bighorn sheep: evaluation of drop-net, drive-net, chemical immobilization and the net-gun. J Wildl Dis 23(4):634–640, 1987.
19. Kock MD, Jessup DA, Clark RK, Franti CE: Effects of capture on biological parameters in free-ranging bighorn sheep: evaluation of drop-net, drive-net, chemical immobilization and the net-gun. J Wildl Dis 23(4):641–651, 1987.
20. Martucci R, Jessup DA, Gronert G, et al: Capture stress: blood gases and catecholamine levels in bighorn sheep. J Wildl Dis 28(2):250–254, 1992.
21. Singer FJ, Whitten K, Nichols L: Experiences darting Dall sheep from helicopters in Alaska during 1983. Proceedings of the Northern Wild Sheep and Goat Council, Whitehorse, Yukon, Canada, pp 499–505, 1984.
22. Snyder SB, Richard MJ, Foster WR. Etorphine, ketamine and xylazine in combination (M99KX) for immobilization of exotic ruminants: significant additive effect. Proceedings of the Joint Conference of the American Association of Zoo Veterinarians and the American Association of Wildlife Veterinarians, Oakland, CA, pp 253–263, 1992.
23. Thorne ET: Agents used in North American ruminant immobilization. *In* Nielsen L, Haigh JC, Fowler ME (eds): Chemical Immobilization of North American Wildlife. Milwaukee, Wisconsin Humane Society, 1982.
24. Wishart W, Smith K, Jorgenson J, Lynch G: The evolution of capturing bighorn in Alberta. Proceedings of the Northern Wild Sheep and Goat Council, Salmon, ID, pp 590–600, 1980.

CHAPTER 104

Medical Aspects of Arabian Oryx Reintroduction

JACQUES R. B. FLAMAND

GENERAL CONSIDERATIONS

The Arabian oryx (*Oryx leucoryx*) is a medium-sized antelope of the sub-family Hippotraginae weighing between 80 and 100 kg. Its habitat was much of the Arabian peninsula, but, by 1972, habitat degradation and excessive hunting led to the extinction of the species in the wild. The creation of the World Herd in 1962 and its success in saving the species from extinction has become a celebrated example of how zoological collections can contribute to the conservation of a large mammal species.[12, 24] Indeed, the Arabian oryx reintroduction programs in the Arabian peninsula have been with captive-bred animals. These reintroduction programs with individuals from the World Herd[20, 41, 42] and a number of other collections in the Middle East have been major successes. To date, Arabian oryx have been returned to four areas in their former range: two fenced areas (Shaumari in Jordan in 1978 and Mahazat As-Sayd in Saudi Arabia from 1990) and two unfenced areas (Jiddat-al-Harasis in Oman from 1982 and 'Uruq Bani Ma'arid in Saudi Arabia from 1995).

As a species, the Arabian oryx has attributes that predispose it to successful reintroduction,[42] including its adaptation to extreme environments and its tolerance of a range of changing habitat conditions. Arabian oryx also tend to form cohesive groups and are explorers. The latter two characteristics could lead to an increased risk of transmission of infectious diseases between conspecifics and of contracting diseases in domestic livestock that share the same habitat. However, the environments where Arabian oryx naturally occur and have been reintroduced are often inhospitable to infectious agents because those areas are arid, hot, and sunlit.[33] Another factor reducing the likelihood of disease transmission is the behavioral reluctance of oryx to be in close proximity of other species.

Reintroduction programs aim to re-establish viable, free-ranging populations of a species back into the wild in areas from which they were extirpated. Generally, the programs are carried out in protected conservation areas where other wildlife and domestic livestock may or may not exist. Reintroduced animals are the founders of future generations and must be the fittest possible individuals, both genetically and medically. Animals infected with contagious diseases should not be reintroduced because they can present a risk to the relocated animals as well as to the existing native wildlife and any resident domestic livestock.[49] Translocation of parasites and diseases must be limited, and their implications have been discussed by numerous workers from various areas of the world.[7, 8, 10, 43, 49, 50, 52] Veterinarians must be involved in disease control before, during, and after any reintroduction program.

This chapter primarily discusses the experience gained during a reintroduction program of Arabian oryx in the Kingdom of Saudi Arabia between 1986 and 1996. The National Wildlife Research Centre (NWRC), near the town of Taif in Saudi Arabia, has been the site of an intensive Arabian oryx breeding program. Disease-free animals were produced for reintroduction, even though bovine tuberculosis was initially present in the founder animals. The production of a healthy herd was the result of a strict tuberculosis monitoring strategy and control program. Although the techniques used to eliminate the tuberculosis were intensive, they were justified by the genetic value of the animals (genetically, the NWRC herd has a higher heterozygosity than other Arabian oryx herds because of the different origins of the founders of the herd and the management of their breeding)[45] and the cultural importance that the Saudis placed on them.

BEHAVIOR

Arabian oryx are a herding species, with social groups numbering from one to 15 individuals.[42] Equal numbers of males and females are normally found in a group, and a dominance hierarchy exists within that group. Moving groups of oryx for management and reintroduction purposes may lead to changes in the established hierarchies and to aggressive and combative behavior that can result in trauma and stress. To avoid creating such conflict, oryx should be kept in large enclosures, and transport in tightly packed communal crates should be avoided. When communal transport is done, plastic piping should be used to cover the horns to prevent the animals from hurting each other.

Arabian oryx are relatively easily kept in captivity, a fact that partially led to their demise. Even adults could easily be caught by being run down with the aid of four-wheel-drive vehicles, leading to a flourishing pet trade in the Middle East. That legacy remains in that Arabian oryx are still found in private collections.

Animals born in captivity are generally tolerant of fairly close approach by humans, but hand-reared adult males can turn aggressive and dangerous to humans.

HANDLING AND RESTRAINT

The periodic handling of individual Arabian oryx is essential for thorough clinical examinations, the collection of diagnostic samples, vaccinations, and treatments. Handling can either be done manually or by using chemical immobilization. At the NWRC, capture myopathy following transport has led to some oryx deaths.[47] Successful reintroductions depend in large part on the atraumatic handling of the animals to minimize stresses and the occurrence of captive myopathy.

The oryx at the NWRC are kept in enclosures varying in size from 25 hectares down to pens 10 × 30 m. In a corner of each larger enclosure is a smaller "capture pen" in which the animals are fed and watered to habituate them to the pen, making it relatively simple to trap them by means of a sliding door. Once trapped, animals can be visually examined, darted, or released. Younger, hand-reared oryx can be manually restrained, but the lack of fear toward humans by adult hand-reared males can make them dangerous.

Manual Handling

A mobile restraint crush, made of wooden paneling, has been used to handle Arabian oryx at the NWRC. The crush has a number of hinged windows cut into the side at strategic levels to facilitate grabbing horns, jugular bleeding, vaccination, and other procedures. Oryx are coaxed into the crush by herding them with wooden boards, which act as shields to the handlers. Although it is a relatively rapid technique, it is labor-intensive. The animals may become nervous or stressed, and some bruising and superficial injuries can be sustained by the animals. Manual handling can be a practical option when the number of animals to be handled precludes chemical immobilization of all the animals. However, the use of chemical immobilization became a preferred method of handling untamed oryx at the NWRC.

For hand-reared oryx up to 1 year of age, manual

handling is practicable in the capture pens. The animals are cornered with a wooden shield or stretched tarpaulin and held by the horns. Even for these smaller oryx, however, chemical immobilization is preferred as a less stressful technique.

Chemical Immobilization

GENERAL POINTS

To avoid the risk of hyperthermia, the immobilization of Arabian oryx, particularly in the Middle East, is best carried out in the cooler times of the day. Stress should be minimized before and after darting. Darts can be placed in any muscle mass, most usually in the hindquarters. Invariably, the dart hitting the animal causes major excitement, so once darted, the animal should remain undisturbed until anesthetized. Then a mask is placed over the animal's eyes to prevent sand or dust from entering them and to reduce visual stimulation. The animals are kept in sternal recumbency to avoid bloating or regurgitation of rumenal contents.

DRUGS USED FOR IMMOBILIZATION

Arabian and other oryx have generally been considered difficult to immobilize because of the extreme excitement that morphine derivatives produce in this species. This excitement and poor relaxation are inadequately suppressed by available tranquilizers.[51] In addition, until the advent of the alpha2-adrenoagonist inhibitors, tranquilizers such as xylazine hydrochloride prolonged recovery excessively.[2, 3, 51] A number of dosage regimens are presented in Table 104–1.[21, 51] As a rough guide, the doses for etorphine hydrochloride calculated for confined animals can be increased by one fourth to one third in free-ranging animals. Underdosing and the consequent prolonged excitation can lead to cases of hyperthermia, exhaustion, myopathy, and death.

Combinations that exclude morphine derivatives have generally been unsatisfactory. To avoid the excitement produced by morphinics in oryx, some workers have used tiletamine-zolazepam combinations in Beisa oryx (*Oryx beisa callotis*).[30] Despite good relaxation and sedation, the lack of an antidote necessitated that the animals recover naturally, a long process with some excitation during the recovery phase.

The preferred dosage regimen currently used in Saudi Arabia is a combination of etorphine, ketamine hydrochloride, and xylazine, based on doses used in other Hippotraginae.[40] The advantages of this mixture are that, compared to other drug combinations, the amount of etorphine is reduced, the mixture is reversible, and relaxation is excellent.

For Arabian oryx to be kept under anesthesia for more than 3 hours (e.g., when they are to be transported while anesthetized), an etorphine-medetomidine combination has been used successfully (see Table 104–1).[3]

TABLE 104–1. Various Dosage Rates for Immobilizing Arabian Oryx

Immobilizing Agents	Antagonist Agents	Notes	Ref.
Unconfined animals: Etorphine (0.04 mg/kg) + xylazine (0.32 mg/kg) *Confined animals:* Etorphine (0.34 ± 0.004 mg/kg) + xylazine 0.32 ± 0.02 mg/kg)	Diprenorphine (1.3 mg per 1 mg etorphine used) + idazoxan (15 mg total).	Depressed respiration, stable cardiovascular system, normal acid-base balance.	51
Etorphine (0.04–0.07 mg/kg) + azaperone citrate (1.0–1.5 mg/kg)	Diprenorphine (2.5 mg per 1 mg etorphine).	Good induction, poor relaxation. (Azaperone useful where animals are required to be fully conscious after release, e.g., when free-ranging oryx are to be released into wild immediately after capture.)	
Etorphine (0.04 ± 0.008 mg/kg) + medetomidine (0.005 ± 0.0002 mg/kg)	Diprenorphine (2 mg per 1 mg etorphine used). + atipamezole (5 mg per 1 mg medetomidine used—two thirds IV, one third SQ).	Useful for long-duration (>3 hours) immobilization.	3
Etorphine (0.012–0.020 mg/kg) + xylazine (0.13–0.27 mg/kg) + ketamine (0.13–0.27 mg/kg)	Diprenorphine (2 mg per 1 mg of etorphine used). + tolazoline (0.4–0.6 mg/kg) *OR* + yohimbine HCl (0.1–0.2 mg/kg).	Good relaxation and reversal, but animal may remain sedated for 2 days after reversal.	40
Tame and confined oryx: medetomidine alone (0.04–0.07 mg/kg, up to 0.08 mg/kg for deeper sedation)	Atipamezole 5 mg per 1 mg of medetomidine used.	No resedation.	21
Hand-reared and tame oryx: xylazine alone (0.5 ± 0.07 mg/kg)	Atipamezole 1 mg per 5.5 mg xylazine used—two thirds IV, one third SQ.	Frequent resedation 2–5 hrs later for 1–2 hours.	2

TAMER AND HAND-REARED ORYX IN CAPTIVITY

The use of alpha$_2$-adrenergic agonist tranquilizers alone has proved a useful immobilization tool in handling hand-reared and confined oryx. Before the advent of antagonists to these tranquilizers, the prolonged recumbency associated with these drugs was potentially hazardous to ruminant animals. Medetomidine has been the most effective of these drugs in tame Arabian oryx.[21] Doses of these drugs and reversal agents are listed in Table 104–1.

Other Tranquilizers

The butyrophenone tranquilizer haloperidol has not been useful in Arabian oryx because of a lack of marked tranquilizing effects and the extrapyramidal effects (usually torticollis) seen in this species.

As in other oryx species, the long-acting tranquilizer perphenzine enanthate is not as effective as in other antelope. In Arabian oryx, it has been administered 3 days before shipment at a dose rate of 4 mg/kg intramuscularly.[4] It can be given while the animal is anesthetized and begins to take effect from 24 to 36 hours after injection. A reduction of anxiety and flight distance was seen in usually nervous animals; the effects usually persist for 6 days. At doses of less than 2.5 mg/kg, the drug appeared to have no effect, whereas at more than 4 mg/kg, extrapyramidal side effects (dyskinesia) occurred, which could be suppressed with intravenous diazepam.

TRANSPORT

Arabian oryx are best transported in individual crates. The usual crate size used at the NWRC is 126 cm long, 132 cm high, and 42 cm wide. Oryx can be crated while anesthetized, and the antagonist administered while the animal is in the crate. The animals should regain complete consciousness before transport.

To prevent myopathy, oryx can be trained to load into a trailer and habituated to rides of increasing length in a communal crate.[4]

When capture myopathy has occurred, infusions of sodium bicarbonate are warranted, but recovery may take several months.[4]

RELEASE

The release of captive-bred animals has been successful and animals rapidly revert to their wild status. Oryx are best placed in a pre-release enclosure of adequate size for at least 2 weeks before release. The pre-release also provides an extended quarantine and allows for a final examination of the animals before release. It is important to be able to handle the animals. When animals are placed in their pre-release enclosure, any piping on the horns should be removed.

Animals are able to acquaint themselves with their new surroundings and gradually begin to eat the prevailing type of vegetation of area.

The release should be done with the least disturbance possible, often by simply leaving a gate open. The process can be expedited by placing the feed closer and closer to the gate in the days before release, and then beyond it. Feed and water should be put out for the animals after their release in case they want it, although the animals rarely return to the pre-release pen.

Once oryx are free-living, control of infectious diseases presents enormous difficulties, so the most important aspect of disease control becomes that in the domestic livestock that share the range. The separation of wildlife and domestic stock with fences is generally impracticable in vast desert areas.

REPRODUCTION

Male oryx are sexually mature by between 470 and 500 days.[48] Females reach sexual maturity at 13 months of age and are polyestrus with an average estrous cycle length of 22 days. Gestation is about 260 days and births in captivity can be at any time of the year. In the wild, females can produce one calf per year, and removal of the calf at birth has no effect on fecundity. Average fecundity of females older than 2 years of age was 0.99 calves per year. Twins were never recorded.[48]

The female reproductive tract can be examined by rectal palpation in immobilized, fully grown adult females.[28] Ultrasonography has been used routinely at the NWRC for pregnancy diagnosis.

The presence of Q fever (*Coxiella burnetii*) caused abortion in one animal and a retained afterbirth in another. In a survey covering 6 years of data on 47 females, five (3.6%) aborted between 2 and 5 months into gestation. One was associated with tuberculosis and one with listerosis. Two other abortions occurred in an old female, and another occurred in an oryx with lumpy skin disease.[48]

CLINICAL

Arabian oryx usually manifest few signs of clinical disease, so hematologic and biochemical samples can be of diagnostic assistance. Hematologic and biochemical analyses, carried out from anesthetized or tranquilized oryx held at the NWRC, which is at an altitude of 1500 m above sea level in semidesert-type habitat, are presented in Table 104–2.[46]

HEALTH

Arabian oryx are susceptible to most infectious and parasitic agents affecting domestic livestock. Preventive medicine strategies for disease prevention in domestic animals can also be applied to Arabian oryx.[23] Agents reported to infect Hippotraginae include the following: foot-and-mouth disease (FMD), malignant catarrhal fever, epizootic hemorrhagic disease, peste des petits ruminants (PPR), rinderpest, bluetongue, parainfluenza 3, *Actinomyces pyogenes, Fusiforum necrophorum, Myco-*

TABLE 104–2. Normal Blood Parameters for Arabian Oryx at the NWRC, Saudi Arabia

	Sample Size	Mean ($\pm$ Confidence Interval at 5%)	Variation Interval for 1 Individual
Hematology			
WBC (1000/mm^3)	63	3.48 $\pm$ 0.32	0.952–6.006
RBC (million/mm^3)	63	7.29 $\pm$ 0.38	4.25 –10.33
Hemoglobin (g/dl)	22	14.5 $\pm$ 1.48	7.54–21.46
Hematocrit (%)	50	41.5 $\pm$ 1.3	32.34–50.66
MCV (fl)	20	44.94 $\pm$ 5.5	20.36–69.52
MCH (pg)	20	14.62 $\pm$ 1.67	7.15–22.09
MCHC (%)	20	32.88 $\pm$ 1.54	26–39.76
Differential white cell count			
Neutrophils (%)	59	75.2 $\pm$ 2.44	56.5–93.91
(1000/mm^3)	59	2.68 $\pm$ 0.278	0.553–4.826
Lymphocytes (%)	59	20.56 $\pm$ 2.3	2.87–38.25
(1000/mm^3)	59	0.70 $\pm$ 0.094	0–1.432
Monocyte (%)	59	1.02 $\pm$ 0.29	0–3.25
(1000/mm^3)	59	0.036 $\pm$ 0.012	0–0.127
Eosinophils (%)	59	2.86 $\pm$ 0.65	0–7.87
(1000/mm^3)	59	0.108 $\pm$ 0.029	0–0.331
Basophils (%)	59	0.37 $\pm$ 0.2	0–1.91
(1000/mm^3)	59	0.013 $\pm$ 0.007	0–0.068
Chemistry			
Total protein (g/L)	73	68.01 $\pm$ 3	42.37–93.65
Glucose (g/L)	73	1.95 $\pm$ 0.15	0.64–3.25
Blood urea nitrogen (g/L)	73	0.51 $\pm$ 0.04	0.14–0.87
Creatinine-kinase (μ/L)	32	303.34 $\pm$ 72.52	0–713.59
Creatinine (mg/dl)	59	1.38 $\pm$ 0.06	0.92–1.83
Bilirubin (mg/L)	43	3.65 $\pm$ 0.54	0.11–1.83
Uric acid (mg/dl)	44	2.07 $\pm$ 0.41	0–4.82
ASAT (μ/L)	69	47.65 $\pm$ 3.29	20.3–75

ASAT, aspartate aminotransferase.
From Vassart M, Greth A: Hematological and serum chemistry values for Arabian oryx (*Oryx leucoryx*). J Wildl Dis 27:506–508, 1991.

bacterium bovis, Corynebacterium pseudotuberculosis, Bacillus anthracis, and *Brucella, Salmonella, Clostridium,* and *Nocardia* species.[23] Additionally, any livestock in the area should be vaccinated and screened.

To prevent the introduction of disease, any captive breeding center should, in effect, be a quarantine facility. In the case of the NWRC, an outbreak of bovine tuberculosis led to the isolation of the entire breeding group of animals and the extraction of non-infected animals only from that group for reintroduction (Table 104–3).

VIRAL DISEASES

Rinderpest

Rinderpest is a highly contagious viral disease of artiodactyla, characterized by necrosis and erosions in the gastrointestinal tract.[37] Gemsbok (*Oryx gazella*) are reported to be moderately susceptible to the disease.[34] This is probably true for Arabian oryx as well. However, there is the possibility that, like in cattle, some virus strains may have varying virulence in wildlife.[34] In camels, which in Arabia often share oryx habitat, the disease has been reported to cause variable signs, from subclinical disease to diarrhea and death.[37]

Middle East countries are regularly infected with rinderpest by the widespread traffic in live animals from Africa and Asia, including sheep and goats in which rinderpest is endemic in southern Asia.[37]

Infected animals shed virus in body secretions and feces, and close contact is necessary for disease transmission. The fragile virus survives for only a few hours outside the host and survives for 1 to 3 days in a carcass. A number of other factors further reduce the chances of oryx becoming infected with rinderpest: the aridity of their natural environment, the low stocking densities of domestic and wild artiodactyls in such habitats, the generally less susceptible species, both domestic and wild, living in such areas, and the lack of water points around which susceptible animals might congregate. Furthermore, dehydration in arid environments would cause rapid death of any affected animals, further reducing the chances of spread.

Despite the low likelihood of infection of wild oryx, reintroduced animals should be vaccinated before release. Both rinderpest attenuated virus vaccine (Kabete strain type 0) and PPR vaccine (which provides cross-immunity) have been used. These vaccines provide lifelong immunity, which is passed on maternally to calves. In the hot conditions of the Middle East, it is important that the freeze-dried vaccine be used within an hour of reconstitution. Arabian oryx older than 3 months of age should be vaccinated and then again after 1 year of age.

Additionally, the regular vaccination of domestic stock in and around captive breeding and release sites is recommended.

TABLE 104–3. Potentially Important Diseases to Which Arabian Oryx Are Susceptible

Disease	Etiology	Principal Hosts	Arabian Oryx Susceptibility
Viral Diseases			
Rinderpest	*Morbillivirus* Family Paramyxoviridae	Cattle	Moderate
Peste des petits ruminants	*Morbillivirus* Family Paramyxoviridae	Goats, sheep	Possibly resistant
Rabies	*Lyssavirus* Family Rhabdoviridae	All mammals	Susceptible, although infection unlikely
Foot and mouth disease	*Aphthovirus* Family Picornaviridae. Many types. In Middle East, types A, O, C, and Asia 1[13]	Artiodactyls, principally cattle and sheep	Probably low susceptibility
Bluetongue	*Orbivirus* Family Reoviridae	African antelopes, inapparent infections; sheep clinically affected	Probably inapparent infections
Malignant catarrhal fever	Alcelaphine *herpesvirus 1*	Alcelaphines, sheep	Probably low susceptibility
Akabane virus	Bunyavidirae	Cattle, sheep	Antibodies found in one Arabian oryx[17] and other Hippotraginae, including *Oryx gazella*[38]
Lumpy skin disease	*Capripoxvirus* Poxviridae	African wildlife, cattle, sheep, goats	Susceptible[19]
Rickettsial Diseases			
Q Fever	*Coxiella burnetii*	Cattle, sheep	Susceptible
Chlamydiosis	*Chlamydia psittaci*	All species	Positive titers found[17]
Bacterial Diseases			
Tuberculosis	*Mycobacterium bovis*		Highly susceptible
Pasteurellosis	*Pasteurella multocida* A, B, and D *Pasteurella haemolytica*		Carriers: disease under stress[17]
Salmonellosis	*Salmonella* species		Susceptible[42]
Clostridial diseases	*Clostridium botulinum*		Susceptible[42]
Parasitic Diseases			
Coccidiosis	*Eimeria saudiya*[29]		Probable
Cryptosporidiosis	*Cryptosporidium parvum*	Young cattle, sheep	Young susceptible
Nematodes			
Ticks			
Other Diseases			
Spongiform encephalopathy	Prion protein	Cattle, sheep	Known susceptibility[27]

Peste des Petits Ruminants

PPR is a disease of goats, sheep, and closely related wild bovidae, and is similar to rinderpest. It occurs on the Arabian peninsula.[1, 16]

An outbreak of PPR was reported from the Al Ain Zoo in Abu Dhabi in which three of four gemsbok died. Arabian oryx and scimitar-horned oryx (*Oryx dammah*) in the same collection were not apparently infected.[16] The susceptibility of Arabian oryx to PPR remains in question.

Vaccination with attenuated rinderpest virus vaccine of all reintroduced oryx will effectively protect them against PPR. However, the immunity conferred against PPR may not be as long lasting as that produced against rinderpest by the vaccine.

Vaccination of domestic stock around protected ar-eas in which oryx are reintroduced is important to safeguard the oryx.

Rabies

Rabies is prevalent in Saudi Arabia,[5] perpetuated by feral dogs and probably foxes. Both occur in the protected areas where oryx reintroductions have been carried out. Although rabies in oryx has not been reported, all Arabian oryx reintroduced in Saudi Arabia to date have been vaccinated prior to release.

Foot-and-Mouth disease

The susceptibility of Arabian oryx to FMD is unknown, but it is likely to be low. The disease does occur in

Arabian domestic stock, so Arabian oryx in captivity are routinely vaccinated annually with serotypes prevalent in the Middle East (i.e., types A, O, C and Asia 1).[13]

The limited period of immunity makes vaccination applicable to captive stock only. Of greater importance to reintroduced animals is the continued vaccination of domestic livestock in and around reserves where Arabian oryx are reintroduced.

Bluetongue

Bluetongue is endemic in tropical and subtropical Africa, the Middle East, and the United States. It is generally confined to areas where the *Culicoides* midges, which transmit the virus, occur.

Oryx from the United States, serologically positive to bluetongue, were only allowed into Saudi Arabia after virus isolation tests proved negative. In a serologic survey of the NWRC herd, only one of the Saudi oryx was positive to bluetongue, compared to 50% of those from the United States.[17]

Athough bluetongue is not considered a threat to Arabian oryx, they act as a reservoir that could pose a threat to sheep where they share habitat. Thus, only oryx that are not shedding bluetongue virus should be considered for release.

Malignant Catarrhal Fever

Malignant catarrhal fever has never been reported in Arabian oryx in the Middle East, although it has been reported in this species from zoos in the United States, and antibodies were found in Beisa oryx in Kenya.[32] The possibility of a carrier state in the Hippotraginae has been suggested.[6]

Lumpy Skin Disease

Lumpy skin disease is a highly infectious cutaneous disease caused by a capripox virus. One isolated case was recorded at the NWRC. It is likely that the disease was transmitted to the animal by a biting insect because the NWRC is completely fenced but is surrounded by sheep that could have been infected.[19]

In that case, a 2-year-old female of the founder generation exhibited lethargy, anorexia, and soft feces with generalized urticaria; a few cutaneous lumps were followed by lumps over the whole body, concentrating on the neck, head, and leg. On day 13, it aborted, either because of the infection or previous corticosteroid therapy.

The cutaneous lesions were numerous. They were round, raised, and nonsensitive, varying in size from 0.5 cm to 4 cm in diameter. Ulcers were also present on the gingival, vulval, and anal mucosae. The nodules persisted for 1.5 months. By 2.5 months after onset, most of the lesions had disappeared, leaving black scars that were still visible as dark hairless patches 2 years later.

Confirmation of diagnosis was by the demonstration by electron microscopy of intracytoplasmic poxvirus particles in the stratum spinosum of the epidermis.

Serum neutralization tests on sera collected 2 months after the onset of clinical symptoms demonstrated virus neutralization at greater than 1:640 dilution. Nine months later, the titer declined to 1:128.

Parainfluenza 3 Virus

In a serologic survey of oryx in Saudi Arabia, significant numbers of animals showed positive titers to parainfluenza 3 virus.[17] The virus, in synergy with *Pasteurella* species, can lead to pneumonia and death. Vaccination against pasteurellosis is important and should be routinely carried out to prevent such mortalities.

RICKETTSIAL AND CHLAMYDIAL DISEASES

Q Fever

Antibodies to *C. burnetii* were found in a few of the NWRC oryx.[17] The clinical manifestations of Q fever were abortion in one female and retained afterbirth in another. The calf of the latter female was also positive for the pathogen. Both had been in the same enclosure, and they were probably infected by ticks.

Good immunity generally follows infection and Q fever is not likely to be significant in a breeding program. Also, problems occur only when females are infected during pregnancy.

Chlamydiosis

Evidence of *Chlamydia psitacci* antibodies were present in 7% of the Arabian oryx tested in most herds.[17] The clinical significance of the presence of such infection in Arabian oryx is not known.

BACTERIAL DISEASES

Tuberculosis

Tuberculosis has been recognized as a serious disease problem in captive and wild artiodactylids. An outbreak of tuberculosis in Arabian oryx in Saudi Arabia was a major setback to the original reintroduction plans. However, the measures taken to deal with the disease were effective in containing it and producing disease-free Arabian oryx suitable for reintroduction.

HISTORY OF TUBERCULOSIS IN THE ARABIAN HERD

The NWRC was established in 1986 to breed indigenous Arabian species in captivity for reintroduction. The Arabian oryx program at the NWRC was initiated in April 1986 when 57 animals were transported in communal crates from the late King Khalid's farm at Thumamah near Riyadh.[39] There a herd of 70 oryx had shared a 600-hectare enclosure with 22 other species.[22]

Two months after the translocation, the first deaths occurred, and *M. bovis* was isolated.[22] It is highly likely that the stresses associated with the capture operation contributed to the apparently acute manifestation of tuberculosis, because most of the deaths occurred in the 6 months following transport. On necropsy, the oryx showed either extensive disseminated miliary lesions or granulomatous lesions of varying size. The lungs of all autopsied animals were involved. Some had an acute illness of short duration and there was often little sign of debilitating disease until the day before death. By September 1987, 16 oryx (25%) had died of tuberculosis. A decision was made to attempt to save the NWRC oryx herd, so it became important to separate positive from negative animals. Difficulties in diagnosis arose when the comparative skin test and enzyme-linked immunosorbent assay (ELISA) test gave variable results. Eventually, a combination of diagnostic tests was used to evaluate each animal, and a strict testing protocol was developed.[15]

DIAGNOSTIC TESTS

The range of tests included the comparative skin test, the indirect ELISA test, the comparative ELISA test, and the lymphocyte transformation test. For interpretation, the tests were ranked in order of value: the lymphocyte transformation test, which is a sensitive indicator of early infections; the ELISA tests; and the comparative skin test. On this basis, animals could be categorized into high, moderate, and low risk.

The protocol initiated in October 1987 consisted of testing all the oryx at 6-month intervals and calves from the age of 2.5 months old, using all the above tests. At that stage, the diagnostic tests had not yet been interpreted with confidence, and therefore, in the interests of caution, all the oryx present at the NWRC were considered tuberculosis-positive and individually penned in a remote area of the NWRC. In an attempt to eliminate tuberculosis from the herd, all of these founders underwent treatment while their calves were hand-reared.[18]

Currently, tuberculosis is monitored annually with the comparative ELISA tests. In this test, the background optical density reading for a known negative tuberculosis reference serum is subtracted from the reading for the test serum. The resultant value is multiplied by 100 to give it an ELISA unit value. Based on experience with the Arabian oryx, interpretation of results is as follows:

Positive: 1. ELISA bovine (Eb) units − ELISA avian (Ea) units = ≥ 15

or   2. Eb − Ea = 10 to 15 and ELISA MBP 70*(EM) ≥ 5

Equivocal: Eb − Ea = 10 to 15 and EM <15

Negative: Eb − Ea = <10

---

*MBP 70 or M peptide 70 is a protein derived from *M. bovis*.

The use of polymerase chain reaction techniques for amplifying certain regions of *M. bovis* DNA may provide a useful diagnostic tool in the future.

TREATMENT

The treatment regimen included a 9-month course of rifampicin (10 mg/kg body weight), ethambutol (15 mg/kg), and isoniazid (10 mg/kg). The tablet form of these was dissolved or suspended by mixing in warm water with a magnetic stirrer. To increase palatability, each animal's dose was diluted with more water, but the volume never exceeded 3 L so that the oryx would finish it. Animals were penned individually to ensure that each animal received its full dose.

Until consumed, the treatment water was the only source of water to the animals. When provided in the drinking water in this way, the three antibiotics attained adequate therapeutic blood levels.

Following treatment of the herd, morbidity and mortality caused by tuberculosis ceased. During treatment, ELISA titers declined. Four months after the end of the treatment period, the ELISA and lymphocyte transformation tests were negative. At necropsy, the lungs showed extensive scarring and numerous fibrotic, nodular, calcified, and apparently inactive tubercles. However, *M. bovis* was isolated from one lung lesion and one lymph node.[36]

HAND-REARING CALVES

At the same time that the founder group received treatment, all calves born of that group (the B generation) were removed from their dams immediately after birth. After removal, the calves were given subcutaneous injections of bovine gammaglobulins, and a broad-spectrum antibiotic was injected for 3 days.[14]

Calves were hand-reared in groups of four to prevent the spread of any potential infection to a larger group. The calves were fed 10% to 15% of their body weight per day, a mixture of evaporated milk and whole homogenized cow's milk in a 1:1 ratio supplemented with multivitamins and trace elements. For the first 19 days, there were six feedings a day, then feedings were gradually reduced to three daily until weaning at 3 months of age. From 3 weeks of age, the oryx were provided with dried alfalfa and grass hay; at 4 weeks, a commercial concentrate pellet containing 14% digestible protein was offered. Water was available anytime.

Nearly all the B-generation calves of the founder group were free of tuberculosis infection.

Brucellosis

Brucellosis has never been detected in any of the Arabian oryx tested from the Middle East. However, both *Brucella melitensis* and *B. abortus* occur in cattle and sheep in Saudi Arabia,[35] so there is a risk of infection to Arabian oryx through close proximity with domestic stock.

Pasteurellosis

A serologic survey of oryx in Saudi Arabia revealed a relatively high number of *Pasteurella multocida* type A seropositive animals.[17] The rareness of clinical manifestations makes it likely that this bacterium is carried freely by Arabian oryx and causes disease only when animals are stressed.

A few hand-reared calves at the NWRC died of pasteurellosis, and some deaths in 1989 in the population of oryx at Shaumari in Jordan were believed to be due to *Pasteurella* pneumonia triggered by nutritional stresses.[29] Four adult oryx at the NWRC died of acute pasteurellosis within 10 days of being translocated.[4]

Vaccination of oryx against pasteurellosis is important, particularly before stressful situations. Primary vaccination consists of two injections given 1 month apart, and an annual booster vaccination is necessary.

Clostridia

Botulism caused by toxins of *Clostridium botulinum* was thought to be the cause of death in three adult zoo-bred Arabian oryx reintroduced in Oman.[42] Oryx at the NWRC are not routinely vaccinated against botulism.

However, oryx released in Saudi Arabia have been routinely vaccinated against *Clostridium chauvei, Clostridium tetani,* and *Clostridium perfringens.*

Anthrax

There are no records of anthrax in Arabian oryx. Other members of the Hippotraginae, such as roan antelope (*Hippotragus equinus*) and gemsbok, are susceptible to anthrax. Where anthrax is a threat, reintroduced oryx should be vaccinated against the disease. Anthrax occurs in these species during times of limited water availability when animals congregate around limited watering points.[11] However, this is not likely to be a factor in the Middle East, where there is rarely any surface water in release areas.

PROTOZOAL DISEASES

The protozoa found in oryx at Thumamah in Saudi Arabia include *Eimeria saudensis*,[25] *Cryptosporidium parvum* in juveniles, and a *Sarcocystis* species found in a single old individual.

Coccidiosis

E. saudensis was isolated from three oryx from Riyadh Zoo.[25] None of them showed clinical symptoms, but coccidiosis could become a problem in crowded and unhygienic conditions, particularly where young animals are concerned.

Cryptosporidiosis

C. parvum infection has been implicated in clinical diarrhea in neonate Arabian oryx calves at Thumamah,

near Riyadh. Typical signs include severe diarrhea, which may lead to death. No treatment is available, although spiramycin has been suggested as being potentially useful.[44] Intravenous infusions can be given to correct any fluid loss.

Toxoplasmosis

Arabian oryx kept in identical conditions and fed the same food as gazelles at Thumamah in Saudi Arabia were all negative to *Toxoplasma gondii* antibodies, whereas 4.7% of the gazelles in their vicinity had positive titers.[31] Despite the high population of *Toxoplasma*-positive feral cats present, this suggested that oryx may be less susceptible to toxoplasmosis than gazelles.

METAZOAN PARASITES

The presence of internal and external parasites has not been a problem and should not become one where oryx densities are kept low and where the animals are kept in good conditions. However, a regular anthelminthic treatment schedule limits the build-up. Injectable ivermectin administered annually at a dose of 0.2 mg/kg has been useful for prevention and treatment.

Nematodes encountered in Arabian oryx include *Camelostrongylus mentulatus, Trichostrongylus* species, *Trichuris cervicaprae,* and *Nematodirus spathiger.*

Ticks found on Arabian oryx have included *Hyalomma dromedarii.* Tick numbers in the arid conditions of the Middle East rarely are a problem, although a build-up in pens at the NWRC has occurred. Arabian oryx should undergo treatment with an acaricide prior to release.

OTHER DISEASES

Spongiform Encephalopathy

Spongiform encephalopathy, a neurodegenerative disease similar to scrapie in sheep and goats and bovine spongiform encephalopathy (BSE) in cattle, has been reported from a number of wildlife species in zoological collections, including gemsbok and Arabian oryx. It is believed that cattle have acquired the disease by consumption of proprietary feeds containing ruminant-derived protein containing the agent. Some zoo ungulates were also fed these feeds.[27]

Symptoms developed in a 38-month-old Arabian oryx at London Zoo 2 years after a diet containing animal meat and bone-meal was discontinued. Eventually, clinical signs progressed from somnolence to a semicomatose state and death.

Most cattle become infected as calves and clinical signs of BSE develop at 4 to 5 years of age. The age of onset in the Arabian oryx and other species suggests that, in wildlife species, the incubation period is shorter than in cattle. Also, the 22-day duration of clinical signs in the Arabian oryx is considerably shorter than in cattle.

Horizontal transmission of the spongiform encephalopathies occurs in sheep and may also occur in cattle. A case in a greater kudu (*Tragelaphus strepsiceros*) suggested maternal transmission, resulting in serious implications for captive breeding programs and reintroductions.[26]

Until more is understood about the epidemiology of the diseases, only oryx from collections known not to have had spongiform encephalopathies in them should be considered for conservation programs.

SURGICAL CONDITIONS

The principal surgical conditions encountered in Arabian oryx are traumatic wounds from impact with fences and posts. Horn wounds are rare if the animal densities and groupings of individuals are carefully managed. Horns broken off or damaged during early growth in calfhood can be common. These are generally not a problem unless abnormal horn growth penetrates the side of the animal's face or neck.

Corneal pitting, particularly in older oryx, is often encountered. This is ascribed to erosion by sand brought about by a life in the desert. It does not appear to adversely affect the animals, and surgical intervention was never contemplated.

GENETIC CONSIDERATIONS

Despite Arabian oryx population bottlenecks at the NWRC (where an outbreak of tuberculosis reduced the number of animals from 57 to 37), the breeding herd at the NWRC is genetically the most diverse to be found anywhere.[45] To further reduce inbreeding and to broaden the genetic base, exchanges with other herds are ongoing. To limit the loss of genetic variability and retain 90% of the genetic characters of the founders, the aim is to increase the breeding herd to 200 individuals.

Although, affected animals show no differences in appearance, health, or reproductive performance, the discovery of a 17/19 Robertsonian chromosomal rearrangement in the NWRC herd has led to a policy of not releasing such animals into the wild until such time as the effects of such characteristics are understood.[9] Approximately 17 out of 250 (6.8%) oryx at the NWRC are affected. All oryx are routinely screened karyotypically to identify such carriers of the condition. Normal Arabian oryx have a diploid chromosome number of 2n = 58, whereas those with the Robertsonian translocation have 2n = 57 or, rarely, 56.

CONCLUSION

There are a number of steps in the reintroduction process of Arabian oryx into the wild:

1. Selection of the animals for release.
   a. Animals for release should be selected to have as broad a genetic base as possible. A wide range of ages should be released together, although older animals are less suitable for release.
   b. Animals should be healthy in all respects and should be screened for appropriate infectious diseases.
   c. Only oryx with a normal chromosome number of 2n = 58 should be considered.
2. Preparation of the animals for release.
   a. Oryx should be constituted into release groups, usually about 10 individuals. This allows social hierarchies to be established within the group and minimizes social friction in pre-release enclosures.
   b. If transport is to be carried out in a communal crate, the animals should be habituated to enter the transport crate and to short preparatory trips in the crate.
   c. Before release, all the animals should be inoculated with rabies, rinderpest, FMD, and pasteurellosis vaccines as well as a *Clostridium* vaccine that incorporates *C. chauvei, C. tetani,* and *C. perfringens.*
3. Selection of a release area. The release area should be in a protected conservation area, with appropriate environmental and sociopolitical prerequisites. Of particular importance is the cooperation of the local people in allowing their livestock to be vaccinated against the contagious diseases of concern and in limiting the entry of their stock into the protected area.
4. Preparation of the release site. The pre-release enclosure site should be within the core of the release area. It should be well vegetated so that the oryx may feed there, allowing adaptation of their rumenal flora before release. Water and feed should be provided.
5. Translocation of the Arabian oryx to the pre-release site enclosure and acclimatization. Arabian oryx can either be transported individually or in communal crates, in which case their horns must be covered with plastic piping. The trip should be made as rapidly as possible. The use of air transport has been particularly helpful in the Saudi Arabian region.
6. Acclimatization.
   a. The animals should be given time to recover from the trip, to re-establish social hierarchies, to habituate to the new environment, and for adaptation of rumenal flora to new vegetation.
   b. The animals should be closely monitored. The local managers of the reserve can learn to recognize individuals.
7. Release. Immediately before their release, Arabian oryx should be visually checked and, if they appear normal, released by opening a gate or dropping the fence around the enclosure. The animals can be encouraged to leave by feeding them in and beyond the mouth of the exit gate. Water and feed should be left available at the pen entrance in the period immediately after release, should any recently released animals feel a need to return for these.

REFERENCES

1. Abu Elzein EME, Hassanien MM, Al-Afeleq AI, et al: Isolation of peste des petits ruminants from goats in Saudi Arabia. Vet Rec 127:309–310, 1990.

2. Ancrenaz M: Use of atipamezole to reverse xylazine tranquilization in Arabian oryx (*Oryx leucoryx*). J Wildl Dis 30(4):592–595, 1994.

3. Ancrenaz M, Ostrowski S, Anagariyah S, et al: Long-duration anesthesia in Arabian oryx (*Oryx leucoryx*) using a medetomidine-etorphine combination. J Zoo Wildl Med 27(2):209–216, 1996.

4. Ancrenaz M, Ostrowski S, Delhomme A: The return of the Arabian oryx, *Oryx leucoryx*, to the Saudi Arabian Empty Quarter: disease monitoring for the reintroduction process. Proceedings of the Joint Conference of the American Association of Zoo Veterinarians/Wildlife Disease Association/American Association of Wildlife Veterinarians, East Lansing, MI, pp 79–84, 1995.

5. Bales JD, Choudury AA, Oertley RE: Rabies in eastern Saudi Arabia. Saudi Med J 3(3):195–201, 1982.

6. Barnard BJH, van der Lugt JJ, Mushi EZ: Malignant catarrhal fever. *In* Coetzer JAW, Thomson GR, Tustin RC (eds): Infectious Diseases of Livestock with special reference to southern Africa. Oxford University Press, pp 946–957, 1994.

7. Bigalke RD. The important role of wildlife in the occurrence of livestock diseases in southern Africa. *In* Coetzer JAW, Thomson GR, Tustin RC (eds): Infectious Diseases of Livestock with Special Reference to Southern Africa. New York, Oxford University Press, pp 152–163, 1994.

8. Bush M, Beck BB, Montali RJ: Medical considerations for reintroduction. *In* Fowler ME (ed): Zoo and Wild Animal Medicine, Current Therapy 3. Philadelphia, WB Saunders, pp 24–26, 1993.

9. Cribiu EP, Asmodé J-F, Durand V, et al: Robertsonian chromosome polymorphism in Arabian oryx (*Oryx leucoryx*). Cytogenet Cell Genet 54:161–163, 1990.

10. Cunningham AA: Disease risks of wildlife translocations. Conservation Biology 10:349–353, 1996.

11. De Vos V: Anthrax. *In* Coetzer JAW, Thomson GR, Tustin RC (eds): Infectious Diseases of Livestock with Special Reference to Southern Africa. New York, Oxford University Press, pp 1262–1289, 1994.

12. Dolan JM: The Arabian oryx—its destruction, captive history and propagation. Int Zoo Yearbook 16:230–239, 1976.

13. Farag MA, Hafez SM: Comparative studies on the status of currently prevalent serotypes of foot-and-mouth disease virus in Saudi Arabia and its neighboring countries during the period from 1981 to 1992. Proceedings of the Fifteenth Annual Meeting of the Saudi Biological Society, Makkah Al-Mukarramah, p 25, 1994.

14. Flamand JRB, Delhomme A, Ancrenaz M: Hand-rearing the Arabian oryx *Oryx leucoryx* at the National Wildlife Research Centre, Saudi Arabia. Int Zoo Yearbook 33:269–274, 1994.

15. Flamand JRB, Greth A, Haagsma J, et al: An outbreak of tuberculosis in a captive herd of Arabian oryx (*Oryx leucoryx*): diagnosis and monitoring. Vet Rec 134:115–118, 1994.

16. Furley CW, Taylor WP, Obi TU: An outbreak of peste des petits ruminants in a zoological collection. Vet Rec 121:443–447, 1987.

17. Greth A, Calvez D, Vassart M, et al: Serological survey for bovine bacterial and viral pathogens in captive Arabian oryx (*Oryx leucoryx* Pallas, 1776). Rev sci tech Off int Epiz 11(4):1163–1168, 1992.

18. Greth A, Flamand JRB, Delhomme A: An outbreak of tuberculosis in a captive herd of Arabian oryx (*Oryx leucoryx*): management. Vet Rec 134:165–167, 1994.

19. Greth A, Gourreau JM, Vassart M, et al: Capripoxvirus disease in an Arabian oryx (*Oryx leucoryx*) from Saudi Arabia. J Wildl Dis 28(2):295–300, 1992.

20. Greth A, Schwede G: The reintroduction program for the Arabian oryx (*Oryx leucoryx*) in Saudi Arabia. Int Zoo Yearbook 32:73–80, 1993.

21. Greth A, Vassart M, Anagariyah S: Evaluation of medetomidine-induced immobilization in Arabian oryx (*Oryx leucoryx*): clinical, hematologic and biochemical effects. J Zoo Wildl Med 24(4):445–453, 1993.

22. Haagsma J, Poilane JF: Tuberculosis in captive Arabian oryx. *In* Abuzinada AH, Goriup PD, Nader IA (eds): Proceedings of the First Symposium, National Commission for Wildlife Conservation and Development [Publication No. 3], Riyadh, pp 349–357, 1989.

23. Heuschele WP: Pathology of oryx and gazelles. *In* Abuzinada AH, Goriup PD, Nader IA (eds): Proceedings of the First Symposium, National Commission for Wildlife Conservation and Development [Publication No. 3], Riyadh, pp 358–369, 1989.

24. Jones DM: The Arabian oryx in captivity with particular reference to the herds of Arabia. *In* Dixon A, Jones D (eds): Conservation and Biology of Desert Antelopes. London, Christopher Helm, pp 47–57, 1988.

25. Kasim AA, Al Shawa YR: *Eimeria saudensis* N. Sp. (Apicomplexa: Eimeriidae) from the Arabian oryx (*Oryx leucoryx*) in Saudi Arabia. J Protozool 35(4):520–521, 1988.

26. Kirkwood JK, Wells GAH, Cunningham AA, et al: Scrapie-like encephalopathy in a greater kudu (*Tragelaphus strepsiceros*) which had not been fed ruminant-derived protein. Vet Rec 130:491–492, 1992.

27. Kirkwood JK, Wells GAH, Wilesmith JW, et al: Spongiform encephalopathy in an Arabian oryx (*Oryx leucoryx*) and a greater kudu (*Tragelaphus strepsiceros*). Vet Rec 127:418–420, 1990.

28. Kock RA: Veterinary aspects of the Hippotraginae. *In* Abuzinada AH, Goriup PD, Nader IA (eds): Proceedings of the First Symposium, National Commission for Wildlife Conservation and Development [Publication No. 3], Riyadh, pp 370–385, 1989.

29. Kock RA, Woodford MH. An outbreak of disease in the Shaumari herd of Arabian oryx in Jordan (abstract). The 6th International Conference on Wildlife Diseases, Berlin, pp 38–39, 1990.

30. Majonica I, Bonath KH, Haller R: Tiletamine-zolazepam-immobilisation of East African oryx antelopes (*Oryx beisa callotis*). Verh ber Erkrg Zootiere 36:321–323, 1994.

31. Mohammed OB, Hussein HS: Antibody prevalence of toxoplasmosis in Arabian gazelles and oryx in Saudi Arabia. J Wildl Dis 30(4):560–562, 1994.

32. Mushi EZ, Karstad L: Prevalence of virus-neutralizing antibodies to malignant catarrhal fever virus in oryx (*Oryx beisa*). J Wildl Dis 17:467–470, 1981.

33. O'Reilly LM, Daborn CJ: The epidemiology of *Mycobacterium bovis* infections in animals and man: a review. Tubercle and Lung Disease 76(suppl 1):1–46, 1995.

34. Plowright W: The effects of rinderpest and rinderpest control on wildlife in Africa. Symp Zool Soc Lond 50:1–28, 1982.

35. Radwan AI, Bekairi SI, Al-Bokmy AM, et al: Successful therapeutic regimens for treating *Brucella melitensis* and *Brucella abortus* infections in cows. Rev sci tech Off int Epiz 12(3):909–922, 1993.

36. Rietkerk FE, Griffin FT, Wood B, et al: Treatment of bovine tuberculosis in Arabian oryx (*Oryx leucoryx*). J Zoo Wildl Med 24(4):523–527, 1993.

37. Rossiter PB: Rinderpest. *In* Coetzer JAW, Thomson GR, Tustin RC (eds): Infectious Diseases of Livestock with Special Reference to Southern Africa. New York, Oxford University Press, pp 735–757, 1994.

38. St. George TD, Standfast HA: Diseases caused by Akabane and related Simbu-group viruses. *In* Coetzer JAW, Thomson GR, Tustin RC (eds): Infectious Diseases of Livestock with Special Reference to Southern Africa. New York, Oxford University Press, pp 681–687, 1994.

39. Seitre R: Mammal breeding programme of the National Wildlife Research Centre, Taif. *In* Abuzinada AH, Goriup PD, Nader IA (eds): Proceedings of the First Symposium, National Commission for Wildlife Conservation and Development [Publication No. 3], Riyadh, 320–326, 1989.

40. Snyder SB, Richard MJ, Foster WR: Etorphine, ketamine and xylazine in combination (M99KX) for immobilization of exotic ruminants: a significant additive effect. Proceedings of the Joint Meeting of the American Association of Zoo Veterinarians/American Association of Wildlife Veterinarians, Oakland, CA, pp 253–263, 1992.

41. Spalton JA: The Arabian oryx (*Oryx leucoryx*) re-introduction project in Oman: 10 years on. Proceedings of the International Symposium "Ongulés/Ungulates 91," Toulouse, France, pp 343–347, 1991.

42. Stanley-Price MR: Animal Re-Introductions: The Arabian Oryx in Oman. New York, Cambridge University Press, 1989.

43. Thorne ET, Miller MW, Jessup DA, et al: Disease as a consideration in translocating and reintroducing wild animals: Western State Wildlife Management Agency perspectives. Proceedings of the Joint Meeting of the American Association of Zoo Veterinarians/American Association of Wildlife Veterinarians, Oakland, CA, 18–25, 1992.

44. Urquhart GM, Armour J, Duncan JL, et al: Veterinary Parasitology. London, Longman, p 226, 1987.

45. Vassart M, Granjon L, Greth A: Genetic variability in the Arabian oryx (*Oryx leucoryx*). Zoo Biology 10:399–408, 1991.

46. Vassart M, Greth A: Hematological and serum chemistry values for Arabian oryx (*Oryx leucoryx*). J Wildl Dis 27:506–508, 1991.

47. Vassart M, Greth A, Anagariyah S, et al: Biochemical parameters

following capture myopathy in one Arabian oryx (*Oryx leucoryx*). J Vet Med Sci 54:1233–1235, 1992.

48. Vié J-C: Reproductive biology of captive Arabian oryx (*Oryx leucoryx*) in Saudi Arabia. Zoo Biology 15:371–381, 1996.

49. Woodford MH: Veterinary aspects of the reintroduction of the Arabian oryx into Saudi Arabia. *In* Abuzinada AH, Goriup PD, Nader IA (eds): Proceedings of the First Symposium, National Commission for Wildlife Conservation and Development [Publication No. 3], Riyadh, pp 393–399, 1989.

50. Woodford MH, Kock RA: Veterinary considerations in re-introduc-tion and translocation projects. Symp Zool Soc Lond 62:101–110, 1991.

51. Woodford MH, Kock RA, Daly RH, et al: Chemical immobilization of Arabian oryx. *In* Dixon A, Jones D (eds): Conservation and Biology of Desert Antelopes. London, Christopher Helm, pp 90–101, 1988.

52. Woodford MH, Rossiter PB: Disease risks associated with wildlife translocation projects. *In* Olney PJS, Mace GM, Feistner ATC (eds): Creative Conservation: Interactive Management of Wild and Captive Animals. London, Chapman and Hall, pp 178–200, 1994.

Note: Page numbers in *italics* refer to illustrations; page numbers followed by t indicate tables.

A

A3080 (synthetic opioid), 430
  in elephants, 526, 527t, 529
Abbot's duiker (*Cephalophus spadix*). See also *Duikers.*
  conservation status of, 669
Abdominocentesis, in sea turtle, 226
Abomasal cryptosporidiosis, 125
Abortion, 319
  due to brucellosis, 621, 627
  in Arabian oryx, 690
Abscesses, in duikers, 679
  in elephants, 536, 539
  in okapi, 648
  in tapirs, 565
Acanthophis antarcticus (death adder), organ location in, 245
Acaricides, for cheetahs, 420, *420,* 420t
  for elephants, 527
  for ranched hoofstock, 589
Acelaphine herpesvirus–1. See also *Malignant catarrhal fever (MCF).*
  in mixed-species exhibits, 27
Acepromazine, in canids, 430
  in duikers, 674t
  in mountain sheep, 684
  in otters, 441
  in sea turtles, 221, 222t
  in suids, 640t, 642t
Acerodon species. See also *Megachiropterans.*
  conservation status of, 344
Acetylpromazine, in cheetah, 418t
  in hippopotamus, 638
Acid-fast staining, for cryptosporidiosis diagnosis, 128–129
Acinonyx jubatus. See *Cheetah (Acinonyx jubatus).*
Acquired immunodeficiency syndrome (AIDS),
    cryptosporidiosis in, 124
  nontuberculous mycobacterial disease in, 146, 147, 148
  toxoplasmosis in, 134
Acral lick dermatitis, in duikers, 679
Acrodont teeth, in lizards, 252, *253*
  histologic examination of, 253–254, *254*
Acrylic polymers, ultraviolet light transmission by, 66
Activated charcoal, for oiled birds, 303
  to improve water quality for fish, 175
Addax (*Addax nasomaculatus*), artificial insemination in, 599
  handling systems for, 659–660
  leptospirosis in, 590
Adder, death, organ location in, 245
Adenocarcinoma(s), biliary, 425
    in macaw, imaging of, 85, *86*
    in ursids, 426
  gastritis due to, in cheetah, 458
  in callitrichids, 375
Adenomas, biliary, in ursids, 426
  hepatocellular, 425
Aders' duiker (*Cephalophus adersi*). See also *Duikers.*
  conservation status of, 669
Adrenal exhaustion, in duikers, 679
Adrenal gland, sonographic assessment of, 47t, *48*
Adrenal myelolipomas, in callitrichids, 375

α_2-Adrenergic agonists. See also specific drugs.
  in birds, 312
  in canids, 430–431
  in crocodilians, 211–212, 213t–214t
  in marsupials, 334t, 335
α_2-Adrenergic antagonists. See also specific drugs.
  in canids, 431, 433
ADTFs (Animal Data Transfer Forms), 20
Aepyceros melampus (impala), tranquilizers in, 579t, 581
Aeration, in water quality maintenance, for waterfowl, 296, *296*
Aeromonas salmonicida vaccine, 173
Afghan pika (*Ochotona rufescens*), iron overload in, 267
Aflatoxin poisoning, hepatic neoplasms and, 425, 426
  in lemurs, 368
African buffalo (*Syncerus caffer*), tranquilizers in, 579t, 580
  tuberculosis in, 103, 104
    clinical signs of, 106
    lesions of, 106, *107,* 107t
    prevalence of, 104, 105t
    transmission of, 102–103
African bush pig (*Potamochoerus porcus*), anesthesia in, 644, 645
African crested porcupines (*Hystrix* species), reproduction in, 363
African elephant (*Loxodonta africana*). See *Elephants.*
African gray parrot (*Psittacus erithacus*), biliary cysts in, 424
African green monkey (*Cercopithecus aethiops*), viral hepatitis in, 378
African hunting dogs (*Lycaon* species), immobilizing drug dosages for, 434t
African marabou (*Leptoptilus crumeniferus*), sonographic sex determination in, *43*
African river hog (*Potamochoerus porcus*), anesthesia in, 644, 645
African spurred tortoise (*Geochelone sulcata*), vitamin D metabolism in, 73–74
African water hog (*Potamochoerus porcus*), anesthesia in, 644, 645
Agamids. See also *Lizards.*
  periodontal disease in, 252–257, 253t
Agkistrodon species. See also *Snakes.*
  antimicrobials in, 192t, 194
Agoutis (*Dasyprocta* species), reproduction in, 363–364
  vitamin D toxicity in, in mixed-species exhibits, 27, 72, 75
AIDS (acquired immunodeficiency syndrome),
    cryptosporidiosis in, 124
  nontuberculous mycobacterial disease in, 146, 147, 148
  toxoplasmosis in, 134
Ailuropoda melanoleuca (giant panda). See under *Pandas.*
Ailurus fulgens (red panda), iron overload in, 267
Air emboli, in fish tissue, 168–169, *170*
Air pollution, marine mammals and, 477
Akabane virus, in Arabian oryx, 692t
Akineton (biperiden), for extrapyramidal symptoms in herbivores, 579, 580, 581, 583
Alarm system, for snakebite, 98, *98*
Albendazole, in fish, 183t, 188
  in hoofstock, 587t, 589

Albumin, in vitamin D transport, 64
Alcelaphus species. See *Hartebeests.*
Alces alces (moose), brucellosis in, 623
  Elaphostrongylus infection in, 632
  Parelaphostrongylus tenuis in, 29, 633
    white-tailed deer and, 635
Alcohols, for disinfection, 176t
Aldrin, in marine mammals, 472
Alexandrium tamarense, marine mammal deaths due to, 477
Alfadolone acetate, alfaxolone with, in cheetah, 416–417
  in marsupials, 335
Alfalfa (*Medicago sativa*), vitamin D in, 63
Alfaxalone/alfadolone acetate, in cheetah, 416–417
  in marsupials, 335
Algogens, 309–310
Allergies, bird-related, 153t, 155
  in black rhinoceros, 554
Alligators. See also *Crocodilians.*
  antimicrobials in, 191t, 193
  gallamine morbidity and mortality in, 206, 210
  respiratory rate of, 216
Alopecia, in lemurs, 367
  in megachiropterans, 352
Alopex species (foxes), immobilizing drug dosages for, 434t
  rabies in, 139
Alouatta species (howler monkeys), herpesvirus infection in, 28
  rickets in, 71, *71*
Alpaca (*Lama pacos*), embryo transfer in, 601
Alpha-adrenergic agents. See *Adrenergic* entries.
Alphaxolone/alphadolone acetate, in cheetah, 416–417
  in marsupials, 335
Alum, for phytoplankton control in waterfowl exhibits, 297
Aluminum hydroxide, for leptospirosis in pinnipeds, 471
Aluminum phosphide, as rodenticide, 118t
Aluminum sulfate, for phytoplankton control in waterfowl exhibits, 297
Alveolitis, allergic, due to bird contact, 153t, 155
Amazon parrot (*Amazona farinosa farinosa*), meningoencephalitis in, imaging of, 87, *87*
Ambylomma species, on cheetah, 419t
  on ranched hoofstock, 589
American alligator (*Alligator mississippiensis*). See also *Crocodilians.*
  antimicrobials in, 191t, 193
  gallamine morbidity and mortality in, 206, 210
  respiratory rate of, 216
American bison (*Bison bison*), brucellosis in, 623, 624
  embryo transfer in, 599, 600–601
  estrous cycle synchronization in, 598
  handling systems for, 660, *660*
  Ostertagia ostertagi in, 588
  tuberculosis in, 101, 102–103, 651
    clinical signs of, 106
    lesions of, 107t
    prevalence of, 105t
American black bear (*Ursus americanus*), hepatic proliferative disease in, 426
American Zoo and Aquarium Association (AZA), cervid tuberculosis regulation in, 655
  quarantine protocol of, 13–17
Amethystine python (*Morelia amethistina*), organ location in, 243, *246*
  case study, 247–248
Amikacin, in chelonians, 191–192
  in crocodilians, 191t, 193
  in elephants, 537
  in lizards, 257
  in manatees, 511
  in reptiles, renal-portal system's effect on kinetics of, 250

Amikacin *(Continued)*
  temperature and, 197
  in sea turtles, 230t
  in snakes, 192t, 194
    in combination dosing, 194–195
  in stranded cetaceans, 489t
  in tree kangaroos, 340
Amino acids, fruit bat requirements for, 356
  in pigeon milk, 271, 272t
  in pigeon milk replacer, 275
Aminoglycosides. See also specific drugs.
  in chelonians, 191–192, 191t
  in elephants, 537
  in reptiles, renal-portal system's effect on kinetics of, 250, 251
  in snakes, 192t, 194
    in combination dosing, 194–195
4-Aminopyridine, as anesthetic antagonist in canids, 431
  as bird repellent, 119
Amitraz, in cheetah, 419, 420t
Ammonia, water contamination with, 169, 170–171, 170t
Ammotragus lervia (aoudad, Barbary sheep), immobilization of, 685
Amoebiasis, in lemurs, 366
  in mixed-species exhibits, 29
Amoxicillin, in cheetah, 459t, 460
  in elephants, 535, 536
  in fish, 183t, 185
Amoxicillin/clavulanic acid, in stranded cetaceans, 489t
Amphibians. See also specific animals.
  attaching telemetry equipment to, 8t
  iron overload in, 264
  minimally invasive surgery in, 36
  quarantine for, 14, 16t
  shipment of, 21, 22
  sonographic assessment in, for sex determination, 42, *43*
    of health, 47t
  vitamin D deficiency in, 74
Amphojel (aluminum hydroxide), for leptospirosis in pinnipeds, 471
Amphotericin B, in fish, 187
  in marine mammals, 483, 483t
Ampicillin, for leptospirosis, 471
  in California condor, 287, 290
  in chelonians, 191, 191t
  in elephants, 535–536
  in koala, 326, 327
Amsinckia intermedia (fiddleneck), toxicity of, 89
Amyloidosis, pancreatic, in primate diabetes, 398
Ana-Kit, for anaphylaxis with snakebite, 100
Analgesia, in birds, 309–313
    agents for, 311–313
    mechanical forms of, 313
  in fish, 184t, 189
  mechanisms of, 310
Anaphylaxis, with snakebite, 100
Anas platyrhynchos (mallard duck), seasonal siderosis in, 264
Ancylostoma caninum, in giant panda, 413
Andean condor (*Vultur gryphus*), anesthesia in, 282
  in California condor management program, 278
Andrias davidianus (Chinese giant salamander), sonographic sex determination in, *43*
Anemia, in oiled birds, 302, 304
Anemones, clown fish and, 171–172
Anesthesia. See also *Immobilization;* specific drugs.
  artificial insemination and, in felids, 454–455, 455t
  in Andean condor, 282
  in California condor, 281–282, *282*
  in chameleons, 204
  in cheetah, 416–418, 418t, 459

Anesthesia *(Continued)*
   in elephants, 526–527, 527t, 528–529
   in fish, 158–163, *160,* 161t
      monitoring of, 162
      waterborne, 159–161, *160,* 161t
   in manatees, 510
   in marsupials, 333–336, 334t
      injectable agents for, 334–335, 334t
      monitoring of, 333–334
      volatile agents for, 335–336
   in megachiropterans, 345, *346*
   in Nile hippopotamus, 638–639
   in otters, 436–442
      agents for, 439–441
      drug delivery for, 437
      in translocation projects, 441–442, 446, 447t
      monitoring during, 437–438, *438,* 438t
      recovery from, 438
   in sea turtles, 221–223, *222,* 222t
   in suids, 639–645
      domestic, 640–642, 640t, 642t
      monitoring of, 641, 643
      nondomestic, 642–645
   in tapirs, 562–563
   in tree kangaroos, 338–339
   in turkey vulture, 282
   in white rhinoceros, 556–561. See also under *Rhinoceroses.*
   local, in birds, 313
   pulse oximetry in monitoring of, 2–3. See also *Pulse oximetry.*
Aneurysm, aortic, in lemurs, 367–368
Anhingas, water retention in feathers of, 306
Anichkov cells, in elephant heart, in flaccid trunk paralysis, 542
Animal and Plant Health Inspection Service (APHIS), 23
Animal Data Transfer Forms (ADTFs), 20
Animal Welfare Act (AWA), behavioral enrichment standards of, 387–391. See also *Environmental enrichment.*
   shipping regulations of, 17, 19, 22, 23
Anoplocephala, in manatees, 514
Antacids, for leptospirosis in pinnipeds, 471
Antagonil. See *Yohimbine.*
Antarctic fur seal (*Arctocephalus gazello*), fungal infections in, 479t
Antelope. See also *Artiodactylids;* specific animals.
   copper deficiency in, in mixed-species exhibits, 27
   embryo transfer in, 600, 600t, 601, 601t
   parasites in, 587–588
   protocol for pre-shipment health screening of, 587
Anthelmintics. See also specific drugs.
   classification of, 589
   for trichostrongyloid parasites, 595–596
   in cheetah, 421t
   in fish, 183t, 187–188
   in hoofstock, in game ranching, 587t, 588–589
   parasite resistance to, 589, 594, 596
   strategies for use of, 594
Anthrax, in Arabian oryx, 695
   in elephants, 536
   in ranched hoofstock, 590
Antibiotics. See *Antimicrobials;* specific drugs.
Antibody detection assays, 57–58. See also *Serologic testing;* specific types.
Antibody transfer, passive. See *Passive antibody transfer.*
Antidorcas marsupialis (springbok), biliary cysts in, 424
   tranquilizers in, 579t, 581–582, *582, 583*
Antigen(s), specific, lymphoproliferative response to, as measure of anamnestic response, 62
Antigen 85 testing, in cervids, 653

Antigen 85 testing *(Continued)*
   in orangutan, 395
   in ranched hoofstock, 590
Antigen detection assays, 56–57. See also *Serologic testing;* specific types.
Antihelminthics. See *Anthelmintics;* specific drugs.
Antilope cervicapra (blackbuck), artificial insemination in, 599
   handling systems for, 660
Antimicrobials. See also specific drugs.
   in ape neonates, for bacterial meningitis, 385
      for diarrheal disease, 386
   in chameleons, 204
   in duikers, 679
   in elephants, 533–540
      clinical application of, 539–540
      dosage calculation for, 534
      pharmacokinetic studies of, 535–539
      routes of administration for, 534–535
   in fish, 182, 183t, 184–187
      during quarantine, 165, 169t
   in koala, for chlamydiosis, 326
      for respiratory disease, 326
   in manatees, 511–512
   in mountain sheep and goats, 686
   in otters, in translocation project, 444–445, 445t
   in reptiles, 190–198
      administration of, 197–198
      combination dosing with, 194–195
      doses for, 191–195, 191t, 192t
      environmental considerations in, 196–197
      metabolic scaling and, 198
      renal-portal system's effect on kinetics of, 249–251
      selection of, 195–196
   in sea turtles, 230, 230t
   in stranded cetaceans, 488, 489t
Antispermatogenics, 317, 318
Antivenom, 96–97, *97, 98*
Antivenom Index, 96
Anubis baboon (*Papio anubis*), tuberculosis in, 105t
   vitamin D transport in, 64
Aonchotheca putorii, in cheetah, 458
Aonyx capensis (Cape clawless otter), anesthesia in, 439
   geographic distribution of, 436t
Aonyx cinerea (Asian small-clawed otter), anesthesia in, 439, 440, 441
   geographic distribution of, 436t
Aonyx congica (Congo clawless otter), geographic distribution of, 436t
Aortic aneurysm, in lemurs, 367–368
Aotus trivirgatus (owl monkey), herpesvirus infection in, 28
   viral hepatitis in, 378
   vitamin D transport in, 64
Aoudad (*Ammotragus lervia*), immobilization of, 685
Apes. See also *Primates;* specific types.
   neonates of, 382–387
      congenital defects in, 386–387
      hand-rearing of, 383–384
      infections in, 385–387
      mother-rearing of, 383
      normal, 382–383
   obstetric complications in, 384–385
Apgar scale, for neonatal apes, 382
APHIS (Animal and Plant Health Inspection Service), 23
Apnea, during anesthesia, in elephants, 529
   in white rhinoceros, 559–560
Apophysomyces elegans infection, in marine mammals, 480t
April Formula, for dolphin milk replacement, 494, 494t
Arabian oryx (*Oryx leucoryx*), 687–696
   behavior of, 688

Arabian oryx (*Oryx leucoryx*) (*Continued*)
  genetic considerations in, 696
  hand-rearing of, in tuberculosis outbreak, 694
  immobilization of, 689–690, 689t
  infectious diseases of, 690–696, 692t
  laboratory reference values for, 690, 691t
  physical restraint of, 688–689
  reintroduction of, 687–696
    steps in, 696
  release of, 690
  reproduction in, 690
  surgical conditions in, 696
  transport of, 690
Arctic fox (*Alopex lagopus*), rabies in, 139
Arctocephalus gazello (Antarctic fur seal), fungal infections in, 479t
Argentine tortoise (*Geochelone chilensis*), herpesvirus infection in, 28
Armenian red sheep (*Ovis orientalis*), embryo transfer in, 599, 600
  estrous cycle synchronization in, 598
Arowana (*Osteoglossum bicirrhosum*), sonographic sex determination in, *43*
Arthritis, degenerative, in lemurs, 367
  rheumatoid, in elephants, 540
  septic, in ape neonates, 386
Arthus-like reactions, in black rhinoceros, 554
Artibeus jamaicensis (fruit bat), energy requirement of, 357
  protein requirement of, 356
Artificial insemination, in artiodactylids, 598–599
  in black-footed ferret, 452, 452t, 454, 461–462
  in carnivores, 451–456
    disease transmission in, 453–454, 454t
    future challenges in, 456
    hormonal stimulation in, 455–456, 455t, *456*
    laparoscopic, 452–453, 452t, *453, 454*
    site of, 452, 452t
    time of, 454–455, 455t
  sonographic support of, 52–53, *53*
Artiodactylids, 575–696. See also specific types.
  assisted reproduction in, 597–602
    using artificial insemination, 598–599
    using embryo transfer, 599–601, 600t, 601t
    using in vitro fertilization, 601–602
  contraception in, using PZP vaccination, 628–631, 629t, 630t
  estrous cycle synchronization in, 598
  free-ranging, *Brucella abortus* infection in, 621–625. See also *Brucella abortus infection.*
    Brucella suis infection in, 626–627
    Elaphostrongylus cervi in, 632, 635–636
    Parelaphostrongylus tenuis in, 632–635
  game ranching of. See *Game ranching.*
  iron overload in, 266
  tranquilizers in, 575–584. See also *Tranquilizers;* specific drugs.
Ascarids, in chameleons, 203
  in giant panda, 413
Ascites, sonographic detection of, 44–47, *47*
Ascorbic acid (vitamin C), for elephant poxvirus infection, 549
  for stranded cetaceans, 491
  in captive lemur diet, iron overload and, 366
  in fish diet, 173, 173t
Asian cobra (*Naja naja*), biliary cystadenoma in, 424
Asian elephant (*Elaphus maximus*). See *Elephants.*
Asian rhinoceros (*Rhinoceros unicornis*). See also *Rhinoceroses.*
  feeding behavior in, 568
  leiomyoma in, sonographic assessment of, *50*

Asian rhinoceros (*Rhinoceros unicornis*) (*Continued*)
  nutrition in, 570t
Asian small-clawed otter (*Aonyx cinerea*), anesthesia in, 439, 440, 441
  geographic distribution of, 436t
Asian tapir (*Tapirus indicus*), 562, 562t. See also *Tapirs.*
  birth weight of, 565
Asian wild dog (*Cuon alpinus*), immobilizing drug dosages for, 434t
  sonographic health assessment in, *47, 50, 51*
Asiatic black bear (*Selenarctos thibetanus*), hepatic proliferative disease in, 426
Aspergillosis, in California condor, 290
  in marine mammals, 479t, 482, 483
  in oiled birds, 302, 304
  zoonotic potential of, 153t, 154
Aspiration, gastric, in stranded cetacean, 487, 488, 490
Aspiration and injection test, 34
Aspiration pneumonia, in ape neonates, 385
  in oiled birds, 302
Assault (bromethalin), 117
Asses. See also *Equids.*
  captive population of, 572t
Ateles species (spider monkeys), herpesvirus carriage by, 28
Atelocynus species (small-eared dogs), immobilizing drug dosages for, 434t
Atipamezole, in birds, 312
  in canids, 431
  in cheetah, 417
  in crocodilians, 214t, 215
  in duikers, 673t
  in marsupials, 335
  in mountain sheep and goats, 685
  in okapi, 649
  in otters, 440, 441, 442
Atlantic bottlenose dolphin. See *Bottlenose dolphin (Tursiops truncatus).*
Atropine, in canids, 431
  in crocodilians, 214t, 215
  in hippopotamus, 639
  in marsupials, 335
  in otters, 441
  in sea turtles, 230t
  in suids, 640t, 642, 642t
    nondomestic, 642, 644
Auks, shipment of, 22
Australian bat virus, 137t, 138
Austrochirus perkinsi, on koala, 330t
Avian botulism, 297–299, *298*
Avian herpesviruses, in mixed-species exhibits, 28
Avitrol (4-aminopyridine), 119
AWA (Animal Welfare Act), behavioral enrichment standards of, 387–391. See also *Environmental enrichment.*
  shipping regulations of, 17, 19, 22, 23
Axis deer (*Axis axis*), handling systems for, 658, 659
  tuberculosis in, 106, 651
Axolotis species, shipment of, 21
AZA (American Zoo and Aquarium Association), cervid tuberculosis regulation of, 655
  quarantine protocol of, 13–17
Azaleas, toxicity of, 89
Azaperone, in Arabian oryx, 689t
  in canids, 430
  in cheetah, 418t
  in duikers, 673t, 675
  in elephants, 527t, 529, 530, 583
  in marsupials, 335t
  in okapi, 649
  in otters, 438t, 441

Azaperone *(Continued)*
  in suids, 640t, 642t
    nondomestic, 642
  in tapirs, 563
  in white rhinoceros, 556t, 557t, 559, 560
    for darting in confinement, 561
    for transport, 583
  in wild herbivores, 577–578
    species guidelines for, 579–584
Azithromycin, in stranded cetaceans, 489t
  in tree kangaroos, 340

B

Babirusa *(Babyrousa babyrussa)*, 639
  anesthesia in, 644, 645
Baboons. See also *Apes.*
  biliary cystadenoma in, 424
  malignant T cell lymphoma in, 380–381
  reproductive tract evaluation in, using minimally invasive
    surgery, *39*
  tuberculosis in, 102, 103, 104
    clinical signs of, 106
    lesions of, 107t, 108, *108*
    prevalence of, 105t
    vitamin D transport in, 64
Babyrousa babyrussa (babirusa), 639
  anesthesia in, 644, 645
Bacdip (quinthiophos), in cheetah, 420t
Bacille Calmette-Guérin (BCG) vaccine, 112
  in cervids, 654
Bacterial dermatitis, in manatees, 514
Bacterial enteritis, in California condor chicks, 286–287, *287*
  in koala young, 331
  in lemurs, 365–366
Bacterial infections. See also specific diseases.
  acquired from birds, 151–154
  in ape neonates, 385–386
  in Arabian oryx, 692t, 693–695
  in callitrichids, 371
  in chameleons, 203
  in chelonians, 240t
  in duikers, 677–679
  in equids, 572t, 573
  in lemurs, 365–366
  in megachiropterans, 347–348
  in mixed-species exhibits, 28
  in reptiles, 190, 195
  in tree kangaroos, 339–341, *340, 341*
Bactrian camel *(Camelus bactrianus)*, equine herpesvirus
    infection in, 27
  leiomyoma in, sonographic assessment of, *50*
Badgers, tuberculosis in, 102, 103
  clinical signs of, 106
  lesions of, 107t
  prevalence of, 105t
Baikal seal *(Phoca sibirica)*, canine distemper virus in, 408,
    497
Baird's tapir *(Tapirus bairdi)*, 562, 562t. See also *Tapirs.*
  neonatal isoerythrolysis in, 565
Baiting, in mountain sheep and goat capture, 682, *683,*
    686–687
  in vermin control, 116
    for birds, 119
    for rodents, 117, 118t
Balantidium infection, in ape neonates, 386
  in lemurs, 366
  in mixed-species exhibits, 29

Bamboo, in giant panda diet, 411
Bandl's rings, 522
Banteng *(Bos javanicus)*, embryo transfer in, 601
  estrous cycle synchronization in, 598
Barasingha deer *(Cervus duvauceli)*, obesity in, 27
Barbary red deer *(Cervus elaphus barbarus)*. See also *Cervus
    elaphus (red deer, elk, wapiti).*
  biliary cysts in, 424
Barbary sheep *(Ammotragus lervia)*, immobilization of, 685
Barbiturates, in crocodilians, 212
Basking, by sea turtles, 219
Bat paramyxovirus, 349
Bats. See *Chiroptera;* specific types.
Bay duiker *(Cephalophus dorsalis)*. See also *Duikers.*
  anesthesia in, 673t
  conservation status of, 669
  iron overload in, 266
  laboratory reference values for, 676t–677t
Baylisascaris species, in callitrichids, 373
  in mixed-species exhibits, 29
Bayticol (flumethrin), in cheetah, 420t
BCG (bacille Calmette-Guérin) vaccine, 112
  in cervids, 654
BCH (benzene hexachloride), in marine mammals, 473
BCV (bovine coronavirus). See *Coronavirus infection.*
Beaked whale, Cuvier's, subcutaneous emphysema in, 490
Bearded pig *(Sus barbatus)*, anesthesia in, 644, 645
Bears, hepatic proliferative disease in, 426
  polar. See *Polar bear (Thalarctos maritimus).*
  sonographic fetal assessment in, *52*
Beaver, North American, reproduction in, 362
Behavioral enrichment, 387–391. See also *Environmental
    enrichment.*
Behavioral fever, in reptiles, 196
Beluga whale *(Delphinapterus leucas)*, antifungal drugs in,
    483t
  hand-reared, dolphin immunoglobulin for, 496
  organochlorines in, 474
Benzene hexachloride (BCH), in marine mammals, 473
Benzodiazepines. See also specific drugs.
  in canids, 430
  in crocodilians, 214t, 215
  in otters, 439–440
  in white rhinoceros, 559
Benzuldazic acid, for ringworm, in cheetah, 418
Bertiella obesa, in koala, 330t
Besnoitiosis, in duikers, 677
Betamethasone, in birds, 312
Big brown bat *(Eptesicus fuscus)*, control of, 118
Bighorn sheep *(Ovis canadensis)*, 681–687, *683, 684*
  capture techniques for, 682–683, *683, 684*
    evaluation of, 685–686
  immobilization of, 684, 685
  Johne's disease in, 616–617, 618, *618*
  physical restraint of, 683–684
Bile duct carcinoma, 425
Biliary adenocarcinoma, 425
  in callitrichids, 375
  in macaw, imaging of, 85, *86*
  in ursids, 426
Biliary adenoma, in ursids, 426
Biliary cystadenocarcinoma, 425
  in felids, 427
Biliary cystadenoma, 424, *424*
  in felids, 427
Biliary cysts, noninfectious, 423–424, *424*
Biochemical reference values, for Arabian oryx, 690, 691t
  for duikers, 675–676, 676t–678t
  for giant panda, 412t
  for koala, 324t

Biochemical reference values *(Continued)*
    for manatees, 512t
    for sea turtles, 224t
    for tapirs, 564t
    for tree kangaroos, 339, 339t
Biopsy, endoscopic, 38–39
    gastric, in cheetah, 459
    gill, *168*
    in fungal infection diagnosis, in marine mammals, 482
    in Johne's disease detection, 614–615
    liver, in iron overload diagnosis, 262, 263t
Biotelemetry, equipment for, suppliers of, 9t–11t
    techniques for attaching, 8t
    in wildlife monitoring, 7–13
Biotin. See also *Vitamin B complex.*
    in fish diet, 173t
Biparietal diameter, sonographic, in dolphin fetal growth
        assessment, 503–504, *504, 505*
Biperiden, for extrapyramidal symptoms in herbivores, 579,
        580, 581, 583
Birds, 260–313. See also specific types.
    analgesia in, 309–313
        agents for, 311–313
    attaching telemetry equipment to, 8t
    cryptosporidiosis in, 125–126, 153t, 155
    in mixed-species exhibits, bacterial infection in, 28
        nutritional problems in, 27
        parasites in, 29
        trauma to, 26, 27
    iron levels in, 261–262
    iron overload in, 264–265, 265t
    minimally invasive surgery in, 37–38
    nontuberculous mycobacterial disease in, 147, 148, 153t,
        154
    oiled. See under *Oil spills.*
    pain in, recognition of, 310–311
        treatment of, 313
    problems associated with contact with, 153t, 155
    quarantine for, 14, 16t, 151
    shipment of, 21, 22–23
    sonographic assessment in, for sex determination, 42, *43*
        of health, 47t
        of sexual maturation, 44, *45*
    uninvited, disease introduction by, 28
    water-related diseases in, 297–299, *298*
    zoonoses acquired from, 151–155, 152t, 153t. See also *Zoo-
        noses;* specific diseases.
Bisdiamine, for contraception, 317, 319
Bismuth subsalicylate, for gastritis in cheetah, 459t, 460
    for oiled birds, 303
    for stranded cetaceans, 489t
Bison. See *American bison (Bison bison).*
Black bears, hepatic proliferative disease in, 426
Black duiker *(Cephalophus niger).* See also *Duikers.*
    anesthesia in, 673t
    laboratory reference values for, 676t–677t
Black racer *(Coluber constrictor),* antimicrobials in, 192t,
        194
Black rat *(Rattus rattus),* control of, 116–117
Black rat snake *(Elaphe obsoleta),* antimicrobials in, 192t,
        193
Black rhinoceros *(Diceros bicornis).* See under *Rhinoceroses.*
Black snake, red-bellied, organ location in, 245
Black wildebeest, tranquilizers in, 579, 579t
Blackbuck *(Antilope cervicapra),* artificial insemination in,
        599
    handling systems for, 660
Black-chested mustached tamarin *(Saguinus mystax).* See also
        Callitrichids.
    vitamin D metabolism in, 71

Black-footed ferret *(Mustela nigripes),* artificial insemination
        in, 452, 452t, 454, 461–462
    conservation program for, 460–462
Black-footed penguin *(Spheniscus demersus),* sonographic sex
        determination in, *43*
Black-tailed deer. See *Mule deer (Odocoileus hemionus).*
Black-tailed marmoset *(Callithrix argentata).* See also
        Callitrichids.
    herpesvirus infection in, 28
Blastomyces dermatitidis infection, in marine mammals, 480t
Blesbok *(Damaliscus dorcas),* copper deficiency in, in mixed-
        species exhibits, 27
    tranquilizers in, 579t, 580
Bloat, in callitrichids, 374
    in stranded cetaceans, 489
Blood collection, in California condor, 281, 281t, 287
    in cheetah, 459
    in fish, 179, *179,* 180t
    in manatees, 510, *511*
    in megachiropterans, 345–346, *346, 347*
    in sea turtles, 224–225, *225, 226*
    in suids, 643, 644
    in tapirs, 563
    in tree kangaroos, 339
Blood python *(Python curtis),* antimicrobials in, 192t, 193
Blood tuberculosis test (BTB), 590–591
    in cervids, 653
Blow pipes, for drug administration, in canids, 432
Blow specimen, cetacean, diagnostic cytology of, 465–466,
        466
Blowflies, on koala, 330t
Blue and gold macaw, biliary adenocarcinoma in, imaging of,
        85, *86*
Blue duiker *(Cephalophus monticola).* See also *Duikers.*
    anesthesia in, 673t
    conservation status of, 669
    laboratory values for, 676t–677t
Blue wildebeest, tranquilizers in, 579–580, 579t
Bluetongue (BT), in Arabian oryx, 692t, 693
    in ranched hoofstock, 591
Boa constrictor *(Boa constrictor),* antimicrobials in, 192t, 194
Bobcats, control of, 118
Boids. See also *Snakes.*
    organ location in, 244–245, *247*
    paramyxovirus infection in, 28
Boiga dendrophila (mangrove snake), antimicrobials in, 192t,
        193, 194
Boiga irregularis (brown tree snake), organ location in, 245
Bolivian red howler monkey *(Alouatta seniculus),* rickets in,
        71, *71*
Bone disease, metabolic, in callitrichids, 374
    in chameleons, 204
    in megachiropterans, 349
Bongo *(Boocercus euryceros),* embryo transfer in, 600, 600t,
        601, 601t
    handling systems for, *661*
    iron overload in, 266
Bonobo *(Pan paniscus),* birth weight for, 383
    herpesvirus infection in, 386
    papillomavirus in, 380
    simian T lymphotrophic virus in, 381
Bontebok *(Damaliscus dorcas),* copper deficiency in, in
        mixed-species exhibits, 27
    tranquilizers in, 579t, 580
Boocercus euryceros (bongo), embryo transfer in, 600, 600t,
        601, 601t
    handling systems for, *661*
    iron overload in, 266
Bordetella bronchiseptica, in koala, 326–327
    in mixed-species exhibits, 28

Bos gaurus. See *Gaur (Bos gaurus).*
Bos javanicus (banteng), embryo transfer in, 601
  estrous cycle synchronization in, 598
Bottlenose dolphin (*Tursiops truncatus*). See also *Cetaceans.*
  caloric requirements of calves, 495
  diagnostic cytology in, *466, 468*
  fetal ultrasonography in, 502–506, *503–506*
  fungal infections in, 479t–481t, 483t
  hand-reared, immunoglobulin for, 496
    weaning of, 496
  morbillivirus infection in, 497, 498
Botulism, avian, 297–299, *298*
  in Arabian oryx, 692t, 695
Bovids. See also *Artiodactylids;* specific animals.
  contraception in, using PZP vaccination, 630, 630t
  cryptosporidiosis in, 122t, 125
  domestic. See *Livestock, domestic.*
  scrapie-like spongiform encephalopathy in, 662, *663, 665,* 665t
Bovine coronavirus (BCV). See *Coronavirus infection.*
Bovine rotavirus (BRV). See *Rotavirus infection.*
Bovine spongiform encephalopathy. See *Scrapie-like spongiform encephalopathies.*
Bovine tuberculosis. See *Tuberculosis.*
Bovine viral diarrhea, in ranched hoofstock, 591
Box chutes. See also *Handling systems.*
  for ungulates, 660
Box turtle (*Terrapene carolina*), antimicrobials in, 191t, 193
Brain, fish, diseases affecting, 178t
  macaw, tumor imaging in, 85–87, *86, 87*
  pigeon, imaging of, 87, *87*
Brainlia species, in koala, 330t
Branta canadensis (Canada goose), control of, 119–120
Brazilian tapir (*Tapirus terrestris*), 562, 562t, 567. See also *Tapirs.*
Breeding. See also *Reproduction.*
  sonographic assessment of potential for, 44–47, *47,* 47t, *48,* 53–54
Breeding facility, for cheetahs, 415–422
Brewer's yeast, with sulfa-pyrimethamine therapy for toxoplasmosis, 133
Brodifacoum, in vermin control, 117, 118t
  poisoning by, in callitrichids, 374
Bromadiolone, 117, 118t
Bromethalin, 117
Bromhexine hydrochloride, in koala, 326
Bronchi, of cetaceans, diagnostic cytology of, 466
Bronchiolitis, allergic, due to bird contact, 153t, 155
Bronchoalveolar lavage, in fungal infection diagnosis, in marine mammals, 482
Brown bats, control of, 118
Brown bear, Eurasian, hepatic proliferative disease in, 426
  sonographic fetal assessment in, *52*
Brown lemur (*Lemur fulvus*), vitamin D toxicity in, 75
Brown snake, eastern, organ location in, 245
Brown tree snake (*Boiga irregularis*), organ location in, 245
Browse, for koala, storage of, renal disease and, 329
  for rhinoceroses, 569, 569t, 570t
  for tree kangaroos, 338
  toxic species in, 89, 389–390
Brucella abortus infection, in Arabian oryx, 694
  in carnivores, 622
  in free-ranging artiodactylids, 621–625
    control and eradication of, 623–625, 624t
    diagnosis of, 622
    epizootiology of, 623
    transmission of, 622
    treatment of, 622
  in ranched hoofstock, 590
  pathogenesis of, 621–622

Brucella abortus infection *(Continued)*
  screening test for, predictive value of, 56, 57t
  vaccination for, 622–623, 624
Brucella melitensis infection, in Arabian oryx, 694
Brucella species, classification of, 621
Brucella suis infection, in free-ranging artiodactylids, 626–627, *627*
  in humans, 626–627
BRV (bovine rotavirus). See *Rotavirus infection.*
BT (bluetongue), in Arabian oryx, 692t, 693
  in ranched hoofstock, 591
BTB (blood tuberculosis test), 590–591
  in cervids, 653
Bubalus bubalis (water buffalo), tuberculosis in, 101, 102–103, 104
  lesions of, 107t
  prevalence of, 105t
Bubbler aerators, in water quality maintenance, for waterfowl, 296, *296*
Buffalo, African. See *African buffalo (Syncerus caffer).*
  American. See *American bison (Bison bison).*
  water, tuberculosis in, 101, 102–103, 104
    lesions of, 107t
    prevalence of, 105t
Bull snake (*Pituophis melanoleucus catenifer*), antimicrobials in, 192t, 194
Bupivacaine, in birds, 313
Buprenorphine, in birds, 311
Burmese python (*Python molurus bivittatus*), antimicrobials in, 192t, 194
Bush dogs (*Speothos* species), immobilizing drug dosages for, 434t
Bush pig (*Potamochoerus porcus*), anesthesia in, 644, 645
Butorphanol, in birds, 311–312
  in canids, 430
  in fish, 162, 184t, 189
  in marsupials, 335
  in otters, 441
  in suids, domestic, 642, 642t
    nondomestic, 644–645
  in tapirs, 562
B-virus, in mixed-species exhibits, 28
  in primates, 380

C

Cabergoline, for abortion, 319
Cadmium, in marine mammals, 475
Cadmium chloride, sterilization using, 317
Cage card, for venomous snakes, *96,* 97, *98*
Cage paralysis, 70–71
Caiman (*Caiman crocodilus*). See also *Crocodilians.*
  respiratory rate of, 216
Calcidiol (25[OH]D₃), 64
  oral supplements of, 69–70
Calciferol in oil (injectable vitamin D₂), 70
Calcijex (injectable calcitriol), 70
Calciol (vitamin D₃), 63–65, *64*
  as rodenticide, 117, 118t
  crystalline, 70
  in chameleon diet, 202
Calcitonin (CT), in calcium regulation, 65
Calcitriol (1,25[OH]₂D₃), 64
  in calcium regulation, 65
  injectable, 70
Calcium, in chameleon diet, 202
  in fish diet, 174t
  plasma concentration of, in duikers, 675, 676, 676t, 678t
  regulation of, vitamin D and, 65

Calcium sulfate, for phytoplankton control in waterfowl exhibits, 297
Calel-D (vitamin D/calcium supplement), 70
Calf diarrhea. See also *Coronavirus infection; Rotavirus infection.*
  clinical signs of, 608
  epizootiology of, 607
  treatment of, 610
Calf Guard, 611
Calicivirus, vaccination for, in cheetah, 418
California condor (*Gymnogyps californianus*), 277–291
  anesthesia in, 281–282, *282*
  annual examination of, 280–281, 281t
  biologic data on, 278–279, *278*
  captive husbandry of, 279
  environmental contaminants affecting, 288
  fatal malposition in, 283, *283, 285*
  infections in, 288–290
  necropsy findings in, 287–288, 289t
  physical restraint of, 280, *280, 281*
  population of, 279t
    causes for decline in, 277–278
  quarantine for, 280
  radiographic imaging in, 282–283, *283, 284*
  released, medical treatment for, 290–291
  reproduction in, 284–285, 284t, *285*
    care of newly hatched chicks, 285–287, *286, 287*
  sex determination in, 287
  sick, clinical evaluation of, 290
  surgery in, 283–284
  transportation of, 279
  yolk sac infection in, 283, 284, *284,* 286, *286*
California gray whale (*Eschrichtius gibbosus*), iron overload in, 267
California sea lion (*Zalophus californianus*), fungal infections in, 479t, 480t
  leptospirosis in, 469–470, *470,* 471
Callicebus moloch (titi monkey), diabetes in, parasite-induced, 398
  treatment of, 399
Callimico goeldii (Goeldi's monkey), 369. See also *Callitrichids.*
  Gongylonema infection in, 372, *372*
  hepatic myelolipoma in, 426
Callithrix argentata (black-tailed marmoset). See also *Callitrichids.*
  herpesvirus infection in, 28
Callithrix jaccus (common marmoset). See also *Callitrichids.*
  iron overload in, 265
  vitamin D metabolism in, 64, 72
Callithrix pygmaea (pygmy marmoset). See also *Callitrichids.*
  callitrichid hepatitis in, 378
Callitrichids. See also *Primates; specific types.*
  classification of, 369
  diseases of, 369–375
    infectious, 370–373, *370, 372, 373*
    noninfectious, 373–375
  hepatitis in, 28, 370, *370,* 377–378
Callorhinus ursinus (northern fur seal), fungal infections in, 479t
  leptospirosis in, 469, *470,* 471
Camel, bactrian, equine herpesvirus infection in, 27
  leiomyoma in, sonographic assessment of, *50*
Camelids. See also specific types.
  New World, artificial insemination in, 599
    embryo transfer in, 601
    estrous cycle synchronization in, 598
Camelostrongylus mentulatus, in Arabian oryx, 695
  in Texas ranch-raised hoofstock, 588

Campylobacter jejuni, 152t, 154
  in California condor chicks, 287
  in callitrichids, 371
  zoonotic potential of, 152t, 154
Canada goose (*Branta canadensis*), control of, 119–120
Canary, pseudotuberculosis in, 154
Candida species, in cetaceans, 466, 467, *467*
  in koala young, 331
  in marine mammals, 479t, 481–482
    diagnosis of, 482
    treatment of, 483
Canids. See also *Carnivores; specific animals.*
  capture of, 432
  immobilization of, 429–434
    animal handling in, 432–433
    drugs for, 430–431
      administration of, 431–432, 433
      doses for, 432, 433–434, 434t
    medical concerns in, 433
Canine anti-lipopolysaccharide antiserum, for septicemia, in koala, 327
Canine distemper virus (CDV) infection, in Antarctic seals, 498
  in Baikal seals, 497
  in black-footed ferret, 461, 462
  in large cats, 407–409
  in primates, 379
  vaccination for, for marine mammal morbillivirus infection prevention, 500
    in black-footed ferret, 461
Canis familiaris dingo (dingo), hepatic cysts in, 424, *424*
Canis lupus (gray wolf), artificial insemination in, 451–452
  weight of, 429
Canis species, immobilizing drug dosages for, 434t
Cape buffalo. See *African buffalo (Syncerus caffer).*
Cape clawless otter (*Aonyx capensis*), anesthesia in, 439
  geographic distribution of, 436t
Cape eland, tranquilizers in, 579t, 580, *580*
Capra falconeri (markhor), immobilization of, 685
Capra hircus (Nubian goat), biliary cysts in, 424
Capra pyrenaica (Spanish ibex), embryo transfer in, 601
  estrous cycle synchronization in, 598
  induced ovulation in, 599
Capreolus capreolus (roe deer), artificial insemination in, sonographically supported, 53
  polycystic liver disease in, 424
  sonographic pregnancy detection in, *48*
Caprids. See also *Artiodactylids; specific animals.*
  contraception in, using PZP vaccination, 630, 630t
Captan, for ringworm, in cheetah, 418
Capture, of canids, 432
  of elephants, 528–529, 531
  of mountain sheep and goats, 681–687, *683, 684*
    evaluation of techniques for, 685–686
  of sea turtles, 221
  of wild herbivores, 576
Capture myopathy, in Arabian oryx, 690
  in bighorn sheep, 682
  in mountain goats, 686
Capuchins (*Cebus* species), diabetes treatment in, 399
  herpesvirus infection in, 28
  vitamin D metabolism in, 64, 70–71
  vitamin D toxicity in, 74
Capybara (*Hydrochaerus hydrochaeris*), reproduction in, 363
Carbamate poisoning, diagnosis of, 477
Carbenicillin, in chelonians, 191, 191t
  in reptiles, renal-portal system's effect on kinetics of, 250
  in snakes, 192t, 193
    in combination dosing, 194
  in stranded cetaceans, 489t

Carbon, activated, for oiled birds, 303
    to improve water quality for fish, 175
Carbon dioxide, as rodenticide, 118t
    for fish anesthesia, 161–162, 161t
Carcinoma, bile duct, 425
    hepatocellular, 425–426
        in felids, 427
Cardiomyopathy, in megachiropterans, 350, *351*
    in tree kangaroos, 342
Cardiopulmonary depression. See also *Respiratory depression.*
    in immobilized crocodilians, 205–206, 208, 214
Cardiovascular system, of fish, diseases of, 178t
    of megachiropterans, 350, *351*
    of prosimians, diseases of, 367–368
    of tree kangaroos, diseases of, 342
    sonographic assessment of, 47t
Caretta caretta (loggerhead sea turtle), anesthesia in, 222
    characteristics of, 217t
    chemical dips for, 195
    nutrition for, 219, 220, *220*
Carfentanil, in canids, 430
    in domestic goats, 685
    in duikers, 672–675, 674t
    in elephants, 526, 527t, 529
    in mountain goats, 685
    in mountain sheep, 684
    in okapi, 649
    in suids, 645
    in tapirs, 562, 563
    in white rhinoceros, 557, 557t
Caribou. See *Rangifer tarandus (caribou, reindeer).*
Carina scutulata (white-winged wood duck), fungal tracheitis in, endoscopic examination of, *39*
Carnivores, 401–462. See also specific animals.
    assisted reproduction in, 449–456
        benefits of, 449–450, 449t
            using artificial insemination, 451–456. See also *Artificial insemination.*
        using in vitro fertilization, 450–451, *450*, 450t, *451*
    Brucella abortus infection in, 622
    hepatic disorders in, 423–428
    iron overload in, 266–267
    quarantine for, 15t, 16t
    uninvited, control of, 118
    vitamin D deficiency in, 70
    vitamin E requirements for, 80–81, 81t
Carollia perspicillata (short-tailed fruit bat), energy requirement of, 357
    protein requirement of, 356–357
Carp pituitary extract, in fish, 184t, 189
Carpet python (*Morelia spilota variegata*), organ location in, 243, *246*
Carpus, elephant, radiography of, 517–520, *518*
Cassowary, helmet, sonographic sex determination in, *43*
Castor canadensis (North American beaver), reproduction in, 362
Castration, 316, 318
    behavioral effects of, 319
    in elephants, antibiotics with, 536
Casuarius casuarius (helmet cassowary), sonographic sex determination in, *43*
Catagonus wagneri (Chacoan peccary), anesthesia in, 643
Catatonia, due to tranquilizers, in herbivores, 579
Caterpillar cells, in elephant heart, in flaccid trunk paralysis, 542
Cathartes aura (turkey vulture), anesthesia in, 282
Cats. See also *Carnivores; Felids;* specific animals.
    domestic, control of, 118
        vitamin and mineral requirements of, 358t

Cats *(Continued)*
    feral, control of, 118
        feline leukemia virus carriage by, 404
        tuberculosis in, 101
Cavies, reproduction in, 363
$CD4^+$:$CD8^+$ ratio, 62
CDC (Centers for Disease Control and Prevention), animal importation regulations of, 24
CDV (canine distemper virus). See *Canine distemper virus (CDV) infection.*
Cebus species (capuchins), diabetes treatment in, 399
    herpesvirus infection in, 28
    vitamin D metabolism in, 64, 70–71
    vitamin D toxicity in, 74
Cefoperazone, in squamates, 192t, 193–194
Cefotaxime, 538
Ceftazidime, in koala, 331
    in lizards, 257
    in reptiles, renal-portal system's effect on kinetics of, 250
    in snakes, 192t, 194
        in combination dosing, 194–195
Ceftiofur, for leptospirosis, 471
    in elephants, 538
Ceftriaxone, in manatees, 511
    in stranded cetaceans, 489t
Cefuroxime, in stranded cetaceans, 489t
Celebes crested macaque (*Macaca nigra*), diabetes in, 398
Cell-mediated immunity, tests of, 60t, 61–62
Centers for Disease Control and Prevention (CDC), animal importation regulations of, 24
Central American tapir (*Tapirus bairdi*), 562, 562t. See also *Tapirs.*
    neonatal isoerythrolysis in, 565
Cephalexin, in stranded cetaceans, 489t
Cephalophus adersi (Aders' duiker). See also *Duikers.*
    conservation status of, 669
Cephalophus dorsalis (bay duiker). See also *Duikers.*
    anesthesia in, 673t
    conservation status of, 669
    iron overload in, 266
    laboratory reference values for, 676t–677t
Cephalophus jentinkii (Jentink's duiker). See also *Duikers.*
    anesthesia in, 674t
    conservation status of, 669
    laboratory reference values for, 678t
Cephalophus maxwelli (Maxwell's duiker). See also *Duikers.*
    anesthesia in, 673t
    conservation status of, 669
    laboratory reference values for, 676t–677t
Cephalophus monticola (blue duiker). See also *Duikers.*
    anesthesia in, 673t
    conservation status of, 669
    laboratory reference values for, 676t–677t
Cephalophus natalensis (red duiker). See also *Duikers.*
    anesthesia in, 673t
Cephalophus niger (black duiker). See also *Duikers.*
    anesthesia in, 673t
    laboratory reference values for, 676t–677t
Cephalophus ogilbyi (Ogilby's duiker). See also *Duikers.*
    conservation status of, 669
Cephalophus spadix (Abbot's duiker). See also *Duikers.*
    conservation status of, 669
Cephalophus sylvicultor (yellow-backed duiker). See also *Duikers.*
    anesthesia in, 674t
    conservation status of, 669
    laboratory reference values for, 678t
Cephalophus zebra (zebra duiker). See also *Duikers.*
    anesthesia in, 673t
    conservation status of, 669

Cephalorhynchus commersonii (Commerson's dolphin), fungal infections in, 479t, 483t

Cephalosporins. See also specific drugs.
in elephants, 538
in squamates, 192t, 193–194

Ceratotherium simum (white rhinoceros). See under *Rhinoceroses.*

Cercopithecine herpesvirus–1, in mixed-species exhibits, 28
in primates, 380

Cercopithecus aethiops (African green monkey), viral hepatitis in, 378

Cercopithecus mitis (guenon), biliary cystadenoma in, 424

Cercopithecus mona (mona monkey), biliary cystadenoma in, 424

Cercopithecus neglectus (DeBrazzas monkey), herpes B virus infection in, 380

Cerdocyon species (foxes), immobilizing drug dosages for, 434t

Cerebrospinal fluid examination, in sea turtles, 228

Cerebrovascular accident, in lemurs, 367

Cervical tuberculin test, in cervids, 652, 653

Cervids. See also *Artiodactylids;* specific animals.
contraception in, using PZP vaccination, 628–630, 629t, 630t
embryo transfer in, 600
estrous cycle synchronization in, 598
free-ranging, *Elaphostrongylus cervi* in, 632, 635–636
Parelaphostrongylus tenuis in, 632–635
in mixed-species exhibits, limiting trauma by, 26, 27
Johne's disease in, clinical signs of, 618
obesity in, 27
ovarian stimulation in, 599
Parelaphostrongylus tenuis in, population dynamics and, 634–635
protein supplements for, 591
shipment of, 21
tuberculosis in, 101, 103, 104, 650–655
diagnosis of, 651–654
disease control measures for, 655
incidence of, 651
lesions of, 106, 107t
prevalence of, 105t
regulatory control measures for, 655
treatment of, 654
vaccination for, 654
zoonotic implications of, 655
uninvited, control of, 118–119

Cervizine. See *Xylazine.*

Cervus duvauceli (Barasingha deer), obesity in, 27

Cervus elaphus (red deer, elk, wapiti), artificial insemination in, 598
biliary cysts in, 424
brucellosis in, 623, 624–625
Elaphostrongylus cervi in, 635–636
embryo transfer in, 599, 600
estrous cycle synchronization in, 598
handling systems for, 659, 661, *661*
Johne's disease in, 616, 617, *618*
management of, 619–620
Parelaphostrongylus tenuis in, 633–634
in mixed-species exhibits, 29
sympatric white-tailed deer and, 635
tuberculosis in, 651
clinical signs of, 106
human infection from, 655
pathology of, 654

Cervus eldi thamin (Eld's deer), artificial insemination in, 598
estrous cycle synchronization in, 598

Cervus nippon (sika deer), artificial insemination in, 598

Cervus nippon (sika deer) *(Continued)*
tuberculosis in, 651
pathology of, 654

Cervus timorensis (rusa deer), handling systems for, 660

Cesarean section, in elephant, *524, 525*

Cestodes. See also *Parasites;* specific genera and species.
hepatic cysts due to, 423
hepatic neoplasms and, 426
in cheetah, 421t
in duikers, 676
in koala, 330t
in manatees, 514

Cestrum diurnam (wild jasmin), vitamin D in, 63

Cetaceans. See also *Marine mammals;* specific animals.
diagnostic cytology in, 465–469, *466–468*
neonates of, 493–497
criteria for intervention with, 493–494
foster mothers for, 496
hand-rearing of, 493–497
nutrition and feeding in, 494–495, 494t
weaning in, 496
toys for, 496
oil's effects on, 476
quarantine for, 15t
stranded, 485–492
death of, 492
holding area for, 486–487
legal issues, 485
live, species of, 486
medical assessment of, 487
on-site assessment of, 485–486, 486t
record keeping for, 491–492
return of, to wild, 492
transport of, 486
treatment of, 487–491, 489t

Chacma baboon (*Papio hamadryas*), biliary cystadenoma in, 424
malignant T cell lymphoma in, 380–381
tuberculosis in, 105t

Chacoan peccary (*Catagonus wagneri*), anesthesia in, 643

Chain of evidence records, in oil spill response, 300

Chamaeleo jacksonii (Jackson's chameleon), 201

Chameleons, 200–204. See also *Lizards.*
anesthesia in, 204
biologic data on, 200–201, *201, 202*
husbandry of, 201–202
infectious diseases in, 203
nutrition for, 202
parasites in, 203
periodontal disease in, 252–257, 253t
reproduction in, 202–203
restraint of, 204
surgery in, 204
therapeutics in, 203–204

Channel-billed toucan (*Ramphastos vitellinus*), iron chelation in, 262

Charcoal, activated, for oiled birds, 303
to improve water quality for fish, 175

Charles Louis Davis, D.V.M., Foundation, educational resources from, 5

Chédiak-Higashi syndrome, 59

Cheetah (*Acinonyx jubatus*). See also *Felids.*
abdominal dropsy in, sonographic assessment of, *47*
artificial insemination in, 452, 452t, *454,* 454t
hormonal stimulation in, 455, 455t, 456, *456*
time of, 455, 455t
biologic data on, 415t
breeding facility for, 415–422
breeding management of, 421–422
diseases of, 418–419

Cheetah (*Acinonyx jubatus*) *(Continued)*
  feline immunodeficiency virus in, 405
  gastritis in, 418, 458–460
  handling of, in breeding facility, 416, *416, 417, 420*
  immobilization of, 416–418, 418t, 459
  in vitro fertilization of, 450t
  iron overload in, 266–267
  nutrition of, in breeding facility, 421
  parasites in, 419–420, 419t, *420,* 420t, 421t
    gastritis due to, 458, 459
  quarantine for, 418
  tuberculosis in, 101, 103, 107t, 418–419
    clinical signs of, 106
Chelation, for iron overload, 262
  for zinc toxicosis, in California condor, 290
Chelonia mydas (green sea turtle), anesthesia in, 222
  characteristics of, 217t
  conservation status of, 218
  nutrition for, 219
Chelonians. See also *Reptiles; specific types.*
  antimicrobials in, 191–193, 191t
  aquatic, soaks and dips for, 195
  health assessment of, 232–235
  infectious diseases of, 240t, 241
  minimally invasive surgery in, 37
  release of, into wild, 232–241
    decision tree for, 235–240, *236, 237*
    philosophical issues in, 240–241
  threats facing, 232
  vitamin D metabolism in, 73–74
Chelonibia manatii, in manatees, 515
Chemiluminescence, 60
Chemistry reference values. See *Biochemical reference
    values.*
Cheque (mibolerone), for contraception, 317
Cherry, wild, toxicity of, 89
Chickenpox, in apes, 386
Chickens, cryptosporidiosis in, 122t, 126
Children's python (*Liasis childreni*), organ location in, 243,
    246
Chimpanzees. See also *Apes.*
  birth weight for, 382–383
  cytomegalovirus infection in, 386
  Ebola Cote-d'Ivoire in, 380
  herpesvirus infection in, 386
  neonatal jaundice in, 383
  pregnancy in, management of, 384
  pygmy, birth weight for, 383
    herpesvirus infection in, 386
    papillomavirus in, 380
    simian T lymphotrophic virus in, 381
    varicella in, 386
    viral hepatitis in, 378
China, giant pandas in, 410–414. See also *Pandas.*
Chinese giant salamander (*Andrias davidianus*), sonographic
    sex determination in, *43*
Chirochis fabaceus, in manatees, 514
Chiroptera, 344–359. See also specific types.
  classification of, 344
  control of, 118
  rabies in, 140, 348–349
    control of, 145
Chlamydiosis, 151–153, 152t
  in Arabian oryx, 692t, 693
  in koala, 324–326, *325*
  in mixed-species exhibits, 28
Chloramines, water contamination with, 170–171
Chloramphenicol, for toxoplasmosis, 134
  in elephants, 538
  in fish, 183t, 185

Chloramphenicol *(Continued)*
  in koala, 326
  in sea turtles, 230t
  in snakes, 192t, 194
Chlordane, in marine mammals, 472
Chlordecone (Kepone), in marine mammals, 473
Chlorhexidine, for disinfection, 176t
  in lizards, 256–257
  in sea turtles, 230t
Chloride, in fish diet, 174t
Chlorine, for disinfection, 176t
  to improve water quality, for sea turtles, 219
  water contamination with, 170
3-Chloro-4-methylbenzenamine, 119
Chlorophacinone, 118t
Choeropsis liberiensis (pygmy hippopotamus), leiomyoma in,
    sonographic assessment of, *50*
Choke cherry (*Prunus*), toxicity of, 89
Cholangiocarcinoma, 425
Cholangioma, 424
Cholecalciferol (vitamin D_3), 63–65, *64*
  as rodenticide, 117, 118t
  crystalline, 70
  in chameleon diet, 202
Choleliths, cystine, in callitrichids, 374
Cholera, fowl, water quality and, 299
Choline, in fish diet, 173t
Choloepus didactylus (two-toed sloth), sonographic sex
    determination in, *44*
Chorioptes panda, in giant panda, 413
Chromium, in fish diet, 174t
Chronic wasting disease, in cervids. See *Scrapie-like
    spongiform encephalopathies.*
Chrysemys picta (painted turtle), antimicrobials in, 191t, 192
Chrysemys scripta elegans (red-eared slider), antimicrobials
    in, 191t, 192
  renal-portal system of, 249–251, *249–251*
Chrysocyon species (maned wolves), immobilizing drug
    dosages for, 434t
Chrysolophus pictus (golden pheasant), parasites in, 29
Chuckwalla, San Estaban Island, vertebral subluxation in,
    imaging of, 85, *85, 86*
Chutes. See also *Handling systems.*
  for ungulate restraint, 658–661, *659–661*
Cimetidine, in stranded cetaceans, 489t
Ciprofloxacin, in elephants, 538
  in koala, 326
  in snakes, 192t, 194
  in stranded cetaceans, 489t
Cirrhosis, iron overload and, 261
CITES (Convention on International Trade in Endangered
    Species), 22, 23–24
  guidelines of, for captive animals, 235–240, *236, 237*
Civet, palm, hepatic neoplasms in, 426
Cladophialophora bantiana infection, in marine mammals,
    480t
Clawed toad, African, vitamin D metabolism in, 74
Clawless otters, anesthesia in, 439
  geographic distribution of, 436t
Clindamycin, for toxoplasmosis, 133
  in stranded cetaceans, 489t
Clostridial vaccination, in Arabian oryx, 695
  in duikers, 680
  in ranched hoofstock, 589–590
Clostridium botulinum infection, in Arabian oryx, 692t, 695
  in waterfowl, 297–299, *298*
Clostridium botulinum type C bacterin-toxoid, for avian
    botulism prevention, 298
Clouded leopard (*Neofelis nebulosa*), adrenal tumor in,
    sonographic assessment of, *48*

Clouded leopard (*Neofelis nebulosa*) *(Continued)*
   artificial insemination in, 455, 455t
   feline leukemia virus in, 402
   ovarian stimulation in, *451*
Clown fish, anemones and, 171–172
Coati (*Nasua* species), iron overload in, 267
Cobalt, deficiency of, iron overload and, 261
   in fish diet, 174t
Cobra, biliary cystadenoma in, 424
   effects of venom of, 97
Coccidia, in Arabian oryx, 692t, 695
   in chameleons, 203
   in koala, 330t
Coccidioidomycosis, in marine mammals, 480t, 482–483
Cochleotrema cochleotrema, in manatees, 514
Cockroaches, parasite transmission by, 29
Coelomic cavity, of pigeon, imaging of, 87, *87*
Cold stunning, in sea turtles, 219
Colic, in tapirs, 565
Colitis. See also *Enterocolitis.*
   in callitrichids, 371
   in lemurs, 365–366
Collagenolytic diseases, in black rhinoceros, 554, *555*
Collared peccary (*Tayassu tajacu*), anesthesia in, 643–644
   canine distemper virus in, 408
Colobus monkeys, amoebiasis in, 29
   herpesvirus simiae infection in, 28
   papillomavirus in, 380
   rickets in, 71–72, *71*
Colonic adenocarcinoma, in callitrichids, 375
Colostrum. See also *Passive antibody transfer.*
   substitutes for, in hand-reared duikers, 672
Coluber constrictor (black racer), antimicrobials in, 192t, 194
Colubrids. See also *Snakes.*
   organ location in, 245, *247*
   paramyxovirus infection in, 28
Columba inornata (Puerto Rican plain pigeon), growth of, 273–274, *274*
Columba livia (white carneaux pigeon), control of, 119
   crop milk composition, 272t, 273t
   growth of, 273–274, *274*
Columbids. See also *Birds.*
   classification of, 269
   control of, 119
   crop milk of, 270–273, *271, 272t, 273, 273t, 274t*
      digestion of, 274, 276
      replacement for, 275–276
   lactation in, 269–270, *270, 271,* 275
   magnetic resonance imaging in, 87, *87*
   young, body composition of, 274
      growth of, 273–274, *274*
      nutrition and feeding of, 269–276
         recommendations for, 274–276
Commerson's dolphin (*Cephalorhynchus commersonii*), fungal infections in, 479t, 483t
Computed tomography (CT), 83–84
   case studies using, 85–87, *85–87*
Computer programs, for carrying capacity of livestock and exotic hoofstock, 586t
Condor, Andean, anesthesia in, 282
   in California condor management program, 278
   California. See *California condor (Gymnogyps californianus).*
Congo African gray parrot (*Psittacus erithacus erithacus*), biliary cysts in, 424
Congo clawless otter (*Aonyx congica*), geographic distribution of, 436t
Conjunctivitis, chlamydial, in koala, 325, *325,* 326
Connochaetes species (wildebeests), herpesvirus carriage by, 27

Connochaetes species (wildebeests) *(Continued)*
   tranquilizers in, 579–580, 579t
Constipation, in manatees, 512, 514
Contrac (bromadiolone), 117, 118t
Contraception, for vermin control, 116
   in artiodactylids, 628–631, 629t, 630t
   in callitrichids, adverse effects of implants for, 374
   in mammals, 316–319
   in tapirs, 567
   steroid, 317, 318
      hepatic neoplasms and, 425, 427
   using PZP vaccine, 317, 318
      adverse effects of, 319, 630–631
      in artiodactylids, 628–631, 629t, 630t
      pregnancy and, 319
Conures, herpesvirus carriage by, 28
Convention on International Trade in Endangered Species (CITES), 22, 23–24
   guidelines of, for captive animals, 235–240, *236, 237*
Cooperative Brucellosis Eradication Program, 623–625
Cooperia species, in ranched hoofstock, 588
Copper, deficiency of, in antelope, in mixed-species exhibits, 27
   in duikers, 670
   in ranched hoofstock, 591
   in tapirs, 564–565
   in fish diet, 174t
   iron levels and, 261
   toxic levels of, in aquarium water, 170
Copper oxide, for duikers, 670
Copper sulfate, for cheetah cubs, 421
   for fish, 169t, 170
   for phytoplankton control in waterfowl exhibits, 296–297
   for ranched hoofstock, 591
Corn, in hoofstock diet, 591
Corn snake (*Elaphe guttata*), antimicrobials in, 192t, 194
   organ location in, 245
Corneal cloudiness, in tapirs, 566
Corneal pitting, in Arabian oryx, 696
Coronavirus infection, agent causing, 605–606
   in ruminants, 605–611
      clinical signs of, 608
      diagnosis of, 609–610
      epizootiology of, 607–608
      pathology of, 608–609
      prevention of, 610–611
      treatment of, 610
      vaccination for, 611
   in okapi, 649
Corticosteroids. See also specific drugs.
   in birds, 312
   in fish, 184t, 188–189
Co-trimoxazole, in ape neonates, 386
   in duikers, 679
   in elephants, 536–537
Cottonmouth (*Agkistrodon piscivorus*), antimicrobials in, 192t, 194
Cotton-top tamarin (*Saguinus oedipus*). See also *Callitrichids.*
   colonic adenocarcinoma in, 375
   vitamin D metabolism in, 71, 72
Cougar. See *Puma (Felis concolor).*
Coxiella burnetti, in Arabian oryx, 690, 692t, 693
Coyotes, control of, 118
   immobilizing drug dosages for, 434t
   rabies in, 139

Crab-eating monkey (*Macaca fascicularis*), Ebola Reston in, 379
  embryo collection in, sonographically supported, 52, *53*
  mixed viral infection in, 381
  Murayama virus in, 379
  prenatal sex determination in, *49*
  viral hepatitis in, 378
Cranial edema, in megachiropterans, 350, 352, *352*
Craniofacial tumors, in koala, 329
Crash gates, in bison handling systems, 660, *660*
Crates, 17–18, *19*. See also *Handling systems; Restraint.*
  animal acclimation to, 18–19, *19*
  for Arabian oryx, 690
  for elephants, 527–528, 527t
    loading animals into, 529–530, 531
  for white rhinoceros, 560, 561
Crested porcupines, African, reproduction in, 363
Creutzfeldt-Jakob disease. See *Scrapie-like spongiform encephalopathies.*
Crickets, parasite transmission by, 29
Crocodilians, antimicrobials in, 191t, 193
  immobilization of, 205–208, *206–210*
    complications of, 213–214
    drugs for, 208–215, 213t–214t
    recommendations for, 215–216
  intubation of, 212
  minimally invasive surgery in, 37
  shipment of, 20
Crocuta crocuta (spotted hyena), sonographic sex determination in, *44*
Crohn's disease, *Mycobacterium paratuberculosis* and, 613
Crop, lactating, histologic changes in, 270, *270, 271*
Crop milk, composition of, 270–273, *271,* 272t, *273,* 273t, 274t
  digestion of, 274, 276
  replacement for, 275–276
Crotalaria species (rattlebox), toxicity of, 89
Crotalids. See also *Snakes.*
  effects of venom of, 97
  organ location in, 245, *247*
Crotalus adamanteus (eastern diamond-back rattlesnake), antimicrobials in, 192t, 194
Crotalus horridus horridus (timber rattlesnake), antimicrobials in, 192t, 194
Crush. See also *Handling systems.*
  for Arabian oryx handling, 688–689
  for cheetah handling, 416, *416, 417, 420*
Cryptocaryon irritans infestation, early signs of, 164
Cryptococcosis, birds and, 153t, 154
  in cheetah, 419
  in koala, 327–328
  in marine mammals, 480t, 482, 483
Cryptomys damarensis (damara mole rat), vitamin D metabolism in, 74
Cryptosporidiosis, 121–130
  causative agents of, 121–122, 122t
    life history of, 122–124, *123–125*
  clinical features of, 124–126
  diagnosis of, 127–130, *129*
  in Arabian oryx, 692t, 695
  in birds, 125–126, 153t, 155
  in chameleons, 203
  in koala, 330t
  in mammals, 124–125
  in mixed-species exhibits, 29
  in reptiles, 126
  management of, 127
  pathogenesis of, 124–126
  transmission of, 126–127
Cryptosporidium baileyi, 122t, *123, 124,* 126

Cryptosporidium crotali, 122
Cryptosporidium felis, 122t
Cryptosporidium meleagridis, 122t, 126
Cryptosporidium muris, 122t
Cryptosporidium nasorum, 122t
Cryptosporidium parvum, 122, 122t
  in humans, 121, 124
  in mammals, 124–125
  life history of, 122–123, *123, 125*
Cryptosporidium serpentis, 122t
Cryptosporidium wrari, 122t
CT (calcitonin), in calcium regulation, 65
CT (computed tomography), 83–84
  case studies using, 85–87, *85–87*
Ctenocephalides species, on cheetah, 419t
  on koala, 330t
Cuban crocodile (*Crocodylus rhombifer*), immobilization of, 206, *206, 207*
Cultures, for *Brucella abortus,* 622
  for *Mycobacterium bovis,* 651
  for *Mycobacterium paratuberculosis,* 614, 615, 619
Cuniculus paca (paca), reproduction in, 363
  vitamin D toxicity in, in mixed-species exhibits, 27, 72, 75
Cuon alpinus (Asian wild dog), immobilizing drug dosages for, 434t
  sonographic health assessment in, *47, 50, 51*
Cuvier's beaked whale (*Ziphius cavirostris*), subcutaneous emphysema in, 490
Cyamoliseus patagonus (patagonian conure), herpesvirus carriage by, 28
Cyanide, as rodenticide, 118t
Cyanocobalamin. See also *Vitamin B complex.*
  in fish diet, 173t
Cyclodiene insecticides, in marine mammals, 472
Cyclohexanes. See *Dissociative anesthetics;* specific drugs.
Cynomolgus. See *Macaques;* specific animals.
Cynomys species (prairie dogs), reproduction in, 362
Cynopteris brachyotis (dog-faced fruit bat). See also *Fruit bats; Megachiropterans.*
  geographic distribution of, 345t
Cystadenocarcinoma, biliary, 425
  in felids, 427
Cystadenoma, biliary, 424, *424*
  in felids, 427
Cystine choleliths, in callitrichids, 374
Cystitis, chlamydial, in koala, 325, *325*
Cystophora cristata (hooded seal), fungal infections in, 480t
Cysts, hepatic, 423–425, *424*
  diagnosis of, 427–428
  in felids, 427
  treatment of, 428
  sonographic assessment of, *50,* 51, *51*
Cytochrome P-450 enzymes, organochlorine effects on, 474
Cytology, diagnostic, in marine mammals, 464–469, *465–468*
Cytomegalovirus infection, in ape infants, 386

D

Dactylis glomerata (orchard grass), vitamin D in, 63
Dall's sheep (*Ovis dalli*). See also *Mountain sheep.*
  capture and handling of, 681–687
  embryo transfer in, 599, 600
  estrous cycle synchronization in, 598
  immobilization of, 684
Dama dama. See *Fallow deer (Dama dama).*
Damalinia cornuta cornuta, on ranched hoofstock, 589
Damaliscus dorcas (blesbok, bontebok), copper deficiency in, in mixed-species exhibits, 27
  tranquilizers in, 579t, 580

Damaliscus lunatus (topi), herpesvirus carriage by, 27

Damara mole rat (*Cryptomys damarensis*), vitamin D metabolism in, 74

Dantrolene (Dantrium), for malignant hyperthermia in suids, 641

Darting, of Arabian oryx, 689
  of canids, equipment for, 432
  of cheetahs, accidents in, 417
  of elephants, equipment for, 526
    procedure for, 528
    treatment of wound from, 529
  of mountain sheep and goats, 684–685, 686
  of suids, 643
  of white rhinoceros, equipment for, 556
    in confinement, 561
    of cow and calf, 560–561
    procedure for, 558
    treatment of wound from, 559

Dasyprocta species (agoutis), reproduction in, 363–364
  vitamin D toxicity in, 27, 72, 75

Databases, 5–6, 7

Davis Foundation, educational resources from, 5

Day gecko (*Phelsuma madagascariensis*), vitamin D metabolism in, 73

Dazzel (diazinon), in cheetah, 420t

D-Con (warfarin), 117, 118t

D-Con II (brodifacoum), in vermin control, 117, 118t
  poisoning by, in callitrichids, 374

DDD (dichlorodiphenyldichloroethane), in marine mammals, 472

DDE (dichlorodiphenyldichloroethylene), in marine mammals, 472

DDT (dichlorodiphenyltrichloroethane), California condors and, 277–278, 288
  in marine mammals, 472, 473

Deadline (flumethrin), in cheetah, 420t

Death adder (*Acanthophis antarcticus*), organ location in, 245

DeBrazzas monkey (*Cercopithecus neglectus*), herpes B virus infection in, 380

Deer. See *Cervids;* specific animals.

Deer mouse (*Peromyscus* species), control of, 116–117

Degenerative arthritis, in lemurs, 367

Dehydration, in oiled birds, 303

7-Dehydrocholesterol (provitamin D₃), 63, *64*

Delphinapterus leucas (beluga whale), antifungal drugs in, 483t
  hand-reared, dolphin immunoglobulin for, 496
  organochlorines in, 474

Delphinus delphis (common dolphin), caloric requirements of calves of, 495
  morbillivirus infection in, 498

Deltaherpesvirus, in mixed-species exhibits, 28

Demerol (meperidine), in manatees, 510
  in otters, 441
  in stranded cetaceans, 489t

Demodex species, on cheetah, 419, 419t
  on giant panda, 413
  on koala, 330t

Dendrolagus species. See *Tree kangaroos.*

Depo-Provera (medroxyprogesterone acetate), for contraception, 317, 318

Dermacentor albipictus, on ranched hoofstock, 589

Dermatitis. See also *Skin diseases.*
  in black rhinoceros, 553–554, *554*
  in duikers, 679
  in manatees, 514, 515

Dermatomycosis, in cheetah, 418
  in giant panda, 413
  in koala, 328

Dermatophytosis, birds and, 152t

Dermochelys coriacea (leatherback sea turtle), 217
  conservation status of, 218
  ketamine/acepromazine dose in, 221

Desert cat, Indian, in vitro fertilization in, 451

Desert gazelle, parasites in, 29

Desert tortoise (*Gopherus agassizii*), vitamin D metabolism in, 73–74

Desferoxamine B, iron chelation with, 262

Detergent, for removing oil from feathers, 304, 304t

Detomidine, in birds, 312
  in crocodilians, 211–212, 214t
  in marsupials, 335
  in suids, domestic, 642, 642t
    nondomestic, 644–645
  in tapirs, 562
  in white rhinoceros, 559

Dexamethasone, in birds, 312
  in elephants, 536
  in fish, 184t, 189

Dhole (*Cuon alpinus*), immobilizing drug dosages for, 434t
  sonographic health assessment in, *47, 50, 51*

Diabetes mellitus, in apes, hypermature fetus in, 385
  in primates, 397–400
    diagnosis of, 398–399
    etiopathogenesis of, 397–398, *397*
    gestational, 398
    parasite-induced, 398
    treatment of, 399–400
  iron overload and, 261

Diagnostic tests. See *Laboratory tests;* specific tests.

Diamond python (*Morelia spilota spilota*), organ location in, 243, *246*

Diamond-back rattlesnake, eastern, antimicrobials in, 192t, 194

Diaphragmatic defects, in callitrichids, 373, *374*

Diaphragmatic hernia, gastritis due to, in cheetah, 458

Diarrhea, in ape neonates, 386
  in callitrichids, 371–372
  in elephants, 539
  in okapi, 647–648
  in ruminants, 591. See also *Coronavirus infection; Rotavirus infection.*
  in tapirs, 565

Diazepam, in birds, 313
  in canids, 430, 433
  in crocodilians, 214t, 215
  in giant panda, 411–412, 411t
  in herbivores, 579
  in koala, 327
  in manatees, 510
  in marsupials, 334t, 335t
  in mountain sheep, 685
  in otters, 438t, 439, 441, 446
  in stranded cetaceans, 489t
  in suids, 640t, 642t

Diazinon, in cheetah, 420t

Dicerorhinus sumatrensis (Sumatran rhinoceros). See under *Rhinoceroses.*

Diceros bicornis (black rhinoceros). See under *Rhinoceroses.*

Dichlorodiphenyldichloroethane (DDD), in marine mammals, 472

Dichlorodiphenyldichloroethylene (DDE), in marine mammals, 472

Dichlorodiphenyltrichloroethane (DDT), California condors and, 277–278, 288
  in marine mammals, 472, 473

Dichlorvos, in fish, 187–188

Dictyocaulus viviparus, in farmed deer, 588, 589

Didelphis virginiana (opossum), control of, 117–118

Didermocerus sumatrensis (Sumatran rhinoceros). See under *Rhinoceroses.*

Dieffenbachia species (dumbcane), toxicity of, 89
Dieldrin, in marine mammals, 472
Diet. See also *Nutrition.*
  in mixed-species exhibits, 27
    disease transmission by, 28
    parasite transmission by, 29
  iron overload and, in birds, 264–265
    in primates, 265
  periodontal disease and, in lizards, 255–256
  shipping and, 20
  vitamin D in, metabolism of, 64–65
    requirements for, 75–76
    sources of, 67–69, 68t, 69t
  vitamin E in, 80–81, 81t
Diethylnitrosamine, hepatic neoplasms and, 425, 426
Diff-Quik stain, for blood specimen, in sea turtle, 225
Dihydrostreptomycin, for leptospirosis, 471
  in elephants, 536
1α,25-Dihydroxycholecalciferol (1,25[OH]$_2$D$_3$), 64
  in calcium regulation, 65
  injectable, 70
24,25-Dihydroxycholecalciferol (24,25[OH]$_2$D$_3$), 64
  in calcium regulation, 65
1α,25-Dihydroxyergocalciferol (1,25[OH]$_2$D$_2$), 65
24,25-Dihydroxyergocalciferol (24,25[OH]$_2$D$_2$), 65
Dik-dik (*Madoqua* species), iron overload in, 266
  tranquilizers in, 579t, 582
Dimethyl sulfoxide, in birds, 313
Dingo (*Canis familiaris dingo*), hepatic cysts in, 424, *424*
Dinoflagellate toxins, manatees and, 476–477, 514
  marine mammals and, 476–477
Dinomys branicki (pacarana), reproduction in, 363
Dioxin (TCDD), in marine mammals, 473
  toxic equivalency factor and, 474–475
Diphacinone, 118t
Dipodomys species (kangaroo rats), reproduction in, 362
Diprenorphine, in duikers, 674t
  in elephants, 526, 529
  in hippopotamus, 638–639
  in okapi, 649
  in white rhinoceros, 557, 560
Diprivan. See *Propofol.*
Direct agglutination test, for toxoplasmosis, 133
"Dirty tail," in koala, 325, *325*
Disease surveillance, in fish care, 177–181, 178t, *179,* 180t
Disinfection, in fish care, 175–177, 176t
Dissociative anesthetics. See also specific drugs.
  in canids, 430, 433
  in crocodilians, 211, 213t
  in marsupials, 334–335, 334t
Ditrac (diphacinone), 118t
Diuretics, in fish, 184t, 189
DMV (dolphin morbillivirus), 498
Dog(s), control of, 118
  rabies in, 141
  vitamin and mineral requirements of, 358t
Dog-faced fruit bat (*Cynopteris brachyotis*). See also *Fruit
    bats; Megachiropterans.*
  geographic distribution of, 345t
Dolichotis patagonum (Patagonian cavy), reproduction in,
    363
Dolphin morbillivirus (DMV), 498
Dolphins. See also *Cetaceans; Marine mammals;* specific
    animals.
  fetal ultrasonography in, 501–506, *503–506*
  milk replacement formulas for, 494, 494t
  milking, 495
  scoliosis in, 491
Domitor. See *Medetomidine.*
Domosedan. See *Detomidine.*

Doppler blood flow meter, in sea turtles, 222–223
Dopram. See *Doxapram.*
Douc langur (*Pygathrix nemaeus*), parasites in, 29
Douroucouli (*Aotus trivirgatus*), herpesvirus infection in, 28
  viral hepatitis in, 378
  vitamin D transport in, 64
Doxapram, in canids, 431, 433
  in crocodilians, 214t, 215
  in hippopotamus, 639
  in manatees, 510
  in stranded cetaceans, 489t
  in white rhinoceros, 559
Doxycycline, for toxoplasmosis, 134
  in chelonians, 191, 191t
  in koala, 326
  in stranded cetaceans, 489t
Drive nets, for mountain sheep and goat capture, 682, *683,*
    685–686
Droncit. See *Praziquantel.*
Drop floor chutes. See also *Handling systems.*
  for ungulates, 658–660, *659*
Drop nets, for mountain sheep and goat capture, 682, *683,*
    685–686
Droperidol, in suids, 640t, 642t
Drowning, in crocodilians, after immobilization, 207
  in sea turtles, during illness, 221
Drug resistance, in parasites, 589, 594, 596
Drymarchon corais couperi (eastern indigo snake),
    antimicrobials in, 192t, 194
Duck(s). See also *Birds; Waterfowl;* specific animals.
  fungal tracheitis in, endoscopic examination of, *39*
  seasonal siderosis in, 264
Duck plague (duck virus enteritis), water quality and, 299
Duikers, 668–680
  biologic data on, 675–676, 676t–678t
  captive management of, 669–672
  classification of, 668–669
  conservation status of, 669
  geographic distribution of, 668–669
  immobilization of, 672–675, 673t, 674t
  infectious diseases in, 676–679
  iron overload in, 266
  manual restraint of, 672
  noninfectious diseases in, 679
  preventive medicine in, 679–680
  tranquilizers in, 579t, 582, 675
  tuberculosis in, 101
  wasting syndrome of, 670
Dumbcane (*Dieffenbachia* species), toxicity of, 89
Durikainema species, in koala, 330t
Dusicyon species (foxes), immobilizing drug dosages for,
    434t
Duvenhage virus, 137t, 348
Dwarf sperm whale (*Kogia simus*), ink in colon of, 467
  subcutaneous emphysema in, 490
Dystocia, in callitrichids, 374
  in chameleons, 203
  in elephants, 522–525, *522,* 523t, *524*
  in manatees, 514

E

Eastern brown snake (*Pseudonaja texlilis*), organ location in,
    245
Eastern diamond-back rattlesnake (*Crotalus adamanteus*),
    antimicrobials in, 192t, 194
Eastern indigo snake (*Drymarchon corais couperi*),
    antimicrobials in, 192t, 194
Eastern king snake (*Lampropeltis getulus getulus*),
    antimicrobials in, 192t, 194

Ebola virus, in megachiropterans, 349
  in primates, 379
EBV (Epstein-Barr virus), in callitrichids, 370
eCG (equine chorionic gonadotropin), in artiodactylids, in
    artificial insemination, 598
  in embryo transfer techniques, 599–600
  in carnivores, in artificial insemination, 455–456, *456*
  in in-vitro fertilization, 450
Echinococcosis, of liver, 423
Echolocation, in megachiropterans, 353
Edema, cranial, in megachiropterans, 350, 352, *352*
  gular, in chameleons, 204
  in California condor chicks, 285–286, *286, 287*
Edetate calcium disodium, for zinc toxicosis, in California
    condor, 290
Egyptian fruit bat (*Rousettus aegyptiacus*). See also
    Megachiropterans.
  energy requirement for, 357
  geographic distribution of, 345t
  protein requirement for, 357
EHD (epizootic hemorrhagic disease), in ranched hoofstock,
    591
Eider ducks, seasonal siderosis in, 264
Eidolon helvum (straw-colored fruit bat). See also *Fruit bats;
    Megachiropterans.*
  geographic distribution of, 345t
  reproduction in, 353
Eimeria species, in manatees, 515
Elaeophora schneideri, in ranch-raised hoofstock, 588
Elands, embryo transfer in, 600, 600t, 601, 601t
  tranquilizers in, 579t, 580, *580*
Elaphe guttata (corn snake), antimicrobials in, 192t, 193, 194
  organ location in, 245
Elaphe obsoleta (rat snake), antimicrobials in, 192t, 193, 194
Elaphostrongylus alces, 632
Elaphostrongylus cervi, 632, 635–636
Elaphostrongylus rangiferi, 632, 635, 636
Elaphurus davidianus (Pere David's deer), induced ovulation
    in, 599
  malignant catarrhal fever in, 27
  parasites in, 29
Elaphus maximus (Asian elephant). See *Elephants.*
Elapids. See also *Snakes.*
  bite of, 97, 99
  organ location in, 245, *247*
  paramyxovirus infection in, 28
Eld's deer (*Cervus eldi thamin*), artificial insemination in,
    598
  estrous cycle synchronization in, 598
Electrocardiography, in fish, 162
  in sea turtles, 222, *222*
Electroejaculation, in lemurs, urethral obstruction after, 367
Electron microscopy, in viral enteritis diagnosis, in ruminants,
    609
Electrophoresis, serum, as test of humoral immunity, 61
Electrosurgery, in endoscopy, equipment for, 32, 34, *36*
Elephant seals, northern, fungal infections in, 480t
  iron overload in, 267
Elephants, 517–549
  anesthesia in, 526–527, 527t, 528–529
  antibiotic therapy in, 533–540
    clinical application of, 539–540
    dosage calculation for, 534
    pharmacokinetic studies of, 535–539
    routes of administration for, 534–535
  artificial insemination in, sonographically supported, 52–
    53, *53*
  body weight determination in, 533–534
  calving of, normal, 521–522
  dystocia in, 522–525, *522,* 523t, *524*

Elephants *(Continued)*
  flaccid trunk paralysis in, 541–544, *542, 543*
  importation of, 23
  leiomyoma in, sonographic assessment of, *50*
  male reproductive assessment in, sonographic, 53–54
  oral and nasal diseases of, 544–546, *545*
  poxvirus infections in, 547–549, *547–549*
  pregnancy monitoring in, sonographic, *49*
  radiography of foot and carpus in, 517–520, *518–520*
  relocation of, 525–532
    capture procedure for, 528–529, 531
    equipment for, 526–528, 527t
    family units in, 531
    loading procedure for, 529–530, *530,* 531
    off-loading paddock for, 530–531
    off-loading procedure for, 532
    travel procedure for, 531–532
  sexual maturation in, sonographic assessment of, 44, *45,
    46*
  social organization of, 531
  tranquilizers in, 579t, 583–584
  vitamin E supplementation in, 80
ELISA. See *Enzyme-linked immunosorbent assay (ELISA).*
Elizabethan collar, for megachiropterans, 346, *347*
Elk. See *Cervus elaphus (red deer, elk, wapiti).*
Emboli, air, in fish tissue, 168–169, *170*
Embryo collection. See also *Reproduction, assisted.*
  sonographically supported, 52, *53*
Embryonic death, sonographic identification of, 52, *53*
Emergency care, for snakebite, 98–100, *99,* 99t, *100*
Emphysema, subcutaneous, in manatees, 516
  in stranded cetaceans, 490
Emus, shipment of, 21
Encephalitis, equine, in duikers, 677–679, 680
  in Japanese macaque, 408
  in lemurs, 367, 380
  in marine mammal morbillivirus infection, 499
Encephalomalacia, nigropallidal, 543–544
Encephalomyeltis, viral, in duikers, 677–679
Encephalomyocarditis virus, introduced by uninvited species,
    28
Encephalopathy, spongiform. See *Scrapie-like spongiform
    encephalopathies.*
Endangered species, shipment of, regulation of, 22, 23–24
Endometrial cyst, sonographic assessment of, *50,* 51
Endoscopy. See also *Minimally invasive surgery (MIS).*
  in dystocia diagnosis in elephants, 524
  in gastritis diagnosis in cheetah, 459
  in sea turtles, 227–228, *228*
  in stranded cetaceans, 490
Endosulfan, in marine mammals, 473
Endotracheal intubation. See under *Intubation.*
Endrin, in marine mammals, 472
Energy requirements, for cetacean neonates, 494–495
  for fruit bats, 357
  for koalas, 322–324
English sparrow (*Passer domesticus*), control of, 119
Enhydra lutris. See *Sea otter (Enhydra lutris).*
Enilconazole, in cheetah, 418
Enrichment. See *Environmental enrichment.*
Enrofloxacin, in chelonians, 191t, 193
  in elephants, 538
  in fish, 183t, 185
  in koala, 326
  in reptiles, renal-portal system's effect on kinetics of, 251
  in sea turtles, 230t
  in snakes, 192t, 194
  in stranded cetaceans, 489t
Entanglement injury, in manatees, 516
Enteric diarrheagenic viruses, classification of, 605

Enteric red-mouth, vaccine for, 173
Enteritis, bacterial, in California condor chicks, 286–287, *287*
    in lemurs, 365–366
    duck virus, water quality and, 299
    hemorrhagic, in giant panda, 412–413
    in koala young, 331
Enterocolitis, in cetaceans, 467
    in manatees, 513
Environmental enrichment, for fish, 171–172
    for hand-reared cetaceans, 496
    for primates, 387–391
        developing plan for, 390
        documenting plan for, 390
        evaluating effectiveness of, 390–391
        regulatory requirements for, 387–388
        risk assessment and control in, 389
        sources on, 389, 389t, 390
        toxicity and, 389–390
        veterinarian's role in, 388–389
Enzyme-linked immunosorbent assay (ELISA), for feline
        immunodeficiency virus, 405
    for feline leukemia virus, 403
    for Johne's disease, 614, 619
    for toxoplasmosis, 133
    for tuberculosis, in Arabian oryx, 694
        in cervids, 653
    for viral enteritis, in ruminants, 609
    limitations of, for antibody detection, 57–58
        for antigen detection, 57
Eosinophil Unopette method, for blood analysis, in sea turtle,
        225
Eosinophilic diseases, in black rhinoceros, 554
Eosinophilic meningoencephalitis, in small cetaceans, 488
Ependymoma, melanotic, in callitrichids, 375
Epidermal exfoliation, in black rhinoceros, 553
Epinephrine, for anaphylaxis with snakebite, 100
    in stranded cetaceans, 489t
Episiotomy, in elephant dystocia, 524, *524, 525*
Episodic hemolysis, acute, in black rhinoceros, 59
Epizootic hemorrhagic disease (EHD), in ranched hoofstock,
        591
Epomophorus wahlbergi (Wahlberg's epaulated bat). See also
        Megachiropterans.
    geographic distribution of, 345t
Epstein-Barr virus (EBV), in callitrichids, 370
Eptesicus fuscus (big brown bat), control of, 118
Equids. See also specific animals.
    calcium regulation in, 74
    captive population of, 572t
    infectious diseases of, 572–574, 572t, 574t
    iron overload in, 266
    quarantine for, 573–574
Equine chorionic gonadotropin (eCG), in artiodactylids, in
        artificial insemination, 598
    in embryo transfer techniques, 599–600
    in carnivores, in artificial insemination, 455–456, *456*
    in in vitro fertilization, 450
Equine encephalitis, in duikers, 677–679, 680
Equine herpesvirus–1, in mixed-species exhibits, 27–28
Equine morbillivirus, 349
Equus grevyi (Grevy's zebra), in mixed-species exhibits, 27
Equus hemionus (onager), equine herpesvirus infection in, 27
    iron overload in, 266
Ercalciol (vitamin D₂), 63–65, *64*
    injectable, 70
Ercalcitriol (1,25[OH]₂D₂), 65
Erethizon dorsatum (North American porcupine),
        reproduction in, 362–363
Eretmochelys imbricata (hawksbill turtle), characteristics of,
        217t

Eretmochelys imbricata (hawksbill turtle) *(Continued)*
    conservation status of, 218
Ergocalciferol (vitamin D₂), 63–65, *64*
    injectable, 70
Ergosterol (provitamin D₂), 63, *64*
Ericaceae, poisonous species of, 92t
Erysipelas, birds and, 152t
Erythrocebus patas (patas monkey), simian varicella infection
        in, 28
    vitamin D transport in, 64
Erythromycin, for leptospirosis, 471
    in ape neonates, 386
    in elephants, 538
    in fish, 183t, 185
        administration of, in food, 184
Escherichia coli, birds and, 152t
    diarrheal disease and, in ape neonates, 386
    vaccine for, in okapi, 649
Eschrichtius gibbosus (California gray whale), iron overload
        in, 267
Estrogens, for contraception, 317
    lactation and, 319
Estrous cycle synchronization. See also *Reproduction,
        assisted.*
    in artiodactylids, 598
Ethambutol, in Arabian oryx, 694
    in tree kangaroos, 340
Ethanol, for fish anesthesia, 161t, 162
Etorphine, in Arabian oryx, 689, 689t
    in crocodilians, 211, 213t
    in domestic goats, 685
    in duikers, 672, 673t, 674t
    in elephants, 526–527, 527t, 529
    in hippopotamus, 638
    in mountain goats, 684, 685
    in mountain sheep, 684
    in okapi, 649
    in suids, 642, 645
    in tapirs, 562
    in white rhinoceros, 556t, 557, 557t, 559, 561
Eublepharus macularius (leopard gecko), vitamin D
        metabolism in, 73
Eumetopias jubatus (Steller sea lion), leptospirosis in, 470
Eurasian brown bear (*Ursus arctos*), hepatic proliferative
        disease in, 426
    sonographic fetal assessment in, *52*
Eurasian otter (*Lutra lutra*), anesthesia in, 439
    geographic distribution of, 436t
European bat viruses, 137t, 348
European ferret (*Mustela putorius furo*), artificial
        insemination in, 452, 452t, 454
    tuberculosis in, 104
        lesions of, 106, 107t, 108
        prevalence of, 105t
European wildcat (*Felis silvestris*), feline leukemia virus in,
        402
Euthanasia, for confiscated chelonians, emotional issues in,
        241
    for fish, 162–163
    for stranded cetaceans, 492
Excitatory neurons, in pain perception, 310
Extracorporealization, with minimally invasive surgery, 39
The Extractor, for snakebite, 99, *100*
Extrapyramidal effects, due to tranquilizers, in herbivores,
        578, 579, 581, 583
Eye, examination of, in megachiropterans, 353
    venom contamination of, 100, *100*

F

Fallow deer (*Dama dama*), artificial insemination in, 598

Fallow deer (*Dama dama*) *(Continued)*
  embryo transfer in, 599, 600
  estrous cycle synchronization in, 598
  handling systems for, 658, 659
  Johne's disease in, 617
  Parelaphostrongylus tenuis in, 634
  Spiculopteragia asymmetrica in, 588
  tuberculosis in, 651, 654
False gharial (*Tomistoma schlegelii*), gallamine mortality in, 206
  immobilization of, 206–207
False killer whale (*Pseudorca crassidens*), fungal infections in, 479t, 481t
False water cobra (*Hydrodynastes gigas*), antimicrobials in, 192t, 193–194
Fascioloides magna, in ranched hoofstock, 588, 589
Fat, vitamin E absorption and, 79
Fatty acids, in fruit bat diet, 357
  in pigeon milk, 271–273, 272t, *273*
  in pigeon milk replacer, 276
  omega-3, in fish diet, 172
  polyunsaturated, vitamin E interaction with, 79, 82
Feather lice, in California condor, 290
Feathers, oil effects on, 301–302, *301*
  removing oil from, 304–305, 304t
  samples of, in oil spill response, 301
  waterproofing of, 305–306, *306*
  wet, causes of, 306t
Fecal culture, in Johne's disease diagnosis, 614, 615, 619
Fecal egg count reduction test, for anthelmintic effectiveness, 595
Fecal examination, in cryptosporidiosis diagnosis, 128–130, *129*
  of ranched hoofstock, 588
Felids. See also *Carnivores;* specific animals.
  artificial insemination in, 452–456. See also *Artificial insemination, in carnivores.*
  emerging viral infections in, 401–409
  hepatic disease in, 427
  in toxoplasmosis transmission, 131, *132*
  in vitro fertilization in, 450–451, *450,* 450t, *451*
  iron overload in, 266–267
  neoplasms in, 427
  scrapie-like spongiform encephalopathy in, 662, 664, *664, 665,* 665t
Feline immunodeficiency virus, 404–407
Feline leukemia virus (FeLV), 402–404
Feline oncornavirus–associated cell membrane antigen (FOCMA) assay, as feline leukemia virus test, 403
Feline retroviruses, 401–407
Felis bengalensis (leopard cat), artificial insemination in, 455, 455t
  feline immunodeficiency virus in, 405
  feline leukemia virus in, 402
Felis concolor. See *Puma (Felis concolor).*
Felis manul (Pallas cat), feline immunodeficiency virus in, 405, 406, 407
Felis pardalis (ocelot), artificial insemination in, 455, 455t
Felis planiceps (flat-headed cat), feline immunodeficiency virus in, 405
Felis silvestris (European wildcat), feline leukemia virus in, 402
Felis silvestris ornata (Indian desert cat), in vitro fertilization in, 451
FeLV (feline leukemia virus), 402–404
Femoral fracture, epiphyseal, in megachiropterans, 346, *347*
  in cheetah, due to darting, 417
Fenbendazole, in callitrichids, 373
  in cheetah, 459t
  in fish, 169t

Fenbendazole *(Continued)*
  in hoofstock, 587t, 589
  in manatees, 514–515
  in megachiropterans, 348
  in otters, 444–445, 445t
  in sea turtles, 230t
  in stranded cetaceans, 489t
Fencing, for deer control, 119
  for elephant paddock, in translocation project, 531
Fennec fox (*Fennecus zerda*), weight of, 429
Fennecus species (foxes), immobilizing drug dosages for, 434t
Fennecus zerda (fennec fox), weight of, 429
Fentanyl, in duikers, 673t
  in giant panda, 411t
  in otters, 438t, 441
  in suids, 640, 640t, 642
  in white rhinoceros, 556–557, 556t, 559
Ferrets, artificial insemination in, 452, 452t, 454, 461–462
  black-footed, conservation program for, 460–462
  European, tuberculosis in, 104
    lesions of, 106, 107t, 108
    prevalence of, 105t
Ferritin, 260
  measurement of, 262
Fetal death, in elephant, 522–524
  sonographic identification of, 52, *52*
Fetal malposition, in elephant, 522, *522*
Fetal ultrasonography, 47–52, *48, 49, 52*
  in dolphins, 501–506, *503–506*
Fever, behavioral, in reptiles, 196
Fibropapillomatosis, in sea turtles, 223, 228
Fibrous osteodystrophy, in primates, 70–71
Fiddleneck (*Amsinckia intermedia*), toxicity of, 89
Filarial infection, in megachiropterans, 348
Filtration, in water quality maintenance, for waterfowl, 296
Final (warfarin), 117, 118t
Finquel (tricaine methanesulfonate), in crocodilians, 212, 214t
  in fish, 160, 161t
First aid, for snakebite, 98–100, *99,* 99t, *100*
Fish, 158–189
  anesthesia in, 158–163, *160,* 161t
    monitoring of, 162
    waterborne, 159–161, *160,* 161t
  attaching telemetry equipment to, 8t
  disease surveillance in, 177–181, 178t, *179,* 180t
  environmental considerations for, 165–172, *170,* 170t, *171*
  euthanasia in, 162–163
  for phytoplankton control in waterfowl exhibits, 297
  in sea turtle diet, 219–220
  Mycobacterium marinum in, 148
  nutrition for, 172–173, 173t, 174t
  pharmacotherapeutics for, 182–189
    dosage regimens in, 182, 183t–184t
    environmental issues in, 182–184
    routes of administration in, 184–185
  preventive medicine program for, 163–181
  quarantine for, 164–165, *166–167,* 169t
    health assessment in, 165, *168,* 179
  records for, 163–164
  sanitation for, 175–177, 176t
  shipment of, 21–22
  sonographic assessment in, for sex determination, 42, *43*
    of health, 47t
  stress in, 164–165, *165*
  vaccinations for, 173–175
Fish and Wildlife Service (USF&W), shipping regulations of, 22–23
Flagyl. See *Metronidazole.*
Flamingos, shipment of, 21

Flat-headed cat (*Felis planiceps*), feline immunodeficiency virus in, 405
Florfenicol, in fish, 183t, 185
Florida manatee (*Trichechus manatus latirostris*). See *Manatees.*
Florida soft-shell turtle (*Trionyx ferox*), chemical dip for, 195
Flotation jacket, for manatee, 512–513
Flow cytometry, for cell-mediated immunity evaluation, 62
Fluconazole, in fish, 187
  in koala, 328
  in marine mammals, 483, 483t
  in sea turtles, 230t
  in stranded cetaceans, 489t
Flucytosine, in fish, 187
  in marine mammals, 483–484, 483t
Fluid accumulation, abdominal, sonographic detection of, 44–47, *47*
Fluid administration, in callitrichids, 371
  in cheetah, 459
  in koala, 322
  in manatees, 512
  in oiled birds, 303, 307
  in pinnipeds, 471
  in sea turtles, 229, *229,* 230t
  in stranded cetaceans, 487–488, 491
Flumazenil, in crocodilians, 214t, 215
  in manatees, 510
  in otters, 440
  in suids, domestic, 640, 641, 642, 642t
    nondomestic, 644, 645
Flumethrin, in cheetah, 420t
Flunixin meglumine, in birds, 312–313
  in elephants, 536
  in koala, 327
Fluorescent antibody tests. See *Immunofluorescent antibody assay.*
Fluorescent lamps, vitamin D and, 66–67, 75
Fluoride toxicity, in fruit bats, 357–359
  in megachiropterans, 349
Fluorine, in fish diet, 174t
Fluoroquinolones. See also specific drugs.
  in chelonians, 191t, 192–193
  in elephants, 537–538
  in snakes, 192t, 194
Flying foxes. See also *Megachiropterans;* specific animals.
  conservation status of, 344
  geographic distribution of, 345t
  nutritional disorders in, 349–350
FOCMA (feline oncornavirus–associated antigen) assay, as feline leukemia virus test, 403
Folic acid, in fish diet, 173t
Folinic acid, with sulfa-pyrimethamine therapy for toxoplasmosis, 133
Follicle-stimulating hormone (FSH), in embryo transfer techniques in artiodactylids, 599–600
  in in-vitro fertilization in carnivores, 450
Foot, elephant, lesions of, 536, 539
  radiography of, 517–520, *519, 520*
Foot pad disease, in tapirs, 565–566, *567*
Foot-and-mouth disease, in Arabian oryx, 692–693, 692t
Forage, for ranched hoofstock, 591–592
  for rhinoceroses, 569–570
  for tapirs, 564
  poisonous plants in, 89
  sun-dried, vitamin D in, 63, 67–69, 69t
  Toxoplasma contamination of, 134
  vitamin E content of, 81
Formalin, hazards of, 176
  in fish, 169t, 187
  soaking chelonians in, 195

Fowl cholera, water quality and, 299
Foxes, control of, 118
  immobilizing drug dosages for, 434t
  rabies in, 139
Fractures, femoral, epiphyseal, in megachiropterans, 346, *347*
  in cheetah due to darting, 417
Freetail bat (*Tadarida brasiliensis*), rabies in, 140
Freight forwarders, for animal shipment, 24–25
Freund's adjuvant, in porcine zona pellucida vaccine, 630
Frog, vitamin D metabolism in, 74
Fructosamine, serum, in primate diabetes diagnosis, 399
Fruit, in fruit bat diet, 355, 359
  nutrient content of, 355, 355t, 356t
Fruit bats. See also *Megachiropterans;* specific animals.
  gastrointestinal system of, 355
  geographic distribution of, 345t
  nutrition of, 354–359
    recommendations for, 359
    requirements of, 356–359
FSH (follicle-stimulating hormone), in embryo transfer techniques in artiodactylids, 599–600
  in in-vitro fertilization in carnivores, 450
Fungal infections. See also specific fungi and diseases.
  acquired from birds, 154
  in California condor, 290
  in chelonians, 240t
  in equids, 572t
  in marine mammals, 478–484, 479t–481t
    clinical features of, 482
    diagnosis of, 482–483
    pathogenesis of, 481–482
    transmission of, 481
    treatment of, 483–484, 483t
  in okapi, 648
  in reptiles, 190, 195
  in small cetaceans, 488–489
Fur seal, Antarctic, fungal infections in, 479t
  northern, fungal infections in, 479t
    leptospirosis in, 469, 470, 471
Furazone green, in fish, 169t
Furcifer pardalis (panther chameleon), 201
Furosemide, in fish, 184t, 189
  in stranded cetaceans, 489t
Furunculosis, vaccine for, 173
Fusarium infection, in marine mammals, 480t, 482

G

Gallamine triethiodide, in crocodilians, 209–210, 213t
  mortality due to, 206, 210
Gallbladder disease, in fish, 178t
Game ranching, 585–586
  contagious diseases in, 589–591
  individual animal medicine in, 586–587
  nutrition in, 591–592
  parasite control program in, 587–589, 587t
  preventive medicine programs for, 585–592
  quarantine in, 587
  regulation of, 586
  sentinel animals in, 591
Gamete rescue, in carnivores, 451
Gamma interferon assay, in tuberculosis diagnosis, 109
  in cervids, 653
Gas bubble disease, 168–169, *170*
Gastric aspirate, in stranded cetaceans, 487, 488, 490
Gastric biopsy, in cheetah, 459
Gastric bloat, in callitrichids, 374
  in stranded cetaceans, 489
Gastric intubation, in elephants, 534

Gastric intubation *(Continued)*
  in hand-reared cetaceans, 495
  in manatees, 512
Gastric ulcers, in stranded cetaceans, 488
Gastritis, in cheetah, 418, 458–460
Gastroduodenoscopy, in gastritis diagnosis, in cheetah, 459
Gastrointestinal tract, damage to, in birds, from nonsteroidal
      anti-inflammatory drugs, 312
    from oil spill, 302
  disorders of, in callitrichids, 374
    in fish, 178t
    in okapi, 648
    in prosimians, 365–366
    in tapirs, 565, 567
    in tree kangaroos, *340,* 341, *342*
  exteriorization of, with minimally invasive surgery, 39
  of fruit bats, 355
  of megachiropterans, 350
  of stranded cetaceans, 488–489
Gastroscopy, in stranded cetaceans, 490
Gaur *(Bos gaurus)*, artificial insemination in, 599
  embryo transfer in, 599–600, 601
  estrous cycle synchronization in, 598
  handling systems for, 660
  malignant catarrhal fever in, 27
Gavage feeding, for ape neonate, 384
Gavialis gangeticus (gharial), immobilization of, 206–207
Gazella spekei (Speke's gazelle), artificial insemination in,
      599
Gazella thomsoni (Thomson's gazelle), equine herpesvirus
      infection in, 27
Gazelles, desert, parasites in, 29
  Speke's, artificial insemination in, 599
  Thomson's, equine herpesvirus infection in, 27
GB agent, primate infection with, 379
Geckos, vitamin D metabolism in, 73
Gelada baboon *(Theropithecus gelada)*, reproductive tract
      evaluation in, using minimally invasive surgery, *39*
Gemsbok, tranquilizers in, 579t, 581
Genitourinary disorders. See also under *Reproductive system.*
  in prosimians, 367
  in tapirs, 566
Genome resource banks, benefits of, 449, 449t
Gentamicin, in California condor chick, 286–287
  in chelonians, 191–192, 191t
  in crocodilians, 191t, 193
  in elephants, 537
  in fish, 183t, 185–186
  in koala, 326, 327
  in reptiles, renal-portal system's effect on kinetics of, 249
    temperature and, 197
  in snakes, 192t, 194
    in combination dosing, 194–195
Gentoo *(Pygoscelis papua)*, sonographic assessment of sexual
      maturation in, *45*
Geochelone carbonaria (South American red-footed tortoise),
      herpesvirus carriage by, 28
Geochelone chilensis (Argentine tortoise), herpesvirus
      infection in, 28
Geochelone elegans (Indian star tortoise), antimicrobials in,
      191t, 193
Geochelone sulcata (African spurred tortoise), vitamin D
      metabolism in, 73–74
Geopetitia aspiculata, in mixed-species exhibits, 29
Gerbils, iron overload in, 267
Gestation. See *Pregnancy; Reproduction.*
Gestational aging, in dolphins, ultrasonography in, 501–506,
      503–506
Gestational diabetes, in primates, 398
Gharials. See also *Crocodilians.*

Gharials *(Continued)*
  false, gallamine mortality in, 206
    immobilization of, 206–207
  immobilization of, 206–207
Giant otter *(Pteronura brasiliensis)*, anesthesia in, 440, 441
  geographic distribution of, 436t
Giant panda *(Ailuropoda melanoleuca)*. See under *Pandas.*
Giant salamander, Chinese, sonographic sex determination in,
      43
Giardiasis, birds and, 153t, 155
  in lemurs, 366
  in mixed-species exhibits, 29
Gibbons. See also *Apes.*
  siamang, iron overload in, 265
  white-handed, testicular cyst in, sonographic assessment of,
      51
    viral hepatitis in, 378
    vitamin D transport in, 64
Gila monster *(Heloderma suspectum)*, sonographic sex
      determination in, *43*
Gill biopsy, *168*
Gills, of fish, diseases affecting, 178t
Gingivitis, in mammals, 252
Giraffe *(Giraffa camelopardis)*, artificial insemination in, 599
  estrous cycle synchronization in, 598
  handling systems for, 660
  induced ovulation in, 599
  tranquilizers in, 579t, 582–583
Glipizide, for primate diabetes, 399
Globicephala species (pilot whales). See also *Cetaceans.*
  antifungal drugs in, 483t
  morbillivirus infection in, 498
α-Globulin, in vitamin D transport, 64
Globulin electrophoresis, as test of humoral immunity, 61
Glomerulonephritis, in callitrichids, 374
  in megachiropterans, 352, *352*
Glucose, serum, in primate diabetes diagnosis, 398–399
Glucose tolerance tests, in primates, 399
Glucosuria, in primate diabetes, 399
Glycopyrrolate, in canids, 431
  in crocodilians, 214t, 215
  in marsupials, 335
  in suids, 642, 642t
Glycosylated hemoglobin, in primate diabetes diagnosis, 399
Goeldi's monkey *(Callimico goeldii)*, 369. See also
      Callitrichids.
  Gongylonema infection in, 372, *372*
  hepatic myelolipoma in, 426
Goiter, in fish, 170, *171,* 173
Golden lion tamarin *(Leontopithecus rosalia)*. See also
      Callitrichids.
  callitrichid hepatitis in, 377–378
  congenital disorders in, 373, *374*
  parasites in, 29
  vitamin D transport in, 64
Golden oat grass *(Trisetum flavescens)*, vitamin D in, 63
Golden pheasant *(Chrysolophus pictus)*, parasites in, 29
Golden-mantled flying fox *(Pteropus pumilus)*. See also
      Megachiropterans.
  cranial edema in, *352*
  Elizabethan collar use in, 346, *347*
  geographic distribution of, 345t
  venipuncture in, *346, 347*
Gonadectomy, 316, 318
Gonadotropin(s), chorionic, in assisted reproduction, in
      artiodactylids, 598, 599–600
    in carnivores, 450, 455–456, 455t, *456*
    in fish, 184t, 189
Gonadotropin-releasing hormone analogs, for contraception,
      317

Gonads. See also *Reproductive system.*
  of fish, diseases affecting, 178t
  pathologic alterations in, sonographic assessment of, *50, 51, 51*
Gongylonema, in callitrichids, 372, *372*
  in lemurs, 366
Goose, Canada (*Branta canadensis*), control of, 119–120
Gopher(s), control of, 117
Gopher snake (*Pituophis melanoleucus*), antimicrobials in, 192t, 194
Gopher tortoise (*Gopherus polyphemus*), antimicrobials in, 191t, 192, 193
Gopherus agassizii (desert tortoise), vitamin D metabolism in, 73–74
Gopherus polyphemus (gopher tortoise), antimicrobials in, 191t, 192, 193
Gorilla (*Gorilla gorilla*). See also *Apes.*
  Balantidium coli in, 29, 386
  birth weight for, 383
  herpesvirus infection in, 386
  iron overload in, 265
  mastoiditis in, imaging of, 85, *85*
  Mycoplasma infection in, 540
  pregnancy in, management of, 384
  varicella in, 386
Gray duiker (*Sylvicapra grimmia*), 668. See also *Duikers.*
  immobilization of, 673t
  tranquilizers in, 579t, 582
Gray parrot, Congo African, biliary cysts in, 424
Gray rat snake (*Elaphe obsoleta*), antimicrobials in, 192t, 194
Gray rhebok, tranquilizers in, 579t, 582
Gray seal (*Halichoerus grypus*), mycobacterial infection in, 148
  phocine distemper virus in, 498
Gray whale, California, iron overload in, 267
Gray wolf (*Canis lupus*), artificial insemination in, 451–452
  weight of, 429
Gray-headed flying fox (*Pteropus poliocephalus*). See also *Megachiropterans.*
  geographic distribution of, 345t
Great Plains rat snake (*Elaphe guttata*), antimicrobials in, 192t, 193
Greater Yellowstone Interagency Brucellosis Committee (GYIBC), 624
Greek tortoise (*Testudo graeca*), penicillins in, 191, 191t
Green iguana (*Iguana iguana*), metabolic bone disease in, 72–73
Green monkey, African, viral hepatitis in, 378
Green sea turtle (*Chelonia mydas*), anesthesia in, 222
  characteristics of, 217t
  conservation status of, 218
  nutrition for, 219
Green sea turtle fibropapillomatosis, 223, 228
Grevy's zebra (*Equus grevyi*), in mixed-species exhibits, 27
Grey. See *Gray* entries.
Grizzly bear (*Ursus arctos horribilis*), hepatic proliferative disease in, 426
Ground squirrels. See *Squirrel(s).*
Groundsel (*Senecio vulgaris*), toxicity of, 89
Guanaco (*Lama guanicoe*), estrous cycle synchronization in, 598
Guenon (*Cercopithecus mitis*), biliary cystadenoma in, 424
Guinea pigs, *Bordetella bronchiseptica* infection in, 28
Gular edema, in chameleons, 204
GYIBC (Greater Yellowstone Interagency Brucellosis Committee), 624
Gymnogyps californianus. See *California condor (Gymnogyps californianus).*
Gypsum, for phytoplankton control in waterfowl exhibits, 297

H

Haemaphysalis species, on cheetah, 419, 419t
  on giant panda, 413
  on koala, 330t
  on ranched hoofstock, 589
Haemonchus contortus, life cycle of, 593
Haemonchus species, in ranched hoofstock, 588
Hairy nightshade (*Solanum sarrachoides*), toxicity of, 88
  in lemurs, 368
Hairy-nosed otter (*Lutra sumatrana*), geographic distribution of, 436t
Haldol. See *Haloperidol.*
Halichoerus grypus (gray seal), mycobacterial infection in, 148
  phocine distemper virus in, 498
Haloperidol, in duikers, 675
  in elephants, 530, *530,* 579t, 583
  in fish, 184t, 189
  in marsupials, 335t
  in okapi, 649
  in wild herbivores, 578, 579
    species guidelines for, 579–584, 579t, *580, 583*
Halothane, in crocodilians, 212, 213t
  in fish, 161t, 162
  in suids, 641
Hamadryas baboon (*Papio hamadryas*), biliary cystadenoma in, 424
  malignant T cell lymphoma in, 380–381
  tuberculosis in, 105t
Handling systems. See also *Crates; Restraint.*
  for Arabian oryx, 688–689
  for cheetahs in breeding facility, 416, *416, 417, 420*
  for ungulates, 657–658, *658,* 658t, *659*
    chutes in, 658–661, *659–661*
Hand-rearing, of apes, 383–384
  of Arabian oryx in tuberculosis outbreak, 694
  of California condor, 284–286
  of cetaceans, 493–497
    nutrition and feeding in, 494–495, 494t
    weaning in, 496
  of columbids, 275–276
  of duikers, 671–672
  of giant panda, 414
  of koala, 331
Hanging drop test, 33–34
Hank's balanced salt solution (HBSS), for *Cryptosporidium* oocyst storage, 128
Harbor porpoise (*Phocoena phocoena*), caloric requirements of calves of, 495
  fungal infections in, 480t
  hand-reared, weaning of, 496
  morbillivirus infection in, 498
  organochlorines in, 474
Harbor seal (*Phoca vitulina*), fungal infections in, 479t, 480t
  iron overload in, 267
  leptospirosis in, 469
  organochlorines in, 474
  phocine distemper virus in, 497
Hares (*Lepus* species), reproduction in, 362
Harp seal (*Phoca groenlandica*), fungal infections in, 481t
  phocine distemper virus in, 498
Harpacticus pulex, in manatees, 515
Hartebeests, herpesvirus carriage by, 27
  tranquilizers in, 579t, 581
Harvest mouse (*Reithrodontomys* species), control of, 116–117
Hawksbill turtle (*Eretmochelys imbricata*), characteristics of, 217t
  conservation status of, 218
H_2-blockers, for gastric ulcers, in stranded cetaceans, 488, 489t

HBSS (Hank's balanced salt solution), for *Cryptosporidium* oocyst storage, 128
HCB (hexachlorobenzene), in marine mammals, 473
hCG (human chorionic gonadotropin), in carnivores, in artificial insemination, 455–456, 455t, *456*
  in in-vitro fertilization, 450
  in fish, 184t, 189
HCH (hexachlorocyclohexane), in marine mammals, 473
Head and lateral line disease, in fish, 171, *171*
Head gates, in ungulate handling systems, 660
Health certificate, for international shipments, 22, 24, 25–26
Hearing loss, human, due to bird sounds, 153t, 155
Heart. See *Cardiovascular system.*
Heart failure, in tree kangaroos, 342
  iron overload and, 261
Heavy metal poisoning. See also *Iron overload; Lead poisoning; Zinc intoxication.*
  in fish, 170
  in marine mammals, 475–476
Hedgehogs, tuberculosis in, 101
Helarctos malayanus (Malayan sun bear), hepatic proliferative disease in, 426
Helicobacter acinonyx, gastritis in cheetahs and, 458, 459–460
Helicobacter heilmannii, gastritis in cheetahs and, 458, 460
Helicobacter hepaticus, hepatic neoplasms and, 425
Helmet cassowary (*Casuarius casuarius*), sonographic sex determination in, *43*
Heloderma species (venomous lizards), bites from, 100
Heloderma suspectum (Gila monster), sonographic sex determination in, *43*
Hemangiosarcoma, hepatic, 426
Hematologic reference values, for Arabian oryx, 690, 691t
  for duikers, 675, 676t–678t
  for giant panda, 412t
  for koala, 323t
  for manatees, 512t
  for sea turtles, 224t
  for tapirs, 564, 564t
  for tree kangaroos, 339, 339t
Hemochromatosis, 260, 261. See also *Iron overload.*
  in lemurs, 366
Hemolysis, acute episodic, in black rhinoceros, 59
Hemolytic syndrome, in chimpanzee neonates, 383
Hemorrhagic enteritis, in giant panda, 412–413
Hemorrhagic enterocolitis, in cetaceans, 467
Hemorrhagic fever, simian, in mixed-species exhibits, 28
Hemosiderin, 260
Hemosiderosis, 260, 261. See also *Iron overload.*
Hepatic. See *Liver.*
Hepatitis, callitrichid, 28, 370, *370,* 377–378
  viral, hepatic neoplasms and, 425, 426
  in primates, 378–379
Hepatocellular adenoma, 425
Hepatocellular carcinoma, 425–426
  in felids, 427
Hepatocutaneous syndrome, in black rhinoceros, 59, 552–553, *553*
Hepatocystis species, in flying foxes, 348
Hepatoma, 425
Heptachlor, in marine mammals, 472
Herbivores. See also *Hoofstock; Ruminants;* specific types.
  capture methods for, 576
  tranquilizers in, 575–584
    effects of, 577, *578*
    guidelines for using, 578–579
    recommended, 577–578
    side effects of, 579
    species guidelines for, 579–584, 579t
Hermann's tortoise (*Testudo hermanni*), antimicrobials in, 191, 191t, 193

Hernia, diaphragmatic defects and, in callitrichids, 373, *374*
  gastritis due to, in cheetah, 458
Herons, vitamin E supplementation for, in mixed-species exhibits, 27
Herpesviruses, in ape neonates, 386
  in black rhinoceros, 555
  in callitrichids, 370
  in mixed-species exhibits, 27–28
  in primates, 380
Heterakis isolonche, in mixed-species exhibits, 29
Heterocephalus glaber (naked mole rat), vitamin D metabolism in, 74
Heterocheilus tunicatus, in manatees, 514
Heterodon platyrhinos (hog nose snake), antimicrobials in, 192t, 194
Hexachlorobenzene (HCB), in marine mammals, 473
Hexachlorocyclohexane (HCH), in marine mammals, 473
Hexamitiasis, in mixed-species exhibits, 29
Hiatal hernia, gastritis due to, in cheetah, 458
"Hiccups," in anesthetized elephants, 529
Hippobosca longipennis, on cheetah, 419, 419t
Hippopotamus, anesthesia in, 638–639
  importation of, 23
  pygmy, leiomyoma in, sonographic assessment of, *50*
Hippotragus niger (sable antelope), copper deficiency in, in mixed-species exhibits, 27
  tranquilizers in, 579t, 581
Histamine$_2$-blockers, for gastric ulcers, in stranded cetaceans, 488, 489t
Histoplasmosis, birds and, 153t, 154
  in marine mammals, 481t, 483
Hog nose snake (*Heterodon platyrhinos*), antimicrobials in, 192t, 194
Holacanthus tricolor (rock beauties), nutritional needs of, 172
Hooded seal (*Cystophora cristata*), fungal infections in, 480t
Hoof disease, in tapirs, 565–566, *567*
Hoof overgrowth, in okapi, 648
Hoofstock. See also *Herbivores; Ruminants;* specific types.
  computer programs for carrying capacity of, 586t
  fecal examination of, 588
  game ranching of. See *Game ranching.*
  in mixed-species exhibits, parasites in, 29
  quarantine for, 15t, 23
  restraint of, systems for, 657–661, *658–661,* 658t
Horse(s). See also *Equids.*
  calcium regulation in, 74
  captive population of, 572t
  domestic, disease transmission from, to non-domestic equids, 573
    diseases of, 574t
    nutrient concentrations in total diets of, 568t
  iron overload in, 266
  morbillivirus infection in, bats and, 349
  nutritional requirements for, 568t
Horse meat, disease transmission by, in mixed-species exhibits, 28
House mouse (*Mus musculus*), control of, 116
  disease introduction by, 28
  lymphocytic choriomeningitis carriage by, 378
House shrew (*Suncus murinus*), iron overload in, 267
House sparrow (*Passer domesticus*), control of, 119
Howler monkeys, herpesvirus infection in, 28
  rickets in, 71, *71*
Human chorionic gonadotropin (hCG), in carnivores, in artificial insemination, 455–456, 455t, *456*
  in in-vitro fertilization, 450
  in fish, 184t, 189
Hummingbirds, shipment of, 21
Humoral immunity, tests of, 60–61, 60t

Hyacinth macaw, tumor imaging in, 85–87, *86, 87*

Hyalomma dromedarii, on Arabian oryx, 695

Hyalomma species, on cheetah, 419t

Hyaluronidase, in crocodilians, 213–215, 214t
  in elephants, 527
  in white rhinoceros, 557t

Hy.D (vitamin D supplement), 69

Hydatid disease, of liver, 423

Hydraulic chutes. See also *Handling systems.*
  for ungulates, 660–661, *661*

Hydrochaerus hydrochaeris (capybara), reproduction in, 363

Hydrocortisone, in fish, 184t, 189

Hydrodynastes gigas (false water cobra), antimicrobials in, 192t, 193–194

25-Hydroxycholecalciferol (25[OH]D$_3$), 64
  oral supplements of, 69–70

Hyena, spotted, sonographic sex determination in, *44*

Hylobates lar (white-handed gibbon), testicular cyst in, sonographic assessment of, *51*
  viral hepatitis in, 378
  vitamin D transport in, 64

Hylobates syndactylus (siamang gibbon), iron overload in, 265

Hyoscine, in white rhinoceros, 556t, 557

Hyperbilirubinemia, in callitrichids, 373

Hyperkinesis, in anesthetized suids, 643

Hypertension, in anesthetized white rhinoceros, 560

Hyperthermia, during anesthesia, in canids, 433
  in hippopotamus, 638, 639
  in suids, 641–642
  in white rhinoceros, 560

Hypervitaminosis D, 74–75
  in pacas and agoutis in mixed-species exhibits, 27, 72, 75
  in primates, 72, 74–75

Hypoglycemia, in callitrichids, 374

Hypotension, in anesthetized white rhinoceros, 560

Hypothermia, in immobilized canid, 433
  in oiled birds, 302, 303

Hyrax, rock, iron overload in, 267

Hystrix species (African crested porcupines), reproduction in, 363

I

IATA (International Air Transport Association), live animal regulations of, 17–18, 20, 21, 22–24

Ibex, Siberian, immobilization of, 685
  Spanish, embryo transfer in, 601
    estrous cycle synchronization in, 598
    induced ovulation in, 599

Idazoxan, in canids, 431
  in mountain sheep, 685

Identification, of California condors, 284
  of hoofstock in game ranching, 587
  of river otters, 446
  of tapirs, 563

Iguana iguana (green iguana), metabolic bone disease in, 72–73

Immobilization. See also *Anesthesia;* specific drugs.
  of Arabian oryx, 689–690, 689t
  of canids, 429–434
    animal handling in, 432–433
    drugs for, 430–432, 433–434, 434t
    medical concerns in, 433
  of crocodilians, 205–208, *206–210*
    agents for, 208–215, 213t–214t
    complications of, 213–214
    recommendations for, 215–216
  of duikers, 672–675, 673t, 674t

Immobilization *(Continued)*
  of giant panda, 411–412, 411t
  of okapi, 649

Immune response, acquired, 58
  evaluation of, 60–62, 60t
  innate, 58

Immunoassays. See also specific techniques.
  in tuberculosis diagnosis, 109
  limitations of, for antibody detection, 57–58
    for antigen detection, 57

Immunocontraception. See *Porcine zona pellucida (PZP) vaccine.*

Immunodeficiency disorders, 58–62
  due to feline leukemia virus, 404
  in koala, 321
  primary, 59
  secondary, 59

Immunodiffusion assays, in fungal infection diagnosis, in marine mammals, 482–483

Immunoelectron microscopy, in viral enteritis diagnosis, in ruminants, 609

Immunofluorescent antibody assay, for cryptosporidiosis, 130
  for feline immunodeficiency virus, 405–406
  for feline leukemia virus, 403
  for toxoplasmosis, 132–133
  for viral enteritis, in ruminants, 609

Immunoglobulin(s), for hand-reared cetacean, 496
  in pigeon milk, 271
  quantitation of, 61

Immunoglobulin G$_1$, in ruminants, 610–611

Immunostimulants, for fish, 175

Impala (*Aepyceros melampus*), tranquilizers in, 579t, 581

Importation of animals, logistics of, 25
  regulation of, 22–24, 25

In vitro fertilization, in artiodactylids, 601–602
  in carnivores, 450–451, *450,* 450t, *451*

Inbreeding, immunodeficiency and, 59

Indian blackbuck (*Antilope cervicapra*), artificial insemination in, 599
  handling systems for, 660

Indian desert cat (*Felis silvestris ornata*), in vitro fertilization in, 451

Indian flying fox (*Pteropus giganteus*). See also *Megachiropterans.*
  geographic distribution of, 345t
  reproduction in, 353

Indian rock python (*Python molurus molurus*), antimicrobials in, 192t, 194

Indian star tortoise (*Geochelone elegans*), antimicrobials in, 191t, 193

Indigo snake, eastern, antimicrobials in, 192t, 194

Infectious diseases. See also specific types.
  diagnostic tests for, evaluation and interpretation of, 55–58, *56,* 57t
  in ape neonates, 385–386
  in Arabian oryx, 690–696, 692t
  in callitrichids, 370–373, *370, 372, 373*
  in chameleons, 203
  in chelonians, 240t, 241
  in duikers, 676–679
  in equids, 572–574, 572t, 574t
  in koala, 324–328, *325, 327*
  in megachiropterans, 347–349
  in mixed-species exhibits, 27–28
  in okapi, 648
  in ranched hoofstock, 589–591
  in tree kangaroo, 339–341, *340, 341*

Infectious rhinotracheitis, vaccination for, in cheetah, 418

Inflammatory response, in marine mammal cytologic specimen, classification of, 464–465, *465*

Influenza, in birds, 152t, 155
Inhalation anesthetics. See *Volatile anesthetics;* specific
  agents.
Inhibitory neurons, in pain perception, 310
Inositol, in fish diet, 173t
Insects, parasite transmission by, 29
Insufflation, for minimally invasive surgery, 31–32, 34
Insular flying fox (*Pteropus tonganus*). See also
  Megachiropterans.
  conservation status of, 344
Insulin, determination of, in primate diabetes diagnosis, 399
  for primate diabetes, 399–400
Integrated pest management (IPM), 114–116
  trichostrongyloid parasite control program using, 593–597.
    See also *Trichostrongyloid parasites.*
Integumentary system. See *Skin.*
γ-Interferon assay, in tuberculosis diagnosis, 109
  in cervids, 653
International Air Transport Association (IATA), live animal
  regulations of, 17–18, 20, 21, 22–24
International Veterinary Pathology Slide Bank video disc, 5
Internunciary neurons, in pain perception, 310
Interstitial pneumonitis, allergic, due to bird contact, 153t,
  155
Intestines. See *Gastrointestinal tract.*
Intoxication. See *Poisoning.*
Intrauterine device, for contraception, 317
Intubation, endotracheal, in California condor, 282, *282*
  in crocodilians, 212
  in hippopotamus, 639
  in manatees, 510
  in marsupials, 336
  in megachiropterans, 345, *346*
  in sea turtles, 222
  in suids, 641
  in tapirs, 563
  in tree kangaroos, 338
  in white rhinoceros, 557–558
  gastric, in elephants, 534
    in hand-reared cetaceans, 495
    in manatees, 512
Invertebrates, for aquaria, quarantine of, 165
Iodine, in fish diet, 173, 174t
Iodophores, for disinfection, 176t
IPM (integrated pest management), 114–116
  trichostrongyloid parasite control program using, 593–597.
    See also *Trichostrongyloid parasites.*
Iron. See also *Iron overload.*
  in fish diet, 174t
  in rhinoceros diet, 570, 570t
  vitamin E interaction with, 82
Iron dextran, for oiled birds, 304
Iron overload, 260–268
  diagnosis of, 261–262, 263t
  in amphibians, 264
  in birds, 264–265, 265t
  in callitrichids, 375
  in fruit bats, 357
  in lemurs, 366
  in mammals, 265–267
  in reptiles, 264
  in rhinoceroses, 266, 570
  in tree kangaroos, 341
  mechanisms of, 261
  prevention of, 264
  treatment of, 262–264
Island flying fox (*Pteropus hypomelanus*). See also
  Megachiropterans.
  cardiomyopathy in, *351*
  geographic distribution of, 345t

Island flying fox (*Pteropus hypomelanus*) (*Continued*)
  intubation of, *346*
  reproduction in, *353*
Isoflurane, in California condor, 282, *282*
  in chameleons, 204
  in crocodilians, 212, 213t
  in duikers, 672
  in fish, 161t, 162
  in manatees, 510
  in marsupials, 335–336
  in megachiropterans, 345
  in otters, *438,* 441
  in sea turtles, 222
  in suids, 641, 642
    nondomestic, 644, 645
  in white rhinoceros, 557
Isoniazid, in Arabian oryx, 694
  in elephants, 539, 540
Itraconazole, in fish, 183t, 187
  in koala, 328
  in marine mammals, 483, 483t
  in stranded cetaceans, 489t
Ivermectin, in Arabian oryx, 695
  in California condor, 290
  in callitrichids, 373
  in cheetah, 420t, 421t, 459t
  in elephants, 527
  in fish, 183t, 188
  in hoofstock, 587t, 589
  in lemurs, 366
  in manatees, 514
  in megachiropterans, 348
  in stranded cetaceans, 489t
Ivomec. See *Ivermectin.*
Ixodes species, on giant panda, 413
  on koala, 330t

J

Jackals, immobilizing drug dosages for, 434t
Jackson's chameleon (*Chamaeleo jacksonii*), 201
Jaguar (*Panthera onca*), feline immunodeficiency virus in,
  405
Japanese macaque (*Macaca fuscata*), canine distemper virus
  in, 379, 408
Jasmin, wild, vitamin D in, 63
Jaundice, neonatal, in apes, 383
Javelina (*Tayassu tajacu*), anesthesia in, 643–644
  canine distemper virus in, 408
Jentink's duiker (*Cephalophus jentinkii*). See also *Duikers.*
  anesthesia in, 674t
  conservation status of, 669
  laboratory reference values for, 678t
Johne's disease, in free-ranging wildlife, 616–620
  clinical signs of, 618–619, *618*
  diagnosis of, 619, *619*
  management of, 619–620
  pathogenesis of, 617–619, *618*
  transmission of, 617–618
  in okapi, 648
  in ranched hoofstock, 590
  in zoo animals, 612–616
    clinical signs of, 613
    diagnosis of, 614–615
    management of, 615
    pathogenesis of, 613
    transmission of, 613
    treatment of, 615–616

Johne's disease *(Continued)*
  species susceptible to, 613
Johnstonema species, in koala, 330t
Juvenile llama immunodeficiency syndrome, 59

K

Kafue lechwe. See *Lechwe.*
Kangaroo(s), tree. See *Tree kangaroos.*
Kangaroo rats *(Dipodomys* species), reproduction in, 362
Kasokero, in megachiropterans, 349
Kemp's ridley turtle *(Lepidochelys kempii)*, anesthesia in, 221, 222
  characteristics of, 217t
  conservation status of, 218
  nutrition for, 220
  sodium pentobarbital morbidity and mortality in, 221
Kepone (chlordecone), in marine mammals, 473
Keratoconjunctivitis, chlamydial, in koala, 325, *325, 326*
Kerodon rupestris (rock cavy), reproduction in, 363
Ketamine, in Andean condor, 282
  in Arabian oryx, 689, 689t
  in canids, 430, 433–434
  in chameleons, 204
  in cheetah, 417, 459
  in crocodilians, 211, 213t
  in duikers, 673t, 674t
  in elephants, 527
  in fish, 161, 161t
  in giant panda, 411t
  in marsupials, 334t, 335
  in megachiropterans, 345
  in mountain sheep, 685
  in okapi, 649
  in otters, *438,* 438t, 439–441, 442, 446
  in sea turtles, 221, 222t
  in suids, domestic, 640t, 641, 642t
    nondomestic, 642, 643, 644, 645
  in tapirs, 563
  in tree kangaroos, 338
  in turkey vulture, 282
  in white rhinoceros, 559
Ketaset. See *Ketamine.*
Ketoconazole, in chelonians, 191t, 193
  in fish, 183t, 187
  in koala, 328, 331
  in marine mammals, 483, 483t
  in stranded cetaceans, 489t
Ketonuria, in primate diabetes, 399
Kidneys, cadmium accumulation in, in marine mammals, 475
  damage to, in birds, from nonsteroidal anti-inflammatory drugs, 312–313
    from oil spill, 302
  disease of, in callitrichids, 374
    in fish, 178t
    in lemurs, 366–367
    in pinnipeds, due to leptospirosis, 470, *470*
  failure of, gastritis due to, in cheetah, 458
  of megachiropterans, 352, *352*
  sonographic assessment of, 47t
Killer whale *(Orcinus orca)*, diagnostic cytology in, *466, 467*
  fungal infections in, 479t, 480t, 483t
  taurine content of milk of, 494
King snake *(Lampropeltis getulus)*, antimicrobials in, 192t, 193
Kinyoun cold technique, for cryptosporidiosis diagnosis, 129
Klipspringer *(Oreotragus oreotragus)*, tranquilizers in, 579t, 582
Koala *(Phascolarctos cinereus)*, 321–331

Koala *(Phascolarctos cinereus) (Continued)*
  anesthesia for, 333
  drug kinetics in, 324
  hand-raising of, 331
  immunodeficiency in, 321
  infectious diseases in, 324–328, *325, 327*
  laboratory reference values for, 323t, 324t
  noninfectious diseases in, 328–329
  parasites in, 330t
  physiologic data for, 322t
  pouch young of, morbidity and mortality of, 331
    normal development of, 330–331
  supportive care for, 322–324
  tooth wear in, 322, *322–323*
Kodiak bear *(Ursus arctos middendorffi)*, hepatic proliferative disease in, 426
Kogia breviceps (pygmy sperm whale), caloric requirements of calves of, 495
  fungal infections in, 479t, 480t
  ink in colon of, 467
Kogia simus (dwarf sperm whale), ink in colon of, 467
  subcutaneous emphysema in, 490
Komodo dragon *(Varanus komodoensis)*, sonographic sex determination in, *43*
Kudu. See also *Artiodactylids.*
  handling systems for, *659*
  malignant catarrhal fever in, 27
  rabies in, 139
  scrapie-like spongiform encephalopathy in, 662, *663,* 664, 665t
  tranquilizers in, 579t, 580
  tuberculosis in, 101, 103
    clinical signs of, 105, *105,* 106
    lesions of, 106, *107*
Kuru. See *Scrapie-like spongiform encephalopathies.*
Kyaroikeus cetarius, in cetacean blow specimen, 465–466, *466*

L

Laboratory tests. See also specific tests.
  evaluation and interpretation of, 55–58, *56,* 57t
  of immune function, 60–62, 60t
  reference values for, in Arabian oryx, 690, 691t
    in duikers, 675t, 676t–678t
    in giant panda, 412t
    in koala, 323t, 324t
    in manatees, 512t
    in okapi, 649
    in sea turtles, 224t
    in tapirs, 563–564, 564t
    in tree kangaroos, 339, 339t
Lacey Act, 22
Lactated Ringer's solution, in sea turtles, 230t
Lactation, contraception during, 319
  in apes, 383
  in cheetah, feeding during, 421
  in columbids, 269–270, *270, 271, 275*
  induced, in cetacean foster mothers, 496
Lactose intolerance, in ape neonates, 386
  in dolphins, 494
  in giant panda, 414
Lagenorhynchus acutus (white-sided dolphin), fungal infections in, 480t
Lagenorhynchus albirostris (white-beaked dolphin), morbillivirus in, 498
Lagenorhynchus obliquidens, fungal infections in, 480t
Lagomorphs, reproduction in, 361–362
Lagos bat virus, 137t, 348

Lama glama. See *Llama (Lama glama).*
Lama guanicoe (guanaco), estrous cycle synchronization in, 598
Lama pacos (alpaca), embryo transfer in, 601
Lama vicugna (vicuna), estrous cycle synchronization in, 598
Lampropeltis getulus (king snake), antimicrobials in, 192t, 193
Landscaping, plant selection for, 90t–94t
Langurs, parasites in, 29
Lantana (*Lantana camara*), toxicity of, 89
Lanya (*Sus scrofa*), embryo transfer in, 601
Laparoscopy. See also *Minimally invasive surgery (MIS).*
    artificial insemination using, in carnivores, 452–453, 452t, *453, 454*
    history of, 30
    in sea turtles, 226–227
    oocyte recovery using, 450–451, *450, 451*
Large Palau flying fox (*Pteropus pilosus*). See also *Megachiropterans.*
    conservation status of, 344
Larva migrans, visceral, in mixed-species exhibits, 29
Lasionycteris noctivagans (silver-haired bat), rabies in, 140
Latex agglutination test, for cryptococcal antigen, in koala, 328
    for toxoplasmosis, 133
Lauryl alcohol (Teepol), sodium hydroxide with, for disinfection, 176t
Lead poisoning, in California condor, 278, 280, 288
    radiographic findings in, 282
    in elephants, flaccid trunk paralysis and, 542–543
    in fish, 170
    in marine mammals, 476
    in waterfowl, 299
    iron storage and, 264
Leatherback sea turtle (*Dermochelys coriacea*), 217
    conservation status of, 218
    ketamine/acepromazine dose in, 221
Lechwe, red, tranquilizers in, 579t
    tuberculosis in, 101
        age and sex predilection for, 104
        lesions of, 106, 107t
        mortality rate for, 104
        prevalence of, 105t
        transmission of, 102–103
Leg chain injuries, in elephants, 539
Leiomyoma, sonographic detection of, *50,* 51
Lemur(s). See also specific animals.
    cholangioma in, 424
    diseases of, cardiovascular, 367–368
        gastrointestinal, 365–366
        integumentary, 367
        musculoskeletal, 366–367, *367*
        nervous system, 367
        respiratory, 366
        systemic, 368
        urogenital, 367
    iron overload in, 265
    toxoplasmosis susceptibility of, 131
Lemur catta (ring-tailed lemur), cholangioma in, 424
    diabetes in, 398
    toxoplasmosis susceptibility of, 131
Lemur fulvus (brown lemur), vitamin D toxicity in, 75
Lemur macaco, cholangioma in, 424
Lentiviruses, 404
Leontopithecus rosalia (golden lion tamarin). See also *Callitrichids.*
    callitrichid hepatitis in, 377–378
    congenital disorders in, 373, *374*
    parasites in, 29
    vitamin D transport in, 64

Leopard(s). See also *Felids;* specific animals.
    canine distemper virus in, 407, 408
    feline immunodeficiency virus in, 405
Leopard cat (*Felis bengalensis*), artificial insemination in, 455, 455t
    feline immunodeficiency virus in, 405
    feline leukemia virus in, 402
Leopard gecko (*Eublepharus macularius*), vitamin D metabolism in, 73
Lepidochelys kempii. See *Kemp's ridley turtle (Lepidochelys kempii).*
Leptoptilus crumeniferus (African marabou), sonographic sex determination in, *43*
Leptospirosis, in duikers, 677
    in marine mammals, 469–471, *470*
    in ranched hoofstock, 590
Lepus species (hares), reproduction in, 362
Leucothoe davisiae (mountain laurel), toxicity of, 89
Leuprolide, for contraception, 317
Levamisole, in callitrichids, 373
    in lemurs, 366
Levonorgestrel, for contraception, 317, 318
Liasis childreni (children's python), organ location in, 243, *246*
Lice. See also *Parasites;* specific genera and species.
    on California condor, 290
    on ranched hoofstock, 589
Lichtenstein's hartebeest, tranquilizers in, 579t, 581
Lidocaine, in birds, 313
    in fish, 161, 161t
Ligatures, for minimally invasive surgery, 35, *36*
Light, artificial, vitamin D and, 66–67, 75
    for fish, 171, *171*
    for sea turtles, 219
    in handling systems, 658, 658t, *659*
    ultraviolet, as vitamin D source, 63, 65–67, 75
        for chameleons, 202
        to improve water quality for fish, 175
Lignonathus species, on ranched hoofstock, 589
Lincosamides, in elephants, 538
Lindane, in marine mammals, 473
Lintex. See *Niclosamide.*
Lion (*Panthera leo*), canine distemper virus in, 407, 408
    feline immunodeficiency virus in, 405, 406, 407
    tuberculosis in, 101, 103
        clinical signs of, 106
        lesions of, 106, 107t
Lipoproteins, vitamin E and, 79–80
Lipoptena mazamae, on ranched hoofstock, 589
Lissodelphis borealis, fungal infections in, 479t
Listeria monocytogenes infection, in megachiropterans, 348
Litomosa species, in flying foxes, 348
Little brown bat (*Myotis lucifugus*), control of, 118
Liver, cystic disorders of, 423–425, *424*
        diagnosis of, 427–428
        in felids, 427
        treatment of, 428
    diseases of, in fish, 178t
    neoplasms of, 425–426
        diagnosis of, 427–428
        in callitrichids, 375
        in felids, 427
        in ursids, 426–427, *426*
        treatment of, 428
    sonographic assessment of, 47t
    veno-occlusive disease of, in cheetah, 458
        in felids, 427
Liver biopsy, in iron overload diagnosis, 262, 263t
Liverpool vervet virus, in mixed-species exhibits, 28
Livestock, domestic. See also specific animals.

Livestock *(Continued)*
    brucellosis in wildlife and, 624–625, 624t
    parasites orginating in, 588
Lizards. See also *Chameleons; Reptiles;* specific animals.
    antimicrobials in, 192t, 193–194
    minimally invasive surgery in, 37, *37*
    periodontal disease in, 252–257, 253t
        causes of, 255–256
        clinical findings in, 252–253
        diagnosis of, 256, *256*
        histopathology of, 253–254, *254, 255*
        treatment of, 256–257
    shipment of, 20
    venomous, bites from, 100
    vitamin D metabolism in, 73
Llama *(Lama glama)*, biliary cystadenoma in, 424, *424*
    embryo transfer in, 601
    equine herpesvirus infection in, 27
    Mycobacterium kansasii in, 148
    primary immunodeficiency in, 59
Loboa loboi infection, in marine mammals, 481t, 482
Loggerhead sea turtle *(Caretta caretta)*, anesthesia in, 222
    characteristics of, 217t
    chemical dips for, 195
    nutrition for, 219, 220, *220*
Long-haired fruit bat, Ruwenzori. See also *Fruit bats;
        Megachiropterans.*
    geographic distribution of, 345t
Loris, slow, herpesvirus-associated lymphoma in, 380
    parasite transmission by, 29
Lowland gorilla. See *Gorilla (Gorilla gorilla).*
Lowland tapir *(Tapirus terrestris)*, 562, 562t, 567. See also
        Tapirs.
Loxodonta africana (African elephant). See *Elephants.*
LRH-A (luteinizing hormone analog), in fish, 184t, 189
Lumisterol$_3$, 63
"Lumpy jaw," in duikers, 679
Lumpy skin disease, in Arabian oryx, 692t, 693
Lung, sonographic assessment of, 47t
Lung cancer, human, birds and, 153t, 155
Lung mite, simian, in mixed-species exhibits, 29
Lupron (leuprolide), for contraception, 317
Luteinizing hormone analog (LRH-A), in fish, 184t, 189
Luteinizing hormone–releasing hormone analogs, for
        contraception, 317
Lutra canadensis. See *North American river otter (Lutra
        canadensis).*
Lutra felina (marine otter), geographic distribution of, 436t
Lutra longicaudis (neotropical otter), anesthesia in, 440
    geographic distribution of, 436t
Lutra lutra (Eurasian otter), anesthesia in, 439
    geographic distribution of, 436t
Lutra maculicollis (spotted-necked otter), geographic
        distribution of, 436t
Lutra perspicillata (smooth-coated otter), geographic
        distribution of, 436t
Lutra provocax (southern river otter), geographic distribution
        of, 436t
Lutra sumatrana (hairy-nosed otter), geographic distribution
        of, 436t
Lycaon species (African hunting dogs), immobilizing drug
        dosages for, 434t
Lymphocystis, in fish, *165*
Lymphocyte blastogenesis, 61–62
    in tuberculosis diagnosis, 109
    in cervids, 652–653
Lymphocyte subsets, in cell-mediated immunity evaluation,
        62
Lymphocyte transformation assay, 61–62
    in tuberculosis diagnosis, 109

Lymphocyte transformation assay *(Continued)*
    in cervids, 652–653
Lymphocytic choriomeningitis virus, callitrichid hepatitis and,
        28, 370, *370,* 378
Lymphoid neoplasia, in koala, 329
Lymphoma, due to feline leukemia virus, 404
    herpesvirus-associated, in slow loris, 380
    malignant T cell, in primates, 380–381
Lymphosarcoma, in callitrichids, 375
Lyssavirus species, 348–349. See also *Rabies.*
    geographic distribution of, 137–138
    survival of, 137
    taxonomy of, 136–137, 137t

M

M99. See *Etorphine.*
Maalox (antacid), for leptospirosis in pinnipeds, 471
Macaca arctoides (stump-tail macaque), viral hepatitis in,
        378
Macaca fascicularis. See *Crab-eating monkey (Macaca
        fascicularis).*
Macaca fuscata (Japanese macaque), canine distemper virus
        in, 379, 408
Macaca mulatta. See *Rhesus macaque (Macaca mulatta).*
Macaca nigra (Celebes crested macaque), diabetes in, 398
Macaques. See also specific animals.
    diabetes in, 398
    parasite transmission by, 29
    simian herpesvirus carriage by, 28
Macaws, tumor imaging in, 85–87, *86, 87*
Macrolides. See also specific drugs.
    in elephants, 538
Madoqua species (dik-dik), iron overload in, 266
    tranquilizers in, 579t, 582
Maggots, in botulism transmission, 297–298
Magnesium, in fish diet, 174t
Magnesium phosphide, as rodenticide, 118t
Magnetic resonance imaging (MRI), 84–85
    case studies using, 87, *87*
Maki (bromadiolone), 117, 118t
Makifilaria inderi, in flying foxes, 348
Malachite green, in fish, 169t
    soaking chelonians in, 195
Malayan flying fox *(Pteropus vampyrus).* See also
        Megachiropterans.
    geographic distribution of, 345t
Malayan sun bear *(Helarctos malayanus)*, hepatic
        proliferative disease in, 426
Malayan tapir *(Tapirus indicus)*, 562, 562t. See also *Tapirs.*
    birth weight of, 565
Malignant catarrhal fever (MCF), in Arabian oryx, 692t, 693
    in duikers, 677
    in mixed-species exhibits, 27
Malignant hyperthermia, in suids, 641–642
Mallard duck *(Anas platyrhynchos)*, seasonal siderosis in, 264
Mammals, 316–696. See also specific types, e.g., *Carnivores;
        Equids; Marine mammals.*
    attaching telemetry equipment to, 8t
    contraception in, 316–319
    cryptosporidiosis in, 122t, 124–125
    iron levels in, 261
    iron overload in, 265–267
    minimally invasive surgery in, 38
    Mycobacterium avium in, 147
    periodontal disease in, 252
    quarantine for, 14, 15t–16t
    shipment of, 21, 22–23
    sonographic assessment in, for sex determination, 42, *44*

Mammals *(Continued)*
  of health, 47t
  uninvited, control of, 117–118
Manatees, 507–516
  anesthesia for, 510
  biologic data on, 507–508, *508*
  diagnostic cytology in, 464–465, *465, 469*
  diagnostic techniques in, 510–511, *511*
  dinoflagellate poisoning of, 476–477, 514
  diseases of, 513–516, 513t
    human-related, 513t, 515–516
    natural, 513–515, 513t
  handling of, 509–510
  morbillivirus infection in, 498, 515
  Mycobacterium chelonae in, 148
  Mycobacterium marinum in, 149
  nutrition for, 508t, 509, 513
  nutritional content of milk of, 507, 508t, 513
  oil's effects on, 476
  restraint of, 509–510
  sedation of, 510
  treatment in, 511–513
  water quality for, 508, 509
Mandibular abscesses, in okapi, 648
  in tapirs, 565
Mandibular osteomyelitis, in duikers, 679
Maned wolves *(Chrysocyon* species), immobilizing drug
    dosages for, 434t
Manganese, in fish diet, 174t
Mangrove snake *(Boiga dendrophila)*, antimicrobials in, 192t,
    193, 194
Mannitol, for septicemia, in koala, 327
Mantoux test, for personnel, 655
Marabou, African, sonographic sex determination in, *43*
Marianas flying fox *(Pteropus mariannus)*. See also
    Megachiropterans.
  conservation status of, 344
Marine Mammal Protection Act, shipping regulations of, 23
Marine mammals, 464–516. See also specific types.
  diagnostic cytology in, 464–469, *465–468*
  fungal infections in, 478–484, 479t–481t
    clinical features of, 482
    diagnosis of, 482–483
    pathogenesis of, 481–482
    transmission of, 481
    treatment of, 483–484, 483t
  iron overload in, 267
  leptospirosis in, 469–471, *470*
  morbillivirus infection in, 497–500. See also under *Morbil-
    livirus infection.*
  quarantine for, 15–16, 15t–16t
  shipment of, 19, 21, 23, 24
  toxicology in, 472–477
Marine otter *(Lutra felina)*, geographic distribution of, 436t
Marinil. See *Metomidate*.
Markhor *(Capra falconeri)*, immobilization of, 685
Marmosets, 369, *369*. See also *Callitrichids;* specific animals.
  herpesvirus infection in, 28
  iron overload in, 265
  wasting syndrome in, 371
    iron overload and, 265
Marmota monax (woodchuck), reproduction in, 362
Marsupials, 321–342. See also specific animals.
  anesthesia in, 333–336, 334t
    monitoring of, 333–334
    volatile agents for, 335–336
  intubation in, 336
  Mycobacterium avium in, 147
  toxoplasmosis in, 131, 132
Marsupostrongylus longilarvatus, in koala, 330t

Mastitis, in koala, 331
Mastoiditis, in gorilla, imaging of, 85, *85*
Matschie's tree kangaroo *(Dendrolagus matschiei)*. See *Tree
    kangaroos.*
Maxwell's duiker *(Cephalophus monticola maxwelli)*. See
    also *Duikers.*
  anesthesia in, 673t
  conservation status of, 669
  laboratory reference values for, 676t–677t
May-Grunwald/Wright-Giemsa stain, for fish blood specimen,
    179, 180t
MBD (methylene blue dye) test, for toxoplasmosis, 132
MCF (malignant catarrhal fever), in Arabian oryx, 692t, 693
  in duikers, 677
  in mixed-species exhibits, 27
Meadow mouse *(Microtus* species), control of, 116–117
Meal worm beetles, parasite transmission by, 29
Measles, in primates, 379
Mebendazole, in callitrichids, 373
  in cheetah, 421t
  in fish, 183t, 188
  in lemurs, 366
Mechanical chutes. See also *Handling systems.*
  for ungulates, 660, *660*
Meclofenamic acid, in birds, 312
Meconium aspiration, in apes, 385
MedARKS (Medical Animal Record Keeping System), 7
Medetomidine, in Arabian oryx, 689, 689t, 690
  in birds, 312
  in canids, 433–434
  in cheetah, 417, 418t
  in crocodilians, 212, 213t
  in duikers, 673t
  in fish, 161, 161t
  in marsupials, 334t, 335
  in mountain sheep and goats, 685
  in okapi, 649
  in otters, *438*, 438t, 440–441, 442
Medicago sativa (alfalfa), vitamin D in, 63
Medical Animal Record Keeping System (MedARKS), 7
Medical Lake macaque virus, in mixed-species exhibits, 28
Medroxyprogesterone acetate, for contraception, 317, 318
  in tapirs, 567
Megachiropterans, 344–353, 345t. See also *Fruit bats;*
    specific animals.
  anesthesia in, 345, *346*
  cardiovascular system of, 350
  common injuries in, 346–347, *347*
  conservation status of, 344
  diseases of, 347–350
  drug administration in, 347
  gastrointestinal system of, 350
  hematology in, 345–346, *346, 347*
  housing of, 344–345
  integumentary system of, 350–352
  musculoskeletal system of, 352
  nutritional disorders in, 349–350
  preventive medicine program for, 347
  quarantine for, 347
  renal system of, 352, *352*
  reproductive system of, 353, *353*
  respiratory system of, 350
  restraint of, 345
  special senses in, 353
  surgery in, 346–347, *347*
Megestrol acetate, for contraception, 317
Melanotic ependymoma, in callitrichids, 375
Melengestrol acetate (MGA) implants, 317, 318
  adverse effects of, 319
    in callitrichids, 374

Melengestrol acetate (MGA) implants *(Continued)*
  in tapirs, 567
  pregnancy and, 319
Melursus ursinus (sloth bear), hepatic proliferative disease in, 426, *426*
Meningeal worm. See *Parelaphostrongylus tenuis.*
Meningitis, bacterial, in ape neonates, 385
Meningoencephalitis, in Amazon parrot, imaging of, 87, *87*
  in small cetaceans, 488
Meperidine, in manatees, 510
  in otters, 441
  in stranded cetaceans, 489t
Mephitus mephitus (striped skunk), control of, 117–118
Mercury, in marine mammals, 475
Mesoplodon carlhubbsi, fungal infections in, 479t
Metabolic bone disease, in callitrichids, 374
  in chameleons, 204
  in megachiropterans, 349
Metabolic limiters, in food concentrates, 591–592
Metabolic scaling, in dose calculation, for elephants, 534
  for reptiles, 198
Metal poisoning. See also *Iron overload; Lead poisoning; Zinc intoxication.*
  in fish, 170
  in marine mammals, 475–476
Methocarbamol, in birds, 313
Methoxyflurane, in suids, 641
Methylanthranilate, 119
Methylene blue dye (MBD) test, for toxoplasmosis, 132
Methylprednisolone acetate, in birds, 312
Metoclopramide, for gastritis in cheetah, 459, 459t
Metomidate, in birds, 313
  in fish, 160–161, 161t
Metronidazole, in cheetah, 459t, 460
  in elephants, 539
  in fish, 169t, 183t, 187
  in lemurs, 366
  in reptiles, 195
  in stranded cetaceans, 489t
MGA implants. See *Melengestrol acetate (MGA) implants.*
Mibolerone, for contraception, 317
Mice, control of, 116–117, 118t
  disease introduction by, 28
  laboratory, vitamin and mineral requirements of, 358t
  neonatal, as carriers of lymphocytic choriomeningitis virus, 370, *370,* 378
Miconazole, in fish, 183t, 187
Microfilaremia, in chameleons, 203
Microsomal enzyme activity, in detoxification, 94
Microsporum canis infection, in cheetah, 418
Microsporum gypseum, birds and, 152t
Microtus species (meadow mouse), control of, 116–117
Midazolam, in birds, 313
  in canids, 430, 433
  in cheetah, 459
  in crocodilians, 214t, 215
  in manatees, 510
  in marsupials, 335
  in otters, *438,* 438t, 439–440, 441, 442, 446
  in suids, domestic, 640, 640t, 642, 642t
    nondomestic, 643, 644–645
Midland water snake (*Nerodia sipedon*), antimicrobials in, 192t, 194
Migratory Bird Treaty Act, 300
Milk, ape, 383
  cetacean, 494, 494t, 495
    replacements for, 494, 494t
  crop (in pigeon), composition of, 270–273, *271,* 272t, *273,* 273t, 274t
    digestion of, 274, 276

Milk *(Continued)*
    replacement for, 275–276
  duiker, 671
  manatee, 507, 508t, 513
  tapir, 565
  vitamin D in, 67
Milk powders, low-lactose, for koalas, 324
Mineral(s). See also specific minerals.
  deficiencies of, in fish, 172, 173, 174t
  in cultivated and native fruit, 356t
  in fruit bat diet, 357–359
  in pigeon crop milk, 273, 273t, 274t
  in pigeon crop milk replacer, 276
  in rhinoceros diet, 569–570, 570t
  requirements for, in domestic and laboratory species, 358t
Mineral oil, in manatees, 512
  in okapi, 648
Minimally invasive surgery (MIS), 30–39
  anatomic variations in, 35–38
  closed technique for, 33–34
  equipment for, 30–32, *31–33,* 32t
  history of, 30
  instrumentation and technique considerations for, 32–35, *34–36*
  open (Hasson's) technique for, 33
  procedures for, 38–39, *39*
Minocycline, in stranded cetaceans, 489t
Mirex, in marine mammals, 473
Mirounga angustirostris (northern elephant seal), fungal infections in, 480t
  iron overload in, 267
MIS. See *Minimally invasive surgery (MIS).*
Mites. See also *Parasites;* specific types.
  in mixed-species exhibits, 29
  on koala, 330t
  on ranched hoofstock, 589
Mitogens, for lymphocyte blastogenesis assays, 61
Mixed-species exhibits, health problems in, 26–29, 72, 75
  sea turtles in, 219
Modified agglutination test, for toxoplasmosis, 133
Mokola virus, 137t, 348
Mole rats, vitamin D metabolism in, 74
Moles, control of, 117
Molybdenum, in fish diet, 174t
Mona monkey (*Cercopithecus mona*), biliary cystadenoma in, 424
Moniligerum blain, in manatees, 514
Monitor lizard, Savannah, minimally invasive surgery in, *37*
Monkeys. See also specific types.
  tuberculin testing in, 393
Moose (*Alces alces*), brucellosis in, 623
  Elaphostrongylus infection in, 632
  Parelaphostrongylus tenuis in, 29, 633
    white-tailed deer and, 635
Morbillivirus infection. See also specific viruses.
  in horses, bats and, 349
  in manatees, 515
  in marine mammals, 497–500
    clinical signs of, 499
    control of, 500
    diagnosis of, 499–500
    epizootics of, 497–498
    organochlorine exposure and, 474
    pathogenesis of, 499
    serologic investigations of, 498
    species susceptibility to, 498
    transmission of, 498–499
Morelia amethistina (amethystine python), organ location in, 243, *246*
  case study of, 247–248

Morelia spilota (diamond python), organ location in, 243, *246*

Mortlock flying fox (*Pteropus phaeocephalus*). See also *Megachiropterans.*
    conservation status of, 344

Mouflon (*Ovis musimon*), embryo transfer in, 599, 600
    estrous cycle synchronization in, 598

Mountain goat. See *Rocky Mountain goat (Oreamnos americanus).*

Mountain laurel (*Leucothoe davisiae*), toxicity of, 89

Mountain lion. See *Puma (Felis concolor).*

Mountain reedbuck, tranquilizers in, 579t, 582

Mountain sheep, 681–687. See also specific animals.
    capture techniques for, 682–683, *683, 684*
        evaluation of, 685–686
        immobilization of, 684–685
        restraint of, 683–684

Mountain tapir (*Tapirus pinchaque*), 562, 562t. See also *Tapirs.*

Mouse. See *Mice.*

MRI (magnetic resonance imaging), 84–85
    case studies using, 87, *87*

MS-222 (tricaine methanesulfonate), in crocodilians, 212, 214t
    in fish, 160, 161t

Mucocutaneous ulcerative disease, in black rhinoceros, 59, 552–553, *553*

Mule deer (*Odocoileus hemionus*), control of, 118–119
    Elaeophora schneideri in, 588
    Elaphostrongylus cervi in, 636
    handling systems for, 658
    Parelaphostrongylus odocoilei, 632
    Parelaphostrongylus tenuis in, 634
    tuberculosis in, 651

Multimilk, in dolphin milk replacement formulas, 494, 494t

Muntjac (*Muntiacus* species), malignant catarrhal fever in, 27

Murayama virus, in primates, 379

Mus musculus (house mouse), control of, 116
    disease introduction by, 28
    lymphocytic choriomeningitis virus carriage by, 378

Musculoskeletal system, disorders of, in fish, 178t
    in okapi, 648
    in prosimians, 366–367, *367*
    in tree kangaroo, 342
    of megachiropterans, 352

Mustela eversmanni (Siberian polecat), artificial insemination in, 452, 452t, 454

Mustela nigripes (black-footed ferret), artificial insemination in, 452, 452t, 454, 461–462
    conservation program for, 460–462

Mustela putorius furo (European ferret), artificial insemination in, 452, 452t, 454
    tuberculosis in, 104
        lesions of, 106, 107t, 108
        prevalence of, 105t

Mycobacteria. See also specific organisms.
    fastidious, 148
    nontuberculous, 146–150
        survival of, 149
    rapidly growing, 148

Mycobacterial infection. See also *Johne's disease; Tuberculosis.*
    in callitrichids, 371
    in orangutan, 392
    in tree kangaroos, 339–341, *340, 341*
    nontuberculous, diagnosis of, 149
        public health concerns, 149–150
        transmission of, 149–150

Mycobacterium abscessus, 148

Mycobacterium asiaticum, 149

Mycobacterium avium complex, 147, 153t, 154

Mycobacterium bovis, 101, 651. See also *Tuberculosis.*
    survival of, 104–105

Mycobacterium chelonae, 148

Mycobacterium flavescens, 149

Mycobacterium fortuitum, 148

Mycobacterium genavense, 148, 153t, 154

Mycobacterium gordonae, 149

Mycobacterium haemophilum, 148

Mycobacterium intracellulare, 147

Mycobacterium kansasii, 147–148

Mycobacterium malmoense, 148

Mycobacterium marinum, 148–149

Mycobacterium microti, tuberculosis vaccine based on, 112

Mycobacterium paratuberculosis, 613. See also *Johne's disease.*

Mycobacterium scrofulaceum, 147

Mycobacterium simiae, 148

Mycobacterium smegmatis, 149

Mycobacterium szulgai, 149

Mycobacterium terrae, 149

Mycobacterium ulcerans, 149

Mycobacterium vaccae, tuberculosis vaccine based on, 112

Mycobacterium xenopi, 149

Mycoplasma infection, in elephants, arthritis and, 540
    in gorilla, 540

Mydriacyl (tropicamide), for pupillary dilatation, in megachiropterans, 353

Myelolipomas, hepatic, 426
    in callitrichids, 375

Mynahs, iron overload in, 263, 265
    protozoal infection in, 29

Myotis lucifugus (little brown bat), control of, 118

N

Naja naja (Asian cobra), biliary cystadenoma in, 424

Naked mole rat (*Heterocephalus glaber*), vitamin D metabolism in, 74

Nalbuphine, in elephants, 529

Nalidixic acid, in fish, 183t, 186

Nalmefene, in canids, 431
    in elephants, 526, 529

Nalorphine, in black rhinoceros, 557
    in white rhinoceros, 557, 559, 560

Naloxone, in canids, 431
    in manatees, 510
    in otters, 441
    in suids, 642, 642t
    in tapirs, 563
    in white rhinoceros, 557, 560

Naltrexone, in canids, 431
    in duikers, 674t
    in elephants, 529
    in hippopotamus, 638–639
    in marsupials, 335
    in okapi, 649
    in suids, 644, 645
    in tapirs, 563
    in white rhinoceros, 557, 559, 560

Nanday conure (*Nandayus nenday*), herpesvirus carriage by, 28

Nandinia binotata (palm civet), hepatic neoplasms in, 426

Narcan. See *Naloxone.*

Narcotics. See *Opioids;* specific drugs.

Nasitrema species, in cetaceans, 466, *466,* 468
    stranded, 488

Nasua species (coati), iron overload in, 267

Nat-Herrick method, for blood analysis, in sea turtle, 225

National Animal Poison Control Center, 389t, 390

National Center for Animal Health Information Systems (NCAHIS), 25

National Marine Fisheries Service, stranded cetaceans and, 485, 492

Natural resources damage assessment, in oil spill, 300–301

Naxcel (ceftiofur), for leptospirosis, 471
  in elephants, 538

NBT (nitroblue tetrazolium) dye reduction test, 60

NCAHIS (National Center for Animal Health Information Systems), 25

Nebraska calf diarrhea virus. See *Rotavirus infection.*

Nebulization, for respiratory disease, in koala, 326, *327*

Necrolytic dermatopathy, superficial, in black rhinoceros, 59, 552–553, *553*

Necropsy, 5, 6–7
  in cervid tuberculosis, 654
  of fish, 177–179, 178t
  of oiled birds, 301

Nectar formulas, in fruit bat diet, 359

Negative staining procedure, for cryptosporidiosis diagnosis, 129–130, *129*

Nematodes. See also *Parasites;* specific genera and species.
  in Arabian oryx, 695
  in California condor, 290
  in callitrichids, 372–373
    diabetes due to, 398
  in cheetah, 421t
  in chelonians, 240t
  in duikers, 676, 677
  in giant panda, 413
  in koala, 330t
  in lemurs, 366
  in manatees, 514–515
  in mixed-species exhibits, 29
  in ranched hoofstock, 588, 589

Nematodirus spathiger, in Arabian oryx, 695

Nemex-H. See *Pyrantel.*

Neofelis nebulosa (clouded leopard), adrenal tumor in, sonographic assessment of, *48*
  artificial insemination in, 455, 455t
  feline leukemia virus in, 402
  ovarian stimulation in, *451*

Neonatal calf diarrhea virus. See *Rotavirus infection.*

Neonatal hemolytic syndrome, in chimpanzees, 383

Neonates, ape, 382–387. See also under *Apes.*
  cetacean, 493–497. See also under *Cetaceans.*
  duiker, 671–672
    examination of, 680
  okapi, 647–648
    examination of, 649
  tapir, 565
    causes of death in, 566–567

Neoplasia, gastritis due to, in cheetah, 458
  hepatic. See under *Liver.*
  in callitrichids, 375
  in felids, 427
  in giant panda, 413
  in koala, 329
  in macaws, imaging of, 85–87, *86, 87*
  in marine mammal cytologic specimen, classification of, 465
  sonographic assessment of, 47, *47, 48*

Neostigmine, in crocodilians, 210, 214t, 215

Neotragus moschtus zeluensis (suni antelope), artificial insemination in, 599
  estrous cycle synchronization in, 598
  induced ovulation in, 600
  tranquilizers in, 579t, 582

Neotropical otter (*Lutra longicaudis*), anesthesia in, 440

Neotropical otter (*Lutra longicaudis*) *(Continued)*
  geographic distribution of, 436t

Nephrolithiasis, in stranded cetacean, 490

Nerium oleander (oleander), toxicity of, 89

Nerodia erythrogaster (red-bellied water snake), antimicrobials in, 192t, 194

Nerodia sipedon (midland water snake), antimicrobials in, 192t, 194

Nervous system diseases, in prosimians, 367

Nets, for mountain sheep and goat capture, 682–683, *683, 684,* 685–686

Neuroleptics. See *Tranquilizers;* specific drugs.

Neuromuscular blocking drugs, in canids, 430
  in crocodilians, 208–210, 213t

Newcastle's disease, 152t, 154

Niacin. See also *Vitamin B complex.*
  in fish diet, 173t

Niclosamide, in cheetah, 421t
  in fish, 183t, 188

Nicotiana glauca (tree tobacco), toxicity of, 88–89

Night monkey (*Aotus trivirgatus*), herpesvirus infection in, 28
  viral hepatitis in, 378
  vitamin D transport in, 64

Nightshade, hairy, toxicity of, 88
  in lemurs, 368

Nigropallidal encephalomalacia, 543–544

Nile crocodile (*Crocodylus niloticus*), immobilization of, 206

Nile hippopotamus (*Hippopotamus amphibius*), anesthesia in, 638–639

Nitrite, water contamination with, 169

Nitroblue tetrazolium (NBT) dye reduction test, 60

Nitrosamines, hepatic neoplasms and, 425, 426

Noah's Arkive, 5

Nociceptors, 309–310

Nodular collagen degeneration, in black rhinoceros, 554, *555*

Noise pollution, in fish environment, 171

Nonachlor, in marine mammals, 472

Nonsteroidal anti-inflammatory drugs (NSAIDs), in birds, 312–313

Norplant (levonorgestrel), for contraception, 317, 318

North American beaver (*Castor canadensis*), reproduction in, 362

North American bison. See *American bison (Bison bison).*

North American porcupine (*Erethizon dorsatum*), reproduction in, 362–363

North American river otter (*Lutra canadensis*), anatomy of, *437*
  anesthesia in, complications of, 439t
    in translocation project, 441–442, 446, 447t
    respiratory depression with, 437–438, *438,* 438t
  geographic distribution of, 436t
  translocation of, 443–448
    daily treatment in, 444–445
    environmental acclimation in, *447,* 448, *448*
    feeding in, 445–446, 446t
    health status assessment in, 446–447
    housing in, 444
    initial assessment in, 444, *444*
    medical problem management in, 447–448

Northern elephant seal (*Mirounga angustirostris*), fungal infections in, 480t
  iron overload in, 267

Northern fur seal (*Callorhinus ursinus*), fungal infections in, 479t
  leptospirosis in, 469, 470, 471

Norway rat (*Rattus norvegicus*), control of, 116–117

Notechis species (tiger snakes), organ location in, 245

Notoedres cati, on cheetah, 419, 419t
  on koala, 330t

NRAMP gene, brucellosis resistance and, 622

NSAIDs (nonsteroidal anti-inflammatory drugs), in birds, 312–313
Nubian goat (*Capra hircus*), biliary cysts in, 424
Nudacotyle undicola, in manatees, 514
Nutrient load, in water for waterfowl exhibits, 294–295, *294, 295*
Nutrition. See also *Diet; specific nutrients.*
  in mixed-species exhibits, 27
  of ape neonates, hand-reared, 384
  of bats, disorders of, 349–350
  of California condor, 279
  of California condor chicks, 286
  of calves with diarrheal disease, 610
  of cetacean neonates, hand-reared, 494–495, 494t
  of chameleons, 202
  of cheetah, in breeding facility, 421
  of columbid young, 269–276
    recommendations for, 274–276
  of duikers, 669–670
  of fish, 172–173, 173t, 174t
  of fruit bats, 354–359
    recommendations for, 359
  of giant panda, 411
  of koala, in illness, 322–324
  of manatees, 508t, 509, 512, 513
  of oiled birds, 306–307
  of otters, in translocation project, 445–446, 446t
  of primates, in diabetes management, 399
  of ranched hoofstock, 591–592
  of rhinoceroses, 568–571, 569t, 570t
  of sea turtles, 219–220, *220,* 221t
  of stranded cetaceans, 491
  of tapirs, 564–565
  of tree kangaroos, 338
Nyala (*Tragelaphus angassii*), handling systems for, 660
  tranquilizers in, 579t, 580
Nyctereutes species (raccoon dogs), immobilizing drug dosages for, 434t
Nycticebus coucang (slow loris), herpesvirus-associated lymphoma in, 380
  parasite transmission by, 29
Nystatin, in koala, 331
  in reptiles, 195

O

Oaks, scrub (*Quercus*), toxicity of, 89
Obesity, in deer, 27
  in megachiropterans, 350
Ocelot (*Felis pardalis*), artificial insemination in, 455, 455t
Ochotona rufescens (Afghan pika), iron overload in, 267
Ochotona species (pikas), reproduction in, 362
Odobenus rosmarus (walrus), antifungal drugs in, 483t
Odocoileus hemionus. See *Mule deer (Odocoileus hemionus).*
Odocoileus virginianus. See *White-tailed deer (Odocoileus virginianus).*
Ofloxacin, in stranded cetaceans, 489t
Ogilby's duiker (*Cephalophus ogilbyi*). See also *Duikers.*
  conservation status of, 669
Oil spills, birds affected by, 300–308
    environmental effects and, 301
    husbandry of, 306–308
    iron storage in, 264
    legalities of handling, 300
    physiologic effects and, 301–302, *301*
    treatment of, 302–306, 304t
  major, resources needed for, 301
  marine mammals affected by, 476
  natural resources damage assessment in, 300–301

Oil spills *(Continued)*
  otters affected by, 442, 476
Okapi (*Okapia johnstoni*), 646–649
Old tuberculosis (OT). See *Tuberculin testing.*
Oleander, toxicity of, 89
Olive baboon (*Papio anubis*), tuberculosis in, 105t
  vitamin D transport in, 64
Ollulanus tricuspis, in cheetah, 458
Omega-3 fatty acids, in fish diet, 172
Omeprazole, for gastritis in cheetah, 459t, 460
Onager (*Equus hemionus*), equine herpesvirus infection in, 27
  iron overload in, 266
Online information sources, 5–6
Ophidian paramyxovirus infection, in mixed-species exhibits, 28
Opiates. See *Opioids; specific drugs.*
Opioid antagonists. See also specific drugs.
  in canids, 431
Opioids. See also specific drugs.
  endogenous, 310
  in Arabian oryx, 689
  in birds, 311–312
  in canids, 430
  in crocodilians, 211, 213t
  in otters, 441
  in white rhinoceros, 559
Opossum (*Didelphis virginiana*). See also *Possums.*
  control of, 117–118
Oral cavity, of cetaceans, diagnostic cytology of, 466–467, *467*
Orangutan (*Pongo pygmaeus*). See also *Apes.*
  birth weight for, 383
  iron overload in, 265–266
  pregnancy in, management of, 384
  Strongyloides stercoralis infestation in, 385–386
  tuberculin testing in, 392–396
    evaluation of response to, 393–394, *394*
    future research on, 395–396
    management of responders to, 394–395
  viral hepatitis in, 378
Orchard grass (*Dactylis glomerata*), vitamin D in, 63
Orcinus orca (killer whale), diagnostic cytology in, *466, 467*
  fungal infections in, 479t, 480t, 483t
  taurine content of milk of, 494
Oreamnos americanus. See *Rocky Mountain goat (Oreamnos americanus).*
Oreotragus oreotragus (klipspringer), tranquilizers in, 579t, 582
Organochlorine compounds, in marine mammals, 472–475
Organophosphate poisoning, diagnosis of, 477
  in California condor, 288
  in callitrichids, 374
Oribi (*Ourebia ourebi*), tranquilizers in, 579t, 582
Ormetoprim, sulfadimethoxine with, in elephants, 537
  in fish, 183t, 186–187
Orthomyxovirus species, birds and, 152t
Oryx. See also *Artiodactylids; specific animals.*
  in mixed-species exhibits, 27
Oryx dammah (scimitar-horned oryx), artificial insemination in, 599
  embryo recovery from, 600, 600t
  estrous cycle synchronization in, 598
  handling systems for, 660
Oryx gazella dammah (scimitar oryx antelope), testicular calcifications in, sonographic assessment of, *51*
Oryx leucoryx (Arabian oryx). See *Arabian oryx (Oryx leucoryx).*
Osteodystrophy, fibrous, in primates, 70–71
Osteoglossum bicirrhosum (arowana), sonographic sex determination in, *43*

Osteomalacia, in primates, 70–71
Osteomyelitis, mandibular, in duikers, 679
   mycobacterial, in tree kangaroos, 340, *341*
   periodontal disease with, in lizards, 253, 253t, 255
      diagnosis of, 256, *256*
      treatment of, 257
Ostertagia ostertagi, in bison, 588
Ostrich (*Struthio camelus*), cryptosporidiosis in, 122t, 126
   in mixed-species exhibits, 27
   shipment of, 21
OT (old tuberculin). See *Tuberculin testing.*
Otocyon species (foxes), immobilizing drug dosages for, 434t
Otters, anatomy of, 436, *437*
   anesthesia in, 436–442
      agents for, 439–441
      drug delivery for, 437
      in translocation projects, 441–442
      monitoring during, 437–438, *438,* 438t
      recovery from, 438
   diagnostic cytology in, 464–465, 469
   fungal infections in, 480t
   geographic distribution of, 436t
   restraint of, 436–437
   sea. See *Sea otter (Enhydra lutris).*
   size of, 436t
   translocation of, 441–442, 443–448. See also *North American river otter (Lutra canadensis).*
Ourebia ourebi (oribi), tranquilizers in, 579t, 582
Ovaban (megestrol acetate), for contraception, 317
Ovariectomy, 316
   behavioral effects of, 319
Ovaries, pathologic alterations in, sonographic assessment of, *50, 51*
Ovariohysterectomy, 316
Ovine follicle-stimulating hormone (FSH), in assisted reproduction in artiodactylids, 599–600
Ovis canadensis. See *Bighorn sheep (Ovis canadensis).*
Ovis dalli (Dall's sheep). See also *Mountain sheep.*
   capture and handling of, 681–687
   embryo transfer in, 599, 600
   estrous cycle synchronization in, 598
   immobilization of, 684
Ovis musimon (mouflon), embryo transfer in, 599, 600
   estrous cycle synchronization in, 598
Ovis orientalis (Armenian red sheep), embryo transfer in, 599, 600
   estrous cycle synchronization in, 598
Owl(s), control of, 120
Owl monkey (*Aotus trivirgatus*), herpesvirus infection in, 28
   viral hepatitis in, 378
   vitamin D transport in, 64
Oxalate crystals, renal, in koala, 328–329
Oxfendazole, in ruminants, 587t
Oximetry. See *Pulse oximetry.*
Oxolinic acid, in fish, 183t, 186
Oxychlordane, in marine mammals, 472
Oxygen therapy, in hippopotamus, 639
   in suids, 644
   in white rhinoceros, 559–560
Oxygenation, of water for waterfowl exhibits, 294
Oxymorphone, in crocodilians, 211
   in otters, 441
Oxytetracycline, for leptospirosis, 471
   in elephants, 536
   in fish, 169t, 183t, 186
   in koala, 326
   in manatees, 511
Oxytocin, for dystocia in elephant, 525
Oxyuranus scutellatus (taipan), organ location in, 245
Ozone, to improve water quality, for fish, 175

Ozone *(Continued)*
   for sea turtles, 219

P

Paca (*Cuniculus paca*), reproduction in, 363
   vitamin D toxicity in, in mixed-species exhibits, 27, 72, 75
Pacarana (*Dinomys branicki*), reproduction in, 363
Pacheco's disease virus, in mixed-species exhibits, 28
Pacific harbor seal. See *Harbor seal (Phoca vitulina).*
Pagophilus groenlandicus, fungal infections in, 481t
Pain. See also *Analgesia.*
   in birds, recognition of, 310–311
      treatment of, 313
   perception of, 309–310
Painted turtle (*Chrysemys picta*), antimicrobials in, 191t, 192
Palau flying fox, large. See also *Megachiropterans.*
   conservation status of, 344
Pallas cat (*Felis manul*), feline immunodeficiency virus in, 405, 406, 407
Palm civet (*Nandinia binotata*), hepatic neoplasms in, 426
Pan paniscus (bonobo), birth weight of, 383
   herpesvirus infection in, 386
   papillomavirus in, 380
   simian T lymphotrophic virus in, 381
Pan troglodytes. See *Chimpanzees.*
Pancreas, amyloidosis of, in primate diabetes, 398
   sonographic assessment of, 47t
Pandas, giant, artificial insemination in, 413, 452
   laboratory values for, 412t
   management of, in China, 410–411
   medical care of, 411–413, 411t, 412t
   reproduction in, 413–414
   red, iron overload in, 267
Panleukopenia, in cheetah, gastritis due to, 458
   vaccination for, 418
Panther chameleon (*Furcifer pardalis*), 201
Panthera leo. See *Lion (Panthera leo).*
Panthera onca (jaguar), feline immunodeficiency virus in, 405
Panthera pardus saxicolor (Persian leopard), artificial insemination in, 452
Panthera tigris (tiger). See *Tiger (Panthera tigris).*
Panthera uncia (snow leopard), artificial insemination in, 455t
   feline immunodeficiency virus in, 405
   iron overload in, 267
Pantothenic acid. See also *Vitamin B complex.*
   in fish diet, 173t
Pap, koala, 330–331
Papillomaviruses, in primates, 380
Papio anubis (olive baboon), tuberculosis in, 105t
   vitamin D transport in, 64
Papio hamadryas (chacma baboon), biliary cystadenoma in, 424
   malignant T cell lymphoma in, 380–381
   tuberculosis in, 105t
Parainfluenza 3 virus, in Arabian oryx, 693
Paralytic agents, in canids, 430
   in crocodilians, 208–210, 213t
Paralytic shellfish poisoning, 477
Paramyxovirus infection, bat, 349
   birds and, 152t, 154
   in mixed-species exhibits, 28
   in primates, 379
Parasites. See also specific types.
   acquired from birds, 153t, 155
   cholangiocarcinoma and, 425
   control programs for, design of, 593–597

Parasites *(Continued)*
    evaluation of, 596
    examples of, 596–597
    management considerations in, 594–595
    types of, 594
  determining clinically important species of, 595
  diabetes induced by, in primates, 398
  drug resistance in, 589, 594, 596
  hepatic cysts due to, 423
  hepatic neoplasms and, 426
  in ape neonates, 385–386
  in Arabian oryx, 692t, 695
  in California condor, 290
  in callitrichids, 372–373, *372, 373*
  in chameleons, 203
  in cheetah, 419–420, 419t, *420,* 420t, 421t
    gastritis due to, 458, 459
  in chelonians, 234, 240t
  in duikers, 676–677
    routine testing for, 680
  in elephants, 527
  in fish, carried by invertebrates or plants, 165
  in free-ranging artiodactylids, 631–636
  in giant panda, 413
  in koala, 330t
  in lemurs, 366, 368
  in manatees, 514–515
  in megachiropterans, 348
  in mixed-species exhibits, 28–29
  in okapi, 648, 649
  in ranched hoofstock, control of, 587–589, 587t
    fecal examination for, 588
  in ruminants, control of, program design for, 593–597
    examples of, 596–597
    species difference, in susceptibility to, 594–595
  in stranded cetaceans, 488
  in tree kangaroos, 341
Parasympatholytic drugs. See also *specific drugs.*
  in crocodilians, 214t, 215
Parathormone, in calcium regulation, 65
Paratuberculosis. See *Johne's disease.*
Parelaphostrongylus andersoni, 632
Parelaphostrongylus odocoilei, 632
Parelaphostrongylus tenuis, ecologic role of, 634–635
  geographic range of, 634
  in farmed game, 588, 589
  in free-ranging artiodactylids, 632–635
  in mixed-species exhibits, 29
Paromomycin, in lemurs, 366
Parrot, African gray, biliary cysts in, 424
  Amazon, meningoencephalitis in, imaging of, 87, *87*
Parson's chameleon, 201
Parturition. See also *Dystocia; Reproduction.*
  in apes, 384–385
  in elephants, 521–522
  in giant panda, 413
  in megachiropterans, 353
  in okapi, 647
Parvovirus, simian, 381
Passer domesticus (house sparrow), control of, 119
Passerines. See also *Birds; specific types.*
  Plasmodium infection in, 29
  trichomoniasis in, 29
Passive antibody transfer, calf diarrhea and, 610–611
  failure of, 59
    tests for, 60–61
  in cetaceans, 496
  in duikers, 671
Pasteurellosis, birds and, 152t
  in Arabian oryx, 692t, 695

Pasteurellosis *(Continued)*
    parainfluenza 3 virus and, 693
  in callitrichids, 371
  in ranched hoofstock, 590
  water quality and, 299
Pasture rotation, for parasite control, 594
  in game ranching, 588
Patagonian cavy (*Dolichotis patagonum*), reproduction in, 363
Patagonian conure (*Cyamoliseus patagonus*), herpesvirus carriage by, 28
Patas monkey (*Erythrocebus patas*), simian varicella infection in, 28
  vitamin D transport in, 64
Pathology program, educational resources for, 5–6
  value of, 3–7
PBBs (polybrominated biphenyls), in marine mammals, 473
PBV (pteropid bat virus), 137t, 138
PCBs (polychlorinated biphenyls), in marine mammals, 473
  toxic equivalency factor and, 474–475
PCDDs (polychlorinated dibenzodioxins), in marine mammals, 473
PCDFs (polychlorinated dibenzofurans), in marine mammals, 473
PCNs (polychlorinated naphthalenes), in marine mammals, 473
PCQs (polychloroquaterphenyls), in marine mammals, 473
PDV. See *Phocine distemper virus (PDV).*
Peccaries, 640. See also *Suids; specific animals.*
  canine distemper virus in, 408
Pedetes capensis (springhaa), reproduction in, 362
Pelicans, vitamin E toxicity in, in mixed-species exhibits, 27
Pemba Island flying fox (*Pteropus voeltzkowi*). See also *Megachiropterans.*
  geographic distribution of, 345t
Penguins, *Plasmodium* infection in, 29
  shipment of, 22
  sonographic assessment in, for sex determination, *43*
    of sexual maturation, *45*
Penicillins. See also *specific drugs.*
  for leptospirosis, 471
  in chelonians, 191
  in elephants, 535–536
  in manatees, 511
  in snakes, 192t, 193
    in combination dosing, 194
Pepto-Bismol (bismuth subsalicylate), for gastritis in cheetah, 459t, 460
  for oiled birds, 303
  for stranded cetacean, 489t
Pere David's deer (*Elaphurus davidianus*), induced ovulation in, 599
  malignant catarrhal fever in, 27
  parasites in, 29
Periarticular hyperostosis, in lemurs, 366–367, *367*
Periodontal disease, in lizards, 252–257, 253t
    bacteria in, 254–255, 255t
    causes of, 255–256
    clinical findings in, 252–253
    diagnosis of, 256, *256*
    histopathology of, 253–254, *254, 255*
    treatment of, 256–257
  in mammals, 252
Perissodactylids, 551–574. See also *specific types.*
  iron overload in, 266
Peromyscus species (deer mouse), control of, 116–117
Perphenazine, in Arabian oryx, 690
  in duikers, 675
  in elephants, 530, 579t, 583
  in marsupials, 335t

Perphenazine *(Continued)*
  in wild herbivores, 578
    species guidelines for, 579–584, 579t, *580*
Persian leopard *(Panthera pardus saxicolor)*, artificial
  insemination in, 452
Peste des petits ruminants, in Arabian oryx, 692, 692t
Phacochoerus aethiopicus (warthog), 639
  anesthesia in, 644, 645
  tuberculosis in, 101
Phagocytosis, tests of, 60, 60t
Phalacrocorax species (cormorants), water retention in
  feathers of, 306
Phantom egg behavior, in California condor, 285
Pharmacokinetics, renal-portal system's effect on, in red-
  eared slider, 249–251, *249–251*
Phascolarctos cinereus. See *Koala (Phascolarctos cinereus).*
Pheasant, golden, parasites in, 29
Phelsuma madagascariensis (day gecko), vitamin D
  metabolism in, 73
Phencyclidine, 430
  in canids, 431
  in suids, 642
Phenobarbital, in lemurs, 367
Phenothiazines, in canids, 430
Phenylephrine, for pupillary dilatation, in megachiropterans,
  353
Philodendron species, toxicity of, 89
Phlebotomy. See also *Blood collection.*
  for iron overload, 262–263
Phoca groenlandica (harp seal), fungal infections in, 481t
  phocine distemper virus in, 498
Phoca hispida (ringed seal), phocine distemper virus in, 498
Phoca sibirica (Baikal seal), canine distemper virus in, 408,
  497
Phoca vitulina. See *Harbor seal (Phoca vitulina).*
Phocine distemper virus (PDV). See also *Morbillivirus
  infection.*
  discovery of, 497
  organochlorine exposure and, 474
  pathogenesis of infection with, 499
  serologic investigations of, 498
  species susceptibility to, 498
Phocoena phocoena (harbor porpoise). See *Harbor porpoise
  (Phocoena phocoena).*
Phocoenoides dalli, fungal infections in, 480t
Phosphorus, in fish diet, 174t
  in rhinoceros diet, 570, 570t
  plasma concentration of, in duikers, 675, 676, 676t, 678t
Physaloptera, in cheetah, 458
  in lemurs, 366
Physiologic fuel value, 357
Phytobezoars, in okapi, 648
Phytoplankton control, in waterfowl exhibits, 296–297
Pied tamarin *(Saguinus b. bicolor).* See also *Callitrichids.*
  parasite-induced diabetes in, 398
Pigeon lung disease, 153t, 155
Pigeons. See *Birds; Columbids.*
Pigs. See *Suids;* specific animals.
Pikas, Afghan, iron overload in, 267
  reproduction in, 362
Pilot whales *(Globicephala* species). See also *Cetaceans.*
  antifungal drugs in, 483t
  morbillivirus infection in, 498
"Pink foam" syndrome, in anesthetized elephants, 529
Pinnipeds. See also *Marine mammals;* specific animals.
  diagnostic cytology in, 464–465, 469
  leptospirosis in, 469–471, *470*
  quarantine for, 16t
Pipa, shipment of, 21
Piperacillin, in lizards, 257

Piperacillin *(Continued)*
  in reptiles, renal-portal system's effect on kinetics of, 250
  in snakes, 192t, 193
    in combination dosing, 194
Pipothiazine palmitate, in marsupials, 335t
Pit vipers. See also *Snakes.*
  effects of venom of, 97
  organ location in, 245, *247*
Pithecia pithecia (white-faced saki), gestational diabetes in,
  398
Pituophis melanoleucus (gopher snake), antimicrobials in,
  192t, 194
Placenta previa, in apes, 384–385
Placental abruption, in apes, 385
Plague, black-footed ferrets and, 461, 462
Plains bison. See *American bison (Bison bison).*
Plant(s), for aquaria, quarantine of, 165
  for zoo landscaping, selection of, 90t–94t
Plant lectins, for lymphocyte blastogenesis assays, 61
Plant poisoning, 88–94, 389–390
  animals' methods for coping with, 89–94
  avoiding, 89
  circumstances associated with, 88–89
  flaccid trunk paralysis in elephants and, 543–544
  sources of information on, 89
Plasma transfusion, for calf diarrhea, 610, 611
Plasmodium species, in lemurs, 368
  in mixed-species exhibits, 29
Pleural effusions, in lemurs, 366
Pleurodont teeth, 252
PMV (porpoise morbillivirus). See also *Morbillivirus
  infection.*
  discovery of, 498
  serologic investigations of, 498
Pneumonia, aspiration, in ape neonates, 385
  in oiled birds, 302
  in ape neonates, 385–386
  in aquatic turtles, 234
  in koala, 326–327, *327*
  in lemurs, 366
  in marine mammal morbillivirus infection, 499
  in stranded cetaceans, 489
  in tapirs, 565, 567
  in tree kangaroos, *340*
Pneumonitis, allergic interstitial, due to bird contact, 153t,
  155
Pneumonyssus simicola (simian lung mite), in mixed-species
  exhibits, 29
Pneumothorax, in manatees, 515–516
Poisoning, aflatoxin, hepatic neoplasms and, 425, 426
  in lemurs, 368
  carbamate, diagnosis of, 477
  fluoride, in fruit bats, 357–359
    in megachiropterans, 349
  in manatees, 514
  in marine mammals, 472–477
  metal. See also *Iron overload; Lead poisoning; Zinc intoxi-
    cation.*
    in fish, 170
    in marine mammals, 475–476
  organophosphate, diagnosis of, 477
    in California condor, 288
    in callitrichids, 374
  plant. See *Plant poisoning.*
Polar bear *(Thalarctos maritimus)*, diagnostic cytology in,
  464–465, 469
  hepatic proliferative disease in, 426
  organochlorine metabolism in, 475
  shipment of, 22
Pole syringe, for drug injection, in canids, 431–432

Polecat, Siberian, artificial insemination in, 452, 452t, 454
Pollution, air, marine mammals and, 477
  noise, in fish environment, 171
  water. See *Oil spills; Water quality.*
Polybrominated biphenyls (PBBs), in marine mammals, 473
Polychlorinated biphenyls (PCBs), in marine mammals, 473
  toxic equivalency factor and, 474–475
Polychlorinated dibenzodioxins (PCDDs), in marine
  mammals, 473
Polychlorinated dibenzofurans (PCDFs), in marine mammals,
  473
Polychlorinated naphthalenes (PCNs), in marine mammals,
  473
Polychloroquaterphenyls (PCQs), in marine mammals, 473
Polymerase chain reaction (PCR) assays, for *Toxoplasma
  gondii* detection, 133
  limitations of, 57
Ponape flying fox (*Pteropus molossinus*). See also
  Megachiropterans.
  conservation status of, 344
Pongo pygmaeus. See *Orangutan (Pongo pygmaeus).*
Ponies. See also *Equids.*
  iron overload in, 266
Pontoporia blainvillei, fungal infection in, 479t
Porcine zona pellucida (PZP) vaccine, 317, 318
  adverse effects of, 319, 630–631
  in artiodactylids, 628–631, 629t, 630t
  pregnancy and, 319
Porcupines, reproduction in, 362–363
Porpoise morbillivirus (PMV). See also *Morbillivirus
  infection.*
  discovery of, 498
  serologic investigations of, 498
Possums, control of, 117–118
  tuberculosis in, 102, 103, 104
    clinical signs of, 105–106
    lesions of, 107t, 108
    prevalence of, 104, 105t
Potamochoerus porcus (red river hog), anesthesia in, 644,
  645
Potassium, in fish diet, 174t
Potassium dichromate solution, for *Cryptosporidium* oocyst
  storage, 128
Potassium permanganate, soaking chelonians in, 195
Povidone-iodine, for propeller wounds in manatees, 515
  in sea turtles, 230t
Poxvirus infection, in Arabian oryx, 692t, 693
  in black rhinoceros, 554
  in elephants, 547–549, *547–549*
  in okapi, 648
PPD (purified protein derivative). See *Tuberculin testing.*
Prairie dogs (*Cynomys* species), reproduction in, 362
Praziquantel, in cheetah, 421t
  in fish, 169t, 183t, 188
  in manatees, 514
  in stranded cetaceans, 489t
Predictive value, 56, 57t
Prednisolone, in koala, 327
  in marine mammals, 483
  in stranded cetaceans, 489t
Pregnancy, contraception during, 319
  in cheetah, 421
  in dolphins, 501–506, *503–506*
  in elephants, 521
  in megachiropterans, 353, *353*
  in primates, diabetes during, 398
  in tapirs, 567
  sonographic detection and monitoring of, 47–52, *48, 49,
    52, 53*
    in dolphins, 501–506, *503–506*

Pregnancy *(Continued)*
  toxoplasmosis risk in, 134
Pressure immobilization technique, for elapid snakebite, 99,
  99
Previtamin D$_3$, 63
PREX online information service, 6
Prey, vitamin E content of, 80–81, 81t
Primates, 365–400. See also specific types.
  behavioral enrichment requirements for, 387. See also *Envi-
    ronmental enrichment.*
  diabetes in, 397–400
    diagnosis of, 398–399
    etiopathogenesis of, 397–398, *397*
    gestational, 398
    parasite-induced, 398
    treatment of, 399–400
  emerging viral diseases of, 377–381
  herpesviruses affecting, in mixed-species exhibits, 28
  importation of, 24
  in mixed-species exhibits, limiting trauma by, 27
    parasites in, 29
  iron overload in, 265–266
  Mycobacterium avium in, 147
  progestin-based contraception in, 318
  quarantine for, 15t
  shipment of, 21, 23
  toxoplasmosis in, 131, 132
  vitamin and mineral requirements of, 358t
  vitamin D deficiency in, 70–72, *71*
  vitamin D toxicity in, 72, 74–75
Primor. See *Sulfadimethoxine/ormetoprim.*
Prion diseases, 662–667. See also *Scrapie-like spongiform
  encephalopathies.*
Priscoline. See *Tolazoline.*
Procavia species (rock hyrax), iron overload in, 267
Procyon lotor (raccoon), control of, 117–118
  parasite transmission by, 29
  rabies in, 139
Progesterone, in pregnancy detection in elephants, 521
Progestins, for contraception, 317, 318
  adverse effects of, 318–319
  behavioral effects of, 319
  pregnancy and, 319
  for estrous cycle synchronization, 598
Projection neurons, in pain perception, 310
Prolactin, in calcium regulation, 65
Promazine, in canids, 430
  in suids, 642
Propeller wounds, in manatees, 515
Propofol, in crocodilians, 212, 214t
  in marsupials, 335
  in suids, 641
Prosimians. See also *Primates;* specific types.
  classification of, 365
  diabetes in, 398
  diseases of, 365–368
    cardiovascular, 367–368
    gastrointestinal, 365–366
    integumentary, 367
    musculoskeletal, 366–367, *367*
    nervous system, 367
    respiratory, 366
    systemic, 368
    urogenital, 367
Prostaglandin F$_{2\alpha}$, for abortion, 319
  for estrous cycle synchronization, 598
Prosthenorchis elegans, in callitrichids, 373
Protein, fruit bat requirements for, 356–357
  serum, in screening for failure of passive antibody transfer,
    61

Protein *(Continued)*
supplemental, for ranched hoofstock, 591
Protein electrophoresis, as test of humoral immunity, 61
Provitamin D₂ (ergosterol), 63, *64*
Provitamin D₃ (7-dehydrocholesterol), 63, *64*
Prunus species, toxicity of, 89
Pseudechis porphyriacus (red-bellied black snake), organ location in, 245
Pseudoephedrine hydrochloride, in koala, 326
Pseudomonas species, birds and, 152t
Pseudonaja texlilis (eastern brown snake), organ location in, 245
Pseudopregnancy, in cheetah, 422
in giant panda, 413
Pseudorca crassidens (false killer whale), fungal infections in, 479t, 481t
Pseudotuberculosis, birds and, 152t, 154
in callitrichids, 371
uninvited species and, 28
Psittacines. See also *Birds; specific types.*
trichomoniasis in, 29
Psittacosis, 151–153, 152t
Arabian oryx and, 692t, 693
in mixed-species exhibits, 28
Psittacus erithacus erithacus (Congo African gray parrot), biliary cysts in, 424
Psoroptes cuniculi, on ranched hoofstock, 589
Pteronura brasiliensis (giant otter), anesthesia in, 440, 441
geographic distribution of, 436t
Pteropid bat virus (PBV), 137t, 138
Pteropus giganteus (Indian flying fox). See also *Megachiropterans.*
geographic distribution of, 345t
reproduction in, 353
Pteropus hypomelanus (island flying fox). See also *Megachiropterans.*
cardiomyopathy in, *351*
geographic distribution of, 345t
intubation of, *346*
reproduction in, 353
Pteropus insularis (Truk flying fox). See also *Megachiropterans.*
conservation status of, 344
Pteropus mariannus (Marianas flying fox). See also *Megachiropterans.*
conservation status of, 344
Pteropus molossinus (Ponape flying fox). See also *Megachiropterans.*
conservation status of, 344
Pteropus phaeocephalus (Mortlock flying fox). See also *Megachiropterans.*
conservation status of, 344
Pteropus pilosus (large Palau flying fox). See also *Megachiropterans.*
conservation status of, 344
Pteropus poliocephalus (gray-headed flying fox). See also *Megachiropterans.*
geographic distribution of, 345t
Pteropus pumilus (golden-mantled flying fox). See also *Megachiropterans.*
cranial edema in, *352*
Elizabethan collar use in, 346, *347*
geographic distribution of, 345t
venipuncture of, *346, 347*
Pteropus rodricensis (Rodrigues Island flying fox). See also *Megachiropterans.*
geographic distribution of, 345t
Pteropus samoensis (Samoan flying fox). See also *Megachiropterans.*
conservation status of, 344

Pteropus tonganus (insular flying fox). See also *Megachiropterans.*
conservation status of, 344
Pteropus vampyrus (Malayan flying fox). See also *Megachiropterans.*
geographic distribution of, 345t
Pteropus voeltzkowi (Pemba Island flying fox). See also *Megachiropterans.*
geographic distribution of, 345t
Pterygodermatites nycticebi, in callitrichids, 372
diabetes due to, 398
in mixed-species exhibits, 29
Ptychodiscus brevis, marine mammal deaths due to, 476–477
Puerto Rican plain pigeon (*Columba inornata*), growth of, 273–274, *274*
Pulse oximetry, 2–3
in California condor, 282, *282*
in elephants, 528
in fish, 162
in marsupials, 334
in otters, 438
in suids, 641, 643
in tree kangaroos, 338–339
in white rhinoceros, 559
Puma (*Felis concolor*), adrenal gland of, sonographic assessment of, *48*
artificial insemination in, 452, 455t
control of, 118
feline immunodeficiency virus in, 405
feline leukemia virus in, 402, 404
in vitro fertilization in, 450t
Pump priming effect, in detoxification, 94
Purified protein derivative (PPD). See *Tuberculin testing.*
Pustular dermatitis, superficial, in black rhinoceros, 553–554, *554*
Pygathrix nemaeus (Douc langur), parasites in, 29
Pygmy chimpanzee (*Pan paniscus*), birth weight for, 383
herpesvirus infection in, 386
papillomavirus in, 380
simian T lymphotrophic virus in, 381
Pygmy hippopotamus (*Choeropsis liberiensis*), leiomyoma in, sonographic assessment of, *50*
Pygmy marmoset (*Callithrix pygmaea*). See also *Callitrichids.*
callitrichid hepatitis in, 378
Pygmy sperm whale (*Kogia breviceps*), caloric requirements of calves of, 495
fungal infections in, 479t, 480t
ink in colon of, 467
Pygoscelis papua (gentoo), sonographic assessment of sexual maturation in, *45*
Pyrantel, in cheetah, 421t
in fish, 183t, 188
in lemurs, 366
Pyridoxine. See also *Vitamin B complex.*
in fish diet, 173t
Pyrimethamine, sulfonamides with, for toxoplasmosis, 133
Pythons, antimicrobials in, 192t, 193, 194
organ location in, 243, *246*
case study of, 247–248
PZP (porcine zona pellucida) vaccine, 317, 318
adverse effects of, 319, 630–631
in artiodactylids, 628–631, 629t, 630t
pregnancy and, 319

Q

Q fever, in Arabian oryx, 690, 692t, 693
Quails, cryptosporidiosis in, 122t, 126

Quarantine, 13–17, 26
  after rabies exposure, 143–144
  for aquarium plants, 165
  for birds, 14, 16t, 151
  for California condor, 280
  for cervid tuberculosis, 654
  for cheetah, 418
  for equids, 573–574
  for fish, 164–165, *166–167,* 169t
    health assessment in, 165, *168,* 179
  for hoofstock, 587
  for imported animals, 23, 24
  for megachiropterans, 347
  for sea turtles, 228
  for tree kangaroos, 342
  for wild-caught mammals, 143
  in parasite control, 595
  testing during, 14–16, 15t–16t
Quaternary ammonium compounds, for disinfection, 176t
Quercus species, toxicity of, 89
Quinaldine sulfate, in fish, 160, 161t
Quinthiophos, in cheetah, 420t
Quintox (vitamin D_3 rodenticide), 117, 118t

R

Rabbits, *Bordetella bronchiseptica* carriage by, 28
  calcium regulation in, 74
  reproduction in, 362
Rabies, 136–145
  causative agent of, 136–138, 137t
  diagnosis of, 139
  epizootiology of, 139–140
  geographic distribution of, 136t
  in Arabian oryx, 692, 692t
  in bats, 140, 348–349
    control of, 145
  in birds, 153t, 154–155
  in humans, bats and, 140
    prevention of, 143, 143t–145t
  pathogenesis of, 138–139
  post-exposure management of, in humans, 143, 145t
    in zoo animals, 143–144
  public health concerns, 143–145, 143t–145t
  small mammal pest control and, 118
  species-specificity of, 141
  vaccination for, during incubation period, 138–139, 142
    in duikers, 680
    in humans, 143, 143t–145t
    in zoo animals, 140–143
Rabies virus neutralizing antibodies, 138, 142
Raccoon (*Procyon lotor*), control of, 117–118
  parasite transmission by, 29
  rabies in, 139
Raccoon dogs (*Nyctereutes* species), immobilizing drug dosages for, 434t
Radial immunodiffusion, immunoglobulin quantitation using, 61
Radiography, in California condor, 282–283, *283, 284*
  in elephants, of foot and carpus, 517–520, *518–520*
  in sea turtles, 226
  in stranded cetaceans, 490
  in tapirs, 563
Radionuclides, in marine mammals, 477
Radiotelemetry, equipment for, suppliers of, 9t–11t
  techniques for attaching, 8t
  in wildlife monitoring, 7–13
Radiotransmitters. See also *Radiotelemetry.*
  on California condors, 284

Ragwort, tansy, toxicity of, 89
Ramphastos vitellinus (channel-billed toucan), iron chelation in, 262
Rana temporaria (frog), vitamin D metabolism in, 74
Rangifer tarandus (caribou, reindeer), *Brucella suis* infection in, 626–627, *627*
  Elaphostrongylus infection in, 632
  iron overload in, 266
  Parelaphostrongylus odocoilei in, 632
  Parelaphostrongylus tenuis in, 633
Ranitidine, in stranded cetaceans, 489t
Raphicerus campestris (steenbok), *578*
  tranquilizers in, 579t, 582
Raptors, control of, 120
  rabies and, 154–155
Rat(s), control of, 116–117, 118t
  disease introduction by, 28
  laboratory, vitamin and mineral requirements of, 358t
Rat snakes, antimicrobials in, 192t, 193, 194
Ratites, shipment of, 21
Rattlebox (*Crotalaria* species), toxicity of, 89
Rattlesnakes. See also *Snakes.*
  antimicrobials in, 192t, 194
Rattus norvegicus (Norway rat), control of, 116–117
Rattus rattus (black rat, roof rat), control of, 116–117
Records, chain of evidence, in oil spill response, 300
  for fish, 163–164
  for stranded cetaceans, 491–492
Rectal prolapse, in tapirs, 565
Rectocolon, of cetaceans, diagnostic cytology of, 467
Recycled materials, in enrichment programs, disease transmission and, 389
Red deer. See *Cervus elaphus (red deer, elk, wapiti).*
Red duiker (*Cephalophus natalensis*). See also *Duikers.*
  anesthesia in, 673t
Red fox (*Vulpes vulpes*), rabies in, 139
Red hartebeest, tranquilizers in, 579t, 581
Red howler monkey, Bolivian, rickets in, 71, *71*
Red lechwe, tranquilizers in, 579t
Red panda (*Ailurus fulgens*), iron overload in, 267
Red river hog (*Potamochoerus porcus*), anesthesia in, 644, 645
Red sheep, Armenian, embryo transfer in, 599, 600
  estrous cycle synchronization in, 598
Red tide. See *Dinoflagellate toxins.*
Red-bellied black snake (*Pseudechis porphyriacus*), organ location in, 245
Red-bellied water snake (*Nerodia erythrogaster*), antimicrobials in, 192t, 194
Red-eared slider (*Chrysemys scripta elegans*), antimicrobials in, 191t, 192
  renal-portal system of, 249–251, *249–251*
Red-footed tortoise, South American, herpesvirus carriage by, 28
Reedbuck, tranquilizers in, 579t, 582
Reference values. See under *Laboratory tests.*
Reindeer (*Rangifer tarandus*). See *Rangifer tarandus (caribou, reindeer).*
Reintroduction, of Arabian oryx, 687–696
  steps in, 696
  of black-footed ferret, 462
Reithrodontomys species (harvest mouse), control of, 116–117
ReJexit (methylanthranilate), 119
Release into the wild. See also *Reintroduction.*
  of Arabian oryx, 690
  of chelonians, 232–241
    decision tree for, 235–240, *236, 237*
    philosophical issues in, 240–241
  of stranded cetaceans, 492
Relocation. See *Translocation.*

Renal disease. See under *Kidneys.*
Renal failure, gastritis due to, in cheetah, 458
Renal lithiasis, in stranded cetaceans, 490
Renal-portal system, of reptiles, 249–251, *249–251*
Reo-like virus. See *Rotavirus infection.*
Repellents, in vermin control, 116, 119
Reproduction, assisted, benefits of, 449–450, 449t
  in artiodactylids, 597–602
    using artificial insemination, 598–599
    using embryo transfer, 599–601, 600t, 601t
    using in vitro fertilization, 601–602
    in black-footed ferret, 452, 452t, 454, 461–462
  in carnivores, 449–456
    using artificial insemination, 451–456. See also *Artificial insemination.*
    using in vitro fertilization, 450–451, *450,* 450t, *451*
    in duikers, 671
    in fish, 184t, 189
    sonographic support of, 52–54, *53*
  control of. See *Contraception.*
  failure of, in marine mammals, organochlorines and, 474
    in pinnipeds, leptospirosis and, 470
  in apes, problems in, 384–385
  in Arabian oryx, 690
  in California condor, 284–285, 284t, *285*
  in callitrichids, problems in, 374
  in chameleons, 202–203
  in duikers, 670–671
  in elephants, normal, 521–522
    problems in, 522–525, *522,* 523t, *524*
  in giant panda, 410, 413–414
  in lagomorphs, 361–362
  in manatees, problems in, 514
  in okapis, 647
  in rodents, 361, 362–364
  in tapirs, 567, 567t
  in tree kangaroos, 338
  minimally invasive surgery applications in, 39, *39*
  ultrasonography applications in, 42–54
Reproductive system, *Brucella abortus* infection of, 621
  Brucella suis infection of, 627, *627*
  chlamydial disease of, in koala, 325
  disorders of, in callitrichids, 374
    sonographic diagnosis of, *50,* 51, *51*
  of megachiropterans, 353, *353*
Reptiles, 190–257. See also specific types.
  antimicrobials in, 190–198
    administration of, 197–198
    combination dosing with, 194–195
    doses for, 191–195, 191t, 192t
    environmental considerations in, 196–197
    metabolic scaling and, 198
    selection of, 195–196
  attaching telemetry equipment to, 8t
  cryptosporidiosis in, 122t, 126
  iron overload in, 264
  minimally invasive surgery in, 36–37, *37*
  quarantine for, 14, 16t
  renal-portal system of, drug kinetics and, 249–251, *249–251*
  shipment of, 20–21, 22
  sonographic assessment in, for sex determination, 42, *43*
    of health, 47t
  vitamin D deficiency in, 72–74
Reserpine, in fish, 184t, 189
Respirators, for working with tuberculosis-infected cervids, 655
Respiratory depression, in anesthetized otters, 437–438, *438,* 438t
  in immobilized canids, 433

Respiratory depression *(Continued)*
  in immobilized crocodilians, 205–206, 208, 214
Respiratory disease, in elephants, 540
  in koala, 326–327, *327*
  in prosimians, 366
  in stranded cetaceans, 489–490
  in tapirs, 565, 567
  in tree kangaroos, 341–342
Respiratory syncytial virus infection, in ape neonates, 385
Respiratory system, of cetaceans, diagnostic cytology of, 466
  of megachiropterans, 350
Restraint. See also *Crates; Handling systems.*
  chemical. See *Anesthesia; Immobilization.*
  for mountain sheep and goats, 683–684, *684*
  of Arabian oryx, 688–689
  of California condor, 280, *280, 281*
  of chameleons, 204
  of cheetah, 416, *416, 417*
  of crocodilians, 207
  of duikers, 672
  of manatees, 509–510
  of megachiropterans, 345
  of otters, 436–437
  of sea turtles, 221
  of suids, 642
  of tree kangaroos, 338
  of ungulates, systems for, 657–661, *658–661,* 658t
  of venomous snakes, 96
Reticulated giraffe (*Giraffa camelopardis reticulata*), artificial insemination in, 599
  estrous cycle synchronization in, 598
  induced ovulation in, 599
Reticulated python (*Python reticulatus*), antimicrobials in, 192t, 193, 194
Retroviruses, feline, 401–407
  simian, type D, 381
Rhebok, gray, tranquilizers in, 579t, 582
Rhesus macaque (*Macaca mulatta*), diabetes in, 398
  Ebola Reston antibodies in, 379
  mixed viral infection in, 381
  papillomavirus in, 380
  viral hepatitis in, 378
  vitamin D toxicity in, 74–75
  vitamin D transport in, 64
Rheumatoid arthritis, in elephants, 540
Rhinitis/pneumonia complex, in koala, 326–327, *327*
Rhinoceros unicornis (Asian rhinoceros, greater one-horned rhinoceros). See under *Rhinoceroses.*
Rhinoceroses, Asian (greater one-horned), feeding behavior of, 568
  leiomyoma in, sonographic assessment of, *50*
  nutrition in, 570t
  black, anesthesia in, 557
    feeding behavior of, 568
    handling systems for, 660
    in mixed-species exhibits, 27
    iron overload in, 266, 570
    nutrition in, 569, 570t
    primary immunodeficiency in, 59
    skin of, diseases of, 551–555, *553–555*
      normal histology of, 551–552, *552*
      response of, to injury, 552
    tranquilizers in, 579t, 583
  importation of, 23
  iron overload in, 266
  nutrition in, 568–571, 569t, 570t
  Sumatran, feeding behavior of, 568
    iron overload in, 266
    nutrition in, 569, 570t
    vitamin E supplementation in, 80

Rhinoceroses *(Continued)*
  white, anesthesia for, 556–561
    drug delivery systems for, 556
    drugs for, 556–557, 556t, 557t
    equipment for, 557
    for cow and calf, 560–561
    in confinement, 561
    planning for, 556–557
    procedure for, 558–560
  feeding behavior of, 568
  in mixed-species exhibits, 27
  loading of, into crate, 560, 561
  nutrition in, 570t
  requirements for physiologic manipulations of, 557–558
  tranquilizers in, 559, 579t, 583
Rhinotracheitis, infectious, vaccination for, in cheetah, 418
Rhipicephalus sanguineus, on cheetah, 419, 419t
Rhododendron species, toxicity of, 89
Riboflavin. See also *Vitamin B complex.*
  in fish diet, 173t
Rickets, in primates, 71–72, *71, 383*
Ridall (zinc phosphide), 117, 118t
Rifabutin, for mycobacteriosis in tree kangaroos, 340
Rifampicin, in Arabian oryx, 694
Rifampin, in stranded cetaceans, 489t
Rinderpest, in Arabian oryx, 691, 692t
Ringed seal *(Phoca hispida),* phocine distemper virus in, 498
Ring-tailed lemur *(Lemur catta),* cholangioma in, 424
  diabetes in, 398
  toxoplasmosis susceptibility of, 131
Ringworm, in cheetah, 418
  in giant panda, 413
  in koala, 328
River otter, North American. See *North American river otter (Lutra canadensis).*
  southern, geographic distribution of, 436t
Roan antelope, tranquilizers in, 579t, 581
Rocaltrol (vitamin D supplement), 70
Rock beauties *(Holacanthus tricolor),* nutritional needs of, 172
Rock cavy *(Kerodon rupestris),* reproduction in, 363
Rock hyrax *(Procavia* species), iron overload in, 267
Rock python, Indian, antimicrobials in, 192t, 194
Rocket nets, for mountain sheep and goat capture, 682
Rocky Mountain bighorn sheep. See *Bighorn sheep (Ovis canadensis).*
Rocky Mountain goat *(Oreamnos americanus),* 681–687
  capture techniques for, 682–683, *683*
  immobilization of, 684–685
  Johne's disease in, 616–617
  Parelaphostrongylus infection in, 632
  physical restraint of, 683–684, *684*
Rodenticides, 117, 118t
Rodents, control of, 116–117, 118t
  iron overload in, 267
  reproduction in, 361, 362–364
Rodrigues Island flying fox *(Pteropus rodricensis).* See also *Megachiropterans.*
  geographic distribution of, 345t
Roe deer *(Capreolus capreolus),* artificial insemination in, sonographically supported, 53
  polycystic liver disease in, 424
  sonographic pregnancy detection in, *48*
Romet 30. See *Sulfadimethoxine/ormetoprim.*
Rompun. See *Xylazine.*
Roof rat *(Rattus rattus),* control of, 116–117
Rotavirus infection, agent causing, 605–606
  in okapi, 648
    prevention of, 649
  in ruminants, 605–611

Rotavirus infection *(Continued)*
  clinical signs of, 608
  diagnosis of, 609–610
  epizootiology of, 607–608
  pathology of, 608–609
  prevention of, 610–611
  treatment of, 610
Rousettus aegyptiacus (Egyptian fruit bat). See also *Fruit bats; Megachiropterans.*
  energy requirement for, 357
  geographic distribution of, 345t
  protein requirement for, 357
Rousettus lanosus (Ruwenzori long-haired fruit bat). See also *Fruit bats; Megachiropterans.*
  geographic distribution of, 345t
Rousettus leschenaulti. See also *Megachiropterans.*
  reproduction in, 353
Rovimix D$_3$, 69
Ruffed lemur *(Varecia variegata),* bone disease in, 367
  cholangioma in, 424
  herpesvirus encephalitis in, 380
Ruminants. See also *Herbivores; Hoofstock;* specific types.
  anthelmintics in, 587t, 595–596
  coronavirus infection in, 605–611
  rotavirus infection in, 605–611
  trichostrongyloid parasites in, designing control program for, 593–597
Rusa deer *(Cervus timorensis),* handling systems for, 660
Ruwenzori long-haired fruit bat *(Rousettus lanosus).* See also *Fruit bats; Megachiropterans.*
  geographic distribution of, 345t
RX821002 (α_2-antagonist), in okapi, 649

S

Sable antelope *(Hippotragus niger),* copper deficiency in, in mixed-species exhibits, 27
  tranquilizers in, 579t, 581
Saddleback tapir *(Tapirus indicus),* 562, 562t. See also *Tapirs.*
  birth weight of, 565
Saffan (alfaxolone/alfadolone acetate), in cheetah, 416–417
  in marsupials, 335
Saguinus b. bicolor (pied tamarin). See also *Callitrichids.*
  parasite-induced diabetes in, 398
Saguinus mystax (black-chested mustached tamarin). See also *Callitrichids.*
  vitamin D metabolism in, 71
Saguinus nigricollis (white-lipped tamarin). See also *Callitrichids.*
  vitamin D metabolism in, 71
Saguinus oedipus (cotton-top tamarin). See also *Callitrichids.*
  colonic adenocarcinoma in, 375
  vitamin D metabolism in, 71, 72
Saiga antelope *(Saiga tatarica),* self-induced trauma in, 27
Saimiri sciureus. See *Squirrel monkey (Saimiri sciureus).*
Saki, white-faced, gestational diabetes in, 398
Saksenaea vasiformis infection, in marine mammals, 480t
Salamander, Chinese giant, sonographic sex determination in, *43*
Salmonellosis, 152t, 153
  in Arabian oryx, 692t
  in California condor chicks, 286–287, *287*
  in cheetah, 419
  in elephants, 536, 539–540
  introduced by uninvited species, 28
Salt, for ranched hoofstock, 591
Saltwater crocodile *(Crocodylus porosus),* immobilization of, 206

Samoan flying fox (*Pteropus samoensis*). See also
    Megachiropterans.
  conservation status of, 344
San Estaban Island chuckwalla, vertebral subluxation in,
    imaging of, 85, *85, 86*
Sand impaction, in tapirs, 565
Sanitation, in fish care, 175–177, 176t
  in vermin control, 115
Sarafloxacin, in fish, 183t, 186
Sarcoptes scabiei, on koala, 330t
Savannah monitor lizard (*Varanus exanthematicus*),
    minimally invasive surgery in, *37*
Sawdust, as rodenticide, 118t
Saxitoxins, marine mammal deaths due to, 477
Scatterhoarding, by agoutis, 363
Sceloporus occidentalis (lizard), vitamin D metabolism in, 73
Scimitar oryx antelope (*Oryx gazella dammah*), testicular
    calcifications in, sonographic assessment of, *51*
Scimitar-horned oryx (*Oryx dammah*), artificial insemination
    in, 599
  embryo recovery from, 600, 600t
  estrous cycle synchronization in, 598
  handling systems for, 660
Sciurus species. See *Squirrel(s).*
Scoliosis, in small cetaceans, 491
Scopolamine, for pupillary dilatation, in megachiropterans,
    353
ScourGuard, 611
  in okapi, 649
Scrapie-like spongiform encephalopathies, 662–667
  clinical signs of, 664–665
  diagnosis of, 665
  epizootiology of, 663–664
  in Arabian oryx, 692t, 695–696
  incubation period for, 664, *665,* 665t
  pathology of, 665–666
  prevention of, 666–667, *666*
  risks to human health from, 667
  species affected by, 662–663, *663, 664, 664*
Scrub oaks (*Quercus*), toxicity of, 89
Sea lions, fungal infections in, 479t, 480t
  leptospirosis in, 469–470, *470,* 471
  Mycobacterium smegmatis in, 149
Sea otter (*Enhydra lutris*), anesthesia in, 439, 440, 441, 442
  fungal infections in, 480t
  geographic distribution of, 436t
  oil's effects on, 442, 476
  shipment of, 21, 22
Sea snake, effects of venom of, 97
Sea turtles, 217–230. See also *Chelonians.*
  anesthesia for, 221–223, *222,* 222t
  blood collection and analysis in, 224–225, 224t, *225, 226*
  capture of, 221
  characteristics of, 217t
  clinical procedures in, 224–228, *225–228*
  conservation status of, 218
  diagnostic imaging of, 226, *226, 227*
  environmental considerations for, 218–219, *218*
  in mixed-species exhibits, 219
  nutrition in, 219–220, *220,* 221t
  physical examination of, 223–224, *223*
  physical restraint of, 221
  quarantine for, 228
  soaks and dips for, 195
  therapeutic considerations for, 229–230, *229,* 230t
  threats to population of, 217–218
Sea World Formula, for dolphin milk replacement, 494, 494t
Seals. See also *Marine mammals; Pinnipeds;* specific
    animals.
  canine distemper virus in, 408, 497

Seals *(Continued)*
  iron overload in, 267
Sedatives. See also *Tranquilizers;* specific drugs.
  for shipping, 20
  in manatees, 510
Seizures, in giant panda, 413
  in immobilized canids, 433
  in lemurs, 367
Selenarctos thibetanus (Asiatic black bear), hepatic
    proliferative disease in, 426
Selenium, in fish diet, 174t
  in rhinoceros diet, 570, 570t
  mercury toxicity and, in marine mammals, 475
  vitamin E interaction with, 82
Senecio jacobaea (tansy ragwort), toxicity of, 89
Senecio vulgaris (groundsel), toxicity of, 89
Sensitivity, 55–56, *56*
Sensitization of nociceptors, 310
Sentinel animals, in aquaria, 181
  in game ranching, 591
Sepsis, neonatal, in apes, 385
Septic arthritis, in ape neonates, 386
Septicemia, in callitrichids, 371
  in koala, 327
Serologic testing, 57–58. See also specific types.
  for brucellosis, 622
  for Johne's disease, 614, 619
  for rabies, 141
  for toxoplasmosis, 132–133
  for tuberculosis, 109–110
Serosal proliferations, in koala, 329
Serum electrophoresis, as test of humoral immunity, 61
Serum neutralization assay, for feline leukemia virus
    antibody, 403
Sesquiterpene lactones, in plants, 543–544
Sewer rat (*Rattus norvegicus*), control of, 116–117
Sex determination, in California condor, 287
  sonographic, 42–44, *43, 44*
    in fetus, 48, *49*
Sexual maturation, sonographic assessment of, 44, *45, 46*
Sharks, goiter in, 173
  shipment of, 22
Sheather's sugar flotation, for *Cryptosporidium* oocyst
    concentration, 128
Shellfish poisoning, paralytic, 477
Ship rat (*Rattus rattus*), control of, 116–117
Shipment, 17–26
  animals' needs during, 18–20
  containers for, 17–18, *19*
  documentation for, 24
  logistics of, 24–25
  of antelope, protocol for health screening before, 587
  of Arabian oryx, 690
  of California condor, 279
  of duikers, 669
  of elephants, crates for, 527–528, 527t
    loading animals for, 529–530, 531
  preshipment testing and medical history for, 25–26
  regulatory requirements for, 22–24
  species requirements for, 20–22
Short-finned pilot whale (*Globicephala macrorhynchus*),
    antifungal drugs in, 483t
Short-tailed fruit bat (*Carollia perspicillata*), energy
    requirement of, 357
  protein requirement of, 356–357
Shrew, house, iron overload in, 267
Siamang gibbon (*Hylobates syndactylus*), iron overload in,
    265
Siberian ibex, immobilization of, 685
Siberian polecat (*Mustela eversmanni*), artificial insemination
    in, 452, 452t, 454

Siberian tiger. See *Tiger (Panthera tigris)*.
Siderosis, 260, 261. See also *Iron overload*.
Sika deer (*Cervus nippon*), artificial insemination in, 598
  tuberculosis in, 651, 654
Silver-haired bat (*Lasionycteris noctivagans*), rabies in, 140
Simian bone disease, 70–71
Simian hemorrhagic fever, in mixed-species exhibits, 28
Simian immunodeficiency virus, 381
  in mixed-species exhibits, 28
Simian lung mite (*Pneumonyssus simicola*), in mixed-species
  exhibits, 29
Simian parvovirus, 381
Simian retrovirus type D, 381
Simian T cell lymphotrophic virus, 381
Simian varicella viruses, in mixed-species exhibits, 28
Simian virus 5, in primates, 379
Sirenians. See also *Manatees*.
  classification of, 507
  oil's effects on, 476
  quarantine for, 16t
Skin, of black rhinoceros, normal histology of, 551–552, *552*
  response of, to injury, 552
  of cetaceans, diagnostic cytology of, 467
  protection of, after stranding, 488
  of megachiropterans, 350–352
Skin diseases. See also *specific disorders*.
  in Arabian oryx, 692t, 693
  in black rhinoceros, 551–555, *553–555*
  in fish, 178t
  in megachiropterans, 352
  in okapi, 648–649
  in prosimians, 367
  in tapirs, 565, *566*
Skunks, control of, 117–118
  parasite transmission by, 29
  rabies in, 139
Slate-gray snake (*Stegonotus cucullatus*), organ location in,
  245
Sling, for stranded cetaceans, 490
Sloth, two-toed, sonographic sex determination in, *44*
Sloth bear (*Melursus ursinus*), hepatic proliferative disease
  in, 426, *426*
Slow loris (*Nycticebus coucang*), herpesvirus-associated
  lymphoma in, 380
  parasite transmission by, 29
Small-clawed otter, Asian, anesthesia in, 439, 440, 441
  geographic distribution of, 436t
Small-eared dogs (*Atelocynus* species), immobilizing drug
  dosages for, 434t
Smooth-coated otter (*Lutra perspicillata*), geographic
  distribution of, 436t
Snakebite, 95–100
  prevention of, 95–96, *96*, 96t
  response to, 97–100, *98–100*, 99t
Snakes. See also *Reptiles; specific types*.
  antimicrobials in, 192t, 193–194
  minimally invasive surgery in, 36–37
  organ location in, 243–248, *244, 246, 247*
    clinical application of data on, 245–248
  paramyxovirus infection in, 28
  shipment of, 20–21
Snow leopard (*Panthera uncia*), artificial insemination in,
  455t
  feline immunodeficiency virus in, 405
  iron overload in, 267
Social environment. See also *Environmental enrichment*.
  for fish, 171
Sodium, in fish diet, 174t
  in rhinoceros diet, 570, 570t
Sodium hydroxide/Teepol, for disinfection, 176t

Sodium hypochlorite, for disinfection, 176t
Sodium pentobarbital, sea turtle morbidity and mortality with,
  221
Sodium thiopental, in cheetah, 417
  in giant panda, 411t
Soft-shell turtle, Florida, chemical dip for, 195
Solacryl SUVT, 66
Solanum glaucophyllum, vitamin D in, 63
Solanum malacoxylon, vitamin D in, 63
Solanum sarrachoides (hairy nightshade), toxicity of, 88
  in lemurs, 368
Solar irradiation, as vitamin D source, 63, 65–66, 75
Sotalia guianensis, fungal infections in, 481t
South Africa, cheetah breeding facility in, 415–422
South American red-footed tortoise (*Geochelone carbonaria*),
  herpesvirus carriage by, 28
South American tapir (*Tapirus terrestris*), 562, 562t, 567. See
  also *Tapirs*.
Southern river otter (*Lutra provocax*), geographic distribution
  of, 436t
Spanish ibex (*Capra pyrenaica*), embryo transfer in, 601
  estrous cycle synchronization in, 598
  induced ovulation in, 599
Sparrows, house, control of, 119
Specificity, 55–56, *56*
Spectacle, in squamates, antimicrobial administration and,
  198
Speke's gazelle (*Gazella spekei*), artificial insemination in,
  599
Speothos species (bush dogs), immobilizing drug dosages for,
  434t
Sperm whales. See also *Cetaceans*.
  dwarf, ink in colon of, 467
    subcutaneous emphysema in, 490
  pygmy, caloric requirements of calves of, 495
    fungal infections in, 479t, 480t
    ink in colon of, 467
Spheniscus demersus (black-footed penguin), sonographic sex
  determination in, *43*
Spiculopteragia asymmetrica, in white-tailed deer, 588
Spider monkeys (*Ateles* species), herpesvirus carriage by, 28
Spilogale putorius (spotted skunk), control of, 117–118
Spirocerca lupi, in cheetah, 458
  in lemurs, 368
Spirochidiasis, in sea turtles, 228
Spleen, of fish, diseases affecting, 178t
  sonographic assessment of, 47t
Spongiform encephalopathies, transmissible, 662–667. See
  also *Scrapie-like spongiform encephalopathies*.
Spotted dolphin (*Stenella* species), caloric requirements of
  calves of, 495
Spotted hyena (*Crocuta crocuta*), sonographic sex
  determination in, *44*
Spotted skunk (*Spilogale putorius*), control of, 117–118
Spotted-necked otter (*Lutra maculicollis*), geographic
  distribution of, 436t
Spraddle legs, in California condor chicks, 286
Springbok (*Antidorcas marsupialis*), biliary cysts in, 424
  tranquilizers in, 579t, 581–582, *582, 583*
Springhaa (*Pedetes capensis*), reproduction in, 362
Spurred tortoise, African, vitamin D metabolism in, 73–74
Spur-thigh tortoise (*Testudo graeca*), penicillins in, 191, 191t
Squamates. See *Lizards; Snakes; specific animals*.
Squirrel(s), control of, 117
  disease introduction by, 28
Squirrel monkey (*Saimiri sciureus*), biliary cysts in, 423
  herpesvirus carriage by, 28
  toxoplasmosis susceptibility of, 131
  vitamin D metabolism in, 70, 71
  vitamin D toxicity in, 74

Staplers, for minimally invasive surgery, 34, *36*
Star tortoise, Indian, antimicrobials in, 191t, 193
Starlicide (3-chloro-4-methylbenzenamine), 119
Starling (*Sturnus vulgaris*), control of, 119
    seasonal siderosis in, 264
Starvation, iron storage and, 264
Steenbok (*Raphicerus campestris*), *578*
    tranquilizers in, 579t, 582
Stegonotus cucullatus (slate-gray snake), organ location in, 245
Steller sea lion (*Eumetopias jubatus*), leptospirosis in, 470
Stenella coeruleoalba (striped dolphin), fungal infections in, 479t
    morbillivirus infection in, 498
    organochlorines in, 474
Stenella species (spotted dolphins), caloric requirements of calves, 495
Stephanofilariasis, in black rhinoceros, 555
Sterilization (contraceptive method), 316–317, 318
Sterilization of equipment, 175–177
Steroids. See also specific drugs.
    for contraception, 317, 318
        hepatic neoplasms and, 425, 427
    in birds, 312
    in fish, 184t, 188–189
Stomach. See also *Gastrointestinal tract.*
    of cetaceans, diagnostic cytology of, 467–468, *468*
Stomoxys calcitrans, on cheetah, 419t
Stool specimens. See *Fecal* entries.
Stranded cetaceans, 485–492. See also under *Cetaceans.*
Straw-colored fruit bat (*Eidolon helvum*). See also *Fruit bats; Megachiropterans.*
    geographic distribution of, 345t
    reproduction in, 353
Streptococcus zooepidemicus infection, in callitrichids, 371
    in mixed-species exhibits, 28
Stress, capture, in bighorn sheep, 686
    in fish, 164–165, *165*
    in rehabilitation of oiled birds, 306
    in small cetaceans, 486
    in translocation, 576–577
Stressnil. See *Azaperone.*
Striped dolphin (*Stenella coeruleoalba*), fungal infections in, 479t
    morbillivirus infection in, 498
    organochlorines in, 474
Striped skunk (*Mephitus mephitus*), control of, 117–118
Strongylids, in chameleons, 203
Strongyloides, in lemurs, 366
    in orangutan, 385–386
Strongylus, in lemurs, 366
Struthio camelus (ostrich), cryptosporidiosis in, 122t, 126
    in mixed-species exhibits, 27
    shipment of, 21
Stump-tail macaque (*Macaca arctoides*), viral hepatitis in, 378
Sturnus vulgaris (starling), control of, 119
    seasonal siderosis in, 264
Subcutaneous emphysema, in manatees, 516
    in stranded cetaceans, 490
Sublimaze. See *Fentanyl.*
Succinylcholine chloride, in crocodilians, 210, 213t
Sucralfate, in cheetah, 459t, 460
    in stranded cetaceans, 488, 489t
Suction, for snakebite, 99, *100*
Sufentanil, in canids, 430
Suggested Protocol for Pre-shipment Health Screening of Antelope Species, 587
Suids. See also specific animals.

Suids *(Continued)*
    anesthesia in, 639–645
        monitoring of, 641, 643
    classification of, 639–640
    domestic, anesthesia in, 640–642, 640t
        vitamin and mineral requirements of, 358t
    feral, tuberculosis in, 101–102
        lesions of, 107t
        prevalence of, 105t
    imported, quarantine for, 23
Sulfadiazine, pyrimethamine with, for toxoplasmosis, 133
    trimethoprim with, for toxoplasmosis, 134
        in reptiles, 195
        in stranded cetaceans, 489t
Sulfadimethoxine/ormetoprim, in elephants, 537
    in fish, 183t, 186–187
Sulfamethoxazole, trimethoprim with, in ape neonates, 386
    in duikers, 679
    in elephants, 536–537
Sulfur, as rodenticide, 118t
    in fish diet, 174t
Sumatran rhinoceros (*Dicerorhinus sumatrensis*). See under *Rhinoceroses.*
Sumatran tiger. See *Tiger (Panthera tigris).*
Sun bear, Malayan, hepatic proliferative disease in, 426
Suncus murinus (house shrew), iron overload in, 267
Suni antelope (*Neotragus moschtus zeluensis*), artificial insemination in, 599
    estrous cycle synchronization in, 598
    induced ovulation in, 600
    tranquilizers in, 579t, 582
Superficial necrolytic dermatopathy, in black rhinoceros, 59, 552–553, *553*
Superficial pustular dermatitis, in black rhinoceros, 553–554, *554*
Surgery, in California condor, 283–284
    in chameleons, 204
    in megachiropterans, 346–347
    minimally invasive. See *Minimally invasive surgery (MIS).*
Sus barbatus (bearded pig), anesthesia in, 644, 645
Sus scrofa, anesthesia in, 644, 645
    feral, tuberculosis in, 101–102
        lesions of, 107t
        prevalence of, 105t
    miniature, anesthesia in, 642, 642t, 644, 645
        embryo transfer in, 601
Sutherland's pressure immobilization technique, for elapid snakebite, 99, *99*
Swim bladder, of fish, diseases affecting, 178t
Swine. See *Suids.*
Sylvicapra grimmia (gray duiker), 668. See also *Duikers.*
    anesthesia in, 673t
    tranquilizers in, 579t, 582
Syncerus caffer. See *African buffalo (Syncerus caffer).*

T

Tachysterol$_3$, 63
Tadarida brasiliensis (freetail bat), rabies in, 140
Taipan (*Oxyuranus scutellatus*), organ location in, 245
Talon (brodifacoum), in vermin control, 117, 118t
    poisoning by, in callitrichids, 374
Tamarins, 369, *369.* See also *Callitrichids; specific animals.*
    herpesvirus infection in, 28
    parasites in, 29
    vitamin D metabolism in, 64, 71, 72
Tammar wallaby, toxoplasmosis vaccines tested in, 134
Tannin, in lemur diet, iron metabolism and, 366
Tansy ragwort (*Senecio jacobaea*), toxicity of, 89

Tapirs, 562–567
anatomy of, 562
anesthesia for, 562–563
causes of mortality in, 566–567
classification of, 562, 562t
clinical disorders in, 565–566, *566, 567*
clinical procedures in, 563
conservation status of, 562
geographic distribution of, 562t
importation of, 23
iron overload in, 266
laboratory reference values for, 563–564, 564t
neonates of, 565
causes of death in, 566–567
nutrition in, 564–565
reproduction in, 567, 567t
Tapirus bairdi (Baird's tapir), 562, 562t. See also *Tapirs.*
neonatal isoerythrolysis in, 565
Tapirus indicus (Malayan tapir), 562, 562t. See also *Tapirs.*
birth weight of, 565
Tapirus pinchaque (mountain tapir), 562, 562t. See also
Tapirs.
Tapirus terrestris (South American tapir), 562, 562t, 567. See
also *Tapirs.*
Taurine, in dolphin milk replacement formulas, 494, 494t
Taxus species (yew), toxicity of, 89
Tayassu pecari (white-lipped peccary), anesthesia in, 643–644
Tayassu tajacu (collared peccary), anesthesia in, 643–644
canine distemper virus in, 408
Tayassuidae (peccaries), 640. See also *Suids;* specific
animals.
canine distemper virus in, 408
TCDD (2,3,7,8-tetrachlorodibenzo-*p*-dioxin), in marine
mammals, 473
toxic equivalency factor and, 474–475
Teepol (lauryl alcohol), sodium hydroxide with, for
disinfection, 176t
Teeth, of duikers, 671, 675
of elephants, diseases of, 545–546, *545*
of koala, 322, *322–323*
of lizards, 252, *253*
histologic examination of, 253–254, *254*
of megachiropterans, 350
of okapi, 648
of tree kangaroos, disease of, 341
TEF (toxic equivalency factor), 474–475
Tegu (*Tupinambis teguixin*), antimicrobials in, 192t, 193
Telazol. See *Tiletamine/zolazepam.*
Telemetry, equipment for, suppliers of, 9t–11t
techniques for attaching, 8t
in wildlife monitoring, 7–13
Telescopes, for minimally invasive surgery, 31, 32, *32*
Telmin. See *Mebendazole.*
Temporal gland disorders, in elephants, 539
Terrapene carolina (box turtle), antimicrobials in, 191t, 193
Testes, pathologic alterations in, sonographic assessment of,
51, *51*
Tests. See *Laboratory tests;* specific tests.
Testudo graeca (Greek tortoise), penicillins in, 191, 191t
Testudo hermanni (Hermann's tortoise), antimicrobials in,
191, 191t, 193
Tetanus prophylaxis, in ranched hoofstock, 590
2,3,7,8-Tetrachlorodibenzo-*p*-dioxin (TCDD), in marine
mammals, 473
toxic equivalency factor and, 474–475
Tetracyclines, for toxoplasmosis, 134
in cheetah, 459t, 460
in chelonians, 191, 191t
in elephants, 536
in gorillas, 540

Tetracyclines *(Continued)*
in pinnipeds, 471
in stranded cetaceans, 489t
Texas, game ranching in, 586
Thalarctos maritimus. See *Polar bear (Thalarctos maritimus).*
Thermotherapy, for python illness, 196
Theropithecus gelada (gelada baboon), reproductive tract
evaluation in, using minimally invasive surgery, *39*
Thevetia peruviana (yellow oleander), toxicity of, 89
Thiabendazole, in fish, 183t, 188
in lemurs, 366
Thiamine (vitamin B₁), for cheetah cubs, 421
for fish, 172–173
for fish-eating birds, 307
for otters, in translocation project, 445, 445t
for sea turtles, 220
for stranded cetaceans, 491
Thiopentone sodium, in cheetah, 417
in giant panda, 411t
Thomson's gazelle (*Gazella thomsoni*), equine herpesvirus
infection in, 27
Thoracic diameter, sonographic, in dolphin fetal growth
assessment, 503–504, *504, 505*
Ticarcillin sodium, for septicemia, in koala, 327
Ticks. See also *Parasites;* specific genera and species.
on Arabian oryx, 695
on cheetah, 419, 419t, 420, 420t
on koala, 330t
on ranched hoofstock, 589
Tiger (*Panthera tigris*), artificial insemination in, 455t
time of, 455
canine distemper virus in, 407, 408
feline immunodeficiency virus in, 405
feline leukemia virus in, 402
in vitro fertilization in, 450t, 451, *451*
sonographic assessment in, *50, 51*
Tiger snakes (*Notechis* species), organ location in, 245
Tiletamine/zolazepam, in Beisa oryx, 689
in canids, 430, 433
oral administration of, 431, 432
in cheetah, 417, 459
in crocodilians, 211, 213t, 215
in duikers, 673t
in giant panda, 411t
in marsupials, 334t, 335
in otters, *438*, 438t, 440, 442
in suids, domestic, 640–641, 640t, 642t
nondomestic, 642, 643–644, 645
in tree kangaroos, 338
Tilmicosin, in duikers, 679
Timber rattlesnake (*Crotalus horridus horridus*),
antimicrobials in, 192t, 194
Timber wolf (*Canis lupus*), artificial insemination in,
451–452
weight of, 429
Tissue banks, creation of, 6
Titi monkey (*Callicebus moloch*), diabetes in, parasite-
induced, 398
treatment of, 399
Toads (*Xenopus* species), shipment of, 21
vitamin D metabolism in, 74
α-Tocopherol, 80. See also *Vitamin E.*
Tocopherol-binding protein (TBP), 79–80
Tolazoline, in birds, 312
in canids, 431
in okapi, 649
in suids, 640t, 641
Tolbutamide, for primate diabetes, 399
Tomistoma schlegelii (false gharial), gallamine mortality in,
206

Tomistoma schlegelii (false gharial) *(Continued)*
  immobilization of, 206–207
Tooth. See *Teeth.*
Topi (*Damaliscus lunatus*), herpesvirus carriage by, 27
Tortoises. See also *Chelonians; specific animals.*
  antimicrobials in, 191–193, 191t
  herpesvirus carriage by, 28
  vitamin D metabolism in, 73–74
Total protein concentration, in screening for failure of passive
    antibody transfer, 61
Toucans, herpesvirus infection in, 28
  iron overload in, 262–263
  pseudotuberculosis in, 154
Toxaphene, in marine mammals, 472–473
Toxic equivalency factor (TEF), 474–475
Toxins. See *Poisoning.*
Toxocara pteropodis, in flying foxes, 348
Toxoplasmosis, 131–134
  agent causing, 131
  clinical findings in, 132
  diagnosis of, 132–133
  human infection with, 134
  in Arabian oryx, 695
  in birds, 29, 155
  in callitrichids, 372
  in koala, 330t
  in lemurs, 368
  in manatees, 515
  in tree kangaroos, 342
  management of, 133–134
  pathogenesis of, 131–132
  prevention of, 134
  transmission of, 131, *132*
Toxotest-MT, 133
Toys, for hand-reared cetaceans, 496
Trachea, of cetaceans, diagnostic cytology of, 466
Trachemys scripta (turtle). See also *Red-eared slider
    (Chrysemys scripta elegans).*
  vitamin D metabolism in, 73
Tragelaphus species. See *Kudu.*
Trailers, for animal shipment, 18
Training, crate, 18–19, *19*
Tranquilizers. See also *specific drugs.*
  for shipping, 20
  in canids, 430–431, 433
  in cheetah, 417–418, 418t
  in duikers, 675
  in marsupials, 334, 335t
  in okapi, 649
  in white rhinoceros, 559, 579t, 583
  in wild herbivores, 575–584
    effects of, 577, *578*
    guidelines for using, 578–579
    recommended, 577–578
    side effects of, 579
    species quidelines for, 579–584, 579t
  long-acting, 577, 578
  short-acting, 577, 578
Translocation, *Elaphostrongylus cervi* and, 636
  of elephants, 525–532
    capture procedure for, 528–529, 531
    equipment for, 526–528, 527t
    family units in, 531
    loading procedure for, 529–530, *530,* 531
    off-loading paddock for, 530–531
    off-loading procedure for, 532
    travel procedure for, 531–532
  of otters, 441–442, 443–448. See also *North American
      river otter (Lutra canadensis).*
  of wild herbivores, capture methods for, 576

Translocation *(Continued)*
    tranquilizer use in, 575–584
    Parelaphostrongylus tenuis and, 634
    stress prevention in, 576–577
Transmissible mink encephalopathy. See *Scrapie-like
      spongiform encephalopathies.*
Transmission electron microscopy, in viral enteritis diagnosis,
    in ruminants, 609
Transportation. See *Shipment.*
Trapping, for vermin control, 115–116
    for birds, 119
    for rodents, 117
    for skunks, 118
Trauma, in ape neonates, 384
  in California condor, 283, 287
  in duiker neonates, 671
  in elephants, 539
  in manatees, 515–516
  in megachiropterans, 346–347
  in mixed-species exhibits, 26–27
  in oiled birds, 303
  in okapi neonates, 647
  in otters, 447
Tree kangaroos, 337–342
  anesthesia in, 338–339
  bacterial infections in, 339–341, *340, 341*
  cardiovascular problems in, 342
  gastrointestinal problems in, 341, *342*
  husbandry of, 337–338
  laboratory reference values for, 339, 339t
  life expectancy of, 342
  musculoskeletal problems in, 342
  nutrition in, 338
  parasites in, 341
  preventive medical procedures in, 342
  quarantine for, 342
  reproduction in, 338
  respiratory disease in, 341–342
  restraint of, 338
Tree squirrels. See *Squirrel(s).*
Tree tobacco (*Nicotiana glauca*), toxicity of, 88–89
Trematodes. See also *Parasites; specific genera and species.*
  hepatic cysts due to, 423
  in chelonians, 240t
  in duikers, 676
  in manatees, 514, 515
Triatrix (amitraz), in cheetah, 419, 420t
Tricaine methanesulfonate, in crocodilians, 212, 214t
  in fish, 160, 161t
Trichechus manatus (West Indian manatee). See *Manatees.*
Trichobezoars, in cheetah, 458
  in lemurs, 366
  in okapi, 648
  in tree kangaroos, *340,* 341, *342*
Trichomoniasis, in lemurs, 366
  in mixed-species exhibits, 29
Trichophyton gallinae, birds and, 152t
Trichospirura leptostoma, in callitrichids, 372
  in monkeys, diabetes due to, 398
Trichostrongyloid parasites. See also *specific organisms.*
  in ruminants, anthelmintics for, 595–596
    control programs for, design of, 593–597
      examples of, 596–597
    determining clinically important species of, 595
    epidemiology of, 593–594
Trichostrongylus species, in Arabian oryx, 695
  in Texas ranch-raised hoofstock, 588
Trichuris species, in Arabian oryx, 695
  in ranched hoofstock, 589
Triglycerides, vitamin E absorption and, 79

Trilafon. See *Perphenazine.*
Trimethoprim/sulfadiazine, for toxoplasmosis, 133–134
  in reptiles, 195
  in stranded cetaceans, 489t
Trimethoprim/sulfamethoxazole, in ape neonates, 386
  in duikers, 679
  in elephants, 536–537
Trionyx ferox (Florida soft-shell turtle), chemical dip for, 195
Triple antibiotic ointment, in sea turtles, 230t
Trisetum flavescens (golden oat grass), vitamin D in, 63
Trocars, for minimally invasive surgery, 34, *34*
Tropicamide, for pupillary dilatation, in megachiropterans, 353
Trucks, for animal shipment, 18
Truk flying fox (*Pteropus insularis*). See also *Megachiropterans.*
  conservation status of, 344
Trunk disease, in elephants, 544–545, *545*
Trunk paralysis, in free-ranging elephants, 541–544, *542, 543*
Trypanosoma cruzi, in callitrichids, 372
Trypanosoma megachiropterorum, 348
Tsessebe, tranquilizers in, 579t, 581
Tubal ligation, 317
Tuberculin testing, 108–109
  for personnel, 655
  in cervids, 651–652, 653
  in monkeys, 393
  in orangutans, 392–396
    evaluation of response to, 393–394, *394*
    future research on, 395–396
    management of responders to, 394–395
  in tapirs, 563
Tuberculosis, clinical signs of, 105–106, *105*
  diagnosis of, 108–110
  differential diagnosis of, 110
  domestic animal health concerns, 112
  in Arabian oryx, 692t, 693–694
  in cervids, 101, 103, 650–655. See also under *Cervids.*
  in cheetah, 101, 103, 107t, 418–419
    clinical signs of, 106
  in elephants, 540
  in free-ranging mammals, 101–112
    control and treatment of, 110–112
    species reported with, 102t
  in lemurs, 366
  in orangutan, 392
  in ranched hoofstock, 590–591
  lesions of, 106–108, *107,* 107t, *108*
  mortality rates for, 104
  pathogenesis of, 106
  population at risk for, 103–104
  prevalence of, 104, 105t
  public health concerns with, 110
  source of infection in, 101–102
  transmission of, 102–103
Tubs, for ungulates, 660
Tubulointerstitial nephrosis, in koala, 328–329
Tule elk (*Cervus elaphus nannodes*). See also *Cervus elaphus (red deer, elk, wapiti).*
  Johne's disease in, 616, 617, *618*
    management of, 619–620
Tumors. See *Neoplasia.*
Tungu penetrans, on cheetah, 419t
Tupinambis teguixin (tegu), antimicrobials in, 192t, 193
Turkey(s), cryptosporidiosis in, 122t, 126
Turkey vulture (*Cathartes aura*), anesthesia in, 282
Tursiops species. See *Bottlenose dolphin (Tursiops truncatus).*
Turtles. See *Chelonians.*
Tusks, in elephants, diseases of, 545, *545*
  injuries to, treatment of, 536, 538, 539

Two-toed sloth (*Choloepus didactylus*), sonographic sex determination in, *44*
Tylosin, for leptospirosis, 471
  in elephants, 538
  in reptiles, 195

U

Ulcerative skin disease, in black rhinoceros, 59, 552–553, *553*
Ulcers, gastric, in stranded cetaceans, 488
Ultrasonography, 41–54
  advantages of, 41
  applications of, 42, *42*
  fetal, 47–52, *48, 49, 52*
    in dolphins, 501–506, *503–506*
    in salt water, 502
  of sea turtles, 226, *226, 227*
  problems in, 41
Ultraviolet light, as vitamin D source, 63, 65–67, 75
  for chameleons, 202
  to improve water quality for fish, 175
Ungulates. See *Hoofstock.*
Uniform Methods and Rules for Tuberculosis Eradication in Cervidae, 655
United States Fish and Wildlife Service (USF&W), shipping regulations of, 22–23
Urethral obstruction, in lemurs, after electroejaculation, 367
Urinary tract infection, chlamydial, in koala, 325, *325*
Urine, collection of, in manatees, 511
  in megachiropterans, 352
  of cetaceans, diagnostic cytology of, 468–469
  of okapi, reference values for, 649
Urocyon species (foxes), immobilizing drug dosages for, 434t
Urogenital disorders. See also under *Reproductive system.*
  in prosimians, 367
  in tapirs, 566
Urolithiasis, in duikers, 670
Ursids. See also *Polar bear (Thalarctos maritimus).*
  hepatic proliferative disease in, 426–427, *426*
Ursodeoxycholic acid (ursodiol), 426–427
Ursus species (bears), hepatic proliferative disease in, 426
  sonographic fetal assessment in, *52*
USF&W (United States Fish and Wildlife Service), shipping regulations of, 22–23
Uterine inertia, in elephant, 522

V

Vaccinations, brucellosis, 622–623, 624, 627
  canine distemper virus, 408–409
    for marine mammal morbillivirus infection prevention, 500
    in black-footed ferret, 461
  clostridial, in Arabian oryx, 695
    in duikers, 680
    in ranched hoofstock, 589–590
  contraceptive. See *Porcine zona pellucida (PZP) vaccine.*
  coronavirus, 611
    in okapi, 649
  equine encephalitis, in duikers, 679, 680
  feline leukemia virus, 404
  foot-and-mouth disease, in Arabian oryx, 693
  in Arabian oryx, 691, 692, 693, 695, 696
  in cheetah, 418
  in duikers, 679, 680
  in fish, 173–175
  in game ranching, 587, 589–590

Vaccinations *(Continued)*
in okapi, 649
leptospirosis, in pinnipeds, 471
in ranched hoofstock, 590
marine mammal morbillivirus, 500
measles, in primates, 379
pasteurellosis, in Arabian oryx, 693, 695
rabies, during incubation period, 138–139, 142
in duikers, 680
in humans, 143, 143t–145t
in zoo animals, 140–143
rinderpest, in Arabian oryx, 691, 692
rotavirus, 611
in okapi, 649
toxoplasmosis, 134
tuberculosis, 112
in cervids, 654
Vagina, of cetaceans, diagnostic cytology of, 468
Valium. See *Diazepam.*
Vancomycin, in stranded cetaceans, 489t
Varanus exanthematicus (Savannah monitor lizard),
minimally invasive surgery in, *37*
Varanus komodoensis (Komodo dragon), sonographic sex
determination in, *43*
Varecia variegata (ruffed lemur), bone disease in, 367
cholangioma in, 424
herpesvirus encephalitis in, 380
Varicella, in apes, 386
Varicella viruses, simian, in mixed-species exhibits, 28
Vas deferens, occlusion of, for contraception, 316, 317
Vasectomy, 316, 318
Vengeance (bromethalin), 117
Venom, of reptiles, effects of, 97
Veno-occlusive liver disease, in cheetah, 458
in felids, 427
Veress needle, for minimally invasive surgery, 33
Vermin, control of, 114–120
for bats, 118
for birds, 119–120
for deer, 118–119
for large mammals, 118
for rodents, 116–117, 118t
for small mammals, 117–118
integrated pest management for, 114–116
diseases transmitted by, 115t
Vertebral subluxation, in chuckwalla, imaging of, 85, *85, 86*
Vesicular and ulcerative dermatopathy, in black rhinoceros,
59, 552–553, *553*
Vesicular skin disease, in tapirs, 565
Veterinary Librarian, 5–6
Veterinary Services Form 17–140, 24, 25
Vibriosis, birds and, 152t
vaccine for, 173
Vicuna *(Lama vicugna)*, estrous cycle synchronization in, 598
Videoimaging system, for minimally invasive surgery, 32, *33*
Vietnamese pot-bellied pigs, anesthesia in, 642, 642t, 644,
645
Vipera ammodytes, organ location in, case study, 246–247
Viperids. See also *Snakes.*
effects of venom of, 97
paramyxovirus carriage by, 28
ViraCHEK/FIV, false negatives with, 405
Viral infections. See also specific viruses and diseases.
acquired from birds, 154–155
emerging, in large cats, 401–409
in primates, 377–381
in ape neonates, 385
in Arabian oryx, 691–693, 692t
in black rhinoceros, 554–555
in callitrichids, 370–371, *370*

Viral infections *(Continued)*
in chameleons, 203
in chelonians, 240t
in duikers, 677–679
in equids, 572t, 573
in megachiropterans, 348–349
in mixed-species exhibits, 27–28
in ranched hoofstock, 591
Viruses, enteric diarrheagenic, classification of, 605
Vision, in megachiropterans, 353
Vital signs monitoring, in immobilized canids, 432–433
Vitamin(s). See also specific vitamins.
deficiencies of, in fish, 172, 173t
in fruit bat diet, 357
in sea turtle diet, 220
requirements for, in domestic and laboratory species, 358t
Vitamin A, in fish diet, 173t
vitamin E interaction with, 82
Vitamin A toxicity, due to fish liver oils, 67
Vitamin B complex. See also *Thiamine (vitamin B₁).*
for fish, 173t
for otters, in translocation project, 445, 445t
for stranded cetaceans, 491
Vitamin C (ascorbic acid), for elephant poxvirus infection,
549
for stranded cetaceans, 491
in captive lemur diet, iron overload and, 366
in fish diet, 173, 173t
Vitamin D, 63–76
assessing status of, 65
deficiency of, 65
in amphibians, 74
in carnivores, 70
in farm animals, 74
in primates, 70–72, *71*
in reptiles, 72–74
for ape infants, 383
in fish diet, 173t
injectable, 70
international standard for, 64
meeting needs for, 75–76
metabolism of, 63–65, *64*
oral supplements of, 69–70
requirements for, in callitrichids, 374
sources of, 65–70, 68t, 69t
Vitamin D toxicity, 74–75
in pacas and agoutis in mixed-species exhibits, 27, 72, 75
in primates, 72, 74–75
Vitamin D₂ (ergocalciferol), 63–65, *64*
injectable, 70
Vitamin D₃ (cholecalciferol), 63–65, *64*
as rodenticide, 117, 118t
crystalline, 70
in chameleon diet, 202
Vitamin E, 79–82
absorption and transport of, 79–80
assessment of status of, 82
in rhinoceros, 570–571, 570t
deficiency of, in megachiropterans, 349, 350, *351, 352,*
357
in rhinoceroses, 569, 570
in tree kangaroos, 338
for duikers, 670
for fish, 172–173
for okapi, 649
for otters, in translocation project, 445, 445t
for sea turtles, 220
for stranded cetaceans, 491
nutrient interactions with, 82
sources of, 80–81, 81t

Vitamin E toxicity, in mixed-species bird exhibits, 27
Vitamin K, in fish diet, 173t
Volatile anesthetics. See also specific drugs.
  in crocodilians, 212, 213t
  in marsupials, 335–336
  in otters, 441
  in suids, 641, 645
Vole (*Microtus* species), control of, 116–117
Volunteers, in care of stranded cetaceans, 492
Vomiting, in cheetah gastritis, 458
  in immobilized canid, 433
Vulpes species (foxes), immobilizing drug dosages for, 434t
  rabies in, 139
Vultur gryphus (Andean condor), anesthesia in, 282
  in California condor management program, 278
Vulture, turkey, anesthesia in, 282

W

Wahlberg's epaulated bat (*Epomophorus wahlbergi*). See also
    Megachiropterans.
  geographic distribution of, 345t
Wallaby, tammar, toxoplasmosis vaccines tested in, 134
Walrus, antifungal drugs in, 483t
Wapiti. See *Cervus elaphus* (red deer, elk, wapiti).
Warfarin, as rodenticide, 117, 118t
Warthog (*Phacochoerus aethiopicus*), 639
  anesthesia in, 644, 645
  tuberculosis in, 101
Wasting marmoset syndrome, 371
  iron overload and, 265
Water, fruit bat requirements for, 356
Water buffalo (*Bubalus bubalis*), tuberculosis in, 101,
    102–103, 104
  lesions of, 107t
  prevalence of, 105t
Water cobra, false, antimicrobials in, 192t, 193–194
Water hyacinths, for phytoplankton control in waterfowl
    exhibits, 297
Water quality, feather waterproofing and, after oil spill,
    305–306, *306*
  for fish, 165–171, *170,* 170t
    drug treatment and, 184
    for anesthesia, 158, 160
    for quarantine, 165
    records of, 164
  for manatees, 508, 509
  for sea turtles, 218–219
  for waterfowl, 292–299
    disease and, 297–299, *298*
    factors in, 293–295, *294, 295*
    maintenance of, *293,* 295–297, *296, 297*
Water snakes, antimicrobials in, 192t, 194
Waterbuck, tranquilizers in, 579t, 582
Waterfowl, causes of wet feathers in, 306t
  in oil spills. See *Oil spills, birds affected by.*
  types of water amenities for, 292–293, *293*
  uninvited, control of, 119–120
  water quality for, 292–299
    disease and, 297–299, *298*
    factors in, 293–295, *294, 295*
    maintenance of, *293,* 295–297, *296, 297*
Weaning, of cetacean, 496
  shipping and, 19–20
Weeds, poisonous, 88, 92t
Weight loss, chronic, in tapirs, 566
West Indian manatee (*Trichecus manatus*). See *Manatees.*
Western blot, for feline immunodeficiency virus, 406
Whales. See *Cetaceans;* specific animals.

White carneaux pigeon (*Columba livia*), control of, 119
  crop milk of, composition of, 272t, 273t
  growth of, 273–274, *274*
White ear-tufted marmoset (*Callithrix jaccus*). See also
    Callitrichids.
  iron overload in, 265
  vitamin D metabolism in, 64, 72
White rat (*Rattus norvegicus*), control of, 116–117
White rhinoceros (*Ceratotherium simum*). See under
    Rhinoceroses.
White-beaked dolphin (*Lagenorhynchus albirostris*),
    morbillivirus infection in, 498
White-faced saki (*Pithecia pithecia*), gestational diabetes in,
    398
White-fronted capuchin (*Cebus albifrons*), vitamin D
    metabolism in, 64, 70–71
  vitamin D toxicity in, 74
White-handed gibbon (*Hylobates lar*), testicular cyst in,
    sonographic assessment of, *51*
  viral hepatitis in, 378
  vitamin D transport in, 64
White-lipped peccary (*Tayassu pecari*), anesthesia in,
    643–644
White-lipped tamarin (*Saguinus nigricollis*). See also
    Callitrichids.
  vitamin D metabolism in, 71
White-sided dolphin (*Lagenorhynchus acutus*), fungal
    infections in, 480t
White-tailed deer (*Odocoileus virginianus*), contraception in,
    using PZP vaccination, 628–629, 629t
  control of, 118–119
  handling systems for, 658, 659, *659*
  induced ovulation in, 599
  Parelaphostrongylus tenuis in, 632–633
    cervid population dynamics and, 634–635
    infection of other species by, 29, 588
  polycystic liver disease in, 424
  Spiculopteragia asymmetrica in, 588
White-winged wood duck (*Carina scutulata*), fungal
    tracheitis in, endoscopic examination of, *39*
Wild boar (*Sus scrofa*), anesthesia in, 644, 645
Wild cherry (*Prunus*), toxicity of, 89
Wild dog, Asian, immobilizing drug dosages for, 434t
  sonographic health assessment in, *47, 50, 51*
Wild jasmin (*Cestrum diurnam*), vitamin D in, 63
Wildcat, European, feline leukemia virus in, 402
Wildebeests (*Connochaetes* species), herpesvirus carriage by,
    27
  tranquilizers in, 579–580, 579t
Wing-tip trauma, in megachiropterans, 346
Winter dysentery. See also *Coronavirus infection.*
  clinical signs of, 608
  epizootiology of, 607–608
  treatment of, 610
Wolves, artificial insemination in, 451–452
  immobilizing drug dosages for, 434t
Wood bison. See *American bison (Bison bison).*
Wood duck, white-winged, fungal tracheitis in, endoscopic
    examination of, *39*
Woodchuck (*Marmota monax*), reproduction in, 362
Wooly monkey disease, 70–71
Wooly tapir (*Tapirus pinchaque*), 562, 562t. See also *Tapirs.*
Wounds, darting, in elephants, 529
  in white rhinoceros, 559
  in elephants, 539
  in immobilized canids, 433
  in sea turtles, 230
  propeller, in manatees, 515
Wrasses, social structure of, 171
Wright-Giemsa stain, for fish blood specimen, 179, 180t

X

Xenopus laevis (African clawed toad), vitamin D metabolism in, 74
Xenopus species (toads), shipment of, 21
Xylazine, for extrapyramidal symptoms in herbivores, 581
    in Arabian oryx, 689, 689t
    in birds, 312
    in canids, 430, 433, 434
    in cheetah, 417, 418t
    in crocodilians, 211, 213t
    in duikers, 673t, 674t
    in elephants, 527
    in fish, 161, 161t
    in giant panda, 411t
    in hippopotamus, 638, 639
    in marsupials, 334t, 335
    in megachiropterans, 345
    in mountain sheep, 684, 685
    in otters, 440, 442
    in suids, domestic, 640, 640t, 641, 642t
        nondomestic, 642, 644, 645
    in tapirs, 562, 563
    in tree kangaroos, 338
    in turkey vulture, 282
    in white rhinoceros, 557

Y

Yeasts. See also *Candida species.*
    in cetaceans, 466, 467, *467*, 468, *468*
Yellow oleander (*Thevetia peruviana*), toxicity of, 89
Yellow rat snake (*Elaphe obsoleta*), antimicrobials in, 192t, 193, 194
Yellow-backed duiker (*Cephalophus sylvicultor*). See also *Duikers.*
    anesthesia in, 674t
    conservation status of, 669
    laboratory reference values for, 678t
Yersinia enterocolitica infection, birds and, 154
    in callitrichids, 371
    uninvited species and, 28
Yersinia pseudotuberculosis infection, birds and, 152t, 154
    in callitrichids, 371
    uninvited species and, 28
Yersinia ruckeri, vaccine for, 173
Yew (*Taxus* species), toxicity of, 89
Yogue, in megachiropterans, 349
Yohimbine, in birds, 312
    in canids, 431
    in cheetah, 417
    in crocodilians, 214t, 215
    in duikers, 674t

Yohimbine *(Continued)*
    in elephants, 527
    in hippopotamus, 639
    in marsupials, 335
    in mountain sheep and goats, 685
    in okapi, 649
    in otters, 440
    in suids, domestic, 640t, 641, 642, 642t
        nondomestic, 644, 645
    in tapirs, 563
Yolk sac infection, in California condor, 283, 284, *284,* 286, *286*

Z

Zalophus californianus (California sea lion), fungal infections in, 479t, 480t
    leptospirosis in, 469–470, *470,* 471
Zebra(s). See also *Equids.*
    captive population of, 572t
    in mixed-species exhibits, 27
    tranquilizers in, 579t, 583
    viral disease in, 573
Zebra duiker (*Cephalophus zebra*). See also *Duikers.*
    anesthesia in, 673t
    conservation status of, 669
Zinc, immune function and, 59
    in fish diet, 174t
    in rhinoceros diet, 570, 570t
Zinc intoxication, in California condor, 290
    in waterfowl, 299
Zinc phosphide, 117, 118t
Zinc sulfate turbidity test, 60–61
Ziphius cavirostris (Cuvier's beaked whale), subcutaneous emphysema in, 490
Zolazepam, tiletamine with. See *Tiletamine/zolazepam.*
Zoletil. See *Tiletamine/zolazepam.*
Zoonoses, 121–155. See also specific diseases.
    from birds, 151–155, 152t, 153t
        bacterial, 151–154
        fungal, 154
        parasitic, 155
        prevention of, 151
        viral, 154–155
    from fish, 177, 177t
    preventing transmission of, in quarantine, 14
Zuclopenthixol, in marsupials, 335t
    in wild herbivores, 578
        species guidelines for, 580–583
Zygomycetes, in marine mammals, 480t, 482
        treatment of, 483

ISBN 0-7216-8664-8

90038